PSYCHIATRIC MENTAL HEALTH NURSING

Faye Gary, Ed.D., R.N., FAAN
College of Nursing and Department of Psychiatry
University of Florida
Gainesville, Florida

Charlene Kate Kavanagh, Ph.D., R.N.

Departments of Psychiatry and Pediatrics
University of Wisconsin Medical School
School of Nursing, University of Wisconsin
Madison, Wisconsin

With 27 contributors

PSYCHIATRIC MENTAL HEALTH NURSING

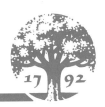

J. B. Lippincott Company

PHILADELPHIA NEW YORK
ST. LOUIS LONDON SYDNEY TOKYO

Compositor: *The Clarinda Company*
Printer/Binder: *The Murray Printing Company*

3 5 6 4 2

Psychiatric mental health nursing/[edited by] Faye Gary, Charlene Kate Kavanagh; with 27
  contributors.
      p.   cm.
    Includes biographical references.
    Includes index.
    ISBN 0-397-54852-4
    1. Psychiatric nursing.   I. Gary, Faye.   II. Kavanagh, Charlene Kate.
    [DNLM: 1. Mental Disorders—nursing.   2. Psychiatric Nursing.   WY
160 P97203]
RC440.P7352   1990
610.73'68—dc20
DNLM/DLC
for Library of Congress   90-6205
                                                                CIP

To the memory of my father and mother, Homer G. and Ollie C. Gary

Faye Gary

To my mentor, Dr. Richard Anderson, who taught me nearly all I needed to know; to my analyst, Dr. Mark Trewartha, who taught me the rest, plus gave me back my self; and to my patient Kristen (September 20, 1980– January 13, 1990), who, in the five short years I knew her, taught me what is *really* important: how to live and how to die.

Charlene Kate Kavanagh

CONTRIBUTORS

LINDA J. BAKER, PH.D.

Assistant Professor of Psychiatry, University of Wisconsin Medical School, Madison, Wisconsin

RICHARD D. BARTHEL, M.D.

Assistant Professor, Division of Child Psychiatry, Medical College of Wisconsin, Milwaukee, Wisconsin

BEVERLY BENFER, M.A., R.N., F.A.A.N.

Consultant, Psychiatric Nursing/Administration, Marion, Iowa

ROGER K. BLASHFIELD, PH.D.

Professor of Clinical Psychology, Department of Psychiatry, College of Medicine, University of Florida, Gainesville, Florida

NANCY BOHNET, M.N., R.N.

President/CEO, Visiting Nurses Association, Butler, Pennsylvania

GEORGE DAWSON, M.D.

Fellow in Biological Psychiatry, University of Wisconsin, Madison, Wisconsin

BURR EICHELMAN, M.D., PH.D.

Clinical Director, Dorothea Dix Hospital, Raleigh, North Carolina

NORMAN FOST, M.D., M.P.H.

Program in Medical Ethics, University of Wisconsin Medical School, Madison, Wisconsin

FAYE GARY, ED.D., R.N., F.A.A.N.

Professor, College of Nursing and Department of Psychiatry, University of Florida, Gainesville, Florida

LOIS GRAU, PH.D., R.N.

Director, Nerken Center for Geriatric Research, Parker Jewish Geriatric Institute, New Hyde Park, New York

MEL HAGGART, M.S., M.D.

Clinical Associate Professor, University of Wisconsin Medical School, Madison, Wisconsin

CHRISTINE HERRMAN, M.S., R.N., C.S.

Certified Specialist, Child and Adolescent Psychiatric and Mental Health Nursing, Rush-Presbyterian-St. Luke's Medical Center, Chicago, Illinois

CHARLES HODULIK, M.D.

Clinical Associate Professor of Psychiatry, University of Wisconsin Medical School, Madison, Wisconsin

NED KALIN, M.D.

Professor of Psychiatry and Director of Research, Department of Psychiatry, University Hospital, University of Wisconsin, Madison, Wisconsin

CHARLENE KATE KAVANAGH, PH.D., R.N.

Clinical Associate Professor, Departments of Psychiatry and Pediatrics, University of Wisconsin Medical School, and School of Nursing, University of Wisconsin, Madison, Wisconsin; Clinical Licensed Psychologist, Shorewood Psychiatric Associates, Madison, Wisconsin

DAVID KEITH, M.D.

Associate Professor of Psychiatry, Pediatrics, and Family Medicine and Director of Family Therapy Program, Department of Psychiatry, Health Science Center, State University of New York, Syracuse, New York

GWEN LAPHAM-ALCORN, PH.D., R.N.

Instructor, Department of Nursing, Central Florida Community College, Ocala, Florida

HANNAH LEE, M.S.S.W., A.C.S.W

Clinical Social Worker, Family-Based Services, Dane County Department of Social Services; Private Psychotherapy Practice, Affiliated Counseling Services, Madison, Wisconsin

KEM B. LOUIE, PH.D., R.N., C.

Assistant Professor, College of Nursing, Lehman College C.U.N.Y., Bronx, New York

LYN MARSHALL, M.S.N., R.N.

Manager, Adolescent Unit and Adult Dual Diagnosis Program, Menninger, San Francisco Bay Area, Peninsula Hospital, Burlingame, California

BOB MCDONALD, B.SC.

Clinical Supervisor, Psychological Treatment Unit, Institute of Psychiatry, London, England

DANIEL SAUNDERS, PH.D.

Associate Scientist, Department of Psychiatry, University of Wisconsin, Madison, Wisconsin

PATRICIA J. SCHRODER, M.A., R.N., C.S.

Psychiatric Nursing Consultant, Marion, Iowa

ELIZABETH SHENKMAN, PH.D., R.N.

Director of Women's Health and Children's Health, Shands Hospital, University of Florida, Gainesville, Florida

FRANCES BLACKWELL SMITH, ED.D., R.N.
Associate Professor, Department of Nursing, University of Central Florida, Orlando, Florida

JONATHAN T. STEWART, M.D.
Associate Professor of Psychiatry, College of Medicine, University of Florida, Gainesville, Florida

DALMAS A. TAYLOR, PH.D.
Dean, College of Liberal Arts, Wayne State University, Detroit, Michigan

BEV WOLFGRAM, PH.D., R.N.
Clinic Director, Affiliated Counseling Services, Madison, Wisconsin

LOUISE B. ZEULI, J.D., ARNP
Attorney-at-law, Orlando, Florida

PREFACE

We believe that nursing care must focus on the whole person, not simply one dysfunctional or diseased part. This makes psychiatric mental health nursing not only a specialty but a vital component of every nurse's practice, regardless of clinical setting. Nurses assess, analyze, and synthesize the data they collect, and plan nursing interventions related to *all* aspects of the individual: physiological, psychological, and sociocultural. However, it is not just this attention to the whole person that gives nursing its unique perspective in the health care field. Nurses, unlike anyone else on the health care team, have the daily access to and frequent contact with the patient and family that allows them to develop a therapeutic relationship, observe subtle deviations from baseline, and *really* get to know the patient and the unique meaning of the illness or injury to him or her. Moreover, "R.N." may inspire a kind of trust and willingness to open up that "M.D." may not. This unique opportunity for establishing a therapeutic, caring relationship with the patient is specific to the psychiatric and nonpsychiatric nurse alike.

Psychiatric Mental Health Nursing addresses that component of nursing that focuses on psychological functioning—mental and emotional health and psychopathology. The goal of this text is to prepare nursing students to work in any number of general nursing or specialty areas, including, but not limited to, psychiatric nursing. For the student who will be working in nonpsychiatric settings such as a pediatric clinic or a medical-surgical service, *Psychiatric Mental Health Nursing* provides a sound basis for the assessment of emotional problems associated with acute or chronic illness or injury and its treatment or those related to the unique stresses in an individual's life and their outcome. It teaches the student how to differentiate between "normal" responses to illness or hospitalization and primary psychological dysfunction. And it prepares the student to provide sensitive, scientific care that always takes the psychosocial dimension of health into account.

For the undergraduate nursing student who will be working in psychiatric health care settings, *Psychiatric Mental Health Nursing* provides the depth of information needed to care for patients suffering from a variety of psychiatric illnesses, in conjunction with the primary therapist and the psychiatric team. It focuses heavily on the importance of good observation and communication skills. In particular, Chapters 5 ("Psychiatric Assessment for the Generalist Nurse") and 7 ("The Nurse as Therapist") provide concrete material on the roles in the therapeutic process available to the nurse. Finally, for the student who plans to continue with advanced study in psychiatric nursing as well as the professional nurse already working in this clinical specialty, this book provides in-depth coverage of the theories that attempt to explain human behavior, especially the etiology of psychological dysfunction, and the theory and research that have led to the development of therapies used to treat psychopathology and rehabilitate affected individuals and families.

In this text, we have strived to present the *realities* of the health care system. We started by inviting contributions from experts in a wide variety of academic disciplines who practice in the field of mental health as clinicians, teachers, and researchers. Psychiatric nurses, nurse educators, psychiatrists, psychologists, social workers, and researchers—all of whom play a vital role in the description and treatment of mental illness—have contributed chapters in their particular areas of expertise. Because of this, each chapter, within the overall framework of the text, has its own flavor and the perspective of the author's discipline along with that of nursing. Chapter 21 ("Psychiatric Mental Health Nursing with Families"), for instance, mirrors the systems approach to family therapy required to define and treat the family when it is defined as the "patient." This chapter's existential-experimental feel reflects this approach as well as the clinical style of its author, a family therapist. Chapter 3 ("Psychiatric Classification") is written by a psychologist who has devoted much of his professional life to the study of the classification systems that have defined mental illness since the concept was first described. Most chapters rely heavily on recent research to guide their contents. Chapter 25 ("Psychiatric Mental Health Nursing with the Patient in Intensive Care"), for instance, describes in detail the research carried out by nurses and physicians to determine just how damaging the critical care environment can be to the patient, and on strategies used to lessen the stress of the critical care experience.

Two classification systems, chosen because of their widespread familiarity in the nursing and mental health fields, are used in *Psychiatric Mental Health Nursing*. The North American Nursing Diagnosis Association's *Taxonomy I, Revised* (1988) provides a framework for describing actual or potential health problems that fall within the scope of nursing practice. NANDA-approved nursing diagnoses are an integral part of the text and, in conjunction with end-of-chapter case studies, form the basis for in-depth nursing care plans. The American Psychiatric Association's *Diagnostic and Statistical Manual of Mental Disorders, Third Edition, Revised* (DSM-III-R [1987]) provides the classification system for the description of psychopathology within the text. Though not ideal, DSM-III-R criteria provide a common language for communication among all mental health professionals—a necessity, given the team approach used in helping individuals with mental illness.

The *reality* of psychological pain and suffering is generally manifested not in a blood sample or x-ray, but in a person's eyes, verbal expressions, or nonverbal behavior. Therefore, observation and empathic listening are probably the most important skills to be developed by the nurse working in the mental health field. To help students practice their observation and analytical skills, we have provided numerous brief case studies, based on the authors' experiences, throughout the text. Of course, nothing can replace the student's own experiences in talking with patients, but the cases can help to prepare the student for the variety and intensity of such interactions. At the end of each chapter, one or two detailed case studies depicting individuals in a psychiatric or a nonpsychiatric health care facility provide the student with an opportunity to delve deeper into the issues of psychiatric nursing. When the case provides enough information, a DSM-III-R diagnosis is given on the five axes. For every case nursing diagnoses are listed, followed by a nursing care plan that includes nursing diagnoses, desired outcomes, interventions, and their rationales. It is our hope that students will spend time reading and evaluating these cases on their own, and consider whether they might handle certain situations differently and why. These detailed cases can also be used effectively as a springboard for classroom discussion of theory, current or needed research, and/or the complexities of clinical practice that considers the individual and that individual's own story first and foremost.

Another example of our focus on the current realities of mental health nursing is our acknowledgment of and attention to the elements of today's society that contribute to psychopathology and, often, make the nurse's job more difficult. These include the prevalence of violence and abuse within families and society as a whole; the growing AIDS crisis; the complex problem of drug abuse and addiction and the violence that has accompanied the drug culture; the increasing incidence of suicide, particularly among adolescents; the growing homeless population, particularly among the chronically mentally ill; and the cutback of governmental programs to adequately handle these pressures. The mental health care system is stretched to its limits, yet the nurse, in a variety of roles and varying responsibilities, can have an enormous positive impact on the lives of individuals who seek help both within and outside this system.

Psychiatric Mental Health Nursing is divided into five major sections. Part One, "Theoretical Foundations and Content of Practice," provides the core of scientific principles and social realities necessary to understand and implement psychotherapeutic nursing care. Chapter 1 describes psychiatric nursing practice in today's world and places the nurse at its center. Chapter 2 defines the three major models of behavior—psychoanalytic, behavioral, and biological—used to describe and understand "normal" human behavior as well as psychopathology and its treatment. Chapters on communication theory, psychiatric assessment, sociocultural issues, and the role of the nurse as therapist provide the clinical focus for the rest of the book.

Part Two, "Psychological Dysfunction and Psychopathology," describes the major types of psychological dysfunction, their assessment, treatment, and nursing care. Each chapter, where relevant, covers the range—from normal to severely dysfunctional—of "psychopathology" involved in the mental disorder discussed. For instance, Chapter 8 ("Anxiety Disorders") discusses both the normal anxiety felt by a patient undergoing surgery and the severe anxiety of the person suffering from one of the anxiety disorders, as well as the associated nursing responsibilities for each.

In Part Three, "Psychiatric Mental Health Nursing Throughout the Life Span," the science and art of psychiatric nursing practice is applied to the problems of women, men, families, children, and the elderly. The most common types of mental illness and special needs of individuals from infancy and childhood to old age are the focus of this section.

Part Four, "Psychiatric Mental Health Nursing with Special Populations," focuses on the unique mental health problems and needs of other special populations—the violent patient (Chapter 24), the critically ill patient (Chapter 25), and the chronically ill or dying patient (Chapter 26).

Part Five, "Psychiatric Mental Health Nursing Practice Issues," addresses legal and ethical issues relevant to psychiatric nursing practice. Patient rights and the associated legal and ethical responsibilities and dilemmas they create for the nurse and other health care professionals, are discussed in these two chapters.

In writing this text, we have taken much care to present both the science and the art of the full experience of psychiatric mental health nursing—the settings, the variety of patients and their problems, the theory and research behind medical treatment, and nursing care in today's world. Since this encompasses a huge amount of information, we have also taken great care to present it in a manner that will be most interesting and useful to the student.

Each chapter follows the same format, beginning with an outline and a list of *Learning Objectives*. Brief *Case Studies* throughout the chapters provide "pictures" of psychopathology and interactions among patients, nurses, and other members of the health care team. At the end of each chapter, detailed Case Studies (whenever appropriate, one for the psychiatric setting and one for the non-psychiatric setting) apply the key concepts discussed in the chapter. These are followed by a *Summary* of the chapter's major concepts, a list of the *Key Terms* that appear in boldface type in the chapter (and are defined in the glossary at the end of the text), *Study Questions,* and *References.*

Psychiatric Mental Health Nursing is also filled with summary tables, illustrations (many done by patients), numerous photographs, and special interest boxes that focus on controversial issues and, often, provide a different perspective (or most current research) on the topics covered in the text. The *Glossary* at the end of the text provides a quick and ready reference for definitions of key terms. We have also developed an instructor's manual for educators using this book. This supplement contains chapter summaries, test questions (both short-answer and essay), and answers to these questions as well as to those appearing in this text.

It is our hope that *Psychiatric Mental Health Nursing* will give students genuine insight into a facet of life they possibly have not seriously considered, an awareness of their own feelings and responses to human pain and suffering, and a growing eagerness and facility to observe, listen to, and effectively communicate with people who are experiencing such pain, whether it is the result of "fragmentation anxiety" or Alzheimer's disease. We further hope that students will come away from the study of this text with an understanding of the importance of caring to healing in all interactions with the patient and family, as well as an understanding of the range of psychiatric disorders and associated treatment modalities, and what is known about the origins of both; and, finally, a sense of confidence about their ability to use themselves and their own experience to practice sensitive and effective psychiatric mental health nursing with *all* their patients.

ACKNOWLEDGMENTS

Many people helped us put this book together, some by supporting us personally and professionally before and while the book was developing, and others by providing direct and much needed help at different steps along the way.

On behalf of Faye, thanks go to her children Michael, Jonathan, William, and Benjamin, who provided her with their unique reality and helped her to understand what is important. Thanks also to her sisters June, Gladys, and Ollie, and brother Homer, and their families for their support and love, and to Lucy Robinson and Zelma Gary, Faye's aunts, who provided her with a vision built on the past, linked to the present, and projected into the future.

On behalf of Kate, thanks go to Sister Charlette, Professor Marshall Sanborn, Ms. Cookie Krol, and Maxine Berlinger, for encouraging her to be the best she could be. Thanks also are due to Norm, Kate's friend and husband (and most severe critic) and her 19-year-old son Matt, whose enthusiasm about his mom's writing a textbook consistently refueled his mother during this long process.

Many individuals helped us prepare and wade through the manuscript drafts. We'd like to especially thank Gretchen Benson for typing the first in a series of "final drafts"; Peggy Wiley for her enormous commitment of time and friendship during the manuscript development phase; Jacquelyn Warren for her enthusiastic diligence; and Laura Davis and Beth Frantz-Browning for getting to the Express Mail box on time when it counted. We would also like to thank Ann West, our Sponsoring Editor, who in her own way made this book happen.

Our colleagues in both academic and clinical circles have provided a tremendous amount of support in the writing process and in helping us pull the whole book together. Their names are too numerous to mention, but we would like to thank our chapter contributors who believed in this book the way we did and the friends and colleagues who reviewed chapters for us. Thanks also to the College of Nursing and Department of Psychiatry at the University of Florida and the Schools of Nursing and Medicine at the University of Wisconsin. In addition, we'd like to thank Professors Stephen Suomi and Susan Mineka, who shared their research with us while it was still in progress; Professor Judy Leavitt for sharing her invaluable slide collection of women and nurses through history; and the University of Wisconsin Primate Center for providing pictures of Harlow's early mother-infant monkey separation research.

Finally, we owe a debt of gratitude to our patients—the children for their drawings, their parents for letting us use family photographs, and all the patients who have shared with us their feelings about and insight into their illnesses and lives and who are always teaching us more about who we are and what we do.

Table of Contents

Part Two
PSYCHOLOGICAL DYSFUNCTION AND
PSYCHOPATHOLOGY

PSYCHIATRIC MENTAL HEALTH NURSING

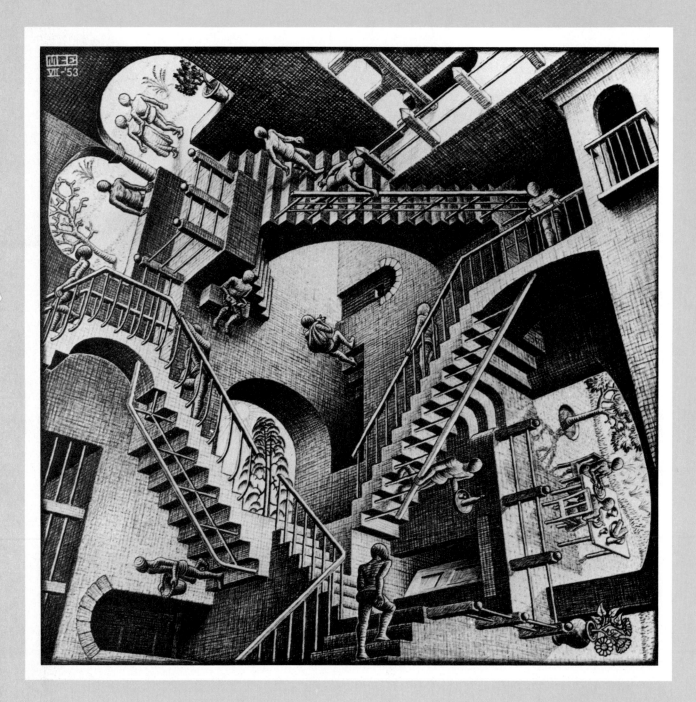

Part One
THEORETICAL FOUNDATIONS AND CONTENT OF PRACTICE

1

PSYCHIATRIC MENTAL HEALTH NURSING PRACTICE

CHARLENE KATE KAVANAGH

LEARNING OBJECTIVES

After studying this chapter, the student will be able to:

- Describe psychiatric mental health nursing in the practice of both the generalist nurse and the psychiatric nurse specialist in the hospital and community.
- Discuss the ethical and sociological issues involved in the definition of psychopathology and mental illness.
- Describe the three models of psychopathology and understand the connections between them.
- Describe the nursing process and its application to psychiatric mental health problems.
- Discuss the nurse's relationship to other members of the mental health care team.

Jason is a 5-year-old boy with cancer who has been on the pediatric unit of University Hospital for eight weeks. He has finished his first course of chemotherapy and is currently receiving radiation therapy. Nausea and vomiting, his reactions to the treatment, have left him irritable and fatigued. He has begun to complain of pain from mouth sores. His mood is depressed.

After Jason has kept breakfast down for the first time since his admission, and has received treatment for his mouth sores as well as some Tylenol and Codeine for his pain, Jason's nurse suggests a visit to the recreation room, where he can play and be with peers. Jason refuses her suggestions and pulls the covers over his head; he says he would rather stay in bed and go back to sleep. The nurse accepts this, explaining to his mother that, whenever possible, Jason should be allowed to make his own decisions in order to keep some control over his environment and to avoid feeling helpless and depressed.

The nurse is correct in her concern about Jason's vulnerability to depression. However, Jason is exhibiting **learned helplessness,** that is, he believes he does not have any control over what happens to him. Jason needs to have control of the events which, when not under his control, leave him feeling anxious and helpless. Giving him control of his feelings of helplessness (letting him give in to his depression by avoiding activity and play) won't help Jason overcome his anxiety and depression. Jason's nurse should insist that he attend recreation therapy so that he is actively involved in play and can again experience a sense of being in control in his environment. In addition, she can look for ways to give him control over the scary and unpleasant or painful events he experiences daily in the hospital. For example, he can be encouraged to watch and participate actively in obtaining his own blood samples and in starting his IV. He can choose the hours for a break in his chemotherapy and then decide how he will spend that time. He can choose whether or not to take an antiemetic to curb nausea, when to do his own twice-daily mouth care, and when he wishes to receive pain medication (within the range established by his physician and nurse).

This book has been written with people like Jason and his nurse in mind. It will provide the knowledge base essential to honoring a commitment to psychiatric mental health nursing for all patients, not just the ones on the psychiatric unit. It will also introduce the process of self-discovery associated with this commitment. Chapter 1 will lay the groundwork for this process.

THE NURSE AND PSYCHIATRIC MENTAL HEALTH NURSING

Regardless of the setting, every practicing nurse knows the symptoms of congestive heart failure and incipient shock; she can immediately formulate appropriate nursing diagnoses, patient outcomes, and interventions. But she may not know the symptoms of depression and incipient suicide and as a result may miss a key opportunity to develop nursing diagnoses and carry through vital interventions. Why is there such a discrepancy? Twenty years ago, nursing students spent one semester or less of their three–four year educational program studying abnormal psychology and/or psychiatric nursing. With few exceptions, the same is true today. But at the same time, the medical, surgical, and pediatric areas of the typical nursing curriculum have expanded. In most nursing programs, specialty courses on cardiopulmonary and newborn intensive care nursing, as well as rehabilitation and geriatric nursing, have been developed to keep nurses abreast of changing technology in medical care. The same is not necessarily true of specialty courses in psychiatric nursing. As a result, both the foundations and more advanced concepts related to psychiatric nursing must often be fit into one or two semesters of work. This text focuses on both levels of knowledge, because, as we will see, both are essential to the practice of generalist nurses and psychiatric nurse specialists.

OBTAINING ACCESS TO PSYCHIATRIC MENTAL HEALTH CARE

NEEDS OF THE PEDIATRIC/ADULT HOSPITALIZED POPULATION

It has been estimated that as much as 75 percent of the U.S. population suffers from mental illness at some point in life, with symptoms ranging from mild (36 percent) to moderate (21 percent) to severe (23 percent) (Srole and Fischer, 1978). (See Box 1–1.) The incidence is no doubt higher in health-care settings, where individuals experience the stress of ill-

Box 1–1 ●
Understanding
Depression

Depression:

1. Is the most common of all mental disorders.

2. Is a more serious condition than normal blues, feeling 'down in the dumps', sadness, or grief.

3. Interferes with one's functioning or causes great personal distress—or both.

4. Is more common in women than in men.

5. Is unrelated to marital and social status.

6. Can occur in people of all ages from early childhood through old age.

7. Is felt to be caused by abnormalities in chemicals in the brain called neurotransmitters which carry messages from one nerve ending to the next in the brain.

8. Needs treatment.

Depression Occurs in:

1. At least 5 percent of the population at any one time.

2. About 10 to 25 percent of the population at some time during their lives.

3. About 20,000,000 Americans.

It Is also Known that:

1. Only about 25 to 50 percent of depressed people seek professional help.

2. At least 10 percent of people with depression also have mania or mood swings.

3. 18 to 23 percent of women and 8 to 11 percent of men have a major depression severe enough to be hospitalized sometime in their lifetime.

4. 1.5 million people are treated for depression each year in the United States, but over 4.5 million others suffering with depression go untreated.

5. Over half of those who have a major depression will eventually have another episode.

Source: Center for Affective Disorders
Department of Psychiatry
University of Wisconsin, Madison

---

ness and its treatment, or are being treated for the physical symptoms of psychological illness such as the anorexia and weight loss associated with depression, or the gastric ulceration associated with chronic anxiety. In ICUs, for example, today's often highly technological medical care frequently places the already psychologically compromised patient under tremendous physical and psychological stress. As a result, many psychological illnesses such as anxiety and severe depression are commonly found on the problem list of today's intensive-care patient. A patient might be a chronic renal patient post-transplant, a child with biliary atresia who receives a liver transplant, or a cancer patient undergoing immunosuppressive therapy in preparation for a bone marrow transplant. Families of patients subjected to such stress also require skilled support.

NEEDS OF THE GERIATRIC POPULATION

Another group vulnerable to psychiatric illness is the geriatric population. This group has the highest incidence of functional and organic psychiatric illness as well as the highest suicide rate. This group also occupies most of the chronic and acute-care hospital beds in the United States (Jarvik & Small, 1982; Larson et al., 1983).

DETERRENTS TO OBTAINING NEEDED PSYCHIATRIC MENTAL HEALTH TREATMENT

Despite their high incidence of psychiatric illness, few geriatric or critical-care patients ever see a psychiatrist or a psychiatric nurse. The lack of psychiatric or

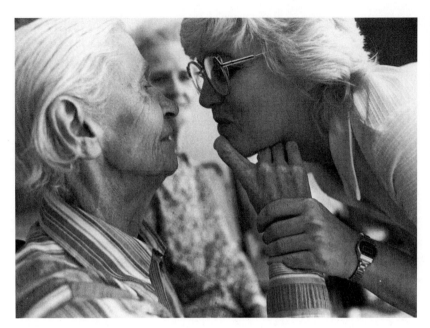

Medicare may not pay for mental health treatment for the elderly, but it does pay for nursing care, and a caring nurse can be worth a lot of psychotherapy.

psychological services for the elderly and/or intensive-care patient can be attributed in part to the gap between traditional psychiatry, which depends on talking about feelings, and today's patient, who may be unable to talk at all because of being intubated and/or immobilized, and who is usually too overwhelmed by the experience of being ill and hospitalized to respond to traditional therapy even if it were physically possible.

In spite of studies which show that providing mental health services for the hospitalized elderly can significantly reduce hospital stays and subsequent care needs (Mumford et al., 1984), it appears that the elderly are seriously underusing mental health services that would benefit them and their communities (Mumford et al., 1984).

It is not just the problem of a traditional system in a high-tech society that prevents people from receiving the psychiatric mental health services they may need. Consulting a mental health professional is still, for many people, embarrassing; they are often afraid of being labeled "crazy" or unable to solve their own problems. This remains the case, despite evidence that nationwide efforts to increase access to mental health care—for example, the establishment of a mental health center in each county—has succeeded in decreasing the number of visits to local physicians for physical complaints (Mumford et al., 1984). (See Box 1–2.)

The most significant deterrent to obtaining adequate psychiatric care, however, is lack of financial resources. Insurance coverage for inpatient and outpatient psychiatric services is becoming more and more limited, even though the nurse who is trained in psychiatric care and other mental health professionals are likely to save the patient and his insurance company the cost of extra medical care. For example, traditional psychiatric care for a burn patient who is hospitalized for two months would cost approximately $2,400 (three therapy or consultation hours per week at $100 per hour). Nursing care that addresses the patient's psychological as well as physiological needs adds no additional cost. But if no psychiatric care is given, the charges for medical care arising from the physical complications of burn injury associated with psychiatric illnesses such as severe anxiety and depression (complications which are likely to occur in the absence of some type of psychiatric consultation for the burn victim) could be astronomical. For instance, if the nurse is unable to debride adequately a burn patient's wounds due to his anxiety, the stage is set for infection. If a patient's anxiety also limits or eliminates physiotherapy, limb contractures are likely to occur. The plastic surgery to release such contractures would add risk as well as cost to the patient's rehabilitation. Complications such as graft loss and gastrointestinal disturbances (decreased appetite, vomiting, ulcer formation, and diarrhea), both associated with anxiety and depression, present similar problems.

Additional impediments to psychiatric services include the decline of federal funding for psychiatric

Box 1–2 ● The Psychological Route to Cutting Costs

Bill Thompson was in bad shape. He had no appetite, could not sleep, and had lost interest in sex. His lower back pain had gotten so bad that he was missing work frequently. Finally he could not go to work at all.

After 18 months of disability, Mr. Thompson was considering surgery to sever nerves in his back. As a last resort, he went to a psychotherapist, and the truth came out.

Mr. Thompson was the controller of the Acme Company, a family-run business that had not changed chiefs in the 23 years he had worked for it. But when the owner's son took over and started to computerize the operations, Mr. Thompson, at age 54, had to face a whole new world. That idea so frightened him that

he literally made himself sick.

After just five therapy sessions, he understood that fact. His back pains and other symptoms vanished.

Between medical bills and lost work days, Mr. Thompson's back episode cost his company $100,000. Had he immediately gone for therapy, the cost would have been a fraction of that amount.

Bill Thompson and Acme are fictitious names—but Nicholas Cummings, the psychologist who tells the story, swears that all the other details are true. And he insists that similar stories abound throughout Corporate America. "Companies are realizing what a tremendous waste of re-

---

care of individuals on welfare, and the proliferation of Health Maintenance Organizations (HMOs) (President's Commission on Mental Health, 1978). Though it has been claimed that Medical Assistance covers psychiatric services, the red tape involved in getting this benefit effectively results in psychiatric services being unavailable or severely limited to Medical Assistance patients who do not also have private health insurance, or who have enrolled in an HMO that does not offer adequate mental health care services. Many HMOs allocate as little as 1 percent of their health care budget for mental health care (Marshall, J., 1986). In addition, HMOs decrease the incentive of affiliated mental health professionals to provide psychiatric care by creating an inverse ratio between length of treatment and reimbursement: the longer the psychotherapist counsels a patient, the less she is paid.

IMPORTANCE OF PSYCHIATRIC MENTAL HEALTH NURSING CARE

It is clear that psychiatric mental health nursing care can save money, and, more important, help restore both physical and mental health more quickly in many kinds of patients. Nurse generalists in the hospital and community as well as psychiatric nurses need to be informed about mind-body phenomena

since they are often responsible for making referrals to and participating in services directed at promoting mental health, detecting and treating the symptoms of mental illness (for example, depression associated with hospitalization), referring patients who require the skills of a psychiatric specialist, and helping patients deal with the associated problems of social stigma and limited financial resources. In addition, the commitment of the nursing profession to treat the "whole person" and/or to provide family-centered care, demands that today's nurse have a working knowledge of psychopathology as well as pathophysiology (ANA, 1982).

The nurse also needs to be familiar with the models and research used in understanding and treating psychiatric illness in addition to the models and theories that guide nursing practice in the area of psychiatric mental health nursing care. Most important, today's nurse must be committed to promoting mental health and working with mental illness with an approach just as scientific as her approach to physical illness.

SCOPE OF PSYCHIATRIC MENTAL HEALTH NURSING PRACTICE

The Standards of Psychiatric and Mental Health Nursing Practice are summarized in Table 1–1 and apply to any setting in which psychiatric and mental

sources it is" to ignore an employee's psychological problems, Mr. Cummings said.

Indeed, health care professionals have long talked about "somatization"—the process by which a psychological problem manifests itself as a physical disability. But now a growing number of insurance companies and their corporate clients are starting to talk about it too, in dollars-and-cents terms. They are finding that they can lower overall health care costs by picking up the tab for psychotherapy, or by offering in-house mental health programs.

It is not hard to document. Preliminary results from the first year of a five-year, $4.3 million study in which some 85,000 Federal employees and Hawaii residents eligible for Medicaid were provided with access to short-term psychotherapy, show a reduction of 37 percent in their total medical bills. That reduction already has translated into a savings to the Government in terms of Medicaid health claims of nearly $16 million.

Other studies have shown even more dramatic cost cuts. As far back as 1967, Mr. Cummings, who is now directing the Hawaii project, published data indicating that as much as 60 percent of visits to physicians are made by people with no physical illness, and that short-term psychotherapy to find the psychological problem behind their ailments could cut down on further medical bills by 75 percent.

An ongoing study of health claims filed by 6.7 million Federal workers, begun in the 1970's, shows that employees who went for mental health treatment had much higher medical costs initially than did those not receiving treatment. After five years, however, even as they got older, their medical costs dropped below that of the second group. The study also found that patients aged 55 and older who received treatment showed the greatest drop in hospital charges.

Source: Mervis, J. (1985) *New York Times,* Sun. Nov. 24, p. 12.

health nursing is practiced, and to both generalists and specialists. In dealing with the patient's psyche, the nurse uses the scientific **nursing process** of assessment, analysis, planning, intervention, and evaluation which provides the context for nursing care. Assessment, the first step, requires not only the ability to differentiate abnormal from normal psychological functioning but also knowledge of the parameters which apply. While the physical assessment includes information on vital signs, respiratory functioning, and so on, the parameters of the **psychiatric/mental-health assessment** include general behavior, cognitive functioning, mood or affect, and thought content. Psychiatric assessment with a psychoanalytic component also includes an appraisal of the nurse's own emotional reactions to the patient (countertransference)[1] in order to complete the data base. Finally, the context of the nursing process when psychological functioning and/or psychopathology is its focus includes the theoretical models that attempt to explain human behavior, as well as the outcome of research regarding the causes and treatment of psychiatric illness.

[1]Countertransference is a controversial concept in psychoanalytic circles. Definitions range from the sum total of the therapist's feelings about and behavior towards the patient, to the therapist's unanalyzed conflicts (Gorkin, 1987) that affect the treatment process. See Chapter 7, "The Nurse as Therapist," for more discussion of this concept.

DEFINING PSYCHOPATHOLOGY

Psychopathology and mental illness are hard concepts to define. Many questions arise. Is it possible to define psychological normality and, thus, mental abnormality without imposing value judgments? Does the label "normal" apply to what we value as good, and the label "sick" apply to what we consider strange, deviant, or bad? Seeking therapy for depression, for example, may be labeled "positive" by some (therapists) and "negative" by others (people who view psychiatric illness as an indication of poor moral character).

ETHICAL ISSUES

Once we define psychopathology and start looking for examples in mental states and behaviors, ethical issues arise. Labeling an individual's behavior may make communication about treatment, prognosis, and research easier, but it also can determine other people's perceptions of that person by setting up expectations. For example, it has been shown that students falsely labeled retarded were perceived as, and in fact, "made" retarded by teachers who expected little of them and encouraged less (Rosenthal and Jacobsen, 1960). This has led some mental health professionals to define "disease" as "that which is called a disease by a disease-caller" (Fost, 1984).

TABLE 1–1 Standards of psychiatric and mental health nursing practice

Professional Practice Standards

Standard 1. Theory

The nurse applies appropriate theory that is scientifically sound as basis for decisions regarding nursing practice.

Standard 2. Data collection

The nurse continuously collects data that are comprehensive, accurate, and systematic.

Standard 3. Diagnosis

The nurse utilizes nursing diagnoses and/or standard classification of mental disorders to express conclusions supported by recorded assessment data and current scientific premises.

Standard 4. Planning

The nurse develops a nursing care plan with specific goals and interventions delineating nursing actions unique to each client's needs.

Standard 5. Intervention

The nurse intervenes as guided by the nursing care plan to implement nursing actions that promote, maintain, or restore physical and mental health, prevent illness, and effect rehabilitation.

Standard 5-A. Intervention: Psychotherapeutic Interventions

The nurse uses psychotherapeutic interventions to assist clients in regaining or improving their previous coping abilities and to prevent further disability.

Standard 5-B. Intervention: Health Teaching

The nurse assists clients, families, and groups to achieve satisfying and productive patterns of living through health teaching.

Standard 5-C. Intervention: Activities of Daily Living

The nurse uses the activities of daily living in a goal-directed way to foster adequate self-care and physical and mental well-being of clients.

Standard 5-D. Intervention: Somatic Therapies

The nurse uses knowledge of somatic therapies and applies related clinical skills in working with clients.

Standard 5-E Intervention: Therapeutic Environment

The nurse provides, structures, and maintains a therapeutic environment in collaboration with the client and other health care providers.

SOCIOLOGICAL ISSUES

Philosophical and ethical issues are complicated by sociological ones. For example, a welfare recipient may be more likely to be harmed rather than helped by being labeled as having a psychiatric illness. The label may stigmatize the person, making it harder for him to find or keep a job. A jobless, single parent suspected of child abuse may be more likely to be sent to jail than to a therapist, because he is more likely to come to the attention of the police than would a community member with high social and economic status.

The sociological perspective has also been used to argue that behavior which is the "norm" or statistically average, understandable, avoidable under other sociological conditions, and/or a "socially appropriate" adaptation (Offer, 1974) warrants neither labeling nor *treatment*. It would follow from this that the high incidence of alcoholism in the American Indian, and the high incidence of depression in the general population (which occurs four times more frequently than cancer [CAD Courier, April, 1985]), should not be attended to. This is difficult to justify considering the financial cost alone of treating the non-stigmatizing *physical illness* associated with many psychiatric conditions, for example, liver failure and organic brain syndrome in the case of alcoholism.

MENTAL ILLNESS: MYTH OR GROWTH-PROMOTING REALITY?

Philosophical, ethical, and sociological issues cannot be avoided in any attempt to identify the presence or absence of mental disorder in a person. Even attempts to be as scientific as possible are fraught with philosophical challenges and value judgments. How do we decide what to measure? An individual's single act or moment of behavior? The whole functioning person? The outcome of an individual's behavior or the process that sets it in motion (Kubie, 1954)? Many mental health researchers and clinical practitioners have wrestled with these questions. The individuals discussed below have been chosen for this text because of their contributions to the field of

Standard 5-F. Intervention: Psychotherapy

The nurse utilizes advanced clinical expertise in individual, group, and family psychotherapy, child psychotherapy, and other treatment modalities to function as a psychotherapist and recognizes professional accountability for nursing practice.

Standard 6. Evaluation

The nurse evaluates client responses to nursing actions in order to revise the data base, nursing diagnosis, and nursing care plan.

Professional Performance Standards

Standard 7. Peer Review

The nurse participates in peer review and other means of evaluation to assure quality of nursing care provided for clients.

Standard 8. Continuing Education

The nurse assumes responsibility for continuing education and professional development and contributes to the professional growth of others.

Standard 9. Interdisciplinary Collaboration

The nurse collaborates with other health care providers in assessing, planning, implementing, and evaluating programs and other mental health activities.

Standard 10. Utilization of Community Health Systems

The nurse participates with other members of the community in assessing, planning, implementing, and evaluating mental health services and community systems that include the promotion of the broad continuum of primary, secondary, and tertiary prevention of mental illness.

Standard 11. Research

The nurse contributes to nursing and the mental health field through innovations in theory and practice and participation in research.

Source: From American Nurses' Association (1982). Standards of psychiatric and mental health nursing practice.

mental health care and because of the significance of their attempts to resolve the philosophical, ethical, and sociological problems cited above.

SZASZ: THE MYTH OF MENTAL ILLNESS

Thomas Szasz (1960) believes that mental illness is a myth. He claims that labels denoting mental disorder reflect the social context of the individual who has been labeled rather than anything that is wrong with the individual (Szasz, 1960). Stating that the concept of illness, whether physical or mental, implies deviation from a norm based on psychosocial, ethical, and legal concepts, Szasz warns that medical remedies are inappropriate. The nature of the defects and their proposed remedies must not be in conflict.

An even greater problem, according to Szasz, is the idea that there are such things as mental defects at all. This relegates "conflicting human needs, aspirations, and values" or "complicated problems in living" (p. 17) to the status of an immoral, impersonal "thing." In fact, Szasz feels that belief in mental illness as something other than man's trouble getting along with his fellow man is the proper heir to the belief in demonology and witchcraft. Szasz feels that the purpose of belief in mental illness is to "render more palatable the bitter pill of moral conflicts in human relations" (p. 118).

ROSENHAN: MENTAL ILLNESS IS IN THE EYE OF THE BEHOLDER

Rosenhan (1973) holds a view similar to that of Szasz: he has attempted to prove that there is no such thing as mental illness. In his famous but controversial experiment, pseudo-patients were admitted to several inpatient psychiatric units where they feigned auditory hallucinations. Once admitted, the pseudo-patients behaved "normally," that is, they were asymptomatic. The majority of these pseudo-patients were discharged with a diagnosis of "schizophrenia, in remission", rather than "recovered", and Rosenhan thus argues that illness is in the eye of the beholder, and labels tend to be "sticky." Rosenhan's critics refute his conclusions, citing that the experimental design was inadequate and led to generalizations about real patients based on the hospital staff's reactions to pseudo-patients. However, even Rosenhan's critics applaud him for demonstrating the associated ambiguities and potential problems of labeling patients with psychiatric diagnoses. Twelve years later the "stickiness" of labels denoting psychiatric illness and associated risk was dramatically demonstrated by one man's bid for the vice-presidential nomination. In 1972, Thomas Eagleton was pressured out of his vice-presidential spot on the Democratic ticket because of a history of being treated for depression. (It should be noted that discouraged supporters countered with the observation that at least *their* man had had *treatment*.)

WHITAKER: CRAZINESS IS WHERE LIFE IS

Carl Whitaker, a well known family therapist (see Chapter 21) is on the other end of the theoretical continuum from Szasz and Rosenhan: he contends that "craziness is where life is" (Neil and Kniskern, 1982). Whitaker, dubbed the "mad hatter" by his colleagues and students, is known for inviting schizophrenic patients to be cotherapists; falling asleep during therapy; and, in general, treating craziness with craziness. More a philosopher than a scientist, Whitaker draws on his personal and professional experience over the last fifty years in arriving at this perspective. At least one scientific study supports his belief that symptoms of psychopathology may reflect a more realistic response to the world than "normal" affect and/or behavior: Alloy and Abramson found that depressives see the world more, not less, realistically than normal controls (1981).

MODELS OF PSYCHOPATHOLOGY

Clearcut causes of psychopathology are even more elusive than definitions. Scientifically rigorous prospective studies are few. Excellent work using animal models of mental illness is bringing researchers significantly closer to understanding, but it is a giant leap to generalize from the rat or the Rhesus monkey to a human being. At the same time, it is important to hypothesize intelligently about the causes of mental illness in order to develop effective treatment. Hypotheses about mental illness typically fall into one of three categories: psychoanalytic (also referred to as psychodynamic), behavioral, and biological (see Chapter 2). No single theory is likely to provide a

wholly satisfactory explanation. Most psychiatric disorders are thought to have several causes. For example, because evidence has accumulated that suggests there are biological correlates of schizophrenia (Gottesman et al., 1972; Kety, 1983), the old hypothesis that schizophrenia is caused solely by lack of affection from "refrigerator mothers" (Haley et al., 1956) during childhood is no longer considered tenable. At the same time, biology isn't "the answer" either. This is clear because even an identical twin of an individual with schizophrenia will not *necessarily* develop the illness. What seems most likely is that schizophrenia, as well as other psychiatric disorders, are caused by a combination of biological and experiential factors.

PSYCHOANALYTIC THEORIES

The **psychoanalytic model** of mental illness had its beginning in the work of Freud. Freud, a neurologist who was a contemporary of Pavlov and Einstein, was unsatisfied with an entirely biological view of man and physical explanations of behavior, especially when none was apparent. He is thought to have been influenced by Einstein's theory of relativity which holds that the universe is composed of matter *and* energy, and is credited with the theory of the unconscious and its structure (id, ego, and superego), drive-theory, and the power of infantile sexuality (Freud, S., 1958). His successors have gone on to expand his ideas through work on defense mechanisms and stages of psychological development (Erickson, 1950; Freud, A. 1966), the effect of early relationships (Mahler, 1975; Masterson, 1981), and the family's, not just the individual's, unconscious (Neil and Kniskern, 1982; Andolfi et al., 1983).

BEHAVIORAL THEORIES

The **behavioral model** of psychopathology draws on the work of Pavlov (1927), Skinner (1938), Wolpe (1973), and other learning theorists. This model is built on the premise that all behavior, normal and pathological, is learned. According to this view, randomly occurring behaviors that are reinforced positively, with rewards, or negatively, through the avoidance of negative consequences, persist. Behavioral theory has become very complex since Pavlov's first conditioning experiment (Pavlov, 1927). The notion of "behavior" has been expanded to include an individual's thoughts (Beck, 1964). Whether or not rewards and punishment are contingent on specific behavior has been shown to be as important to

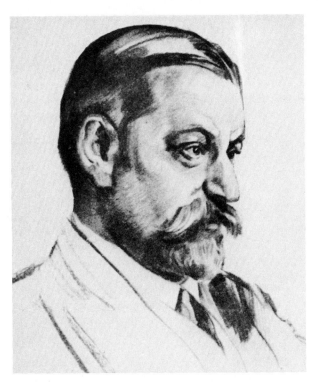

A little known fact about Sigmund Freud: Unlike his male colleagues, Freud fostered aspiring female analysts in their professional pursuits. He tried to get them into the (all male) Psychoanalytic Society, but failed. However, upon his retirement, he turned over his work and clients to his last analysand (patient), a woman who called herself H. D. (Information courtesy of Susan Freidman from an unpublished manuscript, March, 1984.)

outcome as the intensity of the positive or negative consequence itself (if not more so) (Seligman, 1968). The organism's "readiness" to learn at critical periods of development has also proven to be an important variable in the behavioral model.

BIOLOGICAL THEORIES

Biological models of psychopathology, such as depression (see Chapters 2 and 9), have more credence than ever, but, at best, only explain part of the picture. For example, low levels of circulating catecholamines such as epinephrine and norepinephrine are found in some, but not all, depressed patients. They are strongly associated with the learned helplessness-type of depression (Seligman, 1971), at least in animal experimental subjects, but this has been difficult to demonstrate in humans. Drugs that increase the level of circulating catecholamines are often effective in alleviating most of the symptoms of depres-

sion: sleep and appetite disturbances, decreased energy and sex drive. Yet not all victims of depression are found to be catecholamine deficient; and even those who are do not all respond to drug treatment (Kraemer and McKinney, 1979). Studies with animals point to a combination of both low catecholamine levels and certain experiences in the development of depression: for example, separation of an infant from his mother (Suomi et al., 1976). It is difficult, however, to generalize from animal research to the human situation. Mental-health professionals are left with potentially effective but not guaranteed treatments and some treatments, such as antidepressant drugs and electroconvulsive therapy, which have significant side effects.

IF YOU'VE SEEN ONE THEORY . . .

At first glance, these three models appear to be very different; however, upon closer inspection, it is apparent that they have many links. The first researchers to break free from the biological model, Freud and Pavlov, were both neurologists by training, as well as contemporaries. Also, the behaviorists who followed Pavlov examined many of Freud's observations under the lens of the scientific method. Today the behavioral and psychoanalytic models are being brought even closer together through biological links. Endorphins, the endogenous opiates released in the brain under conditions of extreme physical or psychological stress, have been implicated in phenomena ranging from attachment (Herman & Panksepp, 1978), to a manifestation of depression called "learned helplessness," the consequence of lack of environmental predictability and controllability (Maier et al., 1981). And given the genetic links surfacing in research on schizophrenia, alcoholism, and mood disorders, Freud would not be alone today among clinicians and theorists cautioning us to choose our relatives wisely.

While these three models greatly help us understand and deal with pathological human behavior, they do have their limits. Regardless of the model we choose as the context for viewing behavior, we cannot make statements about cause and effect unless we do prospective, controlled studies.

Retrospective data gathering can only illuminate things that vary together. What is cause and what is effect is impossible to sort out, yet we often think about things as if this were not so. The depressed mother of a child who is failing to thrive is typically viewed and treated as the cause of the child's pathology rather than the other way around, probably be-

Box 1—3 ● Is Mental Illness Inherited? Amish Families Offer a Clue to Manic Depression

It is rare to find a chatterbox among the Amish of Lancaster County, Pa. Rarer still is a flamboyant personality, a braggart, a show-off or, at the other extreme, someone who is deeply depressed or suicidal. In this community of quiet-spoken, humble pacifists, such behavior "really stands out against the social landscape," observes Medical Sociologist Janice Egeland, who has spent more than 25 years among the Old Order Amish, as the group is formally known. When it does occur, the Amish often have an explanation: *"Siss im blut,"* they say; the peculiar behavior is "in the blood."

Last week Egeland, who is from the University of Miami School of Medicine, and a group of scientists at Yale and M.I.T. confirmed that traditional Amish explanation. By employing the tools of molecular biology along with the handwritten genealogical records of Amish families, they showed that the mental disorder known as manic depression is indeed at least partly a matter of bloodlines. Their report, published in the journal *Nature,* conclusively linked cases of manic depression in an Amish family to genes in a specific region of human chromosome 11. "This is the first demonstration of a possible genetic basis for one of the major mental disorders," says Dr. Darrel Regier, director of the division of clinical research at the National Institute of Mental Health (NIMH). "The study ushers in a new era of psychiatric research."

Usually beginning somewhere between the ages of 15 and 35, manic depression afflicts about 1 in every 100 people. Because it causes its victims to oscillate between two extreme emotional states, it is also known to psychiatrists as bipolar affective disorder. In the manic phase, victims become expansive and extravagant, are often unable to sleep or eat, and may talk incessantly. Some assume airs of grandeur. The depressive phase plunges them into hopelessness, loneliness and boundless guilt, feelings that sometimes lead to suicide.

Researchers have long suspected that heredity plays a role in some if not all cases, and the Amish present an ideal setting in which to test that hypothesis. Not only does bipolar behavior contrast sharply with the community's quiet ways, making it

cause of our tendency to see the child who appears to be neglected as the "victim." Because of this common error in thinking, one highly respected psychologist, Paul Meehl (1973), has stated:

> . . . Everything that is wrong with anybody is attributable either to having a battle-ax mother, being raised on the wrong side of the tracks, or having married the wrong mate. It is dangerous to be the parent or spouse of a mentally ill person because you will almost certainly get blamed for it, even if he was patently abnormal before you met him and his family tree abounds with food faddists, recluses, perpetual-motion inventors, suicides, and residents of mental hospitals (p. 263).

Models are not just limited in what they can explain. They can limit the nurse or mental-health professional in her work if she attaches herself to one model and behaves as if the others do not exist. As Meehl (1973, p. 264) has said, if genes turn out to have something to do with deviant behavior (See Box 1–3.), the psychodynamics we think we understand don't necessarily have to be abandoned. The notion that something as "mentalistic" as relationship (talking) therapy can help someone with an organic problem does not have to be given up. Thinking otherwise is not logical, but it is common. A case in point: behavioral and psychodynamic therapy for depression, senile dementia, and schizophrenia has been demonstrated in many studies to be effective in decreasing symptoms (Lazarus, 1973; Simpson & May, 1982; and Wetzel, 1984) in spite of the attractiveness that the biological model holds in attempting to understand better the causes of these disorders.

easy to diagnose, but a number of confounding factors that might contribute to such behavior are absent: alcoholism, drug abuse, unemployment, divorce and violence are extremely rare. In addition, the Amish have large families (seven children on average) and keep genealogical records worthy of Mendel. Best of all, they represent a closed genetic pool. All 12,500 Amish in Lancaster County are descended from 20 or 30 couples who emigrated from Europe in the early 1700s, and only a handful of outsiders have ever married in.

Though manic depression is no more common among the Amish than other groups, Egeland's research turned up 32 active cases. All proved to have family histories of the disease going back several generations. Curiously, all of the 26 suicides documented in the community since 1880 occurred in just four of these families.

The study published last week focused on one 81-member clan. Fourteen members had been diagnosed with manic depression and another five with other mental disorders. Thanks to unusual cooperation from the family, the researchers were able to obtain blood from each member and then isolate DNA from each sample. Using so-called restriction enzymes, they "cut" the DNA into segments. When they compared gene segments from manic depressives with those from normal family members, they found a discrepancy in a region of chromosome 11. Their conclusion: a gene or group of genes in or near this region confers a predisposition to manic depression.

The researchers also confirmed that children of individuals with this genetic anomaly have a 50% chance of inheriting it. However, only 63% of those carrying the gene show signs of the disorder, which suggests that other factors—perhaps environmental—also play a role in bringing on the disease.

Does the same genetic defect play a role in all manic depression? Not necessarily. Two studies also published in last week's *Nature* revealed no link between the chromosome 11 site and manic depression in six non-Amish families prone to the disease. Still, these findings do not undermine the important discovery of a genetic basis for the ailment. Instead, observes NIMH Psychiatrist Sevilla Detera-Wadleigh, who led one of the other studies, they suggest that more than one gene may be involved in manic depression.

The next step for scientists will be to identify the particular gene or genes responsible for manic depression. This will enable them to understand the biochemical basis for the disease, which could lead to better treatments. (The drug lithium carbonate is effective in 70% to 75% of cases.) It could also lead to tests for the diagnosis and identification of people at risk for bipolar disorder.

Egeland hopes for a more immediate benefit from her work. "Too often," she says, "personal embarrassment and social stigma are associated with an illness whose cause is beyond the control of the individual." That stigma should be lessened and more people should be encouraged to seek treatment now that scientists have confirmed the source of manic depression can indeed be *im blut*.

Source: By Claudia Wallis. Reported by Andrea Dorfman/New York and Dick Thompson/Washington *Time*, March 9, 1987, p. 67.

THE NURSING PROCESS

The psychodynamic, behavioral, and biological models provide mental health professionals with the means to organize information about human behavior, including abnormal behavior, and to think about it in ways that help formulate plans for treatment. How then, does the nurse initiate the nursing process in an individual case that involves psychopathology, and how does she obtain the information about thoughts, feelings, and behavior needed to do an adequate assessment? When does she stop collecting information? How and when does she develop a treatment plan? How does she follow up (evaluate) the patient's improvement or lack of it? While the steps in the nursing process outlined in the preceding questions are common to all types of nursing, a few aspects of each stage are specific to nursing that involves mental illnesses wherever they are encountered, in the psychiatric or nonpsychiatric setting.

PSYCHOLOGICAL ASSESSMENT

Time is never wasted by collecting data because the process of assessment is in itself therapeutic. That patients' symptoms often remit during the assessment process (Strupp, 1978) may be due to the sincere interest or apparent caring in the nurse or therapist. If her respect for the patient as a unique individual who needs help in understanding and managing some aspect of his experience is conveyed, relief may be associated with feeling that someone is trying to understand and wants to help. In fact, data collection should never stop. The more information the nurse has, the more accurate her assessment is likely to be. Continuing to collect data after treatment has begun enables her to evaluate the effects of treatment as well as refine the psychiatric and nursing diagnoses.

Several guidelines rule the psychiatric assessment:

1. When the initial psychological assessment is conducted during a crisis or when the patient is emotionally distraught, as is frequently the case, the evaluation must be brief as well as accurate in order to avoid adding to the patient's stress, and it must be accompanied by whatever acute intervention the situation demands.

2. Because the initial assessment marks the beginning of a therapeutic relationship, it should help the patient feel that his concerns are understood and labeled as primary, even when the nurse feels that there are more important things to explore.

3. The nurse monitors the process as well as the content of the entire assessment. She attends to the patient's behavioral and emotional responses as well as her own, since both are necessary components of the data base.

4. The nurse monitors her tendency to proceed in a way determined by her own interests and/or personal needs rather than what are perceived to be the needs of the patient.

The case below illustrates these points.

The Baby Who "Rolled off the Bed"

Anthony, a one-month-old infant, was brought to the emergency room by his mother, Maria, a young single parent. Anthony was irritable and crying and had just vomited. There were bruises on his face and head but no sign of other injuries. The mother, who seemed anxious about the baby's condition, described him as an active infant who cried a lot, and said that he rolled off the bed onto the floor when she left the room briefly to get a clean diaper. She added that he often banged his head against the crib rails and wondered if he had sustained brain damage.

As the nurse took the infant's vital signs and did a physical assessment, she got a psychosocial history from Maria and learned that she had recently left the baby's father after he had abused her. New in the area, she was socially isolated. Her parents lived out of state and had a history of alcoholism. She hadn't heard from them since she left home six months ago with her boyfriend, the baby's father.

The nurse emphathized with Maria's anxiety and offered her some coffee while Anthony was taken to radiology for a CT scan to determine the extent of any internal injury. She then talked with the on-call pediatric resident about whether or not Anthony's condition warranted admission. She was concerned that the resident might not understand the seriousness of the situation that her assessment indicated. She recommended admission of the infant, regardless of the results of the CT scan, because she felt there was a need to evaluate more fully this family's social situation and any immediate threat it might pose to Anthony's physical and mental well-being. In addition, the nurse suggested encouraging Maria to stay in the hospital with her child so that the staff would have a chance to offer her the emotional support she needed now as well as determine her need for continuing social and/or mental-health services.

With the physician's agreement, the nurse explained to Maria that it was necessary to keep the child in the hospital through the night so that his physical condition could be monitored. She told Maria that it was unlikely Anthony had brain damage, but his vomiting and irritability might continue for a day or so. For safety's sake, she explained, it was necessary to keep a close eye on him. With nurses around, Maria would be able to get some sleep. In the morning, one of the pediatric nurses and the doctor would talk with her again in order to see how they could help her prevent her child from injury in the future. The nurse noticed that Maria seemed much less anxious, and offered to take her up to pediatrics and introduce her to the night nurse who would watch the baby while she got some needed rest. When Maria asked the nurse if she would see her again, the nurse felt pleased. She had made contact with a woman who could be an abusive parent and, as a result, had paved the way for the potentially life-saving treatment this family could be offered.

This nurse's concern that Anthony, too young to roll off a bed, was shaken or thrown in his crib by his exasperated, needy mother was supported by the X-ray findings of brain contusion. Her empathic, directive approach with Maria set the stage for a complete psychosocial evaluation in the morning and the beginning of a treatment plan directed at preventing further abuse of the child. The nurse's focus on the child *and* the mother's worry about him, rather than on any of their other problems, conveyed that she had taken the mother's concern about the child seriously and wanted to work with the mother in trying to prevent further injury to the infant. The mother, no doubt, felt listened to, respected, and accepted despite the fact that her child had been injured while in her care.*

---

*It should be noted that either the nurse, the physician, the pediatric social worker, or the hospital's child abuse team is required by law in all states to report suspected physical child abuse through the County Social Services Department of Child Protection. Time should be taken, however, to advise the parent of the legal mandate to report, its purpose, the chances of it ultimately being helpful though acutely traumatic, and the primary nurse's and/or social worker's commitment to provide support and consultation through this crisis.

The ER nurse in the example about Anthony did a *brief* psychological assessment. Emergency rooms and ICUs lend themselves to little else. How, then, does the brief assessment provide the nurse with the information she needs?

The psychological assessment, brief or comprehensive, *always* includes an interview with the patient during which the nurse, while asking questions about the **presenting problem** and medical and psychiatric history, attends to the patient's behavioral and affective (or emotional) responses to the interviewer. The nurse also attends to her own inner responses to the patient, asking herself whether she feels, for example, intimidated, rejected, angry, or clung to. These feelings can be a source of information about the patient. They may indicate how he is experienced by others or, possibly, how he himself is feeling.

INTERVIEW FORMAT. The brief-interview format includes a history of the presenting problem and the mental-status exam. The **mental-status exam** includes the assessment of the patient's general appearance and behavior, affective range, thought processes, and thought content.

The extensive interview includes the same information as the brief interview, but adds previous treatment history, family and social history, school and work history, and medical history. The mnemonic "Basic Id" (Lazarus, 1973) offers a guide for conducting an assessment that includes most of this content.

B **B**ehavior during the interview and the patient's report of behavior during a typical day.

A **A**ffect (emotional range) during the interview as well as in general, as reported by the patient.

S **S**ensory: What gives the patient pleasure? What is positive in his life? Has he ever had any unusual sensory experiences (such as hallucinations)?

I **I**nterpersonal relationships: Who is the patient close to in his family, or of his friends? Who is he worried about or angry with?

C **C**ognitive functioning: If formal testing is not practical, what does the patient's general level of cognitive functioning seem to be? How much education does he have and how well did he do in school?

I **I**magery: What are the patient's wishes and fantasies? Does he have any troubling thoughts or feelings?

D **D**rugs: Is the patient under medical supervision of any kind? Does he regularly take prescribed medication? Does he use nonprescription or street drugs of any kind? What is his average daily alcohol and/or caffeine intake? Is the patient a smoker?

OTHER ASPECTS OF ASSESSMENT. Observing the patient in situations other than the one-to-one interview setting can be illuminating. Seeing the patient in the context of his family is especially helpful. Old treatment records should be reviewed by the nurse as soon as possible after seeing the patient. Medical records, therapy case notes, and social service agency files should be requested and reviewed with the patient's written consent. In some cases, neuropsychiatric, intelligence, personality, and/or projective testing (testing of the patient's response to ambiguous stimuli, such as the Rorschach "ink blots") can uncover information that is otherwise difficult to obtain. Psychological testing can also help to validate (or invalidate) impressions formed during the interview.

NURSING DIAGNOSIS

When the assessment has been completed (although the nurse will continue to assess in the course of her interventions), the nurse will make hypotheses about the DSM-III-R diagnosis and will formulate the **nursing diagnoses.** As defined by the ANA Division on Psychiatric and Mental Health Nursing Practice (1982), the nursing diagnoses will be related to actual or potential health problems in regard to:

1. Self-care limitations or impaired functioning whose general etiology is mental and emotional distress; deficits in the ways significant systems are functioning; and internal psychic and/or developmental issues.

2. Emotional stress or crisis components of illness, pain, self-concept changes, and life process changes.

3. Emotional problems related to daily experiences.

4. Physical symptoms that occur simultaneously with altered psychic functioning.

5. Alterations in thinking, perceiving, symbolizing, communicating, and decision-making abilities.

6. Impaired abilities to relate to others.

7. Behaviors and mental states that indicate the client is a danger to self or others or is gravely disabled (ANA, 1982, p. 5).

Box 1—4 ● Integrating Body and Mind with Relaxation Techniques

The stresses associated with illness and hospitalization will often evoke the physiological state termed the "fight or flight response." Fight or flight, characterized by increased oxygen consumption and rises in heart rate, blood pressure, and respiratory rates, usually leaves a person feeling anxious and uncomfortable. Fortunately, the body has another, opposite mechanism, called the **relaxation response,** which is characterized by lowered oxygen consumption and decreases in heart rate, blood pressure, and respiratory rates, with associated feelings of peace and tranquility. The relaxation response may be elicited in a number of ways, such as focused attention on one word or phrase while passively disregarding everyday thoughts as they try to intrude.

Nurses have long recognized the importance of relaxation techniques to people undergoing the stress of illness and hospitalization. But in the past fifteen years, researchers have focused their attention on how this re-

sponse works, how it is elicited, and what specific effects it has on the body; studies suggest that the relaxation response works because it allows the right and left hemispheres of the brain to interact more, increasing cognitive receptiveness and making it easier to think innovatively. It has been found that regular use of the relaxation response may help to reduce both the frequency and intensity of pain and can also be used to increase the effectiveness of psychotherapy. Migraine sufferers, for instance, have experienced less severe and less frequent headaches with regular elicitation of the response. Anxiety and its accompanying hostility has also been relieved (see Chapter 8) with the relaxation response. People who regularly evoke the response say they feel more calm and in better control of their lives (Benson, 1988).

Given the power of this response to help not only people who are suffering from physical or mental illness, but anyone who is subject to the stresses of modern life, it seems

---

Specific nursing diagnoses are cited throughout this text with application to the mental health and illness described.

PLANNING AND IMPLEMENTATION

After formulating the diagnoses, the nurse considers the major models or theories (both psychological and nursing) used to understand the etiology of psychiatric illness and suggest directions for treatment. Treatment may involve psychoanalytic or "talking" therapies, biological, and/or behavioral or learning therapies. While most professionals reserve the term **psychotherapy** for the "talking" therapies, or those that involve exploring thoughts and feelings within a therapeutic relationship directed at increasing self-understanding and healthy adaptation, any treatment or intervention directed at alleviating psychological distress or injury is psychotherapy. Within this framework, psychoanalysis is psychotherapy, but so is a positive reinforcement program or giving a depressed hospitalized child maximum control of painful pro-

cedures. Two biological therapies, electroconvulsive therapy and psychotropic drug therapy, and behavioral therapy, such as biofeedback, should also be considered psychotherapy. Thus while a patient may have only one "talking" psychotherapist, his psychoanalyst, he may have several professionals working with him to preserve or improve his mental health. His nurse may qualify as one of them if she attempts to set up his environment in a psychologically therapeutic way, for example, by increasing the predictability and controllability of painful procedures like dressing changes and wound care; if she administers psychotropic medications in a safe, informed way; and if she focuses on helping the patient develop a psychological support network and/or a therapeutic relationship with a mental health professional. (See Box 1–4.)

Use of one or more of the models is essential to organizing the patient's specific psychiatric symptomatology and concerns, hypothesizing about their etiology, and developing treatment plans. The fol-

reasonable for nurses to understand more about how the response can be elicited. Nurses themselves work in one of the most stress-producing jobs of our time and are likely to experience some form of job burn-out if they are not able to learn skills that will help them achieve a sense of balance and calm in their working life. Evoking the relaxation response is not difficult; it is not necessary to have a lot of time or even a quiet room to bring it about. Some ideas for learning this technique are summarized below.

1. Just focus on rhythmic abdominal breathing. As you inhale and exhale, just be with your breathing. Be mindful of the experience of air moving in and out. It is so simple. Another variation is breath counting. With each exhale, count one.

2. As you sit in a chair while charting or taking a break, imagine that you have an imaginary sky hook coming out of the top of your head. Attach your imaginary sky hook to your imaginary skyline. Allow your shoulders to drop, and feel the relaxation filling your total body as you float freely up into the sky.

3. Feel your body in postural alignment. Scan your body to feel areas of tension. Imagine that those tense muscle fibers are smoothing out.

4. Be aware of special images that you can clearly bring to mind that help you feel peaceful and quiet, to gain an inner calm, such as an ocean, a special place in nature, a meadow, or even a place in your own home.

5. Sit quietly, close your eyes, relax your face muscles, and breathe with your abdomen. Be mindful of focusing your attention. There are several ways of focusing. You can watch your flow of consciousness—all those thoughts that come and go—not trying to hang onto any particular thought. Second, you can focus on one thing, such as a symbol or your breath. Any time your mind wanders, just bring your attention back to focusing on the object. This exercise is also helpful when you feel yourself getting angry at work. Just for a moment, shift your awareness away from the anger. Bring into your mind a relaxing image or bathe yourself in a calming color. Focus on it for a few seconds. Then rehearse in your mind a way to deal with the anger in the least stressful way.

6. Use the quieting response. Imagine that you have breathing holes in the bottom of your feet. (There are no rules in the imagination!) Whenever you feel yourself getting tense, smile to yourself and say, "I can help calm myself" and focus on the breathing holes in your feet. Take a deep breath in through your feet— feel the relaxation move all the way to the top of your head. As you exhale, feel the tension moving all the way down your body and out your feet. This exercise takes only a few seconds and is very helpful during the most difficult situations in critical care, e.g., cardiac arrest and cardiogenic shock. (Kenner et al., 1985)

lowing example illustrates the use of all three models in understanding and treating symptoms of depression in a young child.

Mark: A Burn Patient

Mark, age 3, was a patient on a burn unit, where he was being treated for second and third degree scald burns sustained when he turned on the hot water faucet in the bathtub. His 7-year-old sister had been bathing him while their mother, a single parent, slept. Though his and his sister's screams woke their mother immediately, Mark was seriously burned by the time she pulled him out of the bathtub. Relevant history included the following.

Mark's mother, age 25, was self-supporting but currently unemployed. She had been struggling to keep her family together since they were left by the children's father shortly after Mark's birth. Mark's mother was an adult child of alcoholic parents. She did not have a drinking problem but had trouble with depression, which had been treated successfully in the past with antidepressant medication and psychotherapy. Her current financial and social situation, however, made therapy and antidepressant medication unavailable to her. There was a waiting list at the local mental-health center and she did not have private insurance. She was isolated socially as a result of her financial problems, unemployment, and lack of a support system in her family. The evening Mark was burned, his mother, who had been sleeping poorly at night, had fallen asleep on the living room sofa. As she rode with her son in the ambulance on the way to the hospital, she reproached herself for thinking the children could manage their evening baths alone. They were "good kids" and often able to manage by themselves. This helped when she was too depressed to function—about one week a month on the average. This had been one of those weeks.

Once they arrived in the emergency room at University Hospital, Mark was evaluated by a pediatrician, a surgical resident, and a nurse from the burn unit. While most burn patients do not initially experience a lot of pain, children are usually quite anxious about all the commotion going on around them as well as the series of invasive procedures they experience. Mark, unlike most 3-year-olds, seemed to accept passively his situation. He did not protest actively, but only whimpered and clung to his mother as much as it was possible. The nurse noted his malnourished appearance and sad facial expression along with his passivity. Though she had not yet completed the psychological and social assessments, she had an idea about the type of social situation this mother and her children came from as a result of their appearance and the medical assistance card the mother presented. The nurse was impressed with how fatigued the mother appeared to be, as well as Mark's depressed presentation. As the nurse began the process of assessment, she began organizing the information available to her with the help of the psychoanalytic, behavioral, and biological models of psychopathology. She also began to think about the diagnostic labels, medical and nursing, that the situation warranted and the associated plan of care and treatment.

Mark's psychological problems can be best understood in the context of all three models. The psychoanalytic model would suggest that he, though currently at risk for depression secondary to the gradually increasing pain and loss he has begun to experience, may have a preexisting depression associated with his mother's depression and associated emotional unavailability and social isolation. The hospitalization-induced separation from her, while not total, would be sure to make a bad situation worse for them both.

The behavioral model also applies to Mark's situation. First, since the hospitalization is likely to involve painful daily dressing changes and scrubbing and debriding of open wounds, it is likely to induce learned helplessness (Seligman, 1971), the specific type of depression referred to on page 3 (see also Chapter 7), the result of unpredictable and uncontrollable events, especially those that are aversive. From another behavioral perspective, Mark's now-hampered ability to elicit positive reinforcement from his environment in familiar ways as a result of his burn injury and associated hospitalization is certain to maintain, if not worsen, his depression.

Finally, the biological model would put Mark at risk for depression because of his family history of depression and alcoholism and his mother's responsiveness to antidepressant medication. In addition, the biological model would suggest that Mark's situ-

ation is especially precarious, since depression, regardless of its origin, is associated with appetite, sleep, mood and energy disturbances, and gastrointestinal distress. Thus Mark's physical recovery is certain to be sabotaged by what seems to be an inevitable, serious psychological illness. This, in turn, is likely to result in further physical complications such as infection, graft loss, extensive scarring, and muscle contractures, all of which are associated with longer hospitalization and the anxiety and depression that often accompanies it. A downward spiral can begin that is very difficult to stop.

All three models can be useful in the development of a treatment and care plan for Mark and his family. For example, the psychoanalytic model would suggest play therapy directed at helping him find words to describe his feelings, especially sadness, anger, and fear, obviating the need to act them out, especially in ways that interfere with recovery (for example, by refusing to eat or physically protesting needed treatments). Play therapy would also provide a forum in which Mark, rather than the adults in his life, could be in control. He could also use it to attempt to master his newly acquired fears by identifying with the "aggressor" (medical and nursing staff who are perceived as "attacking" to the extent that they do not or cannot encourage his active involvement with his daily treatment) in his fantasies, in an attempt to overcome his sense of helplessness and victimization. The psychoanalytic model would also support treating Mark's mother's depression with one-on-one psychotherapy, and reinvolving her actively in his life, or, if that isn't possible, providing a mother substitute.

The behavioral model would suggest still other treatment strategies. Learned helplessness theory would emphasize maximizing the predictability and controllability of the aversive aspects of Mark's world, for example, by focusing him on and actively involving him in his daily dressing changes. This theory, along with the theory of associative learning, suggests that "safety signals" (Seligman et al., 1971), stimuli predictably associated with safety (or lack of aversive events), be developed and used to help Mark sort out conditioned stimuli for pain from stimuli associated with neutral events, thus making his world more manageable. For example, the nurse could wear a specific apron for burn care only, making the *lack* of the apron a signal for "safety" (Kavanagh, 1981, 1983a).

From an operant conditioning perspective, it would be important to encourage and help Mark to again elicit positive reinforcement from his world, for example, through active play and renewed attempts to master his environment, as well as pleasant social interactions with his caretakers and peers.

The biological model would prescribe some of the same interventions for different reasons. Active play and play therapy in which anger is experienced and labeled may be therapeutic, according to the biological model, since both are associated with increased levels of serum catecholamines (Low levels of serum catecholamines are associated with learned helplessness as well as other types of depression). Tricyclic antidepressant medication may also increase catecholamine levels; however, the anticholinergic side effects (for example, hypotension, constipation, dry mouth) make this treatment more complicated. Nevertheless, if antidepressants effectively treat the vegetative symptoms of depression (appetite and sleep disturbances, decreased energy, and so forth), as they do in many clinically depressed patients, this particular treatment may be worth the risks in Mark's case, since he needs to eat and sleep to heal, and to be active to recover physical functioning. Finally, since one of the biological correlates of learned helplessness, increased serum beta endorphin is associated with loss of control, as is administration of narcotic analgesics (Maier et al., 1981), these medications should be used with caution, if at all, in young children in intensive care, especially the young burned child (Kavanagh, 1990).

EVALUATION

RESEARCH AND TREATMENT. While all three models suggest potentially therapeutic treatments, the nurse should base her choice of treatment or treatments on research findings when they are available. While research that compares two or more psychological treatments for the same problem is scarce, there are controlled studies that look at the effects of various treatments compared to no treatment. Good case studies can also shed light on potentially useful interventions, though they do not qualify as controlled research. For example, Engel and Reichsman's (1956) classically detailed study of Monica, an infant hospitalized for repair of a tracheal-esophageal fistula, demonstrates dramatically the devastating effect of hospitalization on an infant, namely, psychotic depression and its treatment, substitute "mothering" by nurses.

Some research has provided support for particular treatments and the models from which they spring. In a comprehensive and scientifically rigorous review of research on psychotherapy outcome, it was estimated that the average patient is better off at the end of therapy than 80 percent of peers who are identified as needing therapy but who remain untreated (Smith, Glass, & Miller, 1980). This estimate is based on 475 controlled outcome studies involving all types of therapy and patients, 1,766 measured effects (such as amelioration of symptoms), and tens of thousands of persons.

MENTAL HEALTH NURSING IN THE COMMUNITY

Many people consider the 1960s a pivotal time for community mental health nursing. Federal legislation providing for the establishment of more community outpatient clinics and an increase in federal funding of community-level health services provided new avenues for nursing to participate in mental health care at the community level (Jarvis, 1985). While community mental health initiatives brought some of their own problems (such as those associated with widescale deinstitutionalization, discussed in Chapter 10, Schizophrenia), the major thrust of the legislation passed at this time emphasized the federal role in the prevention and treatment of mental disorders at the community level. Over the last twenty years, those involved in community mental health have worked to clarify the meaning of this objective. The chronically mentally ill are generally considered to have the highest priority in public mental health care, with heightened attention given to creating better support programs for deinstitutionalized patients and attacking the issue of homelessness (Lamb, 1988). However, due to decreased funding and lack of resources most creative and effective programs have been cut. In some cases the mental health centers are so overwhelmed with patients that nurses have very little time to talk to their patients and must use every opportunity available such as when giving medications to establish communication.

ROLES OF THE COMMUNITY HEALTH NURSE

Nursing roles in community mental health are centered around the basic elements of community nursing: health promotion, prevention of disease, and evaluation and research.

MENTAL HEALTH PROMOTION. Mental health promotion can include anything from wellness programs offered in public health nursing and visiting nurse clinics, HMO's, and businesses to stress reduction seminars, to educational programs for children about issues such as divorce, substance abuse, and sexual feelings and behavior.

PREVENTION. Prevention of mental illness may be viewed on the three levels commonly practiced in community health: primary prevention, secondary prevention, and tertiary prevention (Spradley, 1990).

Primary prevention consists of looking for and removing conditions that might contribute to mental illness as well as fostering those positive conditions that contribute to mental health. Primary prevention involves anticipatory planning and requires the nurse to look into the future, envision potential needs and problems, and design programs that can counteract these potential problems (Spradley, 1990). While mental or psychosocial health may be somewhat more difficult to define than physical health, many things can be done to help people cope with their brand of stress; the nurse can help people recognize stress, understand how they cope with it (and whether such coping is adaptive or not), and look at options for eliminating stress, or at least decreasing it in their lives.

Given the high incidence of psychopathology associated with certain types of acute trauma, for example, burn injury requiring hospitalization (Kavanagh, 1981), nurses can do much in the service of primary prevention by educating the public in the basics of accident prevention. Much has been written about what can be done to prevent burn injury of children, the most vulnerable burn victims (Surveyer, 1981), for example, turning down the temperature of hot water heaters (Katcher, 1989). Other types of acute trauma can also be prevented, for example, through routine use of car seats for infants and seat belts for older children and adults. It is the responsibility of nurses committed to primary prevention to be familiar with such important information, help disseminate it, and model its use.

Secondary prevention focuses on detecting and treating existing mental health problems at the earliest possible stage.

Physical abuse in childhood is highly correlated with psychopathology in adulthood, and is something the nurse can try to do something about. Considering the estimated frequency of child abuse (20 percent of parents admit to hitting a child with an object or fist at some point; 13 percent have done so in the previous year) (Gelles, 1978), it is something the nurse is certain to encounter at some point in her profession. The nurse learns to identify the victim of abuse, if not the abuser. Reporting suspected child abuse, which is required in all states, will hopefully lead to treatment and reintegration of the family, which is likely to be split during the crisis of investigation and judgment. The nurse can recommend, design, and implement treatment programs for both the injured child and the adult abuser (who, in most cases, is an untreated victim of child abuse himself). The nurse can also use her influence to educate other health care professionals, legislators, district attorneys, judges, and, in some cases, social workers, that treatment works (Helfer and Kempe, 1976), while punishment without treatment perpetuates the generational cycle of child abuse and the psychopathology associated with it.

Crisis invervention is often used to help people cope with short-term crises or intermittent crises of the chronically mentally ill. However, this service primarily deals with the suicidal individual. The nurse will help to clarify the problem, explore possible solutions, and provide information and reassurance (see Chapter 18, Psychological Crises).

Tertiary prevention is aimed at reducing the severity of a mental health problem and helping a person live at their highest functional capacity. Psychiatric and other nurses who are involved with step-down programs or supportive services for the chronically mentally ill or half-way houses for recovering substance abusers are practicing tertiary prevention.

RESEARCH AND EVALUATION. Community health nurses also need to be involved in research and evaluation of current programs. Research in the area of community mental health might focus on the effectiveness of drug treatment and crisis intervention programs within a community. Spradley (1990) gives one example of the importance of evaluation in the community: when the mental health services in a particular community were evaluated, it was found that if a psychiatric crisis occurred during the night, the only people available to help were police and the only place where a person could be held was jail. As a result of this evaluation, a 24-hour psychiatric emergency service was established in the community mental health center.

THE NURSE'S RELATIONSHIP TO OTHER MEMBERS OF THE MENTAL HEALTH TEAM

In order to function effectively, the nurse must be more than familiar with the assessment and treatment of psychopathology and comfortable with the scientific process. She must understand her role vis-a-vis that of the other professionals, including mental health professionals, involved in the care of her patients. Sometimes the nurse's role is complicated when nurses on several rungs of the "professional ladder" are involved in a patient's care, or when the setting includes nurse practitioners as well as nurse academicians (teachers and researchers). There continue to be struggles throughout the nursing profession over job descriptions of the staff nurse (diploma, associate degree, and baccalaureate), head nurse, nurse clinician, clinical nurse specialist, and nurse practitioner. While the debate over the definition of nursing in all its guises is more heated than ever, fired in part by the increasing need of the nursing profession to differentiate itself clearly from the medical profession, the once obvious boundaries between nursing and medicine are more blurred than ever. Today, nurses as well as physicians have physical assessment skills, and both "diagnose" physical and mental health problems. While the physician still "writes the orders," does the surgery, and prescribes medication, many people realize that it's the nursing care that determines the patient's outcome in many cases—in the high-risk nursery, ICU, burn unit, geriatric unit, cardiac care unit, and the rehabilitation center. Additional confusion is caused by the increasing overlap of clinical responsibility and functioning between physicians and nurses. Competent nurses are able, and often expected, to draw blood, start IVs, manage complicated machinery (ventilators, monitors, laminar flow units, and so on), and participate actively in clinical decision making. At the same time, increased interest among physicians in the fields of family practice, pediatrics, and psychiatry reflects medicine's growing appreciation of the need to treat the whole person and the whole family, an ideal nursing once considered its own, at least during the era of the medical specialist.

For the nurse generalist interested in the psychological well-being of patients, or the psychiatric nurse, whatever her setting, the need for clear delineation of role is greater and more difficult than ever. For psychiatric treatment to be effective, patients and treating professionals need to know who the physician of record, case coordinator, and psychotherapist are. They often are not the same person. In addition, it is very helpful to know whether a primary nurse, clinical psychologist, psychiatric social worker, or any other mental health professional is involved in the case at present, has been in the past, or is likely to be in the future. Since expertise, educational background, professional philosophy, interests, and definition and appreciation of the roles of health and

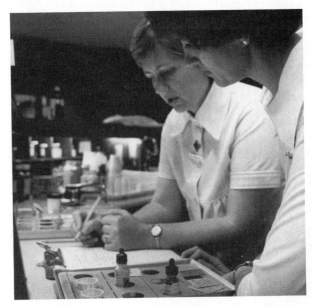

At the end of the shift, the associate nurse reports her most recent assessment of their patients to the primary nurse. The primary nurse will later make rounds with other members of the health care team in order to plan the patients' care for that day.

mental health professionals vary within the disciplines of medicine, nursing, and clinical psychology, nothing can be assumed. All individuals involved in a patient's psychiatric care need to be identified at the outset of the assessment process for the purpose of coordinating the patient's assessment, treatment, and followup; pooling expertise to avoid unnecessary duplication of activity; minimizing patient confusion; and establishing an efficient communication network. Frequent communication among professionals and between the case coordinator and patient is essential to the continuing process of assessment, treatment, and evaluation.

THE PSYCHOTHERAPIST

It is especially important that the patient be clear about who his psychotherapist is, given the intimacy, intensity, and centrality of the relationship between patient and psychotherapist. The psychotherapist (whether physician, nurse, psychologist, social worker, or other) needs to be identified clearly by the patient and all professionals involved in his care. This is not to minimize the roles of the rest of the health care or mental health care team, only to facilitate psychotherapy if it is a part of the treatment plan. Similarly, the professionals responsible for the planning, implementation, and evaluation of environmental,

Box 1—5 ● Mind-Body Phenomena: Feelings

In this society we are confused about the very purpose and value of emotion. We are not sure whether the healthy person is emotion-free, emotionally open, or subject only to certain selected emotions. We are often ashamed of certain emotions; for example, concern for power and assertion makes us overvalue rage and demean guilt. Granted this confusion, emotion is worth re-examination, particularly the elusive, neglected aspect of emotion called feelings. In studying feelings we must fly in the face of expert advice—eschew objective analysis and return to the shadow world of the inexact, the poetic, and the subjective.

Even the nomenclature presents a problem. Psychologists now generally use three terms for feelings. 'Emotion' is the general term which encompasses feeling, the related biophysiological state, and even underlying chemical changes. 'Affect,' introduced by psychoanalysts, is used to describe the dominant emotional tone of an individual as others perceive it. 'Feeling' is the subjective awareness of one's own emotional state.

Since it is emotional imbalance that drives people to psychiatrists and other mental health professionals, one might expect professionals to be absorbed with problems of feeling. Instead, beguiled by the unconscious and psychodynamic processes, they have been most intrigued by ideas and thoughts. 'Insight' has dominated their thinking; 'conflict' has

been the key, and emotions simply a sign of it. When they do think about emotion, psychiatrists are most likely to examine its measurable, observable or physiological aspects rather than the feelings themselves.

Anxiety is a partial exception, but even this emotion was not viewed as central in psychoanalytic theory until very recently. It was seen as a derivative phenomenon, the product, if you will, of repressed sexual appetite. Only in the last creative years of his life did Freud decide that fear and anxiety were primary warning signals that led to repression of sexual drives.

Feelings Often Ignored

Psychologists have also ignored feelings, and they too have rationalized their neglect. In this country, at least, many psychologists are behaviorists who prefer not to think about emotion when doing research and sometimes when treating patients. Some psychologists, especially those who work mainly with animals, have tended to ignore such complex purely human feelings as pride, shame, regret, and grief. B.F. Skinner's pigeons were no more likely to feel hurt or touched than Konrad Lorenz's geese. . . .

Psychotherapists in their everyday work must deal with patients' feelings, whether or not theory allows for them. For that reason the clinical world is in a sense freer of self-deception than the world of the

behavioral, or biological therapies must be identifiable and regularly available for consultation. A nurse may be the primary and responsible professional in any treatment plan, regardless of its theoretical perspective (psychoanalytic or behavioral, individual or family oriented).

ROLE CONFLICTS

Regardless of whether the context of the nurse's practice is the ICU or the community, role confusion and conflicts can and do occur. If, as mentioned, overlap

of role and function occurs in the highly specialized context of the ICU where there may be a different professional assigned to every part of the patient's body, it would be even more likely to occur in less specialized settings. There, several professionals, all generalists, may define their roles as providers of care or treatment of the total patient or the patient and his family.

Role conflict, however, occurs for reasons other than role overlap. It can occur, for example, when one professional perceives another as having a closer, special, or more valued position in the patient's

laboratory or the study. But mental health professionals are also partly to blame for public confusion about the meaning of feelings and the propriety of their public expression. This confusion is exploited by a continuing flow of 'How To' books offering to guide the perplexed and despairing via conflicting pathways. The 'emotions are bad' school sees them as stormy intruders on the tranquil sea of life. Shame and guilt are most frequently denounced as unnecessary and 'neurotic.' But shame and guilt are noble emotions essential to civilized society and vital for the development of some of the most refined and elegant human qualities: generosity, self-sacrifice, and service to others. . . .

Adaptive Value of Emotion

Emotions, even distressing ones, serve adaptive purposes. For example, pain is a message to our intelligence—a signal of danger whose purpose is to direct behavior. In extreme cases we do not need to think and decide because the protective maneuver of withdrawal from pain is reflexive. But even then the experience of pain serves a purpose; it is stored in memory to be recalled in other cases where choices must be made.

The complex and subtle range of human feelings testifies to our capacity for choice and learning. Feelings are the instruments of rationality. Human beings are free of instinctive and patterned behavior to a degree unparalleled in the animal kingdom, and feelings are our guides to using that freedom rationally. Anxiety, boredom, tension, and agitation, for example, send subtly different messages, each of which indicates a certain kind of danger and suggests appropriate adaptive maneuvers. Guilt allows us to measure our behavior against an ideal and register when we fall short. The pain of guilt, like a thermostatic control, initiates the process of moving back toward the ideal.

Feelings Out of Balance

Feelings can also go out of balance. Like every other aspect of our humanity they can be corrupted and lose their original purposes. Freedom allows us to design badly. As hunger drove primitive men and women to the nurture required for life, gluttony can drive modern men and women to the obesity that destroys. So, too, with feelings. Jealousy, which serves the struggle for survival, can deteriorate into the envy that extracts defeat even from victory. We can be overwhelmed by inappropriate guilt, anxiety, or shame. Mental illness is usually a mere disarray of the ingredients of survival.

Emotions are contagious; we respond to the feelings of others. Anxiety moves like a ripple through a crowd. Tears evoke tears, even when the content or cause of the distress is unknown. By allowing others to discern our emotional state, we make individual experience available to the group and thus enhance group survival. Emotional contagion is vital for our species. It allows each of us to warn others and makes the individual an extension of the group. Affects are the 'language' of most herding animals and serve them as an early warning system. While we are not cattle or sheep, we are not isolates either. Other people are nutrients, essential for our survival. Feelings like shame, when they force us to forgo selfish pleasures for the benefit of the group, manifest our unwitting sense that the individual must at times defer to the requirements of group survival.

Thus feelings are, if not all, almost all. They serve utility and sensuality. They are the fine instruments that shape decision-making in an animal cursed and blessed with intelligence and the freedom which is its corollary. They are signals directing us toward goodness, safety, pleasure, and group survival. In addition, they are their own rewards. They are the means and the ends. We measure and value our lives in the balance of daily passions. Now we should also give feelings more serious attention in our research and a more important role in our theoretical evaluations of human behavior.

Source: Gaylin, W. (1988) Feelings. *The Harvard Medical School Mental Health Letter*, Vol. 5, No. 1, pp. 4–5.

world. This frequently occurs in the pediatric setting, when a psychiatric consultation has been obtained and the child is assigned a play therapist. The nurse, who has responsibility for medication administration and painful procedures, may understandably begin to feel that she is associated with the negative aspects of her patient's world while the psychotherapist is associated with the positive aspects, for example, play and comforting. This feeling may intensify if the therapist reports that the patient is expressing anger about injections, dressing changes, and other procedures. If the nurse is not aware of or in control of her feelings of jealousy or has low personal or professional self-esteem, she may unwittingly sabotage psychotherapy. For example, she may not make time for play therapy in the patient's busy day, or she may put off or cut short a needed treatment or nursing care because it is scary or painful for the patient. Neither is in the patient's interest, of course, as the nurse would be first to agree once she sorted out her thoughts and feelings.

SOLUTIONS TO ROLE CONFLICT. The nurse in the above example and in similar situations may be able to carry out her difficult but necessary role *and* preserve her self-esteem by keeping in mind the following:

1. Just as the psychotherapist must consider mind-body connections, for example, the physiological effects of exposure to a feared object or procedure, the nurse must remember the reverse, or body-mind connections. If the nurse structures the patient's environment so that it is predictable, and maximizes the patient's control during the most aversive parts of it, for example, chemotherapy, blood drawing, and physical therapy, she will be working actively against the development of helplessness and depression in the patient, as well as treating his anxiety more effectively than the psychiatric consultant who has a psychotherapy session with the patient once or twice a week.

2. In one study, the majority of intensive care patients and their families often reported feeling that competence in the nursing staff was the most important source of psychological support during hospitalization (May, 1972).

3. In some cases, it may be in the patient's and the nurse's interest to have the person who focuses the patient on feelings (the psychotherapist) be someone other than the nurse, who is closely associated with his medical care. It can be too "loaded" for the patient to feel and express anger directly at the person on whom he feels physically dependent. The nurse is the person who is there in the middle of the night to care for him; she is not someone he wants to alienate. The guilt and anxiety associated with expressing anger directly at her or the physician can make an already difficult situation unmanageable for most patients.

The nurse may also feel guilt; for example, when she makes the patient feel bad instead of good. If she has to bear the brunt of the patient's anger, she might at times be too conflicted to determine objectively what the patient needs. On the other hand, if the psychotherapist takes on the burden by encouraging the patient to tell *her* about his anger, the nurse will be free to allow the patient's physiological state to dictate the direction or aggressiveness of nursing care. If the nurse keeps in mind that psychotherapy is usually not the source of "warm fuzzies" in the patient's life but the place where the patient faces fear, anger, and sadness, she may be better able to see herself as someone potentially able to comfort and soothe the patient after a painful procedure, *and* after a painful psychotherapy session by asking him how he feels, and listening, if he feels safe enough to tell her. (See Box 1–5.)

4. Finally, the nurse who considers herself as much a psychiatric nurse as anything else should see herself and other mental health professionals as having common ground. The first mental health profession, psychiatry, grew out of the medical subspecialty of neurology and the work of Charcot, Janet, and Freud, neurologists who developed an interest in mind-body problems, or physical symptoms or dysfunction in the absence of an observable anatomical lesion. Emphasis on what binds mental health professionals together rather than on what increases the distance between them is more likely to facilitate the achievement of what all would agree is the common goal—the physical and mental health of the patient.

SUMMARY

Psychiatric nursing is often a neglected part of the nurse's education. Yet 75 percent of the U.S. population suffers from mental illness at some point in life. The number is even higher in health care settings where anxiety and depression are common. The pediatric/adult hospitalized population and the geriatric population are both vulnerable to psychiatric illness. Deterrents to obtaining psychiatric mental health treatment include: the gap between traditional "talking" psychiatry and the hospitalized patient's high-tech world and associated difficulty talking; social stigma attached to seeking psychiatric mental health services; lack of financial resources; the decline of federal funding for psychiatric care for welfare recipients; and the proliferation of HMOs.

The scientific nursing process of assessment, analysis, planning, intervention, and evaluation is also used in dealing with a patient's psyche. The parameters of the psychiatric mental health assessment include: general behavior, cognitive functioning, mood or affect, thought content, and an appraisal of the nurse's own emotional reaction to the patient.

Psychopathology and mental illness are hard to define due to ethical and sociological issues. For example, Szasz believes mental illness is a myth, Rosenhan thinks mental illness is in the eye of the beholder, and Whitaker contends that there is something to be learned from "craziness" as it always contains an important message about life.

There are three categories of theories about mental illness: psychoanalytic, behavioral, and biological. Most psychiatric disorders are thought to have several causes, often involving all three theories; thus, they are often used in conjunction with one another to understand and treat mental illness.

The psychological assessment is an ongoing process and involves interviews, a mental-status exam, observation, previous medical records, and, at times, psychological testing. Nursing diagnosis is made by the nurse following the initial assessment and is related to the DSM-III-R diagnosis and actual or potential physical and psychological problems. Nursing interventions involve psychotherapy and any treatment or intervention directed at alleviating psychological distress or injury, preferably, interventions based on research from the disciplines of psychology, nursing, and medicine. Evaluation is ongoing and determines future intervention.

The nurse must understand her role vis-a-vis that of other professionals, including mental health professionals, involved in the care of her patients. The psychotherapist (whether physician, nurse, psychologist, social worker, or other) needs to be clearly identified by the patient and all other professionals involved in his care. Role conflict often occurs and should be identified and resolved before it impedes patient care.

KEY TERMS

learned helplessness
nursing process
psychiatric mental health assessment
psychoanalytic model
behavioral model
biological model

presenting problem
mental-status exam
nursing diagnosis
psychotherapy
primary prevention
secondary prevention
tertiary prevention

STUDY QUESTIONS

1. What role does psychiatric mental health nursing play in the practice of the generalist nurse?

2. What deterrents exist in obtaining psychiatric mental health treatment?

3. Define the psychiatric mental health assessment and describe how it differs from the physical assessment.

4. Why are psychopathology and mental illness so hard to define?

5. Name and describe the three categories of theories that exist to explain psychopathology.

REFERENCES

Alloy and Abramson. (1981). *Journal of Experimental Psychology,* Vol. 110, p. 436.

American Nurses Association Division on Psychiatric and Mental Health Nursing Practice. (1982). *Standards of psychiatric and mental health nursing practice,* p. 5.

Andolfi, M., Angelo, C., and Nicolo-Corifliano, A. M. (1983). *Behind the family mask: therapeutic change in rigid family systems.* N.Y.: Brunner/Mazel.

Beck, A. T. (1964). Thinking and depression: Theory and therapy. *Archives of General Psychiatry, 10,* pp. 561–571.

Benson, H. (1988). The relaxation response: a bridge between medicine and religion. *The Harvard Medical School Mental Health Letter,* Vol. 4, No. 9, pp. 4–6.

Center for Affective Disorders, University of Wisconsin Department of Psychiatry. Center for Affective Disorders Courier, April, 1985.

Engel, G. and Reichsman, F. (1956). Spontaneous and experimentally induced depression in an infant with a gastric fistula, a contribution to the problem of depression. *Journal of the American Psychoanalytic Association,* 4, pp. 428–451.

Erikson, E. H. (1950). *Childhood and Society.* N.Y.: W. W. Norton.

Escalona, S. K. (1974). Intervention programs for children at psychiatric risk. In E. J. Anthony and C. Koupernik (eds.) *The Child in His Family,* Vol. 3. N.Y.: John Wiley and Sons, pp. 33–45.

Fost, N., (1984). Personal communication.

Freud, A., (1966). *The Ego and The Mechanisms of Defense.,* International Universities Press, N.Y.

Freud, S. (1958). Formulations on the two principles of mental functioning. In the *Standard Edition of the Complete Psychological Works of Sigmund Freud,* Vol. 12, pp. 218–226. London: Hogarth Press.

Gelles, R. J. (1978). Violence toward children in the United States. *American Journal of Orthopsychiatry,* 48, 4, p. 580–592.

Gorkin, M. (1987). *The Uses of Countertransference.* Northvale, New Jersey: Jason Aronson.

Gottesman, I. I., and Shields, J. (1972). *Schizophrenia and Genetics, A Twin Study Vantage Point,* N.Y.: Academic Press. Graduate Medical Education National Advisory Commission, 1982.

Haley, J., Bateson, G., Jackson, D., and Weakland, J. (1956). Toward a theory of schizophrenia. *Behavior Science,* 1, pp. 251–264.

Helfer, R. E., Kempe, C. H. (1976). *Child abuse and neglect: the family and the community.* Cambridge, MA: Ballinger.

Herman, B. and Panksepp, J. (1978). Effects of morphine and naloxone on separation distress and approach attachment: evidence for opiate mediation of social affect. *Pharmacology, Biochemistry, and Behavior, 9,* pp. 213–220.

Jarvik, L. F., and Small, G. W. (eds) (1982). *The Psychiatric Clinics of North America,* 5 (1), April.

Jarvis, L. L. (1985). *Community health nursing: Keeping the public healthy,* 2nd ed. Philadelphia, PA: F. A. Davis, pp. 445–457.

Katcher, M. (1989). Liquid crystal thermometer used in pediatric office counseling about tap water burn prevention. In *Pediatrics, 83,* (5), May, pp. 766–771.

Kavanagh, C. (1981). *The concepts of predictability and controllability as applied to the treatment of children with severe burn injury*, (Doctoral Dissertation, University of Wisconsin). Ann Arbor: Dissertation Abstracts International.

Kavanagh, C. (1983a). Psychological intervention with the severely burned child: Report of an experimental comparison of two approaches and their effects on psychological sequelae. *American Academy of Child Psychiatry, 22:* 145–156.

Kavanagh, C. (1983b). A new approach to dressing change in the severely burned child and its effect on burn-related psychopathology. *Heart and Lung: The Journal of Critical Care, 12:* 612–619.

Kavanagh, C. (1990). Learned helplessness and the pediatric burn patient: dressing change behavior and serum cortisol and beta-endorphin. In *Advances in pediatrics*, 37, April.

Kenner, C., Guzzetta, C., and Dossey, B. (1985). *Critical care nursing: body, mind, spirit*, 2nd ed. Boston: Little, Brown and Co., pp. 16–17.

Kety, S. S. (1983). Mental illness in biological and adoptive relatives of schizophrenic adoptees: findings relevant to genetic and environmental factors in etiology. *American Journal of Psychiatry* 140: 6, June.

Kraemer, G. W., and McKinney, W. T. (1979). Interactions of pharmacological agents which alter biogenic amino metabolism and depression. *Journal of Affective Disorders, 1,* pp. 33–54.

Kubie, L. S. (1954). The fundamental nature of the distinction between normality and neurosis. *Psychoanalytic Quarterly,* 23, pp. 167–204.

Lamb, H. R. (1988). Community psychiatry and prevention. In J. A. Talbott, R. E. Hales, & S. C. Yudofsky (Eds.), *Textbook of Psychiatry*. Washington, D. C.: APA Press, Inc., pp. 1141–1145.

Larson, D. B., Whanger, A. D., and Busse, E. W. (1983). Geriatrics, in B. B. Wolman (ed) *The Therapist's Handbook*, N. Y.: Van Nostrand Reinhold Co., pp. 343–388.

Lazarus, A. A. (1973). Multimodal behavior therapy: Treating the "Basic ID." *Journal of Nervous and Mental Disease*. Vol. 156, 6, pp. 404–411.

Mahler, M., Pine, F., and Bergman, A. (1975). *The psychological birth of the human infant*. N.Y.: Basic Books.

Maier, S. F., Drugan, R., Grau, J. W., Hyson, R. A., Maclenna, A. J., and Moye, T. (1981). Learned helplessness, pain inhibition and the endogenous opiates. In M. D. Zeilier, P. Marrem (eds) *Advances in analysis of behavior*. N. Y.: John Wiley & Sons.

Marshall, J. (1986). Personal communication.

Masterson, J. (1981). *The narcissistic and borderline disorders: an integrated developmental approach*. N. Y.: Brunner/Mazel.

May, J. G. (1972) A psychiatric study of a pediatric intensive therapy unit. *Clinical Pediatrics*, 11, 2, pp. 76–82.

Meehl, Paul. *Psychodiagnosis: selected papers*, N. Y.: W.W. Norton and Company, Inc., 1973.

Mumford, E., Schlesinger, J. V., Glass, C. P., and Cuerdon, T. (1984). A new look at evidence about reduced cost of medical utilization following mental health treatment. *American Journal of Psychiatry*, 141, pp. 1145–1158.

Neil, J. R. and Kniskern, David P. (1982). *From psyche to system: The evolving therapy of Carl Whitaker*. London: Guilford Press.

Offer, D., Sabshin, M., Offer, J. (1974). *Normality*. Basic Books, N. Y.

Pavlov, I. P. (1927). *Conditioned reflexes*. (Translated by G. V. Amrep) London: Oxford University Press.

President's Commission on Mental Health (1978). *Report to President, Volume I*. Washington, D.C.: U.S. Government Printing Office, Stock #: 040–000–00390–8.

Rosenhan, D. L. (1973). On being sane in insane places. *Science*, 179, pp. 250–258.

Rosenthal, R. and Jacobsen, L. (1960). *Pygmalion and the classroom*. N. Y.: Holt.

Seligman, M. E. (1968). Chronic fear produced by unpredictable shock. *Journal of Comparative and Physiological Psychology*, 66, pp. 402–411.

Seligman, M. E., Maier, S. F., Solomon, R. I. (1971). Unpredictable and uncontrollable aversive events. In F. R. Brush (ed) *Aversive Conditioning and Learning*. N. Y.: Academic Press.

Simpson, G. M., and May, P. R. (1982). Schizophrenic disorders. In J. H. Greist, J. W. Jefferson, and R. L. Spitzer (eds) *Treatment of Mental Disorders*, pp. 143–176.

Skinner, B. F. (1938). *The behavior of organisms*. N. Y.: Appleton-Century-Crofts.

Smith, M. L., Glass, G. V., and Miller, T. I. (1980). *The benefits of psychotherapy*. Baltimore: The Johns Hopkins University Press.

Spradley, B. (1990). *Community health nursing: Concepts and practice*, 3rd ed. Glenview, IL: Scott, Foresman/Little, Brown, pp. 13–18.

Srole, L., and Fischer, A. K. (eds) (1978). *Mental health in the metropolis: The midtown Manhattan study* (Revised). N. Y.: New York University Press.

Strupp, H. H. (1978). Psychotherapy research and practice: an overview. In S. L. Garfield, and A. E. Bergin, (eds) *Handbook of psychotherapy and behavior change*, pp. 3–22.

Suomi, S. J., Harlow, H. F., and Delzio, R. (1979). Social rehabilitation of separation-induced depressive disorders in monkeys. *American Journal of Psychiatry*, 133, pp. 1279–1285.

Surveyer, J. A. and Halpern, J. (1981) Age-related burn injuries and their prevention. *Pediatric Nursing*, September/October.

Szasz, T. S. (1960). The Myth of Mental Illness. *The American Psychologist*, 5, pp. 113–118.

Wetzel, J. W. (1984). *Clinical Handbook of Depression*, N. Y.: Gardner Press, Inc.

Wolpe, J. (1973). *The practice of behavior therapy*. N. Y.: Pergamon Press.

2

MAJOR MODELS OF BEHAVIOR AND PSYCHOPATHOLOGY

NED KALIN
GEORGE DAWSON
C. KATE KAVANAGH

LEARNING OBJECTIVES
After studying this chapter, the student will be able to:

- Outline the historical development and scientific basis of the psychodynamic, behavioral, and biological theories of behavior and psychopathology.
- Compare the major therapies for psychopathology based on these three theories.
- Understand the interrelationships between the three major theories, especially where they come together.
- Discuss integrated approaches to the understanding and treatment of psychopathology.

UNDERSTANDING HUMAN BEHAVIOR

Although there is still controversy about the definitions of and distinctions between normal and abnormal behavior and certainly about treatment methods, most people would agree that human behavior, both normal and abnormal, results from an interaction of environment and biology. Mental disorder is characterized by behavior that is either maladaptive or inappropriate for the individual's environment. Some of this behavior, such as the auditory hallucination "kill everyone," may be so distinct from everyday experience that it would be considered abnormal in any context. Other kinds of behavior may not be so easy to categorize. A person who reports that he communicates regularly with God would be considered delusional by some, an example of religious fervor by others. (See Box 2–1.) Numerous theories attempt to explain the development of normal and abnormal behavior, and each has its implications for the etiology, diagnosis, and treatment of mental illness. These theories can be grouped in a variety of ways, and there is much overlap among them. Many of the major theories, in fact, are offshoots of others, and the exploration of the roots of these theories can provide an interesting view of the development of the field. Briefly, however, for the purpose of this discussion, the theories can be divided into three major groupings: psychoanalytic theories, biological theories, and behavioral theories.

PSYCHOSOCIAL THEORIES

Psychoanalytic or psychodynamic theory looks at the *unconscious* motivations of human behavior and tries to bring these motivations into conscious awareness. **Behavioral theory** focuses on the relationship between environment and behavior, and the importance of the effect of *conscious* motivation on action (stimulus vs. response).

Other theories which spring from these two theories and which are broadly referred to as "psychosocial" include cognitive, humanistic, and interpersonal theories, all of which have their basis in psychoanalytic or behavioral theory but which have gone in very different directions. An outgrowth of behavioral theory, **cognitive behavior therapy** looks at the internal changes and mental operations people use to process information. The **humanistic approach** stresses the inherent goodness in each individual as well as the potential for maximum growth and fulfillment. Abraham Maslow (1908–1970), whose hierarchy of needs has become a basis for many conceptual models of nursing, was one of the pioneers of the humanistic perspective. Other "humanists" include psychologists Carl Rogers and Fritz Perls, who is best known for the development of confrontation groups. Humanistic theorists talk about feelings and free will in the conscious world and focus on the future rather than on the past. The **interpersonal approach** looks mainly at the relationships, first with parents, and later with others, that the child forms during the socialization process. Personality development occurs in stages, and failure to progress through these stages may affect an individual's ability to form healthy relationships with others later in life. Alfred Adler, Erik Erikson, and Karen Horney are considered early interpersonal psychologists, developing their views directly from the psychoanalytic perspective. Erikson's discussion of stages of development, which expanded on Freud's stages, focuses on important tasks that a child must accomplish within a given stage, such as learning to trust during the oral stage. His work has provided a theoretical framework for nurses who routinely assess developmental stages and needs of their patients. Recent research on infant development, however, indicates that we need to update our thinking on child development. In his research on infants and young children, Stern (1985) has shown that growth is discontinuous, and the process of development is horizontal, not vertical. For example, trust is an issue that is dealt with across the lifespan in different ways, as the psychological organization of shifting domains of experience changes. This occurs as the infant's self, well-formed by about 3 months of age, has more to work with as his genetic capacities for cognitive, affective, and psychomotor development unfold. Stern has also shown that the ability to differentiate self from other is "there from the start." The major goal of early development then is not Separation, as Mahler (1975) would have it, but Attachment. Basch (1988), a psychoanalytic theorist, clinician, and student of "self-psychology," agrees with this view of development. **Self-psychology** is a theory grounded in traditional psychoanalytic theory, which asserts that the primary goal of psychotherapy is to have the patient feel understood. This is accomplished through working with the patient from within (from *his* point of view) and providing affective attunement, all in service of growth of the "self" (Ornstein, 1986).

Box 2–1 ● Popular Views of Abnormal Behavior

Examples of mental disorders that we have heard or read about are apt to be extreme cases that give us a chamber-of-horrors impression of abnormal behavior. In reality, less spectacular maladjustments are far more common. The following are some popular myths and misconceptions concerning mental disorder and abnormal behavior.

1. **Myth:** Abnormal behavior is invariably bizarre.
   Fact: The behavior of most mental patients most of the time is indistinguishable from that of "normal" persons.
2. **Myth:** Normal and abnormal behavior are different in kind.
   Fact: Few if any types of behavior displayed by mental patients are unique to them. Abnormality consists largely of a poor fit between behavior and the situations in which it is enacted.
3. **Myth:** As a group, former mental patients are unpredictable and dangerous.
   Fact: The typical former mental patient is no more volatile or dan-

gerous than people in general. The exceptions to the rule generate much publicity and give a distorted picture.
4. **Myth:** Mental disorder is associated with fundamental personal deficiencies and hence its occurrence is shameworthy.
   Fact: So far as we know, everyone shares the potential for becoming disordered and behaving abnormally.
5. **Myth:** Appropriate attitudes toward mental disorder include awe and fearfulness about one's own foibles and vulnerability.
   Fact: Mental disorders are natural adaptive processes that are comprehensible within this context. The average person has an excellent chance of never becoming disordered and of recovering completely should the unlikely happen.

Source: Adapted from Carson, R., Butcher, J., & Coleman, J. (1988). *Abnormal psychology and modern life,* 8th ed. Glenview, IL: Scott, Foresman, p. 7.

BIOLOGICAL THEORIES

Biological theories propose that neurochemical events in the brain are central in determining behavior. The work of neurologists and neuropsychiatrists in the last 10 years has uncovered a wealth of information about how the brain functions and the relationship of the brain to emotions and behavior. Much is yet to be discovered in this area of behavior.

SOCIOCULTURAL CONTEXT

Since the study of human behavior is in its infancy, the above theories of behavior are supported by limited scientific evidence. It is also important to recognize that any psychological disorder is colored by the individual's sociocultural context, that is, the cultural beliefs, values, and behaviors that comprise the individual's environment. Nonetheless, three of these theories or approaches—psychoanalytic, behavioral, and

biological—have assumed a prominent position in guiding research and treatment of mental disorders. The rest of this chapter will discuss the historical development and scientific bases of these theories. An overview and synthesis is presented, capitalizing on the strengths of each theory and how they apply clinically.

PSYCHOANALYTIC THEORY

Psychoanalytic (or psychodynamic) theory is based on the premise that experiences occurring in infancy and childhood determine an individual's behavior as an adult. Four major concepts are useful in understanding this theory: (1) the unconscious mind, (2) the topographical model of the mind, (3) psychosexual development, and (4) object relations such as attachment bonds and social relationships.

Sigmund Freud (1856–1939) laid the groundwork for the development of the psychoanalytic perspective on behavior, and out of this perspective has grown the treatment process called psychotherapy. Freud initially was a neurologist who became interested in the contemporary French studies of Janet and Charcot on hysteria. Freud quickly moved beyond their ideas, dropped his neurological focus, and developed radical, but exciting, psychological theories of hysteria.

THE UNCONSCIOUS MIND

Before Freud developed his theories, the accepted belief among psychiatric professionals was that individuals were completely aware of the factors motivating their behavior. Using the techniques of hypnosis, free association, and dream analysis, Freud was able to uncover a person's **unconscious mind,** helping patients to understand more completely the factors determining their thoughts, feelings, and behavior.

TOPOGRAPHICAL MODEL OF THE MIND

The basic principles of the psychoanalytic perspective hinge upon Freud's (1923) theory of a **topographical model of the mind.** He divided the mind into three components: id, ego, and superego. The instinctual (sexual and aggressive) drives make up the id. The id is concerned only with immediate gratification without any reference to reality or external considerations. The id is thus considered to operate on the basis of the "pleasure principle." The ego mediates behavior by using reason to modify input from the id in accordance with demands of the external world; thus the ego is said to operate in terms of the "reality principle." Freud hypothesized that the role of the ego is to control sexual and aggressive impulses that would otherwise disrupt appropriate social functioning (1926). The third component in Freud's topography of the mind is the superego, which functions as an inner conscience.

PSYCHOSEXUAL DEVELOPMENT

Freud theorized that individuals go through specific stages of **psychosexual development,** progressing from infantile to mature sexuality. The oral stage, encompassing the first 18 months of life, is characterized by a marked dependence on the mother and the interaction around feeding. The anal stage occurs from age 18 months to 3 years. During this time toilet training is a central issue, and issues of control are prominent for the child. From age 3 to 5, during the phallic stage, the child is focused on his or her sex-

uality and masturbation increases. The latency period extends from age 6 to 10. During this stage the sexual focus diminishes as the child becomes more involved with the world away from home. During adolescence there is a resurgence of genital sexuality, completing the psychosexual stages. It is hypothesized that the normal progression through the psychosexual stages allows the individual to master unconscious sexual feelings directed toward the parent of the opposite sex—the resolution of the Oedipal conflict and the "birth" of the superego. It is during development that the **ego defense mechanisms** are established as they serve to modify the early instinctual drives. Failure to develop adequate defenses results in conflict, which is the basis of neurosis. Through the defense mechanisms, the ego enables a person to function effectively in society. Repression, for instance, is one of the earliest defense mechanisms to develop and one of the most prominent. Repression keeps at the unconscious level certain socially unacceptable impulses generated by the id. If conflicts related to the development of these defense mechanisms persist unresolved, they may lead to the development of psychopathology. While some defense mechanisms, such as repression, are adaptive at one time in an individual's life, they can become maladaptive attempts to deal with reality, resulting in intra- and/or interpersonal conflict. Table 2–1 summarizes some of the defense mechanisms which are often seen in psychopathology. (Also see Chapter 12 on Personality Disorders.)

SOCIAL RELATIONSHIPS AND ATTACHMENT BONDS

The work of the psychoanalytic theorist and clinician, Bowlby, and his associates highlights the importance of **social relationships** and **attachment bonds** in human development (Bowlby, 1969; 1980). Attachment-bond theory suggests a basis for separation anxiety and the grieving and mourning that occur with a loss. Bowlby's observation of the profound effects on the emotional development of young children separated from their parents and placed in nonsupportive environments establishes that attachments early in life are necessary for normal emotional and psychological development. In adulthood, disruption of attachments results in responses that vary among individuals. The intensity and duration of the response to separation depends on the individual's history of separations, the importance of the relationship disrupted, and the availability of other supportive attachment figures.

TABLE 2–1 Summary chart of ego-defense mechanisms

Mechanism	Example
Denial of reality. Protecting self from unpleasant reality by refusal to perceive or face it.	A smoker concludes that the evidence linking cigarette use to health problems is scientifically worthless.
Fantasy. Gratifying frustrated desires by imaginary achievements.	A socially inept and inhibited young man imagines himself chosen by a group of women to provide them with sexual satisfaction.
Repression. Preventing painful or dangerous thoughts from entering consciousness.	A mother's occasional murderous impulses toward her hyperactive two-year-old are denied access to awareness.
Rationalization. Using contrived "explanations" to conceal or disguise unworthy motives for one's behavior.	A fanatical racist uses ambiguous passages from Scripture to justify his hostile actions toward minorities.
Projection. Attributing one's unacceptable motives or characteristics to others.	An expansionist-minded dictator of a totalitarian state is convinced that neighboring countries are planning to invade.
Reaction formation. Preventing the awareness or expression of unacceptable desires by an exaggerated adoption of seemingly opposite behavior.	A man troubled by homosexual urges initiates a zealous community campaign to stamp out gay bars.
Displacement. Discharging pent-up feelings, often of hostility, on objects less dangerous than those arousing the feelings.	A woman harassed by her boss at work initiates an argument with her husband.
Emotional insulation. Reducing ego involvement by protective withdrawal and passivity.	A child separated from her parents because of illness and lengthy hospitalization becomes emotionally unresponsive and apathetic.
Intellectualization (isolation). Cutting off affective charge from hurtful situations or separating incompatible attitudes by logic-tight compartments.	A prisoner on death row awaiting execution resists appeals on his behalf and coldly insists that the letter of the law be followed.
Undoing. Atoning for or trying to magically dispel unacceptable desires or acts.	A teenager who feels guilty about masturbation ritually touches door knobs a prescribed number of times following each occurrence of the act.
Regression. Retreating to an earlier developmental level involving less mature behavior and responsibility.	A man whose self-esteem has been shattered reverts to child-like "show-off" behavior and exhibits his genitals to young girls.
Identification. Increasing feelings of worth by affiliating oneself with person or institution of illustrious standing.	A youth league football coach becomes excessively demanding of his young players in emulation of an authoritarian pro football coach.
Overcompensation. Covering up felt weaknesses by emphasizing some desirable characteristic or making up for frustration in one area by overgratification in another.	A dangerously overweight woman goes on eating binges when she feels neglected by her husband.
Acting out. Engaging in antisocial or excessive behavior without regard to negative consequences as a way of dealing with emotional stress.	An unhappy, frustrated sales representative has several indiscriminate affairs without regard to the negative effects of the behavior.
Splitting. Viewing oneself or others as *all* good or bad without integrating positive or negative qualities of the person into the evaluation. That is, reacting to others in an "all or none" manner rather than considering the full range of their qualities.	A conflicted manager does not recognize individual qualities or characteristics of her employees. Instead, she views them as all good or all bad; seeing most of them as all bad.

Source: From Carson, R. C., Butcher, J. N., & Coleman, J. C. (1988). *Abnormal psychology and modern life,* 8th Ed. Glenview, IL: Scott, Foresman. Based on Anna Freud (1946); DSM-III-R (1987).

THE DEVELOPMENT OF PERSONALITY

Psychodynamic theories have attempted to account for the development of personality. Building on Freud's work, others have suggested that failure of the young child to progress from one psychosexual stage to the next will result in a characteristic adult personality with maladaptive traits. For example, a person with an "oral character" has an intense need to be taken care of and becomes easily frustrated when his dependency needs are not met. Some have emphasized the role of **object** (significant other) **relations.** Melanie Klein (1937) has discussed the importance of the breast as the first object in the infant's life. Klein suggests that when the infant's needs are met, the breast is perceived as a good object; when the infant is unsatisfied, the breast is perceived as bad. An important developmental step for the child is to integrate good experiences and bad ones into one love object, the mother. If this does not occur it is thought that the adult will be able to see objects (people) only as all good or all bad. Margaret Mahler (1975) observed interactions of young children with their mothers and suggested that to become an independent adult, the infant must negotiate various degrees of individuation and separation from the mother. It is important to keep in mind that these concepts are based on anecdotal observations, and empirical data supporting them do not exist. Although different theorists study different aspects of child development, most of them agree on the importance of early mother-infant interaction to functioning in later life.

PSYCHOANALYTIC TREATMENT

Treatments based on psychoanalytic theory range from **classical psychoanalysis** to **brief psychodynamic psychotherapy.** While there are differences in technique, these therapies are aimed at helping patients discover their unconscious motivations for maladaptive behavior. This increased awareness is thought to enable the patient to control disturbing impulses and behavioral patterns. The main vehicle for change in psychoanalytic therapies is the working through of the transference. **Transference** is the development of certain attitudinal and behavioral predispositions as a result of early experiences with significant others. As therapy progresses, the patient begins to experience the therapist as embodying characteristics of important individuals in his life. The patient and therapist reenact old conflicts with these important persons, allowing them to explore and attempt to understand the origins of present conflict. The patient becomes aware of how unconscious assumptions based on earlier events continue to dictate his present, unwanted behavior.

The "working through" aspects of the therapy involve therapist and patient not only examining the patient's previously unknown underlying assumptions, but modifying them. The actual process of psychotherapy may be time-limited or, in the case of classical psychoanalytic therapy, may extend in an open-ended manner. Time-limited techniques are used in cases in which the patient has a history of successful attachments, good cognitive abilities and psychological mindedness, and a problem that can be conceptualized as a focal conflict. Psychoanalysis focuses on alteration of pathological personality structure through long-term, intensive therapy.

Recent research by Strupp (1968) and Luborsky and Spence (1978) has provided insight into the mechanisms of psychoanalytic therapy. For an optimal outcome to occur, a therapeutic alliance must be present; that is, the patient must feel that he is being understood. Barriers to the development of a therapeutic alliance include a diminished capacity of either participant to engage in an intense but structured relationship, for example, a patient's close personal relationship with the therapist, thought disorder, or ongoing substance abuse. Therapist qualities such as the ability to provide an environment for change and to facilitate therapeutic learning while controlling personal reactions to the patient are thought to be important. Research aimed at identifying other therapeutic aspects of psychoanalytic therapy has focused on the use of specific techniques with patients who have diverse DSM-III-R diagnoses. One example is the method of **interpersonal** or **person-centered** (Meador & Rogers, 1979) **therapy** which has been shown to be effective both alone and with concomitant drug treatment for major depressive disorder. It involves focusing on the patient's interpersonal relationships by examining the feelings experienced in his relationship with the therapist. The therapist functions as a participant observer in the patient's life. Psychoanalytic psychotherapy, used by itself, appears to have a limited role in the treatment of many major psychiatric conditions such as most anxiety disorders, psychosomatic illness, and schizophrenia. The efficacy of this method of treatment in the clinical situations in which it is most often prescribed, treatment of severe personality disorders, remains to be established.

BEHAVIORAL THEORY

Behavioral theory is based on the relationship between learning and behavior; that is, an organism's behavior is determined by the environmental contingencies of that behavior experienced in the past. Its emphasis is on the interaction between the person and his environment. Underlying principles that determine both normal and abnormal behavior consider the nature and timing of stimuli, the nature of reinforcements (reward or punishment), schedules of reinforcement, and traumatic conditioning. Work over the last century has distinguished two basic types of learning: associative learning and nonassociative learning. In humans, learning almost always involves elements of both. For example, learning to eat in a socially appropriate manner involves the association of hunger and its expression and observation of other people.

ASSOCIATIVE LEARNING

A now classic study of **associative learning** is the early work of Pavlov (1927), who demonstrated the phenomenon of **classical conditioning.** When dogs are presented with meat (the unconditioned stimulus) they salivate reflexively. Pavlov showed that if a bell is rung (conditioned stimulus) at the same time meat is presented, the dog learns to salivate upon hearing the bell.

Work by Thorndike (1932) and others resulted in the concept of **operant conditioning.** Here an animal learns that one of its spontaneous behaviors is associated with a predictable outcome. For example, if a rat is placed in a cage with a lever, it will explore the cage, randomly pressing the lever. If the rat is rewarded with food every time it accidentally presses the lever, it will rapidly learn to press the lever to obtain food. Thorndike soon realized that behavior learned this way could be enhanced by reinforcers or diminished by lack of reinforcement. Reinforcers are events that will increase the frequency of the learned response. An important variable in maintaining learned behavior is the frequency of the presentation of the reinforcer. When the learned behavior is no longer paired with the reinforcer, the animal forgets the association. This has been termed *extinction.* Aversive events, or punishment, have an unpredictable effect on behavior. They may *increase* or cause undesirable behavior and/or psychological conflict within the individual.

NONASSOCIATIVE LEARNING

Nonassociative Learning is more primitive than associative learning. Habituation and sensitization are two forms of nonassociative learning. After the repeated presentation of a stimulus, one outcome is weakening of the stimulus-induced response (habituation). If the stimulus has significant noxious qualities, another possibility is enhancement of the response (sensitization). Habituation and sensitization occur in all animals and have important adaptive significance since they function to keep the animal from being distracted by unimportant events (such as air temperature), enabling it to respond to critical environmental events (such as the approach of a predator).

The understanding of associative and nonassociative learning in animals has led to the application of the same principles to human behavior. Although many conditioning paradigms have been useful in attempting to understand behavior, more complex learning processes, such as language acquisition, have not been explained. A more comprehensive explanation of behavior has been attempted by Bandura (1977), who has proposed **social-learning theory.** This theory is based on the premise that human behavior cannot be explained in terms of an interaction between a person and the environment, but that the person, environment, *and* behavior are interdependent. Bandura suggests that modeling is the primary way in which human behavior is learned. Modeling occurs when a behavior is observed and processed into a mental image that then serves as a guide for behavior. Humans also have the capacity for delayed modeling, by which memories of observed behavior can be used in the future. Reinforcement for learning in humans also differs from a stimulus-response paradigm. Social learning recognizes that there is a broad range of reinforcers for any given human behavior. Many potential reinforcers may not be observable as environmental events but may occur as thoughts or images. An example would be the anticipated benefits of long hours of study (an "A," or eventually a college degree) which may be a potent reinforcer for studying behavior.

BEHAVIOR THERAPY

Behavioral theory has resulted in numerous specific treatments that are designed to modify specific behaviors associated with various psychiatric syndromes. For example, nocturnal enuresis (bedwetting) is a common problem with children. Classical conditioning has been used successfully to treat this problem. In one such treatment a bell and pad are used (Mowrer and Mowrer, 1938). When the child wets the bed, a sensor in the pad rings a loud bell that awakens and startles the child. One explanation for the efficacy of this method is that the child develops an increasing awareness of a full bladder and eventually is able to use physiological cues to awaken before enuresis occurs.

Phobic avoidance behaviors associated with depression, panic, and phobic disorders as well as other psychiatric syndromes can also be treated with behavioral therapy. Repeated exposure to the fear or phobic situation helps the individual eventually to tolerate the situation (Rachman, Hodgson, and Marks, 1971). With exposure, the individual learns that the fear does not represent a real danger. This frequently is accompanied by a reduction in the physiological fear response. Experience in the treatment of phobic avoidance behaviors has established that exposure to the real situation is more effective than exposure to the mental image of fearful situations. Behavioral treatments that focus on positive thoughts or pleasant mental imagery are useful for patients with depression.

Seligman (1968, 1975) has suggested that "learned helplessness" plays a role in the characteristic negative thinking pattern associated with depression—a pattern characterized by self-criticism and low self-esteem. Depressed patients frequently assume responsibility for negative events occuring in their environment. As a result they become hopeless about their ability to perform in the world. Cognitive behavioral therapy (CBT) attempts to interrupt the illogical thinking pattern responsible for these totally negative attributions. As a patient's thinking becomes more positive, he is able to resume activities for which he will receive social reinforcement.

BIOLOGICAL THEORY AND THERAPY

The underlying premise of **biological theory** is that behavior is determined by biochemical events in the brain. Psychoanalytic and behavioral theory acknowledge some contribution of biological events to behavior but hold that behavior cannot be reduced solely to them. During the late 19th century, postmortem examinations of the brains of patients with marked impairments in motor, sensory, and cognitive function in some cases revealed structural abnormali-

ties. Broca and others attempted to correlate gross lesions in these brains with the behavioral changes noted in the patients. This work established that certain behavioral abnormalities could be linked to damage in specific brain regions. It also became apparent that infections or toxic insults to the brain could result in behavioral changes. When the brains of "insane" patients were examined, neurosyphilis was found to be a common cause of insanity. During the early 20th century it was estimated that 10 percent of patients in state asylums were suffering from this disorder.

Nevertheless, the majority of the brains from insane patients appeared normal. Some scientists felt that abnormalities existed even in these brains, but were undetectable by the technology of the time. However, most of the psychiatric community used this lack of pathophysiological markers or changes as evidence to support psychoanalytic theory regarding etiologies of psychopathology.

It was not until the 1940s that psychotropic drugs and electroshock were used to treat mental illness. It rapidly became apparent that psychotic patients had a reduced number of hallucinations and delusions after they received chlorpromazine. Patients in tuberculosis sanitoriums had improvements in mood after they were treated with the antituberculosis agent isoniazid. This compound was also found to increase levels of norepinephrine, dopamine, and serotonin—brain neurotransmitters. Antidepressants that are structurally similar to chlorpromazine and isoniazid were developed as a result and continue to be the drugs of choice in the treatment of depression. Another major breakthrough was the discovery that lithium salts control the hyperactivity and euphoria associated with manic-depressive illness and prevent recurrences of the manic and depressive episodes. Initially, electroconvulsive therapy was administered to schizophrenics, but with time it became evident that depressed patients were more responsive to this treatment.

These treatment developments strengthened the concept that biochemical changes in the brain are responsible for mental illness. Researchers began to search intensively for altered biochemical systems in patients and also worked to understand the mechanisms of action of effective treatments. Schizophrenia and mood disorders have been the most thoroughly studied of the illnesses. Although specific biological etiologies have not yet been found, there is a consensus that certain neurotransmitter systems are involved. Dopamine systems are thought to be overactive in schizophrenia, so current treatment for this illness usually involves reducing the activity of dopamine systems with medication. Similarly, in depression, since underactivity of norepinephrine and serotonin systems has been demonstrated, tricyclic antidepressants are often used along with psychotherapy in its treatment.

Inheritance studies provide additional support for the role of biology in the etiology of the major mental disorders. Alcoholism, antisocial personality disorder, anxiety disorder, mood disorders, and schizophrenia tend to run in families. While there is debate over whether this is due to genetic transmission or to early learning, evidence from studies of twins supports the concept that the vulnerability to becoming schizophrenic or having a mood disorder is genetic. For example, the concordance rate of schizophrenia in identical twins is approximately 50 percent (as compared to 10 percent in fraternal twins), and the prevalence of schizophrenia in the general population is approximately 1 percent. Studies of adopted individuals, which minimize environmental influences, show that when children of schizophrenic parents are raised by nonschizophrenic parents, they have the same prevalence rate of schizophrenia as those who are raised by their biological parents. There have been similar findings in the study of mood disorders (Rosenthal, 1971).

Currently, investigators are searching for physiological alterations that are associated with specific psychiatric disorders. Studies of endocrine function reveal changes in stress-related hormones that are relatively specific for depressive illness. Sleep studies find abnormal sleep patterns to be associated with mood disorders, schizophrenia, and alcoholism. Newly available brain imaging techniques suggest specific changes in the brains of schizophrenics. At the cellular level, changes in cell membrane receptors for neurotransmitter substances occur in depressed patients. Researchers are using new developments in molecular biology in an effort to identify the genes controlling the vulnerability to these illnesses. Table 2–2 summarizes the biological findings and treatments associated with the major psychiatric syndromes.

INTEGRATED APPROACHES

Clinical work and research employing models of animal behavior have emphasized the importance of integrating aspects of each of these theories in attempts to explain behavior. Engel (1977) has called this approach the **biopsychosocial model,** suggesting that all mental and physical illnesses have biological, psychological, and social components. Three prominent animal models illustrate these relationships.

SEPARATION AND SOCIAL DEPRIVATION

Studies of attachment-bond disruption in infant rhesus monkeys are beginning to illuminate the complex relationships among these variables. (See Mitchell, 1970, for a review. See also Box 2–2.) When infant rhesus monkeys are separated from their

TABLE 2–2 The biology of the major psychiatric disorders

Diagnosis	Hypothetical etiology	Biological markers	Biological treatment
Mood disorders	Brain monoamine dysregulation	Changes in neurotransmitter and metabolite levels; neuroendocrine dysregulation; altered sleep; impaired immune function.	Tricyclic antidepressants; monoamine oxidase inhibitors; lithium; anticonvulsants; ECT; phototherapy
Schizophrenia	Altered brain dopaminergic systems	Altered smooth-pursuit eye movements; increased size of lateral ventricles; enhanced response to amphetamine challenge; decreased metabolic activity in frontal cortex	Antipsychotic drugs
Panic disorders	Altered brain noradrenergic systems	Susceptibilty to lactate-induced panic; altered cerebral blood flow in left brain hemisphere	Tricyclic antidepressants; monoamine oxidase inhibitors; benzodiazepines; β-adrenergic blockers

Box 2–2 ● Animal Use or Abuse in Biomedical Research? A Plea for the Chimps

Chimpanzees and other primates are used in biomedical research because of their physiological and psychological similarities to humans. This justification for what is their abuse in many cases is also an argument against it. Naturalist and author Jane Goodall is one of the many animal rights activists who have spoken out against animal abuse in the name of scientific research. After a visit to the National Institutes of Health primate lab in 1987, she reported:

"It was a visit I shall never forget. Room after room was lined with small, bare cages, stacked one above the other, in which monkeys circled round and round and chimpanzees sat huddled, far gone in depression and despair. . . . And there they will remain, living in conditions of severe sensory deprivation, for the next several years. During that time, they will become insane."

Goodall organized a conference co-sponsored by the N.I.H. which was held in December, 1987 that brought together for the first time administrators, scientists, and animal technicians from primate facilities around the country. Its purpose was to begin to formulate new humane standards for the maintenance of chimps in the laboratory.

Goodall recommends increasing the number of trained animal caretakers selected for their understanding of animal behavior and their compassion and respect for their charges, as the best way to improve the quality of life for lab chimps. She also suggests that researchers provide their animal subjects with a rich and stimulating environment and work to alleviate their pain and stress during experimental procedures, for example, by treating them in the presence of a trusted human friend.

Source: *The New York Times Magazine*, May 17, 1987, pp. 108–120.

---

mothers, a dramatic response occurs. The infants' behavior is characterized by immediate agitation and frequent distress vocalizations. When the mother returns, the response abates. This intense behavioral response is important for survival, since it maximizes the mother's chances of relocating her lost infant. Studies in the laboratory reveal that this characteristic behavioral response is associated with the secretion of stress-related hormones, changes in body temperature, heart rate, blood pressure, and disruption of sleep (Kalin and Carnes, 1984). These physiologic changes help the infant to face the stress of separation through numerous mechanisms, including increasing the availability of glucose, an essential energy source. When antianxiety agents and opiates are administered, the immediate behavioral and endocrine response to separation is blocked. This result suggests that, on a neurochemical level, the response to separation is mediated through brain benzodiazepine and opiate receptors. Work with squirrel monkeys suggests that a specific area of the brain, the cingulate cortex, is responsible for the production of isolation-induced distress vocalizations.

If separation is prolonged, behavioral inhibition and withdrawal frequently occur. (In the wild, prolonged separation frequently results in death of the infant.) Extensive laboratory studies have revealed that the intensity of the separation response varies among individual animals (Kaufman, 1975). When it occurs in its most dramatic form, the animal maintains a characteristic fetal-like position—behavior called huddling. This separation paradigm has been suggested as a model of human depression (Kaufman and Rosenblum, 1967). Catecholamine systems have been implicated in this model since the separation response is made more intense if brain norepinephrine is depleted, and since administration of tricyclic antidepressants prevents separation-induced behavioral inhibition. Analyses of norepinephrine levels in cerebrospinal fluid (CSF) suggest that monkeys with lower levels have a more intense response.

The long-term effects of early separation also vary and depend on numerous factors including the length of time the young animal experiences social isolation. When young monkeys are isolated for long periods of time, they are found to be socially defi-

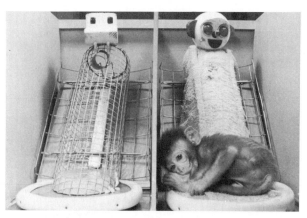

Harlow (1958) showed that when infant rhesus monkeys were separated from their mothers and provided artificial surrogate mothers, the infants preferred to spend their non-eating time with the soft, heated version without food rather than with the wire mesh "mother," which was their food source. He concluded that contact-comfort, not feeding, was responsible for maternal-infant attachment.

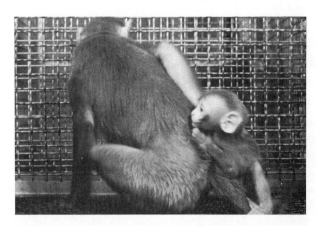

When infant rhesus monkeys were reared in isolation for the first six months of life, they were at best inadequate mothers who ignored their offspring (as is shown in this photo), and at worst, were so abusive that the infants had to be removed from them. This is reminiscent of the strong relationship between social isolation and child abuse demonstrated in humans (Polansky, 1977).

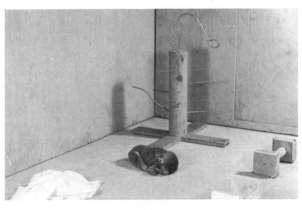

John Bowlby, upon touring Harlow's laboratory, was the first to point out the psychopathology in monkeys reared in isolation. Like the young children separated from their mothers that Bowlby was studying, these monkeys demonstrated increased self-orality and self-clasping, rocking patterns (or hair pulling or head banging), self-directed biting (chewing arms and legs), and passive behavior. This was the birth of the animal model of depression (Suomi, 1978, personal communication).

Right: Suomi (1983) has shown that infant monkeys who display extreme autonomic reactions to mild stressors are likely to display extreme behavioral reactions involving fearfulness, anxiety, and withdrawal when placed in stressful situations. These individual characteristics may only be apparent during stress, but they appear to be stable over time and across repeated experiences and stressful events.

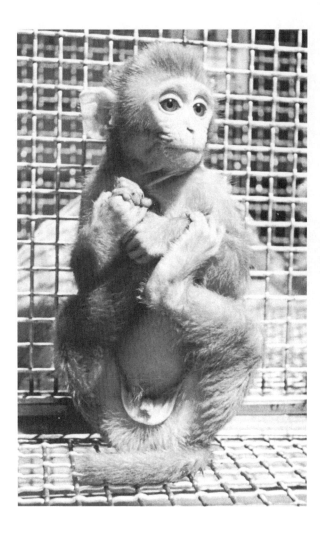

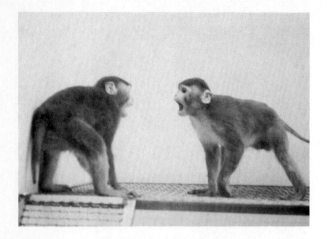
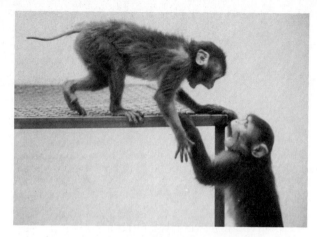
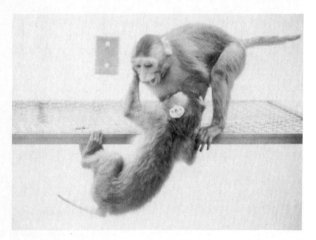
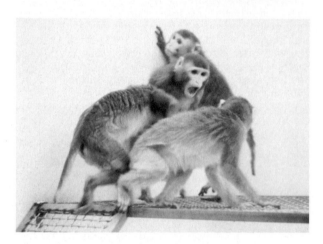

Young rhesus monkeys displaying normal aggression in play.

cient later in life. These monkeys have difficulty interacting with other animals and they display inappropriate aggressive and sexual behavior. However, if they are exposed long enough to younger normal animals ("monkey therapists" who are nonthreatening since they can do little more than cling to the "monkey patient" and engage in simple play), their behavior normalizes. Work by Kraemer and McKinney (1979) has shown that social deprivation of rhesus monkeys during infancy may result in permanent alteration of brain neurochemical systems. Administration of amphetamines to normal rhesus monkeys generally results in behavioral activation and increases in CSF norepinephrine. However, monkeys that have experienced early prolonged social deprivation respond to amphetamines with psychotic-like and aggressive behavior.

STRESS AND LEARNED HELPLESSNESS

Maier (1983), Seligman (1968, 1975), and others have explored issues related to the controllability of stressors in animals. They have found that animals unable to control their exposure to aversive events demonstrate behavioral and physiological changes similar to those seen in depressed humans. The "learned helplessness" paradigm involves exposing rats to mild electrical shock. By rotating a wheel, one rat is able to turn off the shock for both itself and its separately caged partner. The other rat thus receives the same amount and duration of shock but has no control over it. The rat without control develops a number of behavioral deficits, including the inability to learn new tasks, attentional problems, and decreased activity and motivation. Social behavior is also affected in that dominant rats that receive this

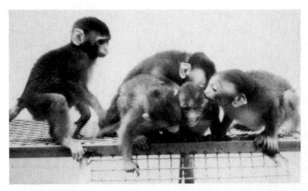

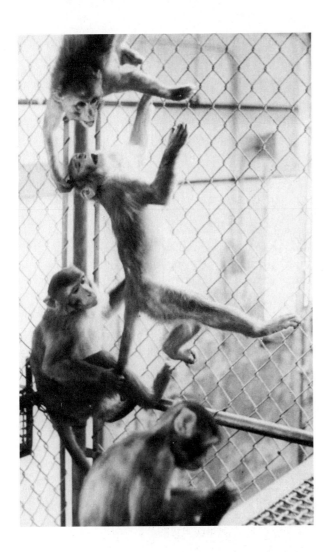

Aggression in one-year-old rhesus monkeys in the service of establishing their territory as a dominance hierarchy. Note the "attacked" monkey's fear grimace, behavior which appears in the first two weeks of life and is mediated in the neuroendocrine system. The fear grimace is also seen when the young monkey is confronted with a stranger, similar to stranger-anxiety in human infants (Kalin, 1988, personal communication).

In the wild, the best fighter would become the dominant male in the group, and have priority access to food and preferred living areas as a result. This dominance would then "run in the family" as the infants of the dominant male share not only their father's biological prowess but also his priority access to food, and so on.

Dominance in a group of monkeys is subject to change, depending on the changing composition of the group. Subordinate males may remain on the group's periphery, form a coalition, and drive out the leader. Adolescents (male and female) are typically on the periphery of the group or in their own group. Among male siblings, the oldest is dominant; in the case of females, it is the youngest. Non-conformist adolescent males, that is, those who don't respect the group's hierarchy are killed by other group members within two to three months unless they are able to leave the group and join another. (Suomi, 1978, personal communication). While it is often difficult to generalize from the animal model to the human situation, in this case, the required "leap" does not seem to be a big one. Think of all the young men who have been sent off to war—and death—the most recent example being Vietnam.

treatment become submissive. Physiologic effects of exposure to uncontrollable shock are dramatic and include gastric ulceration, diminished responsiveness to painful stimuli, and immunological deficits. The effects on the immune system are of particular interest, since it has been shown that malignant tumors grow more rapidly in rats exposed to uncontrollable stress (Laudenslager, 1988). On a biochemical level, specific depletions in brain norepinephrine have been found. Weiss (1968, 1971) has hypothesized that these changes may play a mechanistic role in the behavioral and physiological alterations associated with learned helplessness. Endorphins have also been implicated, since opiate antagonists block the *stress-induced analgesia* associated with uncontrollable shock. There is a striking resemblance between the changes that uncontrollable shock induces in rats and the behavior of depressed humans, and it is of interest that

pretreatment with antidepressants and ECT will prevent learned helplessness in rats.

LEARNING AT THE BIOCHEMICAL LEVEL

To elucidate the cellular and molecular mechanisms of behavior, Kandel and Schwartz (1982) have used the marine snail, *aplysia*. These invertebrates use simple and complex forms of learning similar to those used by vertebrates to adapt to environmental demands. The simplicity of their nervous system allows investigators to identify neuronal pathways that directly mediate learning. The withdrawal reflex has been studied intensively, as it is easy to elicit and plays an important role in the snail's survival. When the snail is stimulated it withdraws its external organs. If presented with a mild stimulus it rapidly learns to decrease the intensity of the withdrawal reflex (habituation). On the other hand, if the stimulus presented is noxious the snail learns to withdraw its external organs into its shell more actively (sensitization). This nonassociative learning allows the snail to discriminate rapidly between potentially dangerous threats and innocuous events and to respond appropriately. *Aplysia* also has been shown to exhibit long-term memory. The snail stores environmental associations that occur with noxious events, allowing it in the future to recognize and respond adaptively to potentially dangerous environmental situations.

The biology of this learning has been studied at cellular and molecular levels. Habituation results from a progressive decrease in the amount of neurotransmitter released from the sensory neuron, leading to a reduction in the withdrawal reflex. When sensitization occurs, another set of neurons releases serotonin onto the sensory neuron. This promotes the enhanced release of neurotransmitters onto the motor neuron, which is seen as an exaggerated withdrawal reflex.

These examples of research in animals demonstrate the complex interactions among learning, social, and biochemical events. Ample data exist suggesting that they are relevant to the development of human behavior. Throughout this text, evidence of the applicability of these studies to human behavior is explored. The case study below about Jamie illustrates the necessity of an integrated approach in understanding psychopathology.

 Case Study: Nonpsychiatric Setting

Jamie, a 20-year-old college student, came to the general medicine clinic worried that he was having a heart attack. In relating his history to the nurse, he stated that he had been under a lot of stress recently. Last evening when he went to bed, he developed chest pain, shortness of breath, lightheadedness, and a rapid pulse. After a physical examination, an ECG was performed and found to be normal. While interacting with the patient, the nurse noted that in addition to appearing anxious, at times his voice quivered and he became teary-eyed. After the evaluation the physician and nurse suggested to Jamie that his chest pain might be related to anxiety. At that point he started to cry and admitted that he had had thoughts of killing himself, which was what made him feel panicked the night before.

A psychiatric consultant was asked to assist in Jamie's evaluation. On further questioning Jamie acknowledged that for the past week he had had recurrent thoughts of suicide and recently he had developed a plan to kill himself. He stated that during the past two months his mood had become progressively worse and now he had frequent crying spells for no apparent reason. He had been unable to sleep, uninterested in food or sex, and socially withdrawn, spending most of his time alone. Three weeks before, he had failed two of his midterm exams because he was unable to concentrate or retain what he had studied. He stated that he was a loser, unattractive to women, and had no future. As evidence, he stated that his most recent girlfriend had broken off their relationship four months earlier. While he felt that this should not still be upsetting him, he continued to ruminate obsessively about his loss and wondered what he had done to drive her away.

This was the first time he had thought seriously about suicide; however, he stated that in high school he had lacked confidence and had been shy, anxious, and mildly depressed until he met his girlfriend. She was outgoing and supportive, bringing a new sense of comfort and happiness to him. During the course of their relationship she was concerned about his dependence and possessiveness and gave this as her reason for breaking up. On further questioning, he revealed that his mother had died when he was three years old, but he denied that this still had any effect on him. His father had been devastated by the death and became depressed and started drinking heavily. Shortly after, his father started bringing home a series of women. Four years later, while attending Alcoholics Anonymous, his father met a woman whom he later married. Jamie was never able to feel close to his stepmother and had feelings of resentment toward her in order to avoid feeling disloyal to his mother. His family history revealed that his maternal grandfather became depressed at the age of 44 and hanged himself. He had an older brother who drank heavily and appeared to be chronically depressed.

It is apparent from this history that Jamie's depressed state was determined by multiple factors. Based on his family history, it is likely that Jamie had a genetic predisposition to become depressed. He lost his mother at a critical developmental phase, and his father was unavailable as an adequate replacement. He saw his father's depression and inability to cope effectively with the loss of his wife. Jamie was unable to feel close to his new stepmother and felt resentment and guilt about this. As a consequence, he had chronically low self-esteem and was unsure of himself in social situations, particularly those involving girls. His close relationship with his girlfriend made him feel more confident and he could not understand how she could be concerned about his dependency on her. The disruption of this attachment was an overwhelming stress for him and activated earlier feelings of depression, anxiety, and insecurity. This, along with his genetic vulnerability, likely triggered a prolonged period of intense depression associated with altered function of physiological systems regulating sleep and appetite.

Jamie was treated with a combination of antidepressants and psychotherapy. He was placed on a tricyclic antidepressant and the dose was gradually increased over the first three weeks. In addition, he met with his therapist twice per week initially, to work on issues related to his low self-esteem. His suicidal ideation diminished after his first session and he felt more hopeful about the future. Within 10 days he noticed that his energy level was beginning to increase, he felt less tense, and he was able to concentrate on his school work and to sleep well. After four weeks it was apparent that he no longer felt depressed. His mood had improved markedly—this was associated with an increase in his self-esteem. He felt like becoming socially active again and even considered asking a girl he did not know very well out to a movie. He continued in psychotherapy for twelve weeks and was able to understand more about why his self-esteem was so dependent on having a girlfriend who loved him. Four months after he began treatment he stated that he hadn't felt this good for as long as he could remember. His antidepressant medication was stopped, and at followup one year later he continued to do well.

SUMMARY

Human behavior results from an interaction of biological and environmental determinants. Although many theories attempt to explain the development of normal and abnormal behavior, the three predominant models are the psychoanalytic, the behavioral, and the biological.

Psychoanalytic theory is based on the premise that experiences occurring in infancy and childhood determine an individual's behavior as an adult. The four major concepts that are helpful in understanding this theory are: 1) the unconscious mind; 2) the topographical model of the mind; 3) psychosexual development; and 4) attachment bonds, social relationships, and object relations. Behavioral theory is based on the relationship between learning and behavior. This theory assumes that an organism's behavior is determined by the environmental contingencies of that behavior experienced in the past. It emphasizes the interaction between the person and his environment. The underlying premise of biological theory is that behavior is determined by biochemical events in the brain.

The major treatments based on psychoanalytic theory are classical psychoanalysis and psychodynamic psychotherapy. Behavioral therapies are designed to modify specific behaviors that are associated with various psychiatric syndromes, for example, avoidance behavior in the phobic patient. Biological therapies, including psychotropic drugs and electroconvulsive therapy, have been shown to be effective in the treatment of a number of illnesses, including schizophrenia and mood disorders.

Clinical work and research employing animals have emphasized the importance of integrating aspects of each of the three theories in attempts to explain behavior. Engel calls this approach the biopsychosocial model, suggesting that all psychiatric illnesses have biological, psychological, and social components.

KEY TERMS

psychopathology

psychoanalytic (or psychodynamic) theory

behavioral theory

cognitive approach

humanistic approach

interpersonal approach

self-psychology

sociocultural theories

unconscious mind

topographical model of the mind

psychosexual development

ego defense mechanisms

social relationships

attachment bonds

object relations

classical psychoanalysis

brief psychodynamic psychotherapy

transference

interpersonal therapy (IPT)

associative learning

classical conditioning

operant conditioning

nonassociative learning

social-learning theory

biological theory

biopsychosocial model

STUDY QUESTIONS

1. What is the basic premise underlying psychoanalytic theory?

2. What is the basic premise underlying behavioral theory?

3. What is the basic premise underlying biological theory?

4. What is the primary aim of psychoanalytic therapy?

5. Name specific ways in which behavioral principles have been applied to the treatment of psychiatric patients.

REFERENCES

Bandura, A. (1977). *Social Learning Theory.* Englewood Cliffs, NJ: Prentice-hall.

Basch, M. (1988). *Understanding Psychotherapy.* New York: Basic Books.

Bowlby, J. (1969). Attachment and loss. *Vol. I. Attachment.* New York: Basic Books.

Bowlby, J. (1980). Attachment and loss. *Vol. III. Loss: Sadness and Depression.* New York: Basic Books.

Dale, A. J. P. (1980). Organic mental disorders associated with infections. In H. I. Kaplan, A. M. Kaplan, A. M. Freedman, and B. J. Saddock (eds) *Comprehensive Textbook of Psychiatry.* Baltimore: Williams and Wilkins.

Dewald, P. A. (1971). *Psychotherapy, a Dynamic Approach.* New York: Basic Books.

Dickinson, A. (1980). *Contemporary Animal Learning Theory.* New York: Cambridge University Press.

Engel, G. L. (1977). The need for a new medical model: a challenge for biomedicine. *Science, 1960,* 129–136.

Freud, S. (1923). The ego and the id. *Standard Edition* 19, 12–66.

Freud, S. (1926). Inhibitions, symptoms, and anxiety. *Standard Edition,* 20, 87–172.

Greenberg, J. R. and Mitchell, S. A. (1983). *Object Relations in Psychoanalytic Theory.* Cambridge, MA: Harvard University Press.

Harlow, H. F. (1958). The nature of love. *American Psychologist* 13: 673.

Harlow, H. F., and Harlow, M. K. (1969). Effects of various mother-infant relationships on rhesus monkey behavior. In B. M. Foss (ed) *Determinants of infant behavior* Vol. 4, London: Methuen.

Kalin, N. H. and Carnes, M. (1984). Biological correlates of attachment bond disruption in humans and nonhuman primates. *Progress in Neuropsychopharmacology and Biological Psychiatry,* 8, 459–443.

Kalisch, P. and Kalisch, B. (1986). *The advance of American nursing,* second edition. Boston: Little, Brown.

Kandel, E. R. and Schwartz, J. H. (1982). Molecular biology of learning: modulation of transmitter release. *Science, 218,* 433–443.

Kaufman, I. (1975). Mother-infant separation in monkeys: an experimental model. In E. Senoy and J. P. Scott (Eds.), *Separation and Depression: Clinical and Research Aspects.* Washington, D.C.: Amer. Association for Advancement of Science.

Kaufman, I. and Rosenblum, L. (1967) The reaction to separation in infant monkeys: anaclitic depression and conservation-withdrawal. *Psychosomatic Medicine, 29,* pp. 648–675.

Klein, D. F., and Gittelman, R., Quitkin, F., and Rifkin, A. (1980). *Diagnosis and Drug Treatment of Psychiatric Disorders: Adults and Children.* Baltimore: Williams and Wilkins.

Klein, M. (1937). Love, guilt, and reparation. In M. Klein and J. Riviere (eds) *Love, Hate, and Reparation.* London: Hogarth Press.

Kohut, H. (1984). How does analysis cure? In Goldberg and Stepansky (Eds.). Chicago: University of Chicago Press.

Kraemer, G. W. and McKinney, W. T. (1979). Interactions of pharmacological agents which alter biogenic amine metabolism and depression. *Journal of Affective Disorders, 1,* 33–54.

Kupfermann, I. (1981). Learning. In E. R. Kandel and J. H. Schwartz (Eds) *Principles of Neural Science.* North Holland, New York; Elsevier.

Laudenslager, M. L., Ryan, S. M., et al. (1983). Coping and immunosuppression: Inescapable but not escapable shock suppresses lymphocyte proliferation. *Science,* 221, 568–570.

Luborsky, L. and Spence, D. P. (1978). Quantitative research on psychoanalytic therapy. In S. Garfield and A. Bergin (eds) *Handbook of Psychotherapy and Behavior Change.* New York; John Wiley and Sons, 331–368.

Mahler, M. S., Pine F., and Bergman, A. (1975). *The Psychological Birth of the Human Infant.* New York: Basic Books.

Maier, S. F. (1983). Learned helplessness, depression, analgesia, and endogenous opiates. *Pharmacology Bulletin,* 19, 531–38.

Meador, B., and Rogers, C. R. (1979) Person-centered therapy. In Corsini, R. (Ed) *Current Psychotherapies,* Itasca, Ill.: F. E. Peacock, pp. 131–184.

Mowrer, O. & Mowrer, W. (1938). Enuresis: A method for its study and treatment. *American Journal of Orthopsychiatry,* 8, 436–459.

Mitchell, G. (1970). Abnormal behavior in primates. In Rosenblum, L. A. (Ed.), Primate behavior: Developments in field and laboratory research, Vol. I. New York: Academic Press.

Ornstein, P. & Ornstein, A. (1986). *Self-Psychology in Psychoanalytic Theory.* Cape Cod Institute of Albert Einstein College of Medicine.

Pavlov, I. P. (1927). *Conditioned Reflexes: An Investigation of the Physiological Activity of the Cerebral Cortex.* London: Oxford University Press.

Pincus, J. and Tucker, G. J. (1985). *Behavioral Neurology.* New York: Oxford University Press.

Rachman, S., Hodgson, R. & Marus, I. M. (1971). The treatment of chronic obsessional-compulsive neurosis. *Behavior, Research, & Therapy,* 9, pp. 237–247.

Rajecki, D. W., Lamb, M. E., and Obsmascher, P. (1978). Toward a general theory of infantile attachment: a comparative review of aspects of the social bond. *The Behavioral and Brain Sciences,* 3, 417–464.

Rosenthal, D. (1971). *Genetics of Psychopathology.* New York; McGraw-Hill Book Company.

Seligman, M. (1968). Chronic fear produced by unpredictable shock. *Journal of Comparative and Physiological Psychology,* 66, 402–411.

Seligman, M. (1975). *Helplessness: On Depression, Development, and Death.* San Francisco: W. H. Freeman and Company.

Spradley, B. (1990). *Community health nursing: Concepts and practice,* 3rd ed. Glenview, IL: Scott, Foresman/ Little, Brown.

Stern, D. (1985). *The Interpersonal World of the Infant.* New York; Basic Books.

Strupp, H. H. (1968). Psychoanalytic therapy of the individual. In J. Marmor (ed) *Modern Psychoanalysis: New Direction and Perspectives.* New York: Basic Books, 193–342.

Suomi, S. J. (1983). Social development in rhesus monkeys: consideration of individual differences. In A. Oliverio and M. Zupella (Eds.), New York: Plenum Press, pp. 71–89.

Thorndike, E. L. (1932). *The Fundamentals of Learning.* New York; Bureau of Publications, Teacher's College.

Weiss, J. M. (1968). Effects of coping responses on stress. *Journal of Comparative and Physiological Psychology,* 65, 251–260.

Weiss, J. M. (1971). Effects of coping behavior in different warning signal conditions on stress pathology in rats. *Journal of Comparative and Physiological Psychology.* 77, 1–13.

3

PSYCHIATRIC CLASSIFICATION
ROGER BLASHFIELD

LEARNING OBJECTIVES
After studying this chapter, the student will be able to:

- Discuss the roles of Kraepelin and Freud in the development of psychiatric classification.
- Discuss the development of the Diagnostic and Statistical Manual of Mental Disorders.
- Identify and describe the major DSM-III-R categories of disorders.
- Describe the multiaxial system of the DSM-III-R.
- Describe the development of nursing diagnosis.
- Identify nursing diagnoses which pertain to psychosocial human needs.
- Discuss the pros and cons of psychiatric classification.

INTRODUCTION

Imagine that a girl is sitting on the beach with a collection of shells, pebbles, and stones. As she sits with her collection, she sorts the objects into piles. Gradually, she forms four groups: one of pretty shells; another of shiny pebbles and stones; another of the broken shells; and finally those she has decided to throw away. As she is sorting, a large wave washes on shore, bringing an interesting new shell with it. The girl spots the shell, examines it, decides it is very attractive, and places it in the group of pretty shells to be taken home.

This chapter is about **classification.** When sorting her collection of shells and pebbles, the girl on the beach classified these objects (cf. Menninger, 1963), using the process of abstraction to organize them. Classification takes place in many areas of human activity. Foods are classified according to their nutritional contents, their taste, their use in the cooking process, and their origins. Baseball players are classified according to the positions they play, their statistics as batters, and their teams.

Psychiatric classification, or classification of psychopathology, is an important aspect of mental health care. Unfortunately, however, it is often described pejoratively by many mental health professionals and others, for example, when it is called "labeling" (see Chapter 28 on Ethics). While this is a legitimate concern, classification of psychopathology creates an essential common language used by a wide variety of mental health care providers, and is critical to assessment, treatment, and prevention of psychopathology. Likewise, the development of specific nursing diagnoses related to mental health and illness is just as critical, for this will provide the nursing profession with a common language and accepted practice for care of patients whose physical disorders create secondary disturbances in mental health as well as those with primary psychiatric illnesses.

THE HISTORY OF PSYCHIATRIC CLASSIFICATION

The classification of psychopathology can be traced back to the Greeks. In their consideration of people who had mental disorders, the Greeks introduced a number of terms, some of which are still used today. *Mania, melancholia, hysteria,* and *paranoia* are all classificatory concepts about psychopathology whose or-

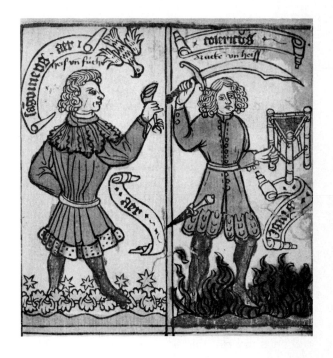

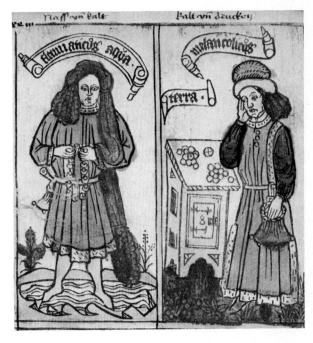

In Medieval times, it was thought that an imbalance in the four humors, which arose from the four basic elements of life (air, fire, water, and earth) adversely affected the physical and psychological well-being of an individual. The individuals portrayed above were intended to illustrate the four disorders that could result from such an imbalance. The types are (from upper left to right): sanguine (blood/air), choleric (yellow bile/fire), phlegmatic (phlegm/water), and melancholic (black bile/earth).

igins can be traced back to the Greeks. *Mania* refers to a condition in which people are extremely agitated and excited. The manic individual's speech becomes very rapid, at times, to the point of incoherence, and he typically has grandiose ideas about his powers and abilities. *Melancholia* refers to what is currently described as depression. Hippocrates described this disorder as being caused by an abnormality in black bile, one of the four basic humors in the body; hence its name, *melan* (black), + *cholia* (bile). Although the term melancholia is no longer synonymous with depression, it is still used in clinical literature to refer to a severe form of depression, most often seen in older adults. *Hysteria* was assumed by the Greeks to occur only among women and to be caused by a "floating uterus," which caused many somatic complaints as it moved about the body. *Paranoia* comes from *para* (abnormal) + *nous* (mind); that is, abnormal mind, deranged, or crazy. Paranoia has come to refer to a disorder in which patients are suspicious and often feel that they are being persecuted or plotted against by others.

DEMENTIA PARALYTICA

Modern views of psychopathology date back to the late 1700s and 1800s and the writings of Philippe Pinel, Rush, and others. During the early 1800s, an important event in the classification of mental disorders occurred in France. At that time, a popular diagnostic term, whose use still continues into the present, was **dementia**. This term, which literally meant "out of one's mind" or "crazy" was used to refer to psychotic (demented) patients. In 1819 in France, a physician named Bayle performed autopsies on a number of patients who had become demented and discovered that all had marked changes in their brains. In addition to their dementia, all these patients developed motor paralysis before they died. The brains of these patients had shrunk to almost half the weight of a normal brain, the "skin" (meninges) of the brains was thickened, and the color of the brains was strikingly different from that of normal brains. Because of the paralysis that normally occurred during the course of this disorder, the condition was named **dementia paralytica.**

The discovery of dementia paralytica was the first instance in which a mental disorder had been shown to be associated with demonstrable changes in the brain. Following the discovery of dementia paralytica, there was a major surge of interest in the mental disorders. Hundreds of new terms were proposed,

largely based upon the experience of physicians who worked in insane asylums. There were many autopsy studies of changes in the brain, followed by retrospective attempts to demonstrate a relationship between observable changes in the brain and a history of disordered behaviors of the individual while alive. During this time, a dictum by Griesinger, a famous German physician, became the guiding principle of most studies of psychopathology: "All mental diseases are brain diseases." Thus, for every new mental disorder that was proposed, investigators attempted to verify its existence through studies of brain anatomy and brain physiology.

KRAEPELIN

An abundance of terms were proposed during the 1800s, and there was a great deal of confusion sur-

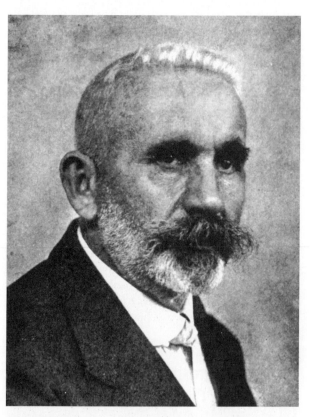

Emil Kraepelin's (1856–1926) classification system for mental disorders was utilized exclusively throughout the world until the American Psychiatric Association, in 1952, introduced the Diagnostic and Statistical Manual of Mental Disorders (DSM–I). His classification, however, serves as the lynch pin for the conceptualization of all subsequent DSM publications.

rounding the classification of mental disorders. Various classifications were proposed but none gained widespread acceptance. At the end of the 1800s, however, the classifications proposed by Emil Kraepelin, a German physician, became dominant throughout the world. Born in 1856, Kraepelin spent a year after medical school working in the research laboratory of one of his professors, Wilhelm Wundt. Wundt directed the first known laboratory devoted to psychological studies. After working with Wundt, Kraepelin left Germany to become the director of an insane asylum in one of the Baltic states (now in the Soviet Union). While there, Kraepelin continued his psychological research, using mental patients as his subjects. Kraepelin also taught medical students about psychiatry and wrote a "textbook of psychiatry." This textbook became popular because of its clear and interesting behavioral descriptions of patients.

There are a number of important points to note about Kraepelin's approach to classification. First, Kraepelin did not set out to create new classifications. He was an author of textbooks, and, like most textbook authors, organized his chapters around the major categories of psychopathology as they were generally accepted by contemporary authorities. What have become known as Kraepelin's classifications were simply the tables of contents to the various editions of his books. Thus Kraepelinian classification systems were not structured with the idea of becoming official nomenclatures for use in institutions or outpatient clinics. Kraepelin organized his books in the way that he felt best helped him to communicate with students and other professionals.

Second, Kraepelin was much more psychological in his approach to mental disorders than were his medically oriented contemporaries. He did believe, along with these colleagues, that most mental disorders had an associated organic etiology. However, he advocated careful behavioral analysis of patients in order to understand their clinical picture. He was also a proponent of using applied research to better understand abnormal behavior and its neurophysiologic bases (Kahn, 1959).

Recall that, before Kraepelin, researchers concerned with the mental disorders attempted to verify the validity of these categories by correlating them with neuropathologic findings on autopsies or with the genetic histories of the patients. Kraepelin, in contrast, believed that the most productive initial step in the study of psychopathology was to make a careful behavioral description of patients in order to

search for systematic patterns of similarities and differences. After a base of descriptive information was created, the search for biological correlates could be undertaken.

The third important point to note about Kraepelin is that his international fame was associated with his introduction of two important diagnoses. These diagnoses were manic-depressive insanity (now called a bipolar mood disorder) and dementia praecox (now called schizophrenia). The first concept was revolutionary because Kraepelin combined two disorders, mania and melancholia, into one (he had noted that the courses of these disorders were very similar). That is, patients who present either manic or depressed symptoms often have a history of acute episodes. During an episode the mood changes gradually wane, with the patient eventually returning to normal functioning; however, additional episodes of mood changes are likely. Because of the similarity of the courses of mania and melancholia, Kraepelin believed them to be opposite sides of the same coin, and so combined them into one disorder: **manic-depressive insanity.**

The other important diagnosis introduced by Kraepelin, **dementia praecox,** means "precocious insanity." Kraepelin used this term to refer to a form of psychosis that occurred relatively early in the life of the patient. Most of the forms of dementia have onset in patients who are 40 years of age and older (for example, senile dementia). Kraepelin called this new disorder "dementia praecox" because an important distinguishing feature was that its onset often occurred during late adolescence. Kraepelin described this disorder as having associated characteristics such as hallucinations, delusions, bizarre behaviors, and markedly disturbed speech patterns. He included the diagnoses of hebephrenia, catatonia, and paranoia as subtypes of this disorder (Boisen, 1938).

Dementia praecox had a number of parallels to the concept of dementia paralytica. The initial clinical pictures (hallucinations, delusions, and so forth) of these patients were often very similar. Moreover, both were associated with a progressive deterioration of functioning. Finally, the names of the two disorders were similar. At this point, however, the similarities stop. The age of onset for dementia paralytica was recognized as the 40s and 50s, while the age of onset for dementia praecox was usually between the ages of 15 and 30. Moreover, dementia paralytica typically progressed to physical paralysis and eventually to death; dementia praecox usually progressed to a chronic form of psychosis but not death.

DEMENTIA PARALYTICA RESOLVED

At the time of Kraepelin's main writings, the cause of dementia paralytica was still undiscovered. Despite much research during the 1900s, the understanding of this disorder had not progressed since Bayle's initial discovery. By the end of the 1800s, there were three theories about its cause: the French, who at that time dominated the medical community, believed it was caused by alcoholism; the Germans, who were an emerging force in medical science, associated it with syphilis, and the American medical establishment, perhaps dominated by the high moral tone of the time, believed it was caused by poor morals. In 1902, the bacteria that causes syphilis was discovered. A blood test for this bacteria was developed in 1906. This test was positive when performed on both the blood and the cerebrospinal fluid of patients with dementia paralytica. In 1912, it was demonstrated that patients with this disorder had the syphilitic bacteria in their brains. The etiological question was resolved. Dementia paralytica (now called **paresis**) was caused by tertiary syphilis of the central nervous system. With the discovery of antibiotics during World War II, this disorder was practically eliminated and is rarely seen in modern clinical practice.

Dementia paralytica was the first major mental disorder that psychiatry was able to recognize, define the etiology for, and treat effectively. In resolving this disorder, psychiatry demonstrated that it was a viable branch of medicine. In the same spirit, psychiatric researchers have turned their focus to the Kraepelinian disorders of schizophrenia and manic-depressive psychoses, but with little success in the areas of etiology and curative treatment.

FREUD

As discussed in Chapter 2, Sigmund Freud, who was born in the same year as Kraepelin, 1856, formulated important theories about the derivation of obsessions, narcissism, sexual disorders, delusions, and anxiety, and he created a new form of treatment for these disorders, called **psychotherapy.** Freud was not interested in the psychoses, such as schizophrenia, which he considered to be primarily caused by physiological changes. Nor was he interested in classification, which he saw as promoting a superficial and physiologically oriented view of mental disorders. Nonetheless, Freud's views have had a major influence on psychiatric classification, in that most psychiatric diagnoses, particularly those in the neurosis and

personality disorder categories, can be traced back to concepts he introduced.

DSM-I AND DSM-II

Despite the benign neglect with which U.S. mental health professionals have viewed classification, various official classification systems have been developed over the last 70 years. Consistently, these systems have reflected the importance accorded to Kraepelin's concepts. In 1917, a classification system was adopted by the newly formed American Psychiatric Association that included Kraepelin's concepts of dementia praecox, manic-depressive disorder, and paranoia (Menninger, 1963). This classification also made the fundamental Kraepelinian distinction among organic brain syndromes, the functional psychoses, and the neurotic/character disorders.

Between World Wars I and II, Americans were uninterested in classification, and focused instead on the expansion of psychoanalytic ideas, the development of personality theories, and the investigation of new forms of psychological therapies.

In 1932, the American Psychiatric Association officially adopted a new classification system as part of the *Standard Classified Nomenclature of Diseases* (American Psychiatric Association [APA], 1933). This classification system contained 24 major categories, 19 of which had appeared in Kraepelin's classifications. This new classification, however, did not attract much attention and never gained popular acceptance in American psychiatry (Menninger, 1963).

World War II led to a renewed emphasis on classification. During the war, nearly 10 percent of all military discharges were for psychiatric reasons. By the time the war ended, there were four major competing classification systems: 1) the "standard" system adopted by the American Psychiatric Association in 1932; 2) the U.S. Army classification; 3) the U.S. Navy classification; and 4) the Veterans Administration system (Raines, 1952). In response to this disorganization, the American Psychiatric Association formed a task force to create a system that would become standard in the United States. The result was the *Diagnostic and Statistical Manual of Mental Disorders* (APA, 1952). This classification is usually known by its abbreviation: **DSM-I.**

The DSM-I was important for a number of reasons. First, the major rationale behind the DSM-I was to create a classification system that represented a consensus of contemporary thinking. Care was taken to include all diagnostic concepts that were popular in American psychiatry during the 1940s and 1950s. Thus, the DSM-I emphasized communication among professionals as the major purpose of classification and emphasized the need for psychiatric classification to be an accepted nomenclature that members of a profession can use to discuss their clinical cases. Consistent with this emphasis on communication, early versions of the DSM-I were revised based on comments elicited in a questionnaire sent to 10 percent of the members of the American Psychiatric Association. The DSM-I was finally adopted by a vote of the membership of the American Psychiatric Association (Raines, 1952).

The emphasis on communication in the DSM-I led to a similar organizing movement in international psychiatric classification. A committee chaired by the British psychiatrist E. Stengel was formed to review the classification systems used by various countries and to make any necessary recommendations for changes to the World Health Organization. What Stengel (1959) found was a hodgepodge of diagnostic systems, among, and sometimes within, different countries. In 1951, the World Health Organization had proposed an international psychiatric classification as part of the *International Classification of Diseases,* sixth edition—**ICD-6** (World Health Organization, 1948). By 1959, only five member countries of the World Health Organization (Finland, Peru, New Zealand, Thailand, and the United Kingdom) had adopted the ICD-6 classification. Stengel despaired over the confused state of international classification, especially because the ICD-6 had not been generally accepted. The only positive note concerned the DSM-I, which Stengel considered an advance over the other national classifications because of its emphasis on representing a consensus within a country.

As a result of Stengel's review, there was an international movement to create a consensual system that would be adopted by the World Health Organization countries. The final product was the mental-disorders section of the *International Classification of Diseases,* eighth edition; that is, the **ICD-8** (World Health Organization, 1967). In the United States, psychiatrists worked with their international movement to help create this system (Kramer, 1968). The American version of the ICD-8 became the second edition of the *Diagnostic and Statistical Manual of Mental Disorders* (APA, 1968), otherwise known as the **DSM-II.** Only small differences existed between the ICD-8 and the DSM-II.

The DSM-II contained nine major categories of disorders:

1. Mental retardation
2. Organic brain syndrome
3. Functional psychoses
4. Neuroses
5. Personality disorders
6. Alcoholism and other addictions
7. Sexual deviations
8. Special symptoms
9. Disorders of childhood

DSM-III AND DSM-III-R

As noted above, the organizing principle central to forming both the DSM-I and the DSM-II was the goal of better communication among professionals. During the 1970s a new psychiatric edition of the DSM was formed using a new organizing principle, scientific utility, employing principles and methods of science for the purpose of developing a systematic method of classifying mental disorders. In particular, the authors of this new edition, **DSM-III,** were concerned with overcoming the relatively poor reliability associated with the earlier editions.

The DSM-III classification, based on 17 categories and 265 separate disorders, was brought out in 1980 after many years of development and field testing of diagnostic criteria. It quickly became accepted as the common language for mental health professionals when referring to psychological disorders. In 1983, however, the American Psychological Association again began work on revising the DSM-III and published in 1987 a revised version based substantially on the DSM-III categories but with more refined descriptive criteria of disorders. The **DSM-III-R,** currently the official classification of the APA, lists 313 mental disorders in 17 major sections:

1. Disorders Usually First Evident in Infancy, Childhood, or Adolescence
2. Organic Mental Syndromes and Disorders
3. Psychoactive Substance Use Disorders
4. Schizophrenia
5. Delusional Disorders
6. Psychotic Disorders Not Elsewhere Classified
7. Mood Disorders
8. Anxiety Disorders

9. Somatoform Disorders

10. Dissociative Disorders

11. Sexual Disorders

12. Sleep Disorders

13. Factitious Disorders

14. Impulse-Control Disorders Not Elsewhere Classified

15. Adjustment Disorder

16. Psychological Factors Affecting Physical Condition

17. Personality Disorders

Each of these categories is described briefly below, and most are covered in more detail in other chapters in this book.

DISORDERS USUALLY FIRST EVIDENT IN INFANCY, CHILDHOOD, AND ADOLESCENCE.

The interest in childhood psychopathology has grown during the last 40 years. This growth is evident in a comparison of the changing emphasis on childhood disorders in each revision of the DSM. The first edition (1952) contained only 2 disorders relevant to children; the DSM-II listed 10, and the DSM-III and DSM-III-R each contain over 40. The major subdivisions of childhood disorders in the DSM-III-R include the disruptive-behavior disorders, and the developmental disorders (which now include mental retardation and are coded on Axis II), and the eating disorders (anorexia, bulimia), because these disorders usually begin in adolescence. See Chapter 14, on Eating Disorders and Chapter 22, on Psychiatric Mental Health Nursing with Children, for a discussion of these disorders.

ORGANIC MENTAL SYNDROMES AND DISORDERS.

Organic mental disorders are those that have a demonstrated neuropathology such as organic mental disorders caused by alcohol and drug abuse and senile dementia (often called the "psychosis of old age"). Senile dementia has the associated behavioral features of disturbed memory and judgment, abstract thought, disorientation, and unstable emotions. The neuropathology of this disorder is fairly well-recognized: 1) cerebral atrophy is usually more predominant in the frontal lobe; 2) there is usually a reduction in the number of healthy cells; 3) the nerve cells demonstrate shrinkage; 4) necrobiosis (physiologic death of cell) can also occur; and 5) senile plaques, small areas of tissue degeneration, are located throughout the cortex (McHugh & Folstein,

1986). Although the neuropathology of this disorder is known, its etiology remains unknown. Recently, however, there has been a substantial amount of research on this disorder, also called "Alzheimer's disease." Chapter 11, on Organic Mental Disorders, deals with these disorders in detail.

PSYCHOACTIVE SUBSTANCE USE DISORDERS.

Persons with disorders in this category are those who become dependent upon or who abuse various substances, such as alcohol, cocaine, opiates, barbituates, amphetamines, and so forth. Chapter 15, on Substance Abuse, covers these disorders in detail.

SCHIZOPHRENIA, DELUSIONAL (PARANOID) DISORDERS, AND PSYCHOTIC DISORDERS NOT ELSEWHERE CLASSIFIED.

Schizophrenia, paranoia, and the other nonorganic psychoses are also sometimes called the functional psychoses. These disorders are called "psychoses" because patients who are diagnosed with these disorders all have significant problems judging reality. Because they have a disturbed view of reality (for example, an individual who believes he is Jesus Christ), these individuals often behave in ways described as bizarre or crazy. For example, the individual above may walk around the hospital unit with a sheet wrapped around him like the garment Christ is usually depicted wearing. These psychoses are called "functional" because they have no known neuropathology. Despite the lack of demonstrable neuropathology, however, most mental health professionals believe that these disorders are caused by, or at least are associated with, disturbances in the biochemistry of the central nervous system. Chapter 10, on Schizophrenia, discusses these disorders in detail.

MOOD (FORMERLY TERMED AFFECTIVE) DISORDERS.

The *mood disorders,* for example, bipolar disorder (manic-depressive) and unipolar disorder (major depression), involve disruptions in the mood states of individuals. Depression and its classification is discussed later in this chapter. Chapter 9, on Mood Disorders, deals with bipolar and unipolar disorders in detail.

ANXIETY DISORDERS, SOMATOFORM DISORDERS, AND DISSOCIATIVE DISORDERS.

Disorders in these categories are often grouped together under the general term "neuroses." The early U.S. psychiatrist Benjamin Rush believed that many of these disorders were caused by the "wearing out" of nerve cells through overuse. Because of the "nervous breakdowns" these patients suffered, Rush argued for their placement in asylums where the relative peace and quiet would allow their nerves to recover. Rush also warned against use of alcohol, too frequent intercourse, and masturbation, since he felt all of these led to overstimulation of the nervous system, which in turn would lead to a nervous breakdown. Rush's theory of neurosis represented the dominant U.S. attitude toward psychopathology during the 19th century.

Freud's theories changed the concept of neurosis. Freud discarded the idea that neurosis was a result of overuse of nerve cells. Instead, he theorized that many patients who had come to be called neurotics had underlying psychological conflicts that were associated with real (or fantasized) sexual traumas in childhood. As Freud developed his structural view of personality (id, ego, superego), he postulated an internal psychological process as the cause of the neuroses.

The DSM-III-R avoids the term *neurosis* because of its historical and theoretical implications. Instead, the DSM-III-R organizes the associated mental disorders into three descriptive sections. The anxiety disorders (such as agoraphobia) include disorders in which patients experience severe and debilitating anxiety; the somatoform disorders (such as conversion disorder, commonly termed hysteria) are those in which patients complain of various somatic problems that have no known organic basis; and the dissociative disorders (for example, the multiple personality) are those in which the patient experiences markedly altered states of consciousness. Chapter 8, "Anxiety and Anxiety Disorders," Chapter 13, "Psychophysiological Disorders," and Chapter 17, "Dissociative Disorders," deal with these subjects in detail.

SEXUAL DISORDERS. This section of the DSM-III-R includes two major subcategories: 1) paraphilias, or deviant sexual behaviors such as exhibitionism; and 2) sexual dysfunctions, such as premature ejaculation. The DSM-III included many more classifications of sexual disorders than did the DSM-I or DSM-II, an increase associated with the proliferation of research on human sexual behavior and with the clinical sophistication associated with this research. The DSM-III-R has added some specifications to make clearer the distinctions between classifications (with important treatment implications) and has also removed the category of ego-dystonic homosexuality. The sexual disorders are discussed in detail in Chapter 16.

SLEEP DISORDERS. This is the only category new to the DSM-III-R, though the classification of sleep and arousal disorders had been included in an appendix of the DSM-III. This category relates to chronic disorders of sleep as opposed to transient sleep disturbances and may be associated with other physical or mental disorders.

FACTITIOUS DISORDERS, IMPULSE-CONTROL DISORDERS NOT ELSEWHERE CLASSIFIED, ADJUSTMENT DISORDER, AND PSYCHOLOGICAL FACTORS AFFECTING PHYSICAL CONDITION. These four sections in DSM-III-R include the factitious disorders, which are disorders characterized by symptoms intentionally produced (for example, patients who fake physical symptoms, also called Munchausen syndrome); the disorders of impulse control (for example, kleptomania or repetitive stealing of relatively insignificant objects); the adjustment disorders (for example, a person who becomes depressed when faced with major change); and psychological factors affecting physical condition (for example, the patient with angina whose symptoms become worse when family conflicts arise). Of these, the adjustment disorders (discussed in Chapter 18, "Psychological Crises") and the psychological factors affecting physical condition (see Chapter 13, "Psychophysiological Disorders") are especially relevant to general nursing because they focus on the biological expression of psychological conflicts and frustrations.

PERSONALITY DISORDERS. The last section of the DSM-III-R includes all the personality disorders which are covered in detail in Chapter 12.

THE MULTIAXIAL SYSTEM IN THE DSM-III AND DSM-III-R. In addition to expanding the categories for classification, the DSM-III instituted a **multiaxial** (five-axis) **system** for evaluation to allow the clinician to keep related factors in mind when making a psychiatric diagnosis. The DSM-III-R is based on the same five axes with some refinement:

Axis I: **Clinical syndrome** (the diagnosis(es) that best describe the presenting clinical features of the patient).

Axis II: **Developmental disorders and personality disorders.**

Axis III: **Physical disorders and conditions** (a verbal description of the person's physical condition or disorder).

Axis IV: Severity of psychosocial stressors (based on a scale from 1 to 6).

Axis V: Global assessment of functioning (based on a scale of 1 to 90). The GAF scale allows the clinician to indicate her opinion of how well the patient functions overall, in psychological, social, and occupational areas (APA, 1987).

Multiaxial diagnoses should only be made by qualified psychiatric specialists after at least several visits with a patient. It is impossible to make a five-axis diagnosis based on an initial impression or a brief interview. Note the criteria used to determine each diagnosis for the five axes in the case of Phyllis.

Phyllis: An Emergency Room Patient

Phyllis, a 38-year-old woman, was brought to the emergency room of a hospital after ingesting an unknown quantity of pills. The pills were described as sleeping medication prescribed for her by her family doctor. According to Mark, her boyfriend, Phyllis was a graduate student in business, and was doing very well in school until a few weeks before the incident with the sleeping pills. Mark reported that he had been living with Phyllis since shortly after her third marriage ended in divorce because of her husband's physical and sexual abuse. At the time of her admission, Phyllis still had one arm in a cast due to a fracture suffered in a fight with her ex-husband when he was drunk. In the assessment interview, she appeared depressed, cried constantly, and expressed no hope for the future. Since separating from her husband, Phyllis had stayed in the apartment with her boyfriend, refusing to leave, and crying whenever he went out. She reported that she had lost 15 pounds during the previous month and had had great difficulty sleeping. Her motor movements were slow, and her latent responses to questions were long. Mark stated that Phyllis had been hospitalized twice in the past for depression and once was given ECT (electroconvulsive therapy, commonly known as "shock treatment").

Phyllis's Axis I diagnosis would probably be the clinical syndrome of "Major Depression, recurrent, moderate" (296.32). This diagnosis of depression, a mood disorder, would be made because it describes the cognitive (no hope for the future) and behavioral (not eating, sleep difficulties) presentation of the patient. Notice that according to the DSM-III, Phyllis would not be diagnosed as having an adjustment disorder because the latter diagnosis is only made when no other psychiatric disorder is present. Since Phyllis's symptoms were sufficiently severe to warrant a diagnosis of depression, the adjustment disorder diagnosis would not be used.

Besides diagnosing the clinical syndrome, the therapist conducting the interview with Phyllis would need to assign diagnoses along the other four axes. Axis II concerns the relatively constant personality style of the patient (generally a characteristic that developed in childhood or adolescence) and her approach to life. For Phyllis, a possible Axis II diagnosis might be borderline personality disorder because of her history of chaotic interpersonal relationships. Much more information about and experience with Phyllis would be necessary, however, to make this or any definitive personality disorder diagnosis. (See Chapter 12 on Personality Disorders).

Axis III concerns any medical disorders the patient may have. As far as we know, the only medical problem that Phyllis had was a broken arm. This problem would be diagnosed under Axis III. Notice that the medical disorders of a patient are diagnosed on Axis III regardless of whether or not these disorders are etiologically related to the clinical syndrome. Thus the broken arm would be noted on Axis III even though it had no etiological significance for Phyllis's depression. If laboratory tests and subsequent physical exam had demonstrated a significant hypothyroidism in Phyllis, that diagnosis would also be made on Axis III. In the latter instance, the Axis I diagnosis would not change, even though the hypothyroidism may be thought to be the major cause of her depression.

Axis IV concerns the severity of the psychosocial stressors in the patient's life. Since Phyllis and her third husband had recently divorced, the extent of her recent stressors would be considered severe. The severity of the stressors has prognostic importance. Patients who present symptoms associated with relatively severe stressors are more likely to recover quickly than patients who present with the same clinical syndrome, but report only minor psychosocial stress. For instance, if the only stress in Phyllis's life involved receiving a B for the first time in one of her graduate courses, her prognosis would be worse since the stress in her life would be considered relatively minor and not likely to stimulate a major depression in a typical graduate student.

Axis V, global assessment of functioning (GAF), relates to the ability the patient has demonstrated over the past year to function in various social, occupational, and overall psychological roles. In the DSM-III-R, a GAF rating is made for both *current* and *past* (highest level in last year) functioning. For Phyllis, these roles had been those of student and spouse. Although her third marriage had failed, the history does not clearly state her level of functioning in her role as wife. As a student, she had done well until recently. Thus, her highest level of *past* adaptive functioning might be rated "no more than slight impairment." Her current functioning, as suggested in the history, would probably be rated as "seriously impaired." As with Axis IV, the primary clinical significance of Axis V concerns prognosis. The more a mental disorder disrupts the standard roles of an individual, the more severe its effects and the harder it will be for the patient to reconstitute.

To summarize, the multiaxial diagnosis of Phyllis would be:

Axis I—Major depression, recurrent (296.32)

Axis II—Borderline personality disorder (301.83) (Provisional)

Axis III—Fracture of the left arm

Axis IV—Severe (marital separation) (4)

Axis V—Current GAF: 20
Highest GAF Past Year: 40

Advantages of the Multiaxial System. There are two major advantages to a multiaxial diagnosis. First, a multiaxial diagnosis provides more information than a standard single-category classification. As Helmchen (1980) points out, "The psychiatrist with human sensitivity for the particular individuality of each of his patients may hesitate to code a patient as a case in a system" (p. 43). To diagnose a patient by assigning him to one category oversimplifies the knowledge about the complexity of the patient. Although a multiaxial system may also oversimplify the issues concerning a patient, the axes permit the representation of several facets of the patient important to his treatment.

The second advantage of a multiaxial system is that it provides a framework for acquiring more complete and useful information about mental disorders. For instance, Rutter and his colleagues (1969; 1975) have suggested that, when diagnosing children, clinicians should code mental retardation on an axis separate from the clinical syndrome (psychiatric disorder). Rutter believed that this separation was important because clinicians tended to diagnose *either* the clinical syndrome *or* the mental retardation. As a result, the meaning of statistics on the prevalence of either mental retardation or the clinical syndromes is uncertain. Rutter, Shaffer, and Shepherd (1975) cited an example at a World Health Organization seminar on child psychiatry in which the clinicians were presented with the case of a mentally retarded, epileptic girl who was also psychotic. Rutter et al. found that even though all the psychiatrists were aware of the three conditions affecting this girl, most assigned only one diagnosis, and the choice of the one diagnosis among the three possibilities varied among the psychiatrists. It is thought that with the multiaxial system, diagnostic reliability will increase. This, in fact, has been demonstrated.

DIAGNOSTIC CRITERIA IN THE DSM-III. The final innovative feature associated with the DSM-III and DSM-III-R is the use of **diagnostic criteria.** To understand the importance of this innovation, consider the following definition for "Hysterical Personality" that was presented in the DSM-II.

> These behavior patterns are characterized by excitability, emotional instability, over-reactivity, and self-dramatization. This self-dramatization is always attention-seeking and often seductive, whether or not the patient is aware of its purpose. These personalities are also immature, self-centered, often vain, and usually dependent on others (APA, 1968, p. 43).

Notice that this prose definition contains nine separate symptoms: excitable, overreactive, self-dramatizing, attention-seeking, seductive, immature, self-centered, vain, and dependent. In the prose definition, the DSM-II does not specify how many or which of the symptoms together would be sufficient for diagnosing hysterical personality. For instance, if the patient only had one of these symptoms, seductiveness, would that be sufficient in order to say that she (the diagnosis is most often made with women) had a hysterical personality? What if the patient had all nine symptoms, or only three of the nine symptoms? These questions are not easily answered, even by experts who have had a great deal of experience working with persons who have hysterical personalities.

Now consider the diagnostic criteria for histrionic personality disorder listed in the DSM-III-R:

**DSM-III-R
Diagnostic Criteria for
Histrionic Personality
Disorder**

A pervasive pattern of excessive emotionality and attention-seeking, beginning by early adulthood and present in a variety of contexts, as indicated by at least *four* of the following:

1) constantly seeks or demands reassurance, approval, or praise

2) is inappropriately sexually seductive in appearance or behavior

3) is overly concerned with physical attractiveness

4) expresses emotion with inappropriate exaggeration, e.g., embraces casual acquaintances with excessive ardor, uncontrollable sobbing on minor sentimental occasions, has temper tantrums

5) is uncomfortable in situations in which he or she is not the center of attention

6) displays rapidly shifting and shallow expression of emotions

7) is self-centered, actions being directed toward obtaining immediate satisfaction; has no tolerance for the frustration of delayed gratification

8) has a style of speech that is excessively impressionistic and lacking in detail, e.g., when asked to describe mother, can be no more specific than, "She was a beautiful person."

This DSM-III-R definition lists a number of symptoms and states explicitly how many and which symptoms are necessary.

As mentioned, the main reason for developing diagnostic criteria in the DSM-III was to improve reliability. A number of research studies have demonstrated that diagnostic reliability of earlier classifications, including the DSM-I and DSM-II, was less than optimal. For instance, in a direct study of diagnostic reliability, Ash (1949) had three psychiatrists independently interview and diagnose a sample of patients. In only 20 percent of the cases did all three psychiatrists give the same diagnosis. Ash concluded that this level of diagnostic agreement among clinicians was less than optimal.

Ash's study had a number of serious methodological problems (Matarazzo, 1978). Nonetheless, most reviewers of the subsequent studies concerning diagnostic reliability agreed with Ash that this aspect of psychiatric classification needed to be improved. For instance, Spitzer and Fleiss (1974) argued that the first two editions of the DSM had problems with reliability because of their vague and poorly specified definitions of categories.

Research using the DSM-III has shown that the level of diagnostic reliability of the DSM-III has increased relative to the DSM-II (APA, 1980). This increase has been attributed to the use of the relatively explicit diagnostic criteria in the DSM-III.

ICD-9. The **ICD-9** (International Classification of Disease, ninth edition) is the official classification of the World Health Organization covering all diseases and disorders, both physical and mental (World Health Organization, 1978). Because the ICD-9 is a classification of all forms of diseases recognized in medicine, all hospitals in the United States are required to submit patient diagnoses using the ICD codes. These codes are four-digit numbers such as 295.1. To help the clinician who works in an inpatient setting, the DSM-III lists the ICD code associated with each diagnosis beside the name of the category. However, the names associated with the same digit code can vary somewhat from one classification to another.

For instance, "Disorganized Schizophrenia," classified as 295.1x in the DSM-III-R, has a somewhat different definition from the ICD-9's definition of 295.1, "Hebephrenic schizophrenia." Roughly, though, the number codes in these two documents do match up. The important point to remember is that as long as the clinician specifies the *four-digit code* (that is, the ICD number) in a diagnosis, she has satisfied the hospital requirement of using the ICD system.

SPECIFIC DSM-III-R CHANGES. As noted earlier, the DSM-III-R (the R means "revised") is structurally the same as the DSM-III, with the addition of one new category, sleep disorders, and some conceptual distinctions made in the multiaxial system, particularly between Axes I and II, with refinements of Axes IV and V. A new scale has been added to Axis V. The most significant changes, however, are in the specific diagnostic criteria that are used to define the categories, with notable alterations in the categories of psychoactive substance use, schizophrenia, mood disorders, anxiety disorders, and personality disorders. For example, the definitions of the personality disorder categories are almost totally new in order to increase the clarity with which these categories are defined (APA, 1987).

NURSING DIAGNOSIS

Ever since Florence Nightingale and her staff of nurses made diagnoses related to nutritional deficits and unsanitary conditions during the Crimean War, nurses have worked to develop a classification system that would define, organize, and describe the specific concerns of the nurse in patient care. Not until the late 1950s, however, did nurses begin to formally classify these concepts. Abdellah's classification of 21 nursing problems in *Patient-Centered Approaches to Nursing* was one of the earliest nursing classification systems aimed at describing patient-centered approaches for use by nurse educators, practitioners, and administrators (Abdellah et al., 1960). This list of problems, shown in Table 3-1, has become an important resource for the conceptualizing of nursing theory.

In 1973 an intensive and continuing effort began to provide a national forum for the classification of nursing diagnoses with the formation of the National Conference Group on Classification of Nursing Diagnoses. Nursing diagnoses have been defined most often as "actual or potential health problems which nurses, by virtue of their education and experience, are capable and licensed to treat" (Gordon, 1976). The purpose of the first conference on nursing diagnosis was to "identify nursing functions and to establish a classification system suitable for computerization" (Carpenito, p. 5, 1987). In the early stages, the inductive-reasoning approach within small groups was used to generate nursing diagnoses and participants voted to approve or disapprove them (Gebbie, 1976). From this organization grew the North American Nursing Diagnosis Association (NANDA) which has convened seven times since 1973 and has approved a total of 50 nursing diagnoses for testing. Currently, nursing diagnoses must be accompanied

by validating research and clinical data in order to be considered at subsequent conferences for addition to the list.

TABLE 3—1 List of 21 nursing problems

---

1. To maintain good hygiene and physical comfort.

2. To promote optimal activity; exercise, rest, and sleep.

3. To promote safety through prevention of accident, injury, or other trauma and through the prevention of the spread of infection.

4. To maintain good body mechanics and prevent and correct deformities.

5. To facilitate the maintenance of a supply of oxygen to all body cells.

6. To facilitate the maintenance of nutrition of all body cells.

7. To facilitate the maintenance of elimination.

8. To facilitate the maintenance of fluid and electrolyte balance.

9. To recognize the physiological responses of the body to disease conditions—pathological, physiological, and compensatory.

10. To facilitate the maintenance of regulatory mechanisms and functions.

11. To facilitate the maintenance of sensory function.

12. To identify and accept positive and negative expressions, feelings, and reactions.

13. To identify and accept the interrelatedness of emotions and organic illness.

14. To facilitate the maintenance of effective verbal and nonverbal communication.

15. To promote the development of productive interpersonal relationships.

16. To facilitate progress toward achievement of personal spiritual goals.

17. To create and/or maintain a therapeutic environment.

18. To facilitate awareness of self as an individual with varying physical, emotional, and developmental needs.

19. To accept the optimum possible goals in the light of limitations, physical and emotional.

20. To use community resources as an aid in resolving problems arising from illness.

21. To understand the role of social problems as influencing factors in the cause of illness.

Source: Abdellah, F. G., Beland, I., Martin, A., Matheney, R. (1960) Patient-centered approaches to nursing. New York: Macmillan Co. pp. 16–17.

The seventh National Conference General Assembly which convened in April, 1986, also approved the Nursing Diagnosis Taxonomy I, a working document providing a beginning classification framework. The taxonomy is based on nine human response patterns: exchanging, communicating, relating, valuing, choosing, moving, perceiving, knowing, and feeling. The taxonomy appears in Table 3-2.

The North American Nursing Diagnosis Association is the official body that develops and publishes information about nursing diagnoses. Its classificatory system provides a language unique to the profession of nursing (Kim, 1982; 1984; 1986).

As defined by NANDA, a nursing diagnosis is composed of: 1) definition; 2) major defining characteristics and minor defining characteristics (if relevant), and 3) related factors. The list of ninty-eight nursing diagnostic categories approved in June, 1988 under Taxonomy I Revised (NANDA, 1987) appear in Table 3-3.

TABLE 3—2   NANDA taxonomy I

---

1. Exchanging. A human response pattern involving mutual giving and receiving.

2. Communicating. A human response pattern involving sending messages.

3. Relating. A human response pattern involving establishing bonds.

4. Valuing. A human response pattern involving the assigning of relative worth.

5. Choosing. A human response pattern involving the selection of alternatives.

6. Moving. A human response pattern involving activity.

7. Perceiving. A human response pattern involving the reception of information.

8. Knowing. A human response pattern involving the meaning associated with information.

9. Feeling. A human response pattern involving the subjective awareness of information.

Source: North American Nursing Diagnosis Association (1987). *Taxonomy I with complete diagnoses.* St. Louis, Mo.: NANDA.

TABLE 3—3   NANDA approved nursing diagnostic categories (June, 1988)

Pattern 1: Exchanging

1.1.2.1	Altered Nutrition: More than body requirements
1.1.2.2	Altered Nutrition: Less than body requirements
1.1.2.3	Altered Nutrition: Potential for more than body requirements
1.2.1.1	Potential for Infection
1.2.2.1	Potential Altered Body Temperature
**1.2.2.2	Hypothermia
1.2.2.3	Hyperthermia
1.2.2.4	Ineffective Thermoregulation
*1.2.3.1	Dysreflexia
1.3.1.1	Constipation
*1.3.1.1.1	Perceived Constipation
*1.3.1.1.2	Colonic Constipation
1.3.1.2	Diarrhea
1.3.1.3	Bowel Incontinence
1.3.2	Altered Patterns of Urinary Elimination
1.3.2.1.1	Stress Incontinence
1.3.2.1.2	Reflex Incontinence
1.3.2.1.3	Urge Incontinence
1.3.2.1.4	Functional Incontinence
1.3.2.1.5	Total Incontinence
1.3.2.2	Urinary Retention
1.4.1.1	Altered (Specify Type) Tissue Perfusion (Renal, cerebral, cardiopulmonary, gastrointestinal, peripheral)
1.4.1.2.1	Fluid Volume Excess
1.4.1.2.2.1	Fluid Volume Deficit (1)
1.4.1.2.2.1	Fluid Volume Deficit (2)
1.4.1.2.2.2	Potential Fluid Volume Deficit
1.4.2.1	Decreased Cardiac Output
1.5.1.1	Impaired Gas Exchange
1.5.1.2	Ineffective Airway Clearance
1.5.1.3	Ineffective Breathing Pattern
1.6.1	Potential for Injury
1.6.1.1	Potential for Suffocation
1.6.1.2	Potential for Poisoning
1.6.1.3	Potential for Trauma
*1.6.1.4	Potential for Aspiration

TABLE 3–3 (continued)

*1.6.1.5	Potential for Disuse Syndrome		6.4.2	Altered Health Maintenance
1.6.2.1	Impaired Tissue Integrity		6.5.1	Feeding Self Care Deficit
1.6.2.1.1	Altered Oral Mucous Membrane		6.5.1.1	Impaired Swallowing
1.6.2.1.2.1	Impaired Skin Integrity		*6.5.1.2	Ineffective Breastfeeding
1.6.2.1.2.2	Potential Impaired Skin Integrity		6.5.2	Bathing/Hygiene Self Care Deficit

Pattern 2: Communicating

2.1.1.1   Impaired Verbal Communication

Pattern 3: Relating

3.1.1   Impaired Social Interaction
3.1.2   Social Isolation
3.2.1   Altered Role Performance
3.2.1.1.1 Altered Parenting
3.2.1.1.2 Potential Altered Parenting
3.2.1.2.1 Sexual Dysfunction
3.2.2   Altered Family Processes
*3.2.3.1   Parental Role Conflict
3.3   Altered Sexuality Patterns

Pattern 4: Valuing

4.1.1   Spiritual Distress (distress of the human spirit)

Pattern 5: Choosing

5.1.1.1   Ineffective Individual Coping
5.1.1.1.1 Impaired Adjustment
*5.1.1.1.2 Defensive Coping
*5.1.1.1.3 Ineffective Denial
5.1.2.1.1 Ineffective Family Coping: Disabling
5.1.2.1.2 Ineffective Family Coping: Compromised
5.1.2.2   Family Coping: Potential for Growth
5.2.1.1   Noncompliance (Specify)
*5.3.1.1   Decisional Conflict (Specify)
*5.4   Health Seeking Behaviors (Specify)

Pattern 6: Moving

6.1.1.1   Impaired Physical Mobility
6.1.1.2   Activity Intolerance
*6.1.1.2.1 Fatigue
6.1.1.3   Potential Activity Intolerance
6.2.1   Sleep Pattern Disturbance
6.3.1.1   Diversional Activity Deficit
6.4.1.1   Impaired Home Maintenance Management

6.5.3   Dressing/Grooming Self Care Deficit
6.5.4   Toileting Self Care Deficit
6.6   Altered Growth and Development

Pattern 7: Perceiving

7.1.1   Body Image Disturbance
**7.1.2   Self Esteem Disturbance
*7.1.2.1   Chronic Low Self Esteem
*7.1.2.2   Situational Low Self Esteem
7.1.3   Personal Identify Disturbance
7.2   Sensory/Perceptual Alterations (Specify) (Visual, auditory, kinesthetic, gustatory, tactile, olfactory)
7.2.1.1   Unilateral Neglect
7.3.1   Hopelessness
7.3.2   Powerlessness

Pattern 8: Knowing

8.1.1   Knowledge Deficit (Specify)
8.3   Altered Thought Processes

Pattern 9: Feeling

9.1.1   Pain
9.1.1.1   Chronic Pain
9.2.1.1   Dysfunctional Grieving
9.2.1.2   Anticipatory Grieving
9.2.2   Potential for Violence: Self-directed or directed at others
9.2.3   Post-Trauma Response
9.2.3.1   Rape-Trauma Syndrome
9.2.3.1.1 Rape-Trauma Syndrome: Compound Reaction
9.2.3.1.2 Rape-Trauma Syndrome: Silent Reaction
9.3.1   Anxiety
9.3.2   Fear

*New diagnostic categories approved 1988
**Revised diagnostic categories approved 1988
Source: North American Nursing Diagnosis Association. (1988) *Nursing Diagnosis Newsletter.* Vol. 15, No. 1.

Following is an example of a NANDA approved nursing diagnosis, anxiety, with its definition, major defining characteristics, and related factors:

9.2.1 ANXIETY

A vague uneasy feeling whose source is often nonspecific or unknown to the individual.

MAJOR DEFINING CHARACTERISTICS

Subjective: increased tension; apprehension; painful and persistent increased helplessness; uncertainty; fearful; scared; regretful; over-excited; rattled; distressed; jittery; feelings of inadequacy; shakiness; fear of unspecific consequences; expressed concerns re change in life events; worried; anxious.

Objective: *sympathetic stimulation—cardiovascular excitation, superficial vasoconstriction, pupil dilation; restlessness; insomnia; glancing about; poor eye contact; trembling/hand tremors; extraneous movement (foot shuffling, hand/arm movements); facial tension; voice quivering; focus "self"; increased wariness; increased perspiration.

RELATED FACTORS

Unconscious conflict about essential values/goals of life; threat to self-concept; threat of death; threat to or change in health status; threat to or change in role functioning; threat to or change in environment; threat to or change in interaction patterns; situational/maturational crises; interpersonal transmission/contagion; unmet needs (NANDA, 1987, p. 107).

*Critical defining characteristic

USING NURSING DIAGNOSIS IN MENTAL HEALTH/PSYCHIATRIC NURSING. The Standards of Psychiatric Mental Health Nursing (ANA, 1982) acknowledges both the DSM-III-R and NANDA systems in Standard III: "Diagnosis: The nurse utilizes nursing diagnoses and/or standard classification of mental disorders to express conclusions supported by recorded assessment data and current scientific premises" (p. 4).

There has been much debate among psychiatric mental health nurses as to which classification system (or for that matter, whether either of the two classification systems) provides the best language for nurses working with psychiatric mental health patients. Although the DSM-III-R has been criticized for a lack of credibility and tendency to stigmatize patients (as discussed later in this chapter), many psychiatric mental health nurses have come to believe, like Wilson and Skodol (1988), that the DSM-III-R is crucial to the advance of psychiatric research and interdisciplinary communication and collaboration. Others feel that the NANDA system, or a NANDA-based system with additional diagnoses formulated as needed, should be the primary classification source because it identifies those diagnoses which are unique to nursing. It is interesting to note that in the current taxonomy, while the majority of the accepted diagnoses currently relate to physical function or dysfunction, 7 of the 9 pattern categories in Taxonomy I relate to patient problems that are cognitive or psychosocial and emotional rather than physical in nature—communicating, relating, valuing, choosing, perceiving, knowing, and feeling. Taxonomy I leaves room for further development of nursing diagnoses which may be more pertinent to the psychiatric mental health nurse.

Clearly there is a need to be familiar with the language of both the DSM-III-R and nursing diagnosis terminology, and it is our belief that psychiatric mental health nurses must be able to communicate clearly with both. In the nonpsychiatric setting the nurse must be able to formulate nursing diagnoses no matter what the primary health care need of the patient may be. And in the psychiatric setting, the nurse will use nursing diagnoses and DSM-III-R diagnoses to help formulate patient care strategies; she must be familiar with and competent at communicating the DSM-III-R diagnoses to confer with the other involved health care professionals, but the nursing diagnosis will allow the nurse to take the holistic view of the patient and address his or her total health care needs (ANA, 1980).

Still, many nurses have found this two-tiered system lacking, and there have been several proposed solutions. In 1984, the Executive Committee of the Division and Council of Specialists in Psychiatric and Mental Health Nursing Practice of the American Nurses' Association authorized the creation of a task force to "develop a comprehensive working list of the phenomena of concern for psychiatric mental health nurses" (Loomis et al. p. 16, 1987). The work of this task force up to now has focused on identifying a classification system based on "human responses to actual or potential health problems" on individual, interpersonal/family, and community/environment levels. The group has so far developed a classification system based on seven major human response patterns on the individual level (Loomis et al., 1987).

Other nurses have proposed the addition of a sixth, nursing-oriented axis to the DSM-III-R. One proposal suggests that a sixth axis focus on the abilities of the patient to handle adequately nutrition, solitude, grooming activities, and elimination (Morrison et al., 1985).

Coler and Vincent (1987) have developed an axial system for prioritizing nursing diagnoses that is adapted from the five axes of the DSM-III. Their work underscores the similarities in the historical development of both the DSM and nursing diagnosis and details the need for a stable diagnostic process in nursing which would allow standardization and computerization of data for further research and reliability testing.

THE PROS AND CONS OF PSYCHIATRIC CLASSIFICATION

CRITICISMS OF PSYCHIATRIC CLASSIFICATION

The criticisms of psychiatric classification fall into three categories: 1) reliability, 2) the medical model, and 3) labeling.

The first of these, reliability, concerns the variability with which mental health professionals use diagnostic terms. This issue was discussed on pages 53–54. The other two criticisms concern the social context of diagnosis, and will be discussed below.

MEDICAL MODEL. Psychiatric classification's association with the **medical model** is troubling to some critics of the classification system. In the mental health field, the people with whom we deal are usually called "patients." Their care is paid for by "health insurance." When these individuals come to see us, we first attempt to ascertain their "symptoms," assign a "diagnosis," and then choose the best "treatment." Some patients are given "medications" as part of their "therapy" while others may be "hospitalized" and receive a variety of treatments. The professional group that is most popularly associated with the care of these individuals are psychiatrists, that is, "physicians" who have specialized in the mental disorders.

Notice that all of the words inside the quotation marks in the preceding paragraph refer to a medical perspective. Basically, the medical model rests on the assumption, similar to the assertion by Geisinger more than a century ago, that all mental disorders are diseases. It is important to note, however, that the medical model is *not* the only model of behavioral deviance. For instance, the theories of Freud and his

followers are psychological theories that emphasize issues occurring in the minds of individuals as well as in their interpersonal relations. Another model of abnormal behavior that has been popular among psychologists is a behavioral model which focuses on the environmental events that shape and maintain deviant behaviors. An interesting, introductory discussion of the models of psychopathology can be found in Price (1971). (Also see Chapter 2 on Major Models of Behavior.)

The medical model has become an issue with regard to psychiatric classification because classification and diagnosis are usually seen as part of the medical perspective of abnormal behavior. Nonphysicians, particularly psychologists, have often attacked the medical model as an unsubstantiated theory of mental disorders and as an inadequate basis for the political dominance of psychiatry among mental health professionals.

As discussed in Chapter 1, Thomas Szasz (1961) has been a major critic of the medical model and his criticisms have often extended to attacks on classification as a central part of the medical model. Szasz believes that most, if not all, mental disorders are better viewed as "problems in living" rather than as behavioral or medical representations of disease. He believes that classification systems are used by clinicians to legitimize their power over individuals who are judged as having mental disorders.

"In the final analysis, whether we classify behaviors that in some way, however obscure or remote, resemble bodily diseases but are in fact not such diseases as "illnesses" or as "nonillnesses," has, of course, the most profound implications not only for the individuals directly affected, but for the whole social and political system which authenticates the classification" (Szasz, 1974, p. 34).

In addition to the issue of whether all mental disorders are diseases, there is another important controversy related to the medical model. This is the interprofessional rivalry that exists in the mental health field. The mental health profession includes persons trained in a number of fields, such as psychiatry (medicine), psychology, counseling (education), social work, nursing, occupational therapy, religion, and recreational therapy. Of these professions, psychiatry is dominant. Psychiatrists generally hold the highest position of authority in any mental health setting; they are usually paid more than other professionals; and they are often the only caregivers whose charges will be accepted by insurance companies. These practices do vary to a significant degree among states. Nonphysicians in the mental health field have been vocal in their attacks on the medical model since the medical model has often been promoted as the reason for physician dominance.

LABELING. The third and final criticism of psychiatric classification is that it results in **labeling.** This criticism expresses the concern that since many psychiatric diagnoses have stigmatizing connotations, they may act as self-fulfilling prophecies that foster deviant behaviors in individuals. Stigmatizing labels can also foster negative behaviors and attitudes among staff and others toward the patient and are also likely to follow the patient into all other areas of his life: marriage, employment, and social activities.

David Rosenhan (1973) demonstrated the problem of labeling in his paper, "On Being Sane in Insane Places." In this study eight normal volunteers of different backgrounds (housewife, lawyer, dentist, and so forth) were directed by Rosenhan to seek admission to twelve different psychiatric inpatient facilities. In the initial interview, all told the truth about themselves with two exceptions. They used fictitious names, and they all reported that they heard the words "thud", "hollow," or "empty" being repeated even though no one was around them. This particular auditory hallucination was chosen because Rosenhan could not find any recorded instance of this hallucination occurring in an actual patient. Despite the fact that these individuals were all normal (except for the manufactured hallucination), all were admitted. In eleven of the twelve admissions, the individuals were diagnosed as schizophrenic. All twelve were discharged with a diagnosis of "schizophrenia in remission".

Once in the hospital, the pseudopatients noted a number of things about their hospitalization. They found that many of their fellow patients recognized that they did not belong there while none of the staff did. Moreover, the pseudopatients felt that they were dealt with in ways determined by the staff's view that they were schizophrenic, despite their normal behavior. For instance, one of the pseudopatients said "Hello" to each of the staff members he saw each day, and kept a log of the responses to him. He was responded to by staff only 40 percent of the time. This same person, a professor, later said "Hello" to people he met as he walked around his campus and found that greetings were returned by 95 percent of those he spoke to. To this pseudopatient, it seemed that he was a nonperson when he was a psychiatric patient.

The dehumanizing effect of being in the hospital was noted by all the pseudopatients. For example, one man was bored while confined to his ward since he had nothing to read, so he started pacing. A nurse approached him and asked him if he was anxious, an attribution related to the nurse's view that this man was schizophrenic. If she thought he was normal, she may have attributed his pacing to boredom.

In another incident, a male pseudopatient sitting in his unit noticed a nurse near him who had partially unbuttoned her blouse and was adjusting her bra strap. This occurred in the open, on a unit of men. Apparently the nurse's assumption was that she was effectively alone, that none of these men, likely to be in their own world, would notice her, feel she was being provocative, and respond accordingly.

The Rosenhan article stimulated a major controversy. After it was published in *Science,* a series of letters followed, debating its importance. One issue of the *Journal of Abnormal Psychology* focused on the question of diagnostic validity raised by the article (see Weiner, 1975; Spitzer, 1975; Farber, 1975). Most of the controversy was directed at the fact that normal individuals were admitted with diagnoses of schizophrenia. The dehumanizing aspect of being a psychiatric patient was ignored by all commentators.

The most important point of the labeling criticism is that it suggests that the process of diagnosis, by its nature, will always have certain negative effects. In the Rosenhan article, the negative effect of depersonalization associated with being placed on a psychiatric ward was emphasized. The negative effect of having a diagnosis, however, is not limited to that occurring in inpatient hospitalization. Suppose, for example, that a college freshman who is lonely and depressed as a result of being away from home seeks counseling. A psychologist diagnoses the young man as depressed and recommends individual therapy. The implicit message to the individual is that he has a serious problem, one that requires professional care. However, other issues involved in this college freshman's efforts to seek counseling include: 1) being referred to the least skilled professional in the agency because his problem is not considered to be as severe as those of others; 2) substituting the label "depression" for "homesickness" which can lead to confusion and misunderstanding of incidents; and 3) a question about the utility of diagnoses: are they used to guide and direct mental health treatment or do they only create more problems than they resolve?

SUPPORT FOR PSYCHIATRIC CLASSIFICATION

Because the labeling criticism charges that making a diagnosis can have a negative effect, it is important to understand the positive aspects of psychiatric classification.

A good classification system can serve five purposes. First, it provides the nomenclature necessary for communication among professionals working in the field. An official classification system is also utilized by medical insurance companies to determine reimbursement schedules. **DRGs (diagnostic-related groups)** are used by insurance companies to determine payment schedules and lengths of stay for patients with specified diagnoses. Thus the economic implications of psychiatric diagnoses for patients and their families can be significant.

Second, classification furnishes a basis for information retrieval. There is a saying in botany that the name of a plant is the key to its literature. If a clinician is told that her new patient has Huntington's chorea, the diagnosis can help the clinician know where to look for information about the disorder's symptoms and course, and the neurophysiological process involved in the progressive degeneration of the central nervous system characteristic of the disease.

Third, a classification system provides useful descriptive information about known diseases. If a nurse knows that her new patient has Huntington's chorea, she has a fair amount of general information about the patient: he has a movement disorder; he will show mild to moderate decrease in intellectual functioning; and he is likely to be depressed.

Fourth, a classification system provides a basis for making predictions about a patient's future. For instance, knowing a patient has Huntington's chorea means that the nurse also knows that he is likely to die within ten years of diagnosis (as do most patients with the disorder).

Fifth, a classification system provides basic concepts essential for developing a theory of psychopathology. The current knowledge about psychopathology is much like the knowledge physicians and surgeons in the 17th century had about medical disease. At that time, there was reasonably good understanding of gross anatomy and the beginnings of a science of physiology. However, as practitioners, most physicians and surgeons had only crude tools at their disposal, such as herbs, leeches, instruments of amputation, and so forth. Similarly, contemporary scientific knowledge about mental disorders is in its infancy. While much is known about gross neuroanatomy and neurophysiology, contemporary ideas about how neuroanatomy and neurophysiology are related to psychology and the interpersonal relationships of human beings are speculative at best. Thus it is important for researchers to be able to communicate about what *is* known to develop theories about what isn't. Creating a useful classification system is like drawing a map of a strange new land. Without the map, the exploration is mysterious and difficult; with the map, the explorer has a better idea of where to go and what to expect.

Case Study: Nonpsychiatric Setting to Psychiatric Setting

Renee is a 32-year-old female who, a short time ago, began practice as a certified public accountant. She was recently separated. She had lived an uneventful life with her husband and one son, age twelve. Renee was perceived by other professionals as ambitious, meticulous, a bit compulsive and, at times, somewhat suspicious. However, all of her associates viewed her as extremely competent and committed to excellence in her work.

Three months ago Renee reported to her office and started accusing the secretaries of trying to poison her by putting arsenic in her coffee. She also stated that her neighbor was having an affair with her estranged husband and that her colleagues and trusted friends were wooing her clients from her business. Renee's behavior interfered with her work, as she was preoccupied with securing food and drink for herself that was free of poisons, and so on. Her weight loss was becoming more obvious; interpersonal relationships with staff were limited; and at times Renee refused to see clients who depended on her services.

While in her office late one evening, Renee complained of a terrible migraine headache. (She was known to have a history of migraines.) The executive secretary took Renee to a nearby emergency room where she was treated for the migraine headache. A psychiatric consult was also ordered by the physician in the emergency room because of Renee's suspicious and uncooperative behaviors. The secretary notified Renee's estranged husband who willingly offered to care for their twelve-year-old son during the course of Renee's hospitalization.

Renee's history revealed that she had a long record of feeling rejected by her parents. Her history also revealed that she had grown up in an upper middle-class family. Her father was a successful businessman whose job necessitated that he be out of town for long periods of time. Renee's mother was a beautiful woman whose role was, as Renee recalled, to look pretty at parties and support her husband's career. However, the mother was an alcoholic and frequently took large quantities of prescription drugs, such as Valium and various sleeping pills. Renee and her mother kept this part of the mother's behavior a secret from the father. The long periods of unavailability, separation, and isolation from Renee, by both mother and father, left Renee feeling lonely and free to create imaginary playmates. She was always worried that her father would one day come home unexpectedly and find her mother intoxicated.

During the psychiatric interview, Renee stated that her formative years were unhappy ones. She remembered crying frequently; feeling insecure about her future; and worried that her father would blame and punish her for her mother's drinking. Renee also did not make friends easily. Currently, most of her time is spent working at her office or home.

DSM-III-R Diagnosis

Axis I: Schizophreniform disorder (295.40)

Axis II: Obsessive-compulsive personality disorder (301.40)

Axis III: Migraine headache

Axis IV: Psychosocial stressors: marital separation; single parent; declining professional productivity. Severity: 3, moderate to severe (acute events)

Axis V: Current GAF: 40
Highest GAF past year: 80

Nursing Diagnoses

*Ineffective individual coping
Impaired verbal communication
Ineffective family coping
Feed self-care deficit
*Social isolation
Altered thought processes

*Nursing diagnoses developed in care plan that follows.

Nursing Care Plan for Renee McAuley

Renee was hospitalized primarily because of her weight loss, dehydration, and recent food refusal. The Mental Health Unit at the hospital recently implemented the case management system of nursing care. A nurse from the unit, who would become Renee's nurse, went to the emergency room to meet Renee, and walked with her to the unit.

Nursing Diagnosis	Desired Outcome	Interventions	Rationale
1. Ineffective individual coping.	Renee will develop a trusting relationship with the nurse, as evidenced by a decrease in suspicious behavior.	The nurse will explain to Renee the reason for and purpose of hospitalization, and the perceived nature of the Nurse-Patient relationship.	Renee needs to know what to anticipate from hospitalization, the staff, and the nurse specifically assigned to her. This approach diminishes her feelings of suspiciousness, decreases anxiety, enhances her self respect and creates a sense that others care about her.
		Orient Renee to the unit; provide her with a schedule of activities; introduce her to staff, and explain treatment program and expectations.	Clarifies the treatment process; gives Renee an opportunity to ask questions and to be active in her treatment at the outset.
		Discuss with Renee her understanding of the problems she consistently experienced. Guide the interview so that nurse has information about Renee's 1) belief that food is poisoned, 2) thoughts about neighbors taking her husband, 3) migraine headaches and so forth.	These areas have been identified as frustrations/ conflicts in Renee's life that are causing extreme problems in occupation, family, and social relationships. Nurse needs to understand Renee's perspective about these conflicts. Provides data for more in-depth planning of nursing care.
		The Nurse might say, "Renee, would you describe your current situation?" Nurse will remain with Renee when (if) she refuses to talk and state: "Renee, I will be here with you for another 30 minutes I am here to listen and help you. Let me know how you think I can help."	Assists in establishing a bond/a commitment between nurse and Renee. Reassures Renee that nurse will not leave her because of her silence, etc. Provides assessment data for planning. Gives Renee an opportunity to ventilate her thoughts and feelings. (Nurse should observe verbal

Nursing Diagnosis	Desired Outcome	Interventions	Rationale
			response and nonverbal behaviors.) Ventilation can relieve anxiety, tension, and reduce the feeling of isolation and abandonment that Renee feels. Too, the nurse's presence (without verbalization) can decrease anxiety, and feelings of aloneness.
	Renee will discuss with nurse previous life problems and her approach to problem solving.	Nurse: "Renee, when you have had problems in the past how did you solve them? Can you discuss this with me?"	Previous behaviors and coping mechanisms can be determined from these data; nurse should explore data for patterns of problem-solving; assists nurse in determining Renee's strengths and weaknesses.
		Ask Renee about suicidal ideation, gesture, and if she has a plan for suicide. Observe.	Essential that nurse and treatment staff know if Renee is suicidal or potentially suicidal; safety is always a priority in treatment. Renee shows signs of depression, has history of loneliness and unhappiness. Place these data in Renee's record. Observe Renee.
		Support Renee as she reveals previous triumphs over difficult situations.	Reassures Renee that she, with help, can overcome her current problems; enhances Renee's self-esteem and self-concept; focuses on Renee's previous successes.
		Discuss with Renee her many achievements such as being a parent, having a career and having been married for numerous years.	The nurse can glean from conversation notions about coping, conflict resolution, feelings/thoughts of happiness, accomplishment, etc. Nurse observes verbal/ nonverbal communication as Renee explores these areas that provided a sense of personal achievement and gratification. Use these data when developing long-range treatment plans with Renee.

Nursing Diagnosis	Desired Outcome	Interventions	Rationale
		Discuss with Renee the onset of her migraine headaches and how she typically gets relief. Include: 1) frequency, 2) duration, 3) situation associated with migraine, 4) thoughts/feelings during time she has migraine, 5) antecedent signs/symptoms, etc.	Migraine headaches can be stress related. When Renee becomes more aware of her thoughts/feelings and stressors, she will increase her chances of "nipping in the bud" the possibility that headaches will occur. Enhances autonomy and self-control.
		Instruct Renee in learning relaxation techniques as a method of stress control.	Relaxation methods are one alternative in problem-solving when individual is not in direct control of a situation, and has little "empowerment".
	Renee will gain 7 pounds within a 30 day period.	Discuss with Renee her weight loss and the need to increase fluids	Do not argue, but present your concerns and plans in a matter-of-fact approach.
		Review with Renee the importance of her gaining weight. Elicit a commitment from Renee.	Knowledge and understanding facilitates patient's cooperation; enhances trust and self respect, etc.
		Ask Renee about measures she believes she could implement that would increase her food intake.	Renee's notions about her care are important and potentially instructive for the nurse; enhances self-care; diminishes feelings of dependency and keeps her actively involved in her treatment.
		Determine the foods Renee likes to eat, how she wishes to have them prepared, etc. Offer Renee a selection of packaged foods that she can prepare in microwave. Provide supply of bananas, oranges and other foods that require minimal handling by others.	Gives Renee a feeling of control; paranoia frequently occurs when person thinks she has no control over a situation. Decreases suspicious behavior and projection (a defense mechanism).
		Encourage Renee to get her own fluids (water from tap; coffee from urn; cola from machine) then open and drink them. Nurse might remain with Renee and support her.	As much as possible, allows Renee to be in control of her own situation. Nurse will be supportive and available to Renee. Nurse should record intake of food and drink.

Nursing Diagnosis	Desired Outcome	Interventions	Rationale
		Reassure Renee that no one will poison her—that she is safe.	Paranoid/suspicious patients find it difficult to experience psychological comfort; support will help develop trust; models positive interpersonal relations, etc.
2. Social isolation.	Renee will evaluate her limited contact with people and determine how she can initiate and maintain relationships.	Identify Renee's feelings that are associated with social isolation.	Validation of feelings of social isolation are useful as it implies that Renee is desirous of increased interpersonal contact; patients sometimes feel powerless to address their social isolation.
		Discuss with Renee the factors/events that occurred to cause the social isolation and its consequences.	Renee's understanding of the relationship between behavior and consequences is useful for future behavior changes.
		Assist Renee in identifying the "lost relationships" that have occurred and then focus on how to "develop new satisfying relationships." Point out to Renee that she is participating in a relationship with the nurse. Compliment her (if deserving of the comment).	Renee can develop insight into how losses create loneliness (she has a history of troubled relationships); it is reassuring for her to know that she can (and will) be supported as she reaches out to initiate new friendships.
		Provide information about community support groups such as "Parents Without Partners" "Adult Children of Alcoholic Parents," etc.	Community self-help groups can potentially provide therapeutic benefits such as: 1) hope; 2) universality; 3) enhancement of social skills; 4) imparting knowledge about self, others, etc. All of these curative factors are useful in diminishing social isolation.
		Offer to assist Renee in making the contacts with self-help groups.	Assisting Renee provides support without fostering dependency; allows Renee to be in control.

Nursing Diagnosis	Desired Outcome	Interventions	Rationale
		Assist Renee in the development of a work schedule that will decrease the demands on her time, and feelings of being overwhelmed, tired, angry, etc.; assist Renee in developing an approach to work, parenting, etc. that is more self-satisfying.	Gives Renee permission to not be so busy; recognizes and acknowledges her feelings, without rejecting or judging her. Renee can, over time, experience a positive self-concept that is not directly dependent on work and the reflected appraisals of others.
		Teach Renee ego observing behaviors; that is, teach Renee how to observe and monitor her own behaviors. Instruct Renee in becoming involved in "self-correcting" her behaviors.	Assists Renee in becoming comfortable with her own feelings and making decisions based on her feelings and self evaluation of her overall level of functioning; increases autonomy, self-esteem, etc. and confidence.
		Support her when she acknowledges: "I am tired" or "I don't want any more responsibilities at the moment."	Women frequently feel compelled to "overfunction." Nurse can serve as a role model for Renee.

The nurse, in planning for Renee's discharge, contacted Mental Health, Inc., a private non-profit community based facility, to assist in arranging continuous care for Renee. The nurse will accompany Renee to the agency, and introduce her to a new case manager at that agency.

SUMMARY

The classification of psychopathology can be traced back to the Greeks. In their consideration of people who had mental disorders, the Greeks introduced a number of terms, some of which are still used today. Later, during the early 1800s, a French physician named Bayle demonstrated through autopsies that a number of patients who had become demented had marked changes in their brains. This was the first instance in which a mental disorder was shown to be associated with changes in the brain. At the end of the 1800s, Emil Kraepelin compiled a classification system based on the tables of contents of his textbooks on psychopathology. While Kraepelin believed that some mental disorders were associated with brain pathology, he also advocated careful analysis of

behavior. Finally, he introduced the important diagnoses of manic-depressive insanity (bipolar disorder) and dementia praecox (schizophrenia).

The *Diagnostic and Statistical Manual of Mental Disorders* (DSM-I) was introduced and adopted by the American Psychiatric Association in 1952. It has been revised a number of times; its most recent edition is the DSM-III-R (revised). The *International Classification of Diseases* (ICD-6) incorporated mental disorders in 1951; this classification is the official system of the World Health Organization. Hospitals in the United States today use the numerical code of diagnosis from the ICD-9.

Nursing diagnosis provides another essential classification system for psychiatric mental health nurses, one which relies on a unique body of knowledge pertaining directly to nursing. Psychiatric mental health nurses need to be able to work with both systems in order to carry out effective strategies for patient care in both psychiatric and nonpsychiatric settings.

There are pros and cons to classifying mental disorders. Critics of classification point to the medical model which assumes that all mental disorders are diseases. They also cite the problem involved in labeling patients, since many psychiatric classifications stigmatize and dehumanize patients. Supporters of psychiatric classification claim that a good system serves five main purposes: 1) it provides the nomenclature necessary for communication; 2) it furnishes a basis for information retrieval; 3) it is useful for description; 4) it provides a basis for making predictions; and 5) it provides the basic concepts for developing theories of psychopathology.

KEY TERMS

classification

dementia

dementia paralytica

manic-depressive insanity

dementia praecox

paresis

psychotherapy

DSM-I

ICD-6

ICD-8

DSM-II

DSM-III

DSM-IIIR

multiaxial system

Axis I—Clinical syndrome

Axis II— Developmental disorders and personality disorders

Axis III—Physical disorders and conditions

Axis IV—Severity of psychosocial stressors

Axis V—Global assessment of functioning

diagnostic criteria

ICD-9

nursing diagnosis

Nursing Diagnosis Taxonomy I

medical model

labeling

DRGs (diagnostic-related groups)

STUDY QUESTIONS

1. Discuss the role of Kraepelin in the development of psychiatric classification.

2. Discuss the development of the DSM and ICD classifications. What is the difference between the two?

3. Define the multiaxial system of diagnosis and name the five axes of the DSM-III system.

4. What is nursing diagnosis, and how does it work?

5. Why should nurses working in psychiatric/mental health care settings be familiar with both DSM-III-R and nursing diagnosis classification systems?

6. Discuss the pros and cons of psychiatric classification. Refer to the medical model and labeling, and the five main purposes of classification.

REFERENCES

Abdellah, F., Martin, A., Beland, I., & Mathevey, R. (1960). *Patient-centered approaches to nursing.* New York: MacMillan.

American Nurses' Association (1980). *Nursing: A social policy statement.* Kansas City: The American Nurses Association.

American Nurses' Association (1982). *Standards of psychiatric and mental health nursing practice.* Kansas City: The American Nurses' Association.

American Psychiatric Association (1933). Notes and comment: Revised classified nomenclature of mental disorders. *American Journal of Psychiatry, 90,* 1369–1376.

American Psychiatric Association (1952). *Diagnostic and statistical manual of mental disorders* (1st ed.) Washington, D.C.: Author.

American Psychiatric Association (1968). *Diagnostic and statistical manual of mental disorders* (2nd ed.) Washington, D.C.: Author.

American Psychiatric Association (1980). *Diagnostic and statistical manual of mental disorders* (3rd ed.) Washington, D.C.: Author.

American Psychiatric Association (1987). *Diagnostic and statistical manual of mental disorders* (3rd ed., revised). Washington, D.C.: Author.

Ash, P. (1949). The reliability of psychiatric diagnosis. Journal of Abnormal and Social Psychology, 70, 361–364.

Boisen, A. (1938). Types of dementia praecox: A study on psychiatric classification. *Psychiatry, 1,* 233–236.

Carpenito, L. J. (1987). *Nursing diagnosis: Application to clinical practice* (2nd ed.) Philadelphia: J. B. Lippincott.

Carson, R. C., Butcher, J., & Coleman, J. C. (1988) *Abnormal psychology and modern life.* Glenview: Scott, Foresman.

Coler, M. S., & Vincent, K. G. (1987). Coded nursing diagnoses on axes: a prioritized, computer-ready diagnostic system for psychiatric mental health nurses. *Archives of Psychiatric Nursing, I,* No. 2, 125–131.

Farber, I. E. (1975). Sane and insane: Constructions and misconstructions. *Journal of Abnormal Psychology, 84,* 589–620.

Gebbie, K. M. (Ed.) (1976). *Classification of nursing diagnoses. Summary of the Second National Conference.* St. Louis: Clearinghouse, National Group for Classification of Nursing Diagnoses.

Gordon, M. (1976). Nursing diagnosis and the diagnostic process. *American Journal of Nursing, 76,* 1298–1300.

Helmchen, H. (1980). Multiaxial systems of classification. *Acta Psychiatrica Scandinavica, 61,* 43–55.

Hurt, H. M. (1881). A plea for systematic therapeutical, clinical and statistical study. *Journal of Insanity, 38,* 16–31.

Kahn, E. (1959). The Emil Kraepelin memorial lecture. In D. Pasamanick (Ed.), *Epidemiology of mental disorders.* Washington, D.C.: American Association for the Advancement of Science.

Kim, M. J. (1986). Nursing diagnoses: A Janus view. In Mary Hurley (Ed.), *Classification of nursing diagnoses.* St. Louis: C. V. Mosby.

Kim, M. J., McFarland, G. K., & McLane, A. M. (Eds.) (1984). *Classification of nursing diagnoses. Proceedings of the Fifth National Conference.* St. Louis: C. V. Mosby.

Kim, M. J., & Moritz, D. A. (Eds.) (1982). *Classification of nursing diagnoses. Proceedings of the Third and Fourth National Conferences.* New York: McGraw-Hill.

Kramer, M. (1968). Introduction: The historical background of ICD-8. In American Psychiatric Association, *Diagnostic and statistical manual of mental disorders* (2nd ed.). Washington, D.C.: Author.

Lewis, E. P. (1975). The stuff of which nursing is made. *Nursing Outlook, 23,* 89.

Loomis, M. E., O'Toole, A. W., Brown, M. S., Pothier, P., West, P, & Wilson, H. S. (1987). Development of a classification system for psychiatric/mental health: individual response class. *Archives of Psychiatric Nursing, 1,* No. 1, 16–24.

McHugh, P. R., & Folstein, M. F. (1986). Organic mental disorders. In J. O. Cavenar (Ed.), *Psychiatry* (revised). Philadelphia: J. B. Lippincott Company.

Matarazzo, J. D. (1978). The interview: Its reliability and validity in psychiatric diagnosis. In B. B. Wolman (Ed.), *Clinical diagnosis of mental disorders: A handbook.* New York: Plenum Press.

Menninger, K. (1963). *The vital balance.* New York: Viking Press.

Morrison, E., Fisher, L. Y., Wilson, H. S., et al. (1985). NSGAE: Nursing adaptation evaluation . . . A proposed Axis VI of DSM-III. *Journal of Psychosocial Nursing & Mental Health Services 23* (8): 10–13.

North American Nursing Diagnosis Association (1987). *Taxonomy I with complete diagnoses.* St. Louis, Mo.: North American Nursing Diagnosis Association.

Price, R. H. (1971). *Abnormal behavior: Perspectives in conflict.* New York: Holt, Rinehart and Winston.

Raines, C. N. (1952). Forward. In American Psychiatric Association, *Diagnostic and statistical manual of mental disorders* (1st ed.). Washington, D. C.: Author.

Rosenhan, D. L. (1973). On being sane in insane places. *Science, 179,* 250–258.

Rutter, M., Lebovici, S., Eisenberg, L., Sneznevskij, A. V., Sadoun, R., Brooke, E., & Lin, T. Y. (1969). A triaxial classification of mental disorders in childhood. *Journal of Child Psychology, Psychiatry and Related Disciplines, 10,* 41–61.

Rutter, M., Shaffer, D., & Shepherd, M. (1975). *A multiaxial classification of child psychiatric disorders.* Geneva: World Health Organization.

Spitzer, R. L. (1975). On pseudoscience in science, logic in remission and psychiatric diagnosis. *Journal of Abnormal Psychology, 84,* 442–452.

Spitzer, R. L., & Fleiss, J. L. (1974). A re-analysis of the reliability of psychiatric diagnosis. *British Journal of Psychiatry, 125,* 341–347.

Stengel, E. (1959). Classification of mental disorders. *Bulletin of the World Health Organization, 21,* 601–663.

Szasz, T. S. (1961). *The myth of mental illness.* New York: Hoeber-Harper.

Szasz, T. S. (1974). *The myth of mental illness: Foundations of a theory of personal conduct, rev. ed.* New York: Harper & Row.

Weiner, B. (1975). "On being sane in insane places": A process (attributional) analysis and critique. *Journal of Abnormal Psychology, 84,* 433–441.

Wilson, H. S., & Skodol, A. E. (1988). DSM-III-R: Introduction and overview of changes. *Archives of Psychiatric Nursing, 2,* No. 2, 87–94.

World Health Organization. (1948). *International classification of diseases* (6th ed.). Geneva: Author.

World Health Organization. (1967). *International classification of diseases* (8th ed.). Geneva: Author.

World Health Organization. (1978) *International classification of diseases.* (9th ed.). Geneva: Author.

4

COMMUNICATION THEORY

GWEN LAPHAM-ALCORN

LEARNING OBJECTIVES

After studying this chapter, the student will be able to:

- Describe intrapersonal and interpersonal communication.
- Explain the effects of self-awareness, including values clarification, on communication.
- Interpret verbal and nonverbal communication.
- Describe three theories of communication.
- Relate theories of communication to nursing practice.
- Apply the principles of therapeutic communication, including listening and responding, to nurse-patient communication.

I know you believe you understand what you think I said, but I am not sure you realize that what you heard is not what I meant.

Anonymous

Because communication is fundamental to human existence, in this chapter we present the process of communication from several perspectives. The process of communication is defined, the variables influencing communication are addressed, the characteristics of communication are identified, and social and therapeutic communication are examined. We also consider the importance of clear communication with the self by looking at the self, self-concept, and values. Also, because insight into communication with others involves understanding language processes and nonverbal communication, we present three theories of communication: paradoxical communication and double bind, pragmatics of communication, and dysfunctional and functional communication patterns. Finally, therapeutic communication is discussed, and techniques for therapeutic listening and responding are suggested. Responses include feedback, mirroring, self-disclosure, informing, and use of the metamodel.

COMMUNICATION DEFINED

Communication is a goal-directed process in which people use a system of symbols and signs to generate and negotiate meanings. We communicate when we talk and when we do not talk. We communicate when we move and when we are still. We communicate within ourselves when we perceive meaning and with others when we negotiate meanings. We cannot *not* communicate—communication pervades our lives. Communication is so much a part of life that we usually communicate without forethought or planning; and we may thus be unaware of the extent to which our communication is ineffective or detrimental. Since communication is something we learn, however, it is possible to examine it and improve it.

Communication has two general purposes, both of which relate to meeting needs. First, people communicate to exchange information in order to promote objective understanding. Second, people communicate to overcome a feeling of separateness. When people feel separate from others, they often feel tension, anxiety, helplessness, shame, and guilt. They reach out to others to relieve these feelings and to replace them with care, responsibility, respect, and knowledge—the basic elements of love (Fromm, 1956).

Communication has been called the matrix of nursing because of the vital role it plays in nursing practice (Pluckhan, 1978). Every aspect of nursing care involves communication, and the nursing process itself is a communication process. Informing, teaching, counseling, and providing emotional support are communication procedures nurses use as therapeutic tools. Technical tasks, such as medication administration or dressing changes, require explanation, and the way a task is carried out—hastily, gently, indifferently, carefully—sends messages to patients. Nurses cannot not communicate. Therefore, nurses must be conscious of their communication and use it effectively in their care of patients.

SOCIAL VERSUS THERAPEUTIC COMMUNICATION

Communication is fundamental to all people—it is the way people influence each other, and it makes possible complex group activity and social life. However, being part of a social situation, a society, or a culture qualifies any communication. Social beings are shaped by society and think and respond in the ways learned within that society (Whorf, 1956). Thus communication is tailored and modified for a specific social situation.

Every human interaction establishes, clarifies, and maintains or changes a relationship. When a nurse interacts with a patient, she establishes a relationship designed to help the patient attain and maintain health. This therapeutic relationship is different in quality and purpose from a superficial or intimate social relationship and is characterized by different communication (Coad-Denton, 1978).

Most social relationships begin at the superficial level with "small talk," which involves little, if any, self-disclosure or sharing of feelings. Topics of conversation are impersonal, may include subjects not directly related to the people involved in the conversation, and may involve present, past, and future events. In this type of social communication, reinforcement of personal worth is not expected or encouraged by either party. Superficial social relationships may develop into intimate relationships in which individuals share responsibilities and rewards. Then they may disclose feelings, validate each other, and meet their own and each other's needs and goals.

In the therapeutic relationship, the role of the nurse is to facilitate the improvement of a patient's physical and mental health (Masson, 1985) by helping him work through uncomfortable feelings while providing support, information, clarification, and/or comfort (Garant, 1980). In therapeutic communication, conversation between patient and nurse is directed at meeting the patient's needs; thus, it is focused on the patient's problems and concerns. Conversation is personal for the patient and includes patient self-disclosure. Self-disclosure by the nurse is limited.

THE COMMUNICATION PROCESS

Communication may be categorized as intrapersonal, interpersonal, or organizational. **Intrapersonal communication** is the processing of information internally or "talking to oneself." **Interpersonal communication** takes place between two people or in a small group. **Organizational communication** is public communication or communication with large groups.

Communication is best understood as an intrapersonal *and* interpersonal transaction because messages originate in the mind of the individual and because meaning is assigned by the person who is interpreting the message. Intrapersonal communication is a prerequisite to interpersonal communication (Pluckhan, 1978). When an individual receives a message that is either verbal or nonverbal, the individual assigns meaning to the message. If the content of the message has been encountered and assigned meaning before, receiving the message and recalling this meaning may seem to occur simultaneously. If the message is unfamiliar, it may be distorted to fit a meaning in memory, the meaning may be sought, or the message may be ignored (Pluckhan, 1978). In communication, it is most important to remember that the ultimate meaning of the message is the meaning assigned by the person interpreting it. This meaning may match exactly the meaning in the mind of the sender or it may differ to varying degrees. (See Box 4–1 and Table 4–1.)

CHARACTERISTICS OF COMMUNICATION

Communication is a process that flows continuously back and forth from within the self to others. Communication reaches into the past, through the present, and into the future without a distinct beginning or ending. Because of the continual flow, communication is characterized by two traits:

1. Redundancy, or repetition, provides a bridge between the known and the unknown (Colby, 1966) and helps the individual define and structure new

---

Box 4–1 ● "Talking" vs. "Communicating"

. . . talking and communicating are not necessarily the same thing. Again and again I have seen people "talking" to each other without giving one another any information, any aspect of self, any aspect of feeling. They each mouthed words, articulated and sometimes enunciated beautifully, without conveying a single idea and without changing one another, in any area, one iota.

. . . I have seen people who hardly talk at all who are obviously in excellent communication. They are open to each other, receive each other, operate on the same wavelength, so that it takes a minimum of verbal symbols—words—to convey meanings, ideas, feelings, and subtle nuances. These people relate—tell each other how they feel—and invariably have enough impact on one another so that both have changed because of their talk (verbal or relatively nonverbal). . . . Communicating is certainly not a black or white activity. There are many gradations and many varieties. But it is certainly the antithesis of compulsive small talk, chatter and the mouthing of many words, which people often mistake for some kind of attempted communication. So, people talk and communicate; people don't talk or talk relatively little and communicate; and people do and don't talk and don't communicate.

THEODORE ISAAC RUBIN,
The Winner's Notebook

Source: Adler, R., & Towne, N. (1975). *Looking Out/Looking In—Interpersonal Communication.* San Francisco: Rinehart Press (pp. 24–25).

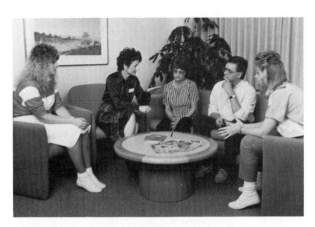

The success of communication is dependent upon the ability to comprehend verbal and nonverbal messages.

ideas or concepts. Without redundancy, the new could not be understood. For example, the unfamiliar term "gyre" can be defined by the redundant terms "a circular or spiral motion; whirl."

2. Feedback, the selective **positive** or **negative** response to one or more aspects of a message (Ruesch, 1957), controls the direction of communication to prevent it from running wild and becoming ineffective.

CODING. To send a message, the individual must **code** it by expressing its meaning in words or in nonverbal language. When coding a message, it is mandatory to consider characteristics of the receiver. Characteristics include physical attributes or problems, age, sex, ethnic background, socioeconomic status, and perceptual frame of reference. The ability to comprehend nonverbal messages and the receiver's social/intellectual level of language affect the success of communication. It is impossible for the nurse to know everything about each person with whom she communicates. However, it is possible, through open and honest effort and the feedback process, to modify or "recode" communication to enhance understanding.

MEANING. Communication has two levels of **meaning**. A receiver may assign meaning to a message at one of two levels. On the first level, meaning is cognitive; it is the literal content of the words of the message. On the second level, the communicators define their relationship by indicating their perceptions of themselves and their listeners. This is the *affective* (emotional) aspect of communication and may reinforce or change the literal meaning of the message. This level has been named **metacommunication** or "communication about the communication" (Bateson, 1966). It is usually nonverbal. On the literal level, the statement "Close the door" has a simple meaning. On the second level, the way the message is delivered gives it an emotional meaning. If it is stated softly as a request, the sender probably sees him or herself as an equal to or a friend of the receiver. If the message is delivered by shouting and demanding, the sender may see him or herself as having authority over the receiver. The way the receiver responds, "Sure, I'll close the door" or "Drop dead," sends a message to the sender about how the receiver sees him or her. These metacommunication messages are always present but are usually not discussed. If the communicators discuss this level of communication (I feel angry when you shout at me to close the door), they are metacommunicating verbally.

The orientation of the individual assigning meaning can range from open to dogmatic. An **open receiver** attempts to take the position of the sender and to understand from that perspective. The **dogmatic receiver** imposes personal needs, values, and feelings on the communication and/or interprets it in a narrow, stereotypical, "right-or-wrong" way. For this receiver, the choice of ways to respond is severely limited. When faced with the statement, "I am going to leave my spouse," the open receiver listens to the individual, tries to understand what is behind the statement, and selects a helpful response from among a variety of possible responses. The dogmatic receiver may have only one reaction—"You got married, that means forever; you cannot leave." Becoming an open receiver is a prerequisite to engaging in therapeutic communication.

COMMUNICATING WITH THE SELF
DEFINING THE SELF

Insight into the internal communication process results in more effective communication. If one can communicate with one's self, one can communicate with others. Self-communication or self-awareness is developed by recognizing one's needs, values, beliefs, motives, and the nature of feelings (Combs, Avila, & Purkey, 1974). The self and self-concept have implications for therapeutic communication because the nurse must understand herself and her own self-concept before she can understand her patient and participate in clear therapeutic communication.

TABLE 4—1 Pathology of communication and predilection age

Age Level	Salient Features of Development	Age-specific Interference with Communicative Behavior
Intra-uterine period: (40 weeks)	Organism responds to thermal, mechanical, and chemical stimuli.	Toxic, infectious, vascular, hormonal, and mechanical **interference with communication apparatus** of foetus.
Neonatal period: (1st 12 wks)	Infant seeks and responds to (as well as begins to categorize) tactile, auditory, visual, and affective stimuli.	**Stimulation exceeding the tolerance limits** of the baby, including neglect and lack of affective attunement.
Infancy: (3 to 24 months)	Mastery of head, eye, and hand movements (second quarter); trunk and fingers (third quarter); legs and feet (fourth quarter); speech (second year).	**Interference with muscular system and locomotion.** Premature training, insufficient exercise; absence of nonverbal exchange, particularly in terms of action, may prevent the establishment of feedback processes.
Early childhood: (2 to 5 years)	Interpersonal communication with one person at a time (mother, father, sibling, or other relative or friend).	**Interference with speech and social action;** selective and tangential responses; extensive or unsupported separation from mother; and interference with perception.
Later childhood: (6 to 12 years)	Group communication with several persons at a time. Learning communication with children of the same age, with emphasis on members of the same sex.	**Interference with group behavior;** separated or divorced families, nonparticipation in school; separation from parent; inappropriate setting of limitations; lack of transmission of social skills at home; lack of responsiveness of parents in verbal terms.
Adolescence: (12 to 18 years)	Interpersonal communication with members of opposite sex resumed; growing attempts to communicate with members of outgroups.	**Interference with participation in autonomous groups,** with pre-mating behavior, with attempts to make decisions and to be independent; inadequate provision for athletic activities and the acquisition of information.

SELF AND SELF-CONCEPT. The self is an elusive concept. According to Rogers (1961), **self** is inherent potential, special individuality, or worth. It is an individual's unique dimensions and purposes, such as true likes and dislikes or athletic or creative potential. Because the self is the "integrator . . . [which] plays the crucial role of finding and making meanings that we grow by" (Perls, Hefferline, & Goodman, 1951, p. 276), it influences perception and interaction with others.

The **self-concept** is an individual's description of his or her "self"; it is what a person means when he or she says "I" or "me." It is an organized pattern of perceptions of the self in awareness (Rogers, 1961).

EXPRESSING AND HIDING THE SELF. Emotions, perceived as feelings, are the bases for order in

a person's life; they help determine what is important to the self. Through life experiences, including interactions with important people (significant others), individuals place values on feelings and on themselves as individuals, and they make decisions about how to behave. When significant others accept an individual's expression of feelings, the self grows and thrives, and the individual feels valued and loved simply for existing. Thus the self and its feelings become part of the developing self-concept, that is, part of the way the individual perceives and describes himself.

Part of the self-concept is an expression of the self; another part of the self-concept actually hides the self. To some extent, most of us have received direct or subtle messages that certain feelings and the behaviors expressing those feelings are "bad" or "wrong." Children who scream in anger are often

Age Level	Salient Features of Development	Age-specific Interference with Communicative Behavior
Young adulthood: (19 to late 20s approx.)	Mastery of the complexity and heterogeneity of adult communication and the multiplicity of roles and diversity of rules. Communication with age superiors. The young adult is often occupationally placed in a position of subservience; observes and follows orders.	**Interference with mating behavior,** with the acquisition of social skills, and the learning of multiple roles. Change-over from family system of communication to other systems may be interfered with by relatives; nonconformance to group practices may jeopardize support from the group.
Middle adulthood: (30 to middle 40s approx.)	Peak of communication with age inferiors and children. Switch from role of perceiver and transmitter to position of greater responsibility.	**Interference with communication vis-à-vis youngsters.** Position between two generations is delicate and ill-defined when pull from either side is too strong.
Later adulthood: (45 to 65, approx.)	Intake of information and learning now displaced in favor of output of information, teaching, governing and ruling. Participation in decision-making groups.	**Interference with independence and decision-making.** Realization of failure to implement self-chosen ideals; collapse of wishful thinking; interference with identification with younger generation.
Age of retirement: (65 to 80, approx.)	Preparation for relinquishment of power and gradual retirement from decision-making. Philosophical considerations after completion of life cycle. Symbolic and global treatment of events.	**Inactivity.** Sudden withdrawal from participation in communication networks. Lack of stimulation.
Old age: (80 +)	Life in retrospect, with emphasis on early memories.	**Interference with equilibrium.** Tolerance limits for over- and understimulation and over- and underactivity quickly reached.

Sources: Adapted from Ruesch, Jurgen, M.D. (1957). *Disturbed communication.* New York: W.W. Norton and Company, Inc., pp. 62–63. Stern, Daniel, M. D. (1985). *The interpersonal world of the infant.* New York: Basic Books, pp. 41–42.

told not to get angry or scream or are told, "You must be tired." Children who touch their genitals may be told they are "bad" or that something bad will happen to them if they masturbate. To be loved and valued, individuals must bury such "unacceptable" feelings and comply with the standards of significant others. To protect themselves from perceived threats, they block the "unacceptable" feelings with "appropriate" counterfeelings and keep both out of their awareness (Perls, Hefferline, & Goodman, 1951). The ways individuals devise to suppress "undesirable" feelings and the behaviors they develop to be loved and accepted combine to form the layers of defenses, masks, or false fronts designed to protect the self. Thus an angry child may no longer recognize that he or she is angry. He or she smiles and is pleasant but seems depressed. The child who was told sex-

ual feelings and behaviors are wrong may grow into a sexually dysfunctional adult.

Events and communications are filtered through a person's self-concept. If the self-concept is the same as or close to the self, the filtering effect is minimal. The individual's **perceptions** are an accurate representation of his or her feelings about outside events (Maslow, 1963). If the self is buried by many masks, the individual selects or distorts perceptions to be consistent with, enhance, and protect the image created by the masks (Combs, Avila, & Purkey, 1974). The individual perceives what the self-concept needs to perceive, and the screening prevents feelings of guilt, anxiety, and unworthiness from surfacing. Through the perception-filtering process, each individual creates a unique reality. The degree to which people have common perceptions is related to the degree of filtering and distorting of perception by the self that goes on.

CREATING PAST AND FUTURE REALITIES. Individuals create reality in the present, but they also create past and future realities. Many details of remembered events were not perceived when they actually occurred; they were filled in by the self-concept (Perls, 1969). Thus memories of the past are, to some extent, distorted abstractions designed to fit the needs of the self-concept. A similar process can occur when individuals think about the future. Rather than face the unknown, take risks, and face new possibilities, people would rather live with sameness; the future can thus become a projection of the present (Rogers, 1961). Perceptions of past and future can be unreliable. Staying in the present minimizes distortion.

CONGRUENT AND INCONGRUENT PERCEPTION. The self-concept influences perception, and it is on that basis that individuals choose their behavior. If perceptions are accurate, behavior will be consistent with and enhance the self. Thus the individual experiences feelings, is aware of this experience, and behaves on the basis of the experience. Ideally, the individual's feelings, awareness, and behavior are **congruent**. Congruence can best be observed in infants: when infants are hungry, they are aware of their hunger and cry. But when individuals' behaviors are based on distorted data, they attempt to convince others (and themselves) that the self-concept is the self. It is behaving according to the distorted self-concept rather than the self.

For example, the owner of a small business projects a self-concept of competitive craftiness and "all knowing." However, the self is a cluster of low self-esteem, insecurity, deficits in knowledge, and so forth. In interpersonal situations, he engages in both non-verbal and verbal communication designed to protect himself from the true feelings within that could emerge. This process is continuous and allows him to convey to others that the projected self-concept (a competitive and competent businessman) is indeed the real self.

When feelings are unrecognized, distorted, or buried, they may express themselves in unhealthy ways, such as psychosomatic illness, and paranoia. They may burst forth unexpectedly, out of control, and hurt others and/or one's self. Although the individual may not be aware of some feelings, they may leak out in behavior and be visible to others. If an individual is not aware of his or her feelings and needs, his or her choices and judgments may not help self-interest; in fact, they may sabotage it. If an individual perceives others inaccurately, relationships may be unsatisfying. For the unaware individual, all these factors may contribute to behavior that, to others, appears confusing, deceptive, controlling, or **incongruent**.

Behavior patterns are learned during childhood. As these patterns are repeated they tend to become fixed (Rogers, 1961). However, the time may come when these patterns are no longer satisfying or adaptive. The self may signal this through confusion, a feeling of being let down, or a sensation that all is not right (Perls, 1969). In this way the self pushes the individual toward a change in the self-concept, and ideally, toward satisfying behavior. "Individuals have within themselves vast resources for self-understanding and for altering their self-concepts, basic attitudes, and self-directed behavior" (Rogers, 1980, p. 115). Growth is the process of changing the self-concept and becoming the true self. It involves integration of all the different aspects of the self that have not been in an individual's awareness and the shedding of masks that lead to unsatisfying behavior and experiences.

SELF-AWARENESS

Growth is accomplished through awareness and congruence (Rogers, 1961). **Awareness** involves "getting in touch" with feelings by allowing experience to come into consciousness. It is not actively *thinking* about the self; rather, it is the spontaneous sensing of what is going on inside (Perls, Hefferline, & Goodman, 1951).

The process of self-awareness begins when individuals become sensitive to clues of incongruity within themselves. Clues include suggestions by other people that they are experiencing a certain feeling when they say they are not; others' responses that catch them "off guard" or surprised; feelings of confusion, discomfort, or unhappiness; and dissatisfaction with the results of personal interactions. Attempts to avoid such observations is an important signal of incongruence (Perls, 1969).

When behavior and feelings (or self-concepts) are incongruent, individuals who want to be self-aware should review their behavior and allow their emotional experience to come into consciousness. Feelings individuals have not been aware of will surface if they are open to them. They should try to identify these feelings which can be used to change behavior to something more congruent and, so, more satisfying whether they are positive or negative.

Next, individuals should identify the behaviors that are congruent with their true feelings. This may not be "typical" behavior or behavior pleasing to others, but it is behavior that expresses the real self. As the individual's awareness of self expands, it encompasses other people—from those closely connected to all of humanity (Combs, Avila, & Purkey, 1974). Thus, behavior that is good for the self is good for others as well.

May Johnson: A Director of Nursing

May Johnson, a director of nursing at a 500-bed hospital, found that the hospital administrator did not listen to her or take her seriously when she presented her ideas. After a meeting, during which her presentation had been disregarded, May examined the events at the meeting. As the events went through her mind, she became aware of feelings of discomfort, anxiety, and fear related to expressing her ideas. She also looked at her behavior and recognized that she became "little girlish," flirtatious, and "cute," in an attempt to hide her feelings and gain attention. May hypothesized that her ideas may not have been taken seriously because of her "childlike" behavior. She began to practice presenting her ideas in a more mature and assertive manner and found that this not only lessened her anxiety, but also got her the recognition she wanted from her associates.

FULLY FUNCTIONING PEOPLE. If by becoming more self-aware, an individual becomes conscious of true feelings, and this experience is reflected in behavior and communication, then the individual is congruent (Rogers, 1961).

Awareness can begin a cycle of growth through which the individual becomes a **fully functioning person** (Rogers, 1961) who is open to experience and has the psychological freedom to be him or herself in this world. This person accepts his or her internal experience and feelings, gives up behavior that is dictated by others but not consistent with the self, sheds behavior that does not satisfy the needs of his or her true self, and risks trying out new behavior which has unknown outcomes but has the potential to satisfy needs.

Behavior that is based on awareness of true feelings is satisfying, results in trusting the self to pre-scribe behavior, and leads to an increasingly positive view of self (increased self-esteem). Such success makes many ego-defenses unnecessary and results in being perceived by others as open, honest, genuine, and worthy of trust.

The self-aware individual recognizes perception as personal and subjective and communicates from this standpoint (Rogers, 1961). (A breakdown of communication occurs when people accept their own perceptions as absolute rather than personal interpretations of reality [Combs, Avila, & Purkey, 1974].) Self-aware individuals verbalize opinions and desires in terms of, "I think," or "I feel"; they do not state their perceptions as facts. The self-aware individual puts the past and the future in perspective. He or she accepts the past as, in part, constructed by the self in order to be congruent with the self-concept, and moves on. The future is seen as a possibility for new experience and growth (Perls, 1969). This individual evaluates him or herself and is open to evaluations from other people; free choice is exercised in terms of, "What is right for me?" The self-aware individual comes to terms with being a *process* rather than a product, realizing that the *perfect* self or perfect personality does not exist.

VALUES

Values are an individual's beliefs about self-worth, behavior, other people, events, and other things that are important in life. They are attitudes that reflect what is desired or held dear. Values guide behavior, eliminating the need to analyze and choose in each situation. They act as a stabilizing force and make people more predictable if their behavior is always consistent with their values. A value system develops along with the self-concept and, as with understanding the self and the self-concept, insight into values can lead to congruence. Values may be freely chosen after considering the alternatives or they may be externally enforced. Externally enforced values are those accepted because significant others have communicated their "rightness." The individual might not have selected these values if given the opportunity to examine and choose. Behavior based on unexamined, externally enforced values—indicated by "should," "must," "you better"—may not be in an individual's best interest nor consistent with the self.

Values clarification is an approach to discovering and developing values. This process, leading to congruence, has three components: thinking about one's values, recognizing true feelings or awareness of the self, and acting. It involves the following steps (Simon, Howe, & Kirschenbaum, 1978):

1. Choose freely: behavior and the values it reflects are examined and alternatives identified.

2. Choose from alternatives: values only exist when there are choices or when there is more than one way to behave. Examine all possible choices.

3. Choose after considering the consequences: the consequences of each alternative and the outcome of behaving in terms of the chosen value should be considered. Can this choice be supported in all situations?

4. Prize and cherish: one must be aware of true feelings as well as being aware of the self and the "rightness" or "fit" of the value.

5. Publicly affirm: personal values should be made known to others, not to be forced on others, but to declare one's position.

6. Act on values: behavior is influenced by identified values.

7. Repeat acting: behavior based on freely chosen values becomes consistent.

Behaviors not meeting the criteria outlined by the seven steps are **values indicators**. Individuals who profess certain values, but who do not consistently behave accordingly, show values indicators. Indicators include beliefs, goals, attitudes, interests, feelings, and aspirations (Raths, Harmin, & Simon, 1966). The individual who professes to value honesty, who finds and returns a wallet, but who does nothing when undercharged at the grocery store is not acting consistently on a value. Rather, honesty is a values indicator. People frequently have more values indicators than values. The value-clarification process can be used to check for values versus values indicators. Values clarification is part of the process of becoming congruent. It is an ongoing process as values form and are affected by changing situations and experience.

COMMUNICATING WITH OTHERS

LANGUAGE

Language makes communication possible. Language has a "time-binding" effect that helps people remember the past, communicate experience, and connect the past to the present. Language allows people to convey new ideas and thoughts. It allows us to solve problems, accumulate knowledge, and record history.

Until recently, the study of language, or linguistics, has been the major focus for understanding communication. Semantics is a branch of linguistics concerned with vocal symbols (words and vocalizations such as "a ha" or "humm"), how symbols relate to "things," and how the mind uses symbols to create meaning. An individual's awareness of the words he or she uses is vital to effective communication.

SYMBOLIZATION. Language is made possible by our ability to create symbols. Creating symbols is a process of abstracting. Through this process, similarities of "events" (people, objects, feelings, actions, and such) are identified. Based on these similarities, the events are placed in categories. The categories are then arbitrarily assigned names which are used to communicate with the self and others.

The process of continuously defining categories from the general (animals) to the specific (*one* Chesapeake Bay retriever named Honey) is ongoing. Language continues to evolve as new categories and words, such as "megabyte" or "mainframe computer," are created.

The structure created by symbolization and language becomes the individual's map for interacting with the world. We have a limited ability to perceive what is going on around us at any given moment. The map simplifies perception, thinking, and acting by reducing and organizing the detail to which we must attend. It is less cumbersome to say one word, such as "freedom," than to list the characteristics of freedom itself. (See also Box 4–2.)

MEANING. People use language to communicate meaning. It is often assumed that everyone assigns the same meaning to a symbol. This is far from the case, for assigning meaning is a personal, internal process, and the symbolic maps that are created as a result can limit effective communication. Three principles described by Korzybski in *Science and Sanity* (1933) address these limitations (Rapoport, 1962).

1. It is impossible to say everything about anything. The categories represented by words leave out many details. The list of details, characteristics, qualities, perceptions, and alternatives is endless, and it makes the choices for assigning meaning to symbols endless, too. The flexibility to define words in terms of different details allows past experience, values, needs, and feelings to affect the meaning assigned. Thus the definition of any symbol rests on the experience the in-

dividual connects to the symbol and the specific details assigned.

2. The symbol is not the event (or person, object, feeling, or such). Meaning may become attached to a word and then generalized to all concrete events symbolized by the word. This is especially true when a word triggers emotion. When people react to words, they may not be reacting to reality.

John: A Nurse Caring for a Cancer Patient

John, an RN, was assigned to care for "the cancer patient" in Room 203. John's father had died of cancer. Upon hearing the words "cancer patient," he conjured up images of suffering, pain, and death. He experienced feelings of fear, dread, and a sense of inadequacy. John put off going to the patient's room and delegated her immediate care to others.

John read the patient's chart and discovered she had had successful surgery for cancer and had a good prognosis for recovery. When he met Marilyn, the patient, he found a happy, friendly, thankful, and vital woman eager to get on with her recovery.

Consider the impact on Marilyn if her care had been based on John's reaction to the label "cancer patient" rather than on her own reality.

---

3. Finally, just as "the thing is not the label," the map is not the territory (Rapoport, 1962). The **mental maps** of the world that all people create in their minds, their perceptions of reality, are not reality itself. They are interpretations of reality.

MAKING BETTER MAPS. If people understand Korzybski's principles of symbolization, they can become aware of their own mental maps. Awareness makes it possible to recognize and deal with discrepancies between words and meanings. Discrepancies occur because mental maps are based on abstractions. Korzybski (1933) identified two levels of abstraction: the extensional and the intensional. The **extensional level of abstraction** is the concrete or nonverbal level. At this level the individual can point to an object or animal, display a feeling, perceive sensations, or see, touch, or experience the "thing" that the symbol stands for directly. The **intensional level of abstraction** is the verbal level. Abstraction at this level can range from close to concrete to generalized. As words become more abstract, detail of discrete events is lost. Thus at the extensional level, Marilyn, the cancer patient, is experienced. Through increas-

ing abstraction, Marilyn may be labeled or referred to as a 56-year-old woman with cancer of the bowel, a woman with cancer, a cancer patient, a patient, and finally Case Number 221. It is essential to effective communication to clarify the meaning of the symbols being used. The best way to do this is to refer or return to the extensional level of abstraction.

Abstraction can be minimized by relating words to concrete events and by using operational definitions that relate specific functions to a word (Steinberg, 1970). Returning to experience involves describing the facts and details of, and the relationships among events, comparing them to something already experienced. Providing such descriptions, or staying as close to the concrete as possible, leads to awareness of the uniqueness of events and avoids stereotyping. The nurse who uses concrete familiar words and symbols rather than medical terms or jargon communicates more effectively with the patient (Byrne & Edeani, 1984). Rather than naming a body part, she points to it; rather than naming a body function, she describes it; and rather than explaining a procedure, she compares it to something the patient has already experienced. When it is difficult to keep conversation at a concrete level, the nurse can take responsibility for abstractions by using qualifiers such as, "I think," or "This is the way I see it."

An operational definition of a symbol describes its function or use, along with how it is experienced and what its criteria are. An operational definition of the word *nurse* might be: "a person who provides specialized health care; or a person with a license to practice nursing."

NONVERBAL COMMUNICATION

While the major focus in communication is language, much communication takes place nonverbally. Within its context, every body movement or expression has meaning (Birdwhistell, 1970). Categories of nonverbal behavior considered here are paralanguage, body language, use of space, and touch.

PARALANGUAGE. Paralanguage includes all aspects of spoken communication except the words themselves. Paralanguage refers to the tone of voice, or the way something is said. Paralanguage includes vocal qualifiers (such as intensity, pitch, patterning, and tempo of the voice) and vocal differentiators (such as laughing, crying, giggling, and quavering) (Pittenger & Smith, 1966). Emotion is often signaled through paralanguage. For example, anxiety may be indicated by a change to a higher pitch, in-

Box 4-2 ● Infant Communication Theory

[A quantum leap in the development of the infant's] . . . sense of self occurs when the infant discovers that he or she has a mind and that other people have minds as well. Between the seventh and ninth month of life, infants gradually come upon the momentous realization that inner subjective experiences, the "subject matter" of the mind, are potentially shareable with someone else. The subject matter at this point in development can be as simple and important as an intention to act ("I want that cookie"), a feeling state ("This is exciting"), or a focus of attention ("Look at that toy"). This discovery amounts to the acquisition of a "theory" of separate minds. Only when infants can sense that others distinct from themselves can hold or entertain a mental state that is similar to one they sense themselves to be holding is the sharing of subjective experience or inter-

subjectivity possible (Trevarthan and Hubley 1978). [What is going on in the infant's mind (non-verbally, of course) is a working notion] . . . that says something like, what is going on in my mind may be similar enough to what is going on in your mind that we can somehow communicate this (without words) and thereby experience intersubjectivity. For such an experience to occur, there must be some shared framework of meaning and means of communication such as gesture, posture, or facial expression.

When it does occur, the interpersonal action has moved, in part, from overt actions and responses to the internal subjective states that lie behind the overt behaviors. This shift gives the infant a different "presence" and social "feel." Parents generally begin to treat the infant differently and address themselves more to the

---

creased nasality (forcing air through the nose by holding the mouth rigid), stumbling over words, increased intensity, and quavering. A depressed person may speak slowly, in a soft monotone, with minimum changes in forcefulness and pitch. An impressive, fluent, and persuasive speaker uses a lower pitch and with greater intensity and minimum nasality; he or she also varies pitch and intensity, ends most sentences, including questions, on a lower pitch, and has a rate of about 170 words per minute.

BODY LANGUAGE. **Body language**, called **kinesics**, includes facial expressions, gestures and posture, and general body movements.

Affective display is the communication of feelings or emotions through body language. Individuals display emotion through changes in voice tone, skin color, lip size, facial muscle tone, and breathing (Cameron-Bandler, 1978). When a change is noted, say by a nurse during a conversation with a patient, she asks about the emotions he seems to be experiencing. If the individual is recalling a frightening experience, his color may pale, breathing may become shallow, tension may develop in the face, and the lips may become thin. By comparison, passionate or sex-

ual feelings are usually indicated by flushing, deeper breathing, soft facial muscle tone, and fuller lips.

Relationships can be defined through nonverbal behavior. People may be open/closed with one another or dominant/submissive. Openness is signaled

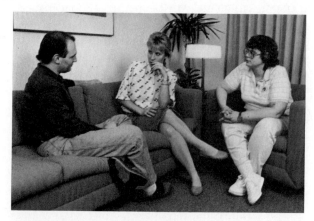

Relationships are identified by the participants' nonverbal behaviors. For example, eye contact, a smile, and arms positioned away from the body and unfolded, signify openness. On the other hand, legs crossed, arms folded across the chest, and infrequent eye contact, signify a closed posture.

subjective domain of experience. This sense of the self and other is quite different from what was possible in the domain of core-relatedness. Infants now have a new organizing subjective perspective about their social lives. The potential properties of a self and of an other have been greatly expanded. Selves and others now include inner or subjective states of experience in addition to the overt behaviors and direct sensations that marked the core self and other. With this expansion in the nature of the sensed self, the capacity for relatedness and the subject matter with which it is concerned catapult the infant into a new *domain of intersubjective relatedness*. A new organizing subjective perspective about the self emerges.

[As a result of this developmental progress, empathy on the part of the caregiver becomes a different ex-perience for the infant.] It is one thing for a younger infant to respond to the overt behavior that reflects a mother's empathy, such as a soothing behavior at the right moment. In the younger infant the empathic *process* itself goes unnoticed, and only the empathic *response* is registered. It is quite another thing for . . . [the infant to sense that an empathic process bridging the two minds has been created. The caregiver's empathy, that process crucial to the infant's development, now becomes a direct subject of the infant's experience. Psychic intimacy as well as physical intimacy is now possible.] The desire to know and be known in this sense of mutually revealing subjective experience is great. In fact, it can be a powerful motive and can be felt as a need-state. (The refusal to be known psychically can also be experienced with great power.)

Finally, with the advent of inter-subjectivity, the parents' socialization of the infant's subjective experience comes to be at issue. Is subjective experience to be shared? How much of it is to be shared? What kinds of subjective experience are to be shared? What are the consequences of sharing and not sharing? Once the infant gets the first glimpse of the intersubjective domain and the parents realize this, they must begin to deal with these issues. What is ultimately at stake is nothing less than discovering what part of the private world of inner experience is shareable and what part falls outside the pale of commonly recognized human experiences. At one end is psychic human membership, at the other psychic isolation.

Source: Stern, D. N. (1985). The sense of a subjective self. The interpersonal world of the infant. New York: Basic Books, pp. 124–126.

---

when one person faces the other, appearing relaxed with feet apart; arms away from the body, showing the palms; a smile or pleasant expression; and frequent eye contact. A closed position would usually involve turning away, general tenseness, arms close to body, arms crossed on chest, legs crossed, feet together, a frown, and infrequent eye contact. Dominance is communicated by a straight body, head high or back, hand on hip, finger waving in air or pointing, fingers steepled, thumb in belt, movement toward other, feet on desk, looking "down the nose," and a constant gaze. Submissiveness is communicated by head down or cocked, slumped posture, "closed" body position, movement backward, and eyes down. Equality in a relationship is signaled by individuals assuming similar open body positions. Such similar or mirror-image positioning may indicate agreement with what is being said and helps to establish rapport.

Nonverbal-behavior patterns can indicate honest/ deceptive or congruent/incongruent communication. For the honest or congruent person, nonverbal behavior will match and support the verbal message. The deceptive person does not want to tell the truth and therefore gives what he or she feels will be an acceptable message verbally. Intentional deception may be difficult to detect because the individual may control or blunt facial expression and body movement in order to control it (Ekman & Friesen, 1969).

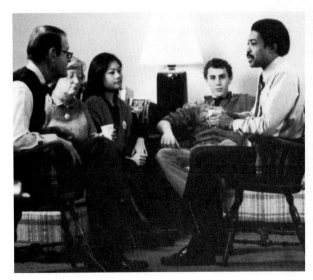

Nonverbal-behavior patterns can signify honest/ deceptive or congruent/incongruent behavior.

Unintentional deception includes self-deception, or unawareness of true feelings. The individual believes a response is truthful but real feelings may leak out in nonverbal behavior, resulting in facial expression and body motion incongruent with the spoken words. Body language may express what the individual cannot express or tries to hold back.

REGULATORS

In our society, people learn what behaviors are considered acceptable and allowable; they also learn what is unacceptable and/or disruptive. These unacceptable and disruptive behaviors induce recalibrations and counterresponses, and will be discussed here. They may be present in the form of kinetic and linguistic behaviors. They serve to forestall or stop an unacceptable behavior, and maintain the expected process of events (Scheflen, 1972).

SELF-MONITORING: Self-monitoring is subtle. The behaviors are not coarse and usually occur outside of the person's conscious awareness. Many times, it is the person who is in violation of certain acceptable standards who serves as his own monitor. For example, consider the person who uses a nose-wiping behavior (monitor) after he has embellished a situation or lied.

Behavior: He brings the index finger under his nose, as he lies.

Behavior: A man who glances at a woman's leg and gets caught, might wipe or rub his eyes to indicate that his eyes are dysfunctional. Too, the offender might avoid eye contact, hang his head, drop his shoulders, and blush. Covering the mouth or face while speaking may indicate embarrassment, a wish to hide or cover what is being said, being unsure or doubtful, or lying (Eibel-Erbesfeldt, 1974).

MONITORS THAT CONTROL OTHER PEOPLE: Monitors are behaviors that can be used to control the behaviors of others. A facial frown is a commonly used monitor that serves to alert the individual(s) that he has behaved in an unacceptable manner (Scheflen, 1974).

Other types of monitors might include flinching, recoiling, and displaying a startled reaction. These types of behaviors occur when others are too loud and aggressive or violate the social order of events (Sheflen, 1974).

There are some common types of monitoring that are expressed by facial displays: contempt, dis-

gust, anger, shame, humiliation, embarrassment, and so forth (Scheflen, 1974).

OVERT CENSURE

Sometimes the behaviors used to regulate unacceptable behaviors are direct, obvious, and well within the person's awareness. Blatant kinesic behaviors that are used in such instances include turning the head from side to side (head shaking) and extending the arm with the palm of the hand open and outstretched.

At times, the person who violates certain codes of behavior might receive non-verbal and verbal censure.

If behavior is not acceptable, and the individual cannot or will not conform to an expected code of behavior, he might be ostracized from a group or an organization; in more extreme instances, the law enforcement agencies, mental health professionals, the military, and so forth, might be called upon for assistance.

QUASI-COURTING

Quasi-courting behaviors, like monitors, are an attempt to regulate communication by keeping individuals attentive, alert, and ready to relate (Scheflen, 1974). Quasi-courting behaviors are seen between individuals and in groups and between members of the same and the opposite sex. Quasi-courting behaviors can promote group cohesion and rapport and can be the impetus for completion of nongratifying tasks (Scheflen, 1974). Quasi-courting must be distinguished from true seductive behavior and sexual advances. Mistaking quasi-courting for these behaviors may result in loss of rapport and forestall group cohesion.

Quasi-courting behavior begins with courting behavior. This includes eyes brightening and increased muscle tone in the body; posture straightens and sagging in the face diminishes. This is accompanied by preening behavior. Individuals may also exchange glances, hold each other's gaze, cock their heads, place a hand on the hip, and show the palm. In actual courtship, this sequence may progress to increasing intimacy. However, in quasi-courting, the courting behavior is accompanied from the beginning by behaviors that indicate nonsexual intentions. In an effort to communicate the intended context of the interaction, a person might verbally indicate a lack of interest in a sexual encounter, and continue to focus on a particular task or some other activity.

A Nursing Group: An Example of Nonverbal Communication

Donna Graham, the newly hired assistant director of nursing, was organizing a quality-control committee. Donna and three other nurses were seated in swivel chairs around a conference table. Donna sat straight up in her chair, leaning forward, with her left hand in her lap her right elbow on the table, and her right hand under her chin. As Donna began to speak she sat even straighter, lowered her right hand, tensed her facial muscles and smiled, and ran her fingers through her hair.

A head nurse, Terry Whit, sat on Donna's left. Terry sat with her back against the chair and her hands folded in her lap.

To Terry's left, across from Donna, sat another head nurse, Helen List. Helen sat straight up in her chair, leaning forward, her right hand in her lap, her left elbow on the table, and her left hand under her chin. As Donna spoke, Helen nodded her head up and down. When Donna spoke to her, Helen cocked her head to the left and looked down. She answered slowly, in a soft voice.

Jean Prince sat to Helen's left. Jean had been day supervisor for eight years; she was the oldest member of the group. As Donna began to speak, Jean left the table to get a cup of coffee from the cart. When Donna asked Jean a question on policy, Jean walked back to the table and stood close enough to Donna so that her leg brushed Donna's arm. As Jean spoke, she lifted her chin and looked down at Donna. She stood with one hand on her hip and the other in the air. She spoke at a fast rate and clipped off the ends of sentences; her voice was louder than necessary for the small group. As Jean was speaking, Donna drew her finger across under her nose twice. When Donna resumed speaking, Jean remained in the same position for two or three minutes longer.

Terry asked Donna two questions about the committee. After Donna explained the function of the committee, she said to Terry, "I would really like you to work on this committee." At the same time, Donna's voice became softer, she crossed her arms and legs, turned her gaze away from Terry by turning her head to the right, and swung her chair to the right, turning her entire body away from Terry.

Each group member was communicating through nonverbal behavior. Donna displayed quasi-courting behavior as she began to speak, thus encouraging the attention and interest of the group. Terry assumed a neutral body-language position. Helen was expressing agreement with Donna through her mirror-image body position and displayed submissive behavior when talking with Donna. Jean, on the other hand, displayed dominance behavior. She was, perhaps, even threatening Donna by violating Donna's personal space and not moving away from her after she spoke. Donna reacted to Jean's behavior with monitoring behavior. Donna's communication with Terry was incongruent; verbally she said she wanted to work with Terry, but nonverbally she turned away and assumed a closed body posture indicating she did not. Terry may have concluded that Donna had some reservations about working with her and that Donna was not aware of these reservations because she did not control her nonverbal behavior to match her dishonest verbal statement.

USE OF SPACE. The study of the perception and use of space is called **proxemics**. The spatial distances individuals find comfortable for communicating depend on cultural background, level of intimacy of the relationship, reason for meeting, available space, and context of the meeting. Hall (1959) identified four space zones used by Americans. The intimate range, zero to twelve inches, is for very personal contact. Discomfort results when anyone but intimate others or children violate this zone. The personal range is twelve to thirty-six inches. This range is comfortable for communicating with close friends and family. The social range, three to eight feet, is for contact with friends and intermediates in business. The public range, eight to twenty feet, is appropriate for small groups and informal gatherings.

Individuals determine comfortable spatial distance by moving toward and away from each other in a "proxemic dance." Certain types of information, especially sensitive or personal information, can only be exchanged within the proper space zone. Thus, in patient interactions, the nurse is aware of the factors determining use of space. The nurse may begin a conversation with a patient standing or sitting within the social range of three to eight feet. As the discussion becomes more personal for the patient, the nurse may move closer. Since the patient frequently cannot move closer to or away from the nurse, the nurse must be sensitive to the patient's reaction to her distance from him. If the patient seems uncomfortable with the nurse's closeness, the nurse may need to move back and vice versa.

Individuals from various cultures perceive and structure space differently (Hall, 1974). Members of some cultures, including Arab, Latin American, and Southern European, are "contact" oriented—they stand close together, face more directly, touch more, gaze more directly, and speak louder than groups such as American, Asian, and Northern European. Misunderstanding occurs when a "contact" person gets too close to a "noncontact" person. The latter may be seen as standoffish and unfriendly; the former as pushy and aggressive. In fact, both individuals are simply behaving according to the dictates of their cultures. When communicating with a patient, the nurse needs to be aware of and sensitive to cultural differences in use of space and other nonverbal behavior in order to avoid misunderstanding.

The concept of territory also relates to the use of space. Individuals desire and attempt to control their surrounding space in order to maintain personal integrity. Public territories, as opposed to private territory such as one's home, are those entered and used freely by people who adhere to public standards of behavior (Lyman & Scott, 1967). People mark, or stake out, public territory as their own by sitting or standing in a space and placing their personal possessions (purse, coat, and such) around them. Individuals react to intrusion by others with feelings of anger and hostility. They defend the territory by using nonverbal behavior (such as avoiding the invader, turning away, or glaring) to communicate to the invader that he or she is unwelcome. If the invader does not leave, the person who first marked the space will probably flee.

For hospitalized patients, the constant invasion of personal and territorial space and the inability to flee may result in feelings of anger, hostility, fear, and helplessness. The nurse can help minimize these feelings by respecting the patient's space, including the intimate space zone and the territories of bed and hospital room, by asking permission to approach and/or touch the patient, and by explaining the necessity to do so. This establishes the patient's control of space and shows the respect to which he is entitled.

TOUCH. Touch is a form of communication which can bring pleasure and satisfaction and is visually associated with caring and concern (Barnett, 1972). In times of stress, adults often communicate through touch. For patients under stress, the most effective means of comforting and quieting the patient has been found to be touch (Rubin, 1963). Kübler-Ross (1969) identified gentle pressure on the hand as the most meaningful communication between nurse and dying patient. McCorkley (1974), in a study of seriously ill patients, found the quickest way to establish rapport was through touch.

Although touch can be an effective nursing measure, some nurses are reluctant to touch. Some have negative associations to touch. Others find that touching triggers anxiety, though this may not be well understood (Ujhely, 1979). The reluctance of some nurses to touch a critically ill and dying patient, one who is often in need of touch, can be ascribed to the nurse's fear of death (Barnett, 1972). Some individuals do not touch because they associate all touch with sex. However, touch with a sexual meaning can be distinguished from touch that is nurturing, comforting, and caring (Satir, 1972).

Because nurses touch their patients, they need to be aware of how they and their patients feel about touching and being touched. A nurse can determine when to use or not use touch with a patient by asking herself the following questions (Ujhely, 1979):

1. Is this patient likely to be comfortable with touch?

2. If I touch this patient, will it be therapeutic?

3. Will touch help the patient experience true feelings and express them? Is this in his best interest at this time?

4. If the patient is experiencing profound feelings, will touch interfere with or facilitate the awareness and expression of feelings?

5. Do *I* want to touch the patient because of my discomfort with the feelings the patient is experiencing or because I feel the patient needs and desires the reassurance of touch?

In summary, the nurse's ability to be empathic will determine her ability to make sound decisions about touch.

THERAPEUTIC USE OF NONVERBAL COMMUNICATION. The blending together and use of various forms of nonverbal communication has been called the therapeutic use of self. "Nursing is based on the use of self: to listen, teach, guide, support, be there" (Masson, 1985, p. 72). All behavior communicates. The many nurturing acts nurses perform—smoothing a sheet, helping with makeup, offering coffee, gently performing procedures—create an environment of emotional support and caring. However, "activity" is not essential to the therapeutic use of self. The nurse should not equate being with the patient, without activity or words, as doing nothing. The nurse's presence alone can be a powerful patient-care tool. In profoundly emotional situations when words fail, the nurse's presence provides support. Standing nearby as parents say goodbye to their dead baby, or holding the hand of a dying patient can convey warmth, strength, and empathy more effectively than any words.

Andrew Jobson: A Myocardial Infarction Patient

Andrew Jobson was a 67-year-old man admitted to the surgical intensive care unit (SICU) with an acute myocardial infarction (MI). He was agitated and moving about in bed. He was shouting at the nurses—complaining that his sheets were covered with blood, that no one had cared for him all night, and that he could not sleep in the SICU. He began throwing objects. The SICU was an open unit, and his voice echoed around the room. When two nurses approached, his shouting increased. The nurses gave Mr. Jobson the necessary care and then retreated quickly.

The literal content of Mr. Jobson's messages at times did not appear to be relevant to the situation and often was not clear. His nonverbal behavior appeared to communicate anger, understandable given his frustration at being dependent (Smith, 1985).

Due to his shouting, it was impossible to use verbal techniques to assist Mr. Jobson. The head nurse, Elaine Jacobson, simply stood next to his bed at a 45-degree angle, with a relaxed posture, arms at sides, and a relaxed facial expression, to listen without comment and provide support through her presence. At first the patient's shouting increased. Elaine became aware of her discomfort with the shouting. However, as she remained in place and slowly turned to face the patient, the shouting diminished. Mr. Jobson became quiet, his head hung, and his body slumped. As this happened, Elaine placed her hand first on the bed-rail, then near his shoulder, and, when he showed no resistance, on his shoulder.

After a few minutes of silence, Mr. Jobson stated, "I don't like this ward." This was followed by an interaction in which he turned toward the nurse, assumed an open posture, and disclosed his fear of dying (this was his second MI in a month) and his feelings of helplessness and insecurity because he was not in a regular medical unit.

THEORIES OF COMMUNICATION

Theories of communication provide a structure for analyzing and improving patterns of communication. The theories presented here are especially applicable to communication in nursing.

DOUBLE BIND

Double-bind theory was developed by Bateson, Jackson, Haley, and Weakland (1956) in the course of their work with schizophrenic patients and their families. Since its inception, double bind has become a general theory of communication (Jones, 1980). It is seen in communication between individuals, family members, groups, and nations (Scheflen, 1972).

Bateson et al. (1956) observed that communication has a literal content which is presented in a qualifying context. The qualification defines the mode of communication. When a message is received, the receiver determines the communication mode (such as play, humor, seriousness, or metaphor) by interpreting highly abstract signals usually delivered nonverbally (Bateson et al., 1956). The individual must be able to identify the mode to understand the message. When a patient states, "The nursing care is terrific," the nonverbal communication with the statement tells the nurse, "I am serious," or it may say, "I am sarcastic." Based on the nonverbal message, the nurse knows whether to be complimented or insulted. When words and nonverbal behavior conflict, an attempt is being made to convey a message without risking repercussions. If the nurse is insulted and confronts the patient, he can deny the nonverbal message and insist he meant to compliment.

The double bind has five necessary ingredients (Bateson et al, 1956):

1. Two or more persons, one of whom is a victim in the interpersonal situation;

2. A victim with repeated experiences which evidence a theme of double bind behaviors;

3. A primary negative injunction that has two possibilities: a) "Do not do so and so, or I will punish you", or, b) "If you do not do so and so, I will punish you." (Bateson et al., 1956, p. 253). The threat of punishment such as withdrawal of love, or in extreme instances, abandonment, is always present.

4. A secondary injunction that conflicts with the first; it is more abstract; and it "is enforced by punishments or signals which threaten survival." (p. 253).

5. The fifth ingredient is "a negative injunction that prohibits the victim from escaping from the field." (p. 253). At times, the individual cannot or will not escape from the situation because of "certain devices which are not purely negative, e.g., capricious promises of love, and the like." (p. 254).

These five ingredients are no longer necessary once the victim has learned to perceive and react with double bind traits and characteristics. Much like Pavlov's experiment in classical conditioning with dogs, in which salivation occurred without the presence of food, the victim of the double bind needs only minimum cues (Foley, 1974; 1986).

Consider this classical example presented by Bateson et al. (1956, p. 259).

> A young man who had fairly well recovered from an acute schizophrenic episode was visited in the hospital by his mother. He was glad to see her and impulsively put his arms around her shoulder, whereupon she stiffened. He withdrew his arm and she asked, "Don't you love me anymore?" He then blushed, and she said, "Dear, you must not be easily embarrassed and afraid of your feelings." The patient was able to stay with her only a few minutes more, and, following her departure, he assaulted an aide and was put in the tubs.

Yet another example with subtleties is from a humorist, Dan Greenberg (1969, p. 16).

> Give your son Marvin two sports shirts as a present. The first time he wears one of them, look at him sadly, and say, "The other one you didn't like?" Marvin has no choice.

The "bound" individual is in a position from which he or she *cannot leave or escape*, frequently because he or she is emotionally dependent on the "binding" individual. Individuals in long-term binding situations are often prohibited from commenting on the binding situation, i.e., metacommunicating, due to the nature of their relationship. Bound individuals do not usually learn to understand nonverbal signals or to use metacommunication.

Those caught in a double bind predictably react in a number of ways (Bateson et al., 1956). They search for the cue for appropriate behavior they think they missed. Their search is futile. Their choice is either to obey the literal content of the message exclusively and compulsively or withdraw from the communication altogether through physical separation or by blocking perception. A person can block perception by withdrawing or through excessive, hyperactive behavior. Hallucinations may occur or the individual may develop amnesia or delusions.

Effective communicators try to avoid double binds. However, a therapeutic double bind[1] may be needed to break the original double bind. A nurse

can respond to a double bind by pointing it out to the patient and confronting the conflicting double message. The objective is to clarify what is desired or needed and to assist the patient in understanding feelings underlying the message. In the example above, the patient felt "Damned if I do, and damned if I don't!". . . there is no escape.

PRAGMATICS OF COMMUNICATION

Watzlawick, Beavin, and Jackson (1967) developed the theory of **pragmatics of communication**. According to their theory, behavior is synonymous with communication because communication implies commitment, influences others, and tells others how the sender rates them. Through these messages, individuals tell how they perceive relationships and how they wish to relate to others. Communication can be understood by analyzing the dynamics of interaction between individuals, focusing on the *sender and receiver relationship* as defined through metacommunication.

Mrs. Debo: The Change Agent

Mrs. Debo is a recently employed head nurse on an adolescent unit. She developed an approach for milieu therapy, which involved expanding roles and expectations of nurses on the unit. She began to implement these changes on the unit by communicating with the nurses in a "drill sergeant" fashion.

The nurses reacted in anger to Mrs. Debo: they were not involved in the planning for change; their work schedule was too heavy to let them be attentive to new changes without more staff; the unit was filled with very disturbed adolescents; and Mrs. Debo was too "junior" to the situation to know what was really needed for effective and therapeutic change to occur.

The nurses determined, through their perceptions of how Mrs. Debo communicated to them, that she had little respect for them, devalued their input, and did not see them as colleagues.

During a staff meeting with Mrs. Debo, the nurses asked that the planned agenda be reordered so that they could "communicate about the communications" (metacommunicate) they had experienced with Mrs. Debo. Their concerns focused on stating how they (each) perceived Mrs. Debo's behaviors and the feelings it generated within them. In fact, they did indeed feel rejection, disconfirmation, and so forth.

Mrs. Debo reacted quickly and stated that she had no intention of creating such negative feelings. Instead, she only wanted to attain a specific goal within a given time frame. She assured the nurses

---

[1]The therapeutic double bind is a technique used by psychotherapists for the purpose of reversing a double bind. It can involve paradoxical instruction (prescribing the symptom or the problem) or an outwardly hostile presentation that carries with it a meta-feeling of warm acceptance that can help to break the "spell" of the original double bind (Felder, Malone, and Warkentin, 1982).

that she would be more sensitive and confirming; too, she would gladly include them in the planning and implementation of the new approach. She asked that the staff nurses commit themselves to the achievement of specific goals for the adolescent unit and work toward its fruition in a timely manner.

The meeting concluded with the nurses identifying their areas of expertise and agreeing to take the lead when their skills were needed.

Communication begins with the metacommunication of the sender, which says, "This is how I see me." The receiver of this message replies with, "This is how I see you," in one of three ways: confirmation, rejection, or disconfirmation (Watzlawick, Beavin, & Jackson, 1967). Confirmation is positive recognition of the other person's existence. It is essential for our mental and emotional health. Rejection, while negative, does have value in that it is at least acknowledgment of the other person's existence. Disconfirmation involves treating the other person as nonexistent or, at best, not important—by ignoring, not hearing, or not addressing the individual. Such a response can be psychologically damaging to the receiver.

Through metacommunication people define their relationships as *symmetrical* or *complementary*. In symmetrical relationships, the communicators are equal, and either can take the lead. In a complementary relationship, one person leads and the other follows. Each individual confirms the role of the other.

PUNCTUATION SEQUENCE. People define and redefine their relationships. Metacommunication is ongoing and involves **punctuation sequence.**

Punctuation sequence is the order of exchanges in communication, or the cause-and-effect relationship between communications. While communicators may perceive a linear cause and effect, punctuation sequence is actually a circular pattern of interacting influences: "I did this because she did that." "No, I did that because he did this." This circular pattern can go on indefinitely. Problems related to punctuation sequence develop when individuals assume that they have all the data needed for the communication and that the other person has reached the same conclusion they have.

DISTURBANCES IN COMMUNICATION. Watzlawick, Beavin, and Jackson have identified the most serious problem in communication as a nearly total inability to communicate about communication (1967, p. 36) and have stated that disturbances in communication can take a number of forms. Disturbed communication results when individuals attempt to *not* communicate. This happens when individuals deny their communication and then deny the denial; when they develop a problem or symptom to avoid communicating; when they state that they do not wish to communicate; or when they engage in disqualifications. Disqualification involves ignoring or avoiding the meaning of a message and can be used either by the sender or receiver to invalidate messages. Disqualification can include sending unclear or contradictory messages, inconsistencies in logic or in statements, listening to either the literal message or metacommunication exclusively, or changing the subject.

Continuous arguing over content may be a symptom of disagreement over the relationship involved. The individuals may not recognize that the problem is a relationship problem or are unable or unwilling to talk about it. In healthy relationships, definition of the relationship falls into the background and tasks or goals of communication are fulfilled.

IMPROVING COMMUNICATION. Resolution of dysfunctional communication rests on communicating about communication. Improvement in communication begins with analyzing interactions to identify patterns and relationships which will allow people to understand, and possibly change, the way they communicate.

One method nurses can use to effect change through communication is putting what is perceived as a negative behavior or situation in a different light. This may result in a change of opinion about the issue. Through "relabeling," what is perceived as negative is described as positive. The new label must fit the facts of the old situation but give it a new perspective. For example, the word "handicapped" is usually associated with finality and limitation. Referring to an individual as "physically challenged" conveys a feeling of strength and growth potential.

PATTERNS OF COMMUNICATION

Virginia Satir uses systems theory to define her method of psychotherapy (Foley, 1986). She believes all behavioral dysfunction results from inadequate communication and thus feels that improving communication is therapy.

Satir is also concerned with feelings. She has said that what happens inside and between people is a function of their self-esteem (Satir, 1972). Furthermore, the ability to function and communicate successfully depends on self-esteem. Without self-esteem a person can neither function nor communicate.

Ineffective communication develops when people do not differentiate between the verbal (denotative) and nonverbal (metacommunication) levels of communication. Communication becomes incongruent when communicators have established "bad" rules for communicating. "Bad" rules are those that impede the expression of feelings and, as a result, lead to pain and dysfunction. The most important "good" rule is "freedom to comment." In a nurturing relationship, anything can be discussed. Both positive and negative feelings are important and need to be expressed.

People may use ineffective communication patterns when they are under stress and when their self-esteem is threatened. They may feel embarrassed, anxious, or incompetent at a task because they think they cannot meet others' expectations of them and fear rejection. Because of a lacking or shaky sense of self-worth, the actions and reactions of others are used to define the self. Therefore, positive relationships with others and associated communication patterns must be maintained to reduce threats to the self. Ineffective communication patterns result when individuals attempt to maintain positive relationships with others at all costs, including giving up the self.

FOUR PATTERNS OF INEFFECTIVE COMMUNICATION. Satir (1972) identified the following as characteristics of individuals who have problems with communication: low self-esteem, fear of hurting others' feelings, concern about retaliation from others, fear of a break in relationships with others, and a desire not to impose on others.

Satir (1972) has also identified four ineffective communication patterns: **placating, blaming, computing,** and **distracting.** Each involves an incongruent double message with the verbal and nonverbal messages saying different things and serving to deny certain feelings. The placater is ingratiating, agrees with everyone, and always tries to please. His or her body language, like that of the submissive individual, says, "I am helpless." The placater blocks feelings about the self or feels worthless. In contrast the blamer disagrees with everything and everyone and is always finding fault with or directing others. The blamer's body language says, "I am dominant," while he or she feels lonely and unsuccessful and blocks feelings about others. The computer is calm, cool, and shows no feelings at all. Everything is logical and reasonable. His or her body language communicates "togetherness," but beneath this facade is an individ-

ual who has separated him or herself from feelings, and feels very vulnerable. Finally, the distractor, who seems to be going in all directions at once, does not make much sense. He or she attempts to cover over feelings with hyperactivity and operates from the position that no one cares.

LEVELING: THE EFFECTIVE PATTERN OF COMMUNICATION. Satir's fifth pattern of communication is termed **leveling.**

Leveling is congruent communication that "represents a truth of the person at a moment in time" (Satir, 1972, p. 73). It involves a whole response with body, senses, thoughts, and feelings working together. It puts people in touch with themselves and has a healing effect. It puts people in touch with each other and opens communication.

Leveling is a functional communication. For Satir, the goal of therapy is for the patient to learn leveling. To achieve leveling, a person must face his or her feelings, including fears about making mistakes, not being liked, being criticized, imposing, being imperfect or not acceptable, and being deserted (Satir, 1972). Next, the individual must accept him or herself and the possibility that his or her fears may come true. Satir's criterion for judging the importance of fears is to ask, "If this fear comes true, will I still be alive?" If the answer is "yes," the individual has an opportunity for growth. By facing and overcoming fear, individuals develop self-esteem and the ability to see fear as the potential for growth. (See Chapter 8 on Anxiety Disorders for more on facing fear.)

THERAPEUTIC COMMUNICATION

Three conditions are basic to any therapeutic relationship: congruence, unconditional positive regard, and empathy (Garfield, 1980; Rogers, 1980). Congruence involves an individual's awareness of his or her true feelings and thoughts which are reflected in behavior and communication. Unconditional positive regard refers to accepting another person without value judgment or prerequisites. It involves accepting the other's feelings, beliefs, and behaviors and valuing the person as a unique, worthy human being. *Accepting does not mean agreeing;* agreeing is a value judgment. Labeling behavior as good or bad, agreeing or disagreeing, making statements about quality, offering solutions or advice, and creating expectations all involve value judgments and are antithetical to unconditional positive regard.

Congruence and unconditional positive regard are prerequisites for empathy. Empathy requires sensitivity to another person's experience (Rogers, 1980). It includes sensing, understanding, and sharing the feelings and needs of the other person, seeing things from the other's perspective, or "walking in another's shoes." An individual's behavior is often the best he or she can do at a particular time in a particular situation. Empathy involves understanding from within the perspective upon which that behavior is based. Empathic people usually have a strong sense of self, which prevents them from becoming "lost" in the experience of the other person (Rogers, 1980).

Empathy has been described as a four-stage process (Reik, 1948). In the first stage, identification, the nurse concentrates on and becomes absorbed in the patient's feelings. In the second stage, incorporation, the nurse takes in the patient's feelings. Through the third stage, reverberation, the nurse draws on her own experience to relate to the patient's feelings. This stage leads to a new understanding of both the patient's and the nurse's experience. Finally, the nurse detaches from the patient's feelings and analyzes the process and results of empathy. The empathy process occurs rapidly and not always consciously. Following this process the nurse communicates the understanding achieved to the patient verbally, seeking his validation, or nonverbally, through her concerned facial expression, touch, and so forth. The nurse cannot experience a high degree of empathy with every patient and in every situation. When she does, her patient experiences something very important, being understood.

In a therapeutic relationship, empathy has a number of positive effects (Rogers, 1980). As a result of feeling understood, the patient begins to trust the nurse and develop a relationship with her. In this relationship, the patient can risk disclosure without fear of rejection, reprisal, or judgment. He is free to reveal material never revealed before and to discover new aspects of himself. The patient feels valued, cared for, accepted, and "blooms" or undergoes personal expansion resulting in increased self-esteem.

The following discussion outlines the major aspects of communicating in therapeutic relationships, integrating the stages of empathic relations outlined above. It is also based on the assumption that the nurse identifies patient characteristics salient to communication and communicates in a language and on a level the patient can understand. Therapeutic communication has two parts: listening and responding.

LISTENING

Empathic listening is fundamental to the nurse-patient relationship and is therapeutic in itself. It allows the patient to ventilate his emotions and, perhaps by doing so, to recognize his own solutions to his problems.

The nurse arranges for a quiet, private environment conducive to interpersonal communication. The best position for the nurse is on the same level as the patient, either sitting or standing, with room to move closer and touch the patient.

The nurse listens with an attitude of openness. The tendency to judge, evaluate, approve, or disapprove emotionally meaningful statements is the major barrier to interpersonal communication (Rogers, 1961). The nurse must be aware of "trigger words" or behaviors that could cause emotional flare-ups in this particular patient. References to the "inefficient nursing staff" and "lousy food" require investigation rather than confrontation.

The patient's nonverbal behavior may say more than he does. "Verbal communication is usually a lie. The real communication is beyond words" (Perls, 1969, p. 57). Attention to the affective component present in all communication may reveal incongruity. Clues to feelings lie in patterns of behavior, subtle changes in emotion or behavior, and in the context of those changes.

The nurse's feelings during an interaction with a patient can provide an important clue to how the patient is feeling and what the patient wants from the

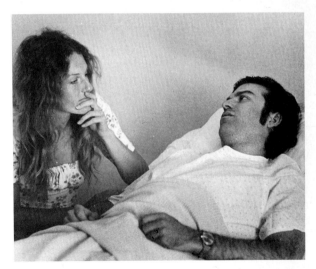

"Verbal communication is usually a lie. The real communication is beyond words." (Perls, 1969, p. 57).

nurse. The nurse needs to attend to her feelings as much as the patient's, and accept both.

The nurse's feelings provide a guide for responding but should not be expressed in a stimulus–response fashion. Some patient feelings, especially anger and hostility, inspire a flare-up of the same feelings in the nurse (Green, 1986). The nurse needs to analyze her reactions before responding by asking herself: How do I feel? What is the patient doing to engender these feelings? What is my or the usual behavioral response to such feelings? What benefit would the patient receive from that response? Is the patient seeking a response as part of a self-fulfilling prophecy or as a defense against feelings he finds threatening? Rather than just responding in kind, the nurse responds based on her understanding of the patient's experience (see Self-Disclosure, below).

People are often uncomfortable with silence because it may be interpreted as a form of rejection. When silence occurs, the nurse must be sensitive to the patient's reaction to it and break the silence if the patient is interpreting it as rejection. However, before speaking, the nurse should consider the ramifications of silence. If the patient is silent because a subject has been exhausted, the nurse may want to provide a lead for continuing the discussion. However, if the patient is "lost in thought" (experiencing anxiety, anger, or sadness), trying to find words for feelings, or struggling between holding back and letting go, the nurse may choose to let the silence continue. This allows time for feelings to surface, to be labeled, and to be expressed.

A patient may refuse to talk for a number of reasons. For example, the patient may be coping with problems through denial. Forcing the patient out of denial may lead to the patient's feeling hopeless despair (Miller, 1985). Or the patient may not be ready, or may not feel comfortable enough with the nurse, to divulge personal information or face certain feelings. The nurse may first need to spend more time developing rapport and a trusting relationship with the patient. Another possibility is that the nurse may have inadvertently created a barrier to communication. The nurse can ask the patient about this. A patient may also refuse to talk due to the disturbing nature of an experience, the profound feeling engendered by it, or shame or guilt associated with it. If the nurse senses the patient has a problem which she cannot help him with, she should not encourage disclosure. As such situations evolve, it may be best to change the direction of the interaction and then consult another professional who is better qualified to help the patient. The nurse must also consider the

potential problems associated with listening to the patient when he requests her promise not to tell anyone. Such promises can lead to ethical dilemmas when the nurse has a moral or legal obligation to report information, yet has an obligation to the patient based on a promise (see Chapter 28 on Ethical Issues in Mental Health Practice). Even without verbal communication, however, the nurse can demonstrate support by, for example, sitting quietly with the patient or checking on him frequently. In summary, the patient's silence should be respected, but the nurse needs to remain available to the patient to try to understand when he is ready to talk.

When listening the nurse must maintain interest. Fatigue, a busy schedule, and other factors can interfere with this. If the nurse is for some reason unable to talk with a patient when he makes the request, she should acknowledge the patient's need and arrange to meet with him at a later time. If the nurse finds her attention waning because she is bored, she should consider why this is happening. The patient may be unconsciously "hypnotizing" the nurse in order to avoid getting in touch with painful or threatening feelings.

On occasion the nurse may need to interrupt the patient to seek clarification or to direct him into a more productive avenue of discussion. The nurse may also interrupt and redirect the discussion if the patient seems to be moving toward potentially harmful behavior (see Chapter 24 on the violent patient). Before interrupting, the nurse should be sure the interruption is not an attempt to talk for the patient by using her experience to fill in data or by making assumptions about what the patient is going to say or what he "should" say (Schmieding, 1984). Generally, the nurse should keep input to a minimum (as little as ten percent of the dialogue [Perls, 1969]).

When the nurse creates an environment in which feelings can be expressed openly and without fear of reprisal, it allows the patient to be himself, or to be congruent with true feelings (Rogers, 1961). The patient learns that expression of feelings is not wrong and does not lead to disaster. Rather, he learns that the expression of true feelings can have a healing effect.

RESPONDING

All communication is goal directed. In the therapeutic relationship the nurse is aware of its goals and responds accordingly. Goal setting is not a rigid process but a fluid one that changes with the situation. While the process is goal directed, responses cannot always be planned and shouldn't be automatic (based on the nurse's assumptions). They must focus on the patient in the present and relate to the patient's perceptions, feelings, and thoughts, confirming or disconfirming the nurse's impressions (Schmieding, 1984). Wondering or worrying about what to say or how to respond to the patient is a distraction to listening. Ideally, the nurse lets her responses come from her empathic self, in the specific situation (Perls, 1969).

The following list of types of responses is intended to help the nurse develop her ability to communicate therapeutically. The nurse uses these techniques in a flexible way, always guided by her ongoing assessment of the patient.

FEEDBACK. All communication is feedback. Here, feedback refers to responses that keep communication flowing, make content and context explicit, build relations, and focus on the here and now. These responses can be means to an end or ends in themselves. Feedback can be provided in the following ways.

1. The nurse listening with full attention focused on the patient encourages patient verbalization. This allows the patient the opportunity for emotional catharsis. The discharge of emotion that has previously clouded the patient's perspective may clear the way for the patient to gain insight into his situation and to prepare to tackle the problems he identifies.

2. The reflective response (Rogers, 1961) helps patients develop the ability to recognize, express, and clarify feelings. With this response, the nurse identifies the feeling underlying the patient's message and its intensity. The nurse labels the feeling and rates its intensity: "You feel very sad because the opportunity to reconcile is gone; it must feel overwhelming" (Henrich & Bernheim, 1981). Or a patient with clenched fists, set jaw, narrowed eyes, and thin lips states, "My husband cannot visit me today." The nurse identifies the anger expressed nonverbally and states, "You seem quite angry about your husband's not coming today."

3. Nonverbal responses, such as nods and gestures, and vocalizations, such as "uh-huh" or "mm-hm," encourage the patient to continue talking.

4. Restatement involves rephrasing what the nurse thinks the patient has said. Using her own words to describe how the patient seems to feel demonstrates attentiveness to the patient and allows him to confirm or correct the nurse's impression.

5. Questioning can be closed or open-ended. Closed-ended questions, which can be answered by "yes" or "no," focus and limit information, and, so, are useful in gathering specific data. Open-ended questions encourage expanding and exploring, for example, "How do you feel about that?" "How" questions are better than "why" questions which can feel like blaming and produce defensiveness (Satir, 1972).

6. Directives point the way for discussion. They include statements such as, "Tell me about. . . ."

7. Illustration and description involve asking the patient for examples or an operational definition to clarify meaning. This ties information to the extensional level of abstraction.

MIRRORING. The nurse can establish rapport by **mirroring** the patient's nonverbal behavior (Bandler & Grinder, 1979). The nurse mirrors by observing the patient and gradually assuming a similar posture, breathing pattern, and voice tone, and by moving her eyes in mirror image of the patient's eye movements (up or down, right to left, or a combination of these, as up-right). The patient's eye movements indicate the way he is remembering information, by seeing mental pictures (up, right, or left), mentally hearing sounds (right, left, or down left), or by reexperiencing body movement or sensations associated with the experiences (down, right) (Bandler & Grinder, 1979). The nurse should mirror slowly (to become comfortable with the changes) and respectfully (to avoid the appearance of mimicking or mocking the patient) (Knowles, 1983). Mirroring can help to build trust and help the nurse gain a new perspective on the patient's experience (Knowles, 1983). Once mirroring is established, the nurse can lead the patient into different feeling states or moods by changing aspects of the behaviors being mirrored at a pace the patient can follow. In this way, patients might be led from a tense state (muscles tight, limbs close to body, fast breathing rate, and so on) to a more relaxed or more open state (muscles relaxed, arms relaxed and away from body, slower breathing).

SELF-DISCLOSURE. **Self-disclosure** involves revealing relevant aspects of one's experience, including personal thoughts, attitudes, feelings, values, and so forth. Self-disclosure must be honest and congruent if the patient is to see the nurse as a fellow human being and someone to whom the patient can relate. It is a tool for building relationships. Self-disclosure encourages patient self-disclosure and often leads to feelings of self-worth in the patient (Hazlewood &

Schuldt, 1977). For both nurse and patient, self-disclosure can become a way to know the self (Jourard, 1974).

The nurse uses self-disclosure with sensitivity and discrimination. When the patient requests disclosure from her, she must first decide if she is comfortable making the disclosure and if doing so is in the best interest of the patient. If asked, "Nurse, do you have a pet?" the nurse may answer, "Yes, I have a dog. I miss him when I am away from him." This disclosure informs the patient and provides a lead for the patient to express his feelings. When the nurse is not comfortable with the request for self-disclosure, for example when a patient expresses interest in her sex life, she can respond to what she feels is behind the patient's need for such information. In this case, it might be the patient's anxiety about his own sexuality or sexual functioning.

Self-disclosure can also be used to inform the patient of how the nurse is experiencing him. Such disclosure, the result of the nurse's insight and empathy, is made in an open, nonthreatening manner, and is a model for self-observation.

The first step in self-disclosure is to check to be sure the feelings to be disclosed are a response to the patient and not to something else. Does the nurse feel warmth toward Mr. Smith because of Mr. Smith or because Mr. Smith reminds the nurse of her father? Is the nurse angry at the patient's behavior or angry because another nurse was twenty minutes late for work? Self-disclosure must always address the patient's needs, and never serve as an opportunity for the nurse to discuss her problems.

The second step is to decide whether the disclosure is relevant to the patient, appropriate in the particular situation, and if the patient is ready to deal with the information at that time. Self-disclosure is most helpful if it reflects an area of difficulty for the patient and thus will assist the patient to resolve the difficulty. A disclosure is most effective if the patient is already somewhat aware of the information. If the disclosure is too far from the patient's awareness, he may have difficulty considering and accepting it.

Finally, the nurse should make disclosures at a rate comfortable for the patient. He needs time to consider what the nurse has said. Too much information given too fast can short-circuit the patient's ability to reflect on what the nurse has said and to use it to solve his problems.

The nurse must remember that self-disclosures are a revelation of the nurse's experience. Thus, they have been filtered through and distorted by the nurse's perceptual screen. The nurse must allow the patient room to correct misconceptions, both the nurse's and the patient's. Self-disclosures are expressed in "I" statements, indicating the nurse takes responsibility for the statement. "I am so happy you made the effort to attend the meeting today." "I feel angry when you shout at me." The nurse offers self-disclosures to allow the patient to experience the results of the patient's behavior and to decide if the results are satisfactory. By facing the consequences of his actions, the patient learns responsibility for himself (Combs, Avila, & Purkey, 1974.).

INFORMING. When the patient requests information, or the nurse perceives such a need, the nurse can respond in a number of ways (Benjamin, 1969).

1. The nurse may determine that the feelings behind the question are more important than the information requested. If the patient says, "Could I wake up during my surgery?" the nurse might reply, "I wonder if you are frightened about anesthesia during your surgery."

2. Rather than just giving information, it may be more helpful for the nurse to take the patient through a problem-solving process to discover answers for himself. Using this approach in the example above, the nurse may help the patient identify his anxious feelings and the source of these feelings. The nurse and patient would then identify a number of possible methods of dealing with the anxiety, perhaps through relaxation techniques, meditation, or discussion and resolution of the patient's myths and fears surrounding surgery. The nurse and patient would then choose one or more of the alternatives, employ them, and assess the results.

3. Finally, if the patient needs information but the nurse is not able to provide it, or feels another health team member would be more helpful, she should state this and arrange for the patient to see that professional: "I am unable to answer your question, but I will ask the dietitian to speak with you."

METAMODEL. The **metamodel** is a linguistic tool used to tie language to experience (Bandler & Grinder, 1975). It can be used to listen to the way people talk, to understand their mental maps, to challenge their verbal representation of experience, and to expand their mental maps (Bandler & Grinder, 1975).

The metamodel addresses the ways people limit and distort experience. These "ways" fall into three categories: data deficits, structure limitations, and semantic ill-formedness (Cameron-Bandler, 1978). In the following discussion each category is defined, and responses are suggested. With each response, the nurse (*N*) challenges the patient's (*P*) mental map.

Responses are questions asking who, what, and how, to draw out specific information and help the patient begin to understand his mental map.

Data deficits result from tendencies to generalize from specific past experience to all experience. People generalize by leaving out information. The nurse focuses on having the patient include information. Responses to data deficits serve to gather specific data which demonstrate the uniqueness of events.

P: "I do not like it." ("It" leaves out information.)

N: "You do not like what?" In response to generalized referents—persons, places, and things—the nurse asks for specific referents.)

P: "No one cares about me." ("No one" is general.)

N: "Who, specifically, does not care?" (In response to generalized verbs, the nurse asks for specifics.)

P: "He hurt me." ("Hurt" can mean feelings or physical pain.)

N: "How did he hurt you?" (Finally, when processes are perceived as events, the nurse focuses on the nature of the process.)

P: "I cannot understand." (Understanding is not a past event; it can still be accomplished.)

N: "How could you understand?"

Model distortions are limitations of the patient's mental map. Responses challenge the limitations the patient assumes exist. Universal qualifiers are generalizations that stop choice. Words used include "always," "never," "all," and "every."

P: "I always get a raw deal."

N: "You always, every time, get a raw deal?" *or* "Have you ever gotten a fair deal?"

Lack of choice is indicated by words such as "have to," "must," "no choice," and "no alternative." The two best responses are, "What is stopping you?" and "What would happen if you did?" The patient might say, "I cannot place my husband in a nursing home." The nurse can respond, "What would happen if you did?"

The final area of map distortion is **semantic ill-formedness.** Sentences which are semantically ill-formed are evidence of a limitation of the mental map (Cameron-Bandler, 1978). By challenging the sentence and having the patient expand verbally, he may also expand his mental map. Responses highlight these distortions. In cause-and-effect distortions

the patient believes that another person's actions have caused his feelings or behavior. The patient sees himself as not having a choice of emotions or behavior, but as one who only reacts. The best response is to ask, "How does one cause the other?" (If the patient says, "She makes me so mad," the nurse can respond, "How does she make you feel mad?")

Mind reading involves using the internal map to fill in data about another person or to read the other's thoughts or emotions. The patient could say, "I know the doctor is worried about my condition." The nurse might respond, "How, specifically, do you know she is worried?"

When a patient practices judging, he takes his rules or values, beliefs, and prejudices and applies them universally. The individual may not be aware of doing this. He might say, "It is wrong to sign a living will." The nurse can respond by asking, "It is wrong for whom to sign?"

Bandler and Grinder (1979) make a number of relevant points about communication. The nurse must have in mind the desired outcome or goal of an interaction and the responses that signal it. She should have enough skill in observing nonverbal behavior to know when desired responses occur. When a response occurs, the nurse must differentiate between the patient's actual response and her personal interpretation of that response based on her own internal map. The nurse must accept that the response received is the response she elicited and be aware of how her internal state elicited that response. *If the nurse continues to use the same behavior, she will be likely to elicit the same response.* If the response received is not the one desired, rather than fighting the response the nurse can use that response to modify her behavior until the desired response is obtained. The nurse can change voice tone, facial expression, body position, words used, and so forth. She needs to have many behaviors available and use them flexibly. With practice, the skills involved in effective communication—observing nonverbal behavior, listening, changing one's behavior, mirroring, asking metamodel questions—must be practiced and so thoroughly integrated that they can be used without conscious effort.

EFFECTIVENESS OF RESPONSES. Any response to the patient may be appropriate or inappropriate, or may be successful to varying degrees, in a given situation. Skill in communicating is the ability to assess situations and use responses appropriately. When the nurse's anxiety about communicating or her hurried schedule leads to avoiding the patient's meaning by using empty reassurances, cliches, or generalizations, it hurts the patient. Through these responses, the nurse ignores the patient's needs, and the message the nurse sends through metacommunication is that the patient is not important. An honest effort at open communication, taking the risk of making errors, and goal-directed practice in communication will lead to increasing ease and success in responding therapeutically.

Marie: A Nurse Who Responds Effectively

Marie entered Karen Rogers' room and found her lying in bed, facing the wall, and crying. Marie pulled a chair between the bed and wall, sat down, and leaned forward so her face was on a level with Karen's. She put her hand on Karen's shoulder and stated, "You're pretty upset." Karen said nothing and continued to cry. Marie felt uncomfortable with the silence; she wondered if Karen would rather be alone. After a couple of minutes had elapsed, Marie stated, "I'd like to try to help with whatever is troubling you, but if you would rather be alone, I understand." Karen was silent for another two minutes, then said, "I'm not sure why I'm crying. Everything seems wrong. My life is a mess with me here in the hospital."

Marie responded, "What is wrong in your life?" Karen listed, "I'm sick and stuck here. My boss is going to fire me, I know. My rent is due, and I left my checkbook at home. My plants haven't been watered in a week."

When Karen stopped talking, Marie waited a few seconds to be sure Karen was finished and then addressed the problems. She asked how Karen knew her boss would fire her. Karen said that she had assumed that would happen. After thinking about it, Karen concluded she could call her boss, explain she was ill, and ask about sick time. Next, Marie asked Karen about people in her life who care about her and might be able to help her now. Karen listed a number of friends and relatives. As she spoke, her face lit up, and she said, "Of course, how dumb that I didn't think of it. My mom has a key to my apartment. She can water my plants and bring me my checkbook. I can call her before she leaves home for the hospital."

Marie responded, "Why don't you call your mom and your boss now and get those things settled? I'll come back a little later. We can talk about how you're doing and how it has been for you to be here." Karen responded that she already felt better than she did a few minutes ago, but she would like a chance to ask some questions about her illness and treatment.

Case Study: Therapeutic Communication

Demographic Data

Name: Matthew Andrews

Age: 27 years

Address: 2000 Clearview Road, #137, Philadelphia, PA

Ethnicity: Caucasian/English

Diagnosis: Schizophrenia, Paranoid, Stable Type

Setting: Stockton Street Community Mental Health Outpatient Clinic

Occupation: Construction Worker

Present Problem

Matt Andrews entered the Stockton Street Clinic, looked around the room, stomped to Mrs. Fernandez's desk in the reception area of the clinic, threw his medications on the counter, and shouted, "This junk doesn't work! Are you trying to poison me? I spent a lot of money in that hospital! This medication costed me $50.00 . . . and I don't feel any better! I have got to feel better! . . . You are all a bunch of rip-off artists . . . money-grabbing quacks!" Matthew was not one of the many patients that the receptionist, Mrs. Fernandez, knew very well.

Mrs. Fernandez stood up, leaned on the desk, pointed her finger to the door, and emphatically stated in a rather loud voice, "You see that door! Well, you either keep your voice down, or I will have security put you out of here! My advice to you is to shut up and sit down!"

Matt leaned toward Mrs. Fernandez, pounded on the desk, and had begun to speak louder when Tim Graham, the nurse in charge of the clinic, walked in. Tim had heard the shouting and came to investigate. He motioned for Mrs. Fernandez to sit down. Slowly and softly, Tim said to Matt, "I'd like to listen to your complaint, but I find it hard to listen when there is shouting. Let's go into my office and talk." Tim turned and walked to the door. When he looked back, Matt was standing still, apparently trying to decide what to do. Tim added, "I know you're angry, and you have no reason to trust me; but, maybe together, we can work on whatever is so upsetting." Matt followed Tim.

As they entered the office, Tim extended his hand, and he and Matt shook hands. Then Tim closed the door. He offered Matt a seat and a cup of coffee. Matt accepted the coffee and sat down.

Tim responded, "How can I help you, Matt?" At this point, Matt began to tell Tim that he had recently been in the hospital, that he thought he was getting better, but now was beginning to have some doubts.

Tim listened attentively to Matt. He positioned himself level with Matt, allowing space between them so that he could move toward Matt if he chose to. Tim listened, but did not become defensive about Matt's negative comments regarding his inpatient treatment. Instead, Tim maintained eye contact and encouraged Matt to describe his feelings. Matt's hostility and anger did not interfere with Tim's genuine interest in trying to understand Matt's thoughts and feelings.

As Matt poured out his emotions, Tim assumed a body position similar to Matt (crossing his legs and placing his arms across his chest), turned his head and body slightly away from Matt, hunched his shoulders, held his head down and tightened his facial muscles, and breathed at the same rate as Matt.

Tim then stated in a calm and empathic manner, "How are you feeling right now?" Matt was silent for nearly five minutes. Then he began to tell Tim that he was frightened and scared: "I'm starting to hear voices again. . . . I got no sleep last night. Tim, I'm very scared! Sometimes I think I'd rather be dead than to go on living like this. . . . Man, this is hell!" Tim commented, "Yes," nodding his head, . . . "go on." Matt continued, "My job is on the line. My boss is beginning to think that I can't handle my job. My buddies, well, they think I'm paranoid and don't want to associate with them. The thing that upsets me the most is how my wife and kid suffer! . . . Tim, I need help! Can you help me!"

When Matt finished talking, Tim asked him to describe how he was taking his medication. Matt responded in a very vague manner, "I take some of the pills." There was silence. Tim concluded that Matt knew very little about his medication. Tim discussed with Matt why he had been prescribed the medication (Thorazine 200 mg bid); the therapeutic benefits of the medication; the possible side effects; and so forth.

Slowly, as Tim talked and changed his body language, Matt began to follow by changing to a more relaxed and open body position. Matt listened carefully to Tim's explanation. Tim then offered to write down the instructions for taking the medication. Matt responded, "It won't do any good; I can't read!"

Tim considered this and suggested, "I wonder if you were so angry before because you were frustrated because you couldn't read the label on your medication and you didn't want to ask for help."

Matt thought for a moment and said, "I get mad a lot and I also think people don't like me . . . I never thought it was because I can't read. I think I probably miss a lot because I can't read and I don't want to ask and look stupid. Maybe that makes me mad."

Tim continued to change his body posture as the situation indicated, and asked, "Have you thought about how you might begin to read?"

Matt stated, "I've heard they have reading classes for adults at the high school. I've thought about going, but I thought I'd feel like a jerk doing that." Tim asked, "How do you see your choices and your future?"

After thinking about this, Matt said, "Well, I guess I can go on not reading and maybe missing out on things, or I can feel like a jerk and go to school."

"Could you go to school and not feel like a jerk, but feel some other way about yourself?" "What do you think?"

Again, Matt thought and responded, "Maybe I'd feel proud of myself if I could read. I think I can learn if I try."

Tim commented in a sincere and genuine manner, "I think you *can* learn to read. I would like to be a source of support and encouragement as you learn. I think it's terrific that you want to learn to read!"

Matt smiled and commented, "I need to take my medication right now." As Tim provided a cup of water, Matt was repeating the information Tim had provided: "Take two pills in the morning, and two pills right before I go to bed." Matt said thanks to Tim as he accepted the water from him. He smiled, stood up, reached to shake Tim's hand, and said, "Thanks, Mr. Graham . . . Thank you!" Matt left Tim's office.

History of Present Problem

After Matthew Andrews had left Tim Graham's office, Tim retrieved Matt's clinical summary and determined the following:

Matthew Andrews has lived and worked in Philadelphia all of his life. He has been employed as a handy-man, construction worker, and a janitor most of his adult life. Matt was able to provide the basic necessities for himself and his family until he began to hear voices and to believe that people were, "out to harm him." During the past three years, he had five brief psychiatric hospitalizations.

Psychiatric History

When Matt was a student in middle school (seventh grade), he was seen by a school psychologist for "temper tantrums, poor academic performance, and poor social adjustment." During that year, he was suspended from school six times for fighting. Matt did not complete the seventh grade.

Family History

Matt's father was a construction worker in the Philadelphia area. His mother died when he was quite young. In fact, Matt had commented that he did not remember his mother but could recall his mother's sister who, on occasion, took him into her home.

Matt has one brother who was raised by foster parents. Matt never got to know his brother and does not know where his brother currently resides.

Matt has been married for eight years. He has one son, age three.

Social History

Matt Andrews spent his early years living with his father. They moved about in the city, seeking better housing, a safer neighborhood, and employment (for his father). Matt stated, "I never felt we stayed any place long. My Dad and I were always on the move. Things were difficult for both of us. I never had many friends . . . used to hang out with my Dad's working buddies . . . actually, a tough life for a kid." Matt felt that he and his father deeply cared for each other. Matt's father died three years ago; Matt experienced his first hospitalization about six months later.

Medical History

Matt has been healthy most of his life. He does complain of a pain in his back and attributes that to the strenuous activity associated with construction work. During the winter months, he "catches colds and has the flu about twice before springtime."

Current Mental Status

General Appearance: Disheveled, loud, upset, and demanding.
Sensorium: Oriented to time, place, and person.
Emotion: Upset, shouting, frightened, flinging arms, accusatory, and so forth.
Motoric Behavior: Constant motion, moving body and arms, looking around room, staring, pounding on desk, etc.
Thought Process: Abrupt, detached, intense.
Thought Content: Suspicious, complaining about medication.

Medications

Thorazine, others not known at this time.

Summary

Matthew Andrews is a 27-year-old man who came to the Stockton Street Community Mental Health Outpatient Clinic complaining that his medications are not helping him. He appeared frightened, suspicious, and demanding.

Five Axes

Axis I: 295.3x, Schizophrenia, Paranoid, Stable Type (from patient's record).
Axis II: Antisocial Personality Disorder (from patient's record).
Axis III: Not known at this time.
Axis IV: Psychosocial stressors: illiteracy; severity: 2 (other stressors not known at this time).
Axis V: Current GAF: 45; Highest GAF in Past Year: Unknown.

Nursing Diagnosis

Impaired verbal Communication
Anxiety
Social Isolation
Ineffective Individual coping

Non-Compliance (not taking prescribed medication; patient cannot read)

Disturbance in Self-Esteem

Knowledge Deficit (does not understand basic information relating to neuroleptic therapy and his psychiatric disorder)

Hopelessness (related to inability to read and thus follow medication instructions)

SUMMARY

Communication is a complex process, closer to weaving a tapestry than shooting an arrow at a target. The skilled communicator constantly weighs and balances many factors to achieve successful communication and does so spontaneously as interactions unfold. Both intrapersonal and interpersonal communication are involved in therapeutic communication.

Self-awareness, a large part of intrapersonal communication, is the foundation for effective interpersonal communication. A clear and stable self-concept, understanding of the communication process, and skill and flexibility in communication techniques are essential for consistent, effective communication, a vital part of nursing practice.

The three theories of communication are: double-bind theory, which places two people in a communication "bind"; pragmatics-of-communication theory, which looks at the dynamics of communication and how relationships are defined through communication; and dysfunctional or ineffective communication, which follows four patterns (placating, blaming, computing, and distracting). A fifth pattern, called leveling, is functional communication.

Listening and responding are important components of therapeutic communication. Feedback, mirroring, self-disclosure, informing, and metamodel questions are types of responses that facilitate therapeutic communication. The challenge to the nurse is to integrate her knowledge of communication theory and technique into practice, creating a growth-enhancing environment for her patients.

KEY TERMS

intrapersonal communication

interpersonal communication

organizational communication

redundancy

feedback

positive feedback

negative feedback

coding

meaning

metacommunication

open receiver

dogmatic receiver

self

self-concept

perception

congruent

incongruent

awareness

fully functioning person

values

values clarification

values indicators

mental maps

extensional level of abstraction

intensional level of abstraction

paralanguage

body language

kinesics

affective display

relationships

regulators

monitors

quasi-courting

proxemics

double-bind theory

pragmatics of communication

punctuation sequence

placating

blaming

computing

distracting

leveling

mirroring

self-disclosure

informing

metamodel

data deficits

model distortions

semantic ill-formedness

STUDY QUESTIONS

1. Define and describe intrapersonal and interpersonal communication.

2. What effect do self-awareness and values have on communication?

3. Name and describe two aspects of verbal communication and two aspects of nonverbal communication.

4. What are the three theories of communication?

5. How do listening and responding work to enhance therapeutic communication?

REFERENCES

Bandler, R., & Grinder, J. (1975). *The structure of magic I.* Palo Alto, CA: Science and Behavior Books.

Bandler, R., & Grinder, J. (1979). *Frogs into princes. Neuro linguistic programming.* Moab, Utah: Real People Press.

Barnett, K. (1972). A survey of the current utilization of touch by health team personnel with hospitalized patients. *International Journal of Nursing Studies, 9,* 125–209.

Bateson, G. (1966). Information, codification, and meta-communication. In A. G. Smith (Ed.), *Communication and culture.* New York: Holt, Rinehart, and Winston, pp. 412–426.

Bateson, G., Jackson, D.D., Haley, J., & Weakland, J. (1956). Toward a theory of schizophrenia. *Behavioral Science, 1,* 251–264.

Benjamin, A. (1969). *The helping interview.* Boston: Houghton Mifflin.

Birdwhistell, R. L. (1970). *Kinesics and context.* Philadelphia: University of Pennsylvania Press.

Buber, M. (1957). Elements of the interhuman. *Psychiatry, 20,* 105–113.

Byrne, T. J., & Edeani, D. (1984). Knowledge of medical terminology among hospital patients. *Nursing Research, 33,* 178–181.

Cameron-Bandler, L. (1978). *They lived happily ever after.* Cupertino, CA: Meta Publications.

Coad-Denton, A. (1978). Therapeutic superficiality and intimacy. In D. C. Longo & R. A. Williams (Eds.), *Clinical practice in psychosocial nursing: Assessment and interventions.* New York: Appleton-Century-Crofts.

Colby, B. N. (1966). Behavioral redundancy. In A. G. Smith (Ed.), *Communication and culture.* New York: Holt, Rinehart, & Winston, pp. 367–373.

Combs, A. W., Avila, D. L., & Purkey, W. W. (1974). *Helping relationships.* Boston: Allyn & Bacon.

Edwards, B. J., & Brilhart, J. K. (1981). *Communication in nursing practice.* St. Louis: C. V. Mosby.

Eibl-Eibesfeldt, I. (1974). Similarities and differences between cultures in expressive movements. In S. Weitz (Ed.), *Nonverbal communication.* New York: Oxford Press, pp. 20–33.

Ekman, P., & Friesen, W. (1969). Nonverbal leakage and clues to deception. In S. Weitz (Ed.), *Nonverbal communication.* New York: Oxford Press, pp. 269–290.

Felder, R. E., Malone, T. P., & Warkentin, J. (1982). First-stage techniques in the experiential psychotherapy of chronic schizophrenic patients. In J. Neill and D. Kniskern (Eds.), *From psyche to system, the evolving therapy of Carl Whitaker.* New York: The Guildford Press, pp. 90–104.

Foley, V. (1986). *Family therapy.* Orlando: Grune and Stratton.

Foley, V. F. (1974). *An introduction to family therapy.* New York: Grune and Stratton.

Fromm, E. (1956). *The art of loving.* New York: Bantam Books.

Garant, C. (1980). Stalls in the therapeutic process. *American Journal of Nursing, 80,* 2166–2169.

Garfield, S. L. (1980). *Psychotherapy: An eclectic approach.* New York: John Wiley & Sons.

Green, C. P. (1986). How to recognize hostility and what to do about it. *American Journal of Nursing,* Vol. 86, #11, 1230–1234.

Greenberg, D. (1964). *How to be a Jewish mother.* Los Angeles: Price, Sloan and Stern, p. 16.

Grinder, J., & Bandler, R. (1976). *Structure of magic II.* Palo Alto, CA: Science and Behavior Books.

Hall, E. T. (1959). *The silent language.* New York: Doubleday.

Hall, E. T. (1974). Proxemics. In S. Weitz (Ed.), *Nonverbal communication.* New York: Oxford Press, pp. 205–221.

Hazlewood, M. G., & Schuldt, W. J. (1977). Effects of physical and phenomenological distance on self-disclosure. *Perceptual and Motor Skills, 45,* 805–806.

Henrick, A. P., & Bernheim, K. F. (1981). Responding to patients' concerns. *Nursing Outlook,* July, Vol. 29, #7, 428–433.

Jones, S. (1980). *Family therapy, a comparison of approaches.* Bowie: Brady Co.

Jourard, S. M. (1974). *The transparent self.* New York: Van Nostrand Reinhold.

Knowles, R. D. (1983). Building rapport through neuro-linguistic programming. *American Journal of Nursing, 83,* 1011–1013.

Korzybski, A. (1933). *Science and sanity.* Lakeville, CT: International Non-Aristotelian Library.

Kübler-Ross, E. (1969). *On death and dying.* New York: MacMillan.

Lyman, S., & Scott, M. B. (1967). Territoriality: A neglected sociological dimension. *Social Problems, 15,* 236–240.

McCorkley, R. (1974). Effects of touch on seriously ill patients. *Nursing Research,* Vol. 23, #2, p. 125–132.

Maslow, A. H. (1963). Self-actualizing people. In G. B. Levitas (Ed.), *The world of psychology.* (Vol. 2). New York: Braziller, pp. 527–556.

Masson, V. (1985). Nurses and doctors as healers. *Nursing Outlook, 33,* 70–73.

Miller, J. F. (1985). Inspiring hope. *American Journal of Nursing, 85,* 22–25.

Perls, F. S. (1969). *Gestalt therapy verbatim.* New York: Bantam Books.

Perls, F. S., Hefferline, R. F., & Goodman, P. (1951). *Gestalt therapy.* New York: Bantam Books.

Pittenger, R. E., & Smith, H. L. (1966) A basis for some contributions of linguistics to psychiatry. In A. G. Smith (Ed.), *Communication and culture.* New York: Holt, Rinehart, & Winston, pp. 169–181.

Pluckhan, M. L. (1978). *Human communication, the matrix of nursing.* New York: McGraw-Hill.

Rapoport, A. (1962). What is semantics? In S. I. Hayakawa (Ed.), *The use and misuse of language.* Greenwich, CT: Fawcett, pp. 11–25.

Raths, L. E., Harmin, M., & Simon, S. B. (1966). *Values and teaching.* Columbus, OH: Merrill.

Reik, T. (1948). *Listening with the third ear.* New York: Grove Press.

Rogers, C. R. (1961). *On becoming a person.* Boston: Houghton Mifflin.

Rogers, C. R. (1980). *A way of being*. Boston: Houghton Mifflin.

Rubin, R. (1963). Maternal touch. *Nursing Outlook,* Vol. 11, p. 829–831.

Ruesch, J. (1957). *Disturbed communication*. New York: W. W. Norton.

Satir, V. (1972). *Peoplemaking*. Palo Alto, CA: Science and Behavior Books.

Scheflen, A. E. (1972). *Body language and the social order*. London: Prentice-Hall.

Scheflen, A. E. (1974). Quasi-courting behavior in psychotherapy. In S. Weitz (Ed.), *Nonverbal communication*. New York: Oxford Press, pp. 182–197.

Schmieding, N. J. (1984). Putting Orlando's theory into practice. *American Journal of Nursing, 84,* 758–761.

Simon, S. B., Howe, L. W., & Kirschenbaum, H. (1978). *Values clarification*. New York: Dodd Mead.

Smith, F. B. (1985). Patient power. *American Journal of Nursing, 85,* 1260–1262.

Stein, D. (1985). *The interpersonal world of the infant*. New York: Basic Books, pp. 41–42.

Steinberg, C. S. (1970). *The communication arts*. New York: Hastings House.

Trevarthan, C., and Hul. (1978). Secondary intersubjectivity: confidence, confiders, and acts of meaning in the first year. In A. Lock (Ed.), *Action, gesture, and symbol: The emergence of language*. New York: Academic Press.

Ujhely, G. B. (1979). Touch: Reflections and perceptions. *Nursing Forum, 18,* 19–32.

Watzlawick, P., Beavin, J., & Jackson, D. (1967). *Pragmatics of human communication*. New York: Norton, p. 188.

Weiss, S. J. (1979). The language of touch. *Nursing Research, 28,* 76–79.

Whorf, B. L. (1956). *Language, thought, and reality*. Cambridge: M. I. T. Press.

5

PSYCHIATRIC ASSESSMENT FOR THE GENERALIST NURSE

ELIZABETH SHENKMAN

LEARNING OBJECTIVES

After studying this chapter, the student will be able to:

- Describe the purpose of psychiatric assessment.
- Explain the relationship between assessment and the psychoanalytic and behavioral models.
- Describe the different nursing models for assessment and understand their function.
- Identify the components of psychiatric assessment.
- Identify and define the five axes of DSM-III-R.
- Describe the different methods of psychological testing and understand their functions.

INTRODUCTION

A **psychiatric assessment** is an examination of both the mind and the body of a patient. The nurse uses the data from the entire psychiatric assessment to make a diagnosis of the patient's presenting problems. In this chapter we first explore the purpose and components of the psychiatric assessment, including the psychiatric interview (within the framework of psychoanalytic, behavioral, and biological models) and physiological assessment; then we discuss assessment for the purpose of making a diagnosis using DSM-III-R and Approved Nursing Diagnoses, North American Nursing Diagnosis Association.

A nurse and patient often make their first contact with each other in the psychiatric interview. The interview may be conceptualized as an art; the clinician employs a set of principles directed by fundamental theory, and applies them to each unique situation. In order to develop the skill of psychiatric interviewing, the nurse must have a thorough knowledge of the purpose and components of the entire psychiatric assessment.

OVERVIEW OF PSYCHIATRIC ASSESSMENT

THE PURPOSE OF PSYCHIATRIC ASSESSMENT

The *psychiatric assessment* elicits information regarding the origin and development of a patient's current behavioral disturbances, current mental status, and past social, psychological, and cultural influences. The assessment also takes into consideration physiological factors.

Throughout the assessment, the interaction between the nurse and the patient is purposeful—it is directed toward a goal. The nurse collects data in a systematic way to gain a basic understanding of the patient's particular problems and behavior. This process in turn leads to the development of a plan for the patient's treatment.

The specific goals of the interview may vary depending on the patient, the interview setting, and the situation surrounding the interaction. Regardless of these specifics, the nurse has the following clearly defined goals: 1) to develop a relationship with the patient; 2) to gather sufficient information about the patient to begin to work therapeutically with him; 3) to assess the patient's past and current level of functioning; and 4) to begin to develop a care plan (Hagerty, 1984).

Unfortunately the patient may not share these same goals. The goals of the patient and nurse may conflict, hindering the development of a therapeutic relationship. For example, the patient may deny having a problem or may tell a vague story that is difficult to separate into specific patterns and feelings. The nurse must help the patient define the problem and decide on a realistic desired outcome. The nurse can help the patient to take the first step toward this goal with a systematic evaluation of the patient's past and current functioning.

THE NURSE–PATIENT RELATIONSHIP

In conducting a successful interview, the nurse carefully manages her interaction with the patient. There are no absolute rules for the adept management of an interview, but there are some general guidelines. First, the nurse should play an active, vital role in the interview process; she should structure and guide the interaction while making an ongoing, objective assessment of the patient's behavior. Second, Kolb and Brodie (1982) recommend that the nurse conduct the initial interview in a private setting to maintain confidentiality and to enhance communication. Third, people who consult a psychiatrist or a psychiatric nurse exhibit anxiety or fear that they will be viewed as "crazy." A calm, matter-of-fact approach by the nurse may do much to allay these fears and increase patient self-disclosure. Kolb and Brodie (1982) note that a simple, yet often overlooked,

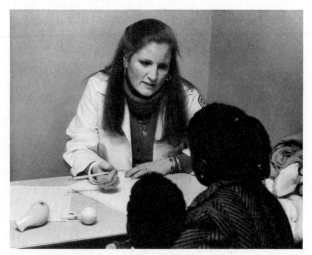

A successful interview incorporates four general principles implemented by the nurse therapist: 1) guide the course of the interview; 2) ensure that confidentiality is maintained; 3) present a calm, direct approach; and 4) provide a certain amount of flexibility.

handshake can bring an element of warmth and respect, thereby setting the tone for the initial relationship between the patient and nurse. The nurse should demonstrate interest and concern for the patient and his problems, regardless of the patient's socioeconomic status, appearance, or degree of personal integration. Fourth, the nurse should remain flexible. If the patient is allowed spontaneity and flexibility, he is more likely to provide detailed information. Fifth, judicious use of guiding questions in an interview is important. Skillful questioning allows the nurse to obtain important details surrounding the patient's life and current problems.

MAJOR MODELS RELATED TO ASSESSMENT

Before discussing the format of the psychiatric interview, it is important to examine the major models that the nurse can use to guide the assessment. Of course, when conducting a psychiatric interview, which is one aspect of the assessment, the nurse must know the manifestations and etiology of various psychiatric disorders in order to recognize their signs and ask intelligent questions. In addition, the nurse can benefit by the use of a conceptual framework, or model, within which to organize data. The use of such a framework also enables her to generate hypotheses about the nature of the patient's problem, test these hypotheses, and plan treatment.

The major models for understanding human behavior discussed in Chapter 2 provide different perspectives related to psychiatric interviewing and assessment. Two of these models, the psychoanalytic and the behavioral, are described here, along with their implications for assessment. In addition, the general categories of nursing models and their relationship to assessment are presented.

The use of models has advantages and disadvantages. When choosing a model to guide her practice, the nurse is aware of the implications the model has for assessment and treatment of the patient. While a model can serve as a tool to guide the practitioner, it can also limit her: the practitioner may fail to see certain dimensions of a patient's problem if the model does not address them. Kuhn (1962) cites a noted historian who stated that different models allow a person to handle "the same bunch of data as before, but placing them in a new system of relations with one another by giving them a different framework." Thus, "the marks on the paper that were first seen as a bird are now seen as an antelope, or vice versa" (p. 85).

Mary: A Patient with Severe Anxiety

Mary was a 60-year-old woman who was hospitalized on an inpatient psychiatric unit for severe anxiety. During the six months before her admission, Mary had refused to leave her home, stating that she was afraid to be around anyone except her husband.

In analyzing this problem and developing an intervention, a behaviorist might focus on events that seemed to elicit the anxiety. The behavior therapist might then have begun a program of systematic desensitization or might have gradually exposed Mary to the feared situation until she was able to function more effectively around other people.

A psychoanalytic therapist might have attempted to understand Mary's personality to determine the source of her current anxiety. This therapist would have placed less emphasis on situational variables and more emphasis on intrapsychic variables. A psychoanalytic therapist may have spent more time discussing Mary's past and its influence on her current problem.

Depending on the model a nurse chooses to use, Mary's case can be viewed as largely internal (intrapsychic) or external (situational). The treatments would vary according to the model used. Mary's nurse should be aware of the theoretical perspective guiding her assessment of Mary while remaining aware that there are other perspectives from which to view the case. And, since one approach might be more successful than another with a particular patient, the nurse should be flexible about the choice of a particular model, perhaps changing from one model to another in order to find the approach that is most effective.

THE PSYCHOANALYTIC MODEL AND ASSESSMENT

All approaches to assessment share the same goal: to elicit reliable, valid, and useful data. However, the methods may vary considerably due to different underlying assumptions. The **psychoanalytic model** emphasizes inner causes. Psychopathology is thought to result from relatively unstable intrapsychic variables or inner causes (Goldfried & Kent, 1972; Mischel, 1968), such as personality and level of psychosexual development.

As early as their first contact the patient and/or nurse may exhibit behavior associated with any of three basic concepts of psychoanalytic theory: resistance, transference, and/or countertransference

(Fromm-Reichman, 1950; Kernberg, 1965; Mischel, 1981).

RESISTANCE. Resistance is a patient's struggle against change. The patient's struggle is both conscious and unconscious and leads the patient, paradoxically, to both seek and reject help. Resistance may manifest itself in many different ways. Perhaps the most obvious is when the patient states that he doesn't have a problem and sees no reason for the interview.

Defense mechanisms are mental attributes that protect the individual against internal dangers that arise because of threatening thoughts, impulses, and affects. They assist the individual in dealing with anxiety. See Table 5–1 for a list of common defense mechanisms.

The resistant patient may become uncooperative *or* excessively compliant; the individual may joke, show hostility or aggression, refuse to discuss problems, or announce that the problems have been resolved. It is important that the nurse recognize resistance when it occurs in the interview. Knowledge of resistance can provide insight into the patient's level of functioning as well as alert the nurse to potential conflicts in developing a therapeutic relationship.

TRANSFERENCE. According to Greenson (1972), **transference** is the experiencing of feelings, drives, attitudes, fantasies, and defenses toward a person in the present that do not befit that person but rather are a repetition of reactions originating with significant others during early childhood, unconsciously

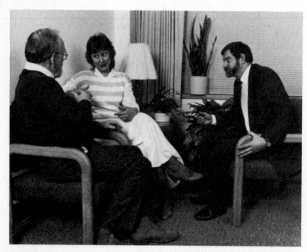

Transference can be utilized to facilitate communication between the patient and the nurse therapist. Transference can also be used by the patient as a defense or resistance to therapeutic change.

TABLE 5–1 Defense mechanisms

Premature Defenses

Denial—unpleasant realities are ignored. Realities are kept out of conscious awareness so that anxiety is reduced.

Projection—a person attributes to another those generally unconscious ideas, thoughts, feelings, and impulses that are in himself or herself undesirable or unacceptable.

Introjection—the unconscious internalization of a mental representation of a hated or loved external object with the goal of establishing closeness to a constant presence of the object.

Regression—a person undergoes a partial or total return to earlier periods of adaptation. Seen in many psychiatric conditions, especially schizophrenia.

Dissociation—the separation of any group of mental or behavioral processes from the rest of the person's psychic activities.

Isolation—the separation of an idea or memory from its associated emotional tone.

Mature Defenses

Sublimation—the energy associated with unacceptable impulses or drives is diverted into personally and socially acceptable channels.

Suppression—conscious act of controlling and inhibiting an unacceptable impulse, emotion, or idea.

Rationalization—irrational, or unacceptable, behavior, motives, or feelings are logically justified or made tolerable.

Identification—a person patterns him or herself after another person.

Source: Adapted from Kaplan, H. I., and Sadock, B. J. (1985). *Comprehensive textbook of psychiatry* (4th ed., Vol. 1). Baltimore: Williams & Wilkins. And from Kaplan, H. I. and Sadock, B. J. (1988). *Synopsis of psychiatry.* Baltimore: Williams & Wilkins, p. 312.

displaced onto figures in the present (p. 155). Transference occurs during psychoanalytic psychotherapy and outside of it, in neurotics, psychotics, and in healthy people. Although all human relationships contain a mixture of realistic and transference reactions, the latter are likely to be more intense in later life toward people who perform a special function that originally was carried out by parents, such as the psychotherapist, physician, or care-giving nurse.

In the psychotherapy relationship, transference can include the defenses (denial, projection, and so on) previously used to cope with wishes and fears related to an important childhood figure. It can in part be used as a defense or resistance to therapeutic change, for example, when the patient puts all his energy into his relationship with his therapist or nurse, thereby avoiding actively dealing with the long-standing wishes or fears revived in that relationship. The development of transference is promoted by psychoanalytically oriented therapists and used as a central theme in psychotherapy. The nurse does not promote positive transference but can take advantage of it if it occurs to facilitate the communication process and assist the patient in modeling the nurse's care-taking behavior in his attitude toward and treatment of himself.

Jane: A Patient Who Developed a Positive Transference Toward Her Nurse

Jane was a 17-year-old woman who was hospitalized in an inpatient psychiatric unit following a suicide attempt (she had ingested a mixture of aspirin, tranquilizers, and alcohol). This was Jane's second suicide attempt. Following her first, Jane had been hospitalized for two weeks and then treated by a psychiatrist in private practice on a weekly basis. Jane was an overweight, unkempt, quiet teenager. Her latest suicide attempt had occurred after her parents transferred her to a new high school. Jane's parents had hoped the transfer to the new school would encourage Jane to make new friends and become involved in school activities. Instead, Jane felt more isolated and lonely than ever.

Kay was assigned as Jane's primary-care nurse. Kay was a 25-year-old, thin, attractive woman who reminded Jane of a favorite teacher whom she had had in high school. Jane and Kay agreed to meet for twenty-minute sessions three times a week. During these sessions, Jane freely discussed her problems with Kay. She reported that she felt comfortable and relaxed with Kay. She also liked to discuss school activities whenever possible with Kay.

Negative transference can manifest itself in a variety of ways, including hostility, contempt, and annoyance. This type of resistance can pose such a tremendous threat to the nurse-patient relationship that the nurse must recognize and address it as early as possible, especially if it occurs in the initial interview. The nurse must acknowledge the patient's emotional reaction to her and, with him, explore its origin; for example, "You seem angry with me for trying to help you. This doesn't make sense. I'm wondering if I or your experience with me so far is reminding you of and stirring up feelings about something else."

COUNTERTRANSFERENCE. Countertransference involves feelings of the *nurse* (positive or negative) toward the *patient,* such as special concern, sexual attraction, anger, impatience, or resentment. Such feelings can lead to a distorted view of the patient. To avoid this problem, it is important for the nurse to have a deep understanding of her own behaviors and needs. Both supervision and consultation as well as psychotherapy can facilitate this understanding. An awareness of both transference and countertransference is essential for the nurse to keep the information obtained in the psychiatric interview in the proper perspective.

Note Kay's problem with countertransference in the following example:

Kay: Countertransference Toward a Patient

During their sessions, Kay felt growing feelings of anger toward Jane. Kay confided to a fellow staff member that she was annoyed because of Jane's self-pitying attitudes and her disheveled appearance. Kay also stated that she wanted to tell Jane to stop trying to be her friend and to stop feeling sorry for herself. The staff member became concerned that countertransference might be the problem and asked Kay if Jane reminded her of a relative or friend. Kay recalled that Jane seemed very much like her younger sister. Kay felt her sister resented her, and their relationship was fraught with tension.

THE BEHAVIORAL MODEL AND ASSESSMENT

In contrast to the psychoanalytic model, the **behavioral model** stresses the relationship between behavior and specific environmental factors. The behavioral approach does not use underlying personality factors to account for overt behavior (Ciminero, 1977; 1986). Skinner argues against a focus on personalogism, or inner causes: "When we say that a man eats because he is hungry, smokes a great deal because he has the tobacco habit, fights because of the instinct of pugnacity . . . we seem to be referring to causes. But on analyses these phrases prove to be merely redundant descriptions" (Skinner, 1953, p. 31). Studying the impact of the environment on the patient can provide objective, quantifiable data for the ongoing assessment and development of a treatment plan.

SORC. The acronym **SORC,** or **stimulus-organism-response-consequence,** summarizes many of the variables that are explored in a behavioral assessment (Goldfried & Sprofkin, 1976). The variables are defined as follows:

1. *Stimulus:* environmental variables that precede the target behavior

2. *Organism:* the person, with all his or her unique variables, such as physiological states, personality, and past experiences

3. *Response:* the target or problematic behavior

4. *Consequences:* events that follow the target behavior

We can look at Jane's case using the SORC format. Jane's transfer to the new high school served as the stimulus that triggered her feelings of loneliness and despair. Jane is the organism or the individual in this case. Some variables unique to Jane that contributed to her feelings of isolation include the fact that she was overweight, unkempt, and quiet. The stimulus, coupled with Jane's quietness and obesity, led to her maladaptive response, a suicide attempt. The consequence of Jane's behavior was hospitalization on a psychiatric unit.

The following guidelines for conducting a psychiatric interview according to the behavioral model are taken from Kanfer and Saslow (1969):

1. The nurse makes an initial analysis of the problem situation, in which problem and other behaviors are specified.

2. The nurse identifies the individuals who object to the problem behavior(s) of the patient, and who may be affected by any behavior change in the patient. This clarification should also help to identify the conditions in which a specific problem behavior occurs.

3. The nurse does a motivational analysis, identifying reinforcers (both positive and negative) that may be maintaining the patient's problem behavior(s) or that may be useful in shaping more appropriate behaviors.

4. The nurse does a developmental analysis, asking questions about the biological, sociological, and behavioral changes in the patient over time that may be pertinent to the problem behavior(s).

5. The nurse analyzes the patient's self-control, alert to any limitations.

6. The nurse examines the patient's social relationships, identifying significant others and their influence on the patient.

7. The nurse analyzes the patient's social-cultural-physical environment, raising questions about cul-

tural norms which may be influencing the patient and his or her behavior as well as various environmental restraints.

Returning to Jane's case, we can use these guidelines to analyze her problems.

1. Kay decided to use a behavioral approach to assess Jane's problems. She identified the following problem behaviors: a) Jane's feelings of loneliness and isolation; b) Jane's appearance; and c) Jane's suicide attempts. Adaptive behaviors included the fact that Jane was a good student and able to talk openly about her problems.

2. Jane's parents objected to the problem behaviors and would be most closely affected by changes in Jane's behavior.

3. Kay observed interactions between Jane and her parents, noting that Jane's parents read magazines and watched television whenever Jane attempted to speak quietly to them. When Jane yelled and cried, she immediately received her parents' attention. Kay identified that Jane's parents were helping to maintain Jane's problem behaviors. Kay also noted that Jane would carry on calm discussions with various hospital staff members when she felt she had their complete attention.

4. Kay reviewed Jane's past medical and social history. Jane had no health problems; however, she was facing the problems associated with adolescence. Jane was conflicted about her body image, making friends, and becoming involved in new activities.

5. Kay identified problems with Jane's self-control. When Jane interacted with her parents, she easily became frustrated and cried if she thought they were not listening to her. Jane also avoided trying to meet new people on the unit. When Jane was introduced to new people, she said "Hello" and tried to leave as quickly as possible.

6. Kay identified Jane's parents as Jane's significant others. Jane reported that she had no close friends.

7. Jane was from a white middle-class family. Her parents expected her to go to college, pursue a career, and eventually marry and have children. They were embarrassed by Jane's behavior and expressed concern regarding any social stigma that might arise because of her suicide attempts.

Useful and comprehensive information can be obtained from a behavioral assessment. However, it is important for the nurse to remember that patients' responses may vary from situation to situation. For example, Jane may behave very differently when her parents are present compared to how she behaves in an individual interview.

NURSING CONCEPTUAL MODELS RELATED TO ASSESSMENT

Nursing models can provide a perspective for the formulation of nursing diagnoses and interventions when the concern or presenting problem is psychiatric or psychological. Nursing theories are influenced by models and paradigms of other theorists and disciplines, the philosophical frameworks of the era, and the educational and experiential experiences of the nurse therapist. Nursing theories/models have premises with underpinnings from psychoanalytic, biological, and systems concepts (Melies, 1985; Fawcett, 1984; 1989).

These models are designed to assist the nurse in explicating the nursing process for the purpose of providing a broad-based approach to health care (Johnston and Fitzpatrick, 1982). Each nursing model suggests a framework for patient assessment and identifies the types of patient problems a nurse may encounter during the assessment process (Riehl & Roy, 1980). Each phase of the nursing process is prescribed by the particular model that the nurse has chosen.

There are a variety of nursing models, each of which provides a different perspective on the patient and integrates nursing process. Nursing models may be organized into the following broad categories which correspond roughly to the three major models described in this book: developmental models (psychoanalytic), systems models (biological), and interaction models (cognitive-behavioral) (Fawcett, 1984).

Developmental models focus on the process of psychological growth and maturation. Actual and potential developmental problems are identified along with appropriate intervention strategies designed to maximize growth and development. Hildegard Peplau's model (1952) is perhaps the most famous of the developmental models.

Systems models emphasize the person in his or her environment. Living organisms are considered to be open systems in constant interaction with the environment. Actual and potential problems are identified that may interfere with the organization and interaction of the parts and elements of the system (Fawcett, 1984). Newman's health care system model, Rogers' system of unitary man, and Roy's ad-

aptation model are three of the best-known models in this category.

Social arts and relationships are emphasized in **interaction models.** The focus is on the individual's perceptions of other people, the environment, situations, and events. Thus when using an interaction model, the key is understanding the individual's definition of the situation. Two theorists who use an interactionist approach in their respective conceptual frameworks are Imogene King and Ida Orlando Pelletier (Meleis, 1985).

Many excellent texts cover the basic assumptions of each model and the associated advantages and disadvantages. The choice of a model depends on a nurse's clinical practice and philosophy of nursing. Only after careful analysis can the nurse determine which model is most applicable to her practice and the patient situations she typically encounters.

COMPONENTS OF PSYCHIATRIC ASSESSMENT
THE PSYCHIATRIC INTERVIEW

The **psychiatric history** and **mental-status examination** comprise the two major components of the traditional psychiatric interview and are used in most settings. However, the nurse may also encounter ego assessment, behavioral assessment, and psychosocial assessment. A **psychosocial assessment** is sensitive to both social and psychological data. A physiological assessment provides information, for example, regarding the presence of neurological disturbances.

THE PSYCHIATRIC HISTORY

The nurse may gather information during the psychiatric history from a variety of sources. Kolb and Brodie (1982) suggest that, when accompanied by other people, the patient should always be interviewed first. The nurse informs the patient of her desire to interview family, friends, police, or other mental health personnel, and asks his permission to do so. This helps to allay a patient's suspicion that the nurse is working in collusion with a family member or some adversary of the patient. The nurse notes variations between the patient's story and that of any other source (Kolb & Brodie, 1982).

The following sequence illustrates the traditional format for preparing a written report of a patient's psychiatric history. As mentioned previously, flexibility and judicious questioning will encourage the patient to reveal the maximum amount of information.

IDENTIFYING INFORMATION. The nurse records the patient's name, age, marital status, gender, occupation, race, and nationality. She also reports the number of previous hospital admissions for a similar condition and the source of the patient's referral.

THE PRESENTING PROBLEM. The nurse usually begins the interview by asking the patient for a statement of the problem. This may be the most difficult aspect of the entire interview (MacKinnon, 1975). Some patients respond with a clear statement, describing an event that has had a negative impact. For example, in response to the question, "What led you to seek help?" the patient may say, "I was divorced recently from my wife and feel very nervous." This statement provides a springboard for further discussion of the patient's current difficulties. Sometimes, however, the patient is so agitated, anxious, depressed, or confused that a concise statement of the problem must be provided by a friend or family member.

Many patients provide vague, nonspecific responses to questions about the chief complaint. Often the patient needs assistance in defining the problem and stating why he is seeking help. A thorough knowledge of major psychiatric disturbances, their etiology and presentation, helps the nurse clarify vague complaints. For example, a patient who complains of fatigue, weight loss, and early-morning awakening is probably depressed. Even if the patient is unable to articulate feelings or describe problematic situations, the knowledgeable nurse is alert enough to the clues and can begin exploring the patient's past and present for possible sources of his depression.

HISTORY OF PRESENT ILLNESS. The nurse obtains a detailed account of the development of the current problem. A description of the current symptoms, including their onset, severity, and duration (that is, persistent or episodic), is included in the report. In addition, the nurse explores any changes in the patient's interest, mood, work or personal habits, social activities, attitudes toward others, and sexual activities.

A careful exploration of the patient's relationships with others is very important. Significant others may have had a strong impact on the patient's present emotional state. The nurse notes any deaths, separations, or losses. Often the patient fails to see the relationship between periods of loss or stress and the onset of his problem. However, the nurse may note such a relationship as she obtains the history.

A complete account of the present physical or psychological illness also takes into consideration the *patient's perception* of the illness. What is the patient's interpretation of the problem, and what are its present and future implications? Does the patient want to get well or is there something to gain from continuation of the illness? This information will help to make sense of immediate and future interactions.

FAMILY HISTORY. The nurse obtains information about genetic, familial, and socioeconomic variables in the patient's life by exploring the family history. Asking the patient about grandparents, parents, and siblings should reveal a picture of family customs, personalities, and support systems. The nurse is sensitive to possible environmental and hereditary influences contributing to the patient's problem and current level of functioning, noting any family history of psychiatric disorders and treatment, substance abuse, or suicide.

PERSONAL HISTORY. The personal history involves an analysis of the maturation of the patient from infancy through childhood, adolescence, and

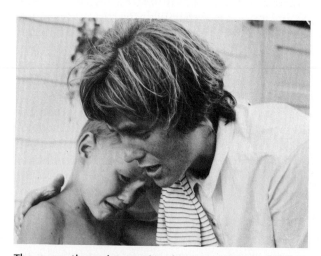

The nurse therapist queries the patient about family and personal history. Obtaining information about the patient's genetic, familial, and personal history helps to shed light on not only those cultural and environmental influences which may contribute to existing problems, but also on important developmental milestones which may yield relevant data.

adulthood. A historical perspective of the patient's personality development and interpersonal relationships may bring the current problem into sharper focus. Ginsberg (1985) and Kaplan and Sadock (1988) caution that patients often use selective perception in retelling past events. They may consciously or unconsciously alter stories to serve current psychological needs. The nurse remembers this problem when interpreting the information she has obtained.

It is useful to note, if possible, conditions surrounding the patient's birth, such as information about the labor and delivery, knowledge of whether he was wanted or unwanted by his parents, and any associated illnesses. Patterns present in infancy and early childhood related to eating, sleeping, and developmental milestones can provide important data.

The nurse obtains an account of the patient's reactions to parental discipline and school during childhood. The nurse also notes childhood injuries, disabilities, and illnesses. It is important for the nurse to obtain this information because early childhood includes the "formative years"—a period when many challenges are faced. Failure to master normal developmental tasks, according to some theorists, may lead to later disturbances (Kolb & Brodie, 1982).

Because adolescence is a time when many problems and conflicts surface, the nurse follows the patient's personal history through his high school experience. Issues such as early sexual experiences, delinquency, obesity, smoking, and alcohol and drug use are addressed. The patient's relationship to peers is crucial to the assessment of adolescent development, for these early associations may provide information related to the patient's struggle for independence and a unique personal identity.

Because adulthood brings with it concerns about primary relationships and work, the nurse asks the patient questions about relationships with partners (that is, the roles established), social contacts, financial concerns, and children. Divorce, separation, and other examples of conflict and/or loss may precipitate changes in the patient, so they deserve special inquiry. Career development is assessed by asking about the patient's expectations for promotions and raises, periods of unemployment, and attitudes toward work.

Finally, when assessing the older adult, the nurse records reactions to retirement, grown children, and the death of significant others. An inquiry into social attitudes, military service, current use of caffeine, alcohol, drugs, and tobacco, and feelings about past accomplishments and failures is essential to the interview regardless of the patient's age.

CURRENT SOCIAL SITUATION. The nurse provides a description of the patient's current residence and neighborhood along with notation regarding the number of individuals in the household, sources of income, and the need for assistance.

THE MENTAL-STATUS EXAMINATION

The mental-status examination provides a summary of the patient's current functioning. Much of the data required for the assessment of mental status may have been elicited during the psychiatric history. The format for the examination varies little from setting to setting; however, aspects of the assessment may be omitted in certain circumstances. The categories below serve as a guide rather than a prescription.

GENERAL DESCRIPTION. A physical description of the patient is written in an objective fashion. The nurse may make a statement about her overall impression of the patient as attractive or unattractive, but these terms are extremely subjective. The nurse notes the patient's age, height, weight, any physical defects, and aspects of personal grooming such as the appearance of hair, skin, and nails. The nurse may also note specific articles of clothing, such as an expensive suit or a torn tee shirt.

The nurse includes the amount and type of the patient's motor activity, as well as any unusual mannerisms in the general description. Table 5–2 lists some typical disturbances of motor activity.

A general description of the patient's attitude during the interview is useful. Adjectives used to describe attitude may include: cooperative, friendly, interested, seductive, hostile, and evasive. The nurse uses caution in writing this description because a patient's response during one particular session may not be representative of an overall attitude. In addition, the nurse must be aware of the kinds of responses she tends to elicit from her patients (MacKinnon, 1975). This sensitivity will help the nurse differentiate between general attitudes revealed by the mental-status exam and personal responses to the nurse.

Speech. This part of the report describes the quality and quantity of the patient's speech. The description may include the words fast, slow, loud, soft, monotonous, pressured, and hesitant. The nurse also reports any speech defects such as lisps and stuttering. Although thought processes are reflected in speech, they are assessed in a separate section of the mental-status exam. However, disordered thought processes

TABLE 5–2 Disturbances of motor activity

Disturbance	Manifestations
Reduction	Decreased activity or retardation; slowing of psychological and physical functioning.
Stupor	A state in which a person does not react to or is unaware of the surroundings; due to neurologic as well as psychiatric disorders.
Negativism	Frequent opposition to suggestions.
Stereotype	Continuous repetition of speech or physical activities.
Catalepsy	A generalized condition of decreased responsiveness, usually characterized by trancelike states.
Tic	An intermittent, involuntary spasmodic movement of a group of muscles, often without a demonstrable external stimulus; may be neurologic or psychologic in origin.
Waxy inflexibility	State in which one maintains the body position into which one is placed.
Echopraxia	Imitative repetition of the movements of another; sometimes seen in patients with catatonic schizophrenia.

Sources: Adapted from American Psychiatric Association, (1980). *A Psychiatric glossary* (5th ed.). Washington, D.C.: American Psychiatric Association. And from Kaplan, H. I., and Sadock, B. J. (1985). *Comprehensive textbook of psychiatry*. Baltimore: Williams & Wilkins. And from Kaplan, H. I., and Sadock, B. J. (1988). *Synopsis of psychiatry*. Baltimore: Williams & Wilkins.

do manifest themselves in language disturbances. Descriptions such as word salad, circumstantiality (a tendency to talk *around* a topic rather than address it directly), and neologisms are included under the section on thought processes (form) (MacKinnon, 1975).

Mood and Affect. Mood is typically defined as a sustained emotion that affects the patient's perception of the world. The nurse notes whether the patient spontaneously describes his mood. If the nurse needs to ask about it, an open-ended question such as, "How would you describe your usual mood?" is preferable to a leading question such as, "Do you feel depressed?" The nurse may use any of the following terms that commonly describe mood: calm, euphoric, anxious, depressed, frightened, labile, agitated, angry, irritable, and apathetic.

Exploring with the patient his feelings about a variety of subjects reveals his capacity for and/or range of emotional experiences and behaviors. The nurse notes the intensity and type of the patient's expressed emotions. Normally, individuals demonstrate variations in facial expressions, gestures, and tone of voice. If the patient shows no signs of affective expression, the nurse can state that the patient is exhibiting flat or blunted affect.

Finally, the nurse makes a statement about the appropriateness of the patient's emotional responses to the situation or thought content. Dissociation or disharmony are terms that describe inappropriate responses. For example, a patient may laugh or smile when talking about a sad or tragic event. MacKinnon (1975) cautions that the appropriateness of the emotion should be judged only within the context of the subject matter. For example, if a patient is describing a delusional system in which he is being followed by a powerful enemy, the patient should express anxiety or fear. A lack of these emotions would be inappropriate within that context.

Thought Process. In this section of the mental-status exam, the nurse observes the characteristics of the patient's thought processes rather than the content of his thought. The nurse also observes the amount of thought and rate of its production. A patient may exhibit unusual rapidity of association, which when extreme is called flight of ideas. Conversely, the patient may exhibit a slowness or poverty of ideas.

The nurse notes any disturbances in the logical progression of ideas. Normally, individuals demonstrate goal-directed thinking and explain events in cause-and-effect context. The nurse reports variations from this norm. Table 5–3 lists some common terms used to describe disturbances in thought.

Thought Content. During the psychiatric interview, the patient is asked about desires, ambitions, and fears. As the patient's story unfolds, the nurse is alert to recurring themes. These central themes reveal important information about thought content. Certain preoccupations, realistic or unrealistic, may emerge in the patient's narrative. Phobias, obsessions, compulsions, and suicidal and homicidal ideas may become apparent. Hypochondriacal or body-image focus are other possible preoccupations. Some patients will readily discuss these things; others, however, can be very evasive.

Many patients learn to conceal unusual thoughts, particularly delusions, unless they are questioned specifically about them. Sometimes an open-ended ques-

TABLE 5–3 Disturbances in thought process

Disturbance	Definition and Manifestations
Circumstantiality	A pattern of speech that is indirect and delayed in reaching its goal.
Confabulation	Fabrication of stories in response to questions about situations or events that the patient does not recall.
Blocking	A sudden obstruction or interruption in spontaneous flow of thinking or speaking, perceived as an absence or deprivation of thought.
Perseveration	Tendency to emit the same verbal or motor responses again and again to varied stimuli.
Tangential	Replying to a question in an oblique or irrelevant way.
Word salad	A mixture of words and phrases that lack comprehensive meaning or logical coherence; commonly seen in patients with schizophrenia.
Clang association	A type of thinking in which the sound of a word, rather than its meaning, gives direction to subsequent associations; punning and rhyming substitute for logic.
Neologisms	A new word or condensed combination of several words coined by the patient to express a highly complex idea not readily understood by others; seen in patients with schizophrenia and organic psychoses.
Loose association	A disturbance of thinking in which ideas shift from one subject to another in an unrelated manner.
Flight of ideas	Verbal skipping from one idea to another; sometimes seen in patients with bipolar disorder.
Condensation	A psychologic process often present in dreams in which two or more concepts are fused so that a single symbol represents the multiple components.

Source: Adapted from American Psychiatric Association (1980). *A Psychiatric glossary* (5th ed.). Washington, D.C.: American Psychiatric Association.

tion such as, "Do you have any unusual experiences that are difficult to explain?" may reveal delusional thinking. This may not be sufficient, however, and the nurse may not find evidence of delusional thinking until she has had repeated conversations with the patient. The nurse describes the content of the delusional system whenever it becomes apparent, noting its importance to the patient and its influence on him.

Somatic delusions require careful assessment. Shortness of breath, facial pallor, headache, weight loss, or insomnia may indicate depression, anxiety, or a physiologic disturbance. Methods for conducting a neurophysiological assessment are discussed in a later section.

The nurse is sensitive to subtle clues that may reflect delusions of alien control, pervasive suspiciousness, or grandiose thinking. Ideas of reference and ideas of influence, or very personal inferences taken from neutral events, should be noted here. (See Chapter 10 on schizophrenia.) Again the nurse includes in the report a description of the delusional content and its importance to the patient. Such disturbances of thought can occur in patients with schizophrenia, mood disorders, and certain organic illnesses. Table 5–4 lists the common symptomatology associated with disturbed thought content.

Perception. Distorted or altered perceptions may be the result of an organic disorder, drug or alcohol abuse, metabolic disturbances, or allergic reactions. Once the nurse has addressed these possibilities, she describes the sensory system involved in the hallucination (for example, auditory or visual). Organic brain syndromes typically involve visual hallucinations, while functional mental disorders usually involve auditory hallucinations.

Occasionally a patient will describe freely the content of a hallucination but usually he has to be prodded. Kolb and Brodie (1982) recommend a direct question for a person who is clearly psychotic or out of touch with reality—for example: "Do you hear voices?" An indirect approach would be to ask the patient if he has had "imaginings" or peculiar experiences of any kind. In her report the nurse describes the circumstances that elicit the hallucinatory experience, along with the exact content of the hallucination.

TABLE 5—4 Disturbances in thought content

Disturbance	Symptoms
Delusions of alien control	Feelings that one is being controlled by others.
Nihilistic delusions	Feeling that the self, others, or the world are nonexistent.
Delusions of grandeur	Feeling unrealistically important or overappraising one's ability.
Somatic delusions	An incorrect fixed belief about one's state of health or bodily functions.
Ideas of influence	Thoughts of being controlled or influenced by outside forces.
Ideas of reference	Incorrect interpretation of casual incidents and external events as having direct reference to oneself; may reach sufficient intensity to constitute delusions.
Delusions of persecution	An incorrect belief that one is being persecuted.
Obsession	A persistent thought that one is unable to control.

Source: Adapted from Packard, K. (1984). The psychiatric interview. In Hagerty, B. K. (1984). *Psychiatric mental health assessment.* St. Louis: Mosby, p. 59.

Illusions are another type of perceptual disturbance. They involve the misrepresentation of real stimuli. For example, a patient in a hospital may think that intravenous tubing is a snake.

Feelings of depersonalization and derealization, both of which involve a sense of being disconnected from or outside of reality, are other perceptual disturbances associated with a wide range of psychiatric disorders (MacKinnon, 1975, and Kaplan & Sadock 1988).

COGNITIVE FUNCTIONING AND ORIENTATION. In this portion of the mental-status exam, the nurse attempts to find if there are any disturbances in the patient's cognition. This part of the exam may not be necessary for every patient—for instance, a young man who relates a clear story of his nervousness and depression following divorce does not need to be asked about his orientation or memory. However, this part of the exam is essential for the assessment of those patients who have shown earlier evidence of disturbances in cognition.

Orientation. If the patient appears confused, the nurse should question him about his orientation to time, place, and person. Cognitive impairments usually occur in this order and improve or disappear in reverse order. Disturbances in orientation are almost always associated with organic mental disorders (see Chapter 11). In addition, orientation may fluctuate according to the time of day. The nurse notes these variations in the report.

Memory. Since memory disturbances are a common feature of organic brain syndrome, the nurse carefully assesses this area. Her assessment includes asking about and testing recent and remote-past memory as well as immediate recall. The nurse may become aware of deficits in these areas that are not reported in the psychiatric history.

The nurse can examine the patient's recent memory by asking how he spent the last twenty-four hours or what he last ate. It is helpful if the nurse can verify the accuracy of these statements. Some patients with impaired memories have a tendency to fill in the gaps with fabrications (confabulation). The only way the nurse can determine whether confabulation is going on is by checking the patient's story (with his permission) with a family member. Remote memory can be evaluated by asking the patient about important events in his life (such as children's birthdates or his first wedding anniversary) or by asking the patient to name the current and past three presidents. The nurse observes and notes the patient's attitude toward any impairment. For example, the patient may not notice mistakes or may demonstrate anxiety over a failure to remember.

The nurse may assess retention and recall ability with the digit-span test. The patient is asked to repeat three digits after the nurse and then to state them in reverse order. This process is repeated with up to seven digits. Most healthy people can recall seven digits forward and four to five digits in reverse. Another way to test retention and recall is to give the patient the names of some objects to remember. After a certain time period (for example, fifteen to thirty minutes), the nurse asks the patient to recall the items.

Abstract Thinking. The nurse may test the patient's capacity for abstract thinking in a variety of ways. A common method is to read or recite a proverb to the patient and ask him to explain what it means. The nurse might recite the following proverb: "People who live in glass houses shouldn't throw stones." A concrete response from the patient might be: "The glass will break." A response that requires abstract thinking would be: "Don't criticize others for faults you may have." This method of testing may result in a false positive, however, since a patient might give a concrete answer to a proverb out of boredom or failure to see the relevance to his own problem (MacKinnon, 1975). Variations in cultural and educational background may also affect the patient's response.

Exercises in analogic reasoning can be an alternative to proverb interpretations. For example, the nurse could ask how a guitar and a violin are alike. Or the nurse may ask the patient to perform some simple arithmetic calculations. Disturbances in the ability to reason appear in patients with both functional and organic psychotic disorders (see Chapters 10 and 11 on schizophrenia and organic mental disorders).

Insight. Insight refers to the patient's awareness and understanding of his illness or problems. Often the nurse has already obtained this information during discussions of the presenting problem. The nurse asks the patient about his reasons for seeking help. The patient may have only partial insight into the nature of his problem; he may not realize the seriousness or ramifications of his disorder. Or the patient may acknowledge the problem but assign the blame to someone else. True insight occurs only when a patient has a full awareness of his motives and feelings. This awareness will, in turn, lead the patient to seek alternative behavior patterns. The nurse defines the patient's level of insight by degree; for example, she may report that a patient admits to a drinking problem but denies that it has any effect on his family.

EGO ASSESSMENT

In this section of the mental-status exam, the nurse will observe ego functioning in certain settings. The use of a systematic ego assessment will depend on the philosophy of the psychiatrist, psychologist, or nurse. The theoretical underpinning for this type of assessment is grounded in psychoanalytic theory and practice. Hence, a behavioralist, for example, would probably not use the ego assessment model as presented in this chapter. A thorough assessment of ego functions may provide more information about the patient. This section describes major functions that

are generally considered to be the most fundamental processes of the ego (Meissner, 1985).

DEFINITION OF EGO. According to MacKinnon (1975):

> The ego is the executive apparatus of the mind; it mediates between the internal demands of biologically determined motives (the id), the socially determined values and behaviors (the superego), and the external demands of reality. All ego functions serve the basic task of the organism's adaptation to the environment to ensure survival while allowing for the gratification of needs (p. 914).

Bellak, Hurvich, and Gediman (1973) and Bellak and Loeb (1969), identified twelve **ego functions** that are present in normals, neurotics, and schizophrenics. Ego functions are those elements in the ego's part of the psychic apparatus that are responsible for helping the individual with overall adaptation to the environment. Bellak's premise was that these functions exist in all people and that the clinician should be able to distinguish the degree of pathology within the different types and configurations of pathology. Knowledge about ego functions will help the nurse to conceptualize and determine the theoretical underpinnings associated with a variety of syndromes and disorders, evaluate the variety of symptoms that the patient displays, assess the patient's behavior for specific strengths and weaknesses, develop a treatment plan and nursing care plan for the individual, determine the patient's prognosis, conduct clinical research to advance knowledge about specific mental disorders, and refine the definitions of pathology.

The twelve ego functions are: reality testing; judgment; sense of reality of the world and of the self; regulation and control of drives, affects, and impulses; object relations; thought processes; adaptive regression; defensive functioning; stimulus barrier; autonomous functioning; synthetic-integrative functioning; and mastery competence.

The following descriptions of the ego functions focus on their use in clinical practice. An interview format designed to assess the ego functions is included in Table 5–5.

REALITY TESTING. **Reality testing** consists of the ability to determine whether a particular stimulus is external to or within the self. A person must be able to draw some conclusion about what is causing a stimulus, the significance of the stimulus, and whether the stimulus has a logical relationship to other previous stimuli from inside and/or outside the

TABLE 5–5 Ego functions, interview questions, and possible disturbances

Ego Function	Interview Questions	Possible Disturbances
1. Reality testing A. A sense of self and the world as real	Are you sometimes confused as to whether things are real or imaginary? Do you sometimes feel that things are happening as if in a dream?	Narcissistic personality disorders (disorder of self); psychosis
B. Accurate perceptions and ability to distinguish between the self and the external environment	Do you have trouble determining the time and place that events occurred?	Disorientation to time, place, person; perceptual disturbance; limited awareness of environment
2. Judgment; understanding of the consequences of one's behavior	What would you do if you found a wallet with $1000 in it? What would you do if you found a stamped, addressed envelope lying in the street?	Failure to learn from previous experiences; unacceptable behavior by social definition; unconcerned about severe danger to life and limb
3. Sense of self as separate from others, stable body image and self-esteem	Have you felt that you are merged with someone else or in special communication with someone else? Do you have strange sensations on different parts of your body?	Alienation, dissociation, identity diffusion, emotional isolation, lack of object-constancy (see Ch. 2 on object-relations theory.)
4. Regulation and control of drives, affect, and impulses; ability to delay gratification	Are you active or do you find it hard to get going? Do you tend to be emotional and excitable or are you calm? Do you have rapid mood changes? What kinds of things make you angry and how angry do you get?	Impulsive self or other destructive acting out; sociopathy
5. Object relations; mature object relationships involve the ability to attach and separate without losing sense of self or other	What were your father and mother like? How is your homelife? How well do you get along with girlfriend/boyfriend, spouse, boss? Do you find it difficult to get close to people? Do you ever feel that you've been rejected or abandoned? How well do you understand others? And how well do you think they understand you?	Schizoid withdrawal; projective identification (see Ch. 12, the defense mechanism); dependency; detachment; narcissism
6. Thought processes; ability to conceptualize and use appropriate abstract thinking	Do you feel that your thoughts get confused? Do you have trouble stating your ideas so that others understand you?	Magical thinking; autistic thinking; difficulty with concentration, memory, and logic; limited to concrete ideation
7. Adaptive regression in service of the ego (ARISE); ability to be creative and demonstrate flexibility	What do you do when you're alone and have nothing to do? Do you daydream? What about? Have you ever been able to let go and think strange thoughts without being frightened?	Rigid character structure and defense; stereotyped thinking; inability to tolerate ambiguity; prejudice; intolerant of fantasy and play; difficulty relaxing; lacks imagination, creativity

Ego Function	Interview Questions	Possible Disturbances
	What is one of the most creative things you've ever done?	
8. Defensive functioning; flexible use of defense mechanisms in order to protect the self from psychological conflict or trauma	What kinds of things upset you? Do you think that you are an anxious person? Have you ever felt that you were falling apart? Do you ever have strange thoughts or nightmares? Are you concerned about what other people are saying about you?	Extreme anxiety, rigidity, obsessions, withdrawal, emotional isolation; feels overwhelmed; fear of not being able to cope, losing it (fragmentation of self)
9. Stimulus barrier; adaptation to external and internal stimuli	Are you especially sensitive to light, sound, temperature? Are you irritable or jumpy when there is too much noise around you? Do you get bored easily? Does excitement upset you?	Extreme sensitization to pain, lights, temperature; unresponsive to stimuli in the environment; limited aesthetic appreciation
10. Autonomous functioning; habit patterns, hobbies, interests, learning	What kinds of hobbies do you have? What kinds of jobs have you held? How much formal education have you had?	In extreme instances, inability to perform activities of daily living; tremendous effort is needed to carry out simple/routine duties
11. Mastery competence; how effectively the person interacts with his environment; how the person perceives himself and his abilities to cope with internal and external stress	Do you function as well as you believe you are capable of functioning? Do you live up to your own expectations of yourself? Do you think you are missing out on life? Why? Do you feel at the mercy of events or do you feel you are in control of your life?	Passivity, helplessness, incongruity between objective abilities and perceived abilities; limited interaction with the environment; withdrawn; limited self-confidence
12. Synthetic integrative functioning; integration of a variety of ego functions that allows for thinking, learning, and judgment	Do you adapt easily to change or does it confuse you? Do you think it's possible to do only one major thing well? Do you find yourself doing or saying things that seem unlike you? Are you bothered by having bits and pieces or loose ends around? How did you do in school? Higher level of education?	Identity diffusion, confusion, fear of dissolution, a sense of fragmentation; disorganization; conflicts between thoughts, feelings, actions; no sense of future; feeling overwhelmed by thoughts and feelings

Source: Adapted from Bellak, L., Hurvich, M., and Gedmen, H. (1973) *Ego functions in schizophrenics, neurotics, and normals.* New York: John Wiley and Sons, pp. 351–372.

self. In order to have good reality testing, an individual must perceive, feel, remember, anticipate, form concepts, reason logically, and concentrate (Bellak, 1975; Schafer, 1968). This ego function is believed to be basic to mental health (Bellak, 1975). When fantasies and daydreams interfere with reality, the person will have extreme difficulty functioning.

JUDGMENT. Judgment includes the ability to determine a course of action that is based on an assessment of available alternatives. It also includes the individual's ability to anticipate, develop, and implement plans that are realistic; it requires that the individual take the initiative, act in a socially acceptable manner, and so forth. Judgment also encompasses the ability to compare and contrast ideas and draw correct inferences and conclusions from facts and observations.

This ego function is usually assessed by asking patients about their awareness of their difficulties, facts that might have led to their problems, insights into their difficulties, and methods by which their problems might be confronted.

Judgment is closely related to reality testing in that good judgment is dependent on adequate reality testing. If one's reality testing is faulty (inability to form concepts, remember, reason logically, concentrate, differentiate internal and external stimuli, and so forth), then one's judgment will also be impaired.

SENSE OF THE WORLD AND SENSE OF SELF. Sense of the world and **sense of self** require that a person have a basic knowledge about two entities: the world (the external environment) and the self (the internal environment). People must understand their world in the context of reality testing. Objects, other people, and meanings of words must be understood as being external to the self but still part of the dynamic forces with which the self communicates. If this separateness exists, a person is considered to have a well-developed sense of self. In other words, a person should be able to say, "I am here, and the chair begins there."

People with a firm sense of self have a clearly defined idea of who they are. Their identities are well formulated, and their self-definitions have been developed and tested out in the external world. They feel comfortable with their age, sex, race, body image, and roles and functions in life. Their self-esteem helps to maintain their sense of self; their own perceived worth as people is validated by other people (Bellak, 1975; Erikson, 1950/1963).

REGULATION AND CONTROL OF DRIVES, AFFECTS, AND EMOTIONS. Regulation and control of drives, affects, and emotions is directly related to a person's capacity to control anxiety, frustration, disappointment, and delay gratification. Sexual and aggressive impulses are kept under control. Many psychiatric disorders, including sociopathic personality, sexual perversions, compulsive shoplifting, gambling, and eating disorders are characterized by the patient's difficulties with impulse control.

OBJECT RELATIONS. Object relations involve the ability to develop and maintain meaningful interpersonal relationships with a minimum of hostility over a long period of time. Object relations can be measured by assessing one's ability to individuate from another person without losing a sense of caring and feeling for that person as well as the ability to recall significant things about the other (appearance and important interactions). The ability to distinguish between the thoughts, feelings, and psychomotor activity of oneself and another person is also part of object relations. Though there is interaction, there is still separation; the individual has an understanding that there are good and bad qualities in all people and hence no need to classify some as all good and some as all bad (Bellak, 1975).

THOUGHT PROCESS. Thinking is trial action (Freud in Bellak, 1975). Thought process is a complex ego function involving logic, interpretation of symbols, language (a systematic set of symbols), cause-and-effect relationships, memory, and judgment. Disturbances in thought process may indicate schizophrenia or an organic disorder. Thought processes in the schizophrenic usually lack a sense of purpose. Highly personal meanings, disjointed thoughts, and other types of pathological methods of communicating seem to be substituted for purposeful thought.

Language must reflect secondary-process thinking. There must be evidence of a cause-and-effect relationship, logic, appropriate sense of time, accurate sequencing, attention, adequate reality testing, and so forth. Thought processes also involve the ability to use abstract and concrete forms of thinking or to conceptualize (Bellak, 1975).

ADAPTIVE REGRESSION IN SERVICE OF THE EGO (ARISE). Adaptive regression in service of the ego (ARISE) provides the individual with a method of relaxing the ego and getting in touch with semiconscious materials for the purpose of creating new methods of problem solving and/or developing new ideas and ideals for the advancement of science, the arts, and so on. It also assists in problem solving of common everyday conflicts that people encounter. The three parts of the ARISE function are:

1. The ego is sufficiently relaxed to allow for a "letdown" of traditional defenses. When the defenses are relaxed, the materials in the semiconscious are brought to the surface and felt and conceptualized by the individual. During this time, logic is temporarily suspended and replaced with thinking that may be illogical, timeless, barren of cause-and-effect relationships, without consequences, and so forth.

2. The new ideas and insights generated during this process (when the defenses are relaxed) may provide new and creative methods of conceptualizing and thinking about problems, people, and objects and symbols in the world.

3. The ego returns to the level of functioning at which all defenses are in place once again; the world of reality is intact. All other ego functions remain undisturbed by this process, enabling the person to apply the newly created insights and information to the task at hand.

Thus an individual may utilize ARISE temporarily to suspend logic and secondary-process thinking to solve an annoying problem. For example, Naomi Robinson, nursing instructor, had to combine the contents of two separate courses into one. Mrs. Robinson confronted this problem by (1) relaxing her defenses and (2) allowing all possibilities to come into her mind; strange and unusual configurations were allowable. After approximately twenty to thirty minutes, she emerged from the thought process with all of the possible images and alternatives still available to her. Using secondary-process thinking (logical, sequential, cause-and-effect related), she designed the new course, a new approach to teaching certain material.

This process is also used to describe the methods of thinking used by creative people such as artists, musicians, entrepreneurs, nurses, scientists, and inventors of technological advancements such as computers and biomedical equipment.

DEFENSIVE FUNCTIONING. Defensive functioning involves specific defense mechanisms and the methods and frequency with which they are utilized. Some common defense mechanisms include repres-sion, denial, sublimation, suppression, conversion reaction, and projection. All the defense mechanisms (also referred to as coping mechanisms) are extremely important. Defense mechanisms protect the individual from impulses, affects, and anxiety that might arise from internal or external sources. The nurse should, however, examine the defenses according to how frequently a patient uses them, their situation-specific appropriateness, the extent to which the defenses are able to protect the person from anxiety, and the ability of the defenses to facilitate adaptive behaviors associated with appropriate goals and objectives.

STIMULUS BARRIER. Stimulus barrier is an ego function that allows the individual to censor and block out external and internal stimulations. It is important because it helps to explain how a person can survive in an environment permeated with continuous excitation and various types of stimuli.

The stimulus barrier acts like a protective shield for the individual against a variety of noxious stimuli, both internal and external. Examples of internal stimuli consist of the individual's responses to bodily pain, temperature changes (fever), premenstrual tensions with bloating, and general feelings of irritability, palpitations, gastrointestinal disturbances, and so forth. External stimuli might consist of noises, bright lights, and temperature changes that occur in the environment.

This ego function was examined with much interest during World War II when clinicians and researchers were studying combat survival. Servicemen were constantly bombarded with noises and the threat of death when on the battlefield. Some survived without enormous side effects while others were labeled as "shell-shocked." Perhaps the latter individuals did not have adequate "protective barriers" or stimulus barriers against the noxious stimuli associated with battle.

A patient with stimulus barrier defects might complain of internal sensations such as hearing, seeing, or smelling things that others do not. He or she might be extremely sensitive to therapeutic drugs, encounter feelings of agitation, or be susceptible to bodily pain. The individual might also complain of stimuli in the external environment such as thunderstorms and crowds. It is possible for a person with these defects to experience a sense of disorganization or chaos within the personality.

Mothers, therapists, and nurses are persons who absorb or deflect stimuli and protect individuals from overwhelming amounts of stimulation. In other words, they act as shock absorbers and actually soak up or divert some of the stimulation overload from the internal and external environment. The degree of adequacy of stimulus barriers can be determined, retroactively, when the clinician assesses the ability of the patient to be adaptive, resilient, and capable to continue working toward life goals despite environmental resistance and interference.

AUTONOMOUS FUNCTIONING. Autonomous functioning includes the ability of the ego to participate in specific tasks and thought processes with a limited expenditure of energy. "Habits take care of themselves" is a particular method of conceptualizing this ego function. The healthy individual executes skills and routines with a high degree of efficiency and effectiveness. The autonomous nature of the ego has a distinct economic, energy-conserving advantage in that the individual does not have to develop new techniques each time specific tasks are required. A person's previous learning and performances help him or her achieve goals with a minimum of energy.

SYNTHETIC-INTEGRATIVE FUNCTIONING. Synthetic-integrative functioning has two basic functions: it assists in reconciling conflicting demands among the id, superego, and ego; and it aids the individual in coming to terms with the many diverse opinions, demands, and frustrations confronted in daily life. Synthetic-integrative functioning allows the healthy person to "integrate" or "synthesize" external and internal experience into a unified whole—that is, it aids the individual in achieving a balance in life, permitting a harmonious coexistence of potentially conflicting feelings, thoughts, opinions, and behaviors.

A deficit in this ego function might result in experiencing life in a disorganized fashion. For example, a woman who is involved in numerous roles might encounter some or all of the following: demands at work that are challenging; child-care responsibilities that are extensive and time consuming; and communication problems with her husband and other family members. Without synthetic-integrative functioning, she might experience mood fluctuations that range from euphoria to depression. Encounters in situations will not provide insights into how activities could be better coordinated. She will experience life as fragmented (a series of crises), accompanied by

a variety of moods and thoughts that do not harmoniously fit within her personality.

MASTERY COMPETENCY. Mastery competence gauges how people approach tasks and demands placed on them in the environment. It is important to know how a person feels about his or her behavior. For example, the nurse will need to determine if the patient's sense or perceived sense of competence is congruent with his actual level of competency. An individual's mastery and competency can be determined if the growth and development history is examined. In each epoch or benchmark there are specific competencies that should be mastered according to developmental theorists. (See Chapter 2 on major models of behavior for other views.) For example, some theorists hold that during the infancy or oral stage of growth and development, the major task is the development of basic trust; during the anal or childhood stage, the child's major task is the development of autonomy, the postponement of gratification, and so forth (Roediger, Rushton, Capaldi, & Paris, 1987).

PHYSIOLOGICAL ASSESSMENT

A thorough physical examination, particularly a neurological evaluation, is an essential aspect of psychiatric assessment. Ignoring the possibility of an organic problem can lead to disastrous consequences. The steps for conducting a neurological examination are easily learned and should be utilized routinely in the assessment process.

HISTORY. A thorough history is a key component of the physiological assessment. It can provide important clues to the presence of neurological disturbances. The nurse first encourages the patient to describe the problem in his own words. Mention of any symptoms requires careful evaluation. The nurse must elicit a clear description of each symptom, the date of onset, whether the onset was sudden or gradual, constant or intermittent in nature, and whether there have been any apparent precipitating factors. She also pays careful attention to any mention of excessive physical or emotional strain or physical trauma.

The nurse is alert for clues of any possible hereditary or congenital illness and records the history of childhood diseases as well as any known instances of convulsions or unconsciousness. The nurse can also ask the patient's relatives to describe the patient's past history and any recent changes in memory, cognition, mood, or behavior.

NEUROLOGICAL EXAMINATION. The neurological examination is organized into five steps (Bates, 1983; Malasanos, et al. 1986) which involve testing the nervous system from higher to lower levels of integration. These simple screening procedures help to assess the patient for organic problems.

Step I—Tests for Cerebral Function. The mental-status examination is the first test of general cerebral functioning. The information discussed in the preceding sections can be applied here. Brief versions of the mental-status exam may be used when the patient is unlikely to be able to tolerate the long version due to impaired physical condition or mental state.

Specific cerebral functions need to be tested, for example, that area of the cerebral cortex necessary for the recognition of objects by sight, sound, and feeling. **Agnosia** refers to the inability to recognize stimuli through any of the senses typically involved in doing so. The varieties of agnosia relate to the specific sense (auditory, visual, and so forth). Auditory agnosia is the inability to recognize a familiar sound such as a doorbell, or a person's voice, while tactile agnosia is the inability to recognize an object by touch or feel. Agnosia can be determined by asking the patient to name familiar objects such as a pen or a book. The inability to carry out purposeful movements in the absence of paralysis is called **apraxia**. Any deficiencies in motor strength or ability to carry out a skilled act should be noted. The nurse also records any deficit in language function **(aphasia).** Mild deficits can be seen in the presence of diffuse brain damage or in the early stages of a progressive lesion. See Table 5–6 for a description of common abnormalities of speech.

Step II—Tests of Functioning of the Cranial Nerves. Nerves that emerge from the central nervous system within the brain are called the **cranial nerves** (Bates, 1983). Frequently, neurologic lesions can be localized by testing the function of the cranial nerves. Table 5–7 provides a summary of the twelve cranial nerves, their functions, and assessment techniques.

Step III—The Motor System. The **cerebellum** is important for balance and coordination. The nurse

TABLE 5–6 Common speech abnormalities

Aphasia or dysphasia	Defects in word formulation or power of expression. Ranges from uncertainty or error in choice of words and syllables (dysphasia) to complete inability to speak (aphasia) despite adequate motor function of mouth and larynx.
Aphonia or dysphonia	A disorder of volume, quality, or pitch of voice secondary to disease of the larynx. Ranges from raspy, hoarse voice (dysphonia) to whisper (aphonia).

Source: Adapted from Bates, B. (1983). *Physical examination* (3rd ed.). Philadelphia: Lippincott.

observes the patient's gait as he walks into the room. Normally, posture, balance, and swinging of the arms are smooth and coordinated. If the nurse suspects a problem, she asks the patient to walk around the room. She also asks the patient to walk in tandem fashion (heel to toe). Any clumsiness may indicate cerebellar disease or an intoxicated state. The limbs and trunk should be assessed for any atrophy, fasciculations, involuntary movement, and weakness. Involuntary movements may indicate a disturbance of the extrapyramidal tract. If abnormalities are determined in this screening process, the patient should be referred to a physician for a more detailed neurological examination.

Step IV—The Sensory System. For a patient with no neurologic symptoms, Bates (1983) recommends using only a few screening procedures to test the sensory system. Superficial tactile sensation can be assessed by using a wisp of cotton. Hands, forearms, upper arms, trunk, lower legs, and feet are compared bilaterally. If abnormalities such as hypersensitivity are detected, sensitivity to pain and temperature should also be assessed. Sensory disturbances may indicate polyneuropathy or peripheral neuropathy. Some common causes for these conditions include diabetes and alcoholism.

Step V—Reflexes. There are many tests for reflexes; however, the major ones are listed in Table 5–8. Re-

TABLE 5–7 A summary of function and assessment techniques for the cranial nerves

Nerve	Function	Test
I. Olfactory	Smell	Apply odor to nostril
II. Optic	Vision	Show eye chart
III. Oculomotor	Upward, downward, medial eye movement Lid elevation	Observe eye movement Observe lid movement
	Pupil constriction	Observe pupil reaction to light and accommodation
IV. Trochlear	Downward, medial eye movement	Observe eye movement
V. Trigeminal	*Sensory* Face Scalp Nasal and buccal mucosa	Check corneal reflex Check stimulation of face, scalp, nasal, and buccal mucosa
	Motor Muscles of the face	Ask patient to bite down with sharp force; press jaw against examiner's hand
VI. Abducent	Lateral eye movement	Observe eye movement
VII. Facial	*Sensory* External ear Taste in anterior 2/3 of tongue Deep facial	Touch with: cotton Offer: sweet, salty, sour Sensation
	Motor Muscles of face	Observe corneal reflex; have patient frown, wrinkle forehead, show teeth
VIII. Acoustic	Hearing	Whisper to patient and have him repeat the phrase.
IX. Glossopharyngeal	Taste in posterior 1/3 of tongue	Taste: sweet, sour, salty, gag test, give patient water to drink and watch swallow
X. Vagus	Phonation	Speech
XI. Accessory	Swallowing Elevation of shoulders Turn head	Give drink and watch swallow; have patient shrug shoulders; have patient turn head.
XII. Hypoglossal	Muscles that move tongue	Observe facial muscles and listen to speech

Source: Adapted from Malasanos, L.; Barkauskas, V.; Moss, M.; Stoltenberg-Allen, K. (1986). *Health assessment,* 3rd ed. St. Louis: Mosby.

TABLE 5–8 Reflex assessment

A. Deep tendon reflexes (DTRs)
  1. Jaw closure
  2. Biceps
  3. Triceps
  4. Bronchio radialis
  5. Patellar
  6. Achilles
B. Superficial reflexes
  1. Plantar (Babinski)
  2. Abdominal

flexes are elicited by tapping briskly on a tendon or bony prominence, such as the knee. The rapidity and strength of contractions are compared bilaterally. Diminished reflexes are seen in patients with diseases that involve neuromuscular damage or dysfunction.

PSYCHOSOCIAL ASSESSMENT

In some settings, a psychosocial assessment is made instead of or in addition to the traditional psychiatric interview. Nurses practice a holistic approach to health care, and perform psychosocial assessments to determine the patient's sociologic and psychologic status (Francis & Munjas, 1976). In a psychosocial assessment, the nurse explores the patient's current difficulties in living. A psychosocial assessment can provide information related to deficiencies in an individual's social-support system or coping abilities (Pearlin & Schooler, 1978). Often individuals arrive at a clinic with a variety of physical complaints, ranging from mild to severe. A trained nurse may quickly discern a relationship between the somatic complaint and stressors in the patient's environment. A complete picture of the patient can lead to a more comprehensive understanding and treatment strategy.

A psychosocial assessment focuses on the patient's current functioning and living situation. Discussion of family relationships and communication patterns generally forms the initial portion of the assessment. Family cohesiveness and resources for a crisis resolution should be assessed and recorded.

The social support that is available to an individual is a crucial area for assessment. Interest in the social environment grew in the mid 1970s when researchers found a link between social support and psychosocial stress and health states (Kessler, Price, & Wortman, 1985).

Social support can be conceptualized in two major ways: structurally and functionally. Structural aspects of social support typically include such characteristics as the size, density, and degree of connection within the patient's social network. Size refers to the number of people who are available for social support (Mitchell & Trickett, 1980). Density refers to the extent to which individuals in the network know and contact one another independently of the patient. The degree of connection, or the amount of advice and information typically shared within the social-support system, is also important (Bott, 1971). Some of the major structural dimensions along which social networks can be described are listed in Table 5–9. A good conceptualization of social support can guide this aspect of psychosocial assessment.

Social support has also been conceptualized functionally. House's (1981) categorization is perhaps the

TABLE 5–9 Structural characteristics of social networks

Characteristic	Definition	Interview Questions
A. Size of range	The number of individuals with whom the patient has direct contact. Often specified as a focal person that has an ongoing personal relationship with the patient in question.	List the people to whom you feel close. Who are the people that are most important to you?
B. Network density	The extent to which members of a patient's social network contact each other independently of the patient.	Look for dense clusters of individuals that the patient describes as support providers (i.e., family cluster, coworker cluster, recreational cluster).
C. Intensity	The strength of the tie.	Ask the patient to rate the strength of his or her thoughts or feelings toward each member of the network.
D. Durability	The degree of stability of the patient's links with others in his or her network.	How long have you known the people that you have named in your network? Do you think these relationships change often or are they stable?
E. Dispersion	The ease with which the patient can make contact with members of his or her network.	How accessible are the people that you have listed in your network?
F. Frequency	The frequency with which the patient makes contact with members of his or her network, variously defined to include phone as well as face-to-face contact.	How often do you have contact with the people in your network? Is this contact face to face, by phone, or what?

Source: Adapted from Mitchell, R. E., and Trickett, E. J., (1980). Social networks as mediators of social support. *Community Mental Health Journal, 16,* 27–44.

best known and most complete. House describes four basic functional supports. The first is **esteem support,** that is, feedback from others that a person is valued and accepted. Self-esteem is enhanced when an individual knows that he or she is valued and accepted despite faults and problems. Second, **informational support** refers to help that the individual receives in defining, understanding, and coping with life's difficulties. The third function, **social companionship,** encompasses an individual's need for affiliation and contact with others, and how that need is met. Asking about the time spent with others in leisure and recreational activities is one way to explore this aspect of an individual's life. Finally, **instrumental support** refers to the adequacy of material and financial aid. An example of an instrument designed to measure social support functionally, the Interpersonal Support Evaluation List (ISEL) (Cohen, et al., 1985), is illustrated in Table 5–10.

House and Kahn (1985) recommend the exploration of both structural and functional aspects of social support in the psychosocial assessment. The content and quality of an individual's relationships can also provide insight into an individual's current problems, as well as increase the nurse's ability to mobilize the patient's available resources for support and treatment planning.

THE DSM-III AND AXES I THROUGH V

In order to practice effectively, the nurse needs to be familiar with *The Diagnostic and Statistical Manual of the American Psychiatric Association* Revised or the DSM-III-R (1987). This universally used guide for psychiatric assessment involves five axes.

AXIS I (CLINICAL SYNDROMES AND CONDITIONS NOT ATTRIBUTABLE TO A MENTAL DISORDER THAT ARE A FOCUS OF ATTENTION OR TREATMENT) AND AXIS II (DEVELOPMENTAL DISORDERS AND PERSONALITY DISORDERS)

Axis I and Axis II together provide for the classification of a disorder as well as those conditions which are not attributable to a mental disorder but which are a focus of attention or treatment. Axis I represents the prominent condition or problem. Axis II helps direct the practitioner to the presence of other disorders that might otherwise be overlooked. Axis II can also be used to assess and record personality traits of the patient in the absence of a specific personality disorder.

The distinction between the episodic disorders that come and go with treatment and progressive disorders (both coded on Axis I) and the early onset of

---

TABLE 5–10 The general population form of the ISEL

For clarity, each subscale is listed separately. The scale presented to subjects consists of all 40 items in random order. T or F indicates response coded as social support.

Instructions

This scale is made up of a list of statements each of which may or may not be true about you. For each statement we would like you to circle (T) *probably* TRUE if the statement is true about you or (F) *probably* FALSE if the statement is not true about you. Although some questions will be difficult to answer, it is important that you pick one alternative or the other. Remember to circle only one of the alternatives for each statement.

Please read each item quickly but carefully before responding. Remember that this is not a test and there are no right or wrong answers.

Appraisal

T   1. There is at least one person I know whose advice I really trust.

F   2. There is really no one I can trust to give me good financial advice.

F   3. There is really no one who can give me objective feedback about how I'm handling my problems.

T   4. When I need suggestions for how to deal with a personal problem I know there is someone to whom I can turn.

T   5. There is someone to whom I feel comfortable going for advice about sexual problems.

T   6. There is someone I can turn to for advice about handling hassles over household responsibilities.

F   7. I feel that there is no one with whom I can share my most private worries and fears.

F   8. If a family crisis arose, few of my friends would be able to give me good advice about handling it.

F   9. There are very few people I trust to help solve my problems.

T   10. There is someone I could turn to for advice about changing my job or finding a new one.

disorders with a more stable course (coded on Axis II) emphasizes the need to consider disorders involving the development of cognitive, motor, and social skills in children and allows for recognition of learning disabilities, mental retardation, and other developmental disorders (APA, 1987). This distinction was made clearer in the 1987 DSM-III Revision.

AXIS III (PHYSICAL DISORDERS OR CONDITIONS)

Axis III allows for the notation of current physical conditions that are important in the understanding and management of the patient. For example, any abnormalities found in the neurological examination would be noted here.

Belonging

T 1. If I decide on a Friday afternoon that I would like to go to a movie that evening, I could find someone to go with me.

F 2. No one I know would throw a birthday party for me.

T 3. There are several different people with whom I enjoy spending time.

   4. I don't often get invited to do things with others.

T 5. If I wanted to have lunch with someone, I could easily find someone to join me.

F 6. Most people I know don't enjoy the same things that I do.

T 7. When I feel lonely, there are several people I could call.

T 8. I regularly meet or talk with members of my family or friends.

F 9. I feel that I'm on the fringe in my circle of friends.

F 10. If I wanted to go out of town for the day I would have a hard time finding someone to go with me.

Tangible

T 1. If for some reason I were put in jail, there is someone I could call who would bail me out.

T 2. If I had to go out of town for a few weeks, someone I know would look after my home (the plants, pets, yard, etc.).

F 3. If I were sick and needed someone to drive me to the doctor, I would have trouble finding someone.

F 4. There is no one I could call on if I needed to borrow a car for a few hours.

T 5. If I needed a quick emergency loan of $100, there is someone who would lend it to me.

F 6. If I needed some help in moving to a new home, I would have a hard time finding someone to help me.

F 7. If I were sick, there would be almost no one I could find to help me with my daily chores.

T 8. If I got stranded ten miles out of town, there is someone I could call to come get me.

T 9. If I had to mail an important letter at the post office by 5:00 and couldn't make it, there is someone who could do it for me.

F 10. If I needed a ride to the airport very early in the morning, I would have a hard time finding anyone to take me.

Self-Esteem

F 1. In general, people don't have much confidence in me.

T 2. I have someone who takes pride in my accomplishments.

F 3. Most of my friends are more successful at making changes in their lives than I am.

T 4. Most people I know think highly of me.

F 5. Most of my friends are more interesting than I am.

T 6. I am more satisfied with my life than most people are with theirs.

F 7. I have a hard time keeping pace with my friends.

F 8. I think that my friends feel that I'm not very good at helping them solve problems.

T 9. I am closer to my friends than most other people.

T 10. I am able to do things as well as most other people.

Source: Cohen, S., Mermelstein, R., Kamarck, T., and Hoberman, H. M. (1985). Measuring the functional components of social support. In I. G. Sarason and B. R. Sarason (Eds.), *Social support: Theory, research and applications.* Boston: Martinus Nijhoff Publishers. pp. 92–94.

AXIS IV (SEVERITY OF PSYCHOSOCIAL STRESSORS)

Axis IV provides for the classification of psychosocial stressors that may have contributed to the development of the patient's condition or exacerbated it. The year preceding the onset of the current illness is re-viewed for potential stressors, with separate ratings for acute and enduring stressors. The rating scale used with Axis IV is displayed in Table 5–11.

In rating the severity of the stressor, several variables need to be considered. First, the clinician should evaluate the stressor with respect to the pa-

TABLE 5–11 Severity of psychosocial stressors scale: adults

Code	Term	Examples of Stressors	
		Acute events	Enduring circumstances
1	None	No acute events that may be relevant to the disorder	No enduring circumstances that may be relevant to the disorder
2	Mild	Broke up with boyfriend or girlfriend; started or graduated from school; child left home	Family arguments; job dissatisfaction; residence in high-crime neighborhood
3	Moderate	Marriage; marital separation; loss of job; retirement; miscarriage	Marital discord; serious financial problems; trouble with boss; being a single parent
4	Severe	Divorce; birth of first child	Unemployment; poverty
5	Extreme	Death of spouse; serious physical illness diagnosed; victim of rape	Serious chronic illness in self or child; ongoing physical or sexual abuse
6	Catastrophic	Death of child; suicide of spouse; devastating natural disaster	Captivity as hostage; concentration camp experience
0	Inadequate information, or no change in condition		

Severity of psychosocial stressors scale: children and adolescents

Code	Term	Examples of Stressors	
		Acute events	Enduring circumstances
1	None	No acute events that may be relevant to the disorder	No enduring circumstances that may be relevant to the disorder
2	Mild	Broke up with boyfriend or girlfriend; change of school	Overcrowded living quarters; family arguments
3	Moderate	Expelled from school; birth of sibling	Chronic disabling illness in parent; chronic parental discord
4	Severe	Divorce of parents; unwanted pregnancy; arrest	Harsh or rejecting parents; chronic life-threatening illness in parent; multiple foster home placements
5	Extreme	Sexual or physical abuse; death of a parent	Recurrent sexual or physical abuse
6	Catastrophic	Death of both parents	Chronic life-threatening illness
0	Inadequate information, or no change in condition		

Source: The American Psychiatric Association. (1987). The Diagnostic and Statistical Manual of Mental Disorders. (Third Edition-R). Washington, D.C.: Author.

tient's circumstances and sociocultural values. For example, how would a similar person with a similar background be affected by the stressor? In assigning a rating code, however, the clinician should only record the severity of the stressor itself, not the perceived vulnerability of the patient to it. Second, the number of stressors, their impact on the patient's life, and the extent to which they have been under the patient's control should be evaluated. Finally, the clinician may want to record any specific events that have been major concerns for the patient. All this information will be useful in planning nursing interventions as well as psychiatric treatment.

AXIS V (GLOBAL ASSESSMENT OF FUNCTIONS [GAF SCALE])

Axis V addresses the individual's psychological, social, and occupational functioning. The Global As-

sessment of Functioning Scale (GAF Scale) is used and appears in Table 5–12. Two separate time periods are considered when making ratings with the GAF Scale. First, the clinician must consider the patient's level of functioning at the time of the evaluation. Second, the clinician must consider the highest level of functioning for at least a few months during the past year. For children and adolescents, a month during the school year must be assessed.

Peggy: An Example of Assessment

Peggy Smith was a 27-year-old woman who was studying law at an Ivy League university. She was doing quite well until her husband left for an overseas tour with the Navy. Shortly after his departure, she began to experience palpitations and shortness of breath. Peggy complained that her husband had been sending secret codes to the Justice Department and

---

TABLE 5–12 Global assessment of functioning scale (GAF Scale)

Consider psychological, social, and occupational functioning on a hypothetical continuum of mental health-illness. Do not include impairment in functioning due to physical (or environmental) limitations.

Note: Use intermediate codes when appropriate, e.g., 45, 68, 72.

Code

90 **Absent or minimal symptoms** (e.g., mild anxiety before an exam), **good functioning in all areas, interested and involved in a wide range of activities, socially effective, generally satisfied with life, no more than everyday problems or concerns** (e.g., an
81 occasional argument with family members).

80 **If symptoms are present, they are transient and expectable reactions to psychosocial stressors** (e.g., difficulty concentrating after family argument); **no more than slight impairment in social, occupational, or school functioning** (e.g., temporarily fall-
71 ing behind in school work).

70 **Some mild symptoms** (e.g., depressed mood and mild insomnia) **OR some difficulty in social, occupational, or school functioning** (e.g., occasional truancy, or theft within the household), **but generally functioning pretty well, has some meaningful inter-
61 personal relationships.**

60 **Moderate symptoms** (e.g., flat affect and circumstantial speech, occasional panic attacks) **OR moderate difficulty in social, occupational, or school func-
51 tioning** (e.g., few friends, conflicts with co-workers).

50 **Serious symptoms** (e.g., suicidal ideation, severe obsessional rituals, frequent shoplifting) **OR any serious impairment in social, occupational, or school func-
41 tioning** (e.g., no friends, unable to keep a job).

40 **Some impairment in reality testing or communication** (e.g., speech is at times illogical, obscure, or irrelevant) **OR major impairment in several areas, such as work or school, family relations, judgment, thinking, or mood** (e.g., depressed man avoids friends, neglects family, and is unable to work; child frequently beats up younger children, is defiant at
31 home, and is failing at school).

30 **Behavior is considerably influenced by delusions or hallucinations OR serious impairment in communication or judgment** (e.g., sometimes incoherent, acts grossly inappropriately, suicidal preoccupation) **OR inability to function in almost all areas** (e.g.,
21 stays in bed all day; no job, home, or friends)

20 **Some danger of hurting self or others** (e.g., suicide attempts without clear expectation of death, frequently violent, manic excitement) **OR occasionally fails to maintain minimal personal hygiene** (e.g., smears feces) **OR gross impairment in communica-
11 tion** (e.g., largely incoherent or mute).

10 **Persistent danger of severely hurting self or others** (e.g., recurrent violence) **OR persistent inability to maintain minimal personal hygiene OR serious sui-
1 cidal act with clear expectation of death.**

0 Inadequate information

Source: The American Psychiatric Association. (1987). The Diagnostic and Statistical Manual of Mental Disorders. (Third Edition-R). Washington, D.C.: Author.

the CIA (Central Intelligence Agency). She became increasingly suspicious of neighbors and friends. She spoke with caution when she discussed her husband's military career and on occasion used a series of neologisms such as "My husband is on a tracterntery and selemopentary." She deteriorated quickly: her sleep pattern was disrupted, she experienced loss of appetite, she imagined things, and she heard voices that told her the CIA "was watching." During the psychiatric interview, it was revealed that Peggy had a long history of being impulsive, anxious, and easily stressed. Her husband had catered to her needs in an effort to keep her functioning and "happy." Peggy was brought to a community clinic by a neighbor after her speech become so incomprehensible that the neighbor felt she was "losing control."

Axis I: Schizophreniform disorder, 295.40

Axis II: Borderline personality characteristics

Axis III: Cardiac palpitations
Shortness of breath

Axis IV: Code 3: Moderate
(Separation from spouse)

Axis V: Current GAF-37
Highest GAF past year: 70.

PSYCHOLOGICAL TESTING

Psychological tests can help to validate or clarify a clinical impression and so can aid the diagnostic process. They are not substitutes for competent informed clincal assessment and judgment (Wiggins, 1973). The tests, which involve assessment of intelligence and personality, are administered by experienced clinical psychologists and are used by all mental health professionals at one time or another in the clinical setting. Thus an understanding of the use and meaning of psychological testing can not only enhance the nurse's understanding of a patient's problems, but can facilitate her communication with other mental health professionals.

TESTS OF INTELLECTUAL FUNCTIONING

A variety of tests assess intellectual and cognitive functioning, often picking up any subtle deterioration that could be associated with some mental disorder. These tests include the Wechsler Adult Intelligence Scale (WAIS), the Wechsler Intelligence Scale for Children (WISC), and the Stanford-Binet Test. The clinician needs to remember, however, that a high score on these psychometric tests does not preclude the possibility of serious psychopathology.

On the other hand, a low score or one that has deteriorated significantly from previous ones may in-

dicate the presence of schizophrenia as the schizophrenic's intellectual functioning is typically in the lower range, especially if the material being considered is affect laden. Disparity between the verbal and performance scales (on the Weschler Adult Intelligence Test [WAIS]) may indicate the presence of an organic mental disorder of some type. Especially difficult to interpret would be the test results of a schizophrenic patient with organic problems. Nevertheless, information obtained from these tests can provide insight into the patient's current level of functioning and can be used in psychiatric treatment and nursing care planning, as long as it is kept in mind that no psychological test *alone* should be used to determine the diagnosis or treatment planning for any patient, or to predict the outcome of that person's illness (Wiggins, 1973).

PERSONALITY TESTS

Personality tests can be either objective or projective. Objective tests are usually paper-and-pencil tests, whereas projective tests use visual stimuli to elicit a response from the patient (and sometimes verbal stimuli are used to engage the person in the test-taking process). Visual stimuli tests include the Rorschach Personality Test, the Thematic Apperception Test (TAT), and the Bender-Gestalt Test. Pencil-and-paper tests include the Sentence Completion Test (SCT), the Draw-a-Person Test, and the Minnesota Multiphasic Personality Inventory (MMPI). Regardless of the type of personality test, it should be administered and interpreted by a licensed clinical psychologist specially trained in personality testing, with the possible exception of the MMPI (described later) which can be computer-scored.

RORSCHACH PERSONALITY TEST. The **Rorschach Personality Test** consists of ten cards, each containing a complex, standard "ink blot" picture. Five cards are gray and white, three are multicolored, and two are gray and red. The purpose of the test is to uncover tendencies within the patient that reflect fundamental personality characteristics. During the test, patients are asked to describe what they see in the blot, what it makes them think of, and what it means to them. In this projective technique, clues are obtained regarding underlying psychopathology. The scoring system for this test is very complex, so it should be administered and interpreted *only* by a clinician highly skilled in its use.

THEMATIC APPERCEPTION TEST (TAT). The **Thematic Apperception Test (TAT)** was developed by Henry A. Murray of Harvard University. Murray's (1951) test consists of twenty pictures showing

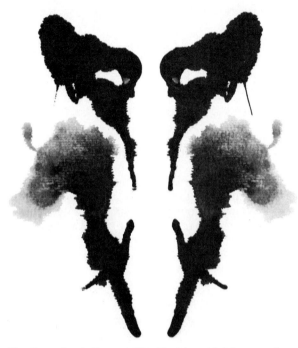

The Rorschach Personality Test is a highly complex analysis of an individual's various personality characteristics. This particular tool is helpful in sorting those personality characteristics which may be considered pathological.

individuals in ambiguous but striking circumstances. It is designed to provoke psychologically significant content. Currently clinicians use fewer than the twenty pictures, depending on the areas they want to explore and the time allotted for testing. In the procedure, patients are asked to describe what seems to be happening in the pictures. Often a patient will identify with a certain character and project his or her own concerns and feelings about self and others onto the characters in the pictures. Central issues and conflicts can be revealed by the stories the patient creates.

BENDER-GESTALT TEST. The **Bender-Gestalt Test** consists of nine patterns that are presented to a patient, one at a time. The patient is then asked to copy what was just seen. A variation is to ask the patient to recall as many patterns as possible after a short time interval. Inferences about personality functioning are then made, based on the organization and distortions in the patient's drawing. Since this test is highly dependent on visual and motor functioning, it can be helpful in the detection of organic brain disease.

SENTENCE COMPLETION TEST (SCT). The **Sentence Completion Test (SCT)** consists of 75 to 100 sentence stems, such as "I like _____," "My greatest fear _____," "Dancing _____." Patients are requested to complete the sentence with the first response that comes to mind. Clinicians review the responses for major patterns and affective tone. Omissions or special attention to detail are also of interest. The individual's reactions to these thoughts about love, goals, failure, and frustration can provide additional understanding of or insight into a patient's unique situation.

DRAW-A-PERSON TEST. In the **Draw-a-Person Test** patients are simply asked to draw a person. Information regarding the patients' body images and their feelings about themselves are often revealed.

MINNESOTA MULTIPHASIC PERSONALITY INVENTORY (MMPI). The **Minnesota Multiphasic Personality Inventory (MMPI)** is very different from the previously described tests. This test is a questionnaire containing 550 items in 26 categories. Nine clinical scales are involved: hypochondriasis, depression, hysteria, psychopathic deviation, masculinity-femininity, paranoia, psychasthenai, schizophrenia, and hypomania. Various indices have been built into the test to provide a measure of the subject's evasiveness, frank or self-critical behavior, and tendency to lie. One of the most commonly used personality tests, the MMPI can provide a great deal of information about the patient when used by a highly skilled clinician. Computer scoring may be available.

NURSING DIAGNOSES

After the nurse has completed the psychiatric assessment, she formulates a care plan based on it and the nursing diagnoses. Quality patient care is facilitated when nursing diagnoses do not simply repeat the psychiatric ones but apply them to or expand them for a particular patient. Care plans based on both psychiatric and nursing diagnoses facilitate continuity of care by serving as a written record of the goals and approaches designed for a particular patient. Based on the information contained in the psychiatric assessment, the nurse must choose those nursing diagnoses that reflect the patient's concerns and problems. A nursing care plan that reflects one patient's major problems and needs follows the case example below. The list of nursing diagnoses does not include every single nursing diagnosis; however, it is an example of the kind of care plan that might be developed for the patient.

Case Study: Psychiatric Setting

Identifying Information

Jane is a 17-year-old, white, single, female high school student. This is her second admission to the psychiatric unit for attempted suicide. Jane resides with her mother and father.

Presenting Problem

Jane was brought to the emergency room after she was found unconscious in her bedroom by her mother. Jane had ingested a mixture of aspirin, tranquilizers, and alcohol. She was treated in the emergency room initially and was then transferred to the medical intensive care unit, where she was observed for twenty-four hours. Subsequently she was transferred to the inpatient psychiatric unit. Jane says that she attempted suicide because "No one cares about me" and "I don't have any friends."

History of Present Illness

Jane reports that she has always had difficulty making friends. She is approximately thirty pounds overweight and states that this has contributed to her problems. She further reports that her parents are always fighting about her and that she feels she is unable to live up to their expectations. Jane first attempted suicide by ingesting barbiturates and alcohol one year ago (due to the previously mentioned problems). She was treated for depression for two weeks on an inpatient basis and has been on outpatient treatment for the past year. In addition to the previously discussed difficulties with her parents and peers at school Jane had just been transferred to a new school. Her parents had hoped that she would become involved in school activities if she were in a new environment. Instead, Jane reports that the transfer has made her feel more lonely and isolated. Jane is unable to report any specific instances that have created difficulties for her in making friends. She states that she feels "nervous and upset" around the students in her school and is afraid to talk to them. She is only able to state clearly that her obesity is a problem.

Jane states that she wants to feel better about herself and make friends. She also says that she wants her parents to stop pushing her into joining clubs and engaging in social activities. She states that her parents' constant mentioning of her lack of friends makes her feel worse. Jane denies any regular alcohol or drug use.

Family History

There is no history of depression or suicide attempts on either maternal or paternal sides of the family. Jane has no siblings. Jane's mother is an elementary school teacher and her father is an insurance salesman. Both her mother and father deny any drug use and report only occasional drinking during social events. Jane's mother reports that she chose not to have other children because Jane required so much attention while she was growing up. She states that she didn't think she could care for more than one child while working fulltime. Jane's father reports that he wanted no more children because Jane had required so much of her mother's time. He felt that two children would have interfered with the marital relationship.

Personal History

1. *Prenatal history:* Jane's mother reports a normal pregnancy, labor, and delivery. The pregnancy was planned and occurred two years after marriage.

2. *Infancy:* Jane's mother reports that Jane had difficulty sleeping and awoke frequently during the night. Jane was two years old before she slept through the night. Jane also had feeding difficulties until she was six months old. She would drink her bottle of milk and then almost immediately vomit approximately one-third of it. Her mother reports that she felt responsible for the vomiting episodes because she felt so "nervous and uncertain" about caring for a new baby. Ages six months through five years were problem-free as far as Jane's parents could recall.

3. *Childhood years:* Her parents state that Jane was extremely frightened about starting school. Although she overcame her fears she remained isolated and never played with other children. Her grades were average to above average during childhood but Jane began to gain weight during this period.

4. *Adolescence:* Jane and her parents report that Jane felt increasingly lonely and upset as she began high school. While her peers were beginning to date and engage in other social activities, Jane did not. Jane's grades declined from average to poor and her weight gain continued.

5. *Current social situation:* Jane's parents own their own home and describe their income as "comfortable." They state that they live in a nice neighborhood and can afford to send Jane to good private schools.

Mental Status Examination

1. *General description:* Jane is an obese teenager sitting slumped in a chair, wearing a wrinkled tee shirt, blue jeans, dirty sneakers, and no socks. Her nails and the skin around her nails are bitten. Her hair is dirty and hangs around her face and eyes. She looks down at the floor or at her hands during the entire interview. She occasionally shifts from side to side in her chair, slowly demonstrating a reduction in activity. Jane seems to respond to the questions in an uninterested manner, although she answers all questions posed.

2. *Speech:* Jane speaks in a soft, hesitant voice. She speaks slowly and answers each question briefly.

3. *Mood and affect:* Jane states that she feels "depressed and lonely." Jane does not gesture when she talks, nor does she change her facial expression. Her affect remains the same during the entire interview. When discussing her loneliness and fears, she stares at the floor and speaks softly. No frowning or crying are evident.

4. *Thought process (form):* Jane speaks only in response to specific questions. Her responses answer the questions and are logical. No impairments are noted.

5. *Content of thought:* Jane spontaneously talks about her obesity and her parents' fighting about her on four different occasions throughout the interview. She states that she will try to kill herself again if she has the opportunity. No delusional thinking is evident. No hallucinations or illusions are present.

6. *Cognitive functioning and orientation:*
   A. Orientation—Jane is oriented to time, place, and person.
   B. Memory—since no deficits are noted in this area during the psychiatric history and subsequent assessment, formal tests of memory are not necessary.

7. *General intelligence:* Jane is a poor to average senior student in high school. There are no specific problems related to intelligence.

8. *Abstract thinking:* When Jane is asked to describe various analogies, such as how an apple and a pear are alike, she does so without error.

9. *Insight and judgment:* Jane states that she would like to feel better but sees "no way out" of her present problems. She says her obesity and her parents are to blame for her current difficulties.

DSM III-R Diagnosis

Jane was diagnosed as having a recurrent major depression, specifically, using a DSM-III-R code, Recurrent major depression, severe, without psychotic features. Using the 5 axes in the DSM-III-R, Jane's full diagnosis is as follows:

Axis I: 296.33   Recurrent Major Depression, Severe, without psychotic features

Axis II: 301.82 Avoidant Personality Disorder

Axis III: Obesity

Axis IV: Psychosocial Stressors: Change to a new school; parents' marital discord related to patient's problems; no friends
Severity: 4 (predominantly enduring circumstances)

Axis V: Current GAF: 18
Highest GAF past year: 25

Nursing Diagnoses

Potential for violence
Social isolation
Self esteem disturbance
Body image disturbance

Nursing Care Plan for Jane

Nursing Diagnosis	Desired Outcomes	Interventions	Rationale
1. Violence, potential for: Self-directed or directed at others; suicidal behavior	Jane will be free of self-destructive behaviors and thoughts.	Determine the presence of suicidal ideation and behaviors. Determine if Jane has developed a plan for her suicide. Record findings in Jane's chart.	Jane's suicide potential/behaviors may vary at any time. Continuous observation and recording are essential for planning and implementing safe and effective care.

Nursing Diagnosis	Desired Outcomes	Interventions	Rationale
		Determine if Jane can enter into a suicide prevention contract with nurses and other staff for a specific time period, for example, 8 hours or one working shift.	This is a basic assessment function that will determine if Jane is able to be free of self-destructive behaviors, or if she needs to be placed on one-to-one suicide precautions.
		Explain the terms of the contract to Jane.	This is a method of involving Jane in her care; it demonstrates the nurse's concern for her, and is indicative of nurse's expectations that Jane is capable of expressing her thoughts and feelings.
		Continue to observe and record any changes in Jane's mood such as euphoria, withdrawal, sense of resignation, or giving up.	Jane's suicidal potential may vary abruptly. Mood/behavioral changes might be indicative of increased risk for suicide.
		Jane's room should be centrally located to enhance opportunities for observation and intervention.	Depending upon the degree of lethality, Jane could use an innocuous object to harm herself.
		Nurse should check Jane's room throughout the night at frequent intervals.	Determines Jane's whereabouts, and ensures her safety
		Encourage Jane's verbal expression of anger and rage.	The identification and verbalization of feelings and thoughts can help Jane work through her conflicts; the nursing staff can provide support.
		Jane and nursing staff should examine the events and relationships that combined to create Jane's suicidal behavior.	Jane's family might need assistance in understanding and appropriately responding to her.
		Discuss the future with Jane: include significant relationships, emotional frustrations, and conflicts and how she might manage them.	These activities can assist Jane in preparing for coping with problems and crises that might occur in the future.

Nursing Diagnosis	Desired Outcomes	Interventions	Rationale
		Assist Jane in identifying the potential impact of her suicide on (1) family (2) friends.	This is a method of further assessing her level of anger and disappointment; it helps her to express anger toward significant others; Nurse can help her to gain insight about potential negative outcome of her behavior, for example, the possibility that her death wouldn't change anything except that *she* would be dead.
2. Social isolation	Jane will develop and maintain meaningful interpersonal relationships as evidenced by increased communication and socialization with others.	Encourage Jane to participate in individual and group therapy.	Jane will become more comfortable in verbalizing feelings through therapy.
		Encourage Jane to talk about feelings of loneliness and isolation; explore with Jane why she thinks these feelings exist.	This assists her in learning useful methods of seeking and maintaining friends.
		Plan social skills training for Jane when her symptoms/behaviors indicate that this is appropriate.	Jane will learn acceptable methods of engaging in meaningful relationships with family and friends.
		Discuss with Jane methods of broadening social contacts and interpersonal relations after hospitalization, such as possibility of joining a community-based group for adolescents, such as her church teen club.	Jane might tend to isolate herself after hospitalization and reinforce her own feelings of isolation and loneliness.
		Encourage Jane to participate in ongoing outpatient therapy.	This provides for the continuation of a meaningful relationship for Jane, a vehicle for support while Jane works on developing and maintaining meaningful relationships.
3. Self esteem disturbance	Jane will experience an increase in self-esteem as evidenced by the development of confidence in herself to achieve her goals and an assessment of (a) her attributes and (b) her limitations as related to her defined goals.	Encourage Jane to express her feelings and thoughts about herself.	These thoughts and feelings must be recognized, labeled, and dealt with. Provides Jane with opportunity to express her thoughts/ feelings and receive feedback that might assist her in acknowledging her attributes and limitations.

Nursing Diagnosis	Desired Outcomes	Interventions	Rationale
		Provide assertiveness training for Jane, preferably in a group format.	Jane will learn how to express her feelings and attitude to others without continuously compromising her wishes.
		Recommend on-going outpatient therapy.	Continuous work in this area will be needed as Jane (a) explores new ways of relating to others, and (b) employs different methods of meeting her own needs.
4. Body image disturbance	Jane will demonstrate behaviors that confront methods of developing the type of body image she desires.	Assess the meaning of Jane's weight gain and explore with her (a) the thoughts, events, and feelings that existed at the time the weight gain occurred and (b) possible alternative behaviors to eating.	Expression of feelings of frustration, conflict, and depression should be explored to help Jane develop impulse control surrounding food consumption.
		Assist Jane (a) in relating excessive eating behavior to affect and thoughts, and (b) in determining an agreed-upon plan for weight reduction.	Understanding of emotions and alternative methods of expressions should assist in weight control.
		Monitor Jane's food and drink intake to determine her level of compliance to an agreed-upon plan.	Involving Jane in her care encourages Jane to take responsibility for her eating and weight gain.
			Jane should be encouraged to assume responsibility for her behavior when she becomes more competent in this area.

SUMMARY

A psychiatric assessment involves the examination of both the mind and the body of a patient. This assessment elicits information about the origin and development of a patient's emotional, cognitive, or behavioral disturbances, current mental status, and the social, psychological, and cultural influences in his or her life. The assessment also takes into account physiological factors.

The two major models used in making psychiatric assessments are the psychoanalytic and behavioral models. The psychoanalytic model emphasizes inner causes. The behavioral model emphasizes the relationship between behavior and specific environmental factors. There are also three broad categories of nursing models of assessment: developmental, systems, and interaction. Developmental models focus on the process of growth and maturation. Systems models emphasize the person in his or her environment. Interaction models focus on the individual's perceptions of other people, the environment, situations, and events.

The psychiatric assessment consists of several components. The largest component, the psychiatric interview, includes the psychiatric history and the mental-status examination, as well as the psychosocial assessment. Ego assessment, physiological assessment, and psychological testing are also part of the psychiatric assessment.

The nurse needs to be familiar with the use of DSM-III-R in many clinical settings. The DSM-III-R uses five axes to evaluate a psychiatric patient.

Psychological tests may be used to clarify a clinical impression and to aid in the diagnostic process. These tests include examinations of both intellectual functioning and personality.

Nursing diagnoses facilitate the provision of quality care to patients. Based on the information gained in a psychiatric assessment, the nurse must choose those diagnoses that reflect the individual patient's concerns and problems, and then base nursing interventions on those diagnoses.

KEY TERMS

psychiatric assessment

psychoanalytic model

resistance

transference

countertransference

behavioral model

stimulus-organism-response-consequence (SORC)

developmental models

systems models

interaction models

psychiatric history

mental-status examination

psychosocial assessment

physiological assessment

ego functions

reality testing

judgment

sense of the world

sense of self

regulation and control of drives, affects, and emotions

object relations

thought process

adaptive regression in service of the ego (ARISE)

defensive functioning

stimulus barrier

autonomous functioning

synthetic-integrative functioning

mastery competence

agnosia

apraxia

aphasia

cranial nerves

cerebellum

esteem support

informational support

social companionship

instrumental support

Rorschach Personality Test

Thematic Apperception Test (TAT)

Sentence Completion Test (SCT)

Draw-a-Person Test

Bender-Gestalt Test

Minnesota Multiphasic Personality Inventory (MMPI)

STUDY QUESTIONS

1. What is the purpose of a psychiatric assessment?

2. Name and describe briefly the two major models used in psychiatric assessment.

3. Name and describe briefly the three categories of nursing models for assessment.

4. Name and describe briefly the major components of a psychiatric assessment.

5. What are the five axes of DSM-III-R?

REFERENCES

American Psychiatric Association. (1980). *A Psychiatric Glossary* (5th ed.). Washington, D.C.: American Psychiatric Association.

Bates, B. (1983). *A guide to physical examination* (3rd ed.). Philadelphia: Lippincott.

Bellak, L. (1975). *Overload: The new human condition*. New York: Human Services Press.

Bellak, L., Hurvich, M., and Gedimen, H. (1973). *Ego functions in schizophrenics, neurotics, and normals*. New York: John Wiley and Sons.

Bellak, L., and Loeb, L. (eds.) (1969). *Schizophrenic Syndrome*. New York: Greene and Stratton.

Bott, E. (1971), *Family and social network: Roles, norms, and external relationships in ordinary urban families*. New York: Free Press.

Ciminero, A. R. (1977). Behavioral assessment: An overview. In A. R. Ciminero, K. S. Calhoun, & H. E. Adams (eds.), *Handbook of behavioral assessment*. New York: Wiley, pp. 3–46.

Ciminero, A. (1986). Behavioral assessment: An overview. In *Handbook of behavioral assessment*. Ciminero, A.; Calhoun, K.; Adams, H. New York: Wiley Co.

Cohen, S., Mermelstein, R., Karmarck, T., and Hoberman, H. M. (1985). Measuring the functional components of social support. In I. G. Sarason and B. R. Sarason (eds.), *Social support: Theory, research and applications*. Boston: Martinus Nijhoff Publishers.

Erikson, E. (1950). *Childhood and society*. New York: W. W. Norton Co.

Erikson, E. (1963). *Childhood and society*. New York: W. W. Norton Co.

Fawcett, J. (1978). The relationship between theory and research: A double helix. *Advances in Nursing Science*, *1* (1) pp. 49–62.

Fawcett, J. (1984). *Analysis and evaluation of conceptual models in nursing*. Philadelphia: Davis.

Fawcett, J. (1989). *Analysis and evaluation of conceptual models in nursing.* 2nd ed. Philadelphia: Davis.

Francis, G., and Munjas, B. (1976). *Manual of social-psychologic assessment.* New York: Appleton-Century-Crofts.

Fromm-Reichmann (1950). *Principles of intensive psychotherapy.* Chicago: University of Chicago Press.

Ginsberg, G. I. (1985). Psychiatric history and mental status examination. In H. I Kaplan and B. J. Sadock (eds.), *Comprehensive textbook of psychiatry: Vol. 1* (4th ed.). Baltimore, MD: Williams & Wilkins, pp. 487–494.

Goldfried, M. R., & Kent, R. (1972). Traditional versus behavioral assessment: A comparison of methodological and theoretical assumptions. *Psychological Bulletin, 77,* 409–420.

Goldfried, M. R., & Sprofkin, J. N. (1976). Behavioral personality assessment. In J. T. Spence, R. C. Carson, & J. W. Thibault (eds.), *Behavioral approaches to therapy.* Morristown, NJ: General Learning Press.

Greenson, R. R. (1972). *The technique and practice of psychoanalysis, Vol. I.* New York: International Universities Press, Inc.

Hagerty, B. (ed.) (1984). *Psychiatric mental health assessment.* St. Louis: C. V. Mosby Co.

Hall, C. S., and Lindzey (1970). *Theories of personality.* 2nd ed. New York: Wiley Co.

House, J. S. (1981). *Work, stress and social support.* Reading, MA: Addison Wesley.

House, J. S., & Kahn, R. L. (1985). Measures and concepts of social support. In S. Cohen and S. L. Syme (eds.), *Social support and health.* Orlando, FL: Academic Press, pp. 83–108.

Johnston, R., and Fitzpatrick, J. (1982). *Relevance of psychiatric mental health nursing theories to nursing models and their psychiatric mental health application.* J. Fitzpatrick, H. Whall, R. Johnston, and J. Floyd (eds.) Bowie: Robert Brady Co.

Kanfer, F. H., & Saslow, G. (1969). Behavioral diagnoses. In C. M. Franks (ed.), *Behavior therapy: Appraisal and status.* New York: McGraw-Hill, pp. 310–315.

Kaplan, H. I., and Sadock, B. J. (1985) *Comprehensive textbook of psychiatry* (4th ed.), vol. 1. Baltimore: Williams and Wilkins.

Kaplan, H. I. & Sadock, B. J. (1988). *Synopsis of psychiatry: Behavioral sciences/clinical psychiatry.* 5th ed. Baltimore, MD: Williams and Wilkins.

Kernberg, O. (1965). Notes on countertransference. *J. Am. Psychoanal. Assoc., 13,* 38–56.

Kernberg, O. (1984). *Severe personality disorders.* New Haven, CT: Yale University Press.

Kessler, R. G., Price, R. H., and Wortman, C. B. (1985). Social factors in psychopathology: Stress, social support, and coping processes. *Ann. Neo. Psychol., 36,* 531–572.

Kolb L., and Brodie, K. (1982). *Modern clinical psychiatry.* Philadelphia: W. B. Saunders Co.

Kuhn, T. S. (1962). *The structure of scientific revolutions* (2nd ed.). Chicago: University of Chicago Press.

MacKinnon, R. A. (1975). Diagnosis and psychiatry: Examination of the psychiatric patient. In H. I. Kaplan and J. J. Sadock, *Comprehensive textbook of psychiatry: Vol. 1* (3rd ed.). Baltimore: Williams and Wilkins, pp. 906–926.

MacKinnon, R. A., & Michels (1971). *The psychiatric interview in clinical practice.* Philadelphia: Sanders Co.

Malasanos, L., Barkauskas, V., Moss, M., Stoltenberg-Allen, K. (1986). *Health assessment.* St. Louis: Mosby Co.

Meissner, W. W. (1985). Theories of personality and psychopathology: Classical psychoanalysis. In H. I. Kaplan and B. J. Sadock (eds.), *Comprehensive textbook of psychiatry: Vol. I* (4th ed.), pp. 337–418.

Melies, A. (1985). *Theoretical nursing: Development and progress.* Philadelphia: Lippincott Co.

Mischel, W. (1968). *Personality and assessment.* New York: Wiley Co.

Mischel, W. (1981). *Introduction to personality* (3rd ed.). New York: Holt, Rinehart and Winston.

Mitchell, R. E., and Trickett, E. J. (1980). Social networks as mediators of social support. *Community Mental Health Journal, 16,* 27–44.

Murray, H. A. (1951). Uses of thematic apperception test. *Am J. Psychiatry, 107,* 577–581.

Nicholi, A. (1978) History and mental status. In A. Nicholi (ed.), *The Harvard guide to modern psychiatry.* Cambridge: The Belknap Press of Harvard University Press.

Packard, K. (1984). The psychiatric interview. In B. K. Hagerty (Ed.) *Psychiatric mental health assessment.* St. Louis: Mosby.

Pearlin, L., and Schooler, C. (1978). The structure of coping. *J. Health Soc. Behav., 19,* 2–21.

Peplau, H. (1952). *Interpersonal relations in nursing.* New York: G. P. Putnam's Sons.

Riehl, J., & Roy, C. (1980). *Conceptual models for nursing practice.* New York: Appleton-Century-Crofts.

Roediger, H.; Rushton, J. P.; Capaldi, E.; Paris, S. (1987). *Psychology.* (2nd ed.) Boston: Little, Brown and Co.

Schafer, R. (1968). *Aspects of internalization.* New York: International Universities Press.

Skinner, B. F. (1953). *Science and human behavior.* New York: Free Press. p. 31.

Wiggins, J. (1973). *Personality and prediction, principles of clinical assessment.* Reading, Mass.: Addison-Wesley.

6

SOCIOCULTURAL DIVERSITY AND PSYCHIATRIC MENTAL HEALTH NURSING

FAYE GARY

LEARNING OBJECTIVES

After studying this chapter, the student will be able to:

- Define the concepts of culture, values, culture contact, predominant culture, and ethnocentrism.
- Develop and identify a sense of her own cultural self-awareness.
- Describe general guidelines for providing mental health care for a person of a cultural background different from her own.
- Identify the attitudes and beliefs of the specific cultural subgroups.
- Describe the relationship between culture and mental illness and treatment.
- Describe the implications of cultural differences for mental health nursing practice.

INTRODUCTION

Each student enters the nursing profession with a unique social and cultural background. Such individual distinctiveness can often be an asset in psychiatric nursing, as a patient's outlook on health problems can improve when others enable him or her to see the problems from different perspectives. But our variations in outlook can also serve as a barrier to understanding, appreciating, and respecting people from different ethnic and racial groups. In this chapter, we provide information about ethnic and racial minority groups in American society. The chapter's goal is to stimulate understanding and respect for the rich array of cultural backgrounds and perspectives that are found in contemporary American society.

Information in this chapter also has clinical implications. Nurses and other mental health professionals have been accused of often giving health care that emphasizes what is important to the professional rather than what is important to the patient and his or her family (Harwood, 1981). Providers of mental health care are more likely to represent Anglo backgrounds than those they serve. Understanding the needs of the patient and the family must include an understanding of, and respect for, the patient's social and cultural background. Thus, we hope this chapter will provide a resource for psychiatric nurses and others who are concerned with developing better methods for treating mental illness and for providing culturally sensitive care for people who represent minority ethnic and racial heritages.

SOCIOCULTURAL DIVERSITY

Some societies, such as Norway, Sweden, and Denmark, are composed of populations that share large degrees of racial, historical, religious, and cultural characteristics. Such societies are referred to as culturally homogeneous. But not all nations are so internally similar. At the other end of the continuum are societies that are culturally heterogeneous; that is, their citizens differ greatly in their beliefs, values, races, histories, and cultures. Examples include the Soviet Union (with over 200 different cultural groups), Yugoslavia, South Africa, Great Britain, and the United States.

Cultural groups in heterogenous societies can usually be arranged in power hierarchies, forming dominant groups and minority groups. The dominant group is not necessarily larger. For example, in South Africa, the white dominant group is made up of less than 2 percent of the population. In the United States, the dominant group is the "WASPS" (White, Anglo-Saxon Protestants), although they make up a numerical minority. Dominant groups are defined by their control over material (for example, money) and non-material (for example, the power to define beauty and self-worth) resources. Hence, the central defining characteristic of minority group status is relative powerlessness: the inability of a group, relative to the whole, to determine its own fate in political, social, or economic activities.

There are four additional elements that characterize minority group status (Hess et al., 1989, p. 244):

1. Visible ascribed traits, by which most minority group members can be recognized.

2. Differential treatment on the basis of possessing these traits.

3. The organization of self-image around this identity.

4. An awareness of shared identity with others in the same group.

The United States contains many large ethnic and racial groups. Minority groups are usually defined along racial and ethnic lines, but can also be defined along religious lines (for example, Jewish Americans or the Amish) or lifestyle differences (for example, gays and lesbians). But despite the importance of race and ethnicity in defining minority group status, the terms are not precise. The significance of race, for example, is based more on sociocultural attitudes than on scientific data; with much intermarriage through history and cross-racial fertility there is no agreement on how many races there are or how those with mixed racial backgrounds should be classified. In broad terms, racial groups are traditionally collapsed into three categories: Negro, Caucasian, and Mongoloid. Similarly, ethnic groups are loosely defined as groups that are characterized by national origin, language, or cultural patterns. Ethnicity often correlates with race and religion. Ethnic and racial groups become minority groups only when they are typified by a history and current status of relative powerlessness.

Given the centrality of powerlessness in defining minority group status, the status also tends to correspond with social class differences in American society. Blacks, Hispanics, and Native Americans are disproportionately represented among the lower economic classes. Some of the constraints placed upon these minority groups (such as denial of opportunities for upward mobility), as well as some of their behaviors (for example, health care practices), may be as much a function of social class as it is of minority group status. Dominant and minority groups share at least one thing in common: a national identity, or, at least, geographic proximity under the same flag. This proximity requires that both groups adopt various strategies to relate to each other. In theory, two different outcomes of minority/dominant group relations are possible: the melting pot and the cultural pluralism models.

The melting pot model is well named; it suggests that immigrants and other minority groups, over time, will gradually lose their differences with the dominant group and come to share a common language, culture, and worldview. The parents and grandparents of some of today's college students, for example, may have strong Irish, Italian, or Polish identifications that the college students themselves no longer emulate or value. In short, the melting pot model suggests that differences between groups will melt down and eventually cease to exist. Whether because of lack of opportunity or because of resistance by particular minority groups, the melting pot model is a more accurate description of some groups' experiences (for example, Irish) than of others' (for example, African or Native Americans).

The cultural pluralism model, on the other hand, values the diversity of various minority groups in American culture, and seeks to preserve them. The model is like a tossed salad, where every ingredient remains unique while contributing to the salad as a whole. To be sure, contemporary American culture falls short of this model, as some minority groups are treated as less important ingredients of the salad. The cultural pluralism model is one in which racial and ethnic group differences are understood, appreciated, respected, and preserved.

MINORITY/DOMINANT GROUP INTERACTION

Minority and dominant groups can have a variable degree of contact, ranging on a continuum from near isolation (segregation), to accommodation, acculturation, assimilation, and finally to intermarriage and the complete melting pot, or amalgamation.

Accommodation involves the recognition of group differences, but no efforts to remove or diminish the differences. An example of accommodation is seen in the relationships between Cubans and Anglos in Miami, Florida.

To a large degree the business and social communities of the two groups are separate, while at the same time the Cubans have learned to deal effectively with the mainstream Anglo social institutions, such as the schools and government, and vice versa. Such accommodation in Miami has not spread, however, to incorporate relations between blacks and Anglos.

Acculturation involves "phenomena which result when groups of individuals having different cultures come into continuous first-hand contact, with subsequent changes in the original cultural patterns of either or both groups" (Redfield et al., 1936 p. 149). Here, the minority group begins to adopt (and influence) the values and culture of the dominant group. Often this process occurs without design or conscious awareness. The process of acculturation requires continuous interaction among individuals from the different cultural groups. The result is a change in cultural patterns in one or both groups, but almost always it is the minority group that changes the most.

Some tensions can arise within cultural groups as acculturation occurs (Olmedo, 1979; Bernal et al., 1983). Among those points of tension are differences in language, social class, and subcultural behavioral norms. For example, white Anglo cultural conceptions of individualism tend to portray Hispanics as group-dependent. The Hispanic may respond by developing behavioral patterns consistent with those of white Anglos, and thereby risk losing the support, understanding, and continuous ties with his or her kinship group. On the other hand, the Hispanic might rebel against the Anglo society and reject many of its values, attitudes, and beliefs.

Assimilation is the end of the process of acculturation. It occurs when groups and individuals replace their original culture with another culture. Minority groups lose their distinctiveness and are absorbed into the dominant population. For assimilation to occur, two things must happen: 1) the individual must want to become part of the dominant culture, and 2) the dominant cultural group must be willing to absorb that individual or group.

Minority groups can learn to vary their behavior, appearing to be assimilated only in specific situations. At school, a student might act "acculturated and assimilated," but upon return to his or her neighborhood, manifest all the behaviors accorded that minority group with little regard for the dominant culture. Such bicultural adaptive techniques often *must* be learned to avoid tension and conflict.

Minority/dominant group interactions may result in mutual acceptance, adaptation, or reaction. When acceptance occurs, the groups assimilate each others' values, attitudes, and languages into the existing culture. When adaptation occurs, the groups combine

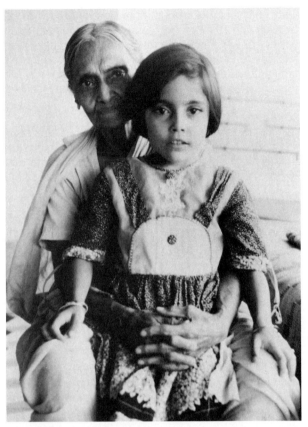

Minority groups learn to vary their behavior in accordance with their situation: they may appear to be assimilated to the dominant culture in one situation until they return to their own neighborhood whereupon they manifest all those behaviors concomitant to their own minority culture or ethnic group.

the original and foreign traits, attitudes, and values into a harmonious whole; conflicts may be resolved over time during interaction with others in the dominant culture. Reaction occurs when contra-acculturative movements arise, either because of oppression or because of unforeseen results of the acculturation process (Redfield et al., 1936).

SOCIAL CHANGE AND MENTAL HEALTH

Minority groups have had to adapt to numerous cultural changes, and the rapid rate of social change may in some cases produce stresses that result in mental health problems. Consider the language problems for Hispanics and Asians: most are concerned with continuing use of their own language, but realize that learning English is essential for upward mobility in American society. Also, values and attitudes about se-

lected components of American society must be learned. This may be particularly difficult for older people. For example, a re-definition of the meaning of time is important for minority groups. Much of America's business is conducted within a framework of deadlines, structured appointments, and prescribed behaviors in organizations. Henderson and Premeaux (1981, p. 14) have written that language shapes the philosophy of a particular ethnic group. With regard to time, in English, the clock "runs"; in Spanish, the clock "walks" (el reloj anda); and for the Native American the clock "just ticks."

The case study of Ann Goren is presented to highlight conflicts in 1) health-care beliefs, 2) rural/urban orientation, 3) North/South behaviors, and 4) minority/dominant group value differences. This vignette describes the conflicts that developed between a black nurse applying for graduate studies and the faculty admissions team at a prestigious university in the Northeast.

Ann Goren: A Graduate Nurse

Ann Goren, a graduate of a nursing school in the South, applied for graduate admission to a prestigious university in the Northeast. She dressed well and prepared for the interview. During the interview Ms. Goren spoke of assisting her grandmother in the preparation of a "secret concoction" that contained natural herbs and other portions from plants and animals that was used for her practice of "root medicine." Ms. Goren had for years been very proud of her relationship with her grandmother and of the great service the two of them had provided for the community. In fact. Ms. Goren had developed an excellent reputation in her community for working with women who were experiencing difficulty with husbands and/or children (a family-therapist role). Her aspiration for being accepted into graduate school at this university was abruptly halted when she responded to the interviewer's questions about her "philosophy and beliefs about mental health care." Ms. Goren described her beliefs about the supernatural, how the alteration of consciousness of her patients was achieved through instructing them to engage in a special chant and hold their breath while keeping their eyes closed. She explained that the concoction was made from a secret formula that she and her grandmother shared. Ms. Goren also stated that the integration of theory and practice of Western scientific knowledge would be most useful in her healthcare practice back home.

The interview committee, predominantly white Anglos, did not share the same views of mental health care. They politely dismissed Ms. Goren from the interview and indicated that she would not "fit" with the goals and objectives of the program. Some months later, Ms. Goren was still unsure about why she was not admitted to the university. After all, she was an honor graduate from a black southern university with an excellent reputation.

RURAL TO URBAN ACCULTURATION AND ASSIMILATION. The study of rural culture and the immigration of its people to urban centers can be systematically accomplished in a way similar to the study of acculturation and assimilation of minority and dominant groups. In fact, all of the dynamics of acculturation and assimilation discussed above occur in this situation as well.

Urbanization can create psychiatric conflicts for those individuals leaving a rural society—the traditional rural cultural values, attitudes, and language may conflict with those in modern urban centers. For instance, behaviors that emphasize bartering, close family ties, and obligation are paramount in the rural dweller's life but are in sharp contrast to the self-reliance and independence stressed in cities. As illustrated by the case of Dr. Maria Tavares, a rural Hispanic physician trying to adapt to city life, individuals who fail to adapt to the demands of the metropolis either return to rural life or experience personal defeat and psychological value conflicts in the form of physical and/or mental problems (Kiev, 1972).

Maria Tavares: A Hispanic Doctor

Dr. Maria Tavares, a Hispanic woman, age 30, had lived in a small town in Texas for most of her life. She enjoyed extended family ties—the sharing of familial responsibilities with numerous siblings, aunts, cousins, and uncles. After graduation from high school, she had attended a small Catholic college in a nearby town and received her undergraduate degree. During this time, she had lived at home and received continuous support from her family. After graduation, Maria worked for two years and then applied to the medical school at a large state university, located in a sprawling, urban city in Texas.

Maria reluctantly left home and moved to the city. She was without family support, felt forced to change her dietary habits, and could communicate only in English. She did not understand the "hustle and bustle" of the city, complained of the "crowded-in feeling" she experienced as a resident in the university dormitory, and missed the usual social gatherings and neighborhood activities of her hometown.

Maria experienced inner anxieties and continuous psychological discomfort but felt forced to identify with the majority group standards. This was extremely difficult and affected her study habits and the ease with which she communicated with others. She felt isolated and alienated but did not want to let her family down by failing in medical school. Since Maria was the first person in her family to pursue advanced study, she felt a family obligation to remain in the school at all costs.

Finally, Maria graduated. By that time, however, she had lost approximately 50 pounds, and was withdrawn, suspicious, depressed, and anxious. The tensions of urban living had proved to be quite stressful.

PREJUDICE AND DISCRIMINATION

Prejudice and discrimination are forms of hostility directed primarily by members of dominant groups towards members of minority groups, although the process can work in reverse. *Prejudice* is a state of mind, including a prejudged set of feelings and attitudes, based on emotions rather than rationality, about an entire group. *Discrimination* involves overt and observable action that results in unfavorable and disenfranchising treatment against a group because of race, ethnicity, or religion. It is disenfranchising because it deprives people of political, economic, and/or social opportunities. Knowledge and information about the individual and/or group does not always dispel prejudicial attitudes (Vander Zanden, 1972). Prejudice can be conceptualized on three levels: cognitive, emotional, and action oriented (Kramer, 1949). The cognitive level involves the mental pictures that a person holds about an individual or group; the emotional components include an individual's feelings and internal states that are aroused by a minority individual or group; the action level involves the propensity or likelihood that an individual will act in a hostile way toward members of a minority group (Kramer, 1949; Bettelheim & Janowitz, 1964; Vander Zanden, 1972; Vontress, 1979).

Many studies of prejudice have examined the psychological characteristics of prejudiced people. From a psychoanalytic view, prejudice can be seen as fulfilling "personality needs." One of the early studies in this vein posited that a particular personality type, the authoritarian personality, was related to prejudice (Adorno et al., 1950). Prejudice against minority groups can create cohesion among dominant groups through its ability to define good guys (dominant groups) and bad guys (minorities). It improves the position of the dominant group when competing with minorities for wealth, jobs, power, and prestige. It also suggests to the individuals in the dominant group that they are better people than members of minority groups, and serves as a method of projecting onto others those characteristics and attributes that are intolerable within oneself (Bettelheim & Janowitz, 1964).

An individual can be prejudiced while not showing any overt expression of that prejudice. Overt behavioral expressions of prejudice are referred to as discrimination. A white nursing student might have strong negative feelings toward black (or other minority) faculty, but never act on those feelings. The student might hold his or her feelings in abeyance because of a fear of reprisal from the faculty member, because of denial, or simply because of an overriding desire to treat everyone with respect regardless of an inner dislike or paternalism for them.

An individual might also discriminate against individual members of a minority group but have little or no prejudice against the group as a whole. Such discrimination is likely to occur if the individual feels that accommodation to members of a minority group might disenfranchise his or her own status with the dominant community. For example, a nurse might elect not to place a Native American, Asian, or a black patient in the same hospital room with a white patient. The nurse may not be prejudiced against these minority groups; the behavior may be based on the fear of reprisal from people perceived to be prejudiced—nursing administrators, hospital officials, the patient, or the patient's family. A person can also discriminate without being consciously prejudiced; for example, a misogynic male professor may unconsciously treat women as subordinates, even though he is not conscious of his implicit biases. Table 6–1 illustrates the relationships between attitude and behavior in minority/dominant group interactions.

Still today, some individuals will not accept minority nurses as qualified care providers. The following experience illustrates how prejudiced attitudes can lead to discriminatory behavior in the health care field. In a recent case, a black home-health nurse was refused entry to a white patient's home. After rejecting her, the patient quickly telephoned the agency and demanded that a white nurse be sent to care for him. Although the agency personnel attempted to reassure him of the minority nurse's qualifications, the patient continued to refuse to allow the nurse to enter his home. Even though the agency had an Equal Opportunity Employer policy, it could not force the patient to accept this particular nurse. So, the agency's administration had to make a decision either to provide a white nurse or to refuse to provide services for the patient. They chose to provide service with a white nurse, leaving the black nurse without employment for the hours allocated for the white patient. In the end, the black nurse was angry and hurt, and the service coordinator felt responsible for having subjected the nurse to such poor treatment by the patient and for not being able to provide employment for such an excellent employee simply because she was black.

TABLE 6–1 An illustration of the relationship between attitudes and behavior

		Attitude	
		Prejudiced	**Accepting**
Behavior	**Discriminatory**	not only hates having strangers next door but actively attempts to prevent having them (e.g., by crossburning and retaining exclusionary zoning laws).	does not care who lives where but will not fight institutional racism/inequality.
	Nondiscriminatory	does not want strangers next door but will not do anything to prevent their moving in or their continued residence.	does not object to and may even welcome strangers' moving into neighborhood.

Source: Hess, B. B., Markson E. W., & Stein, P. J. (1989). *Sociology,* 3rd ed. New York: Macmillan, p. 251.

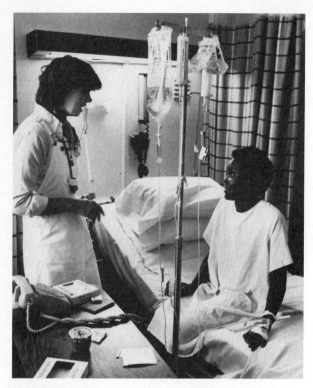

A cultural identity development model may be helpful in exploring those individual cultural and ethnic differences which may hamper the nurse-therapist/patient relationship.

CULTURAL IDENTITY: WHO SHOULD CARE FOR WHOM?

Are there situations when a white therapist cannot provide adequate mental health services to a minority patient, or when a minority therapist can not provide adequate mental health services to a white patient? Given the racial barriers that are still present in American society, there is no easy answer to such questions, or at least to how these barriers can be best surmounted. But there are times when racial (or cultural) homogeneity might be preferable. To illustrate, consider the case of a minority person who is grappling with problems relating to his or her cultural or racial identity. A cultural identity development model is useful in understanding these issues. This model describes transformations in the identity of individual minority group members over time and helps shed light on individual differences within the minority group. It can be applied to nurse therapists, other mental health professionals, and/or patients.

Atkinson, Morten, and Sue (1989, pp. 39–44) have developed the *Minority Identity Development Model (MID)*, which delineates five stages:

Stage One (Conformity Stage): During this stage, the minority person is likely to reject his or her own culture in favor of identification with the dominant (white Anglo) culture. The minority prefers the dominant culture's behaviors, values, and attitudes more than his or her own cultural perspectives.

Stage Two (Dissonance Stage): Confusion and conflict about previously accepted (dominant) cultural beliefs and values are pervasive. New information and experiences tend to lead the individual to question or challenge the beliefs and perspectives that dominated his/her thought during the Conformity Stage.

Stage Three (Resistance and Immersion Stage): The individual begins to reject the dominant culture's beliefs, values, and behaviors. He or she endorses the minority group's views, behaviors, and beliefs, working toward the eradication of racism, prejudice, and oppression. The minority group's history and culture take on a highly significant meaning. The minority individual begins to distrust and reject the dominant (white Anglo) society.

Stage Four (Introspection Stage): The individual begins to feel uncomfortable with the rigid and constraining perceptions about the minority and dominant cultures held in the Resistance and Immersion Stage. Personal autonomy and loyalty to one's own minority group vs. the partial acceptance of the dominant group's outlook are in conflict. Complete distrust for members of the dominant group begins to be replaced by selective trust.

Stage Five (Synergistic Articulation and Awareness Stage): Here, questions of cultural identity are resolved, leading to a sense of self-fullment. The resolution of conflict begun during the Introspection Stage provides feelings of self-control, autonomy, and flexibility. The minority can objectively assess, accept, or reject the cultural values, beliefs, and behaviors of his or her own group as well as other cultural groups, though not all minority group perspectives are automatically accepted. The desire to eliminate oppression remains within the individual, and individual distinctiveness within the minority group is more fully appreciated.

This model is summarized in Table 6–2. Now, it can be used to address the above questions relating to cross-cultural provision of mental health services. The model is useful in understanding variations in minority patients and behavior and individual differences among minority mental health workers them-

TABLE 6–2 Summary of minority identity development model

Stages of Minority Development Model	Attitude Toward Self	Attitude Toward Others of the Same Minority	Attitude Toward Others of Different Minority	Attitude Toward Dominant Group
Stage 1—Conformity	Self-deprecating	Group deprecating	Discriminatory	Group appreciating
Stage 2—Dissonance	Conflict between self-deprecating and appreciating	Conflict between group deprecating and group appreciating	Conflict between dominant held views of minority hierarchy and feelings of shared experience	Conflict between group-appreciating and group-deprecating
Stage 3—Resistance and Immersion	Self-appreciating	Group appreciating	Conflict between feelings of empathy for other minority experiences and feelings of culturocentrism	Group deprecating
Stage 4–Introspection	Concern with basis of self-appreciation	Concern with nature of unequivocal appreciation	Concern with ethnocentric basis for judging others	Concern with the basis of group deprecation
Stage 5–Synergetic Articulation and Awareness	Self-appreciating	Group appreciating	Group appreciating	Selective appreciating

Source: Atkinson, D. R., Morten, G., & Sue, D. W. (1989). *Counseling American Minorities: A Cross-Cultural Perspective,* 3rd ed. Dubuque, Iowa: W. C. Brown, p. 44.

selves. If problems relating to cultural identity are present, for example, minority patients would be more likely to respond to services provided by other minority group members at the Dissonance Stage than at the Conformity Stage. At the Synergistic Articulation and Awareness Stage, cultural group similarity is rarely a problem between the patient and therapist (see Atkinson et al., 1989; Sue, 1981, pp. 66–69). But in practice this model is dynamic, so a particular person may move through different stages at various times during his/her lifetime.

MINORITY GROUPS IN THE UNITED STATES

The two largest minority groups in the United States today are blacks and Hispanics. Table 6–3 gives the distribution of the American population for whites, blacks, Hispanics, and "Others" according to the 1980 census. In 1980, the American population was approximately 226.5 million; estimates are that by 1990 the population had increased by 25 million. Note that the 1980 figures show that there are approximately 6.5 million more females than males, a difference attributable to varying life expectancies. The median age of Hispanics (23.3 years) and of blacks (24.9 years) is lower than that of whites (31.6 years). The West has the largest minority population—14.5 percent of its residents are Hispanic.

BLACK AMERICANS

No understanding of the current status of black Americans is possible unless one first studies the history of brutalization and exploitation that blacks have suffered throughout American history. Whites "systematically closed schools, churches, stores, restaurants, and public places to blacks or made insulting provisions for them. For one hundred years every program of public and private white America was de-

TABLE 6–3 Percent distribution of persons by ethnic/racial background and sex, age, and geographical area United States, 1980

Characteristic	Ethnic/Racial Background				Total
	White	Black	Hispanic Origin	Other	
Total	79.5	11.5	6.4	2.5	226,545,805
Sex					
Male	79.7	11.2	6.6	2.5	110,053,161
Female	79.5	11.8	6.3	2.4	116,492,644
Age					
Median age*	31.6	24.9	23.3	26.5	30.0
Under 15**	73.0	15.0	9.0	3.0	51,290,339
15–44**	79.0	12.0	7.0	3.0	105,203,337
45–64**	84.0	9.0	4.0	2.0	44,502,662
65 + **	88.0	8.0	3.0	1.0	25,549,427
Geographic area					
Region					
Northeast	83.4	9.6	5.3	1.7	49,135,283
North central	87.5	9.0	2.2	1.3	58,864,670
South	74.3	18.4	5.9	1.3	75,372,362
West	73.5	5.1	14.5	6.9	43,172,490
Urban	76.1	13.3	7.9	2.8	167,050,992
Rural	89.4	6.5	2.5	1.6	59,494,813

*Note that the median age is given in years for each racial/ethnic group (and total) and is not a percent distribution.

**Percent distribution is rounded to nearest whole number.

Source: *Report on the secretary's task force on black and minority health*, vol. I. (1985). Washington, D. C.: U.S. Department of Health and Human Services, p. 48.

voted to the exclusion of the black" (Deloria, 1979, p. 37). It was only in 1954 that the United States Supreme Court, in the *Brown* v. *Board of Education* case, officially outlawed the "separate but equal" doctrine that had legitimated virtually total segregation in all aspects of American life during the first half of the twentieth century. It took years before states began to reluctantly heed the Supreme Court's orders, and still today the generation born after the 1950s is faced with struggles in repairing the damage done by America's legacy of racism.

The Supreme Court's orders to desegregate in 1954 were directed at educational institutions. By 1986, black American adults had completed a median of 12.3 years of education, compared to 11.7 years for Hispanics and 12.7 years for white Americans (1988 *Statistical Abstract,* Table 22). Thus, while there are some race differences that remain in education, the difference between whites and blacks is less

than a half year. But this similarity in education is not reflected in economic statistics. In 1986, median income for black families was $17,604, while for Hispanics it was $19,995 and for white families the median income was $30,809. Whereas 11 percent of the white population is below the poverty level (22.2 million citizens), 31.1 percent of the blacks (9 million) and 27.3 percent of the Hispanics (5.1 million) are in poverty (1988 *Statistical Abstract,* Tables 702 and 713). Note that while blacks have a higher median education than Hispanics, a lower proportion of Hispanics fall below the poverty level.

Table 6–4 shows that the number of births to teenage and unwed mothers differs greatly by race and ethnic group. Almost one of every four Americans born today (22 percent) is born to a single mother. But while this figure is 14.5 percent among Anglos, it is 29.5 percent for Hispanics, 40.7 percent

TABLE 6—4 Live births by race and ethnicity, 1985

Race and Hispanic Origin	Number of Births (1000)	Births to Teenage Mothers, % of Total	Births to Unmarried Mothers, % of Total
Total	3761	12.7	22.0
White	2991	10.8	14.5
Black	608	23.0	60.1
Asian and Pacific Islander	116	5.5	10.1
Filipino	21	5.8	12.1
Chinese	18	1.1	3.7
Japanese	10	2.9	7.9
Hispanic Origin	373	16.5	29.5
Mexican	243	17.5	25.7
Puerto Rican	35	20.9	51.1
Cuban	10	7.1	16.1
American Indian	43	19.1	40.7

Source: 1988 *Statistical Abstract of the United States,* Table 86, p. 62.

for Native Americans, and 60.1 percent for blacks. Infant mortality rates in 1985 were nearly twice as high for blacks (18.2) as for whites (9.3). Suicides, however, remain lower for black males (1.08 per 100,000 population) than for white males (21.5). For blacks born in 1986, life expectancy was 69.6 years, while for whites born that year it was 75.4 years (1988 *Statistical Abstract,* Tables 86, 16, 116, and 124).

Health care providers must be sensitive to the fact that not all Americans with African ancestry prefer the term "black." Terms of respect for this group have changed from "colored" (in the early twentieth century), to "Negro," to "black," to "Afro-American," to "people of color." In some circles, the term "minority group" may also be problematic, as, after all, blacks are a majority worldwide. While use of the term "black" is offensive to none, many minorities would agree that the term "people of color" might be preferable in situations where a heightened sensitivity to racial preferences would want to be conveyed. The low income status of black Americans, coupled with the inadequacy of an overburdened health care delivery system, has led to the endurance of a viable folk medical system among some segments of the black population. This folk medical system is more prevalent among lower class blacks who have been socialized in the rural South, but folk medicine also thrives in other rural populations, including

among rural whites, throughout the country (see Table 6–5).

Three themes are common in folk medicine: that the world is a hostile and dangerous place, that the individual can be attacked by external sources, and that the individual needs outside aid to combat these attacks (Snow, 1981). Those who turn to folk medicine for relief often feel a great deal of distrust toward others, emptiness, and helplessness. A recurring theme in witchcraft is that animals have been introduced through magical means into the body. Animal intrusion into the body usually occurs through accidental ingestion—for example, animal eggs may be swallowed while swimming. The victim is thought to be possessed, with lizards, worms, frogs, and snakes thought to be living in his or her body (Whitten, 1962; Snow, 1981). In witchcraft practices, animal parts are dried, pulverized, and sprinkled on an enemy's food or drink; after ingestion they reconstitute in the victim's body.

The ability to cure in most systems of folk medicine is seen as a supernatural gift. While it can be learned, the healers with the greatest abilities are born with it. To be born with such healing powers is seen as God's greatest gift (Snow, 1981).

The adjoining vignette describes Jacquelyn Gaboyd, a person who was helped by witchcraft. If nothing else, the folk remedies can have a calming result through a placebo effect and anxiety reduction.

TABLE 6–5 Selected characteristics of six American ethnic groups

Ethnic Group	Approximate Time of United States Population Influx	Estimated Population (1979)	Traditional Family Structure	Expression of Pain	Folk Healers
Black Americans	1600s	25,000,000	Extended/ matriarchal and egalitarian	Open, public	Hoodoo men and ladies Root doctors Blood doctors
Mexican Americans	400 B.C.	7,000,000	Extended/ patriarchal	Open, public	Curanderos
Puerto Ricans	1900s	1,700,000	Extended/ patriarchal	Open, public	Espiritistas
American Indians	13,000–18,000 B.C.	900,000	Extended/ patriarchal and matriarchal	Closed, private	Medicine men
Chinese Americans	1700s	500,000	Extended/ patriarchal	Closed, private	Herbalists Herb pharmacists Acupuncturists
Japanese Americans	1800s	700,000	Extended/ patriarchal	Closed, private	Herbalists

Source: Henderson, G., & Primeaux, M. (1981) The importance of folk medicine. In G. Henderson & M. Primeaux (Eds.), *Transcultural health care*. Menlo Park, CA: Addison-Wesley, p. 67.

In fact, in its ability to elicit cures through a reduction of anxiety, folk medicine is not all that different from modern psychotherapy (Frank, 1974). Of course, it is possible that Mrs. Gaboyd's problems with her husband would have disappeared without any therapeutic intervention at all.

Jacquelyn Gaboyd: A Patient "Helped" By Witchcraft

Jacquelyn Gaboyd, a 30-year-old professional black woman, became suspicious that her husband was having an affair with a woman in their neighborhood. She sought assistance for her distress (depression, suspicion, worry, difficulty sleeping, loss of appetite) at the local mental health center. Several months of treatment passed but she received no satisfactory help from professional mental health counselors. Jackie discussed her problem with her grandmother who immediately made an appointment with a witch-craft healer in a city approximately 100 miles away. During the first session, the healer requested that Mrs. Gaboyd bring to the next session a piece of her husband's hair, a sample of his urine, and a shirt that he frequently wore. Jackie arrived at the next session with these items. The healer performed a secret ritual that consisted of chanting, praying, going into a trance-like state, and making special requests on behalf of Mrs. Gaboyd. When the session was over, the healer told Jacquelyn to go home, to pray continuously, not to nag her husband, and to wait for the change in her husband's behavior to come. The healer cautioned Jacquelyn that continuous prayer, fasting one day a week, and being mild mannered were essential for her to practice. A month later, Jackie reported that she was feeling better, that there had been no quarrels or disputes in the house, that she was getting her work done on the job and at home, she had lost weight, and her husband seemed to be paying more attention to her and staying home more.

When a member of a cultural minority decides to seek professional health care, the provider should assess for 1) frequency and duration of possible home health remedies, 2) the specific types of folk treatment employed to combat the illnesses, and 3) whether the professional's prescribed treatment is compatible with the folk medicine. When appropriate and when there is concern about the home remedy, the health professional should utilize this opportunity to discuss with the individual and family any immediate and potential dangers associated with a specific home remedy. Alternative suggestions should be provided that do not clash with the individual's health belief system (Snow, 1981). Frequently, a patient's symptoms are acute and management by family and other support systems can no longer control behaviors. It is at this juncture that the family might seek help as a "last ditch effort" to secure symptom relief.

Some researchers have suggested that there must be emphasis on the development of coping mechanisms that will assist the black person (and other people of color) to survive, and "change" as they are confronted with different demands in a basically hostile society (Smith, 1981).

Mental health professionals are challenged to not only treat mental illness among black people, but to seek the causes of their mental illness (Nobles, 1976). When addressing the causes of mental illness, one is again forced to reflect on the institution of slavery and confront the current aftereffects of such a devastating experience (Nobles, 1976; Jones & Rice, 1987).

COUNSELING AFRICAN AMERICANS: A WORLDVIEW. Nobles (1976) submits that the African worldview consists of characteristics and behaviors that support a groupness and commonality of purpose; cooperation and collective responsibility; cooperation and interdependence; survival of the tribe; a oneness with nature; and experiential approaches to life.

On the other hand, Nobles proposes that the European orientation consists of characteristics that reinforce individuality, uniqueness, and differences, competition and individual rights, survival of the fittest, and control over nature. But, mental health concerns have not been given a high enough priority for blacks, whites, Asians, Hispanics, and Native Americans in the United States (Jones & Rice, 1987). Jones and Rice purport that the two prevalent approaches in the literature that addresses preventive

mental health—the proactive and reactive—can be further delineated in our efforts to understand blacks and mental health issues. First, the proactive approach to mental health problems: this tactic underscores the decrease and/or avoidance of stressful situations that might lead to the development of mental symptoms and disorders. It endorses changing deleterious elements in the environment and/or the individual's perceptions of the environment. This approach would allow for such conditions as poverty, poor housing, underemployment and unemployment, and limited educational opportunities to be addressed within the mental health structure. Currently, these approaches are beyond the theoretical and conceptual bases of mental health delivery as it is practiced.

Second, the reactive approach to mental health problems employs tactics that advocate coping and adapting to whatever events that occur in the individual's life. This has been the modus operandi of most mental health delivery systems, and it implements a slow and deliberate exertion directed toward confronting the causative factors that negatively impact on the mental health of minority populations (Jones & Rice, 1987). The astute reader will quickly recognize that neither approach provides an effective conceptual model for addressing mental health difficulties that confront minority groups in our society. It is, however, a place to begin our public debate about change in mental health delivery.

It is important to point out that the dominant culture developed theoretical and practical content that applied to all people of color, seemingly, without much sensitivity about its appropriateness for that particular group (Bell, Bland, Houston, & Jones, 1983; U.S. Department of Health and Human Services, 1985; Smith, 1981; Hall, 1976; Fabrega, 1989). For example, Carl Jung, a noted practitioner and theorist, developed abstract explanations about why blacks should be segregated and controlled by other groups (Jung, 1960).

Deutsch (1944) has demonstrated that numerous writers purported that slavery was a viable institution for Americans. Assumptions about African Americans' inability to care for themselves were prevalent in the psychiatric literature. Too, the human conditions within which African Americans lived were extreme and severe. Interestingly, an effective mental health program for the Negro should consist of "Equal rights. Equal opportunity." (Deutsch, 1944, p. 482). Szasz (1971) wrote that Cartwright, an American physician, thought that enslavement of African Americans was a therapeutic necessity and the medical responsibility of the white master. Furthermore, Cartwright identified two diseases that were characteristic of African American slaves: Drapetomania (evidenced by the escape of the African American slave from the white master) and Dysaesthesia Aethiopis (as evidenced by an African American slave neglecting or ignoring his work or refusing to work) (Szasz, 1971). (See chapter 3, Psychiatric Classification, for more information on labeling.)

Bell, Bland, Houston, and Jones (1983) suggest that the mental health professional must become more sensitive to the historic, economic, social, political, and cultural factors associated with individual and institutional racism; these professionals must also become active in dispelling negative myths, stereotypes, and other damaging perceptions about growth and development, mental health, and the overall functioning of black people. Smith (1981) goes further, delineating a dozen points that a culturally sensitive nurse should know:

1. Blacks have developed certain perspectives about life (religious orientation; nature is powerful and rhythmic as with the seasons) that have assisted with the creation of an identity.

2. "Oral tradition" remains a predominate method of communication. Information is transmitted through stories, religious song, and the "blues". Black humor is definitely a component of the oral tradition, and is sometimes utilized by blacks to express the senselessness of racism, prejudice, and discrimination.

3. Blacks (and other minorities) have developed an unusual ability to observe, unobtrusively, the behaviors of whites and others, and have used this mechanism as a survival strategy (Hall, 1976; Smith, 1981).

4. Blacks traditionally do not give the nodding approval with an accompanying "uh-hm," nor do they feel that they need to have eye contact with the person as do their white counterparts (Hall, 1976). The absence of nods and "uh-hms" does not indicate disinterest or inattention.

5. Blacks generally believe that service to the family and community is a natural phenomenon of life, and is seldom perceived as a burden.

6. Despite many mitigating factors and hardships, black families have remained a strong and powerful force in the lives of black people.

7. Kinship structures are extensive and expansive at almost any time. For example, fictitious kinspeople might be treated the same as actual kinspeople. Moreover, multigenerational families might be living

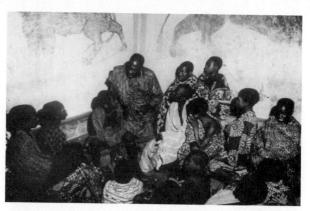

One form of the black Americans' "oral tradition" is story-telling. Shown here is an elder of the Abouré tribe relating a tribal legend to boys of the Yaou village in the Ivory Coast.

in one household, and key individuals in that family system hold powerful positions within their structure (Thomas, 1981).

8. Black women have a long history of being employed outside of the home, and do not tend to experience the same level of conflict about their careers as white women. It should be remembered, however, that black women have a 39 percent greater chance of sustaining job related diseases and serious work related injuries than non-minorities (U.S. Department of Health and Human Services, Vol. 11, 1985).

9. Some blacks might feel that mental health intervention (its theories and strategies) is a part of the problem and not the solution.

10. Traditional forms of mental health care might not take into consideration the historical and life experiences of black people.

11. Blacks can mislead the nurse therapist, and conceal psychopathology by focusing on "blackness" while the mental health problem remains unidentified and untreated.

12. Language usage can be formal as well as highly culturally specific (a vernacular). The nurse therapist should not pretend to understand the vernacular; for example, she should not enter into a "laid-back cool" mode of communication unless she is extremely knowledgeable about that specific subset of the culture and its nuances.

The case study of Rebecca Harding reveals how religious beliefs may in some cases influence the willingness to seek mental health care and to comply with prescribed treatment.

Rebecca Harding: The Community Leader

Mrs. Rebecca Harding is a 60-year-old woman who lives in an "old section" of Chicago. She lost her husband during World War II, and reared two sons as a single parent. Both of her sons attended universities and became successful professionals. One son, a lawyer, became active in politics and owned a lucrative law practice; the other son became a well-known journalist. Mrs. Harding was very proud of her sons, and was frequently used as a role model by other families, on "how to successfully rear good sons." She was always quick to say, "If it were not for the Lord . . . what would I do?" In fact, Mrs. Harding felt that her constant communication with a Supreme Being had provided her with answers about how to manage her affairs and her young sons' affairs for the duration of her life.

In recent years, Mrs. Harding began to experience "mild depression." Her son, the journalist, suggested that she see a mental health professional. Reluctantly, Mrs. Harding visited the mental health nurse at a community health center. When asked why she was there, Mrs. Harding commented ". . . my son wanted me to come . . . he thinks I am getting too tired and too slow." The mental health nurse gently questioned Mrs. Harding, and determined that Mrs. Harding might benefit from seeing a psychiatrist, who could possibly prescribe a mild antidepressive medication, and perhaps something that would give Mrs. Harding a little more "pep." The nurse therapist referred Mrs. Harding to a psychiatrist in the clinic, who prescribed Elavil 30 mg. per day.

Mrs. Harding told the psychiatrist that before she would take the medication, she would need to talk with Jesus and the angels, and depending on the outcome of that "conversation," she would decide whether or not to take the medication. The psychiatrist was astounded and suggested to her that perhaps she needed a stronger medication to help control the "voices" and to lessen her delusional activity. Mrs. Harding listened attentively, accepted the medication, and left the clinic.

The nurse's follow-up contacts occurred in the home and revealed that Mrs. Harding had not received "answers" from Jesus, and was not contemplating taking the medication at this time. She only commented to the nurse, "You must learn to be patient and wait on the Lord . . . I will let you know when the time comes for me to take these pills. Meanwhile, I will continue to pray and lean on Jesus."

From this case study, six lessons emerge that have relevance for the nurse therapist as she plans and implements treatment:

1. Nurse therapists must be thoroughly familiar with the role of religion in the lives of many black people.

2. Differentiation between religious and cultural practices and symptoms of pathology must be clearly understood (there are no delusions or difficulties with reality testing in this instance).

3. The nurse therapist and psychiatrist should explore with Mrs. Harding her decision-making process regarding the medication regimen.

4. "Feeling tired and being slow," as observed by the son, should be further investigated. Mrs. Harding should be asked to describe how she feels.

5. Follow-up contact should offer support, observation, and a plan for Mrs. Harding (and her son) to contact specific professionals at the community clinic whenever she needs information or wants to "talk" and/or reminisce. This follow-up contact could include a home visit, which would assist Mrs. Harding in feeling secure in her own environment.

6. The nurse should query Mrs. Harding about her physical health, and make the appropriate referrals as necessary.

Discussions of how to counsel racial and ethnic minorities run the risk of promoting stereotypes that misrepresent and oversimplify the cultures involved. They also risk missing the cultural diversity that characterizes any particular group (see Table 6–5). What textbooks and teachers cannot fully convey is an understanding and appreciation for the life conditions under which different groups struggle. A black in Harlem, a Mexican migrant in Texas, a Native American in Arizona, and a white nurse in Minneapolis all develop perspectives on the world that are shaped by the life conditions under which they have been raised. Appreciation of these differences is a first step—and often not an easy one—in delivering high-quality care.

How to address the mental health needs of black Americans is a problem that has not attracted much research attention. The specific research agenda regarding blacks recommended by Osborne et al. (1983) should include: 1) The study of institutional racism and its forestalling effect upon the psychological, social, and cultural development of African Americans. 2) The systematic investigation of African Americans who have survived and in many instances thrived, despite the hostile and racist environment within which they lived. 3) The recognition of African Americans who have become emotionally damaged and handicapped because of racism along with the exploration of their many psychopathological responses; identification of effective and useful therapeutic intervention; and determination and documentation of the impact of mental illness upon the individual, family, community, and society.

HISPANIC AMERICANS

Hispanics are Spanish speaking immigrants from Central and Latin America. They are the fastest growing minority group in America, with a growth rate five times that of the rest of the nation. Their 1988 population was estimated at approximately 19.4 million, nearly 60 percent of whom live in Arizona, California, Colorado, New Mexico, and Texas. This includes approximately 12.1 million Mexican Americans, 2.5 million Puerto Ricans, 2.2 million Central and South Americans, and 1 million Cubans (half of whom live in Florida). Hispanics are usually classified as an ethnic rather than a racial minority, and are often classified in statistical summaries as white, thus making efficient and accurate data compilation difficult (U.S. Department of Health and Human Services, Vol. I and II, 1985). Chicanos are Hispanics with Mexican ancestry. Many are descendants of Mexicans who lived in territories annexed by the United States in the nineteenth century. Like Native Americans, the Spanish settled in what is now the United States long before New England was colonized. Today, most Chicanos live in the Western and Southwestern United States. Many live in rural poverty as migrant farm laborers; others live in urban neighborhoods known as *barrios*.

The second largest group of Hispanics in the United States today hails from Puerto Rico. The United States acquired Puerto Rico in 1898, and in 1917 all Puerto Ricans became American citizens. In 1952, the island became a self-governing commonwealth. The 2.5 million Puerto Ricans on the United States mainland today live predominantly in and around New York City; of this number, about 40 percent live below the poverty line.

Ruiz (1981) and Bernal, Bernal, Martinez, Olmedo, & Santisteban (1983) posit that acculturation and assimilation are very important concepts for mental health professionals to understand (see page 138). Despite various degrees of acculturation, however, Hispanics have retained some basic characteristics and patterns. For example, the "English only" rule has been debated for years, but Spanish is still spoken in all areas of American life, especially in the Southwestern region of the United States. Too, the nurse therapist needs to be sensitive to the fact that, despite the extent of acculturation of Hispanics into

American society, this population receives limited education, income, health care, and other socioeconomic opportunities (Ruiz, 1981; U.S. Department of Health and Human Services, Vol. II, 1985).

Assimilation of Hispanics into the American society varies widely. Some Hispanics prefer to be an integral part of the Anglo culture, others may reject the Anglo culture, and still other Hispanics prefer to be bicultural and adapt their ideology and behaviors to their specific circumstances (Bernal, Martinez, et al., 1983). Generally, this latter group prefers to maintain some degree of ethnic identity. Acculturation and assimilation are, however, correlated with social class, and are not fully understood when applied to health behaviors (Schreiber & Homiak, 1981).

Hispanics in general, like other people of color, are faced with having to confront poverty, discrimination, prejudice, high unemployment and underemployment, and acculturation and assimilation pressures. It would seem to follow that such harsh demands would produce high frequencies of mental illness. When one examines available data, however, it is found that Mexican Americans (and other Hispanics) are 1) under-represented in the mental health facilities, and 2) tend to have low rates of psychotic-type illnesses (Meadows & Stoker, 1965; Schreiber & Homiak, 1981; U.S. Department of Health and Human Services, Vol. II, 1985).

Current research suggests that Hispanic Americans do not have especially high rates of mental disorders when compared to rates in the Anglo community (Cockerham, 1989). This may be because Hispanic culture, particularly Mexican American, stresses the importance of close interpersonal ties with family and friends (Mirowsky & Ross, 1984). On the other hand, individuals with Mexican ancestry, compared with Anglos, tend to have a relatively strong belief that events in life are controlled by forces external to the individual; a belief associated with psychological distress insofar as it reduces the individual's will and ability to deal with any problems that may develop (Mirowsky & Ross, 1984). Belief in external control can lead to passiveness and a tendency to accept things as they are—not to a desire to control. But while this belief in external control would lead to the expectation of high distress among Mexican Americans, Mirowsky and Ross (1984) report that the belief increases only rates of depression; it actually reduces anxiety. Overall rates of distress are lower among Mexican Americans because of the effects of close interpersonal relationships (see also Padilla & Ruiz, 1973; Vega & Miranda, 1985).

Murillo-Rohde (1981) has written that Hispanic people tend to be very expressive and emotive. While these behaviors are accepted within the Hispanic culture, they can sometimes be very disturbing to Anglo people who tend to be less expressive. The nurse therapist should be cautious about labeling and interpreting these expressive types of behaviors. Moreover, Murillo-Rohde (1981) points out the Hispanic people do not freely share information about themselves and/or their families with others (especially strangers, to include nurse therapists). This type of attitude about self-disclosure can (and does) provide a base for therapists to perceive the Hispanic patient as a poor candidate for the "talk therapies" (that is, individual and group therapy).

There are some strong cultural patterns that tend to be found among Hispanic groups. The use of **curanderos** remains prevalent; they perform a "spiritual cleansing" ceremony. While this practice is common, the nurse therapist must be extremely cautious about referring or suggesting that Hispanic patients seek intervention from the **curandero**. This is of extreme importance especially if the nurse therapist, or other mental health professional, is *not* thoroughly familiar with these practices, their assets, and limitations. Too, the decision of whether to use traditional healers must be made on reference to the patient's overall physical health and mental health condition. Whether to encourage or discourage traditional healing methods requires extensive knowledge about the patient and family, the Western theoretical formulations about the illness and possible outcomes, and the folklore and theoretical constructs about the traditional approach. Even with extensive experience, skill, and knowledge, the nurse or any other mental health practitioner should proceed with extra caution (Kiev, 1972; Schrieber & Homiak, 1981; Ruiz, 1981).

Other popular types of traditional mental health care include the use of herbs (the "herbalist" or **yerberos**), the folk "chiropractor," and the senoras, or "wise women" (Schrieber & Homiak, 1981). When providing service to the Hispanic population, the nurse therapist needs to know that at some point, the patient might refer to some or all of these practitioners.

COUNSELING HISPANICS: WORLDVIEW. According to Kiev (1972), the Hispanic patient's worldview consists of assumptions that:

1. Man and woman should live in harmony with nature.

2. Hispanics accept life without attempting to alter it (this view can create dependency and/or security).

3. Hispanics believe that there is a natural order of all events and that illness is a part of the larger order.

4. An individual's life condition is of paramount importance to the family and community (see also U.S. Department of Health and Human Services (1985), Report of the Secretary's Task Force on Black and Minority Health, Vols. I and II).

5. Suffering is viewed as a test of one's faith in a supreme power.

6. Emphasis is on living within the framework of tradition, and on living in harmony with nature.

7. Men and women possess components of both good and bad characteristics.

8. Health is a state of equilibrium between (a) a person and God (nature), and (b) a person and his/her family.

The following nine propositions will assist the nurse who provides mental health care to Hispanic individuals and their families:

1. Hispanic individuals and family members depend upon each other for support, information, protection, and crisis resolution (Kiev, 1972; Schrieber & Homiak, 1981; Vega & Kolody, 1985).

2. Hispanic individuals are likely to contact relatives first for assistance in times of upheaval and upset (Vega & Kolody, 1985).

3. There is an interaction between economic, cultural, individual, and other social forces that determines stress in the individual and family (Navarro & Miranda, 1985).

4. The degree to which the Hispanic individual considers himself to be "very Hispanic," "moderately Hispanic," or "Anglo" cannot be determined by simply knowing that the individual is Hispanic. Instead, the nurse therapist must have some sense of the individual's perceived identity and his conceptualization of the external world and his position within it.

5. Family relationships are of supreme importance.

6. There are numerous types of traditional healers (*curandero, yerberos,* and so on) within the Hispanic community. The nurse therapist should know about them, and aggressively seek additional information when necessary.

7. Language barriers are a major setback in the assessment of mental health care needs (U.S. Department of Health and Human Services, Vols. I and II, 1985).

8. The nurse therapist should take a personal interest in the individual/family and display warmth, sincerity, reassurance, and a genuine concern for the patient and family (Schrieber & Homiak, 1981).

9. Avoid intense eye contact and/or the use of confrontational phrases and behaviors.

The case study about Antonio Martinez is provided to highlight a youth's and his family's assessment of his own illness and preferred methods of treatment. It emphasizes the need for the nurse therapist to be aware of Hispanics' traditional methods of treating certain illnesses and the nurse's role in providing information, and facilitating communication, understanding, and good will regarding specific cultural behaviors between the Anglo and Hispanic communities.

Antonio Martinez: An Outstanding Student

Antonio Martinez is a 15-year-old boy who lives with both parents. His parents are employed as migrant laborers, and they live in a small town in Texas contiguous to Mexico.

Antonio is an outstanding student. His father expects that he will complete high school and receive a scholarship to college. This aspiration is very important to Antonio and his parents, neither of whom can read or write English. They rely heavily upon Antonio to communicate with the Anglo population in their community.

Antonio reported to school with vague complaints of headache, vomiting, and stomach pains. He was observed to be generally irritable and agitated, with tremors in his hands and arms. These symptoms persisted for several days. His teacher became very concerned when Antonio could not concentrate in class and complained of being too tired to do his work. Antonio's general movements were also observed to be slow and retarded. His teacher, a concerned, knowledgeable, and gentle Anglo woman, thought she needed to "get help" for Antonio quickly, and she did.

When the teacher questioned Mr. and Mrs. Martinez about their son's condition, they commented . . . "We do not know why he so sick . . . he no sleep at night . . . he got **susto**."

Antonio's behavior did not improve. His teacher sought help for him, and took Antonio to the public health clinic where he was interviewed by a public health nurse. The public health nurse took Antonio's vital signs and completed a health assessment. The nurse commented, "You seem to be fine, Antonio. . . . Your pulse is slightly elevated, however." Antonio asked, "What do you mean?" The nurse commented in a kind but matter-of-fact fashion, ". . . Your heart is beating faster than normal, and it is pumping blood through your body at an unusually forceful pace."

Antonio was startled. ". . . My heart! . . . Does that mean I will die? Is my heart going to leave me? Can you slow it down right now? My mama must take me to see **curandero** in our village. . . . She will know what to do. . . ." Antonio continued, ". . . Let me go . . . I must see **curandero**. . . ."

Antonio left the clinic with his teacher, who returned him to his home where he found his mother preparing dinner. Mrs. Martinez listened with great fear as Antonio told her what the nurse had said, and immediately prepared to take him to the village **curandero** for treatment for **susto**.

Antonio and Mrs. Martinez were sure that the **curandero** would know what to do. The next day, Antonio was at school and was feeling and looking much better. Antonio thanked his teacher for helping him, and commented, "I feel great. . . . My treatment came in time." The teacher did not completely understand how **susto** began, but she was glad that Antonio was feeling fine.
NOTE:

Susto is a term for an anxiety reaction which is believed to be brought about by the evil eye, witchcraft, bad air, or black magic and may result in "soul loss" (Kiev, 1972). Symptoms such as headaches, vomiting, malaise, insomnia, tremors, sweating, and motor retardation characterize this syndrome (Kiev, 1972). Treatment must be started quickly; once the "anxiety" reaches the heart, the patient will die (Kiev, 1972). **Curandero** refers to the community folk-healer, male or female, who practices a combination of popular and scientific medicine along with traditional folk-healing practices, which include the therapeutic use of various herbs and roots to cure specific illnesses (Foster, 1981).

In the case of Antonio, the teacher was very sensitive to his needs, and sought to provide care, at first, with the employment of contemporary medical approaches. Yet, when Antonio expressed his desire to see a curandero, she facilitated that request by not interfering with the decision made by him and his mother. The nurse skillfully completed a health assessment. Her approach, not to offer additional Anglo intervention, served to promote compassion and empathy between the two cultural groups. She knew that health care for low-socioeconomic Hispanic patients should be directed toward short-term goals, and be action orientated (Sue, 1981). She also was aware that folk medicine and the healing arts of the curandero play a fundamental role in the treatment of many illnesses in the Hispanic community (Kiev, 1972; Sue, 1981).

There are numerous areas in psychiatric mental health nursing that need to be researched, and among those priority areas are mental health and Hispanic Americans. Specific research focus, according to Gonzales, Wilson, Gilde-Rubio, and Mejia (1983) should include inquiries about nursing education and psychiatric and mental health practice. Specifically, they recommend studies that are directed toward faculty in educational settings where cultural sensitivities are taught to students, with specific measures designed to quantify student outcomes. Moreover, practice outcomes and attitudes of health care providers that service the Hispanic patient and family should be thoroughly investigated. Additional recommendations include that practice outcome studies be devised to document that the mental health needs of Hispanic patients are being met by nurses and other mental health care professionals.

ASIAN AMERICANS

Although Asian Americans, like Native Americans, are extremely heterogenous, there is a tendency to classify them together. Table 6–6 shows the foreign-born population of various Asian communities in the United States.

Asian Americans enjoy higher levels of employment, income, and education than other minority groups, and often even higher levels than whites. The main reason for this is, simply put, that Asians work harder (Hess et al., 1989, p. 265). Their mental health status generally also surpasses that of other minority groups and whites. Japanese Americans in particular have low rates of mental problems, no doubt reflecting the strength and stability of Japanese family structures (Cockerham, 1989).

The most recent influx to American shores of Asians came shortly after the end of the American war in Vietnam in the mid-1970s. Examining the treatment needs of this population will give readers a taste of challenges encountered with other minority groups in general and other Asian minorities in particular.

According to Sue (1981) the basic sociocultural components in Asian families, age, sex, and generational status, are the major variables that determine role function/behavior. These defined roles are seen as having little tolerance for deviation. The father, in this patriarchal type family, is revered and respected, and is seen as the ultimate authority within the family system. Sons are expected to grow up and function like their fathers; daughters are expected to grow up, marry, and support their husbands' household. The Asian family emphasizes conservatism, a subtle approach to conflicts, avoidance of offending others, and the submergence of aggressive tendencies (Wright, 1964). Individuals must strive to bring credit to the family, and problems such as juvenile delinquency, school failure, or mental illness should be managed (whenever possible) within the family context, with limited involvement from others (Wright, 1964; Sue & Sue, 1987). Methods used to reinforce these behaviors are shame, guilt, and reminders to the specific family member of his/her obligations to the family (Kiev, 1972). Obedience, conformity, high achievement, and honor for the family name are paramount to the Asian individual.

Asian Americans are likely to experience three types of conflicts that have relevance for the nurse in mental health care. They include loyalty and obligatory relationships to their family and community; oversensitization to American values and folkways, thereby rejecting Asian traditions; and intense concern about racism and civil rights (Sue, 1981).

COUNSELING ASIAN AMERICANS: WORLD-VIEW. The nurse therapist must have an understanding of the Asian patient's culture, history, and lifestyle. The nurse therapist should know something about the Asians' worldview.

Primarily, the Chinese American, for example, believes that harmony or balance is a central concept

---

TABLE 6—6 Asian American ethnic groups, 1980

Chinese	894,000
Filipinos	795,000
Japanese	791,000
Koreans	371,000
Indians	312,000
Vietnamese	215,000
Hawaiians	202,000

Source: Hess, B. B., Markson, E. W., & Stein, P. J. (1989). *Sociology,* 3rd ed. New York, Macmillan, p. 255.

in traditional medicine. Health represents a state of homeostasis that exists between two extreme and dangerous forces; it is not merely the absence or presence of disease. If a person is in a state of equilibrium, there is harmony and freedom from disease (Gould-Martin & Ngin, 1981).

This view of health and illness is derived from the Eastern philosophy that purports that the "elemental forces controlling the universe pervade all aspects of human endeavor. Each universe is thought of as a vast entity, each organism in it conceived as an open system that interacts and is affected by others in the universe" (Campbell & Chang, 1981, p. 162).

Specific terminology follows this philosophy. For example, the Yin and Yang forces (the female and male forces that are, ideally, in perfect balance, and therefore, keep the organism disease free). Excess of Yang can cause fever and dehydration. On the other hand, the Yin embodies the strength of life. Too much Yin, nonetheless, predisposes a person to colds, nervous tensions, and gastrointestinal disorders (Campbell & Chang, 1981).

Sue (1981) and other researchers have suggested that low rates of psychiatric hospitalization, juvenile delinquency, and crime have helped to support the Asian American's "Success Myth." This myth suggests that Asians are relatively free of mental health problems, and have successfully been assimilated and acculturated into the larger society. Psychological problems are not easily owned; instead, psychic conflict and pain tend to be expressed through physical complaints (Sue 1981; U.S. Department of Health and Human Services, Vols. I and II, 1985).

Minority and disadvantaged groups who do enter mental health treatment tend to receive somatic treatments (medications, and so on) and less lengthy interpersonal therapies than their white counterparts (Hollingshead & Redlich, 1958; U.S. Department of Health and Human Services, Vol. II, 1985). Perhaps Asians and other people of color feel as if white therapists are symbols of a white society, whose task it is to assist them in adjusting to a racist/prejudiced community without objection (Sue, 1981). Also, Asian Americans and other people of color may think that white people do not understand their problems.

The case of Kim Lu Wu highlights some of the difficulties that Asian Americans experience when they interact in American society. Pay particular attention to the expression of her psychological conflicts that are presented in the form of a physical ailment. Also, even though Kim Lu Wu is living in America and is desperately trying to adapt to the

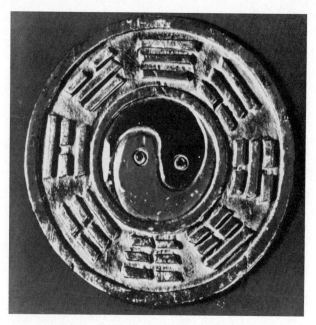

The Chinese symbol for Yin and Yang, the male and female forces in the universe which ideally are maintained in a state of equilibrium. Disequilibrium of these two forces results in diseases in an individual.

American way of life, she is still very much an Asian woman with values, customs, and philosophical beliefs deeply rooted in her Asian culture. In this example, it is imperative that the nurse therapist be informed about physical and mental health problems and their behavioral expressions in Asian Americans.

Kim Lu Wu: An Asian American in Conflict

Kim Lu Wu is a 30-year-old Chinese woman who recently immigrated to the United States for the purpose of receiving an advanced degree in early childhood education. Her family had saved money for many years for Kim's advanced education in the United States.

Kim is known to her family as an obedient, hardworking, and loyal daughter. She was expected to complete her education, return home, marry, and work in her community.

Kim's studies began to be problematic for her during her second year at school. She received several low grades on tests, could not successfully complete class presentations, and had difficulties working with young children in the practice teaching program. She began to complain of headaches. Kim's advisor suggested that she see a physician in the student health center. She was given a mild medication, but the general nagging headache got worse. Physical findings were all negative. Her school work continued to suffer. She seemed to struggle to get to class; appeared sad and depressed, and eventually began to cry, commenting ". . . I am not well. . . . My head needs fixing."

Her advisor recognized that she knew little about Chinese culture, but had enough insight to know that she needed help in assisting Kim. A Chinese American mental health nurse was located in the community, and agreed to interview Kim. The nurse asked Kim about 1) her family at home in China and their expectations for her, 2) the family's time frame for Kim to complete school, 3) the tensions being experienced in school, and 4) how she felt about coming to a mental health professional for assistance. The nurse also completed a mental status examination several visits later.

Kim was very concerned about confidentiality. It was important that her family back home and other Chinese friends in her immediate environment did not know about her mental problems, and that they should never know that she visited a mental health professional. Once confidentiality was established, Kim and the therapist were able to focus on Kim's fear of failure, and the anticipated reactions from family and friends. Discussions revealed that Kim was dating an Asian American, and they had discussed not returning to China. Her fiancee had broached the idea of living together and possibly marriage within a year.

From this case study, we can see that:

1. Kim has traditional Chinese values even though she is in a Western society.

2. Shame and guilt about seeking mental health care are intense and long lasting.

3. Admitting to psychological problems can be tantamount to admitting to complete failure.

4. Stressor/problems that should be addressed include: failure/anticipated failure; conflict between traditional family obligations and her own personal desires for love/intimacy; her interrupted time frame for completing her studies and returning home, vis-á-vis her desire to remain in the United States and create a life of her own, independent of her family of origin; the conflict she experienced about teaching small children, when she really wanted to study physics and work as a university professor. The vocational conflicts could be extreme in Kim's instance, and should be explored thoroughly.

5. The less conflictual issues would need to be explored at first; then, after trust and a sense of psycho-logical safety is established, more conflictual areas can be discussed.

6. Counseling therapy techniques must accommodate Kim, and not the therapist.

7. Openness, verbal catharsis, and "psychological mindedness" may sometimes cause major problems in the nurse/Asian patient relationship (Sue, 1981; Kitano & Matsushima, 1976).

8. At times, it might be useful to provide medications for Kim and other Asian American patients. This action is based on the belief that psychological conflict is so alien to the patient, that communication and treatment can best come by addressing the physiological manifestation of the psychological conflict (Kitano & Matsushima, 1976; Sue, 1981).

9. The employment of a therapy technique that is logical, sequential, directive (at times), and structured, in contrast to an approach that is affective, ambiguous, or reflective (Sue, 1981), is more effective.

10. Language barriers exist among the majority of Asian immigrants, and create barriers to mental health care delivery where most of the services are provided by English speaking personnel. As a result, services are inaccessible to many Asian Americans who do not speak English (U.S. Department of Health and Human Services, Vol. II, 1985).

11. Traditional Chinese values are very much a part of Kim's perspective. Yet, when they are challenged, it causes extensive psychological discomfort.

Only a small portion of Asian Americans who are experiencing some form of mental illness may seek psychiatric help, no matter how intolerable or uncontrollable the disorder becomes. In fact, Lin and Lin (1978) note that, from their past experiences, many Chinese patients may wait 25 years or more before obtaining psychiatric assistance. Knowledge about these kinds of circumstances lead one to believe that mentally ill Asian Americans are assimilated within the family system, thereby causing severe and intolerable stress that family members are expected to cope with.

In his clinic, Kinzie (1985) finds that many Southeast Asian refugees, like other minorities, often suffer from fragmented and incomplete services. Their material needs being so great and accessibility to services lacking, patients often wait until crises develop before they present themselves for services. Hence, emergency services are needed, and frequently both psychiatric and physical needs interact in their presenting complaints. Obviously, language differences present a problem, and therapists need experience with such groups to be able to interpret nonverbal signs as well.

Southeast Asians often stigmatize the mentally ill, caring for them in the home for long periods before, as a last resort, finally seeking professional intervention. They are often reluctant or unable to differentiate among physical, psychological, and supernatural causes for the problem. As shown in Table 6–7, the values of Southeast Asians often differ from those of American psychotherapists. Central to these differences is that whereas the former group has an interdependent orientation to the world, emphasizing the family and proper social relationships, American psychotherapists are usually trained in models emphasizing the centrality of individual autonomy and independence.

TABLE 6–7 Value conflicts between Indochinese patients and American psychotherapists

Indochinese Asian Patient Values	American Psychotherapist Values
Interdependence and traditional family values	Autonomy and independence
"Correct" social relationships	Relativity in values; situational ethics; rejection of authority
Holistic culture, that is, people living in harmony with nature	People versus nature; the need to master or control nature
View of mental illness as imbalance of cosmic forces or supernatural events	View of mental illness as result of psychological and biological factors
No cultural analogy of extended psychological therapy	Belief that psychotherapy is valuable and promotes "growth"
Belief that cure should be rapid, healer active; little history of maintenance therapy	Awareness that cure will be extended and time consuming, and therapist will often be passive
Fear of mental illness	Comfortable attitude about handling mental illness and symptoms
"Refugee" status—insecure in language, vocation, position in society	Secure status in "society," language, vocation, and position

Source: Kinzie, J. (1985). Overview of clinical issues in the treatment of Southeast Asian refugees. In T. Owan (Ed.), *Southeast Asian mental health: Treatment, prevention, services, training, and research.* Washington, D.C.: National Institute of Mental Health. p. 118.

The value conflicts that exist between Asian American patients and American psychotherapists are grounded in the differences between philosophical concepts in the Eastern and Western worlds. Table 6–7 clearly demonstrates that Asian patient values have as their infrastructure the concepts of "interdependence, holistic, and psychosocial orientation that strongly emphasize correct social relations, particularly in the family" (Kinzie, 1985, p. 117). Conversely, American psychotherapists are oriented in Western science, psychology, and metapsychology, and are dominated by a value system that embraces "self-aggrandizement and satisfaction, autonomy, rejection of authority, relativity in values, situational ethics, and avoidance of long-term relationships and responsibility (Kinzie, 1985, p. 117).

American psychotherapists and nurses tend to take an active role in diagnoses, explanation, and treatment. As shown in Table 6–8, this mode is very compatible with the expectations and needs of Southeast Asians.

We hasten to point out that the Asian patient prefers a model for health care that, from a social and interpersonal perspective, does not blame anyone for his illness; is based on the physician (health-care provider)–patient relationship; and allows for the legitimate confirmation of the sick role, which, in turn, excuses the patient of all responsibilities and obligations for a period of time. Moreover, from the health care delivery perspective, the American medical model has definite characteristics which are also attractive to the Asian patient and family. It provides the framework for the enhancement and maintenance of social and interpersonal relationships. Specifically, the features of the American medical model that are most attractive to the Asian American are "symptom reduction, alleviation of pain, and curing of illnesses" (Kinzie, 1985, p. 119).

RESEARCH NEEDS. The critical areas in psychiatric mental health nursing research include inquiry about Asian and Pacific Americans' experiences in the American culture; needed also are descriptive and experimental studies that will provide for the development of measures that test nursing strategies and methods in mental health care delivery. Other specific research recommendations include the development of: mental status assessment instruments that are specific to the Asian and Pacific American individual and family; methods for determining early signs of familial stress and maladaptive behaviors; and knowledge about culturally sanctioned behaviors in the American society that create stress, conflict, and frus-

TABLE 6—8 Indochinese expectation of healers and roles of American physicians

Indochinese Expectations and Needs of Healer/Physician	American Physician's Roles and Duties
Expects healer to understand illness or problems	Actively involved in diagnosis
Needs explanation of illness in understandable terms	Gives firm concept of etiology and education
Wants active treatment to reduce symptoms or cure	Actively involved in treatment, often with medicine
Expects rapid cure—hope in medicine	Goal: to reduce symptoms or cure illness
Often needs to have sick role confirmed	Confirms the sick role
Needs to have family stress, fear, and guilt reduced	Prevents anyone from being blamed for misfortune

Source: Kinzie, J. (1985). Overview of clinical issues in the treatment of Southeast Asian refugees. In T. Owan (Ed.), *Southeast Asian mental health: Treatment, prevention, services, training, and research.* Washington, D.C.: National Institute of Mental Health, p. 119.

tration for the Asian and Pacific American individual (Fujiki, Chin, Hansen, Cheng, & Lee, 1983).

NATIVE AMERICANS

Three basic sources of strength have been observed among Native Americans: the family, the tribe, and the land (Kiev, 1972; Deloria, 1979; U.S. Department of Health and Human Services, Vol. I, 1985). But, consider the following facts:

1. Life expectancy is 44 years.

2. One out of every two Native American families has a relative who has died in jail.

3. Every third Native American will experience being jailed during his or her lifetime.

4. Twenty-five to 35 percent of Native American children are separated from families and live in foster homes or other types of institutions.

5. The average annual family income is $1500.

6. Unemployment ranges from between 4 to 8 percent.

7. Approximately 45 tribes are not recognized by the American government.

8. Indian suicide rates are seven times higher than those of the rest of American society.

9. Until 1975, the Bureau of Indian Affairs was administered by white Anglos (Richardson, 1981).

Native Americans are the poorest minority group in America. At the time of European settlement, there were approximately 1 million Native Americans, but by the end of the nineteenth century their population had dropped to around 300,000. It has rebounded back to a figure of about 790,000 today. Not much is known about the exact prevalence of mental disorders among Native Americans. Their high rates of alcoholism (two to three times the national average) and suicide (20 percent above the national average), however, indicate widespread problems. Although there is great variation within the Native American community, the value systems of the group as a whole show many differences from Anglo beliefs that have direct implications for nursing care. These are summarized in Table 6–9.

Much of the history of Native American-Anglo relations has been a history of cultural oppression and outright genocide. The facts presented in Table 6–9 clearly indicate that Native Americans are in need of comprehensive health services. The nurse therapist who provides care to the Native American and his family will surely be confronted with patients who have a variety of physical health, mental health, and social needs. She should be prepared to address, as much as possible, all of the patient's presenting needs.

Approximately one-half of the American Indians live in the western or southwestern sections of the United States. Twenty-five percent live on reservations, and another 8 percent live on historic tract areas in Oklahoma. Most of these reservations have fewer than 1000 residents; only one reservation has a population of greater than 100,000 (U.S. Department of Health and Human Services, Vol I, 1985, p. 58). The nurse therapist must be mindful that each Native American tribe has its own unique customs, languages, and other characteristic behaviors.

Another issue that is of equal importance to the nurse therapist is this question: Is the behavior that I observe 1) a component of the patient's culture; 2) unique to this patient/family/community; or 3) is this expressed behavior psychopathological? There is no simple answer to these questions. The nurse therapist must grapple with and assess for herself what she knows about her very own culture and specific behaviors, as well as what she knows/does not know about

TABLE 6–9 Differences in Indian and Anglo values

Indians	Anglos		
1. Happiness—this is paramount! Be able to laugh at misery; life is to be enjoyed	1. Success—generally involving status, security, wealth, and proficiency	9. Be carefree—time is only relative. Work long hours if happy. Don't worry over time; "I'll get there eventually"	9. Be structured—be most aware of time. "Don't put off until tomorrow what you have to do today." Don't procrastinate
2. Sharing—everything belongs to others, just as Mother Earth belongs to *all* people	2. Ownership—indicating preference to own an outhouse rather than share a mansion	10. Discreet—especially in dating. Be cautious with a low-key profile	10. Flout an openness—"What you see is what you get." Be a "Fonz" character
3. Tribe and extended family first, before self	3. "Think of number one" syndrome	11. Religion is the universe	11. Religion is individualistic
4. Humble—causing Indians to be passive-aggressive, gentle head hangers, and very modest	4. Competitive—believing "If you don't toot your own horn then who will?"	12. Orient yourself to the land	12. Orient yourself to a house, a job
5. Honor your elders—they have wisdom	5. The future lies with the youth	13. Be a good listener—and it is better if you use your ears and listen well	13. Look people in the eye—don't be afraid to establish eye contact. It's more honest
6. Learning through legends; remembering the great stories of the past, that's where the knowledge comes from	6. Learning is found in school; get all the schooling that you possibly can because it can't be taken away from you	14. Be as free as the wind	14. Don't be a "boat rocker"
7. Look backward to traditional ways—the old ways are the best ways; they have been proved	7. Look to the future to things new—"Tie Your Wagon to a Star and Keep Climbing Up and Up"	15. Cherish your memory—remember the days of your youth	15. Don't live in the past—look ahead. Live in the here-and-now
8. Work for a purpose—once you have enough then quit and enjoy life, even if for just a day	8. Work for a retirement—plan your future and stick to a job, even if you don't like it	16. Live with your hands—manual activity is sacred. "Scratch an Indian—you'll find an artist." (Natives are also intelligent)	16. Live with your mind—think intelligently. Show the teacher how well you know the answer to the questions he/she might ask of you. Good at books
		17. Don't criticize your people	17. A critic is a good analyst

the patient's culture. Also, one's definitions of behaviors determine how she and other mental health professionals will conceptualize, label, and treat the patient. Harwood (1981) has pointed out that professionals are poorly trained to confront the patient's reaction to, and concern for, the illness. That is, the patient's cultural, ethnic, personality, socioeconomic, environmental factors, and psychological aspects, along with the conceptualization of the illness, and what it means to himself, his family, and community, are seldom explored (Kiev, 1972; Kleinman, 1973; Campinha-Bacote, 1988; Fabrega, 1989). The astute nurse therapist must advance one step further and determine how to employ appropriate specific communication and intervention strategies in a therapeutic and "ethno-sensitive" manner (Kiev, 1972; Trimble, 1976; Fabrega, 1989).

Yet, the Native American population continues to struggle with effective methods of coping with the numerous crises, stressors, and disruptions that have invaded their traditional lifestyles.

COUNSELING NATIVE AMERICANS: WORLD-VIEW. Native Americans are unlike any other minority group in that they have been defined in legal terms by the Bureau of Indian Affairs (BIH) which concluded that a person with at least one-quartum of Indian Blood is "Indian" (Trimble, 1976), and such determinations were made by the government. Such criteria do not address the question of identity. Who, then, is the Native American? This issue remains debatable . . . and the answer is probably reflected in one's customs, belief systems, folklore, religion, and spirit (Primeaux & Henderson, 1981).

18. Don't show pain—be glad to make flesh sacrifices to the Spirits

18. Don't be tortured—don't be some kind of a masochistic nut

19. Cherish your own language and speak it when possible

19. You're in America; speak English

20. Live like the animals; the animals are your brothers and sisters

20. "What are you—some kind of animal? A Pig or a Jackass?"

21. Children are a gift of the Great spirit to be shared with others

21. "I'll discipline my own children; don't you tell me how to raise mine!"

22. Consider the relative nature of a crime, the personality of the individual, and the conditions. "The hoe wasn't any good anyway"

22. The law is the law! "To steal a penny is as bad as to steal 10,000! Stealing is stealing! We can't be making exceptions"

23. Leave things natural as they were meant to be

23. "You should have seen it when God had it all alone!"

24. Dance is an expression of religion

24. Dance is an expression of pleasure

25. There are no boundaries—it all belongs to the Great Spirit. "Why should I fence in a yard?"

25. Everything has a limit—there must be privacy. "Fence in your yard and keep them off the grass!"

26. Few rules are best. The rules should be loosely written and flexible

26. Have a rule for every contingency, "Write your ideas in detail"

27. Intuitiveness

27. Empiricism

28. Mystical

28. Scientific

29. Be simple—eat things raw and natural. Remember your brother the fox and live wisely

29. Be sophisticated—eat gourmet, well prepared, and seasoned. Be a connoisseur of many things

30. Judge things for yourself

30. Have instruments judge for you

31. Medicine should be natural herbs, a gift of Mother Earth

31. Synthetic medicines—"You can make anything in today's laboratory"

32. The dirt of Mother Earth on a wound is not harmful but helpful (Sun Dance, mineral intake)

32. Things must be sterile and not dirty and unsanitary.

33. Natives are used to small things, and they enjoy fine detail (Indian fires)

33. Bigness has become a way of life with the white society (compulsion for bigness)

34. Travel light, get along without

34. Have everything at your disposal

35. Accept others—even the drinking problem of another Indian

35. Persuade, convince, and proselytize—be an evangelist/missionary

36. The price is of no concern

36. "You only get what you pay for"

37. Enjoy simplifying problems

37. "Nothing in this world is simple"

Source: Richardson, E. (1981). Cultural and historical perspectives in counseling American Indians. In D. Sue (Ed.) *Counseling the culturally different, theory and practice.* New York: John Wiley and Sons. pp. 225–27.

Native Americans do not share the white Americans' heritage, which is so predominant in our culture. They have little or no experience with the industrial revolution or the rise of the American democratic process (Deloria, 1979). Rather, Native Americans are remembered for the role they played during the settling of the Old West, and for their sometimes violent struggles against the "white man" during the last century (Deloria, 1979). Hence, they have little identification with "this land or the people who live here."

Assimilation and acculturation have not been easy for Native Americans. Limited degrees of acculturation and assimilation may, in part, account for the various social forces such as poverty, limited access to health and education, and poor sanitation that provide a fragile backdrop for the enhancement of the human condition (Primeaux & Henderson, 1981; Kekahbah, Pamburn, Silk Walker, & Wood, 1983; U.S. Department of Health and Human Services, Vol. I, 1985).

Native Americans tend to believe that man, nature, and the supernatural are one. Man should strive to live in harmony with nature (Primeaux & Henderson, 1981). Religious themes are predominant throughout the culture. In fact, there is nothing that can be labeled as non-religious. Perhaps this orientation has helped to sustain the Native Americans despite phenomenal odds (Primeaux & Henderson, 1981).

Illness represents a state of disharmony among these three variables: man, nature, and the supernatural. Many Native Americans have developed ceremonials and rituals that are highly relevant to health care (Primeaux & Henderson, 1981; Kunitz & Levy, 1981).

Healing ceremonies differ among tribes, but all tend to represent some basic components of Indian healing. Native Americans have used holistic health care for centuries. This approach recognizes all factors/forces that affect an individual's life (Primeaux & Henderson, 1981; Kekahbah, et al., 1983). Kunitz and Levy (1981) have written that the Navajos, for example, believe that: 1) The healing system is sacred, representing the very core of Navajo religion; and 2) The aim of healing ceremonies is to remove the cause of disease, not to alleviate symptoms (p. 356). These beliefs might have created an impenetrable protective barrier from external forces, such as Anglo-Christian approaches and other types of faith healers.

When providing care to this diverse population, the nurse should have some basic notion about the foundation of Native American culture. Specifically, it would be helpful to know that:

1. Mental illness is perceived as an imbalance among nature, man, and the supernatural.

2. Indian medicine and religion cannot be separated (Primeaux & Henderson, 1981, p. 244).

3. Tribal healing services are religious and sacred ceremonials and should be perceived as methods of dealing with sickness and death (Trimble, 1976; Kunitz & Levy, 1981; Primeaux & Henderson, 1981).

4. Native Americans who do not initiate or maintain eye contact with the nurse therapist or other health care providers should not be labeled as "shy, bashful, inattentive, or indifferent." In Native American culture, to look into another's eyes is like looking into his soul (Primeaux & Henderson, 1983).

5. There is a tendency not to share personal information about others; obtaining information from others about an individual (patient) is not appropriate.

6. Time has no beginning and no end. When the nurse therapist and others prescribe and teach the patients about medication that has a rigid schedule (take one pill three times a day) they need to know that this approach is not congruent with the culture. Rather, medications that can be taken once daily and whenever the individual chooses within the time frame should be considered. This practice fits with the patient's culture, because it allows for spontaneity.

7. The family is considered one of the Native American's greatest resources. "To be poor in the Indian

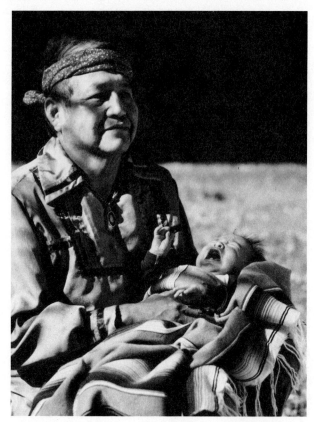

"To be poor in the Indian world is to be without relatives." (Primeaux and Henderson, 1981, p. 242).

world is to be without relatives" (Primeaux & Henderson, 1981, p. 242).

8. Ceremonials are sacred and revered. The nurse therapist should always listen attentively to discussions about ceremonials and when not informed about the subject, remain silent.

9. Languages vary considerably among different Native American tribes, as do customs and other cultural practices. Knowing about one tribe's cultural practices and customs seldom means that other tribes are well understood. Do not be anxious to generalize.

10. The western or Anglo health care system is distinctly different from the Native American's health care system. Yet, in the custody of sensitive, reasonable, and knowledgeable professionals, the two systems can work in harmony with man, nature, and the supernatural for the facilitation of better health care for Native Americans.

11. Native Americans had traditionally been educated away from the reservations because it was the thinking that effective education could not possibly occur on the reservation. Native Americans learn by

example rather than precept (the Anglo method of learning) (Primeaux & Henderson, 1981).

The case study of Billy Red Wolf highlights the conflict that this young Native American experienced when he was thrust into a different cultural world. It also demonstrates how a culturally sensitive therapist can effectively assist other professionals and Native Americans in understanding and respecting each other's cultures and values while finding constructive methods for mental health treatment.

Case Study: Billy Red Wolf

Billy Red Wolf is a 13-year-old male Native American who is enrolled in an Anglo school during the day, and returns home at night to his traditionalist family on the reservation. Billy Red Wolf was considered an academically promising Native American student, who had come to the attention of the Anglo school principal and teachers. The teachers and principal grew very fond of Billy, but they were also extremely concerned that his ancestral tribal habits would interfere with his overall progress in the Anglo society. The teachers and principal would frequently caution Billy about his behaviors (extreme quietness which was labeled as "withdrawn"; easily distracted by external stimuli; fighting; the inability to interact well with other children; excessive fidgeting with hands; shying away from intense verbal exchanges and eye contact; and shifting around in his chair when approached by teacher and peers). He was also observed shifting from one task to another, without giving much attention or thought to any of them. He spoke in a soft voice; the teachers and students would often state, "Billy Red Wolf, you will need to speak up!" To this response he would stare downward, and continue to fidget with his hands and fingers. Billy was uncomfortable, but continued to try and conform to the wishes of his teachers and the other students.

According to the teacher and principal, Billy began to show extreme fidgeting behaviors and was obviously restless. He was beginning to fail most of his homework assignments, and did not seem too interested in his school work. His attention and interest seemed to be elsewhere. The concerned teacher and principal requested a psychological evaluation, and one was completed by the psychologist who served that particular school district. It was suggested that Attention-Deficit Hyperactivity Disorder (ADHD) DSM-III-R (1987), be ruled out.

Billy's parents were extremely disconcerted when they learned that their son had been referred to an Anglo healer (psychologist). Billy's father expressed doubt that Billy would receive the "appropriate healing" from an Anglo therapist, and insisted that Billy receive "proper treatment" from the **peyotist** on the reservation. Billy's father further explained that the tribal healer would know where the "outside influences" causing Billy's illness came from, and would know what to do to get rid of them.

The psychologist, teacher, and principal agreed that Billy Red Wolf should be treated by a Native American healer and remain in school if at all possible. After it was established that Billy Red Wolf was in treatment on the reservation, the psychologist requested that an inservice education workshop be held for staff at the Anglo school, and invited the nurse who lived and worked on the reservation to conduct the workshop. The nurse presented the workshop, and used their recent experiences with Billy Red Wolf and his family as a central focus in her discussion. She covered the following salient points:

1) The teachers and staff should address Billy Red Wolf with a soft voice and a quiet manner, with their faces turned away from him to prevent any eye contact; they role-played culturally relevant methods of communicating with Billy.

2) Teachers and staff should avoid discussing Billy with any family members or other faculty and staff as that practice is considered inappropriate and insulting.

3) Competitive games or methods of reinforcing learning through competitive methods, such as spelling bees or moving to the head of the class, probably makes Billy feel relatively uncomfortable. To participate or not should be Billy's decision.

4) The teachers should request a visit with Billy and his family in the home. Billy, his family, and members of the tribe would then get to know his teachers, and his teachers would know the family, as well as the extended kinship ties associated with Billy and their significance to Billy/family/tribe.

5) The teachers should explore with Billy and his family, in a subtle and indirect fashion, their aspirations for Billy's impending manhood.

6) The teachers should express gentleness, kindness, and their fondness for Billy in a way that is appreciated and accepted by Billy, his family, and tribal members.

7) The nurse would discuss with the teachers how difficult it is for anyone to live in two distinctly different cultures that require one to change behaviors so abruptly and distinctly in order to "fit in"; a role-play situation was constructed so that the teacher and principal could experience being students in a Native American school on the nearby reservation. They learned a lot.

8) Request that there be an Indian school established on the reservation that would utilize general Native American guiding principles of learning, rather than Anglo, and would include members of the tribe, family, and children as part of the educational system.

The case study of Billy Red Wolf emphasizes the necessity of the nurse to know something about a patient's cultural background. It details differences in "expected and normal behavior" as determined by two different cultural groups (Anglo and Native Americans). It also suggests that treatment is conceptualized and administered in very different ways. The two cultures are different; there is not a right or a wrong method of diagnosing and treating Billy Red Wolf. It does, however, frequently become the task of the nurse therapist to "bridge these two vastly different worlds, and provide health care to individuals and families." In order for the nurse to be effective, she must be culturally sensitive to the Native American's culture, as well as her own culture. Of extreme importance, too, is the fact that the nurse should feel relatively comfortable with herself before she begins assessments and interventions.

RESEARCH NEEDS. Kekahbah et al. (1983) suggest the following nursing research needs with regard to Native Americans and Alaskan natives:

1. The extent to which various treatment modalities of psychotherapy and other approaches to mental health care are applicable to Native Americans and Alaskan natives.

2. The relative success rate of psychotherapists who are of the same culture as patients compared to those who are not.

3. The effect of the therapist's cultural values on her ability to function as a therapist.

4. Epidemiological variables by specific tribes and a definition of mental illness as developed by the various tribes.

A FINAL THOUGHT

Mental health practitioners must realize that their job is to treat stresses regardless of their sources. While removing the sources of the stress is usually considered to be beyond the scope of therapeutic intervention, the practitioner must realize that mental problems often have social roots. Consider the following story told by Irving Zola, involving a physician trying to explain the dilemmas of the modern practice of medicine:

You know, sometimes it feels like this. There I am standing by the shore of a swiftly flowing river and I hear the cry of a drowning man. So I jump into the river, put my arms around him, pull him to shore, and apply artificial respiration. Just when he begins to breathe, there is another cry for help. So I jump into the river, reach him, pull him to shore, apply artificial respiration, and then just as he begins to breathe, another cry for help. So back in the river again, reaching, pulling, applying, breathing, and then another yell. Again and again, without end, goes the sequence. You know, I am so busy jumping in, pulling them to shore, applying artificial respiration, that I have no time to see who in the hell is upstream pushing them all in (McKinlay, 1979, p. 9).

SUMMARY

Recognition of sociocultural diversity among both patient and health care professional is a crucial component of psychiatric mental health nursing practice. Variations in outlook can serve as barriers to understanding, while respecting cultural differences can provide important clues to an individual's background—crucial in providing sensitive mental health nursing care.

The purpose of this chapter is to provide information about ethnic and racial minority groups in American society, a society in which many different beliefs, values, and traditions exist in both harmony and, in some cases, disharmony. Concepts of minority/dominant group interaction, social change and mental health, prejudice and discrimination, and cultural identity are discussed. Descriptions of the most common minority groups in America today—Black Americans, Hispanic Americans, Asian Americans, and Native Americans are presented. These include a discussion of the "world view" of each group, with specific applications to mental health counseling and areas for future research.

STUDY QUESTIONS

1. Define the following terms: minority group, melting pot, cultural pluralism, prejudice, discrimination.

2. Define and discuss the major types of minority/dominant group interaction. What model best typifies the direction of interaction between blacks and whites in America, through history and today? What model best typifies relations with Native Americans?

3. What is the relationship between culture, mental health, and its treatment?

4. List five things that the culturally sensitive nurse therapist should know when providing care to: black Americans, Hispanic Americans, Asian Americans, and Native Americans. Discuss why this knowledge is essential in mental health delivery.

5. Read Irving Zola's statement about the practice of modern medicine and discuss the relevance of this statement to the practice of mental health with ethnic/racial minorities. Then construct two research hypotheses that relate his dilemma to one of the ethnic/racial minority groups.

KEY TERMS

accommodation

acculturation

assimilation

discrimination

minority group

melting pot

prejudice

folk medicine

world view

susto

culturally sensitive

REFERENCES

Adorno, T. W., Frenkel-Brunswick, E., Levinson, D. J., & Sanford, R. N. (1950). *The authoritarian personality.* New York: Harper and Brothers.

American Psychiatric Association (1987). *Diagnostic and statistical manual of mental disorders,* 3rd ed., revised. Washington, D.C.: Author.

Atkinson, D. R., Morten, G., & Sue, D. W. (1989). *Counseling American minorities: A cross-cultural perspective.* Dubuque, Iowa: W. C. Brown.

Bell, C., Bland, I., Houston, E., & Jones, B. (1983). Enhancement of knowledge and skills for the psychiatric treatment of black populations. In J. Chunn II, P. Dunston, & F. Ross-Sheriff (Eds.), *Mental health and people of color: Curriculum development and change.* Washington, D.C.: Howard University Press, pp. 205–238.

Bergin, A. E. (1980). Psychotherapy and religious values. *Journal of counseling and clinical psychology, 48,* 95–105.

Bernal, G., Bernal, M. E., Martinez, A. C., Olmedo, E. L., & Santisteban, D. (1983). Hispanic mental health curriculum for psychology. In J. C. Chunn II, P. J. Dunston, & F. Ross-Sheriff (Eds.). *Mental health and people of color: Curriculum development and change.* Washington, D.C.: Howard University Press, pp. 65–94.

Bettelheim, B., & Janowitz, M. (1964). *Social change and prejudice.* New York: The Free Press.

Campbell, T., & Chang, B. (1981). Health care of the Chinese in America. *Transcultural Health Care,* 162–171. American Journal of Nursing Company.

Campinha-Bacote, J. (1988). Culturological assessment: An important factor in psychiatric consultation-liaison nursing. *Archives of Psychiatric Nursing, 11*(4), 244–250.

Cockerham, W. C. (1989). *Sociology of mental disorder,* 2nd ed. Englewood Cliffs, N.J.: Prentice Hall.

Copeland, E. (1983). Cross-cultural counseling and psychotherapy: A historical perspective—Implications for research and training. *The Personnel and Guidance Journal, 62*(1), 10–14.

Deloria, V. (1979). Indians today, the real and the unreal. In D. R. Atkinson, G. Morten, & D. W. Sue (Eds.), *Counseling American minorities: A cross-cultural perspective.* Dubuque, Iowa: W. C. Brown, pp. 33–35.

Deutsch, A. (1944). The first U.S. census of the insane (1840) and its use as pro-slavery propaganda. *Bulletin of the History of Medicine, 15,* 469–482.

Fabrega, H. (1989). An ethnomedical perspective of Anglo-American psychiatry. *American Journal of Psychiatry, 146,* 588–596.

Foster, G. M. (1981). Relationships between Spanish and Spanish-American folk medicine. In G. Henderson & M. Primeaux (Eds.), *Transcultural Health Care.* Menlo Park, CA: Addison-Wesley, pp. 115–135.

Frank, J. D. (1974). *Persuasion and healing.* New York: Schocken Books.

Fujiki, S., Chin Hansen, J., Cheng, A., & Lee, Y. M. (1983) Psychiatric-mental health nursing of Asian and Pacific Americans. In J. C. Chenn II, P. J. Dunston, & F. Ross-Sheriff (Eds.), *Mental health and people of color: Curriculum development and change.* Washington, D.C.: Howard University press, pp. 335–375.

Gonzalez, H., Wilson, J., Gilde-Rubio, E., & Mejia, B. (1983). In J. C. Chunn II, P. J. Dunston, & F. Ross-Sheriff (Eds.), *Mental health and people of color: Curriculum development and change.* Washington, D.C.: Howard University Press, pp. 431–449.

Gould-Martin, K., & Ngin, C. (1981). Chinese Americans. In A. Harwood (Ed.), *Ethnicity and medical care.* Cambridge: Harvard University, pp. 130–171.

Grier, W., & Cobb, P. (1968). *Black rage.* New York: Basic Books.

Hall, E. T. (1976). How cultures collide. *Psychology Today, 10,* 66–74.

Harwood, A. (1981). *Ethnicity and medical care.* Cambridge: Harvard University Press.

Henderson, G., & Primeaux, M. (1981). Health care. In G. Henderson, & M. Primeaux (Eds.), *Transcultural health care.* Menlo Park, CA: Addison-Wesley, pp. 3–17.

Hess, B. B., Markson, E. W., & Stein, P. J. (1989). *Sociology,* 3rd ed. New York: Macmillan.

Hollingshead, A., & Redlich, F. (1958). *Social class and mental illness.* New York: John Wiley.

Jackson, J. (1981). Urban black Americans. In A. Harwood (Ed), *Ethnicity and medical care.* Cambridge: Harvard University Press, pp. 37–129.

Jones, W., & Rice, M. (1987). Promoting mental health: The potential for reform. In W. Jones, & M. Rice

(Eds.), *Health care issues in black America.* New York: Greenwood Press.

Jung, C. (1960). *Psychology and alchemy.* Princeton: Princeton University Press.

Kekahbah, J., Pamburn, A., Silk Walker, P., & Wood, R. (1983). Development of American Indian and Alaskan Native curricula content in psychosocial nursing. In J. C. Chunn II, P. J. Dunston, & F. Ross-Sheriff (Eds.), *Mental health and people of color: Curriculum development and change.* Washington, D.C.: Howard University Press, pp. 405–430.

Kiev, Ari. (1972). *Transcultural psychiatry.* New York: The Free Press.

Kinzie, J. D. (1985). Overview of clinical issues in the treatment of Southeast Asian refugees. In T. C. Owan (Ed.), *Southeast Asian mental health: Treatment, prevention, services, training, and research.* Rockville, Md.: National Institute of Mental Health, pp. 113–135.

Kitano, H., & Matsushima, N. (1976). Counseling Asian Americans. In P. B. Pedersen, J. G. Druguns, W. J. Lonner, & J. E. Trimble (Eds.), *Counseling across cultures.* Hawaii: University of Hawaii Press, pp. 163–180.

Kleinman, A. (1973). Some issues of a comparative study of medical healing. *International Journal of Social Psychiatry, 19,* 159–165.

Kramer, B. M. (1949). Dimensions of prejudice. *The Journal of Psychology, 27,* 389–451.

Kunitz, S. (1983). *Disease change and the role of medicine: The Navajo experience.* Berkeley, CA: University of California Press.

Kunitz, S., & Levy, J. (1981). Navajos. In A. Harwood (Ed.), *Ethnicity and medical care.* Cambridge: Harvard University, pp. 337–396.

Lin, T. Y., & Lin, M. C. (1978). Service delivery issues in Asian-North American communities. *American Journal of Psychiatry, 135,* 454–456.

McKinlay, J. (1979). A case for refocussing upstream: The political economy of illness. In E. G. Jaco (Ed.), *Patients, physicians, and illness,* 3rd ed. New York: The Free Press, pp. 9–25.

Meadows, A., & Stoker, D. (1965). Symptomatic behavior of hospitalized patients: A study of Mexican-American and Anglo-American patients. *Archieves of General Psychiatry, 12,* 267–277.

Mirowsky, J., & Ross, C. E. (1984). Mexican culture and its emotional contradictions. *Journal of Health and Social Behavior, 25,* 2–13.

Murillo-Rohde, I. (1981). Hispanic American patient care. In G. Henderson & M. Primeaux (Eds.), *Transcultural health care.* Menlo Park, CA: Addison-Wesley, pp. 224–238.

Navarro, J., & Miranda, M. (1985). Stress and child abuse in the Hispanic community: A clinical profile. In *Stress and Hispanic mental health—Relating research to service delivery.* Washington, D.C.: U.S. Government Printing Office.

Nobles, W. (1976). Black people in white insanity: An issue for black community mental health. *The Journal of Afro-American Issues, IV,* Winter, 21–27.

Olmedo, E. L. (1979). Acculturation: A psychometric perspective. *American Psychologist, 34,* 161–17.

Osborne, O., Carter, C., Pinkleton, N., & Richards, H. (1983). Development of African American curriculum content in psychiatric and mental health nursing. In J. C. Chun II, P. J. Dunston, & F. Ross-Sheriff (Eds.), *Mental health and people of color: Curriculum development and change.* Washington, D.C.: Howard University Press, pp. 335–375.

Owan, T. C., Ed. (1985). *Southeastern Asian mental health: Treatment, prevention, services, training, and research.* Rockville, Md.: National Institute of Mental Health.

Padilla, A. M., & Ruiz R. A. (1973). *Latino mental health: A review of the literature.* Rockville, Md.: National Institute of Mental Health.

Primeaux, M., & Henderson. G. (1981). American Indian patient care. In G. Henderson, & M. Primeaux (Eds.), *Transcultural health care.* Menlo Park CA: Addison-Wesley, pp. 239–254.

Redfield, R., Linton, R., & Herskovitz, M. J. (1936). Memorandum for the study of acculturation. *American Anthropologist, 38,* 149–152.

Richardson, E. H. (1981). Cultural and historical perspectives in counseling American Indians. In D. W. Sue (Ed.), *Counseling the culturally different: Theory and practice.* New York: John Wiley & Sons.

Ruiz, R. A., (1981). Cultural and historical perspectives in counseling American Indians. In D. W. Sue (Ed.), *Counseling the culturally different: Theory and practice.* New York: John Wiley & Sons.

Schreiber, J., & Homiak, J. (1981). Mexican Americans. In A. Harwood (Ed.), *Ethnicity and medical care.* Cambridge: Harvard University Press, pp. 264–336.

Smith, E. J. (1977). Counseling black individuals: Some stereotypes. *Personnel and Guidance, 55,* 39–396.

Smith, E. J. (1981). Cultural and historical perspectives in counseling blacks. In D. W. Sue (Ed.), *Counseling the culturally different: Theory and practice.* New York: John Wiley & Sons, pp. 141–185.

Snow, L. F. (1981). Folk medical beliefs and their implications for the care of patients: A review based on studies among black Americans. In G. Henderson, & M. Primeaux (Eds.), *Transcultural health care.* Menlo Park, CA: Addison-Wesley, pp. 78–101.

Statistical Abstract of the United States (1988). Washington D.C.: United States Department of Commerce.

Sue, D., & Sue, S. (1987). Counseling Chinese Americans. *Personnel and Guidance Journal, 50,* 637–643.

Sue, D. W. (1981). *Counseling the Culturally Different:* Theory and practice. New York: John Wiley & Sons.

Szasz, T. (1971). The sane slave: A historic note on the use of medical diagnosis as justicatory rhetoric. *American Journal of Psychotherapy, 25,* pp. 228–239.

Thomas, D. (1981). Black American patient care. In G. Henderson, & M. Primeaux (Eds.), *Transcultural patient care.* Menlo Park, CA.: Addison-Wesley, pp. 209–223.

Trimble, J. (1976). Value differentials and their importance in counseling American Indians. In P. Pederson, J. Draguns, W. Lonner, & J. Trimble (Eds.), *Counseling across cultures.* Honolulu: University of Hawaii Press, pp. 203–26.

U.S. Department of Health and Human Services. (1985) *Report of the Secretary's task force on black and minority health*. Vols. I & II. Washington, D.C.: U.S. Department of Health and Human Services.

Vander Zanden, J. (1972). *American minority relations,* 3rd ed. New York: Ronald Press.

Vega, W., & Kolody, B. (1985). *The meaning of social support and the mediation of stress across cultures*. Department of Health and Human Services Publication No. (ADM) 85–1410. Washington, D.C.: U.S. Department of Health and Human Services.

Vega, W., & Miranda, M. R. (1985). *Stress and Hispanic mental health: Relating research to service delivery*. Rockville, Md.: National Institute of Mental Health.

Vogel, V. (1981). American Indian medicine. In G. Henderson, & M. Primeaux (Eds.), *Transcultural health care*. Menlo Park: Addison-Wesley, pp. 136–147.

Vontress, C. (1979). Racial differences: Impediments to rapport. *Journal of Counseling Psychology, 18,* 7–13.

Vontress, C. (1981). Racial and ethnic barriers in counseling. In P. Pedersen, J. Draguns, W. Lonner, & J. Trimble (Eds.), *Counseling Across Cultures*. Honolulu: University of Hawaii Press, pp. 87–106.

Wilson, W. (1987). *The truly disadvantaged—The inner city, the underclass, and public policy*. Chicago: The University of Chicago Press.

Wright, B. R. (1964). Social aspects of change in the Chinese family pattern in Hong Kong. *Journal of Social Psychology, 63,* 31–39.

Whitten, N. (1962). Contemporary patterns of Malign Occultism among Negrocs in North Carolina. *Journal of American Folklore, 75,* 311–325.

7

THE NURSE AS THERAPIST

FRANCES BLACKWELL SMITH

LEARNING OBJECTIVES

After studying this chapter, the student will be able to:

- Identify and describe three levels of psychiatric mental health nursing.
- Identify and describe nine therapeutic roles of the nurse.
- Identify four guidelines for the nurse to use in goal-setting.
- Identify characteristics that make a nurse an effective therapist.
- Describe approaches to common clinical challenges in psychiatric nursing.
- Describe challenges in the development of the nurse's role as therapist.

INTRODUCTION

In defining the role of the nurse as therapist, one must ask what skills every nurse should possess in order to work effectively with patients in all areas of nursing practice. What are the goals of the nurse's work with patients? What is the difference between a therapeutic nurse-patient relationship and psychotherapy conducted by a nurse? What roles are appropriate for the nurse to assume in the treatment of psychiatric patients?

In considering these issues, we acknowledge this premise: All nurses should be therapeutic, but all nurses are not therapists. The theories and principles of psychiatric mental health nursing are applied at different levels. These differences are due not only to the nurse's knowledge, skill, and experience, but also to personal characteristics and individual choices, such as work setting, learning experiences, and career goals. Some nurses may also choose to function at different levels with different patients in the same work setting or assignment (described more fully later). (Also see Box 7–1.)

The purpose of this chapter is to identify, compare, and contrast three levels at which the theories and principles of psychiatric mental health nursing may be applied. This chapter describes therapeutic roles and characteristics of therapy goals applicable to all levels, and discusses factors that influence the nature and depth of therapy. Qualifications and personal characteristics that facilitate the nurse's role in therapy are discussed. We conclude with common problems that arise in nursing practice and suggestions for responding to them therapeutically.

LEVELS OF APPLICATION

The theories and principles of psychiatric mental health nursing may be applied at three levels:

1. In the **therapeutic nurse-patient relationship,** which is applicable to all nurses, all patients, and all practice settings;

2. In **basic therapy,** in which the nurse, the basic therapist, works with selected patients in structured, goal-directed sessions as part of an overall treatment program, most frequently within a psychiatric mental health setting over a period of time; and

3. In **primary therapy,** in which the nurse (the primary therapist) has major responsibility for the patient's therapy, most frequently as a psychotherapist in private practice or in a clinical specialist role.

Each level of functioning requires the application of psychiatric nursing knowledge and skill. On occasion, some nurses may choose to function at different levels with different patients. A team leader might strive for a therapeutic nurse-patient relationship with all of her patients but conduct basic therapy with certain ones; a clinical specialist might function as a primary therapist with her own caseload, but also see psychiatric patients who are referred to her for specific needs as part of their overall treatment plan (for example, group therapy led by the nurse or a contract for certain services). Each level of application is described in the following section.

THE THERAPEUTIC NURSE-PATIENT RELATIONSHIP

The therapeutic nurse-patient relationship applies to all nurses, all patients, and all practice settings, *not* merely to work with diagnosed psychiatric patients. Psychiatric nurses should provide patient care in accordance with the A.N.A. Standards of Psychiatric and Mental Health Nursing Practice (American Nurses' Association [ANA] 1982), and every patient has the right to expect the nurse to relate to him in a professional, therapeutic manner. This requires that the nurse:

1. Present herself to the patient in a professional manner (as opposed to a social, sexual, or totally subservient manner), including style of dress, decorum, and explanation of her role in his care.

2. Focus on the patient (instead of talking about herself or about irrelevant subjects such as the weather).

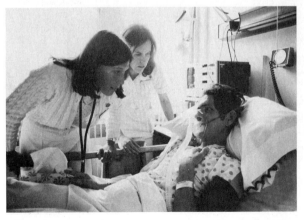

The therapeutic nurse-patient relationship focuses on the patient, and encourages the patient to express his or her feelings.

Box 7–1 ● The Concerns of Psychiatric Mental Health Nursing

Psychiatric mental health nursing is concerned with:

–the principles and laws that govern the recipient's well being and optimum functioning in various states of mental health and mental illness.

–the patterning of behavior during normal life events and in critical life situations.

–the processes by which positive changes in the mental health sta-

tus of persons, families, groups, and communities may be affected.

Source: Wahl, A. (1986). The phenomena of concern to psychiatric-mental health nursing practice: Implications for the 21st century. *Psychiatric-mental health nursing: Proceedings of a conference defining the discipline for the year 2000.* Rockville, MD: U. S. Department of Health and Human Services, p. 47.

---

3. Encourage the patient to express his feelings (via application of basic communication principles and techniques).

4. Listen attentively to the patient.

5. Respond to the patient in an appropriate and supportive manner, both verbally and nonverbally.

6. Observe and report the patient's behavior (for example, his response to the nurse's approaches, medication, and environmental stimuli; any changes in behavior, physical complaints, and so forth).

7. Maintain confidentiality by exercising special caution in discussing the patient's history (using his name, sharing data with family members).

8. Provide a supportive atmosphere and therapeutic milieu for the patient, fostering group support and cooperation; monitoring physical conditions of the environment, activities of daily living, and safety.

9. Encourage the patient's participation in appropriate modes of treatment, such as recreational activities, patient meetings, and group therapy.

10. Demonstrate awareness and appreciation of the patient's culture and values and their implications for treatment (for example, race, ethnic background, religion, sexual orientation, lifestyle, education, socioeconomic status, and family values).

11. Apply relevant theory to patient care, utilizing the nursing process appropriately to plan, implement, and evaluate quality nursing care.

12. Function collaboratively with others on behalf of the patient (for example, communicate with staff, demonstrate respect for organizational policies and roles of others, and facilitate appropriate referrals).

13. Seek further help when needed (that is, recognize her own limitations and request another opinion, consultation, or supervision).

14. Practice within the legal and ethical guidelines of the nursing profession.

These functions are basic to the therapeutic nurse-patient relationship and will be described in further detail throughout this chapter. It is important to note at this point that, although the nurse-patient relationship is designated as the most basic of the three levels of application, it is also the basis for therapy at any level, including brief counseling, crisis intervention, and psychotherapy (Lego, 1980).

The development of the therapeutic nurse-patient relationship is conceptualized in stages, in which the nurse has specific aims and responsibilities (Campaniello, 1980; Bellak, 1979; Doona, 1979; McCann, 1979). For a summary of the stages in a therapeutic nurse-patient relationship, see Table 7-1.

THE NURSE AS BASIC THERAPIST

Although therapy goals for the nurse's participation in therapy with patients are defined and described in greater detail on pages 176 through 178, *therapy* in its broadest sense is simply another word for *treatment*, and a therapist is "one trained in methods of treatment and rehabilitation other than the use of drugs or surgery." (*Webster's,* 1986). The term *therapist* is commonly used for many professionals who work with patients: occupational therapists, physical therapists, respiratory therapists, music therapists, art therapists, and recreational therapists. However, if

---

TABLE 7–1 Summary of stages in the therapeutic nurse-patient relationship

---

I. Orientation Phase
  A. Orients patient to
    1. Physical environment (tour of unit)
    2. Personnel and patients (introductions, roles)
    3. Daily routine (schedule, activities, visiting hours)
    4. Expectations (rules, chores, behavior, participation)
    5. Treatment regime (explanation, purpose, schedule)
  B. Structures relationship with nurse
    1. Clarifies roles
      a. Nurse's functions with patient
      b. Expectations of patient
      c. Limits
    2. Establishes therapy contact, as applicable (time, place, duration, purpose, and so on)
  C. Establishes trust
    1. Establishes rapport
    2. Reduces anxiety
    3. Encourages expression of feelings
    4. Reviews confidentiality (nurse's notes, communication with staff, others)
  D. Assesses patient
    1. Observes and collects data
    2. Performs specific physical and/or mental assessments as appropriate
    3. Identifies major problems, goals

II. Working Phase
  A. Identifies and interprets recurrent patterns
    1. Conversational themes
    2. Behavioral patterns
  B. Develops and refines treatment plan
    1. Specific goals and approaches
    2. Plan of evaluation
    3. Periodic revision of plan
    4. Discharge planning
  C. Works on problems identified
    1. Goal achievement
    2. Problem solving with patient
    3. Development of insight and/or behavioral change
  D. Resolves problems arising in the nurse-patient relationship
  E. Conducts patient education; refers for ongoing psychotherapy

III. Termination Phase
  A. Resolves separation anxiety; dependency
    1. Patient expresses fears, feelings re:
      a. Loss of relationship with nurse
      b. Loss of security of treatment setting.
      c. Prognosis or future plans
    2. Nurse and patient share positive feelings
  B. Reviews accomplishments; progress
  C. Completes discharge planning

---

the term "therapist" is used to refer to a nurse, it usually requires explanation.

One might argue that nursing is so synonymous with nurturing, communicating, caring, and promoting health that the term **nurse therapist** seems redundant. However, questions about "a nurse who calls herself a therapist" often indicate a lack of awareness or acceptance of the nurse's preparation for many of the more fundamental roles, such as performing assessments, structuring a therapeutic relationship, conducting goal-directed interviews, leading patient and family meetings, or planning discharge of patients. For example, employers in mental health settings often associate nurses primarily with medically oriented functions (such as administering medication) without recognizing their education in other areas (such as management, child care and development, family systems, group dynamics, and conducting various types of therapy).

Many nurses can—and do—function as basic therapists. The term *basic therapist* is used here to de-

note an intermediate level of functioning that incorporates, but goes beyond, the therapeutic nurse-patient relationship described previously yet does not require that the nurse function independently as the primary therapist in charge of the patient's treatment. Nurses may function as basic therapists in a variety of settings as part of an overall plan of treatment, working with selected patients in structured, individual sessions to meet specific goals over a period of time.

The basic therapist demonstrates a good understanding of psychopathology and has the ability to use selected tools for assessing mental health status effectively (for example, mental-status exams and nursing histories). The nurse who functions at this level understands and uses at least one basic therapy modality well, such as interpersonal theory or learning theory, and practices its basic methods appropriately. She demonstrates good interpersonal skills in communicating with patients and deals with common psychiatric problems in a therapeutic manner, seeking supervision in unusual or unprecedented situations. As the nurse gains experience and exposure to additional treatment modes, she will evaluate them and select some ideas, reject some ideas, refining and integrating them into a more definite style of therapy.

In addition to observing and reporting, the basic therapist synthesizes and interprets data, makes nursing diagnoses, guides patients in goal setting, and generally uses the **nursing process** of planning, implementing, and evaluating the effectiveness of the therapy. The ability to make some judgments rapidly and independently, especially during the interaction, is crucial, as every possibility cannot be anticipated in supervision and planning sessions. This requires that the nurse have knowledge and be able to use it in order to assume responsibility for long-term effects of therapy (Peplau, 1978). The nurse who is functioning as a basic therapist assumes the responsibility for communicating and collaborating with the primary therapist and agency responsible for her patients, and for obtaining consultation or supervision as needed or required. Therapy goals are discussed later in this chapter.

THE NURSE AS PRIMARY THERAPIST

A nurse may achieve a level of preparation that equips her to function as a primary therapist, assuming the major responsibility for directing and/or conducting a patient's treatment and/or psychotherapy. Primary therapists often conduct psychotherapy in independent, private practice, or in specialized roles designed for nurses with graduate education and/or extensive experience, such as the clinical nurse specialist.

In addition to clinical practice, the nursing profession looks to the nurse with advanced preparation for the development of research and theory in psychiatric mental health nursing. This challenge has been described as the most urgent task of psychiatric nursing (Dumas, 1981; O'Toole, 1981) and is crucial to the profession of psychiatric nursing (Dumas, 1981; O'Toole, 1981) as well as to the profession of nursing as a whole (McBride, 1986; Hoeffer & Murphy, 1982; Mellow, 1982).

THERAPEUTIC ROLES OF THE NURSE

To apply the basic concepts of psychiatric mental health nursing to the nurse-patient relationship at any of the three levels described, the nurse may as-

sume a number of different roles and fulfill a variety of functions in her work with patients. We will discuss the following roles: **healthy role model** (Maloney, 1983; Peplau, 1964); **nurturing parent** (an expansion of the *mother-surrogate* by Peplau, 1982b); **reality base** (Committee on Psychiatric Nursing, 1982a), **technician**, **socializing agent**, **manager**, **teacher** (Peplau, 1982b); **patient advocate** (Smoyak, 1986; Ettlinger, 1973); and **counselor** (Peplau, 1982b).

HEALTHY ROLE MODEL

The nurse seeks to serve as an example of good mental health, demonstrating a positive, realistic attitude and presentation of self. In particular, the nurse who works with psychiatric patients needs to be a mature model of good mental health (Maloney, 1983; Peplau, 1964). Patients notice the nurse's physical appearance and dress, work ethic, and response to frustration and fatigue, and at times, through various means of disclosure, patients become cognizant of crises in the nurse's personal life and her conflicts with patients and other staff. Whether the nurse's self-disclosure is purposeful (Anvil & Silver, 1984) or occurs inadvertently, she may be able to use such occasions therapeutically. Observing the nurse coping with everyday stress or a particular problem, such as bereavement, can provide an important example for the patient, whose own family members may have failed to demonstrate healthy responses to life's problems.

NURTURING PARENT

Peplau (1982b) used the term *mother-surrogate* to describe functions the nurse might perform as a substitute mother, such as bathing, feeding, dressing, protecting, and comforting the patient. The term *nurturing parent* is borrowed from Transactional Analysis (Berne, 1972) and seems more appropriate in today's society than *mother-surrogate*, because fathers and male nurses have also demonstrated the ability to assume a nurturing parent role. *Nurturing parent* is a broad term, referring to a nonthreatening, accepting approach to patients and to the support and caring vital to all patients, rather than to a restricted view of mothering associated primarily with meeting the dependency needs of the very regressed patient.

REALITY BASE

The nurse acts as a reality base for the patient on three levels: 1) she distinguishes what is objectively

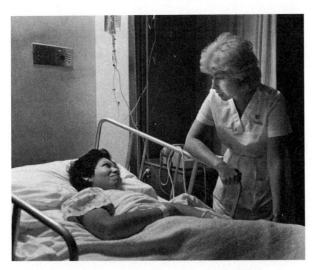

The nurse-therapist may serve as an example of how one demonstrates healthy responses to stress and anxiety.

real from what is not (objective reality); 2) she validates normal feelings and experiences; and 3) she represents social reality to the patient. All three of these levels are applicable to all levels of nursing practice.

DISTINGUISHING OBJECTIVE REALITY. Distinguishing objective reality involves distinguishing internal and external stimuli—determining which perceptions are subjective and originate from one's own feelings and needs (for example, hallucinations) and which are objective, based on external stimuli that can be validated with the five senses and experienced by others within the environment (Bellak, Hurvich, & Gediman, 1973). In using herself as a reality base at this level, the nurse may say to a psychotic patient who is hallucinating, "I know this is real to you, although I don't see what you are describing"; "I believe I heard a car backfiring, but I did not hear a shot"; or "The voices are part of your illness . . . I will stay here with you."

VALIDATING NORMAL RESPONSES. Validating normal responses is an extension of Sullivan's concept of consensual validation (Mullahy, 1973). It refers to a consensus of opinion or agreement between/among two or more persons that a patient's perceptions or one's interpretations of feelings or experiences are valid or well-founded (Wallace, 1983).

Some patients perceive events factually, but misinterpret their meaning, assume motives or intent that is not accurate, or personalize and draw erroneous

conclusions from the data. For example, one patient whose husband arrived late to see her in the hospital assumed that he was being unfaithful and plotting to kill her. Although he was late and his whereabouts were unknown, there was no evidence that he would ever harm her physically. Patients may attempt to mask their own true feelings, playing a guessing game to find out what others are thinking; then they imitate the others in order to gain acceptance by appearing more normal.

Validating normal feelings and experiences with the patient is one of the most important interventions in psychiatric nursing because it helps foster the patient's communication, rational thought, and identity with healthy role models. Many patients are unsure of themselves and cannot differentiate their normal emotions and thoughts from those that have been labeled as symptoms of mental illness. This causes them to feel rejected or restricted in their freedom in some way. The patient's natural reaction is to withdraw—to stop sharing his thoughts and feelings. His reluctance to validate his interpretations with others then results in his sinking deeper into his own private thoughts (Mullahy, 1973). Therefore, it is vital that the nurse validate the healthy aspects of the patient's thinking, feeling, and responding, letting him know that they are indeed normal. For example, the nurse might say, "Everyone feels that way to some degree occasionally"; or "I can see why you are uneasy around that man. He does come on very strong"; or "Wishing you had done something differently is a part of most grief reactions." The nurse may offer comments such as these frequently to encourage the patient to communicate honestly. As long as the patient shares his ideas, there is a potential for reexamining distortions (Peplau, 1964).

If the nurse is consistent with this positive validation of what is normal, the patient is much more likely to trust the nurse's judgment should it become necessary to point out what is pathological (for example, "I can see that the nursing attendant frightened you, but he really is not a spy. He works here, and he was trying to guide you back to your bed. This is someone else's bed.")

Validation of normal emotions and thoughts also improves the patient's self-image and promotes identification with healthy role models. No one likes to focus only on his weaknesses; the success enjoyed by mentally healthy people may be due more to capitalizing on strengths than overcoming weaknesses. Validation of normalcy makes the patient feel more normal, accepted, and understood, more willing to risk the relationships and solutions associated with living a normal life. Wallace (1983) reminds us that anything that reconnects the patient to the healthy community is therapeutic.

Some patients may be in touch with reality but be embarrassed or fearful about how they are coping with the problems in their life. For example, a patient in a crisis or with a post-traumatic stress syndrome associated with rape or war may apologize for emotions or express fears of "going crazy," "falling apart," or "losing it." The nurse can alleviate this additional burden by validating the patient's responses with such comments as, "Your reaction is understandable, considering what you have been through"; "Many veterans report this type of experience"; or "It's O.K. for you to cry. That was a frightening experience."

Some individuals may experience their unique interests or abilities as isolating or interpret any differences in themselves as psychopathology. Validation from the nurse, who represents authority and expertise in judging what is normal, and from others with similar interests, can be very helpful (for example, "Being the only boy in the class who likes violin and hates baseball may set you apart at times, but it does not make you a 'sissy.' Is there a music club for kids your age?").

Frankie Johnson: A Woman in Crisis

Frankie Johnson is a 42-year old woman who was admitted to a crisis stabilzation unit. She had recently received information that her husband had been killed in an automobile accident. When she entered the crisis unit, she was screaming, "Help me . . . I can't stand this . . . I can't live without him . . . help me, nurse, help me."

The nurse responded: "This is a terrible experience and it is normal for you to be upset and feel that your life will never be right again. I will be with you and assist you in dealing with this tragedy." (The nurse remained with Mrs. Johnson . . . and encouraged her to ventilate her feelings, and express her fears and doubts about her own ability to function).

REPRESENTING SOCIAL REALITY. Another way in which the nurse functions as a reality base is by representing to the patient society's values, possible responses to his behavior by others, and alternatives to meet his needs in appropriate, socially acceptable ways. Since this task reflects individual and cultural values, the nurse must be familiar with the current laws or customs of society and the rules and philosophy of the treatment setting in order to define appropriate behavior. Other patients may help to provide a realistic social microcosm by expressing their attitudes, which may be different from those of the nurse or patient. They may react to unusual behavior in ways very similar to the responses the patient encounters in the community. The nurse can help patients use these experiences to develop insight and prepare for discharge.

Sullivan states that if a patient were about to do something that was almost certain to be disastrous, he would say, "Let us consider what will follow that," and then depict the probable course of events (Mullahy, 1973). Examples of comments that the nurse might make in representing social reality to the patient are:

You may express your feelings, but you are not allowed to hit.

It makes me uncomfortable when you try to pinch me . . . that is not appropriate here, and I will not allow it.

Women will often react to comments such as yours in the same way that Mary reacted to you. Can you think of another way to tell Mary you'd like to get to know her better?

What you are doing is against the law. Do you understand the consequences of what you are involved in?

Perhaps you should wear long pants—instead of shorts—to the job interview.

I understand that in your own country people urinate in public, but here you must use the bathroom . . . I will show you where it is.

Such interventions are not designed to coerce the patient into adopting certain values, but to assist him in anticipating consequences, appreciating the impact of his actions on others, and making informed, realistic choices that promote his ability to function and achieve satisfaction in society.

TECHNICIAN

In a world of rapidly developing technology, the nurse's role as technician is necessary and highly valuable; accuracy in technical functions is vital to the patient's overall treatment program and to his life. The nurse must know how to perform technical procedures competently, efficiently, and correctly (Peplau, 1982b). These functions include preparing and administering medication and assisting with diagnostic or treatment measures, such as the use of restraints, electroconvulsive therapy, operation of a biofeedback machine, or performing the technical aspects of physical assessment, such as taking vital signs or testing vision. The extent to which a nurse is involved in the technical aspects of a patient's treatment depends on the philosophy of the treatment setting and the nurse. For example, some nurses who act as primary therapists choose not to assume a technical role with their patients, while others have built a practice around a combination of counseling and technology, such as stress management and biofeedback training.

SOCIALIZING AGENT

Peplau (1982b) described this role as giving the patient an opportunity to test his social skills in a relationship with the nurse, by taking walks, playing games, and engaging in conversation about current events. The nurse's role as socializing agent also includes encouraging the patient's participation in interactions with others, group activities, and recreational therapy; facilitating social activities such as parties or outings by helping the patient to plan them; and participating directly with the patient to improve specific social and interpersonal skills (for example, appearance, table manners, conversational skill, and overcoming shyness). Since the goal of rehabilitation is resocialization of the patient within the community, this is an important role, applicable to all levels of nursing practice.

MANAGER

The role of the nurse as manager has progressed beyond housekeeping and clerical management to include facilitating patients' active participation in decisions about their treatment (Corey et al., 1986; Peplau, 1982b). In addition to the basic functions of unit management, which may include managing supplies, records, staff assignments, and interdepartmental communication, it is primarily the responsibility of the nurse to maintain the therapeutic milieu or environment in the treatment setting (Fagin, 1967; Gregg, 1982). Historically, nurses have also been responsible for management (control) of their patients' behavior. In fact, it has been the nurse's responsibility to determine how to manage combative behavior, despite the lack of human and material resources (Fox, 1986).

The therapeutic environment has been described as one in which the patient has the opportunity to develop new behavior patterns that will enable him to make a more mature adjustment to life (Gregg, 1982). This includes a safe, comfortable, pleasant physical facility and a supportive living environment in which

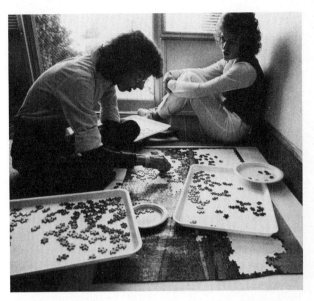

The nurse-therapist may function as a socializing agent by encouraging the patient to participate in recreational and therapeutic activities, as well as helping the patient to improve and practice specific social and interpersonal skills.

the patient can relax, express himself, socialize, and test new behaviors. Such an atmosphere requires nursing management of the patient's daily schedule to avoid conflicts and provide a balance in social stimulation and solitude, rest, and exercise. In order to protect the milieu for all patients, a nurse may remove a patient from a volatile situation, interrupt inappropriate sexual activity, and protect patients from unwelcome visitors. The nurse manages specific aspects of a patient's therapy, such as suicide or escape precautions, seclusion, limit-setting, group and family meetings, referrals, and discharge planning.

In recent years, nurses have become proficient in the use of behavior therapy. Nurse researchers are studying behavior therapy principles and have applied their findings to a variety of patient populations (alcoholism, eating disorders, enuresis, chronic pain, among many others). Many nurses in all areas of nursing practice have found that the behavioral perspective is especially useful in patient teaching where they employ positive feedback for appropriate behavioral responses. This approach concentrates on behavioral change rather than the patient's psychological dynamics.

The psychiatric nurse in independent practice is responsible for managing a patient caseload as well as the business component of the practice: staffing, marketing, fiscal management, and care of the physical plant. See page 184 for a more detailed description of case management.

TEACHER

The role of the nurse as patient educator—or teacher—has become commonplace in other areas of nursing service but is still rare on a psychiatric unit, because of questions about some patients' ability to use information appropriately. However, there are ways in which the nurse on the psychiatric unit can and does act as teacher. The nurse should check legalities and agency policies, making sure the patient is informed of anything he has a legal and ethical right to know. Misconceptions may arise when a patient seeks information about his condition or treatment from other patients, libraries, or television without the guidance necessary to put the information into proper perspective. The risks accompanying informed consumerism are minor in comparison to the problems associated with a lack of understanding (fear, suspicion, poor judgment, overdependence, or noncompliance). Misinformation—or misinterpretations—can have serious, even tragic, consequences for the patient. He may suddenly develop symptoms that he reads about or have a negative reaction to his medication. In one tragic case, a patient misinterpreted the side effects of his medication as permanent brain deterioration and committed suicide.

The following are some useful ways in which the nurse can educate her patient:

1. By teaching him the early signs and symptoms of a problem or its recurrence; by helping him create a plan of action or by giving him suggestions for preventing or reducing its impact (for example, teaching a manic to keep a sleep graph or a child abuser to monitor signs of mounting tension; rehearsing alternative actions).

2. By explaining the effects of psychiatric treatment measures (for example, the therapeutic and side effects of psychotropic medication or electroconvulsive therapy; adverse reactions or possible complications; the incompatibility of some drugs with alcohol, some foods, or other drugs; precautions).

3. By teaching him skills that promote socialization and/or enrich his leisure time. Sports, games, crafts, music, and other interests can foster confidence and provide an entree to interaction with others, both on the treatment unit and in general society. Classes in makeup, hairstyles, or fashion may motivate the patient and increase self-esteem. These activities are less passive and solitary than passing time in the dayroom smoking and watching television.

4. By helping him develop interpersonal skills. Classes in assertiveness training, parent effectiveness training, or the basics of any therapy modality that is appropriate to the patient are beneficial.

Role playing various situations with a patient allows him to experiment with new ways of relating in a protected environment, where feedback is available, as does more formal group therapy or psychodrama. For example, the nurse might simulate a job interview with a patient, then review with him how he presented himself, his response to questions about his hospitalization, and his feelings during the interaction.

5. By informing him of other resources. The patient and his family need information about treatment options, hotlines, self-help or support groups related to his particular problem; emergency facilities; and how to avail themselves of these services (their cost, general purpose, location, and so forth).

All levels of nursing practice may involve some form of teaching. Nonprofessional staff members have been effective in teaching in specific areas, such as guitar lessons or assertiveness training, and experienced psychotherapists report some overlap between the counseling role and the type of experiential teaching that involves helping a patient to analyze and learn from a life experience or problem (Peplau, 1982b). The teaching-learning process is extremely important in helping the patient move toward increasing responsibility for his own health and care (Moscovitz, 1984).

PATIENT ADVOCATE

The patient needs to experience the nurse as a person who is allied with him in his struggle for health (Nicholi, 1988)—someone who will advocate for his welfare. The role of patient advocate is one of the most important and difficult roles in the nursing profession. The nurse speaks for the patient because 1) the nurse's knowledge of the patient's condition and treatment, how the system works, and how his case is being handled is much greater than that of the patient; 2) the nurse's position on the treatment team and relationship with the staff permit the nurse to ask questions and explore possibilities in a way that the patient cannot; 3) a nurse is usually accessible to the patient and his family twenty-four hours a day, is willing to listen, and is able to sort out significant data and concerns; and 4) the patient often feels intimidated by other professionals in the health care system (Smith, 1985), lacking the ego strength to assert himself or the communication skills to make himself understood.

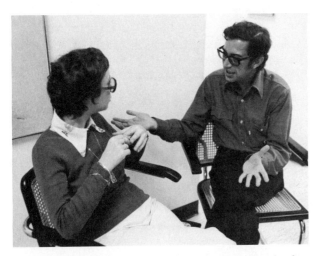

As a patient advocate, the nurse-therapist speaks for the patient, and helps to ensure that the patient's rights are not being violated.

When a nurse observes something that she feels is not in the patient's best interest, and that lies within the direct responsibility of nursing service, she should discuss it with her supervisor or the appropriate nursing administrator. For example, admitting a suicidal patient may affect nursing staff coverage. If the nurse's concerns lie outside the area of direct care, which would be the case if she disagreed with the patient's psychiatrist about the choice of treatment for the patient, the nurse must then decide whether or not to advocate for the patient. (See Chapter 28 on ethics.) She may begin by posing a simple question, such as, "Have you thought about how to ensure that Johnny will get his medication after discharge?" rather than challenging a decision directly, for example, "You can't just discharge him without setting up an out-patient treatment!" Persistent questioning is often useful; so is offering information (for example, "Have you seen this article?" "Several years ago, we tried a method that seemed to work well with this type of patient.") The nurse can also appeal to her supervisor or to others on the staff who may have more influence with those making the decisions on the case.

If no action appears to be forthcoming, the nurse determines what steps to take next: whom to approach, what to do or say, and whether or not to "push it." The consequences of advocacy must always be considered in view of the potential effects on the patient. However, there are also consequences for the nurse (Witt, 1983), who must sometimes weigh the potential benefits that can be achieved for one patient against her continued ability to function effectively in her particular treatment setting. The effective advocate is well-informed about the issues of agency policy and politics and the rights of nurses and patients. In functioning as a patient advocate, the nurse may be guided by the Patient's Bill of Rights (Carnegie, 1974), guidelines of the American Civil Liberties Union (Ennis & Seigel, 1978), and laws pertaining to nursing (Creighton, 1981) and psychiatry, such as the patient's right to refuse medication (Oriol & Oriol, 1986; Feather, 1985), or to be maintained in the least restrictive setting (Garritson & Davis, 1983).

COUNSELOR

Counseling is verbal support and guidance, the principal tool of the primary therapist and the most important tool of psychiatric nursing (Peplau, 1964; 1982a; 1982b). There are very few methods of psychiatric treatment that do not rely heavily on counseling skills (for example, behavior therapy, psychotropic medication, or somatic therapies such as electroconvulsive treatments).

Although counseling with the primary therapist is conducted in a number of sessions over a period of time, it is possible for a nurse to take on a counseling role in a single contact with a patient. For example, a preoperative patient might be counseled regarding his fear of surgery, or a noncompliant patient may be assisted in resolving his concerns about his medication; such cases do not necessarily indicate long-term psychotherapy. Counseling in crises such as a suicide attempt is limited in scope but can be very effective: it can save a life.

Table 7-2 shows an excerpt from a nurse's conversation with her patient and demonstrates the use of the nine therapeutic roles described.

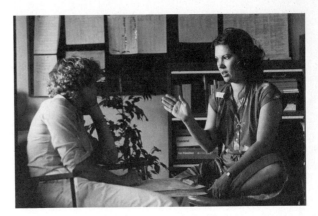

Counseling is the principle tool of the primary therapist and the most important tool of psychiatric nursing (Peplau, 1964; 1982a; 1982b).

TABLE 7–2 The nurse's nine therapeutic roles

Patient	Nurse	Nurse's Role
(John takes pill cup and walks away.)	(Administers medication) "I need to see you swallow it."	Technician
"I don't think I need this stuff anymore."	"You may not remember, but the last time you stopped taking your medication against your doctor's advice, your auditory hallucinations, the voices that told you to kill yourself, came back."	Reality base
"Why do I have to take it?"	"It will help you to feel calmer and regain control of your behavior so you can go back home."	Teacher
(Spits toward nurse)	"John, that is unacceptable and not necessary."	Socializing agent
"I thought you would get mad and leave."	"No, I think we should talk things out."	Healthy role model
"I want to see my doctor, but he hasn't been by today."	"He's on the unit now. I'll ask him if he can see you."	Patient advocate
"I was supposed to see the social worker now."	"The social worker is here all morning. Perhaps she can see you later."	Manager
"Did she tell you my grandpa died?"	"No, I hadn't heard that. I'm very sorry, John."	Nurturing parent
	(Goes over to him and sits down) "Tell me about your grandpa."	Counselor

THERAPY GOALS

The process of formulating nursing diagnoses, goals, and approaches is usually covered extensively in basic nursing textbooks. Therefore, a brief explanation of the process as it relates to psychiatric mental health nursing is presented here. Four characteristics of goals for the nurse's work with a psychiatric patient are: 1) the goals are within the scope of nursing practice; 2) they are compatible with the patient's overall treatment plan; 3) they are culturally relevant and based on the patient's current needs and problems; and 4) they are formulated to measure short-term progress of the patient. (Also see Box 7–2.)

GOALS ARE WITHIN THE SCOPE OF NURSING PRACTICE

Nursing has been defined by the American Nurses' Association's policy statement as the diagnosis and treatment of human responses to actual or potential health problems (ANA, 1980). The scope of psychiatric mental health nursing encompasses a wide variety of conditions (such as emotional disturbances, hallucinations, and problems in relationships) that are responsive to the application of psychiatric mental

health nursing knowledge and skills. When setting goals for a patient's therapy, the nurse considers whether she would be acting within her legal role (Shoemaker, 1984) and whether the nursing intervention she selects addresses the problem presented for treatment.

For example, a nurse does not set the goal of stabilizing a patient's medication (it is not a direct nursing intervention). However, the nurse could be very instrumental in stabilizing the patient's *behavior* (such as helping him handle anger appropriately) by acting within nursing roles such as manager, reality base, socializing agent, and/or counselor.

GOALS ARE COMPATIBLE WITH THE TREATMENT PLAN

Nursing theorists have recommended that the nurse-patient relationship be consistent with the patient's overall treatment plan (Gregg, 1982). However, perhaps it is more appropriate to suggest that goals for nurse-patient interactions be compatible with the overall goals of the treatment as they may complement or supplement the focus of the primary thera-

**Box 7–2 ●
Characteristics of
Psychiatric Mental
Health Nursing**

1. A holistic focus that includes assessment of physical state as well as emotional state.

2. A holistic focus that includes considering environmental, community, and cultural factors.

3. A flexibility that accepts multiple sites appropriate for the conduct of therapy, for example, the home, the community, the hospital, or the office.

4. An approach that focuses more on health than pathology, and on ed-

ucation and environmental manipulation to bring about health.

Source: Wahl, A. (1986). The phenomena of concern to psychiatric-mental health nursing practice: Implications for the 21st century. *Psychiatric-mental health nursing: Proceedings of a conference defining the discipline for the year 2000.* Rockville, MD: U.S. Department of Health and Human Services, p. 49.

---

pist rather than attempting to replicate it. Goals for nurse-patient interactions may be *different* from, but not in *conflict* with, the primary treatment goals. The nurse does not always need to feel compelled to "ask the doctor what to work on," but may independently formulate goals within the scope of nursing practice or collaborate with other members of the treatment team. In many cases it can be very useful for the nurse to deal with issues other than the presenting problem or precipitating event (for example, working on appearance and self-esteem with a phobic patient; utilizing observations from group therapy to enhance the growth of a patient admitted for violent behavior; discussing job satisfaction with a patient admitted for alcoholism).

GOALS ARE BASED ON CURRENT NEEDS AND PROBLEMS

Peplau (1968) described the aim of nursing care in psychiatry as assisting patients toward the full development of their potential for living productively in the community. When conducting an interview with a patient, the nurse focuses on the patient's current needs and problems, rather than childhood history and unconscious motives. For example, the nurse might work with a patient to help him assert himself during his mother's visits to the hospital rather than analyzing his unresolved Oedipal conflict. The nurse could explore with a paranoid patient what might make him feel more comfortable and secure, rather than focusing on his lack of basic trust. With a violent patient, she might demonstrate acceptable outlets for discharging anger, rather than tracking his developmental deficits. Attempts at coping with the problems in daily living that recur in dealing with

others often involve counselling as well as psychotherapy (Mullahy, 1973); the nurse can play an important role in helping her patients learn how to cope.

GOALS ARE FORMULATED TO MEASURE SHORT-TERM PATIENT PROGRESS

Goals for the nurse's work with patients are patient-oriented, measurable, realistic, and usually short-term.

PATIENT-ORIENTED GOALS. The nurse sets goals that focus on the patient. To avoid assuming all of the responsibility for the outcome or confusing the evaluation of the patient's outcome with whether or not a nurse performed a particular intervention properly, the patient rather than the nurse should always be the subject of the goal (for example, not "To confront the patient with his denial," as the nurse does the confronting, but "Joe will acknowledge his drinking problem," which is the desired outcome; not "To reduce the patient's anxiety," but "John will sit and talk with me for ten minutes, which he has not been able to do, due to his anxiety.")

MEASURABLE GOALS. The nurse sets goals that are measurable by the patient's behavior rather than goals that refer to feelings or attitudes that cannot be measured. For example, the nurse would *not* state as a goal, "Mrs. Lee will experience increased ego strength." Rather, she would state, "Mrs. Lee will report her day without making any self-derogatory comments." The work of Mager (1984) and others provides more information about this criterion of nursing goals.

REALISTIC GOALS. The nurse sets goals that are realistic for the patient, the nurse, and the setting. The nurse guards against unrealistic goals for the patient (Campaniello, 1980) to prevent failure, frustration, and possible damage to the patient's self-esteem. The nurse also considers her own ability and level of comfort in working with the patient to reach his goal. Some goals may be realistic for the patient but not appropriate for a particular nurse at a particular time. For example, a beginning student requires time and experience to work effectively with a violent patient.

SHORT-TERM GOALS. The nurse sets realistic, short-term goals. Even in long-term therapy, a series of intermediate, short-term goals allows both patient and nurse to enjoy some degree of intermediate success and ensures periodic evaluation of progress toward the overall treatment goal while change is still possible. For example, in working with a long-term problem such as low self-esteem, a patient might benefit from combining a short-term goal, such as participating in a group exercise program each day, with a long-term goal, such as identifying and changing self-defeating attitudes. Due to changes in health-care economics and changing treatment philosophy, short-term treatment is replacing long-term psychotherapy in many treatment settings, and some professionals trained in long-term treatment methods are making adjustments in their practices.

THE NATURE AND DEPTH OF THERAPY

The nature and depth of the nurse's work with patients is determined by the setting, the supervision available, the patient, and the nurse.

THE SETTING FOR THERAPY

The nurse's function varies according to the clinical setting in which she works (Redmond, 1982), whether she works with inpatients, outpatients, clients in various community agencies, or patients in their homes. Her approach is influenced greatly by the **locus of control**; that is, the center of power and decision making. This determines the amount of control the nurse has over the patient and his environment. A patient has more control of environmental stimuli and reinforcement in his own home; the nurse has more control of these things on an inpatient unit. In addition, the policies of the health care agency may determine or eliminate certain ap-

proaches. For example, a doctor's order may be required for a patient to attend group therapy, or this may be a nursing judgment. Factors for the nurse to consider include: the philosophy of the health care agency and the primary therapist, frequency and duration of contact with the patient, use of medication, methods of payments, and ethical-legal issues.

SUPERVISION OF THE THERAPY

Supervision is the process in which a nurse conducting therapy reviews her efforts with a supervisor who provides consultation and supports her professional development (Platt-Koch, 1986). This type of supervision is different from administrative supervision, which is designed to ensure quality of care and implementation of agency philosophy and policy.

Methods of supervision include case discussion; direct observation; use of a two-way mirror, videotape, or audiotape; analysis of conversational notes; role playing; patient simulations; and individual and group discussions. Proper procedures are followed to protect the patient's confidentiality and other ethical and legal rights.

Supervision of the nurse's therapy with patients is extremely important for the patient and for the nurse. Supervision can help correct bias, validate impressions, offer insights and suggestions for patients' problems, and stimulate the therapist's professional development. Supervision for the nurse conducting therapy should be provided on a regular, ongoing basis by a therapist with more advanced education and/or experience. Some nursing leaders state that the supervisor of a nurse's therapy should also be a nurse (Gregg, Bregg, & Spring, 1976), while others recommend an interdisciplinary approach (Platt-Koch, 1986). In any case, the supervisor should be a good role model, preferably one whose attitudes, style, and methods of treatment the nurse admires and finds compatible with her own. Availability of supervision is another important consideration. This is particularly true for a novice nurse who may need to confer more frequently and more immediately than a more experienced therapist.

If ongoing supervision is not available, the nurse therapist can use other resources available for consultation and/or education on a formal or informal basis. For example, because of the specialization of health care, nurses can improve their general knowledge of psychiatry by consulting with colleagues in more specialized areas such as cocaine abuse, premenstrual syndrome, or the management of panic disorder.

The process of supervision and how it differs from therapy is covered later in this chapter, in the section on "Awareness and Acceptance of Self and Others."

THE PATIENT'S NEEDS IN THERAPY

Knowing that strong affect often produces growth and change in a patient, the inexperienced therapist may feel pressure to try to "get a lot out of the patient." In doing so, she may use interventions or modes of therapy that are not appropriate for her patient in order to prove her own skills as a therapist. Pushing too hard, too fast, or in the wrong direction can be damaging to a patient, while a seemingly simple approach may provide a basis on which to build.

The nurse therapist is guided by the patient's needs. The nurse may ask herself the following five questions to determine accurately which therapies or interventions are most appropriate for the patient's needs.

INITIAL QUESTIONS.
1. *Is exploring this issue the highest priority for this patient at this time?* For example, aspects of the patient's history may be significant in terms of the overall problem, but less urgent for the patient than his immediate need or presenting problem. It might be more useful to one patient to focus on alternative methods of relaxation and socialization than to have him describe in detail his experiences with drugs.

2. *Am I using this approach in order to meet my own needs?* The nurse might have natural curiosity about unusual lifestyles or histories; she may perceive pressure to produce relevant data or to demonstrate insight, ability, or proficiency in a specific technique for the purposes of supervision and evaluation; or she may have a desire to hasten a patient's progress. When personal ambition overrides the patient's needs, therapeutic usefulness is lost or greatly minimized (Committee on Psychiatric Nursing, 1982b).

3. *Am I viewing the patient's problem in proper perspective?* The nurse therapist may overreact to data with which she identifies, or that relates to something she has recently read, discussed, or experienced. For example, a nurse who has been embarrassed by being manipulated by a patient may become overly strict and cautious in dealing with a similar situation later on.

4. *Am I tempering my questions to the patient with adequate support?* Reviewing the therapist's input often reveals a series of questions in succession, unbroken by any statement of support or validation of the patient's feelings, which can make the patient feel like a dartboard. The patient will ultimately share more and gain more benefit from the session if the nurse responds to what has been said with a positive comment before asking another question. Some examples of supportive comments include:

"That must have been frightening (painful, upsetting)."

"I'm glad you were able to share these feelings with me."

"What you described is really not so unusual. I believe you can overcome it."

5. *If the patient answers my questions, am I prepared to deal with the feelings and problems he expresses?* While there is inherent value to the patient in clarifying his thoughts and ventilating his feelings by simply expressing them to another human being and feeling accepted and understood, this can also become a crutch for the nurse therapist who fails to take the next step. The therapist must deal with whatever she has uncovered. It is unfair for the therapist to ask the patient to endure the pain of self-revelation and relive past traumas unless she is prepared to help him gain a new perspective or to deal with these experiences and feelings in a healthier way. Activating strong emotions with no forethought for how they may be resolved may lead the patient to greater despair. For example, if the nurse asks about incest, she must be ready to deal with whatever the patient tells her (or be sure that a good referral source is readily available).

ADDITIONAL PATIENT CRITERIA FOR THERAPY. The additional criteria for determining appropriate therapy for a patient are: (1) the patient's history, mental status, and diagnosis, (2) his level of anxiety, (3) therapeutic match, and (4) the timing of the interventions.

Diagnosis and History. The patient's diagnosis and his history are good indicators of the type of therapy that will be appropriate for him. The psychotic individual generally requires short, supportive interactions focusing on reality, activities of daily living, and behavior that fosters his return to the community, rather than lengthy, in-depth psychotherapy designed to promote insight. A direct, confrontive approach is apt to be more useful with patients who have been admitted for substance abuse, violence, or acting out through other antisocial behaviors. Family and/or group therapy in a controlled, therapeutic environment is often the primary method of treatment for this group of patients. Such programs often rely heavily on the principles of behavior modification and reality therapy, with limit setting, peer pressure, and support as important components. The nurse therapist can apply these principles to her own interactions with patients as well as participate directly in these therapies.

John: A Patient Who Needed Limits and Support

John was a 24-year-old patient admitted to the hospital. Alicia, the basic therapist assigned to John's care, had begun to hear reports that John was using vulgar language around other patients and staff in the dayroom. Alicia approached John about this.

"John, I understand that several patients have complained about your language in the dayroom."

John replied, "Oh, go_____yourself!"

"How do you expect me to react when you say that, John?"

"I don't give a damn."

Alicia countered, "I do. You can express your feelings but that sort of language is not acceptable on this unit." John did not respond. Alicia then asked, "How do people usually respond when you use that kind of language?"

John shrugged. "Walk away, I guess. My old man, he'd knock me around, for sure. And Mrs. Jones on the evening shift locks me up in seclusion."

Alicia asked, "Is that what you want?"

"Hell, no! I hate it! I've got to move around."

"But you just told me that's what happens when you use bad language. Why don't we go to your room and talk about what else you can do instead."

In the case of John, the nurse might explore his problem further, instituting the limit-setting process in relation to John's behavior. However, by following up on the response that the patient elicits from others rather than his actual feelings, the nurse has already used principles consistent with behavioral and milieu therapy rather than a traditional insight-oriented approach to the patient's anger.

Patients who are anxious or depressed with no thought disorders are usually considered the best candidates for insight-oriented psychotherapy, although their treatment is by no means limited to this approach. Many other patients are also candidates for psychotherapy.

In addition to diagnosis, the patient's history may offer clues as to what approaches might be most

effective. Does the patient have a history of signing out against medical advice, doctor shopping, litigation, or violence? If so, these issues should be explored. If there are any indications that a particular approach has been effective with this patient in the past it should be followed up as well.

Patient's Level of Anxiety. The patient's level of anxiety (Peplau, 1963) is perhaps the best indicator of the nature and depth of therapy necessary for treatment. Too little anxiety will not motivate the patient to grow, leading to chronic problems, while a very high level of anxiety creates distorted perception and communication, an inability to examine and learn from problems, and a general resistance or even aversion to therapy. The nurse notes the patient's anxiety level during every contact. Unlike diagnosis, which is more stable, anxiety level may fluctuate day to day, hour to hour, or moment to moment. Behaviors that indicate the patient is ready to progress include:

Asking questions or reading about his diagnosis or treatment;

Following up on suggestions or assignments made by the therapist;

Introducing problems or initiating topics;

Decreasing the usual avoidance maneuvers;

Answering questions more honestly and spontaneously;

Being on time and dressed for the session; or

Decreasing random motor movements and/or other signs and symptoms of anxiety.

Therapeutic Match. The therapeutic process is enhanced when the type of therapy and the therapist chosen are compatible with the patient's personality, manner of thinking and relating, values, and culture. A thorough understanding of the patient's background and way of thinking and relating can be as valuable as selecting appropriate approaches. For example, the nurse therapist may feel that an inhibited intellectual would benefit most from a type of group therapy designed to encourage openness, total honesty, and spontaneity, to help him to be more in touch with his gut-level feelings. However, if this approach is too threatening to him, he may reject therapy totally; he might have been more successful with individual therapy that emphasized attitudes and thought processes.

In considering a patient's personality and background, the nurse therapist anticipates how these factors may influence his reaction to her. Although authorities contend that a good therapist can overcome cultural barriers (Wallace, 1983), some patients seem comfortable only when they are absolutely certain that the therapist not only appreciates, but shares, their particular background (religion, values, race, language, sexual orientation, or personal experience with a particular problem). Some patients fear being "brainwashed" to relinquish their beliefs or lifestyle (Nicholi, 1988), and this prevents them from responding to the nurse's competence, empathy, and training in dealing with their concerns. If this happens, it is better for the nurse to refer the patient to another therapist than to risk having him withhold feelings, discount the therapy, or terminate it altogether. A nurse does not need to feel apologetic about not being "all things to all people," or feel any less competent when referral seems indicated.

Sometimes economics limits the amount of time available to resolve a patient's resistance, and it is important then to find an alternative solution as soon as possible. Many religious and minority groups now offer their own counseling services or are represented somewhere within the mental health delivery system. These services can be helpful in facilitating rapport, offering a greater degree of empathy, providing practical suggestions for dealing with specific aspects of the problem, and differentiating psychopathology from cultural biases (for example, healthy faith versus sick religion, paranoia versus the realities of racism [Mitchell, 1976] or homophobia [Douglas, Kalman, & Kalman, 1985]). Substance abuse programs have long been recognized to be effective on this basis (for example, "You can't con a con. I've been there; I know what you're going through."). Groups that have been identified as having special needs include blacks (Mitchell, 1976), Hispanics (Reeves, 1986), Arab-Americans (Meleis & LaFever, 1984), Vietnam veterans (Keltner, Doggett, & Johnson, 1983), homosexuals (Anthony, 1982; Rochlin, 1982), impaired professionals (Jefferson & Ensor, 1982), battered wives, and others. It is interesting to note that research shows a number of similarities between nurse psychotherapists and their clientele, which is predominantly female and includes many well-educated professionals (Hardin & Durham, 1985; Pelletier, 1984).

Timing of Therapy. Knowing *when* to apply an intervention or employ a particular mode of therapy is as important as knowing how. Timing refers to the stage of the nurse-patient relationship, the progress of a particular therapy session, and the patient's readiness to examine his problems and change his behavior, which may vary with his mood or ability to handle input on a given day.

The goals of the beginning or **orientation phase** of a therapeutic relationship include assessment, structuring the relationship and therapy contract, and establishing rapport, while developing insight and changing behavior is reserved for the **working phase** of the relationship, when the patient feels more comfortable and the therapist has a better understanding of the patient. Later, during the **termination phase,** the nurse avoids introducing new problems that time does not permit the nurse and patient to work through adequately. (See Table 7–1.)

Similar principles apply in each individual therapy session. It helps if the nurse "warms up" (for example, "How have you been since we last talked?") and "winds down" (for example, "This sounds important. Could we focus on it tomorrow when we have more time?"), with enough time in the middle to do justice to the problem at hand.

A patient's readiness for therapy or for progressing in the work of therapy varies, and it does not progress steadily or remain stable just because the therapist has completed the initial assessment. Following a session that the therapist views as beneficial, or even a "breakthrough experience," it is not unusual for the patient to retreat—avoid the nurse, put up distance maneuvers, or in other ways regress to the orientation phase, so that the nurse feels they must start all over again. The patient must be reassured (sometimes over and over again) that the nurse has the ability to help him, will not push him beyond the limits of his tolerance, and asks him to do what is difficult only because it is in his own best interest to do so.

A therapist may be accurate in her interpretation of a situation but wrong in sharing it with the patient before he is ready to hear it. Premature interpretations heighten anxiety and resistance, possibly eliciting silence, anger, denial, or panic from the patient. Asking the patient to give up his defenses while he still needs them has been described as destructive or harmful to the patient (Mellow, 1968), a cruel imposition (Wallace, 1983) that is risky, viciously irresponsible, and futile or therapeutically useless (Mullahy, 1973). Sullivan recommended that when in doubt about a particular intervention, the therapist should refrain from using it, as themes that are important to the patient will be repeated and can be dealt with later (Mullahy, 1973).

THE NURSE'S ROLE IN THERAPY

Just as each patient is different, so each nurse is different; and nowhere are patients more perceptive of and sensitive to these differences than in the psychiatric nurse-patient relationship. It is not always easy to determine whether a patient's response to his therapist is due to transference (and should be worked through on that basis) or to the particular attitudes, actions, and methods of the therapist (see "Automatic Reactions"). Given the brevity of treatment today, the nurse therapist needs to move through any impediments as quickly as possible.

Each person's interactional style is different and will require greater modification for some patients than for others (for example, a nurse who overwhelms one patient may be very effective with another). Due to their own background, values, and experiences, some nurses are more comfortable with certain content than others. For example, one student selected a patient but considered dropping him when she learned that he had a history of child molestation. With support, she continued working with him and focused on preparing him for an impending jail sentence, a subject that she was more comfortable discussing and with which she was very effective with this patient. Nurses and other professionals on the treatment team who were more comfortable discussing sexual abuse talked with him about this major problem.

It is appropriate, then, for the nurse to consider her own strengths and limitations as well as the patient's needs, in determining the nature and depth of therapy. Qualifications and personal characteristics that facilitate the nurse's role in therapy are discussed in the following section.

WHAT MAKES A NURSE EFFECTIVE IN THERAPY

What makes a nurse an effective therapist? Regardless of the level at which she is functioning, the nurse's education, experience, and personal qualities all contribute to her effectiveness in the patient's therapy.

NURSING EDUCATION AND EXPERIENCE

KNOWLEDGE AND SKILL. Knowledge of the content taught in psychiatric mental health nursing education programs is vital to the nurse's functions as a therapist, as are the opportunities for its application in the clinical setting and the development of competencies and skills. (See "Levels of Application" pages 167–170.)

The task of differentiating the levels at which psychiatric mental health nursing theory and principles may be applied and describing the knowledge and skill needed for each level is made more difficult by the problems which the profession of nursing has experienced in differentiating levels of competency and practice in relation to formal education degrees, titling, and licensure. Since each individual nursing education program is allowed considerable freedom in developing its own curriculum and standards, the content and quality of learning experiences in psychiatric mental health nursing vary, even among institutions offering the same degree and accreditation status. Graduates of any particular program also have individual interests, abilities, and learning goals, resulting in considerable variance in performance in a specialty area such as psychiatric mental health nursing.

This lack of standardization in our product results in a reluctance to equate particular degrees in nursing with the levels of application described in this chapter. For example, graduate study is recommended for the primary therapist, but a recent study indicated that only forty percent of nurse psychotherapists felt that their graduate programs prepared them for their role. Although many of these practitioners reported that their programs provided a good foundation, continued supervision was regarded as essential, supplemented by continuing education (Hardin & Durham, 1985). Certainly this is understandable and does not imply that graduate programs failed to fulfill their mission; however, it illustrates the difficulty in attempting to equate formal degrees with levels of functioning in psychiatric mental health nursing, or in failing to recognize that routes other than formal education (good supervision and continuing education over a long period of time) can assist in promoting these competencies.

In addition to the psychiatric nursing content and skills that are directly related to practice, there are also certain general characteristics of nursing education and experience that facilitate the nurse's role in therapy. These include extensive patient contact and the nursing perspective.

EXTENSIVE PATIENT CONTACT. Among all members of the treatment team, the nurse usually has the most contact with the patient (Committee on Psychiatric Nursing, 1982; Lewis, 1982). Staff nurses' observations of patients extend around the clock, seven days a week, in a variety of situations. Nursing personnel have been described as living with their patients (Fagin, 1967). Observant nurses note patterns, reactions to specific stimuli, social deficits, and recurrent themes in conversation and behavior, then synthesize this data in a way that really clarifies the patient's problems and needs.

THE NURSING PERSPECTIVE

The Holistic Approach. Nurses are taught a **holistic approach**—an appreciation of the "whole person" interacting with his environment. The nurse's ability to perceive patients in a holistic manner (Lego, 1973) and to care for both their physical and emotional needs is extremely helpful to them (Fagin, 1967). For example, one new psychiatric nurse observed an experienced therapist telling a patient who was undergoing a myocardial infarction to stop hyperventilating and trying to manipulate her to get another dose of Ativan (lorazepam). The same nurse saw patients with metastatic cancer, electrolyte imbalance, an allergic reaction, and a learning disability, each misdiagnosed as functionally psychotic. In every case, she did not know what was wrong, but realized that the patient was "different." Such "nursing instincts" are actually derived from a knowledge of pathophysiology and psychopathology, which helps the nurse to differentiate functional from organic disorders. Nurses are not medical diagnosticians; rather, they take a holistic approach, checking the patient's diet, vital signs, and physical health along with his psychosocial needs.

An Eclectic Approach. In recent years, nursing and psychiatric nursing have resolved that a component of knowledge basic to nursing practice is also a common or generic knowledge that is shared by and with numerous other disciplines (such as psychiatry, biology, and anthropology). The challenge to nurses, then, is how to take this body of common knowledge and transform it so that it addresses the theoretical and practical aspects of psychiatric mental health nursing (Critchley, 1985).

For example, the biological-medical model advances numerous assumptions about behavior and treatment. The model has some distinct and highly useful features. For one, it provides a framework for the conceptualization of biological treatments such as psychopharmacology and other somatic treatments, e.g. electric shock. The nurse must be conversant with this model so that she can bridge the gap that is likely to exist between physicians, patients, and numerous other nonmedical colleagues (Critchley, 1985).

Yet just as important is the nurse's awareness of the limitations of the biological-medical model; she must use her knowledge about holistic health care to assess, treat, and evaluate the physical, social, and mental needs of patients and their families (Critchley, 1985).

A major limitation of this model is its potential for forestalling the "autonomy and accountability of the behavior of those individuals who interact with the physician as patients or colleagues" (Critchley, p. 20). This limitation can be overcome and "psychiatric nursing practice can be strengthened if nurses clearly understand that theories borrowed from other disciplines must be assessed, evaluated, and reformulated so that they are logically consistent with nursing theory and practice" (Critchley, p. 20).

Whether she is a primary therapist or a basic therapist, the psychiatric nurse is familiar with and competent in practicing at least one theoretical mode of therapy. Sometimes an experienced professional will follow *only* one theory and practice its methods to the extent that she becomes more committed to that particular mode of therapy than she is to her patient. If the patient fails to respond to this mode of therapy, the therapist may dismiss the failure with such comments as, "I really do believe that this therapy is correct"; or "the literature indicates that certain patients do not respond to this approach," rather than asking "might another approach be beneficial to this patient?" To be effective, therapy requires a certain flexibility, as all patients simply do not respond well to a single approach. So, the nurse therapist adopts an **eclectic approach** if she is not already responding to her patient's needs.

Since nurses do not prescribe medication and cannot admit patients to the hospital without being associated with a physician who has admitting privileges, nurses have, of necessity, developed verbal skills to manage patients' behavior, and have learned to experiment with modern, alternative modes of treatment that they can use more independently.

Nurses have become active in the "wellness" movement, with its emphasis on the prevention of illness and the accompanying opportunities for expanding the nurse's role to assist the patient throughout the wellness/illness continuum rather than just during the acute phase during which he is hospitalized (Colliton, 1971). Now nurses in many wellness centers, as well as those in private practice, can capitalize on this trend to provide a stable relationship and point of reference for the patient—to be the one person who knows that patient thoroughly, and whom he trusts, who is willing to help him explore and evaluate various treatment options (either directly or in conjunction with referral resources), and to whom he can always return. (See Figure 7–1.)

Whether the nurse has the opportunity to develop stable relationships can depend upon the nursing model used within a given institution or agency. For example, if primary nursing is employed, the nurse is likely to have an opportunity to provide continuity of care to patients and family in a variety of settings. If, on the other hand, the team approach is used, she will probably have less opportunity for continuous contact with patients because of the shifts in assignments and her other priorities.

In recent years, nurses have assumed the role of case manager, providing a continuing resourse to patients as they move through the mental health system and the community. (See Figure 7–1.) The American

Nurses' Association (1988) has described the concept of case management as a "system of health assessment, planning, service procurement, delivery, coordination, and monitoring through which multiple service needs of patients are met" (p. 1). The population thought to benefit most from this system are high risk patients with complex health care problems. Chapter 10, "Schizophrenia" provides an in-depth discussion of case management in psychiatric mental health care.

A Nurturing Role. Nursing education emphasizes caring, communication, and the family, community, and psychosocial aspects of patient care. Physicians focus on diagnosis and treatment; psychologists study etiology, and perform testing and research; social workers deal primarily with families, social histories, and agency referrals. The nurse, on the other hand, maintains close contact with the patient. Nurturing functions are an established aspect of the nurse's role and a vital part of her success with therapy. (See the sections on "Therapeutic Roles" and

FIGURE 7–1 Core Components of Case Management

Source: *Case Management: A Challenge for Nurses,* Draft Document. The American Nurses Association, February 24, 1988.

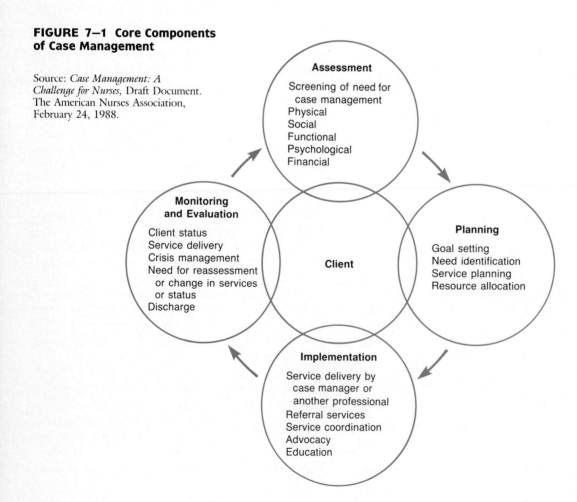

"Nurturing Parent.") The need for nurturance has been recognized as important in motivating patients to seek treatment (Burgess & Burns, 1973) and to remain in therapy (Nicholi, 1988).

PERSONAL CHARACTERISTICS

The teaching-learning process can make every nurse a more effective therapist, but each nurse also brings to the experience various personal qualities, habits, skills, and patterns of interaction that affect the process. Personality and character traits of the individual have generally been recognized as legitimate considerations in educating and selecting therapists or psychiatric personnel (Chapman, 1983; Redmond, 1982; Peplau, 1982b).

> I am as concerned with fostering a set of attitudes as with disseminating a body of knowledge and procedures. The former is the matrix in which the latter must occur if it is to be effective . . . . The relationship is the most important . . . whatever the school. The power of the relationship is carried . . . above all, by your personal characteristics. (Wallace, 1983, pp. 231, 235)

The personal characteristics of nurses considered to be effective in therapy are: genuine concern and caring; an analytical mind; a therapeutic use of self; and an awareness and acceptance of oneself and others.

GENUINE CONCERN AND CARING. Patients have a strong ability to read nonverbal messages—they know who really cares about them and who does not. If a nurse demonstrates genuine caring, a patient will forgive her for a multitude of mistakes. The caring nurse does not really need to be afraid that she will "say the wrong thing" or be "unprofessional." By the time nursing students complete their basic courses and their orientation to psychiatric nursing, most have incorporated enough healthy respect for professional behavior and potential problems with patients into their demeanor to prevent erring too far in this regard. This is especially true with extensive clinical experience and the close supervision provided by most nursing education programs.

The nurse demonstrates genuine concern and caring when she makes eye contact with the patient (unless it is contradicted by extreme paranoia or a cultural taboo in a particular patient); listens attentively to the patient; and follows up on concerns expressed in prior contacts with the patient.

Empathy. Empathy has been defined as the ability to put oneself in another person's shoes, to feel one's

way into his psyche (Wallace, 1983). The nurse may tell the patient she is sorry he is feeling so much pain or say that she cares. If the nurse finds that she *doesn't* feel empathy toward the patient, this should be explored in supervision. If a nurse consistently experiences difficulty in empathizing with patients, she may be happier and more successful in another role. Wallace (1983) states that if empathy is present, the patient will know it and be better for it, but if it is not, he will know that, too, and the therapy will be useless (Wallace, 1983). Mansfield (1973) correlated high levels of empathy with patient improvement and low levels with increased disturbance. The nurse's caring is the vehicle with which the patient learns to tolerate the therapy process—the pain, tears, and fears—all of which are accepted only to the extent that the patient trusts the nurse and believes that the therapy is designed for his ultimate welfare.

In therapy, the nurse's relationship with the patient must be strong enough to sustain the patient's confrontation with truth. Confronting unpleasant truths about oneself in therapy is always difficult and anxiety producing, and the patient's bond with the primary therapist—and his basic trust in the nurse and the support she offers—is the glue that keeps the therapy and the patient intact.

A nurse may experience problems in overidentification with her patient: she may have difficulty separating her own feelings from those of the patient; she may have "rescue fantasies," in which she loses perspective and increases a desire to cure the patient quickly (Mellow, 1968). However, Mellow (1968)

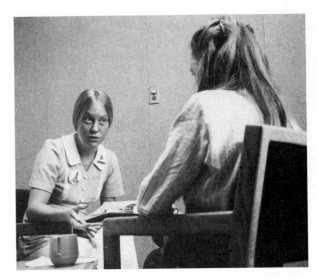

The nurse-therapist maintains eye contact with the patient to demonstrate genuine concern and caring. But first, she must determine if this action is culturally appropriate.

also speaks positively about the fact that a patient "stirs up within you the conviction that something of worth within him is going to waste before your eyes" (p. 2365). Good supervision will assist the nurse in differentiating overinvolvement from the genuine concern and caring that is so vital to therapy. The nurse's own psychotherapy may also be helpful (see p. 187).

Commitment. Although the caring nurse is usually a committed nurse, the inexperienced therapist or student nurse may fail to appreciate the responsibilities of her role (Mellow, 1968). When the nurse therapist selects a patient, she commits herself to that patient and accepts responsibility for her work and the obligation to complete it (Finkelman, 1975; Peplau, 1982b). It is not unusual for a patient to remember a particular student nurse and express disappointment when she is absent, although the student may think that her contact with the patient was too brief and uninformed to be significant.

AN ANALYTICAL MIND. To be effective in working with patients, especially those who are mentally ill, the nurse must develop a talent for "psychological mindedness," which includes the ability to spot themes, patterns, and parallels, and make connections (Wallace, 1983). The one attitude common to all therapists is the consistent attempt to understand what patients are communicating (Wallace, 1983). To be effective in therapy, the nurse must always wonder what the patient meant, why he did something, how it connects with other experiences, what he's really thinking.

The therapist always reexamines the data about her patient; she also thinks analytically "on her feet." Observing and interpreting is basic to the nurse's role (Gregg, 1982). Nightingale stated, "A conscientious nurse is not necessarily an observing nurse, but life or death may lie with the good observer" (Crawford, 1982, p. 3). Some years later Crawford (1982) wrote, "With what emphasis we teach this principle to the psychiatric nurse! She must be trained to the keenest observation of her patient . . ." (p. 3).

THERAPEUTIC USE OF SELF. The phrase **therapeutic use of self** (Committee on Psychiatric Nursing, 1982a) refers to the fact that the nurse uses herself—all her own resources—in a therapeutic relationship with her patient. In the process of therapy, the nurse is her own instrument: there are few

procedures, and the importance of everything the nurse says and does is heightened. This concept includes dress, nonverbal behavior or body language, personal mannerisms, vocal tone, inflection and rate of flow, as well as choice of words. The nurse therapist strives to be flexible, shockproof, and "unflappable." She is in control of her verbal/nonverbal behavior, responding therapeutically to the patient with serene acceptance of most situations (Wallace, 1983). Anticipating problems, planning approaches, and knowing (or establishing) policies for how things should be handled helps, as does experience.

AWARENESS AND ACCEPTANCE OF SELF AND OTHERS. Self-awareness is a key component in psychiatric mental health nursing (Krikorian & Paulanka, 1982). Self-acceptance requires self-awareness—of how the nurse comes across, how others perceive her, why she feels the way she does. The nurse makes efforts at self-improvement, but she also has a basic acceptance of herself. In turn, she accepts the patient as he is at the time of therapy; this is paramount to helping him, even helping him change. Accepting the limitations of doctors and staff helps also, for as Sullivan (1953) says, "We are all much more simply human than otherwise" (p. 32).

An open mind, a sense of humor, and a willingness to make some mistakes is helpful. The beginning nurse therapist may be relieved to discover that she is not alone in the difficulties she experiences with a certain type of patient; many specific behaviors in patients elicit predictable responses from other people. For example, patients who are unpleasant, long-term, hypochondriacal, or mentally ill were identified in one study as generally unpopular with nurses (Nelson, 1973). Knowing some of these pitfalls, or receiving validation that others have experienced similar problems, may encourage the beginning nurse therapist. The nurse therapist develops her skills through feedback—from patients, peers, instructors, supervisors, and consultants. The more open the nurse is in sharing her feelings and problems in working with patients, the more help she can receive. The nurse who is willing to present her patient in a group conference, participate in role play, videotape a session for supervision, or try an unfamiliar approach to therapy will learn from these experiences. If, on the other hand, the nurse is too defensive about her actions with patients and cannot accept suggestions from others, her growth as a nurse may be blocked.

Those who offer feedback to the nurse therapist must remember that her identification with her interactions with patients and her role as a therapist are much more closely related to her sense of self than are other, more technical, interventions. For example, a supervisor who corrects a nurse's aseptic technique is not likely to expect any repercussion from the nurse; but a supervisor who suggests that a nurse rephrase a comment or reexamine her motives for selecting a particular patient may elicit a defensive response from the nurse. The nurse may feel that her supervisor has made a personal attack. Despite this, feedback does help increase the nurse's self-awareness, enhancing her professional growth (Committee on Psychiatric Nursing, 1982a).

Supervision vs. Therapy. What is the difference between therapy and supervision? When is the supervisor "doing therapy" with the nurse rather than offering appropriate supervision? The supervisor is to be a teacher, not a therapist. The goal of supervision is the nurse's professional growth, not personal growth (Platt-Koch, 1986; Feather & Bissell, 1979; Gregg, Bregg, and Spring, 1976).

Although supervision and therapy are both learning processes that promote self-awareness, the difference in their basic purpose suggests that the supervisor focus on the nurse in relation to her nurse-patient interaction. The nurse shares her experiences and attitudes pertaining to her professional role, and the supervisor assists her in identifying and working through problems in order to develop new insights and skills for use in the therapeutic relationship (Lewis, 1982). The supervisor does not expect the nurse to make personal revelations unless they relate to this process; and she should avoid probing deeply into the nurse's personal conflicts unless they clearly interfere with the patient's therapy (Platt-Koch, 1986). For example, if a nurse is abrupt with a patient, the supervisor will discuss it with her; but if the nurse is overheard being abrupt with a friend in the cafeteria, the supervisor will not. If a student reveals that she was sexually abused by her father, she might be referred to appropriate counseling services. However, if she has selected a patient who reminds her of her father and is having difficulty relating to him therapeutically, it becomes an issue for supervision.

Since the patient-therapist relationship differs in intent and focus from a teaching-learning relationship, it is ill-advised to combine or blur these roles. Some potential problems include role confusion, transference/countertransference, carryover into group situations, and questionable objectivity in the supervision and evaluation process. For example, a supervisor who knows the nurse therapist's biases and history too well may look for problems that do not exist, or do not interfere with therapy; or the supervisor may become overprotective of the therapist.

No one is perfect; but if the nurse's bias or pathology interferes with the patient's therapy, it becomes the responsibility of the supervisor to intervene, either by assisting the nurse directly in dealing with those aspects of the problem that are impacting her role in therapy, or by referring the nurse for therapy. When a nurse's needs are not being met, they require attention (Lewis, 1982). If the nurse enters therapy, she can expect the focus to shift from the needs of the patient to her own needs and personal growth. Certainly, it is not usually necessary for students to experience intensive introspection or to undergo psychotherapy to learn to be therapeutic with patients. In fact, focusing heavily on the student may provoke anxiety at a level which actually interferes with the learning process.

When a primary therapist conducts intensive therapy over the years, she needs to be aware of her own mental health—thinking processes, values, motives, biases, patterns of interaction, and coping. Good therapists continue to seek and utilize regular supervision and usually involve themselves in growth groups, experiential learning situations, and continuing education. Some also choose to seek therapy as a means of personal development or assistance with personal conflicts and problems. Some nurses are able to function in the alternate roles of therapist and patient appropriately, while others become "drained" and prefer to drop out of work while in therapy, at least until they are able to function as a healthy role model and devote their full energy and attention to the patient's needs.

Nursing is a high-stress profession, with certain stresses specific to psychiatric nursing (Trygstad, 1986). Psychiatric nursing has generally demonstrated one of the highest burnout and attrition rates in nursing, and the number of nurses who choose this field and remain in it through their career is small in comparison to other areas (ANA, 1985). Yet it is experienced by many as the greatest challenge and reward in the nursing profession.

CHALLENGES AND CHOICES

The nurse encounters many problems in seeking to apply his/her psychiatric mental health nursing knowledge and skills. Some of these problems pertain to the development of the nurse's role in therapy, while others are clinical problems commonly experienced by all those working with psychiatric patients.

CHALLENGES IN CLINICAL PRACTICE

The nurse therapist encounters many challenges in psychiatric nursing. Some of the clinical challenges occur so frequently that they are routine. These clinical challenges are: patients' ambivalence about therapy; silence; automatic reactions; social/sexual overtures; and the use of touch, gifts, and humor.

PATIENTS' AMBIVALENCE TOWARD THERAPY. The term *ambivalence* is used here rather than the term *resistance*, because mixed or conflicting feelings regarding therapy are actually more common among patients than complete opposition to therapy. Most patients do know, on some level, that they are different or unhappy, and they wish to be understood, accepted, and self-actualized.

Some common signs of ambivalence toward therapy are:

1. Reluctance to enter therapy.

2. Problems in scheduling (for example, because therapy is not high among the patient's priorities, he is unwilling to rearrange other commitments).

3. Excessive complaints or questions about the fees and/or policies of the therapist.

4. Frequent verbalizations indicating a lack of confidence in the methods or benefits achieved by therapy, challenging or discounting the therapist or her suggestions.

5. Frequently arriving late for sessions or leaving sessions early.

6. Repeated cancellations and missed appointments.

7. Threats of termination prior to the end of the contractual arrangements.

8. Indications that the patient has entered therapy for reasons other than his own internal motivation for growth and change, such as:
   (a) Involuntary admission
   (b) Court referral, conditions of probation, and so forth
   (c) Legal purposes (for example, documentation of pain and suffering, desire to obtain the therapist's advocacy for a child custody hearing)
   (d) Insurance purposes (for example, validation of injury, damages, and so on)
   (e) Pressure from others (for example, employer, school system, parents, spouse)
   (f) Preoccupation with obtaining medication.

9. Minimal participation or consistent efforts to control the session. (Although these phenomena appear to be opposites, they may both be maneuvers to minimize personal involvement in the therapy process by, for example, answering questions briefly without volunteering information, avoiding eye contact, trying to maintain conversation on a superficial level, joking, flirting, or focusing away from his own personal feelings and problems.)

10. Marked increase in anxiety in response to a particular topic or action of the therapist.

11. Noncompliance in any area of treatment (for example, not following up on an agreement or "homework assignment").

The nurse can address and help decrease a patient's ambivalence toward therapy in the following ways:

1. The nurse can acknowledge the patient's ambivalence and bring it out in the open.

2. The nurse can accept the patient's ambivalence and interpret it to the patient as normal and understandable. The nurse may then take the patient off the defensive by letting him know that this is a common hurdle and that it does not mean he is a bad or undesirable patient. Unconsciously, a therapist may have set the tone by encouraging the patient to pretend to be something he is not (what the therapist wants him to be) and so set the stage for him to be dishonest or less than open, or to mask his true feelings, which is not a good basis for therapy. If, instead, she acknowledges that there is a natural fear or anxiety in the sharing of feelings, she will, in fact, help reduce the patient's anxiety.

3. The nurse can explore with the patient his attitudes toward therapy, his feelings about the pressures that brought him into therapy, and his fears regarding what may happen in therapy. The nurse corrects any misconceptions the patient has about therapy and validates the patient's accurate perceptions about therapy.

4. The nurse can explain that everyone can grow, become happier, and be more fulfilled—that he does not have to be "mentally ill" to benefit from therapy. The nurse emphasizes any strengths the patient has and shows him how they may help him in the therapy process.

5. The nurse can ask the patient about his own goals in life. What would he like to achieve? What makes him happy? How would he change his life?

6. The nurse can talk with the patient about what she feels she can offer him. The nurse tries to use the

same terms that the patient has used, making a connection with his stated goals whenever possible. If the patient expresses no motives other than, "I just want to get everybody off my case," or "I wish my wife would be more sexy," the nurse may honestly say, "I think I may be able to help you with that, if you will work with me." This is a true statement; therapy includes heightened awareness of the consequences of behavior, how others react to one, and how one manages to meet one's own needs in ways that produce the most satisfaction. The nurse therapist deals with the patient at his current level of functioning, while trying to help him progress toward a more responsible and mature level of thinking.

7. The nurse can stress the concept of mutuality in the therapy process. It is the patient's prerogative as a consumer to participate actively in decisions regarding his care and to accept, modify, or refuse a particular treatment (Burgess & Burns, 1973; Feather, 1985; Oriol & Oriol, 1986).

The nurse may ask the patient what he would like to be different about his life as a result of the therapy. She allows the patient to negotiate the goals and conditions of therapy, to understand that he can let the nurse know when he is not ready to talk about something, to answer a particular question, or to try a particular technique. This may appear to be a compromise, but it is necessary to establish or maintain an operable level of trust and comfort in the therapy. The nurse may begin by asking, "Do you think you could tell me if you were uncomfortable with a question or suggestion I might offer?" If the patient says, "No," or "I don't know," or "I'm not sure," the nurse can begin to work here in order to help the patient build his trust in her and in the process of therapy itself. If the patient agrees to let the nurse know when he is feeling uncomfortable, he will be more relaxed. Knowing he has some control of the situation, he may never actually exercise this privilege at all. However, if the patient does signal to the nurse therapist that he feels uncomfortable, the nurse may then offer him extra support until he feels ready to continue.

8. The nurse can establish immediately some sort of contract. If possible, the nurse establishes a contract for a reasonable goal and time frame in which to accomplish the work of therapy. If this seems too much to ask of this patient at this time, the nurse may focus on short-term goals, or simply ask him to agree to return, even for one or two sessions, at which time they can reevaluate the situation.

9. The nurse can respond to the patient's presenting problem. It is often advisable to defer a lengthy his-tory and assessment in order to move directly to the area that has prompted the patient to seek treatment. Patients rarely feel that they are receiving any immediate benefits from "answering a lot of questions" and need to experience the relief and hope that accompany a discussion of the presenting problem on some level, even though the therapist will need to return to a more thorough treatment of the issue throughout the therapy process. Bellak (1979) recommends that the initial contact should create hope based on an understanding of the problem and what can be accomplished in brief therapy. Wallace (1983) describes the restoration of hope as *informed* hope that does not minimize the problem or the struggle that lies ahead, but conveys that, if the patient will work with the therapist, it will be possible for him to recover.

10. The nurse can utilize alternative roles and/or approaches to therapy. If resistance continues, the nurse may have better success by temporarily employing roles other than that of counselor, such as socializing agent. Some patients "open up" more easily while taking a walk or after playing a game of ping-pong. Others are more comfortable sharing feelings with their peers through group therapy, or through indirect methods of self-disclosure, such as art, music, occupational therapy, or psychodrama. Later, they may explain verbally what they were trying to express in other ways.

SILENCE. One of the greatest fears of the beginning therapist is that her patients will not talk to her. Even when a student selects her own patient (often because the patient does talk, initially), it is not unusual for the patient to withdraw and become silent. Silence usually indicates resistance to therapy. The nurse can address and deal with this issue in the following ways:

1. The nurse can accept the patient's silence and sit quietly with him until the session is over; this may be necessary with a very regressed patient.

2. The nurse can tell the patient that she will be available in a specified place whenever he is ready to talk, and allow him to approach her in his own time if he so desires. By dealing more actively with the patient's silence in this way, the nurse may reduce the tension between the patient and herself (Floyd, 1973).

3. The nurse can suggest less threatening activities until the patient becomes more comfortable (for example, playing a game, taking a walk, listening to music, or looking at a magazine).

4. The nurse can empathize with the patient. For example, the nurse might say, "It's hard to talk, isn't it? Do you feel that I don't understand you? I want to understand, if you will try to tell me."

5. The nurse can question and/or comment on observations of nonverbal behavior. For example:

> "You seem to be saying that you don't want to talk."
>
> "Is that a hard question to answer?"
>
> "You look angry (frightened, bored, or sad)."
>
> "Can you tell me what you are thinking about, right now?"

6. The nurse can move slowly to the patient's eye level and say his name. In cases where it is not contraindicated, the nurse may try touching the patient's arm or shoulder gently, asking a simple question to break the silence. If there is no response, the nurse may try asking simple questions that require only a yes or no answer; if she eventually elicits some response, she may progress to more open-ended questions. If she does not get a response to the yes-or-no questions, she may simply make nonthreatening comments to the patient about the environment—such as the weather, or his surroundings—thus making no demands for a response. This helps keep the interaction alive (Mellow, 1968).

AUTOMATIC REACTIONS. A person's response to and interactions with others are influenced by **automatic reactions**, which are reactions based on previous experience.

Transference/Countertransference. Transference/countertransference is a concept derived from the psychoanalytical model. **Transference** refers to the tendency of patients to displace feelings from past experiences and relationships onto current ones (Schroder, 1985). This is especially true when the person the patient must now deal with is an authority figure and/or has some features similar to a significant person in the past (Nicholi, 1988). For example, a patient might be inappropriately hostile to a particular nurse because the nurse reminds him of his mother (that is, he transfers his strong anger toward his mother to the nurse and expects her to behave toward him as his mother did).

Countertransference refers to the response that the nurse then makes to the patient's transference, which involves attitudes and feelings from the nurse's own past history (Schroder, 1985). If the nurse does not know the source of the patient's feelings toward her, she may begin to manifest countertransference reactions, such as demonstrating bias toward the patient, preoccupation with the patient, sexual or aggressive fantasies, anxiety, guilt, embarrassment, or withdrawal (Johnson, 1967; Vidoni, 1975; Schroder, 1985).

The nurse may want to ask the patient any of the following questions to help her differentiate transference from the need for alternative approaches to the patient:

> "Do I remind you of anyone? What was that person like? In what way do you see me as similar? How am I different? What is different about our relationship?"
>
> "When was the last time you felt this way?"
>
> "What did you think I would say?"
>
> "Who gave you the idea you were stupid?" (hopeless, ugly, incompetent)
>
> "Tell me about your experience with therapy. What was your last therapist like?"

Transference/countertransference can be positive or negative; it usually operates on an unconscious level to some extent in all nurse-patient relationships, especially in long-term, intensive therapy (Hall, 1977; McCann, 1979). The nurse's supervisor can provide valuable assistance in recognizing and dealing with transference/countertransference.

The I-P Reflex. The **I-P reflex** or interpersonal reflex, is based on the idea that people generally react automatically and predictably to specific stimuli, as in a knee-jerk reflex. For example, if one person smiles and greets another person, the second person usually returns the greeting; by the same token, when a person is criticized, his most natural and spontaneous reaction is to become angry or defensive. Patients develop patterns of behavior that elicit predictable responses from other people and thus confirm their view of themselves (Leary, 1957). Even though these responses may be negative, familiar patterns of behavior are less anxiety producing to the patient than learning new ways of relating and changing their behavior (Johnson & Miller, 1967).

This interpersonal concept of reciprocity places a dual responsibility on the nurse: 1) she must examine her own actions to determine her role in eliciting a particular reaction from a patient, rather than merely attributing it to the patient's past; and 2) she must consciously control her own reactions to the patient's behavior in order to avoid reinforcing maladaptive patterns with a predictable, reflexive response (Johnson & Miller, 1967).

A nurse can identify the operation of an I-P reflex by observing and analyzing patterns in her interaction with her patient. She may also notice how the patient responds to other, similar situations and ask him, "What set you off?—What did you expect to happen when you behaved that way?—What usually happens right beforehand?" The nurse also uses her own feelings and those of her peers diagnostically. She may ask other nurses, "How do you feel toward this patient?" When one or more nurses acknowledge honestly that the patient has elicited a reaction from them that is nontherapeutic, the nurses can examine what the patient did to trigger this response. For example, a patient who is very perceptive and manipulative may focus on each nurse's particular weakness or vulnerability, making everyone feel uncomfortable. Variations of this concept have led to the identification and naming of certain patterns frequently observed in therapy as "games people play" (Berne, 1972).

SOCIAL/SEXUAL OVERTURES. The role confusion that appears to occur most frequently and seems to be the most difficult for the beginning therapist to handle is the "I-want-you-to-be-my-girlfriend" that the patient often directs at the nurse. The nurse therapist can deal with this in the following ways:

1. The nurse can realize that social or sexual overtures by the patient do not necessarily indicate that the nurse has done something wrong. The beginning nurse may believe she has unknowingly elicited an overture from the patient and lose her composure; this may compound the problem. (For example, the patient may think, "When she started blushing and stammering, I knew I was right—she's crazy about me.") A patient who is mentally ill usually has few close relationships. Few people in this patient's life consistently care about him or demonstrate the amount of interest in him shown by the nurse (Wallace, 1983). So, romantic feelings may develop in the patient, even when the nurse has done everything correctly (she has clarified roles, presented in professional demeanor, and so forth). A homosexual advance by a patient does not necessarily indicate that the nurse is also homosexual, nor does an advance by an attractive patient indicate that the nurse feels mutually attracted or has encouraged the advance in any way.

The nurse's own degree of comfort and skill in dealing with this situation *is* an important determinant in how the patient will ultimately feel about himself, his sexuality, and his relationship with the nurse. If the nurse is uncomfortable with her own sexuality, or is, in fact, attracted to the patient, she may have difficulty in dealing with an overture from the patient. If she reacts with embarrassment or anger, the patient may conclude that his sexual feelings are in general unacceptable, and that it would be inappropriate for him to talk about them in therapy. If the nurse therapist can anticipate these overtures and deal with them comfortably, without anger or embarrassment, and without humiliating the patient, their relationship will continue to be therapeutic.

2. The nurse can accept the patient's sexual desire as a normal, healthy phenomenon that can be used therapeutically, for example, to help the patient to learn appropriate and inappropriate sexual objects, approaches, and outlets; to initiate discussion about the patient's previous social/sexual history, attitudes, and feelings; and to motivate the patient to develop relationships and social skills. The nurse might say to the patient, "You are a young, healthy man. It is natural that you are preoccupied with these thoughts at times. Do you have a girlfriend? Would you like to have a girlfriend? Do you ever talk to any of the female patients here?"

3. The nurse can clarify roles by restating her role and purpose for meeting with the patient. If the patient is quite ill, blurring of roles and ego boundaries is not unusual. If the patient is testing the limits of the relationship by attempting to flirt with the nurse or manipulate her, the nurse sets specific limits for behavior, along with consequences for violating them. In the latter case, the nurse also tells the patient that she is uncomfortable with his behavior and finds it unacceptable. She may also discuss with the patient whether or not his behavior would be acceptable in a social setting or intimate relationship. The nurse may make the following comments in clarifying roles: "I do care about you, but I am your nurse, not your girlfriend. A girlfriend is different, and I'm glad you are thinking about that. We can talk about that again later. But you also need someone you can be honest with (and not have to worry about being the boyfriend), someone who knows more about your problems and how to help you. That is what I am here to do."

4. The nurse can reassure the patient. Even a patient who appears to be arrogant may feel embarrassed that he has been "turned down," and a shy patient who has developed a genuine "crush" on the therapist may feel humiliated. The therapist then exercises special precautions to protect the patient's self-esteem and to reassure him that the relationship will continue. For example, she may say, "No, you aren't stupid to think that anyone could ever want to go out with you, but I am your nurse. Certainly, I will be back tomorrow to continue our talks."

Often a patient is actually relieved to be "off the hook," and may have been extremely threatened if the nurse had accepted his advances; yet, he is still aware that a boundary has been crossed and may worry that this relationship, which is so significant to him at this time, has been ruined.

Less frequently, a nurse may be attracted to a patient. She should acknowledge and discuss these feeling with her supervisor, not the patient; this will only burden the patient. The nurse-patient relationship is designed to focus on the needs of the patient rather than the nurse. Unfortunately, in some cases therapists have initiated detailed discussions of their patients' sexual fantasies and experiences beyond what was appropriate; and this becomes part of a seduction of the patient. Some therapists have even engaged in sexual relationships with their patients. This is a form of exploitation and abuse that is condemned by professional organizations and has been classified as a felony in many states. Sullivan warns that there is no telling how much damage has been done by the small minority of so-called therapists who act out sexually with their patients (Mullahy, 1973). Possible negative effects include reinforcing the patient's poor impulse control, redirecting the therapy toward sexual issues, the therapist's loss of objectivity, and destruction of the respect and trust on which a therapeutic relationship is based (Nicholi, 1988). The therapist also risks damage to her professional reputation and that of her colleagues and profession, censure by her professional organization and licensing board, and legal charges by the patient, as the consent of a psychiatric patient can easily be questioned (Nicholi, 1988; Mullahy, 1973). If the therapist is unable to resolve feelings of attraction to the patient through supervision, the patient should be referred to another therapist.

In some cases, the line of demarcation between what is appropriate or therapeutic in a patient-therapist relationship and what is not is less clear. A patient and her husband may invite the nurse to a large, informal party at their home. Even though the invitation seems casual, the nurse must apply some of the same concerns she would if the patient made a more intimate overture. If the patient is in need of friends, she may overburden the relationship, extending more and more invitations. Sooner or later, the nurse will have to refuse these invitations, which will be more difficult than if she had stated at the outset that it was her policy not to see patients socially.

There are a number of reasons for these guidelines. Can the patient always tell the therapist everything when the therapist sees his wife or friends socially? Can the patient be completely relaxed in a social situation when the therapist is there observing his behavior? Can the therapist really meet her own needs when she knows how it may affect the patient? Is the therapist as free to say "no" to this patient when he calls in what he regards as a crisis, but the therapist does not? The patient-therapist relationship is not a social relationship, and both parties need the freedom of a mutual, reciprocal relationship of equality to meet other types of needs.

TOUCH. In the past, nurses were taught never to touch psychiatric patients, and to be very careful in using touch with other patients, unless it was a part of physical care. For example, backrubs were rarely given on psychiatric units, even if the patient was bedridden. These policies developed because of problems (some legal) experienced with the use of touch, including violent reactions and accusations of child abuse or sexual exploitation of patients. Touch is an ambiguous communication that can be easily misinterpreted and raise anxiety, especially by a patient who tends to distort data or fantasize about the intent of the nurse (for example, that she is grabbing him aggressively or making an intimate or sexual gesture) (DeAugustinis, 1963; Jourard & Rubin, 1968).

Psychiatric patients—especially schizophrenics—can be very territorial and threatened by invasion of their personal space, even if physical proximity does not actually result in touch (Parks, 1966; Roberts, 1969). However, research has not always demonstrated a significant increase in anxiety as a result of invasion of personal space by the nurse (Ricci, 1981), and the taboos on touching have been challenged as the benefits of touch as a part of therapy are explored (Barnett, 1972; DeThomaso, 1971). Psychiatric patients have responded well to being able to touch pets. The number of elderly patients and young children admitted to psychiatric units has further weakened the taboo in touching. As nurses began touching these patients, other patients also reached out for physical contact, particularly depressed patients, but also some who were anxious, dependent, or even psychotic. For example, one young woman who screamed in terror during her hallucinations was able to sit quietly during these experiences when allowed to hold onto her nurse's arms.

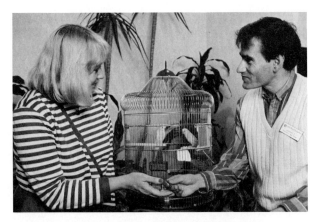

Pet therapy has helped many psychiatric patients to overcome their fear of touch. (Kasmarik & Lester, 1984)

The "seemingly simple matter of when to touch a patient and when to refrain is important, and requires precise professional judgment" (Maloney, 1982 p. 147). "Touch is an integral part of nursing intervention and is to be used judiciously between nurse and patient . . . a vital part of communication" (Barnett, 1972, p. 109). Response to touch is both an individual and cultural phenomenon. How, then, does the nurse exercise good judgment?

1. The nurse observes who initiates the touch—does she initiate it herself or does the patient? If the patient initiates touch, it is safe for the nurse to assume that he is obviously seeking it. In this case, the nurse is concerned primarily with whether touch will be appropriate and therapeutic for the patient, and whether she herself is comfortable with touch. If the nurse fears legal entrapment, sexual connotations, or undue dependency on the part of the patient, these issues should be explored in supervision. If the nurse feels that touch will be therapeutic for the patient, but she is not comfortable with touch herself, the patient will sense this discomfort. In this case, the nurse may explain to the patient that she does not practice touch in therapy so that the patient does not misinterpret her discomfort as a personal rejection. The nurse may then find other ways to demonstrate concern and reassure the patient (she may want to explore this in supervision). If she initiates touch, she assumes a greater responsibility in the other actions described below.

2. The nurse assesses the patient's potential reaction to touch. In anticipating possible responses, the nurse is aware of the patient's history of aggression or violence, sexual expression, and tendency to distort his experiences. It has been suggested that the need for touch is greater in patients who experience loneliness (DeThomaso, 1971), isolation, sensory deprivation, altered body image, depersonalization, regression, self-concealment, low self-esteem, rejection, and fear of death (Barnett, 1972). Greater caution is indicated for patients who are very anxious, dependent, private, territorial, schizoid, or schizophrenic (Barnett, 1972; Roberts, 1969; Parks, 1966). Since the indicators both for and against the use of touch may exist in the same patient, individual assessment, observation, and judgment remain the key. Maloney (1982) recognized early that diagnosis alone was not a sufficient indicator, stating that touch would distress some schizophrenics measurably, while others needed to touch people and things to assure themselves that they really existed, to establish boundaries between their bodies and the world, or to relieve anxiety through a ritualistic pattern of touching certain things.

3. The nurse observes carefully the patient's reaction to touch. Patients who are extremely aversive to touch are often observed to overreact to accidental physical contact on the unit, such as bumping into someone, or to a routine physical examination. If no such "red flags" have alerted the nurse and she touches the patient, the patient's reaction should be observed very closely. (Nonverbal responses, especially, should be monitored, as body language is generally a more accurate indicator of true feelings than what the patient verbalizes.) The nurse takes her cue from the patient. Some patients start, step back, withdraw into their physical space, or even lash out at the nurse, in which case a quick "I'm sorry," or "I'll be more careful to respect your space," is in order. Many patients show no visible reaction, which can, in fact, be a negative reaction, and is a sign of caution to the nurse. Other patients respond immediately in a very positive manner by smiling, reaching out to take the nurse's hand, or returning the touch, seeming to feel a rapport (which is not always possible on a verbal level) through this form of communication.

4. The nurse ensures that if she uses touch, it will be appropriate in a therapeutic, professional relationship. Touch is usually less threatening, less likely to be misinterpreted, and more appropriate to the nurse-patient relationship when it is brief, light, involves an impersonal part of the body, and is offered facing the patient, preferably in the presence of others. A light touch on the arm or a brief goodbye hug across the shoulders in the dayroom, where the patient and others can see clearly, is quite different from close, sustained contact to the face, waist, or full

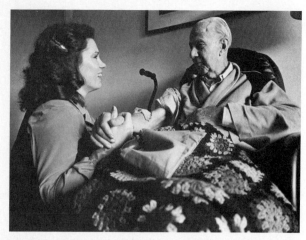

Always observe the patient's reaction (nonverbal and verbal) to touch very closely.

body, which tends to be more personal and has greater sexual connotation. Firm pressure can be painful or perceived as coercive and demanding. Other considerations, such as the stage of the nurse-patient relationship and the particular goals of the therapy, guide the nurse in her decision about whether or not to use touch. For example, the nurse is more cautious with a flirtatious patient who has not yet accepted her role as therapist than she might be after the patient has worked through some of these issues and is terminating. Clark (1984) suggests that the nurse tell a psychotic patient that she is going to touch him before doing so.

In summary, touch has the capacity for increasing or decreasing anxiety and should be used cautiously in the nurse-patient relationship.

GIFTS. Decisions regarding giving and receiving gifts frequently arise in the nurse-patient relationship. Moving cautiously from the historical rule advising against it (Peplau, 1964), nurses are encouraged to examine the motives and implications for both nurse and patient, using nursing judgment (Clancy, 1968; Gordy, 1978). The nurse considers the following questions before accepting or declining a patient's offer of a gift: Why is this patient giving me this gift? What is he trying to express? Could I help the patient to verbalize his thoughts and feelings instead? Does this patient try to "buy" friendship or special favors? Does he feel he owes me something for fulfilling my professional role? Is he afraid of being forgotten by me? Is he attempting to undo or atone for negative behavior? Does the patient have no one else to honor with this special gift? Would his offering the gift in-

stead to a visitor or relative help to foster a needed relationship? What is the general monetary value of the gift and its relationship to the assets of this patient? Is it appropriate? How does the gift affect my feelings and level of comfort with this patient, as well as my obligations to him?

The nurse also examines her own rationale for giving a gift to a patient. In doing so, she considers not only the questions above, but the following questions as well: What are the policies of the treatment setting regarding gift-giving? How will the other staff members feel if I give this patient a gift? How will the other patients feel? How will the patient who receives the gift feel? Will he feel obligated to me in some way? Will he misinterpret the gift in a personal or romantic way? Does buying this patient something really solve his problem, or would it be better to help him find a more long-term solution? Can I, instead, role play a job interview or contact a social worker about his finances? Is helping this one patient the best use of my efforts, or should I invest my energy in seeking changes in the system that would benefit all patients? What needs does this gift meet in me personally and professionally?

If the nurse and her supervisor determine that the timing and intent of gift giving are appropriate (Gordy, 1978), it can, in some circumstances, significantly enhance the nurse-patient relationship (Clancy, 1968). For example, the patient may offer the nurse something that he has made or a small gift that has special significance in terms of the therapy. Once when a patient tried to explain his feelings of regression to his therapist, the therapist assured the patient that she understood, because she herself found a certain comfort in eating stewed tomatoes when she was sick. Although she knew tomatoes were not particularly good "sick food," her mother had always served her stewed tomatoes when she was sick as a child. Much later, when the therapist became ill, the patient sent her a can of stewed tomatoes, symbolizing that they had understood each other well. Certainly the therapist need not refuse such a gift. However, it is usually best to share such transactions with the supervisor in order to avoid any misunderstandings.

HUMOR. The use of humor as a therapeutic tool has received increasing emphasis in recent years (Robinson, 1977; Snidman, 1984; Warner, 1984) and has always been incorporated into certain therapy modalities. Its effectiveness does, of course, depend a great deal on the therapist and on the patient's particular pathology. A psychotic—especially a schizophrenic—may laugh inappropriately due to anxiety, misinterpret a joke, not "catch on" because of his literal interpretations of words, or feel that the nurse is laughing *at* him, rather than *with* him. A depressed patient may not appreciate attempts to make him laugh or may resent that anyone can be so jovial when he feels so terrible. Patients without normal social inhibitions may tell jokes that are very vulgar, or use humor as a way to avoid the serious topics of therapy. In general, frivolity, flippancy, irony, and the inappropriate use of humor can have a destructive effect on a patient's therapy (Mullahy, 1973; Nicholi, 1988).

While considering these precautions, the sensitive therapist who knows her patient and observes his reactions closely may on occasion find humor to be an effective therapeutic tool (for example, to help a patient develop a lighter perspective on his problems, or simply to offer a moment of reprieve from the serious work of therapy). Sullivan acknowledged humor as a mark of maturity that has the capacity for helping people maintain a sense of place in the tapestry of life (Mullahy, 1973).

CHALLENGES IN THE DEVELOPMENT OF THE NURSE'S ROLE AS THERAPIST

HISTORICAL BARRIERS. Historically, the nursing profession has focused on good hygiene, cleanliness, and continuous and systematic observations of patients. Nurses also dispensed medications and provided physical care to patients; the care was custodial, physically oriented, and directed by physicians (Critchley, 1985). There have been many barriers to the further development of the nurse's role as therapist, especially as primary therapist. Chief among these are legal and economic issues, such as the territoriality of other professionals who view the nurse as a rival for their market, inadequate funding for graduate education in psychiatric mental health nursing, and obstacles to third-party payment (that is, government and insurance regulations that will not pay for therapy by a nurse) (Carter, 1986; Dumas, 1983; Lego, 1980; Peplau, 1982b).

Nurses have developed a healthy respect for the preparation, skill, and responsibilities of a psychotherapist, and of their accountability in using these terms judiciously (Pelletier, 1983). Within the profession, the issue of whether or not psychiatric nurse specialists should function as psychotherapists was debated for decades. However, growing numbers of nurses are now practicing psychotherapy successfully, with the focus of debate shifting to other areas (for example, the type of practice and clientele that are most appropriate; the quality and relevance of the therapy; the nurse's particular contribution to psychotherapy; and ways of promoting the nurse therapist's practice for the individual practitioner, the specialty group, and the nursing profession) (McBride, 1986; Hardin & Durham, 1985; Pelletier, 1984; Lego, 1973; 1980).

PAYMENT AND CONTROL. In addition to the nurse's actual income, there are a number of other implications surrounding the issue of payment, including the nurse's degree of freedom and control in practice (Hardin & Durham, 1985; Redmond, 1982). When a nurse is employed by an agency or psychiatrist she is responsible to that employer and must reconcile her personal needs with philosophy, methods, and priorities of her employer. The nurse who wishes to define her own role may establish a private practice to permit increased freedom in functioning, but she usually experiences a reduction in income, at least for several years, while she builds a practice. The nurse therapist in private practice must establish a reputation and referral sources, make arrangements for an office and a secretary or answering service, engage the services of a supervising physician or licensed psychologist if she wishes to meet state certification requirements or obtain third party reimbursement and finance her own Social Security, retirement, vacations, sick leave, and insurance, including professional liability.

Since many insurance carriers do not pay a nurse therapist directly, even persons who prefer the nurse's services may not be able financially to utilize them. For example, a nurse usually charges less than a psychiatrist, but if the insurance policy specifies payment to a physician and will not reimburse the patient for the nurse's fee, the patient is in effect paying more to see the nurse therapist. Nurse psychotherapists have sometimes had difficulty getting clients to pay (Hardin & Durham, 1985). Changes in third-party payment policies are being lobbied nationwide by nursing organizations and private practitioners.

MEDICATION AND HOSPITALIZATION. Legally, nurses cannot prescribe medication. Occasionally nurses work out a special contract whereby a consulting physician assumes the responsibility of allowing the nurse greater freedom with specified routine medications through a variety of arrangements, or the physician may simply write prescriptions and provide medication consultations for the nurse's patients, based on the nurse's input and recommendations and his own brief consultation with the patient. Such arrangements are rare due to competition, territoriality, the physician's concern about the nurse's preparation and judgment in this area, and serious legal implications. Such arrangements may also be awkward if the nurse and physician disagree about a patient's medication needs or if the nurse is unable to reach the consulting physician promptly.

Similar problems exist with hospital privileges (that is, the nurse's right to admit a patient to the hospital and retain the role of primary therapist, continuing to see the patient and/or direct the therapy while he is hospitalized). If the patient requires hospitalization or inpatient therapy, the nurse may lose the patient to another therapist altogether, obtain permission to continue seeing him along with his attending psychiatrist, or arrange to resume his therapy after he has been discharged. Again, this may be awkward if treatment or philosophies differ widely, such as when the nurse feels that the patient is overmedicated at the hospital, or when the methods used by the nurse are criticized by the agency staff.

PROFESSIONAL REPUTATION. The nurse must establish credibility as a therapist in order to develop and maintain a practice. The nurse's professional reputation depends on how her role and work are perceived by her patients and their families, nursing peers, and other professionals, especially within the mental health field. The nurse's choice of a supervisor or cotherapist is very important because professional reputation is affected by such associations.

At this level of practice, it is crucial for the nurse to market her services: participate in professional organizations and lay groups associated with mental health issues; use business cards, brochures, or other forms of advertisement; accept speaking engagements; and visit or send letters of introduction to various target groups and potential referral sources explaining what she has to offer. Pediatricians, general practitioners, social workers, and ministers may be more likely to refer a patient to a nurse therapist than to a psychiatrist or psychologist. Serving as a consultant to various agencies can also generate clientele and increase the name recognition of the nurse.

However, in the long run, perhaps the best referral source is the satisfied client or family member. Word of mouth is excellent advertisement, as the real test of competence always lies in the results. "She really helped me" is the ultimate compliment to the therapist. Research indicates that those who have been served by nurse psychotherapists feel very positively about their experiences and would recommend the therapist to others (Hardin & Durham, 1985; Meldman et al., 1971).

Nursing's Social Responsibility. Sills (1986) has challenged psychiatric nursing to make a difference in mental health care delivery. She suggests that nurses develop a national agenda and include, among others, the nursing needs of the chronically mentally ill, the homeless, and other unserved and underserved populations. Nurses should be cautious about competing with physicians for a certain segment of the population; indeed, there are people in this society who receive little or no care. The unserved and underserved groups offer nurses a challenge and an opportunity for professional autonomy (Sills, 1986). Nurses have always served (and continue to serve) patients in their homes, the community, and other appropriate settings.

Fox (1986) has suggested that psychiatric nurses must assume their own leadership and define its knowledge, role, and practice. Psychiatric nurses must also "cease taking directions from other disciplines ("primarily psychiatry") (p. 58). Moreover, Fox thinks that nurses should explicate the differences between psychiatric nursing and other mental health disciplines, and delegate those tasks to others that are better suited to manage them. Then, perhaps, nursing can focus on a national agenda and excel in specific areas of health care delivery.

Case Study: Psychiatric Setting

Demographic data:

Name: Anthony Ryane
Age: 43
Ethnicity: Caucasian (Scottish)
Religion: Church of God
Referring Agency: Self/family
Occupation: Medical technician,
                   Public Health Dept.
Address: Terre Haute, Indiana

Present problem

Anthony Ryane reluctantly entered the neighborhood health clinic with his family. He admitted to having had a bit too much to drink, but felt that he could "sleep the thing off." Anthony's wife, Jackie, stated that Anthony had increased his drinking ever since their 8-year-old son had been diagnosed as having an inoperable brain tumor. Their son died six weeks ago.

Jackie also stated, "I fear that his drinking will cause him to have another 'breakdown' and he might have those terrible spells again."

Mr. Ryane was sobbing and saying, "Why my son? Why?" At times his face was tense, and he looked extremely agitated and withdrawn.

History

Anthony Ryane is a soft-spoken, gentle man. He had worked as a medical technician at a veterans hospital for about seven years. At work, he is considered diligent, careful, and very knowledgeable about new techniques and tests that are possible in the hematology laboratory. He keeps to himself and does not socialize easily with others.

The couple's 8-year-old child underwent surgery and radiation therapy for a brain tumor. Anthony was very involved with his son's hospitalization. He worked all day at the hospital and spent each night with his son, who was in the pediatric unit. He also phoned the nurses several times during the day to check on his son's status. Anthony was at work when his son died; he immediately came to the unit when phoned by the physician.

The nurses, physicians, Mrs. Ryane, and Anthony met at the hospital to discuss the son's death. The parents saw the child before he was moved from the room, and Anthony demonstrated a dramatic display of emotions. He cried, paced, and asked "Why? Why my son?" The nurse and physician who provided care for the son stayed with the parents for quite some time. The staff nurse gave Mr. and Mrs. Ryane a list of community agencies that could provide help with their grieving; the parents went home to prepare for their son's final rites.

Psychiatric History

Anthony Ryane was hospitalized for a brief period of time (four weeks) approximately 15 years ago with a diagnosis of paranoid schizophrenia. This hospitalization occurred when his mother died immediately after he returned from Vietnam.

Family History

Anthony's mother was an elementary school teacher. She was a kind and supportive woman who demanded loyalty and excellence in performance. Anthony has vivid memories of his mother working at a school in the community and maintaining an excellently kept home.

Anthony's father is a retired hardware store manager. He is described as a kind worker, a disciplinarian, and a good money manager. When Anthony was younger, his father also worked a second job (a small office cleaning business) to supplement the family income.

Siblings

Anthony is the second of six children, four boys and two girls. Three of his brothers are in good health and have their own families. One sister is a physician and is employed with the World Health Organization (WHO). The younger sister resides in a foster home for mentally retarded adults, and Anthony frequently visits her.

Children

Anthony and Jacquelyn Ryane are the parents of three sons (ages 8, 12, and 15). The twelve- and fifteen-year-old sons are well and live with their parents.

Education

Anthony received his first degree from a community college in Indiana. He then enlisted in the Army where he became interested in medical technology. After discharge from the military, utilizing government aid and other educational financing supplements, he attended a university where he received a B.S. degree in medical technology. He has gained the reputation of being precise and thorough in his work.

Health History

Anthony is in good physical health. He has an old military injury, a "knee problem," that bothers him on occasion, for which he receives medical care at the veterans hospital.

Current Mental Status

General Appearance: Anthony was unshaven, wore torn clothes, and had uncombed hair when he and his wife entered the waiting room at the Parkside Neighborhood Health Clinic. He was observed to have an unsteady gait, flushed face, and slurred speech. He was pacing, stating that he needed help immediately, and, seconds later, threatening to leave the center.

Sensorium: Judgment, impaired: family stated that he wanted to go to work today.

Coherence: Time, poor: did not know date and missed time by 3 hours.

Place, poor: thought he was in another clinic across town. Person, good: gave full name and occupation.

Mood: Sadness with outbursts of tears; demands to see the doctor; followed by extreme sobbing and repeating, "Why my child? Why my child?"

Motor Behavior: Pacing, sitting, jumping up, pacing, quiet.

Thought Content: Anger, sadness, guilt.

Thought Process: Disorganized and overcome with grief.

Medications: None known at this time.

Potential for Violence: Suicide, not known; observe and assess. Homicide, not known; observe and assess.

Other significant data: Anthony was taken home by a friend who spotted Anthony at a local bar. Apparently Anthony began drinking at the bar and became intoxicated. The friend took Anthony's car keys and drove him home. According to Mrs. Ryane, Anthony was not a drinker. This behavior shocked her and caused her to worry about Anthony's health.

Summary

Anthony Ryane is a 43-year-old medical technologist who recently lost an 8-year-old son because of a brain tumor. He is obviously intoxicated and verbally expressing grief and pain associated with the death of his son. He is accompanied by his wife, Jacquelyn Ryane. Mr. Ryane was assessed and assigned to a nurse in the clinic. The nurse interviewed Mr. Ryane and developed the following Nursing Care Plan. He will be treated on an outpatient basis. The nurse has scheduled appointments for Mr. Ryane.

DSM-III-R Axes

Axis I: 305.00 Alcohol abuse.

Axis II: None at this time.

Axis III: Inflammation, right knee.

Axis IV: Psychosocial stressors: death of child; severity: 5—extreme.

Axis V: Current GAF: 32

Highest GAF past year: 80

Nursing Diagnoses

*Ineffective individual coping

*Dysfunctional grieving

*Social isolation

  Potential for violence

  Alteration in thought processes

  Anxiety

  Alteration in family process

*Nursing care plan that follows was developed for short-term hospitalization (5–10 days) using these nursing diagnoses.

Nursing Care Plan for Mr. Ryane

Nursing Diagnosis	Desired Outcome	Nursing Interventions	Rationale
1. Ineffective individual coping	Mr. Ryane will not act out feelings by abusing alcohol, but will express his feelings in non self-destructive ways.	Discuss with Mr. Ryane the effects of his drinking (how he behaves, how he feels afterward, reactions of family, implications for health, job, finances, etc.	Fosters insight; links use of alcohol with its natural consequences (loss of health, job, money, and so forth).
		Ask Mr. Ryane to describe the events/thoughts/feelings he experiences just prior to drinking, or acting out his anger.	Fosters insight; links feelings with relief sought through alcohol, a maladaptive coping mechanism.
		Discuss with Mr. Ryane other alternatives for dealing with these feelings: a) Arrange for him to participate in physical activities at least once daily. (Discuss the use of a pillow as a punching bag, hammering in O.T., hitting a ball, and so on) b) Explain to Mr. Ryane the procedure(s) for initiating additional sessions with the doctor or nurse and/or requesting staff assistance for dealing with anger and associated violent or drinking episodes.	Physical exercise helps to sublimate anger and aggressive energy in acceptable ways; it also helps overcome depression by increasing catecholamines in the brain.
		Refer Mr. Ryane to appropriate self-help groups such as Alcoholics Anonymous.	AA offers peer understanding and support and good results in maintaining sobriety for those who attend regularly.

Nursing Diagnosis	Desired Outcome	Nursing Interventions	Rationale
		Discuss with Mr. Ryane any fears he has of not being able to cope. Explain the benefits of stress management. Demonstrate techniques for reducing stress to Mr. Ryane (for example, assertiveness, pacing of work and exercise, planned time for relaxation, social activities, hobbies, regular meals, and at least 7 hours of sleep nightly) and help him find ways to integrate these techniques into his life, encouraging him to practice these methods of reducing stress. Follow-up is essential.	Identifies additional sources of patient's apprehension. Reduces physiological results of stress as well as providing immediate relief.
		If Mr. Ryane continues to express his feelings in an unhealthy manner (by abusing alcohol), institute limit-setting, offering alternatives. The nurse can state: "Mr. Ryane, it makes no sense for you to continue in this program if you are not going to cooperate with your treatment plan. Perhaps you and I can discuss why you have had so much trouble with this so far."	Assists patient in learning to connect behavior with consequences. Provides opportunity for patient to be successful in controlling his own maladaptive behavior.
		When Mr. Ryane appears uncertain or indecisive in daily decisions, ask him to express his ideas and feelings—what he perceives as the options, advantages, disadvantages of his treatment plan. ("Which do you think would be best for you this weekend, to follow your treatment plan or not to follow it? What would be the consequences of each course of action?")	Reinforces his self-confidence and problem-solving ability. Thought is trial action: provides opportunity for him to think through a situation and develop notions about consequences, alternatives, feeling states, and so on.

Nursing Diagnosis	Desired Outcomes	Interventions	Rationale
2. Social isolation relative to alcohol abuse	Mr. Ryane will identify and begin using opportunities to broaden his support system.	Ask Mr. Ryane about his relationships with persons or groups that might be available to offer support (extended family, work colleagues, neighbors, organizations of which he is a member, including his church).	Increases social support system. Prevents feelings of separation; withdrawal; and/or over-burdening a few close relationships. Religious faith offers comfort in grief as well as a social network.
		Share information about local support groups for bereaved parents (benefits, meeting time, place). Discuss any reluctance he expresses about participating.	Self-help groups such as AA and ALANON offer acceptance, understanding, and suggestions specific to problem, and opportunities to form new relationships.
		Refer Mr. Ryane for individual or group psychotherapy, telling him what he can expect from each.	Therapy offers a way for Mr. Ryane to understand his self-defeating behavior and, ultimately, be able to get control of it. Group therapy offers peer support and feedback.
		Encourage him to begin sharing his feelings with other members of his support system. Discuss any fears about this experience.	Sharing with others allows him to receive support and overcome his sense of isolation.

Nursing Diagnosis	Desired Outcomes	Interventions	Rationale
3. Dysfunctional grieving	Mr. Ryane will express his feelings about the death of his son, acknowledging the meaning or impact of his son's death on himself and his family. (Long-term goal: healthy resolution of the grief process.)	Validate with Mr. Ryane his feeling of grief over the loss of his son. (Indicate it has been a difficult time; explain that it is normal to feel guilt, anger, sorrow.)	Decreases anxiety and resistance; facilitates open expression of feelings; helps to focus the patient on the grief process.
		Assure him that you will support him through the crisis ("I am concerned . . . I will work with you until you feel you are able to function well without my help.").	Conveys empathy, concern and caring; helps to define the relationship.
		Ask him to tell you about his son. ("I did not know him; what was he like?") Comment on nonverbal reactions observed and give permission to express any feelings. Support feelings expressed. ("You seem to be fighting back tears. It's O.K. to cry. . . . I'm glad you can tell me how sad you feel.")	Encourages ventilation of feelings; is less threatening initially than direct questions regarding feelings; Clarifies thoughts and feelings for Mr. Ryane and provides nurse with additional information about the relationship.
		Ask him directly about his feelings. ("How have you been feeling? How did you feel when you realized he was dying? When do you miss him most?")	Assists patient in identifying and clarifying his feelings; integral part of grief-work.
		Discuss the reality of his son's death and how it has affected him and his family. (What is it like to lose a son and one's dreams for him? What have been the changes in family life so far? Have physical/psychosocial symptoms been experienced by anyone else in the family?)	Supports reality; facilitates process of "letting go" by acknowledging impact, which is necessary for resolving grief and re-investing in the future.

SUMMARY

There are three levels of psychiatric mental health nursing: the therapeutic nurse-patient relationship, basic therapy, and primary therapy. All nurses should be therapeutic, but all nurses are not therapists. The therapeutic relationship is the basis for therapy at all levels. Many nurses function at the level of a basic therapist. The basic therapist works with selected patients in structured, goal-directed sessions as part of an overall treatment plan, usually in a psychiatric mental health setting over a period of time. Some nurses have achieved a level of preparation that equips them to function as primary therapists. The primary therapist assumes responsibility for directing and/or conducting the patient's therapy, frequently as a psychotherapist in private practice or in a clinical specialist role. The level at which a nurse applies psychiatric mental health nursing principles is not only a function of her knowledge, skill, and experience, but also of the nurse's personal characteristics and individual choice as well as agency policies.

Nine therapeutic roles may be assumed by nurses in applying psychiatric nursing principles to patients' needs: healthy role model, nurturing parent, reality base, technician, socializing agent, manager, teacher, patient advocate, and counselor. Each role is applicable in varying degrees to all areas and levels of nursing practice.

Patient goals developed by nurses are designed to be: 1) within the scope of nursing practice; 2) compatible with the patient's overall treatment plan; 3) based on the patient's current needs and problems; and 4) formulated to measure short-term progress of the patient. Primary therapists may also utilize these guidelines, but they can be more independent in the nature and depth of their therapy with patients.

The nature and depth of the nurse's work with patients' therapy is determined by the setting, the supervision available, the patient, and the nurse. Each nurse is also a unique individual and should acknowledge her own current limitations while working to increase effectiveness with a wider variety of patients and problems. Personal characteristics that facilitate the therapeutic process include: genuine concern and caring, commitment, an analytical mind, "therapeutic use of self," and awareness and acceptance of self and others.

Nursing education and experience provide a good foundation for various roles in therapy through knowledge and skill, extended patient contact, and the nursing perspective, which is holistic, eclectic, and nurturing.

Nurses encounter a number of challenges in applying the knowledge and skills of psychiatric mental health nursing: patients' ambivalence about therapy, silence, social/sexual overtures, automatic reactions such as transference/contertransference and the interpersonal reflex, and the use of touch, gifts, and humor in the therapeutic process.

Four challenges in the development of the nurse's role as primary therapist are historical barriers, the issue of payment and control, the question of medication and hospitalization, and professional reputation.

KEY TERMS

therapeutic nurse-patient relationship
basic therapy
primary therapy
nurse therapist
nursing process
healthy role model
nurturing parent
reality base
technician
socializing agent
manager
teacher
patient advocate

counselor
locus of control
therapeutic match
orientation phase
working phase
termination phase
holistic approach
eclectic approach
therapeutic use of self
automatic reactions
transference
countertransference
I-P reflex

STUDY QUESTIONS

1. Name and describe three levels at which psychiatric mental health nursing principles may be applied.

2. What are nine therapeutic roles of the nurse?

3. What are the four main criteria used by a nurse in formulating goals with patients? Why is each important?

4. What four main characteristics help make a nurse effective in therapy? Why is each important?

5. Name and describe at least four of the clinical challenges frequently encountered when applying the principles of psychiatric mental health nursing in clinical practice.

REFERENCES

American Nurses' Association. (1980). *A social policy statement*. Kansas City, MO: The American Nurses' Association.

American Nurses' Association. (1982). *A.N.A. standards of psychiatric and mental health nursing practice*. Kansas City MO: The American Nurses' Association.

American Nurses' Association. (1985). *Facts about nursing*. Kansas City, MO: The American Nurses' Association.

Anthony, B. D. (1982). Lesbian client—lesbian therapist: Opportunities and challenges in working together. *Journal of Homosexuality, 7*(⅔), 45–57.

Anvil, C. A., & Silver, B. W. (1984). Therapist self-disclosures: When is it appropriate? *Perspectives in Psychiatric Care, 22*, 57–61.

Barnett, K. (1972). A theoretical construct of the concepts of touch as they relate to nursing. *Nursing Research, 21*, 102–110.

Bellak, L. (1979). The therapeutic relationship in brief psychotherapy. *American Journal Of Psychotherapy, 33*, 564–571.

Bellack, L., Hurvich, M., & Gediman, H. K. (1973). *Ego functions in schizophrenics, neurotics, and normals—a systematic study of conceptual, diagnostic, and therapeutic aspects*. New York: John Wiley & Sons.

Berne, E. (1972). *What do you say after you say hello?* New York: Grove Press, Inc.

Burgess, A. C., & Burns, J. (1973). Why patients seek care. *American Journal of Nursing, 73*, 314–316.

Campaniello, J. A. (1980). The process of termination. *Journal of Psychiatric Nursing and Mental Health Services, 18*(2), 29–32.

Carnegie, M. E. (1974). The patient's bill of rights and the nurse. *Nursing Clinics of North America, 9*, 557–562.

Carter, E. W. (1986). Psychiatric nursing: 1986. *Journal of Psychosocial Nursing and Mental Health Services, 24*(6), 26–30.

Chapman, N. W. (1983). An essay on the art of nursing. *Perspectives in Psychiatric Care, 21*, 66–69.

Clancy, K. M. (1968). Concerning gifts. *Perspectives in Psychiatric Care, 6*, 169–175.

Clark, B. (1984). What to do when your patient lets slip his grip on reality. *Nursing, (Horsham)*(Canadian edition) *14*(7), 50–56.

Colliton, M. A. (1971). Symposium on the use of self in clinical practice. *Nursing Clinics of North America, 6*, 691–694.

Committee on Psychiatric Nursing, Group for Advancement of Psychiatry. (1982a). Therapeutic use of the self: A concept for teaching patient care. In S. A. Smoyak & S. Rosuelin (Eds.), *A collection of classics in psychiatric nursing literature*. Thorofore, N.J.: Charles B. Slack, Inc., pp. 68–81. (Reprinted from the Committee on Psychiatric Nursing of the Group for Advancement of Psychiatry, Report No. 33, 1955.)

Committee on Psychiatric Nursing of the Group for Advancement of Psychiatry. (1982b). Toward therapeutic care: A guide for those who work with the mentally ill. In S. A. Smoyak & S. Rouslin (Eds.), *A collection of classics in psychiatric nursing literatire*. Thorofare, N.J.: Charles B. Slack, Inc., pp. 68–81. (Reprinted from the Committee on Psychiatric Nursing of the Group for Advancement of Psychiatry, Report No. 33, 1955.)

Corey, L. J., Wallace, M. A., Harris, S. H., & Casey, B. (1986). Psychiatric ward atmosphere. *Journal of Psychosocial Nursing and Mental Health Services, 24*(10), 10–16.

Crawford, A. L. (1982). Psychiatry: A nursing essential. A paper originally read at the South Carolina State Nurses' Association Annual Convention, October 6, 1934. In S. A. Smoyak & S. Rouslin (Eds.), *A collection of classics in psychiatric literature*. Thorofare, N.J.: Charles B. Slack, Inc. pp. 2–7.

Creighton, H. (1981). *Law every nurse should know*. Philadelphia: W. B. Saunders Co.

Critchley, D. L. (1985). Evolution of the role. In D. L. Critchley & J. T. Maurin (Eds.). *The clinical specialist in psychiatric mental health nursing: Theory, research, and practice*, New York: John Wiley & Sons, pp. 5–22.

DeAugustinis, J. (1963). Ward study: The meaning of touch in interpersonal communication. In S. F. Burd & M. A. Marshall (Eds.), *Some clinical approaches to psychiatric nursing*. New York: Macmillan Co., pp. 271–306.

DeThomaso, M. T. (1971). "Touch power" and the screen of loneliness. *Perspectives in Psychiatric Care, 9*, 112–118.

Doona, M. E. (1979). *Travelbee's intervention in psychiatric nursing* (2nd ed.). Philadelphia: F. A. Davis Co.

Douglas, C. J., Kalman, C. M., & Kalman, T. P. (1985). Homophobia among physicians and nurses: An empirical study. *Hospital and Community Psychiatric, 36*, 1309–1311.

Dumas, R. (1981, September). *What does the future hold for psychiatric/mental health nursing?* Paper presented at the meeting, Psychiatric Nursing Dimensions, New York.

Dumas, R. G. (1983). Social, economic, and political factors and mental illness. *Journal of Psychosocial Nursing and Mental Health Services, 21*(3), 31–35.

Ennis, B. J., & Siegel, L. (1978). *The rights of mental patients: The basic ACLU guide to a mental patient's rights*. New York: Richard W. Brown Publishing Co., Inc.

Ettlinger, R. A. (1973). Advocate informs patients of rights and responsibilities. *Hospital and Community Psychiatry, 24*, 465–470.

Fagin, C. M. (1967). Psychotherapeutic nursing. *American Journal of Nursing, 67*, 298–304.

Feather, R. B. (1985). The institutionalized mental health patient's right to refuse psychotropic medication. *Perspectives in Psychiatric Care, 23*, 45–68.

Feather, R., & Bissell, B. (1979). Clinical supervision vs. psychotherapy: The psychiatric-mental health supervisory process. *Perspectives in Psychiatric Care, 17*, 266–272.

Finkelman, A. (1975). Commitment and responsibility in the therapeutic relationship. *Journal of Psychiatric Nursing and Mental Health Services, 13*(1), 10–14.

Floyd, G. J. (1973). Managing member silence in family therapy. *Journal of Psychiatric Nursing and Mental Health Services, 11*(4), 20–24.

Fox, J. (1986). Essential and critical knowledge for psychiatric-mental health nursing in the twenty-first century.

In *Psychiatric-mental health nursing: Proceedings of a conference defining the discipline for the year 2000*. U.S. Department of Health and Human Services, National Institute of Mental Health, Rockville, MD, pp. 56–67.

Garritson, S., & Davis, A. (1983). Least restrictive alternatives: Ethical considerations. *Journal of Psychosocial Nursing and Mental Health Services, 21*(12), 17–23.

Gordy, H. E. (1978). Gift giving in the nurse-patient relationship. *American Journal of Nursing, 78,* 1026–1028.

Gregg, D. E. (1982). The psychiatric nurses' role. In S. A. Smoyak & S. Rouslin (Eds.), *A collection of classics in psychiatric nursing literature*. Thorofare, NJ: Charles B. Slack, Inc. pp. 207–211. (Reprinted from the *American Journal of Nursing,* July 1954.)

Gregg, D. E., Bregg, E. A., & Spring, F. E. (1976). Individual supervision: A method of teaching psychiatric concepts in nursing education. *Perspectives in Psychiatric Care, 14,* 115–129.

Hall, B. A. (1977). The effect of interpersonal attraction on the therapeutic relationship: A review and suggestions for future study. *Journal of Psychiatric Nursing and Mental Health Services, 15*(9), 18–23.

Hardin, S. B., & Durham, J. D. (1985). First rate: Exploring the structure, process, and effectiveness of nurse psychotherapy. *Journal of Psychosocial Nursing and Mental Health Services, 23*(5), 9–15.

Hoeffer, B., & Murphy, S. (1982). The unfinished task: Development of nursing theory for psychiatric and mental health nursing practice. *Journal of Psychosocial Nursing and Mental Health Services, 20*(12), 8–14.

Jefferson, L. F., & Ensor, B. E. (1982). Help for the helper—confronting a chemically impaired colleague. *American Journal of Nursing, 82,* 574–577.

Johnson, B. S. (1967). The blotting paper syndrome. *Perspectives in Psychiatric Care, 5,* 228–230.

Johnson, B. S., & Miller, L. C. (1967). The interpersonal reflex in psychiatric nursing. *Nursing Outlook, 15,* 60–63.

Jourard, S. E., & Rubin, J. E. (1968). Self-disclosure and touching: A study of two modes of interpersonal encounter and their interrelation. *Journal of Humanistic Psychology, 8*(1), 39–48.

Kasmarik, P. E. & Lester, V. C. (1984). A hard decision: Where institutionalization is the best answer. In B. A. Hall (Ed.), *Mental health and the elderly*. New York: Grune & Stratton (pp. 165–184).

Keltner, N. L., Doggett, R., & Johnson, R. (1983). For the Vietnam veteran the war goes on. *Perspectives in Psychiatric Care, 21,* 108–113.

Krikorian, D. A., & Paulanka, B. J. (1982). Self awareness—the key to a successful nurse-patient relationship? *Journal of Psychiatric Nursing and Mental Health Services, 20*(6), 19–21.

Leary, T. (1957). *Interpersonal diagnosis of personality*. New York: Ronald Press Co.

Lego, S. (1973). Nurse psychotherapists: How are we different? *Perspectives in Psychiatric Care, 11,* 144–147.

Lego, S. (1980). The one-to-one nurse patient relationship. *Perspectives in Psychiatric Care, 18,* 67–89.

Lewis, E. W. (1982). Identifying some concepts nursing personnel need to understand in relation to the nature

of therapeutic functions. In S. A. Smoyak & S. Rouslin (Eds.), *A collection of classics in psychiatric nursing literature*. Thorofare, NJ: Charles B. Slack, Inc., pp. 82–87. (Original paper presented at National League for Nursing Conference Project Washington, D.C., 1956.)

McBride, A. B. (1986). Present issues and future perspectives of psychosocial nursing theory and research. *Journal of Psychosocial Nursing and Mental Health Services, 24*(9), 27–32.

McCann, J. (1979). Termination of the psychotherapeutic relationship. *Journal of Psychiatric Nursing and Mental Health Services, 17*(10), 37–46.

Mager, R. T. (1984). *Preparing instructional objectives* (2nd ed.). Belmont, CA: Pitman Management and Training.

Maloney, E. M. (1982). Does the psychiatric nurse have independent functions? In S. A. Smoyak & S. Rouslin (Eds.), *A collection of classics in psychiatric nursing literature*. Thorofare, NJ: Charles B. Slack, Inc., pp. 272–275. (Original work published 1962.)

Maloney, E. M. (1983). Therapy for whom? *Perspectives in Psychiatric Care, 21,* 147.

Mansfield, E. (1973). Empathy: Concept and identified psychiatric nursing behavior. *Nursing Research, 22,* 525–530.

Meldman, M. J., Newman, B., Schaller, D., & Peterson, P. (1971). Patients' response to nurse-psychotherapists. *American Journal of Nursing, 71,* 1150–1151.

Meleis, A. I., & LaFever, C. W. (1984). The Arab-American and psychiatric care. *Perspectives in Psychiatric Care, 22,* 72–76; 85.

Mellow, J. (1982). Research in nursing therapy. In S. A. Smoyak & S. Rouslin (Eds.), *A collection of classics in psychiatric nursing literature*. Thorofare, NJ: Charles B. Slack, Inc., pp. 251–255. (Reprinted from *The improvement of nursing through research,* The Catholic University of America Press, Washington, D.C., 1958.)

Mellow, J. (1968). Nursing therapy. *American Journal of Nursing, 68,* 2365–2369.

Mitchell, A. C. (1976). Barriers to therapeutic communication with black clients. *Nursing Outlook, 24,* 109–112.

Moscovitz, A. D. (1984). Orem's theory as applied to psychiatric nursing. *Perspectives in Psychiatric Care, 22,* 36–38.

Mullahy, P. (1973). *The beginning of modern American psychiatry—the ideas of Harry Stack Sullivan*. Boston: Houghton Mifflin Co.

Nelson, B. K. (1973). The unpopular patient: Study indicates which patients nurses don't like: The unpleasant, the long-term, the mentally ill, the hypochondriacs, and the dying. *Modern Hospital, 121,* 70–73.

Nicholi, A. M. (1988). The therapist-patient relationship. In A. M. Nicholi (Ed.), *The new Harvard guide to modern psychiatry*. Cambridge, MA: The Belknap Press of Harvard University Press, pp. 3–22.

Oriol, M. D., & Oriol, R. D. (1986). Involuntary commitment and the right to refuse medication. *Journal of Psychosocial Nursing and Mental Health Services, 24*(11), 15–20.

O'Toole, A. (1981). When the practical becomes theoretical. *Journal of Psychosocial Nursing and Mental Health Services, 19*(12), 11–19.

Parks, S. L. (1966). Allowing physical distance as a nursing approach. *Perspectives in Psychiatric Care, 4*(6), 31–35.

Pelletier, L. R. (1983). Interpersonal communications task group. *Journal of Psychiatric Nursing and Mental Health Services, 21*(9), 33–36.

Pelletier, L. R. (1984). Nurse-psychotherapists: Whom do they treat? *Hospital and Community Psychiatry, 35,* 1149–1150.

Peplau, H. E. (1963). A working definition of anxiety. In S. F. Burd & M. A. Marshall (Eds.), *Some clinical approaches to psychiatric nursing.* New York: Macmillan Co., pp. 323–329.

Peplau, H. E. (1964). *Basic principles of patient counseling* (2nd ed.). Philadelphia: Smith, Kline & French Laboratories.

Peplau, H. E. (1968). Psychotherapeutic strategies. *Perspectives in Psychiatric Care, 6,* 264–270.

Peplau, H. E. (1978). Psychiatric nursing: Role of nurses and psychiatric nurses. *International Nursing Review, 25,* 41–47.

Peplau, H. E. (1982a). Interpersonal techniques: The crux of psychiatric nursing. In S. A. Smoyak & S. Rouslin (Eds.), *A collection of classics in psychiatric nursing literature.* Thorofare, NJ: Charles B. Slack, Inc., pp. 276–278. (Reprinted from *American Journal of Nursing,* June 1962.)

Peplau, H. E. (1982b). Therapeutic concepts. In S. A. Smoyak & S. Rouslin (Eds.), *A collection of classics in psychiatric nursing literature.* Thorofare, NJ: Charles B. Slack, Inc., pp. 91–108. (Reprinted from National League for Nursing, *Aspects of Psychiatric Nursing,* League Exchange Pamphlet No. 26, Section B, 1957.)

Peplau, H. E. (1982c). The work of clinical specialists in psychiatric nursing. In S. A. Smoyak & S. Rouslin (Eds.), *A collection of classics in psychiatric nursing literature.* Thorofare, NJ: Charles B. Slack, Inc., pp. 47–49. (Paper presented May, 1959.)

Platt-Koch, L. M. (1986). Clinical supervision for psychiatric nurses. *Journal of Psychosocial Nursing and Mental Health Services, 26*(1), 7–15.

Redmond, M. M. (1982). The nurse as a clinical specialist. In S. A. Smoyak & S. Rouslin (Eds.), *A collection of classics in psychiatric nursing literature.* Thorofare, NJ: Charles B. Slack, Inc., pp. 293–295. (Reprinted from *Military Medicine,* November 1957.)

Reeves, K. (1986). Hispanic utilization of an ethnic mental health clinic. *Journal of Psychosocial Nursing and Mental Health Services, 24*(2), 23–26.

Ricci, M. S. (1981). An experiment with personal-space invasion in the nurse-patient relationship and its effect on anxiety. *Issues in Mental Health Nursing, 3,* 203–218.

Roberts, S. L. (1969). Territoriality: Space and the schizophrenic patient. *Perspectives in Psychiatric Care, 7*(1), 28–33.

Robinson, V. M. (1977). *Humor and the health professions.* New Jersey: Charles B. Slack, Inc.

Rochlin, M. (1982). Sexual orientation of the therapist and therapeutic effectiveness with gay clients. *Journal of Homosexuality, 7*(2/3), 21–29.

Schroder, P. J. (1985). Recognizing transference and counter transference. *Journal of Psychosocial Nursing and Mental Health Services, 23*(2), 21–26.

Shoemaker, J. K. (1984). Essential features of a nursing diagnosis. In M. J. Kim, G. K. McFarland, & A. M. McLane (Eds.), *Classification of nursing diagnoses.* St. Louis: The C. V. Mosby Co., pp. 104–115. (Paper based on the *Concept of nursing diagnoses,* unpublished doctoral dissertation, Teachers College, Columbia University, 1982.)

Sills, G. (1986). The (w) Holly Trinity Revisited, In National Institute of Mental Health, *Psychiatric mental health nursing: Proceedings of a conference defining the discipline for the year 2000.* U. S. Department of Health and Human Services, Rockville, MD. 20–29.

Smith, F. B. (1985). Patient power. *American Journal of Nursing, 85,* 1260–1262.

Smoyak, S. A. (1986). Ethical perspectives. *Journal of Psychosocial Nursing, 24*(11), 7.

Snidman, E. M. (1984). Reflections of a humorist therapist. *Perspectives in Psychiatric Care, 22,* 143–144.

Sullivan, H. S. (1953). *The interpersonal theory of psychiatry.* New York: W.W. Norton & Co., Inc.

Trygstad, L. N. (1986). Stress and coping in psychiatric nursing. *Journal of Psychosocial Nursing and Mental Health Services, 24*(10), 23–27.

Vidoni, G. (1975). The development of intense positive countertransference feelings in the therapist toward a patient. *American Journal of Nursing, 75,* 407–409.

Wallace, E. R. (1983). *Dynamic psychiatry in theory and practice.* Philadelphia: Lea & Febiger.

Walt, A. P., & Gillis, L. S. (1979). Factors that influence nurses' attitudes toward psychiatric patients. *Journal of Clinical Psychology, 35,* 410–414.

Warner, S. L. (1984). Human and self-disclosure within the milieu. *Journal of Psychosocial Nursing and Mental Health Services, 22*(4), 17–21.

Webster's Ninth New Collegiate Dictionary, Unabridged. (1986). Springfield: Merriam-Webster, Inc.

Witt, P. (1983). Dilemmas in practice: Notes of a whistle blower. *American Journal of Nursing, 83,* 1649–1651.

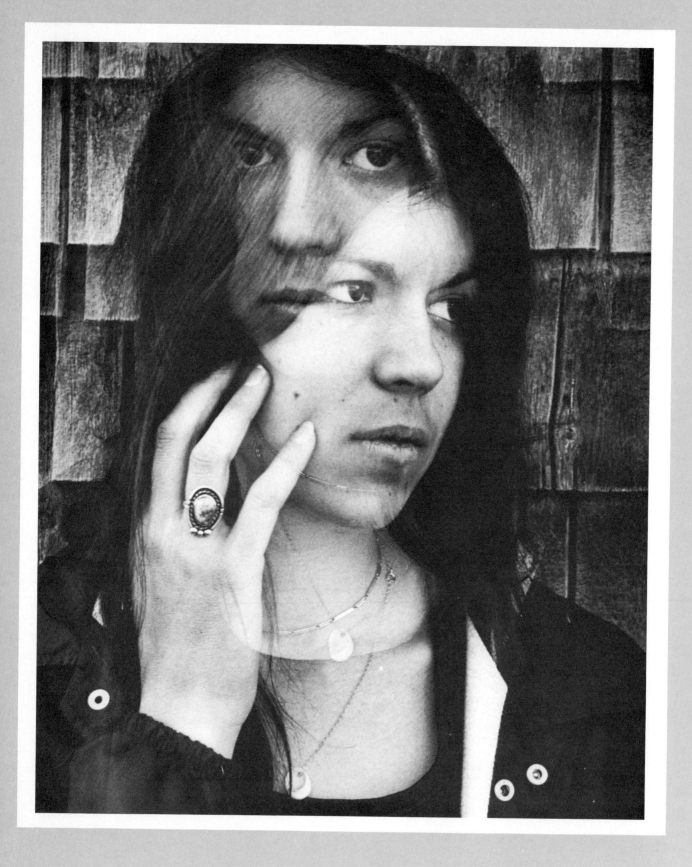

Part Two

PSYCHOLOGICAL DYSFUNCTION AND PSYCHOPATHOLOGY

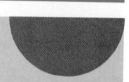

LEARNING OBJECTIVES

After studying this chapter, the student will be able to:

- Identify the three major components of anxiety.
- Identify the only effective criterion for differentiating between anxious feelings and anxiety disorder.
- Identify the two forms of anxiety state, or anxiety neurosis, and describe their symptoms.
- Identify the four other major anxiety disorders and describe their symptoms.
- Define treatment by exposure and explain how it works.

ANXIETY DISORDERS

BOB MCDONALD

DESCRIPTION OF ANXIETY AND ANXIETY DISORDERS

Anxiety is an experience everyone has. Certain objects, people, and situations provoke anxious feelings in all of us. These anxious feelings can, at different times, be minor irritations, cause better or worse performance, prevent us from doing things we want to do, or inhibit us from doing things that we shouldn't do.

For most of us, anxious feelings are a mixed blessing; in some instances, they enhance our performance (for example, in examinations, where it doesn't pay to be *too* calm), and in other instances they cause a small amount of interference (for example, when we get too anxious at a job interview and don't say the necessary things). We all attempt, in different ways, to cope with anxious feelings and most of us are pretty adept at managing them.

However, for some of the population (around eight percent), the anxiety they experience makes them dysfunctional; anxiety represents a serious impediment to daily life. These are people of all ages, both sexes, and all social classes (see Table 8–1), and it is this group with which this chapter is concerned.

ASSESSMENT OF ANXIETY

Anxiety has three major components: **behavior, cognitions,** and **autonomic responses.** An accurate assessment of anxiety takes all three into account. Behavioral aspects, such as avoidance in the case of anxiety specific to certain situations (for example, test anxiety), are probably easiest to measure. In this discussion the number of activities the individual is unable or unwilling to undertake is emphasized. (In clinical research the individual is usually asked to approach a particular object until he or she feels unable to go any closer.)

Assessment of the cognitive component of anxiety is more difficult, but the Fear Questionnaire (Marks & Mathews, 1979) and the Semantic Differential (Osgood, 1956) are instruments commonly used for this purpose. Further details of these and other measures for anxiety and other problems can be

TABLE 8–1 Epidemiology of *DSM-III* anxiety disorders*

Parameter	Lifetime Prevalence in Percent			
	Agoraphobia†	Simple Phobia†	Panic Disorder	Obsessive Compulsive Disorder
Total	4.9	2.5	1.4	2.5
Sex				
Male	1.5	3.9	0.9	2.0
Female	6.0	9.0	2.0	3.0
Race				
Black	4.4	8.0	1.3	2.5
Nonblack	3.7	6.2	1.3	2.6
Education				
College graduate	2.2	4.5	1.1	2.0
Other	4.4	7.2	1.5	2.6
Location				
Central city	4.6	6.6	1.7	1.5
Suburbs	4.3	7.6	0.8	2.4
Small town/rural	3.7	6.3	2.1	1.7

*This table synthesizes information from Robins et al. (1984), Goodwin & Guze (1984), Blazer et al. (1985), and Liebowitz et al. (1985).

†These columns indicate the prevalence of phobic disorders, which disable, as opposed to phobic *symptoms,* which although more common, are usually not disabling.

found in Marks (1986). Both approaches have limitations, and a simple alternative is to ask the individual to rate him or herself on an imaginary scale from 0 to 100 where 0 represents no anxiety and 100 represents the most anxiety ever experienced.

Most patients can do this without difficulty, and it can provide a useful means of arranging feared situations into a hierarchy or "league table" of severity. It can also serve as a means of measuring change. For example, an individual with test anxiety may report a level of 10 a month before an anticipated exam, 25 a week before, 50 the night before, 80 the day of the exam, and 100 when he enters the room where the test will be taken. The goal of treatment would be to decrease the intensity of anxiety in the twenty-four hours prior to the exam so as not to interfere with performance. It would not be desirable to eliminate *all* the anxiety. In fact, reported levels of 10 and 25 are probably necessary for the individual to be motivated to study for the exam.

The easiest autonomic responses to measure in assessment of anxiety are heart and respiration rate. Both increase in direct relationship to anxiety and can serve as useful adjuncts to subjective ratings.

None of the above measures differentiates between "normal" and pathological anxiety. Children, for instance, often develop fears and phobias at different ages that will in most cases resolve without becoming pathological (see Box 8–1). The only effective criterion for distinguishing between "normal" and "pathological" anxiety in adults is interference with personal, social, or occupational functioning. When pathological anxiety is present, nurses should assess for secondary problems, as summarized in the list of nursing diagnoses in Table 8–2. Care of non-psychiatric patients with anxiety is discussed later in this chapter.

Box 8–1 ● Childhood Fears and Anxieties

A child's world is magical and menacing—full of mysteries and dangers, real and imaginary, that most of us forget as adults. In one survey of a thousand children, 90 percent had some specific phobia between the ages of 2 and 14. In another study, 43 percent of children between the ages of 6 and 12 had "many fears and worries." Most of these anxieties are not associated with psychiatric disorders or psychopathology. It can be difficult to decide when a child's fears are so serious that they need treatment. The categories used for adult anxiety disorders, like most adult psychiatric diagnoses, are inadequate when applied to the constantly growing and changing bodies and minds of children. Fears that are normal at one age become incapacitating a few years later; and chronological age is not decisive, since different children have different rates of development.

Judging which fears are abnormal demands a knowledge of which ones are normal. Newborns fear loss of support and loud noises. Fear of strangers begins at six months to a year and normally persists until the age of two or three. Fear of separation from parents begins about the age of one and may last until seven or eight. Preschool children often fear animals, large objects, dark places, changes in the environment, masks, 'bad' people, supernatural creatures, and sleeping alone. Older children may worry about death, examinations, and events in the news such as kidnappings and wars. Teenagers have many social and sexual anxieties.

Most of these fears are mild and transient. Fear becomes a problem only if it interferes with activities normal at a given age, and in most cases it presents a mental health problem only if this situation lasts at least a month. By one estimate, 8 percent of boys and 11 percent of girls have clinically significant anxiety of some kind before the age of 18. A survey in the province of Ontario, Canada found that 6 percent of children aged 4 to 6 and 2.5 percent of children aged 12 to 15 might be in need of treatment for fears and anxi-

THEORIES OF ANXIETY DISORDERS

According to classic psychoanalytic theory, anxieties and phobias are defenses against unconscious conflicts rooted in early upbringing. Certain feelings and impulses may be so painful that they are repressed and displaced onto an object that symbolically represents the real source of the anxiety. According to this theory, it is easier to fear a specific object than to suffer an anxiety that cannot be consciously acknowledged.

Although this model has dominated thinking about anxiety for most of this century, it has failed to provide effective therapeutic strategies (Rachman, 1971). Its one testable idea, that the removal of phobias would lead to the emergence of other psychopathology, has been demonstrated to be completely without foundation. A number of biological theories

---

TABLE 8–2 Common nursing diagnoses in anxiety disorders

Activity intolerance

Altered health maintenance

Anxiety

Decisional conflict

Inability to cope

Fear

Impaired home-maintenance management

Self-care deficit: feeding, bathing/hygiene, etc.

Self-esteem disturbance

Sleep-pattern disturbance

Social isolation

Alteration in thought processes

Post-trauma response

---

eties. Perhaps 2 to 3 percent of children at some time have enough fear of school to worry their parents and teachers.

Researchers have never agreed on how to classify children's fears. General anxiety or specific phobias can be symptoms of many severe childhood psychiatric disorders, including autism, major depression, schizophrenia, and conditions involving brain damage. Anxiety disorders in a narrower sense fall into several distinct patterns. Most of these are exaggerated, prolonged, or disabling versions of normal childhood fears, and some are similar to adult anxiety disorders. The boundaries of the disorders are disputed; any child who has some of the anxiety symptoms discussed here is likely to have others as well.

One type of symptom is a simple phobia. Any of the common childhood fears, and many others, can become clinically significant phobias if they are severe enough, persist long enough, or occur at an inappropriate age. Phobias in children come and go

rapidly up to the age of 10, and they do not usually require treatment unless there are other symptoms, such as excessive general anxiety or refusal to go to school.

Separation anxiety is a more serious matter. It is a disabling fear of being apart from one's parents or away from home that lasts for several weeks or more. It may develop either spontaneously or under stress (a move, a death in the family) and sometimes lasts for several years, waxing and waning. Children with separation anxiety fear going to school or camp or even sleeping in a friend's home. They demand excessive attention from their parents, cling to them, follow them around, even try to climb into their beds at night. When separation threatens, they may develop headaches and stomachaches. They often fear that if they are apart from their parents, either they or the parents will come to harm. This fear may take the form of vague anxiety (in young children) or specific fantasies of accidents, illness, disappearance, torture, or murder

(especially in older children). Children with separation anxiety may become withdrawn, apathetic, depressed, and unable to concentrate. . . .

. . . Fortunately, most childhood fears are treatable or fade by themselves, and most children with troubling anxieties are reasonably healthy as adults (although boys and girls over 11 are harder to treat, and their fears are more likely to be symptoms of deeper problems). Shy, avoidant children sometimes become adults with personality disorders, but usually they do not. Children with problems of school refusal ordinarily do not have agoraphobia as adults, although they may be somewhat sensitive and cautious. Even the effects of traumatic stress can be attenuated over the years. This is an area in which mental health professionals and their patients and clients can afford to be optimistic.

Source: *The Harvard Medical School Mental Health Letter.* Vol. 5(2), August, 1988, pp. 1–5.

have also been developed to explain anxiety. Most of these propose that there may be an adrenal imbalance in the nervous or endocrine system of persons suffering from pathological anxiety, though clearly this can explain only part of the problem. Recently, the behavioral model of anxiety has provided much useful information on the origins and treatment of anxiety and anxiety disorders.

LEARNING THEORY AND THE BEHAVIORAL MODEL

Learning theory is at the heart of all behavioral treatment and research. As a result, behavioral treatment methods are based on observable and replicable findings. Since it currently incorporates data from the neurosciences (particularly neuropsychology, psychopharmacology, and ethology), it is gradually gaining stature as a biological model.

According to learning theory, anxiety is widespread because it has biological and survival value. First, all living things demonstrate specific responses to particular dangerous stimuli; there is conclusive evidence that these responses, usually referred to as "species-specific defense reactions," are innate. Second, in all animals, fear responses are remarkably consistent. In humans, the standard response to threat is known as the fight-or-flight mechanism, and its autonomic responses include tachycardia, increased blood pressure, sweating, and raised muscle tone and respiration rate. These are, of course, the effects that most ideally prepare us for either fighting or fleeing. It is the fight-or-flight response that causes us to tremble and feel faint when an anticipated threat fails to materialize. Third, common irrational fears in humans can be perceived as falling into a very few broad categories. These are:

- the presence or absence of other people
- some small animals
- open or enclosed spaces
- injury and illness

All the above can be perceived as long-standing threats to humans, and it has been argued (Seligman, 1971) that these fears have a biological survival value in that they trigger behaviors which result in survival for a given individual or group when it may be jeopardized. This phylogenetic selectivity of fears has been termed "preparedness," a concept which suggests that, because of innate characteristics of the central nervous system, we are much more prone to develop fears of the above four situations and objects than any others.

Hebb (1946) demonstrated that infant chimpanzees who were reared in isolation showed no fear of snakes when they were younger than three months old. As they got older, the chimpanzees showed considerable alarm when exposed to snakes. Since no social or other influences could have been occurring, the only reasonable conclusion is that a fear of snakes in chimpanzees is innate and dependent on the level of maturity of the central nervous system. Clearly it is impossible to carry out similar experiments with human infants, although most parents will be familiar with the sudden emergence of minor fears in their offspring and the equally rapid disappearance of those fears. (See Boxes 8–1 and 8–2.)

By far the most useful definition of anxiety (in terms of theoretical and clinical applicability) is provided by Lang (1967), who emphasizes three separate but connected response systems to fear-provoking stimuli. These are:

1. *Behavioral responses:* the readiness of the individual to approach or avoid an object, animal, person, or situation.

2. *Cognitions:* those thoughts and attitudes a person has about objects, animals, people, and situations.

3. *Autonomic effects:* the involuntary bodily responses to anxiety, which include increased heart rate, respiration, and sweat-gland activity.

These three systems are usually congruent with one another in the sense that negative cognitions about a situation are accompanied by autonomic arousal and the behavioral response of avoidance. However, in some situations this congruence or "synchrony" breaks down. For example, it would be difficult to account for important but underresearched issues such as courage without recourse to a model that allows synchrony and desynchrony between response systems. It would also be difficult to account for the effects of both pharmacological and psychological interventions. For example, it would appear that antianxiety drugs such as benzodiazepines have an effect on physiological indices of anxiety and appraisal of threat but not on the behavioral measure of approach and avoidance. Similarly, the process of change during psychological treatment of phobic anxiety seems to involve an initial behavioral change that is followed by autonomic changes (such as reduction in heart rate) and finally, sometimes after considerable delay, by attitudinal and other cognitive changes.

It would also be useful at this point to attempt to account for the fact that some people appear to be more prone to fear and anxiety than others. Since the

Box 8–2 ● Animal Models of Psychopathology: The Acquisition of Fear

In her work with an animal model of the acquisition of fear, Mineka (1987) has shown that anxiety and fear can be learned through the observation of a fearful model. She has also found support for the "preparedness hypothesis" for certain fears. That is, it is biologically adaptive (and so, more likely) for an animal to fear a snake than a flower.

Mineka has demonstrated learning of fear with fear-relevant stimuli such as snakes and spiders. She has also shown that despite the likelihood of her animal subjects (rhesus monkeys) developing intense and lasting fear of snakes through vicarious conditioning (watching *another* animal behave fearfully when exposed to a snake), they can be "immunized" against the development of fear of snakes. She has done this by first exposing the monkey subject to another animal behaving non-fearfully in the presence of a snake.

Mineka's findings support the idea that many human fears and phobias have their origins in observa-tional learning. Her findings also lend credence to the idea that viewing certain unpleasant situations or fearful behaviors on television can affect the psychological state and behavior of a viewer, especially a younger viewer who may not have previously been exposed to a similar but more pleasant or positive situation. For example, a young child who has had no prior positive contact with a dog is vulnerable to developing a phobic fear of dogs after even brief, vicarious exposure to an aggressive, attacking dog on television. He might also develop such a phobia after seeing a parent frightened by even a non-threatening animal.

Research on treatment of laboratory induced fears and phobias using the animal model is in progress.

Source: Mineka, Susan (1987). A primate model of phobic fears. In H. Eysenck & I. Martin (Eds.) *Theoretical Foundations of Behavior Therapy.* New York: Plenum Press.

---

degree of propensity to anxiety seems to be a durable characteristic of individuals, it is worth considering whether innate personality factors could account for this. (See Box 8–3.)

Eysenck (1967) proposed a two-dimensional model of personality with two unrelated scales (neuroticism/stability and extraversion/introversion) which, if correct, does account for individual differences in proneness to fear. By *neuroticism*, Eysenck means the extent to which the autonomic nervous system is reactive to incoming stimuli in terms of extensity and intensity of response.

Everyone knows people who seem to respond minimally to quite intense stimulation (such as a sudden loud noise) and others who show dramatic responses to minor stimuli (the proverbial pin dropping). **Neuroticism,** therefore, refers to the *lability of the autonomic nervous system*—how readily and intensely an individual responds to events. It is important to be clear about this, since the word neurotic has at least two other usages. Formerly, in psychiatry, neurotic served as a global classificatory term for a group of psychological disorders for the purpose of distinguishing them from another group, described as psychotic. This classification was dropped in DSM-III, although the term is still used in practice by many professionals. In lay terms, neuroticism is also used, often pejoratively, to describe behavior that is considered to be in some way maladaptive or annoying to others.

Extraversion, in this context, also has a meaning different from its everyday usage. Here it indicates a normally distributed variation in basal levels of cortical arousal. The implications of this are that those at one end of the scale—extraverts—with very low levels of internal arousal will tend to be stimulus seeking in their interaction with the environment, while those at the other end—**introverts**—will tend to be stimulus avoiders, due to high levels of internal arousal. The more important implication of extraversion/introversion for our current purpose, however, is the finding (Eysenck, 1967) that introverts more readily acquire conditioned responses to stressful stimuli than do extraverts.

Box 8–3 ● The Roles of Temperament and Environment in the Development of a Predisposition to Fearfulness

Suomi (1983) has used an animal model to study the roles of intrinsic temperament and environment on social development and the development of a predisposition to fearfulness, as measured behaviorally (through observation of a subject's distress) and physiologically (through plasma cortisol and indices of autonomic reactivity).

In his studies of rhesus monkeys, Suomi found that:

1. Different measures of autonomic reactivity appear to correlate with each other when subjects are exposed to stressful situations but not under baseline conditions.

2. Individual differences on these measures appear to be quite stable during development: monkeys who display extreme reactions early in life are also likely to display extreme reactions as juveniles.

3. Young monkeys who display extreme autonomic reactions to mild stressors are also likely to display extreme behavioral reactions involving fearfulness, anxiety, wariness, and withdrawal when placed in stressful situations.

4. Individual differences in these behavioral reactions to stress also appear to be stable over time and across repeated experiences with stressful events.

5. These individual differences in expressions of fearful and anxious behavior are masked under stable social-environmental conditions, so that monkeys at high risk for extreme physiological and behavioral reactions to stress appear to be totally "normal" in the absence of stress.

The results of Suomi's rhesus-monkey studies carry some interesting implications for human development. The very same factors emphasized in the above analyses of rhesus-monkey social development have been long viewed as important factors in human social development by numerous theorists (Thomas et al., 1968; Bowlby, 1969; Macoby, 1980; Rutter, 1981). Conceptually

the emphasis has usually been on single factors rather than on possible interactions among them (Suomi, 1981). Indeed, if anything, it seems likely that the interactions of these various factors would be even more complex for young humans than they apparently are for young monkeys.

Nevertheless, it can be argued that the conceptual framework for describing and understanding individual differences in monkey development could be readily applied to analysis of individual differences in human social development. Although human infants and children are not usually appropriate or practical subjects for controlled prospective developmental research (and it takes much longer for them to grow up than it does for monkey infants), some generalizations about the two species can be made. If, for example, the same type of autonomic indices of fearfulness and anxiety are stable throughout development for human children as they apparently are for monkey youngsters, they could provide valuable assessment tools for clinical investigators dealing with problems of human social development, for example, the development of fearfulness.

Thus the study of individual differences in monkey development carries with it some promise of extending our conceptual and practical knowledge of social development in human children. The degree to which this promise is realized will ultimately depend not only on the nature and outcome of future primate studies but also on the degree to which they are accepted and utilized by those researchers, educators, and clinicians who deal directly with the children themselves.

Source: Suomi, S. J. (1983). Social development in rhesus monkeys: consideration of individual differences. In A. Oliverio and M. Aupella (Eds.), *Behavior of human infants*. New York: Plenum Press.

If an individual happens to score high on neuroticism and low on extraversion, then he or she will be more likely to have difficulties with anxiety symptoms because of the combination of arousability and conditionability (see Figure 8–1). According to Eysenck, individuals prone to experiencing fear and anxiety would fall in the right upper quadrant, rating high on neuroticism and introversion.

Four main sets of ideas have been presented in this discussion of a behavioral model of anxiety and anxiety disorders. Preparedness accounts for the selectivity of fearful stimuli; individual differences in genetically determined personality dimensions account for variations in susceptibility to anxiety; synchrony and desynchrony explain response patterns in anxiety-provoking situations; and, of course, life experiences account for why an individual develops a particular disorder at a given time in life.

CLINICAL SYNDROMES OF ANXIETY

In our discussion of clinical syndromes of anxiety, we will follow the DSM-III-R classification and examine the diagnostic criteria for each, illustrate each with a detailed case study, and consider the clinical, theoret-

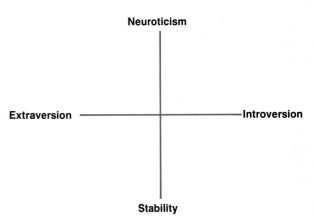

FIGURE 8–1 Eysenck's Model of Personality

ical, and nursing implications of each disorder, using the concepts discussed above.

First, some general points about the treatment of anxiety.

TREATMENT OF ANXIETY

MEDICATION. Though widely debated in psychiatric literature, there is little evidence that psychoactive drugs play a useful role in the treatment of any anxiety disorder. This assertion may seem surprising in view of the widespread use of drugs for treatment, but the evidence from clinical research indicates that their therapeutic usefulness has not been proved (Sartory, 1984). There may be value in administering psychoactive drugs for a short period (a few days), when anxiety is related to a situational crisis, but drugs should not be given over the long term in view of the high risk of addiction and the fact that the anxiolytic or anti-anxiety effects diminish as tolerance develops.

The most commonly prescribed drugs are members of the benzodiazepine group, such as the tranquilizers diazepam (Valium) and chlordiazepoxide (Librium). Other agents that are often prescribed include different kinds of antidepressant medication. Again there is no solid evidence of effectiveness to support this practice. Some evidence indicates that certain antidepressant drugs, MAO inhibitors, are better than placebo drugs for agoraphobics, and that another antidepressant, clomipramine (Anafranil), benefits compulsive ritualizers as long as the drug continues to be taken (Marks, 1982). Beta-blockers (such as propranolol) have also been used, but in one study (Gaind, 1976), these had a *negative* effect in phobic patients (for more information on the use of anti-anxiety medication, see Box 8–4).

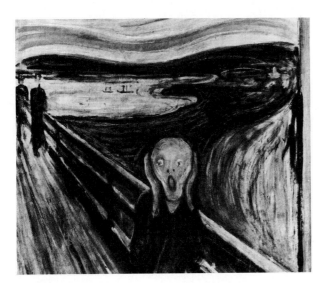

Detail of "The Scream." This very disturbing painting by Edvard Munch seems to reflect the worst kind of anxiety, disintegration anxiety (McDougall, 1985) or the experience of dissolution of the self. This type of anxiety can occur in severe panic states associated with borderline personality disorder, the psychoses, and some of the anxiety disorders, for example, post-traumatic stress disorder in some individuals.

Box 8–4 • Anti-anxiety Medications and Their Use
C. Kate Kavanagh

Medications used to treat anxiety include the sedative-hypnotics (sedative or sleep-inducing drugs), the anti-histamines (used to counteract allergic reactions), and the minor tranquilizers (also referred to as the anxiolytics or antianxiety drugs). These drugs act on the central nervous system to reduce feelings of anxiety, muscular tension, and related physiological symptoms. They tend to produce a calming effect in part by inducing a state of sedation and drowsiness. This feature also makes them useful for treating insomnia caused by tension and worry. While the sedatives and anti-histamines are sometimes used to relieve anxiety, they have significant problems (they are potentially habit-forming and may be lethal if taken as an overdose) which generally make then less useful than the minor tranquilizers.

Indications and Administration

The benzodiazepines are among the most often used anti-anxiety medications. This class of drugs includes two closely related chemical compounds, chlordiazepoxide (Librium) and diazepam (Valium) (See Table A).

Although diazepam is more potent on a milligram-for-milligram basis, they otherwise possess effects and properties which are quite similar. Both are useful for relieving the feelings and physical symptoms of mild to moderate anxiety as described pre-

TABLE A Summary of anti-anxiety medications (minor tranquilizers)

Indications	Drugs	Adult Dosage Range	
Conditions: feelings of tension, anxiety, apprehension muscle tension restlessness insomnia	chlordiazepoxide (Librium)	Initial: 10–25 mg bid–qid Maintenance: 25–50 mg/day Upper Limits: 50–75 mg/day IM or IV 25–50 mg	Contraindications: hypersensitivity; glaucoma; psychosis comatose state; other drugs; liver disease Common Side Effects: drowsiness; unsteady gait; decreased coordination Complications: cumulative effects; withdrawal seizures; drowsiness; drug dependence
	diazepam (Valium)	Initial 2–10 mg bid-qid Maintenance: 10–20 mg/day Upper Limits: 20 mg/day IM or IV 2–10 mg	

Source: *Basic Psychotherapeutics: A Programmed Text*, by C. Warner Johnson, M. D., John R. Snibbe, Ph.D., and Leonard A. Evans, Ph.D., (1980). Jamaica, NY: Spectrum Publications, Inc.

viously. In addition, they also possess muscle relaxant and anti-convulsant properties. For this reason, they are of particular value in the treatment of muscle spasms, muscle tension and in drug and/or alcohol withdrawal states in which seizures may occur. These minor tranquilizers also relieve rest-lessness associated with a variety of medical illnesses. Both medications can be used to induce sleep and com-monly are employed for presurgical relaxation and analgesia. Chlordiaze-poxide and diazepam are *not* recom-mended for the treatment of func-tional psychoses (for example, schizophreniform disorder or schizo-phrenia) (Johnson et al., 1980, pp 161–162).

These drugs generally are ad-ministered in oral form and have an onset of therapeutic effect within two to four hours. Minor tranquilizers are most effective when taken for short

TABLE B Characteristics of benzodiazepines used in the United States

Administered Drug (Year Introduced)	Approved Indications	Rate of Appearance After Oral Dose	Active Substances in Blood*	Overall Rate of Elimination
Chlordiazepoxide (1960)	Anxiety Alcohol withdrawal Preoperative sedation	Intermediate	Chlordiazepoxide Desmethylchlordiazepoxide Demoxepam Desmethyldiazepam	Slow
Diazepam (1961)	Anxiety Alcohol withdrawal Muscle spasm Preoperative sedation Status epilepticus	Rapid	Diazepam Desmethyldiazepam	Slow
Oxazepam (1963)	Anxiety Anxiety-depression Alcohol withdrawal	Intermediate to slow	Oxazepam	Intermediate to rapid
Flurazepam (1970)	Insomnia	Rapid to intermediate	Hydroxyethyl flurazepam [Flurazepam aldehyde] Desalkylflurazepam	Slow
Clorazepate (1972)	Anxiety Seizure disorders Alcohol withdrawal	Rapid	Desmethyldiazepam	Slow
Clonazepam (1974)	Seizure disorders	Intermediate	Clonazepam	Intermediate
Lorazepam (1977)	Anxiety Anxiety-depression Preoperative sedation	Intermediate	Lorazepam	Intermediate
Prazepam (1977)	Anxiety	Slow	Desmethyldiazepam	Slow
Temazepam (1981)	Insomnia	Intermediate to slow	Temazepam	Intermediate
Alprazolam (1981)	Anxiety Anxiety-depression	Intermediate	Alprazolam	Intermediate
Halazepam (1981)	Anxiety	Intermediate to slow	[Halazepam] Desmethyldiazepam	Slow
Triazolam (1983)	Insomnia	Intermediate	Triazolam	Rapid

*Brackets indicate compounds of minor quantitative importance.

Source: Greenblatt, D. J., Shader, R. I., & Abernathy, D. R. (1983). New England Journal of Medicine, Vol. 309:6, p. 355.

periods (days to a few weeks) and intermittently when symptoms are problematic. The therapeutic potency decreases and the likelihood of drug dependency increases if either of these medications are used at constant dosages for longer than a few weeks. The oral route is the usual mode of administration. See Table A for dosage, contraindications, and side effects (Johnson et al., 1980).

Nursing Considerations

The nurse needs to be familiar with the clinical indications for the benzodiazepines (See Table B), widely prescribed for nighttime sedation, delirium tremens, anxiety related to pain, and anticonvulsant use as well as for the reduction of acute anxiety in some cases. The nurse needs to stress to the patient that tolerance develops rapidly to the anti-anxiety effects of these drugs, and, if unusual circumstances require their administration beyond several weeks, drug-free intervals can be helpful in avoiding a regular stepwise increase in dosage (Abrams, 1983). The slow rate of elimination of many of these drugs requires the nurse to point out the potential danger of combining any of them with alcohol or other central nervous system depressants, especially when driving or operating machinery (Greenblatt et al., 1983). Patients with chronic disabling anxiety with associated insomnia, depression, phobias, obsessions/compulsions, depersonalization/derealization, hypochondriasis or somatic symptoms need to know that treatment with the benzodiazepines may make their situation worse as increasing dosages (and associated physical addiction) will be required to maintain the status quo (Abrams, 1983). Special care should be taken when administering anti-anxiety medications to the elderly, debilitated, those with impaired renal or liver functions or those with compromised respiration, as these drugs tend to accumulate in the body producing an overdose effect (Johnson et al., 1980).

Generally, large oral overdoses of benzodiazepines taken alone are almost never lethal. They should be withdrawn gradually after prolonged or excessive use to avoid withdrawal symptoms (insomnia, nausea, twitching, sweating, irritability, and, in some instances, convulsions) that may pose serious risk in some cases (The Medical Letter, May 13, 1983).

Abrams, R. (1983). Psychopharmacology and ECT. In B. Wolman (Ed.) *The Therapist's Handbook, Treatment Methods of Mental Disorders*. New York: Van Nostrand Reinhold, pp. 31–33.

Greenblatt, D. J., Shader, R. I., & Abernathy, D. R. (1983). Current status of benzodiazepines. *The New England Journal of Medicine*, August 11, 1983, pp. 354–357.

The Medical Letter on Drugs and Therapeutics, May 13, 1983, Vol. 25, (635), pp. 45–46.

Johnson, C. W., Snibbe, J. R., & Evans, L. A. (1980). Pharmacologic therapy. *Basic Psychotherapeutics*. New York; S. P. Medical and Scientific Books, pp. 161–163.

OTHER THERAPIES. Various kinds of group, individual, family, and milieu or environmental therapies have their adherents, but there is no clear evidence that these play a useful role in the management of anxiety disorders. However, it is probably true that some support can help the sufferer from chronic anxiety to cope with everyday life. Rachman (1971) has provided a detailed and authoritative review of the evidence for and against various psychotherapies and his conclusion that their use cannot be justified has so far not been seriously challenged.

In discussing the various clinical disorders, we will consider treatments that have been subject to rigorous clinical evaluation and that have demonstrated their usefulness in dealing with anxiety disorders. This is not to argue against the use of all psychoactive drugs nor the use of some psychotherapies that have not been proven effective in clinical research using the experimental method. It simply happens that there is solid evidence that supports approaches with a basis in the behavioral model for treatment of anxiety disorders.

ANXIETY STATE OR ANXIETY NEUROSIS

Anxiety state, or **anxiety neurosis,** takes two forms: panic disorder and generalized anxiety disorder.

PANIC DISORDER

Symptoms and Manifestations of Panic Disorder. Panic disorder is characterized by unpredictable, acute attacks of anxiety that are not specific to a particular situation. The individual suffering from panic disorder tends to experience both intense apprehension, often described as a feeling that he or she is about to die, and a number of physical manifestations that include:

- dyspnea
- palpitations
- choking sensations
- dizziness or vertigo
- depersonalization or derealization
- sweating
- shaking

DSM-III-R Diagnostic Criteria for Panic Disorder

A. At some time during the disturbance, one or more panic attacks (discrete periods of intense fear or discomfort) have occurred that were (1) unexpected, i.e., did not occur immediately before or on exposure to a situation that almost always caused anxiety, and (2) not triggered by situations in which the person was the focus of others' attention.

B. Either four attacks, as defined in criterion A, have occurred within a four-week period, or one or more attacks have been followed by a period of at least a month of persistent fear of having another attack.

C. At least four of the following symptoms developed during at least one of the attacks:

1) shortness of breath (dyspnea) or smothering sensations
2) dizziness, unsteady feelings, or faintness
3) palpitations or accelerated heart rate (tachycardia)
4) trembling or shaking
5) sweating
6) choking
7) nausea or abdominal distress
8) depersonalization or derealization
9) numbness or tingling sensations (paresthesias)
10) flushes (hot flashes) or chills
11) chest pain or discomfort
12) fear of dying
13) fear of going crazy or of doing something uncontrolled

Note: Attacks involving four or more symptoms are panic attacks; attacks involving fewer than four symptoms are limited symptom attacks (see Agoraphobia without History of Panic Disorder).

D. During at least some of the attacks, at least four of the C symptoms developed suddenly and increased in intensity within ten minutes of the beginning of the first C symptom noticed in the attack.

E. It cannot be established that an organic factor initiated and maintained the disturbance, e.g., Amphetamine or Caffeine Intoxication, hyperthyroidism.

Note: Mitral valve prolapse may be an associated condition, but does not preclude a diagnosis of Panic Disorder.

Attacks vary in length—most last only a few minutes, but some can continue for hours. Typically, the person who is prone to panic attacks lives in dread of them and may be reluctant to be alone or far away from medical aid. If this becomes very marked, the individual's functioning can become quite impaired and his or her lifestyle restricted.

Onset of panic disorder is usually in early adult life, although later onset is not uncommon. The natural history of the disorder can consist of a single episode lasting several weeks, recurrences from time to time, or chronicity. Panic disorder appears to be slightly more common in women than in men and a frequent complication is tranquilizer or alcohol dependency.

Treatments for Panic Disorder. Several classes of psychotropic drugs have been used to treat panic disorder, including the benzodiazepines (Alprazolam) and antidepressants such as imipramine (Tofranil). Because of the risks of dependence and other limitations associated with the benzodiazepines, behavioral therapies such as differential relaxation (Goldfried & Davison, 1976) and other coping strategies such as supported exposure and pleasant mental imagery have been used with success in individual cases (see Ost, 1985). To date no controlled evaluation has taken place that clearly indicates a useful and generally applicable approach to the treatment of panic disorder. It may be helpful to consider the person's lifestyle in an effort to either reduce stress or remove possible contributory factors (McDonald et al., 1979). Some people find exercise, preferably aerobic, useful in reducing the frequency of panics. Anyone who ingests more than a minimal amount of caffeine (see Greden, 1974) should be encouraged to stop completely.

It is important to encourage the individual to deal with any situational avoidances that have occurred by asking him or her to practice entering these situations in a systematic way.

Allan: A Panic-Disorder Victim

Allan was 42 years old at the time of his referral to the mental-health center. He complained of panic attacks that occurred five to six times a week, without predictability. These were characterized by a feeling of apprehension, tightness in the chest, tremor, sweating, and dyspnea. The panic attacks could last anywhere from ten minutes to twenty-four hours. He usually left whatever situation he was in at the onset of a panic episode but could identify no triggers for the episodes and had no way of terminating them. This problem had been present for nineteen years and had not responded to previous treatments, including hypnosis and relaxation training.

Allan avoided social situations such as parties and eating in company because he was afraid he would panic and embarrass himself. His intake of alcohol and caffeine was moderate and his drug use was restricted to 1 mg of lorazepam (Ativan) at the onset of panic.

Allan had no other emotional problems and there was no family history of anxiety or other psychiatric disorders. His personal history was unremarkable. He was an average scholar and had spent twelve years in the Navy after leaving school. Since leaving the Navy he had been employed in public transport in a supervisory post. Allan married at age twenty-five, had two children, and, at the time of his referral, had been separated from his wife for just over two years because they "argued too often." He continued to see his family regularly and they got along better after the separation.

Allan was advised to discontinue the use of lorazepam and to remain in social situations when his symptoms appeared. To help him do this, he was trained in simple relaxation techniques involving breathing control and was given a detailed explanation of the mechanisms of anxiety to help him understand the phenomena he was experiencing. He found that this regime reduced the duration and intensity of his attacks. After two months, the frequency of his attacks had dropped to once every two weeks and he rated himself as being ninety percent improved. This improvement was maintained throughout followup.

GENERALIZED ANXIETY DISORDER

Symptoms of Generalized Anxiety Disorder. The second type of nonsituational anxiety disorder is **generalized anxiety disorder.** The patient usually experiences a diffuse feeling of apprehension and physiological symptoms which can be virtually constant but which lack the intensity of panic attacks. The symptoms are usually as follows:

1. *Motor tension:* shakiness, tension, restlessness, fatigue, ease in startling, and sighing respiration.

2. *Autonomic hyperactivity:* sweating, palpitations, dry mouth, dizziness, paresthesia, gastric irritation, frequency of urination, pallor or flushing, and rapid breathing.

3. *Apprehension:* a sense of impending doom, excessive worry about trivial matters or potential mishaps, and undue concern about health of self and significant others.

4. *Vigilance:* constant watchfulness for possible dangers, irritability and impatience, and difficulty in getting to and maintaining sleep.

Generalized anxiety disorder may start at any point in an individual's life, although a history of excessive worry and responsivity is common. There seems to be a fairly equal distribution between the sexes and no consistent familial patterns have emerged.

Generalized anxiety can pose a difficult diagnostic problem because many physical disorders can mimic an anxiety state: hyperthyroidism, Cushing's syndrome, hypoparathyroidism, pheochromocytoma, hypoglycemia, mitral valve prolapse, paroxysmal tachycardia, temporal lobe epilepsy, food and chemical allergies, caffeinism, and hyperventilation. McCue and McCue (1984) provide a useful review of this area.

Since both caffeinism and hyperventilation are common, the patient should be checked routinely for these. A straightforward way of testing for hyperventilation as a cause of anxiety symptoms is to use a provocation test in which the individual voluntarily

DSM-III-R Diagnostic Criteria for Generalized Anxiety Disorder

A. Unrealistic or excessive anxiety and worry (apprehensive expectation) about two or more life circumstances, e.g., worry about possible misfortune to one's child (who is in no danger) and worry about finances (for no good reason), for a period of six months or longer, during which the person has been bothered more days than not by these concerns. In children and adolescents, this may take the form of anxiety and worry about academic, athletic, and social performance.

B. If another Axis I disorder is present, the focus of the anxiety and worry in A is unrelated to it, e.g., the anxiety or worry is not about having a panic attack (as in Panic Disorder), being embarrassed in public (as in Social Phobia), being contaminated (as in Obsessive Compulsive Disorder), or gaining weight (as in Anorexia Nervosa).

C. The disturbance does not occur only during the course of a Mood Disorder or a psychotic disorder.

D. At least 6 of the following 18 symptoms are often present when anxious (do not include symptoms present only during panic attacks):

Motor tension

1) trembling, twitching, or feeling shaky
2) muscle tension, aches, or soreness
3) restlessness
4) easy fatigability

Autonomic hyperactivity

5) shortness of breath or smothering sensations
6) palpitations or accelerated heart rate (tachycardia)
7) sweating, or cold clammy hands
8) dry mouth
9) dizziness or lightheadedness
10) nausea, diarrhea, or other abdominal distress
11) flushes (hot flashes) or chills
12) frequent urination
13) trouble swallowing or "lump in throat"

Vigilance and scanning

14) feeling keyed up or on edge
15) exaggerated startle response
16) difficulty concentrating or "mind going blank" because of anxiety
17) trouble falling or staying asleep
18) irritability

E. It cannot be established that an organic factor initiated and maintained the disturbance, e.g., hyperthyroidism, Caffeine Intoxication.

---

overbreathes for two to three minutes. If symptoms recognizable as those attributed to anxiety are produced, then hyperventilation is probably playing a causal role in symptom production. The provocation test and techniques for correcting hyperventilation are fully described by Lum (1977).

Excessive amounts of caffeine, usually derived from coffee and tea but also present in cola drinks and nonprescription analgesics, can also cause symptoms that are indistinguishable from generalized anxiety disorder. Withdrawing caffeine from the person's diet is an easy test. Caffeine-dependent individuals

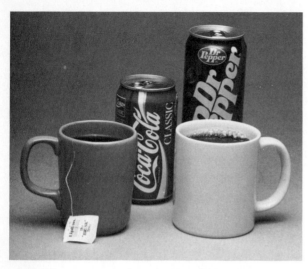

Coffee isn't the only popular beverage containing caffeine. Tea contains as much caffeine as coffee, and some soft drinks contain more than both.

typically respond to withdrawal by developing a moderate to severe headache approximately eighteen hours after cessation. Greden et al. (1980) demonstrated a positive correlation between caffeine intake and anxiety and depression. The correlation existed also for anxiolytic medication.

It is also worth considering whether short-term **withdrawal** from central nervous system depressants such as alcohol and tranquilizers may be contributing to an individual's anxious feelings. Onset of benzodiazapine withdrawal is sometimes delayed for as long as two weeks after the last dose.

Assuming that all the above can be ruled out, no current stressor can be identified, and no other psychiatric disorder is present, then the mental-health professional can consider the appropriate treatment for generalized anxiety disorder.

Treatment for Generalized Anxiety Disorder. Relaxation training, usually based on Jacobson's (1938) method, has been widely employed with a number of variants. Jacobson noted that in some emotional states there is an increase in striate muscle tension. He developed a technique that aimed to teach the individual to relax major muscle groups. Wolpe (1958) used this relaxation method in a technique he termed "systematic desensitization," based on the notion that pairing an anxiety-producing stimulus with a competing one—in this case, deep muscle relaxation—would lead to a reduction in the amount of anxiety produced. Though Wolpe developed his approach as a means of treating phobic and situational problems, other researchers have since attempted to apply a modified approach to generalized anxiety disorder.

Goldfried (1971) taught his patients relaxation skills and then coping skills—responding to the first sign of anxiety by relaxing. While this approach does seem to have some value in experimental volunteers who are moderately anxious, there is no firm evidence that patients with generalized anxiety disorder can be helped. A similar problem has been encountered by Suinn and Richardson (1971), who used a very similar approach called **anxiety management training.** This, too, appears to be useful when applied to nonclinical populations but, apart from single-case reports, there is no convincing evidence that significant numbers of patients can be helped. Other researchers (Townsend, House, & Addario, 1975) used relaxation with biofeedback (some type of electronic signal that indicates the level of muscle tension present) with chronically anxious patients. While the short-term results seemed to show that tension was significantly reduced in the experimental situation, there was no convincing evidence of lasting benefit.

Another treatment that has been employed is **stress inoculation** (Meichenbaum & Turk, 1976). This treatment involves instruction on mechanisms of anxiety, teaching coping skills (particularly coping statements, which the individual practices by saying to himself, "I can cope; anxiety can't hurt me"), and rehearsing the use of these coping skills while faced with artificial stressors (such as the threat of electric shock). While this approach seems promising, there is no clear evidence of its wide-scale applicability. The lack of a proven method of dealing with generalized anxiety disorder is particularly disappointing since this disorder probably outnumbers all other clinical anxiety disorders and could account for as much as thirty percent of visits to primary-care physicians.

Betty: A Victim of Generalized Anxiety Disorder

Betty is a 35-year-old, married woman who was referred by her primary physician to the mental-health clinic for treatment of anxiety that she had been experiencing for over a decade. She complained of fluctuating levels of apprehension, insomnia, palpitations, giddiness, lethargy, and an inability to concentrate.

She was often tearful and unhappy but was not clinically depressed. She had been taking benzodiazepines of various kinds for eight years and, when referred, was taking 30 mg diazepam in divided doses daily. She led a rather restricted life, spending most of her time at home, but there were no situations she could not enter if absolutely necessary.

Betty comes from a stable, working-class background and there is no family history of psychological disorder. She was nocturnally eneuretic (a bedwetter) until the age of eight, and sucked her thumb until age eleven. When she was thirteen, she refused to go to school for several weeks.

Betty was a below-average student and left school at age fifteen with no specific work skills; she worked in a department store for two and a half years before marrying. She had three children during the first five years of her marriage and has not worked since the birth of the first. Her marriage appeared stable but her relationship with her husband seemed distant and lacking in warmth.

Betty's main reason for seeking treatment was her concern about recent publicity about the dangers of long-term benzodiazepine use and, as she told the nurse, her own feeling that she was "living in a dream."

Betty was gradually weaned from diazepam over a period of three months. (Gradual weaning is essential when there has been daily use for one month or longer to avoid life-threatening central nervous system decompensation.) She found this difficult and, for a time, experienced an upsurge in her symptoms, especially insomnia. However, she persevered and eventually became drug free and reported a sharpening of her senses and a greater feeling of well-being than she had experienced for some years.

At the same time, the nurse encouraged Betty to make some changes in her lifestyle. Since she had been a keen swimmer when she was a teenager, she was encouraged to swim an hour a day as part of her daily routine. She found part-time employment working in a sandwich bar, which afforded her a wider range of social contacts. She found this new regime helpful and, although still experiencing some anxiety symptoms, she rated herself as being seventy-five percent improved after one month of treatment.

Betty's improvement was stable at her one-year followup, although she had a brief relapse when an illness prevented her from undertaking her daily swim.

AGORAPHOBIA

There are two DSM-III-R categories of **agoraphobia,** depending on whether panic attacks are part of the clinical presentation or not. The main characteristic of both categories is fear and avoidance of busy public places, particularly if escape or assistance is not immediately available. In addition, other characteristics of agoraphobia are: excessive dependence on others, episodes of depersonalization (the perception

that the body is unreal, floating, or dead) or derealization (the perception that the environment is unreal), concern that some physical or social catastrophe will occur, mild depression, an emphasis on physical manifestations of anxiety (such as giddiness, dyspnea, and cardiac phenomena), and use of anxiolytic agents sometimes to the extent of addiction. Usually, the person's life is markedly restricted and fewer and fewer activities are undertaken as time goes on.

Onset is typically in the early twenties and women are more likely to be affected than men. The course of agoraphobia is unpredictable: sometimes the handicap is minimal and other times the symptoms are particularly severe. There may be a relationship between adult agoraphobia and childhood difficulties in separating from parents. Many agoraphobics find that they are considerably more mobile when a parent (or, later, spouse) accompanies them in public. A remarkably incapacitating disorder, it is not uncommon for an agoraphobic to find him or herself housebound for many years, or even decades, with the resulting social and interpersonal impairment that this entails.

The onset of agoraphobia tends to be associated either with an attack of panic in a public place or a series of events in which the person feels distinctly uncomfortable in a public setting, followed by increasing avoidance of similar situations over a period of months or years. Unless there is intervention, chronicity is the likely endpoint, with fluctuations in severity merely affording a slightly increased range of mobility.

SAFETY SIGNALS. Current theoretical models of agoraphobia emphasize the importance of **safety signals** (Gray, 1972) and neuroticism (that is, susceptibility to stressors). The concept of safety signals is interesting as a possible explanation of onset and of some of the observed phenomena of the syndrome. Safety signals are environmental cues that indicate the absence of danger. They can be external (for example, the presence of a trusted person or the sight of familiar territory) or internal (as in the case of particular feeling states). It is noteworthy that the onset of agoraphobia is frequently associated with loss of a significant person, either by death, change in social circumstances, or a change in lifestyle. Fluctuations in symptomatology frequently can be attributed to changes in the availability of such safety cues. Since everyone uses safety signals in daily life, it has been suggested that deprivation of these familiar cues will provoke anxiety in the same way that the appearance of a novel stimulus (Sokolov, 1960) will provoke increased attention and arousal.

Rachman (1984) has explicated in some detail the possible contribution of safety signals to the genesis and maintenance of agoraphobia and has concluded that a safety-signal model accounts for 1) the persistence of agoraphobic symptoms; 2) fluctuations in degree of fear; 3) the delineation of anxiety in space and time; and 4) the consistent theme of a search for safety. The first of these points is worth exploring further.

Agoraphobia is an example of unusually persistent avoidance behavior. Clinicians who have treated many agoraphobics are familiar with the phenomenon of people who have been housebound for many years discovering, with treatment, that they are not nearly as afraid of the outside world as they had expected. The safety-signal theorist would attempt to explain this phenomenon by saying that although *avoidance* of fear-provoking situations may have been instrumental in initiating the phobic behavior, the continuation of the behavior is dependent on the *positively reinforcing* effects of signals of safety.

Alice: An Agoraphobic

Alice was an agoraphobic who had not left her home for twenty years. When a mental-health professional visited her and suggested that they walk together to the local shops, she agreed with some reluctance. To her surprise, she experienced minimal anxiety and was able to walk around with ease. Then they got on a downtown bus, something Alice could not imagine doing at the assessment interview, and wandered round the major department stores, which were, as always, extremely busy. Again, Alice experienced very low levels of anxiety. Alice was extremely puzzled by this as she had long believed that these were things she could not do. She was sad and disappointed about the time she described as her "wasted years." What accounts for the wasted years is not primarily the aversive (anxiety-provoking) events that initiated her avoidance of public places, but her need for places of safety and the feeling of confidence found there. This, of course, is not a universal experience. It remains true that the vast majority of agoraphobics suffer marked anxiety when first trying to increase their boundaries.

TREATMENT FOR AGORAPHOBIA. Treatment for agoraphobia may differ depending on whether or not the agoraphobia is accompanied by panic attacks. When agoraphobia exists without panic attacks, the usual treatment consists entirely of behavioral psychotherapy that encourages exposure to the phobic situation. When panic attacks accompany agoraphobia, however, one common approach is to use medication to block the attack so that patients can be encouraged to reenter the phobic situation and demonstrate to themselves that they will no longer have attacks (Hollander, Liebowitz, Gorman, 1989 p. 467). But because drugs may in fact exacerbate the condition by creating dependency and symptom rebound upon withdrawal, others feel it is best to rely completely on behavioral psychotherapy; in a review of this area, Marks has recommended that the behavioral approach be used for any sufferer of agoraphobia (Marks, 1981).

Christine: An Agoraphobic

Christine was 29 years old at the time of her referral to the Mental-Health Center. She had been afraid of walking alone through open spaces, shopping centers, and streets for fourteen years in case someone attacked her or she became ill and no assistance was available. The problem had worsened during the previous year after her relationship with her husband became strained. She had spent six years in individual and group psychotherapy, during which time her symptoms worsened. She was taking 30 mg of the tranquilizer chlordiazepoxide (Librium) a day and always carried her bottle of capsules with her.

There was nothing in Christine's background to indicate a predisposition to the disorder. She was married to a telephone engineer, and, although anorgasmic, she was happy with their sexual relationship. She had two children.

Christine was treated by **graded** or gradual **exposure** in real life in conjunction with cessation of her medication. Graded exposure involved her entering crowded shopping areas and similar fear-provoking situations, initially accompanied by her therapist and then alone, remaining in these situations until her anxiety reduced. She had nine sessions of treatment, with each session taking an average of an hour and a half. By the end of treatment, she was able to enter any situation she desired with only minimal and occasional unease. She maintained her improvement during followup and went on to organize a self-help group for other agoraphobics.

Consider how this seemingly very simple treatment works. Using the cognitive-behavioral-autonomic model proposed by Peter Lange (1978), the nurse or therapist would be creating initial desynchrony between these three response systems by initially altering overt behavior from avoidance to approach. The patient experiences a decrease in autonomic responses via the process termed habituation. Finally, perhaps after some delay, the patient experiences changes in attitudinal and other cognitive aspects that combine to form a new, and less fearful, synchrony. Consider the case of Christine.

Initially, Christine's therapist encouraged her to enter all situations that she had previously avoided. Christine experienced the autonomic concomitants of anxiety which, in her case, included giddiness and palpitations. Eventually these experiences waned, accompanied by a reduction in her subjective rating of anxiety.

Within an hour of the start of the first session, which involved Christine traveling on a bus accompanied by her therapist, she reported herself as calm; her heart rate had dropped from 120 to 75 beats per minute. When a patient has experienced this virtually universal sequence of events a few times, she becomes much more confident that it will work and becomes able to take on more of the treatment herself. Indeed, recent work (Ghosh, Marks, & Carr, 1984) suggests that as many as sixty percent of agoraphobics may be able to treat themselves successfully with the aid of detailed therapy instruction, whether provided by a therapist, a book, or a computer program.

Twenty to thirty hours of exposure practice in previously fear-provoking situations is sufficient to generate confidence that avoidance is no longer necessary in the typical agoraphobic. This leads to a change in attitude about herself, her abilities, and the outside world, with associated beneficial changes in mood state and functioning in social and work situations. Occasionally, marital difficulties can arise because of the problems the patient's spouse has in adjusting to such changes, but the likelihood and impact of this can be limited by involving the spouse in treatment as a therapy aide. Upon improving, most agoraphobics show no sign of symptom recurrence when followed up for periods of years. When relapses do occur, they are usually precipitated by changes in circumstances or spontaneous dysphoric episodes and can usually be overcome rapidly by reintroducing exposure treatment.

SOCIAL PHOBIA

Social phobia is characterized by fear and avoidance of situations in which the individual may be scrutinized by others or expected to perform a particular social role or activity. The fear is often complicated by deficiencies in social-skill performance, either because avoidance of contact with others has led to lack of opportunity to acquire or practice these skills or because the individual's anxiety is sufficiently high to have a detrimental effect on performance.

We are all, to some extent, socially anxious in that certain situations frighten the vast majority of us, such as addressing large groups of prestigious strangers or being the center of attention at formal social gatherings. For the social phobic, however, many everyday situations generate anxiety. Sometimes the fears are quite specific (such as writing in front of others because of a fear of being embarrassed by a possible tremor), but more often fears tend to be diffuse and therefore cause marked impairment in social functioning.

Onset usually occurs in adolescence and is associated occasionally with parental overprotectiveness or limited social opportunity. Social phobia seems to be about equally common in both sexes, although men may seek help more frequently, perhaps because social role expectations of males have been higher.

Social phobia is usually chronic, with a tendency for the cycle of anxiety, experience of failure, and avoidance to create greater impairment with time. Some social phobics complicate these problems by using anxiolytic agents, particularly alcohol, to combat anxiety. Mood disturbances can occur, particularly in cases that involve diffuse fears, and widespread avoidance leads to loneliness and isolation.

The most common circumscribed social anxieties seem to be associated with public speaking, eating or drinking with others, interactions with people of the opposite sex, sitting facing a stranger on public transport, vomiting in public, blushing, tremors, and maintaining eye contact. The person with diffuse social anxiety is likely to experience several of these.

TREATMENT FOR SOCIAL PHOBIA. Treatment of specific social anxieties is very similar to that described above for agoraphobia. The therapist determines carefully the characteristics of the feared situation and then creates practice situations that are graded by difficulty so the person can work through them, moving to the next level of difficulty when he or she can tackle the previous level with minimum discomfort.

David: A Victim of Social Phobia

David was a 21-year-old accounting student in his third year of study. He was completely unable to eat in the company of others due to a fear of vomiting. This problem had been present for five years and the onset was related to an episode when he had vomited while eating at a friend's house. The episode was due to gastrointestinal illness, and David had felt acutely embarrassed about this. David was an attractive and personable young man who had many friends and

DSM-III-R Diagnostic Criteria for Social Phobia

A. A persistent fear of one or more situations (the social phobic situations) in which the person is exposed to possible scrutiny by others and fears that he or she may do something or act in a way that will be humiliating or embarrassing. Examples include: being unable to continue talking while speaking in public, choking on food when eating in front of others, being unable to urinate in a public lavatory, hand-trembling when writing in the presence of others, and saying foolish things or not being able to answer questions in social situations.

B. If an Axis III or another Axis I disorder is present, the fear in A is unrelated to it, e.g., the fear is not of having a panic attack (Panic Disorder), stuttering (Stuttering), trembling (Parkinson's disease), or exhibiting abnormal eating behavior (Anorexia Nervosa or Bulimia Nervosa).

C. During some phase of the disturbance, exposure to the specific phobic stimulus (or stimuli) almost invariably provokes an immediate anxiety response.

D. The phobic situation(s) is avoided, or is endured with intense anxiety.

E. The avoidant behavior interferes with occupational functioning or with usual social activities or relationships with others, or there is marked distress about having the fear.

F. The person recognizes that his or her fear is excessive or unreasonable.

G. If the person is under 18, the disturbance does not meet the criteria for Avoidant Disorder of Childhood or Adolescence.

Specify generalized type if the phobic situation includes most social situations, and also consider the additional diagnosis of Avoidant Personality Disorder.

---

shared a rented house with a group of fellow students. He had had a girlfriend for three years and enjoyed all social situations that did not involve eating, although he would always fast twelve hours beforehand. There was nothing of note in his history, he had no other psychological difficulties, and he had had no previous treatment.

David was treated during six sessions by graded exposure, initially eating a snack in a very quiet restaurant with his therapist, who then gradually introduced more people and larger meals over succeeding sessions. Within a few sessions David's habituation was rapid and reliable and he was asked to practice similar situations with his girlfriend between sessions. His progress was rapid and, by the end of treatment, he was able to eat with friends with ease and was attending one dinner party and having one meal in a restaurant each week. David's only remaining problem was discomfort and reluctance to eat with his girlfriend's parents, but by his six-month followup he was achieving this regularly and no longer felt anxious.

Social-Skills Training. Treatment of more diffuse social anxieties takes a different form because of the frequent complication of problems in skill performance. The established approach is group **social-skills training.** An impressive literature (Falloon et al., 1977; Trower, Bryant, & Argyle, 1978) attests to its superiority over alternative treatment approaches.

The key components of social-skills training are:

1. *The group setting:* frequently, individuals with severe social anxiety are very isolated socially. The other members of the group can serve as the initial social contacts with whom to practice social skills. It is important that the group be reasonably balanced in sex distribution. Six to eight group members and a male and female cotherapist team are the optimal arrangement.

2. *Role play and modeling:* the group practices relevant social behavior following modeling (such as a demonstration of the behavior the patient is about to attempt). This involves rehearsing social situations that members of the group find difficult in everyday life, beginning with simple behaviors such as exchanging greetings and maintaining eye contact and working up to more complex situations such as job interviews and conversing with strangers.

3. *Homework assignment:* in order to incorporate skills gained in the group setting into real life, it is important for the individual to complete homework tasks relevant to the material covered in the session. These tasks are usually agreed upon by the group at the end of each session with a plan to review them at the beginning of the next. Positive reinforcement by the group for success with experiences serves as a powerful enhancer of motivation.

Eric: Successful at Social-Skills Training

Eric was 31 years old at the time of his referral to the Mental-Health Center. He described himself as having been shy and anxious in all social situations since he was fourteen years old. He found it particularly difficult to interact with women and had only two male friends, whom he saw only once every two to three months. He felt strongly that he could not converse with people because he had nothing to say and because people would think him stupid and unattractive. He was, in fact, an intelligent man who had been very successful academically and who worked as an engineer. His career had been affected by his difficulties because he was unable to speak in the few meetings he attended and he was unable to refuse difficult, even unreasonable, requests made of him.

Eric was unhappy about his social isolation and felt the future was gloomy, but there was no evidence of depression or any other psychiatric abnormality. There was nothing unusual in his personal and medical history and his only previous treatment had been an unsuccessful course of hypnotherapy.

Eric attended nine sessions of group social-skills training, by the end of which he was going out with people his own age two or three times a week, had a girlfriend for the first time in his life, and was able to negotiate improved conditions at work. When seen at followup, Eric maintained his improvement and reported that the only remaining difficulty was some anticipatory anxiety before social situations, but he had noticed that this was beginning to decrease.

Outcome in group treatment of diffuse social anxieties and skills deficits is generally good, although dropouts seem to be a familiar problem and some individuals need continuing encouragement to practice social behaviors over a period of months after treatment.

SIMPLE PHOBIA

Simple phobia is defined as the persistent, irrational fear and avoidance of a particular object or situation. All phobics who do not meet the diagnostic criteria for agoraphobia or social phobia fall into this category. Simple phobia is by far the most common anxiety disorder. Indeed, most people have irrational fears of one kind or another that don't interfere with their lives sufficiently for them to seek therapy.

The very common simple phobias are those involving animals, such as snakes, spiders, rodents, and dogs. Unless these fears are very intense, they are unlikely to interfere with life, and only a small percentage require treatment. However, for some people these fears are so intense that treatment is justified. Examples include a spider phobic who leapt from a moving car when a small spider appeared on the windscreen; a needle phobic who was diabetic and who had been hospitalized in a coma three times in two months because she was unable to allow herself to be injected; and a dog phobic who became virtually housebound as her fear worsened.

More problematic simple phobias, and those for which people are therefore more likely to seek treatment, are claustrophobia and fear of heights (acrophobia). Both involve avoidance of a large number of situations and can easily impair an individual's functioning.

People also seek treatment for fear of flying, usually because of an occupational handicap. Most people who suffer from simple phobias are otherwise well-adjusted individuals and seldom have the accompanying mood disturbances (anxiety and possibly some degree of depression) seen commonly in agoraphobia and social phobia.

Another common phobia that falls into the simple category and deserves separate mention because of important differences in its clinical presentation is blood/injury phobia. The physiological response of the sufferer distinguishes this phobia from others. Initially, someone who is afraid of injections will respond like other phobics by showing increased heart rate and blood pressure. However, this is followed by a sudden drop in both, which frequently results in fainting. While other phobics may fear fainting in anxiety-provoking situations, they very rarely do. An estimate of the prevalence of such fears and the vagal response to them is provided by the incidence of fainting recorded as being as high as 17 percent in blood-donor clinics. This, of course, excluded those who are so afraid of blood or injury that they avoid giving blood.

TREATMENT OF SIMPLE PHOBIAS. Simple phobias were the first phobias to be treated by a behavioral approach. Joseph Wolpe (1958) developed a technique that he termed **systematic desensitization,** which was based on teaching the individual to relax and then asking him or her to imagine the compo-

DSM-III-R Diagnostic Criteria for Simple Phobia

A. A persistent fear of a circumscribed stimulus (object or situation) other than fear of having a panic attack (as in Panic Disorder) or of humiliation or embarrassment in certain social situations (as in Social Phobia).

Note: Do not include fears that are part of Panic Disorder with Agoraphobia or Agoraphobia without History of Panic Disorder.

B. During some phase of the disturbance, exposure to the specific phobic stimulus (or stimuli) almost invariably provokes an immediate anxiety response.

C. The object or situation is avoided, or endured with intense anxiety.

D. The fear or the avoidant behavior significantly interferes with the person's normal routine or with usual social activities or relationships with others, or there is marked distress about having the fear.

E. The person recognizes that his or her fear is excessive or unreasonable.

F. The phobic stimulus is unrelated to the content of the obsessions of Obsessive Compulsive Disorder or the trauma of Post-traumatic Stress Disorder.

---

nents of the phobia on a very graded hierarchy working from least fearful to most fearful. For example, an acrophobic might begin by imagining himself standing on a box two feet high as the first scene and, after around twenty gradations, imagine himself on top of a cliff. The patient would be asked to carry out the activity imagined in the session in real life between sessions.

This approach does work although, compared with current treatments, it is rather slow, since more than twenty sessions are frequently required for very specific fears. In fact, the evidence indicates (McDonald et al., 1979; Greist, Marks, & Noshirvani, 1980) that the most likely reason for improvement in patients treated with systematic desensitization is the between-session practice they undertake rather than the relaxation training or the imagining of feared scenes during a session. The importance of real-life practice in the treatment of phobias has, in fact, been long recognized. Freud made this a part of his treatment of phobics. He wrote:

> One can hardly ever master a phobia if one waits till the patient lets the analysis influence him to give it up . . . one succeeds only when one can induce them by the influence of the analysis to . . . go about alone and to struggle with their anxiety while they make the attempt (1919, pp. 399–400).

In more recent years it has become clear that the most effective treatment for phobias is some variant of graded exposure to the cues that trigger anxiety, either in real life or in imagination, and that additional components such as psychotherapy or relaxation make no measurable contribution to the outcome. This area is reviewed in greater detail by Emmelkamp (1982).

The nurse or therapist must consider which of the many variants of exposure treatment to use in different clinical situations. By and large, real-life exposure seems preferable (Watson, Mullett, & Pillay, 1973), but there may be some patients for whom imagined exposure is indicated when, for example, the patient needs to be alone for fear to be provoked and is unable to initiate real-life experiences. The most common imagination technique uses long exposure time and asks the patient to provide a narrative about the event he is imagining. The therapist intervenes only to keep the material relevant and fear provoking and, for this reason, the approach is usually referred to as a **guided fantasy.**

Most phobic patients, with the general exception of agoraphobics and social phobics, are able to imagine vividly anxiety-provoking stimuli and to respond to this imagery by generating high levels of anxiety that habituates in the same way as real-life exposure to similar stimuli. Current practice with real-life exposure grades the approach in a way that the individual finds tolerable but that also achieves rapid enough results to ensure that the individual achieves benefits from treatment at each session.

Fiona: A Simple Phobic Who Was Treated by Graded Real-Life Exposure

Fiona was a 52-year-old bank clerk who had been unable to use the subway or elevators for seven years. Onset of her phobia was associated with Fiona's having been stuck in a tunnel in a crowded subway for a few minutes. Fiona feared that she would suffocate if she was trapped in an elevator or a subway and had changed residences to avoid the need for subway travel and had turned down jobs where using an elevator was difficult to avoid. Fiona had more recently begun to avoid shops and other places she feared might become crowded.

Fiona's only relevant history consisted of two periods in the past when she had been prescribed tranquilizers following traumatic life events. There was nothing of note in her family or personal history and she took no medication regularly.

Fiona was treated by graded real-life exposure. During the first session, she entered an elevator that had its doors locked in an open position. She learned rapidly to tolerate this and was soon able to cope with the doors being closed. Following this, Fiona traveled for an increasing number of floors until, by the end of the first session, she was able to travel eight floors and back with minimal anxiety. The second session followed a similar pattern, with a smaller elevator being used. During the third session, Fiona began to tackle subways; first she got used to being in the station and then she traveled on an uncrowded train that was on a section of the line that was above ground. At the end of this session Fiona had her first experience of traveling underground and was able to take the elevator out of the station. Progress continued in this way until Fiona was able to tolerate crowded subways and elevators without anxiety. She was encouraged to practice these situations between sessions, and by the end of treatment, which consisted of seven sessions, Fiona reported no anxiety in these or other similar situations. Her improvement was maintained throughout followup.

POST-TRAUMATIC STRESS DISORDER

Post-traumatic stress disorder (PTSD) is usually considered to take three forms. The first is the Acute form, which begins soon after the trauma and tends to resolve spontaneously within six months. The second is Chronic, where such spontaneous resolution does not occur. The third is Delayed, where the onset of symptoms occurs more than six months after the trauma. Individuals with the Delayed form of the disorder rarely recover without intervention. By and large, the events leading to PTSD are outside such usual life experiences as the death of a significant other, job and relationship difficulties, or illness. They are more likely to take the form of assault, natural or man-made disasters (earthquakes or battle), or such deliberate malevolence as rape or torture. It may be the case, however, that particularly vulnerable individuals will respond to the more common life events with PTSD symptoms.

ACUTE DISORDER. The most typical response pattern in the Acute disorder, which might follow an incident such as an automobile accident, involves the more diffuse symptoms like sleeplessness, nightmares, and phobic-like avoidance.

Often, a brief period of tonic immobility, tremor, and post-immobility aggression may be observed immediately after the incident. Usually, these symptoms resolve within a relatively short time but the process may well be assisted by psychological intervention. It would seem, from the largely anecdotal data available, that any approach that encourages the individual to recall and relive the events that have occurred is likely to accelerate the recovery period. If this is not attempted, or something interferes with the recovery process (such as the use of sedative or tranquilizing drugs or further trauma), the result may be Chronic PTSD.

CHRONIC DISORDER. In the chronic form, there is an apparent failure of the resolution process seen regularly in the Acute form. This may occur for the reasons given above or may occur for no obvious reason. There does not seem to be any clear relationship between the severity of the trauma and development of the Chronic Disorder, although personal vulnerability may well be implicated. Here, recollections and intrusive thoughts, unpleasant dreams, depression, generalized anxiety, and impaired cognitive function are the most common symptoms. It is not clear how long they are likely to continue in the absence of active treatment. This treatment should, in any case, take the same form as intervention in Acute PTSD but will need to be much more intensive and protracted. Imaginal recall under the influence of a powerful sedative (sometimes called "abreaction") has been widely used at various times in treatment, but there is no firm evidence that it has any distinct advantage over drug-free interventions involving repeated recall of the traumatic events. It is possible that abreaction may be useful where amnesia is almost total. (See Box 8–5.)

DSM-III-R
Diagnostic Criteria for
Post-Traumatic Stress
Disorder

A. The person has experienced an event that is outside the range of usual human experience and that would be markedly distressing to almost anyone, e.g., serious threat to one's life or physical integrity; serious threat or harm to one's children, spouse, or other close relatives and friends; sudden destruction of one's home or community; or seeing another person who has recently been, or is being, seriously injured or killed as the result of an accident or physical violence.

B. The traumatic event is persistently reexperienced in at least one of the following ways:

1) recurrent and intrusive distressing recollections of the event (in young children, repetitive play in which themes or aspects of the trauma are expressed)

2) recurrent distressing dreams of the event

3) sudden acting or feeling as if the traumatic event were recurring (includes a sense of reliving the experience, illusions, hallucinations, and dissociative [flashback] episodes, even those that occur upon awakening or when intoxicated)

4) intense psychological distress at exposure to events that symbolize or resemble an aspect of the traumatic event, including anniversaries of the trauma

C. Persistent avoidance of stimuli associated with the trauma or numbing of general responsiveness (not present before the trauma), as indicated by at least three of the following:

1) efforts to avoid thoughts or feelings associated with the trauma

2) efforts to avoid activities or situations that arouse recollections of the trauma

3) inability to recall an important aspect of the trauma (psychogenic amnesia)

4) markedly diminished interest in significant activities (in young children, loss of recently acquired developmental skills such as toilet training or language skills)

5) feeling of detachment or estrangement from others

6) restricted range of affect, e.g., unable to have loving feelings

7) sense of a foreshortened future, e.g., does not expect to have a career, marriage, or children, or a long life

D. Persistent symptoms of increased arousal (not present before the trauma), as indicated by at least two of the following:

1) difficulty falling or staying asleep

2) irritability or outbursts of anger

3) difficulty concentrating

4) hypervigilance

5) exaggerated startle response

6) physiologic reactivity upon exposure to events that symbolize or resemble an aspect of the traumatic event (e.g., a woman who was raped in an elevator breaks out in a sweat when entering any elevator)

E. Duration of the disturbance (symptoms in B, C, and D) of at least one month.

Specify delayed onset if the onset of symptoms was at least six months after the trauma.

Box 8–5 ● Post-Traumatic Stress Disorder and the Vietnam Vet

Post-traumatic stress disorder afflicts about 500,000 Vietnam veterans. One of these psychological casualties of the Vietnam war, Bob Rheault, has, since his recovery, founded an innovative Outward Bound program for other afflicted veterans (Heron, 1988). He describes it as "a deliberate re-creation of the combat experience," a supervised journey back into the emotional realm of Vietnam with assigned gear, ground to cover, rations, maps, and fear, but no guns (p. 34).

The Veterans Administration didn't recognize post-traumatic stress disorder as a combat-related condition until the American Psychiatric Association did in 1980. Since then, post-traumatic stress disorder has been linked to Vietnam in the way that "shell shock" and "battle fatigue" were connected with World Wars I and II. Also specific to Vietnam is that it was a "teen-age war" with the average age of a soldier 19 as opposed to 26 in World War II, a war without clear objectives, and a war so unpopular that public animosity was often directed at individuals who served in it (p. 65). Also, because each combatant fought on his own 12–13 month schedule, friendships were made and dissolved rapidly. The intense psychological isolation that resulted from all this for Vietnam veterans may help explain the high incidence and persistence of post-traumatic stress disorder among them, as well as the enormity of their difficulty with post-war adjustment.

Source: Heron, Kim (1988). The long road back. *New York Times Magazine*, March 6, p. 32–68.

DELAYED DISORDER. This is probably the most serious presentation of PTSD. The individual seems unaffected for a considerable period ("abnormally normal," perhaps) and then produces symptoms such as marked phobic avoidance, sleep disturbance, generalized anxiety, depression, and cognitive impairment. No satisfactory explanation exists for this delay in onset of symptoms, although it may be associated with the phenomenon of "denial" seen so frequently in bereavement. Treatment in this instance, which typically consists of imaginal rehearsal and real-life exposure to evocative cues, is likely to be more difficult and protracted than for the Acute and Chronic disorders.

It should be noted, however, that there is no controlled data in the field of PTSD. Virtually all accounts consist of descriptions of "mopping-up" operations after particular disasters or of reports from agencies dealing with specific traumas such as rape counseling agencies.

While these accounts are valuable in their own way, they do not allow us to generalize readily about PTSD. Thus, the comments made so far need to be regarded as more impressionistic than those in other sections of this chapter. The distinction between Acute, Chronic, and Delayed is similarly less than clear-cut as the following case example, typical of the author's experience, should illustrate:

Peter: A Patient with Post-Traumatic Stress Disorder

Peter was 39 when he was referred for treatment. He was about to be retired from his job as a policeman because of ill health because he had not been able to do his work effectively for the previous five years. He was quite unable to enter any situation, such as a bar, where groups of people might congregate, and this seriously impaired his functioning as a patrolman. He had been treated by graded, real-life exposure two years previously but this had been largely ineffective. He could offer no explanation for his difficulties.

His history revealed that Peter had been involved in a serious crowd-control problem eight years previously. He had been crushed against a wall, suffered difficulty in breathing, and had two months of disability leave because of a spinal injury. When questioned about this reasonably well-documented event, he was vague about details and claimed never to think about it. On closer questioning, it became clear that he had experienced mild anxiety symptoms during the three years between the accident and the apparent onset of his difficulties which had not been present before.

On the basis of this rather circumstantial evidence, we decided to treat this as PTSD.

Accordingly, we began by asking him to relate the events of the day eight years earlier. Again the account was vague and lacked detail and emotion. We then asked him to relax and to imagine himself leaving the police station, to tell us what he remembered as if it were happening in the here-and-now, and to provide as much detail as possible, particularly about his behavior, thoughts, and feelings. After a couple of attempts, he was able to supply significantly more detail.

We then encouraged him to continue his imaginal recall and verbalization of the traumatic incident. The amount of detail remained very high compared to his previous account, and as soon as he began to recall the beginning of the trauma, he became very upset and wanted to terminate the session. We dissuaded him from doing this because of the danger of sensitization, and he began to relate more and more detail about the trauma. This was continued for two-and-a-half hours. We saw him again the following day because we were concerned about the possibility of depression following the elicitation of this material. Now, he was able to recall even more of the incident and, although tearful and upset, continued through several presentations during which his distress became less marked. Four further prolonged sessions of imaginal recall later, he was able to relate the whole incident (which was much more traumatic than we had previously thought) with little discernible discomfort. He confirmed that, as a result of treatment, he could now remember the incident with dramatically more detail than before and also reported that his generalized anxiety had almost disappeared. After a little encouragement, he was able to go into crowds and, on our instruction, attended several football games where he experienced only mild unease. By followup six months later, he had resumed normal police duties and was experiencing no difficulties. Interestingly, he now had full recall of the crushing episode but said he could put it out of his mind at will.

This kind of case would appear to support the idea that PTSD is caused by incomplete "processing" of a traumatic event in the sense that it is not incorporated into memory and so remains a live issue, causing the multiplicity of symptoms associated with the disorder. Effective treatment would seem to consist of any approach which encourages the individual to recall and rehearse the event. This may be achieved by simply talking about it again and again or, probably more powerfully, by the kind of imaginal rehearsal described above.

OBSESSIVE-COMPULSIVE DISORDER

Obsessive-compulsive disorder is, in some ways, the most notorious of the anxiety disorders. Obsessive-compulsive disorder can be extremely handicapping and it is the only major psychiatric disorder in which the prognosis has been radically altered in the past fifteen years.

There are two essential features of the disorder. The first is obsession, which can be defined as recurrent, persistent thoughts, ideas, or images which feel alien to the individual, but which are not attributable to an external source. These are thoughts that frequently invade consciousness and are experienced as unpleasant by the individual who tries, and almost invariably fails, to prevent their reoccurrence. Examples of obsessions include preoccupation with cleanliness or safety.

The second feature of obsessive-compulsive disorder is compulsion, or an act that the individual feels compelled to undertake despite feeling that it is senseless. Such acts tend to be stereotyped and repetitive and, although usually resisted by the person, create high levels of anxiety if not performed. An example is handwashing, a compulsion of some obsessive-compulsive individuals preoccupied with ideas about germs and illness. Usually completion of a compulsion leads to temporary relief of anxiety but this is short-lived and the compulsion soon recurs.

Glynis: A Patient with Obsessive-Compulsive Disorder

Glynis was 35 years old at the time of her referral to the Mental-Health Center. A therapist visited her at home for assessment because she was unable to leave her home, and, indeed, on most days was unable to leave her bed due to her obsession with being "contaminated." Her boyfriend, who had suffered several schizophrenic episodes but currently was functioning reasonably well on antipsychotic medication, provided for her basic needs and kept her company. She had been incapacitated with obsessive-compulsive disorder for fourteen years and had been admitted to hospitals on twenty-three occasions. She had had just about every psychiatric intervention possible, including electroshock therapy (ECT), various psychotherapies, antidepressants of every kind, major and minor tranquilizers, and had been recom-

DSM-III-R Diagnostic Criteria for Obsessive Compulsive Disorder

A. Either obsessions or compulsions:

Obsessions: (1), (2), (3), and (4):

1) recurrent and persistent ideas, thoughts, impulses, or images that are experienced, at least initially, as intrusive and senseless, e.g., a parent's having repeated impulses to kill loved child, a religious person's having recurrent blasphemous thoughts

2) the person attempts to ignore or suppress such thoughts or impulses or to neutralize them with some other thought or action

3) the person recognizes that the obsessions are the product of his or her own mind, not imposed from without (as in thought insertion)

4) if another Axis I disorder is present, the content of the obsession is unrelated to it, e.g., the ideas, thoughts, impulses, or images are not about food in the presence of an Eating Disorder, about drugs in the presence of a Psychoactive Substance Use Disorder, or guilty thoughts in the presence of a Major Depression

Compulsions: (1), (2), and (3):

1) repetitive, purposeful, and intentional behaviors that are performed in response to an obsession, or according to certain rules or in a stereotyped fashion

2) the behavior is designed to neutralize or to prevent discomfort or some dreaded event or situation; however, either the activity is not connected in a realistic way with what it is designed to neutralize or prevent, or it is clearly excessive

3) the person recognizes that his or her behavior is excessive or unreasonable (this may not be true for young children; it may no longer be true for people whose obsessions have evolved into overvalued ideas)

B. The obsessions or compulsions cause marked distress, are time-consuming (take more than an hour a day), or significantly interfere with the person's normal routine, occupational functioning, or usual social activities or relationships with others.

mended for leucotomy (a neurosurgical procedure that involves severing connections between the prefrontal lobes and the thalamus, which can afford relief from intractable pain or anxiety, to which, however, she had refused consent). She looked disheveled and dirty, and her speech was slurred but, although repetitive in content, was coherent.

Glynis had been raised in London by strict but kind parents and was one of five siblings, the rest of whom were in good physical and mental health. She had been popular and successful at school and had gone to a university for a degree in literature, which she passed with honors. Shortly after she finished at the university, a long-standing relationship with a boyfriend was abruptly terminated by him. Within a week, she became profoundly depressed and had to

be hospitalized. Besides the usual biological signs of depression (psychomotor retardation, sleep and appetite disturbance, and so forth), she developed the idea that she had become contaminated by radiation and that anyone she touched would die of cancer. This seemed to be related to a newspaper report she had read about leaks from nuclear power stations.

Glynis failed to respond to antidepressant medication and was eventually given ECT, following which she improved. However, although the major biological signs of depression were no longer present, she continued to express the view that she was contaminated and a danger to others. She conceded that this was perhaps illogical (an obsession), but would wash her hands up to 100 times a day (compulsion) in an effort to rid herself of contamination.

Glynis would not touch anyone and felt extremely anxious if anyone attempted to touch her. She walked around with her hands in the air in case she inadvertently touched something that someone else might touch and repeatedly asked people if she might have touched them without noticing.

OBSESSION AND DEPRESSION. Glynis became depressed and we know there is a relationship between depression and obsessive-compulsive disorder, though quite a complicated one. First, some obsessive disorders start during a period of dysphoria, although the majority do not. If someone already has an obsessive disorder, then depression will make it worse although very severe depression may eliminate symptoms for as long as the depression lasts. Also, obsessives are more prone to depression than the general population, though it remains unclear whether this is simply due to the depressing effects of being obsessive or a predisposition to both disorders in the same individuals. Finally, if someone is both depressed and obsessional, treating the depression has little effect on the obsessions (Marks et al., 1980).

OBSESSION AND DELUSION. It is essential to be clear about the important distinction between an obsession and a delusion. If someone with a delusion is questioned about the veracity of the belief, he or she will insist on its absolute accuracy. Someone with an obsession, on the other hand, will be prepared to acknowledge at least the possibility of being wrong and will say something like, "I feel as though it's true and I can't afford to take the risk." Clinically, obsessive ideas do not respond to antipsychotic medication, although delusions may.

Glynis continued to behave obsessively, despite further ECT and both tricyclic antidepressant and antipsychotic medication. Group and individual psychotherapy were tried with no effect, and finally, after about six months, she discharged herself from the hospital. The next thirteen years were extremely chaotic and therefore difficult to chronicle. She had many hospital admissions, some of them compulsory; was arrested by the police on six occasions (she had discovered that large amounts of alcohol gave her temporary relief); attempted suicide; alienated herself from her family, who found her behavior inexplicable; and ended up living an extremely squalid and limited existence in an attempt to minimize her rituals. When a therapist finally saw her, she had been prescribed

daily doses of 300 mg of the antipsychotic chlorpromazine (Thorazine) and 30 mg of diazepam (Valium) by two of the many physicians she consulted about her problems. She abused both of these substances in an effort to stay asleep most of the day. Glynis agreed to admit herself to a hospital after assurance that the hospital had something different to offer her.

On admission, Glynis weighed over 220 pounds, was dyspneic, and urgently needed a bath. Assessment and measurement of her obsessive behavior was started. During the first three days, she washed her hands an average of 83 times a day and sought reassurance 54 times a day that she had not accidentally touched someone. She was anxious and tearful but not clinically depressed.

TREATMENT FOR OBSESSIVE-COMPULSIVE DISORDER. Prior to 1972, the only realistic treatment options for individuals incapacitated by obsessive-compulsive disorder were psychosurgery and long-term hospitalization. Fortunately, the situation today is completely different: about seventy-five percent of obsessive-compulsive patients can now be treated to the point where their symptoms are absent or at a level that allows them to live normal lives. This almost certainly represents the most dramatic prognostic change for any severe psychiatric disorder since the introduction of phenothiazines made such a difference to the management of schizophrenia during the 1950s.

BEHAVIORAL THERAPY. Meyer (1966) reported the first successful treatment of a severe obsessive disorder using an approach that provided the basis for the more sophisticated approaches practiced today. Meyer's approach was simply to prevent the patient from ritualizing on a twenty-four-hour-a-day basis. After a few days, the patient experiences a marked decrease in the urge to ritualize. This approach has become known as **response prevention.**

Meyer's attempts were brave at the time because conventional wisdom was that the one thing a person should never do with an obsessional was to interfere with his or her ritualizing in any way. Further experience with this approach indicated that it possibly had general value. Treatment methods have been further refined by Rachman and his colleagues (Rachman, Hodgson, & Marks, 1971; Rachman, Marks, & Hodgson, 1973; Roper, Rachman, & Marks, 1975; and Rachman et al., 1979) in a series of carefully controlled experiments and clinical trials. The treatment approach now consists of three main components.

1. *Graded real-life exposure:* similar to the approach for phobics, this approach allows gradual exposure to the stimuli that evoke the obsession. In the case of someone who is obsessed with a fear of being contaminated by everyday dirt and germs, he would be asked to touch objects which he considers sources of contamination (such as chairs and the floor).

2. *Modeling:* before asking the patient to expose himself to possible contamination, the therapist demonstrates the activity, acting as a "model." This appears to make it easier for the patient to carry out exposure exercises.

3. *Response prevention:* after modeling and exposure to the cues that evoke the obsession, the patient is asked to refrain from carrying out the compulsive ritual (for example, handwashing) for a period after the session. Most patients are able to do this on their own, but occasionally someone with severe compulsion will need to be admitted to a hospital so that the staff can monitor prevention of the ritual.

These three components are the essential ingredients for successful treatment of obsessive-compulsive disorder. In practice, they are combined with social reinforcement for achievement and, equally important, a ban on reassurance seeking. For an obsessive, receiving reassurance is functionally equivalent to ritualizing in that it affords temporary relief from anxiety and increases the frequency of reassurance seeking. Another part of treatment is the involvement of significant others in the treatment. This can be important for a number of reasons.

First, many obsessives will have very carefully "trained" those around them to behave in a way that accommodates their obsessive behavior. It is clearly important that those others be helped to readopt a more conventional lifestyle in order for the obsessive to improve. Second, the cooperation of the family in encouraging and assisting the patient to carry out treatment exercises can be of great value in achieving and consolidating gains. Third, the family must be taught a way of resisting demands for reassurance. This can be difficult for them because of the intense emotional responses that refusal of reassurance can produce. Shifting this responsibility to the therapist or hospital can be helpful in reducing family tensions. For example, if the patient repeatedly asks whether he has washed his hands, the family members would be taught to say, "I'm sorry, but hospital instructions are that I'm not allowed to answer that kind of question."

OTHER THERAPIES. Pharmacotherapy is also used to treat obsessive-compulsive disorder, though with varying degrees of success. Psychotherapy has generally proven ineffective in the treatment of obsessive-compulsive disorder, though it may have some use in acute cases (Hollander, Liebowitz, Gorman, 1989 p. 478). (See Box 8–6).

NURSING CARE OF THE PATIENT WITH ANXIETY IN A NONPSYCHIATRIC SETTING

This chapter has been describing all along the nursing care of anxiety disorders. All the patients described in this chapter were treated by nurses. It is clear that, given appropriate training and supervision, nurses can autonomously deliver appropriate care to anxious patients (see Marks et al., 1977). However, even without specialized training, nurses must constantly deal with varying degrees of anxiety in their patients. Illness is in itself a frightening and stressful experience—a person may lose the feeling of control over their life, particularly if the illness is life-threatening or chronically debilitating. The nurse generalist will often make assessments that lead to anxiety-related nursing diagnoses (see Table 8–2)—and there are a number of strategies nurses may use to help the patient overcome anxious feelings. Signs of anxiety in the hospitalized patient include disturbances in sleep and eating patterns, irritability, unwillingness to cooperate, inability to communicate with staff or family, and decreased awareness of feelings. More severe symptoms may include a wide variety of physical symptoms, as we have seen earlier in this chapter, such as sweating, headache, gastrointestinal problems, or insomnia (Boyd & Citro, 1988).

Depending on the nursing diagnosis, possible nursing interventions may include providing a safe and secure environment for the patient; promoting development of the patient's insight into the illness or treatment process; helping the patient find alternative ways to handle the stress that may be accompanying anxiety; promoting the patient's self-esteem; and promoting a balance of rest, sleep, and activity. Specific strategies for helping critically ill patients overcome stress are discussed in Chapter 25.

It would be fair to say that people become anxious in two situations: (1) when they perceive a danger and (2) when they are facing uncertainty. Everyone is familiar with the unease that accompanies waiting to know the outcome of an examination or

Box 8–6 ● Current Research on Anti-anxiety Drugs
C. Kate Kavanagh

While behavioral treatment for anxiety disorders has a successful history and much research to recommend it, as well as no potential for toxicity, some clinicians prefer to use medication as well, especially with patients who do not respond to behavioral treatment alone.

According to University of Wisconsin psychiatrists Greist and Jefferson (1988), a combination of behavioral therapy and medication is the most helpful treatment for many individuals with anxiety disorders. They recommend the minimum effective dose of one of the antidepressants that affect the noradrenergic system (e.g., imipramine) for panic disorder, and beta-blockers such as propranalol or a benzodiazepine such as Valium for the acute anxiety symptoms associated with exposure therapy for agoraphobia (a single dose one hour prior to the treatment sessions is suggested). Beta-blockers, as well as MAO inhibitors, are also useful for the treatment of the sleep disturbance and nightmares associated with post-traumatic stress disorder.

Greist and Jefferson also state that clomipramine, a serotonin reuptake blocking agent, is an antidepressant which has been shown to have anti-obsessive-compulsive properties.

They report that Buspirone, a new antianxiety agent that does *not* have sedative effects, and does not interact with alcohol or lead to dependency, is currently being evaluated as safer than the benzodiazepines for symptomatic treatment of generalized anxiety disorder.

Perse et al. (1987) reported that fluvoxamine, a 2-amenoethyloxine aralkylketose and a more potent serotonin reuptake blocker than clomipramine, has been shown in preliminary double-blind studies to be effective for the treatment of obsessive-compulsive disorder. As with clomipramine, the absence of depression in the patient does not affect its anti-obsessive-compulsive effect. Given that behavioral therapy is at times not effective or poorly tolerated, they say that further study of the usefulness of fluvoxamine is warranted.

Greist, J., Jefferson, J. (1988). Anxiety disorders. In *Goldman's Review of General Psychiatry,* East Norwalk: Appleton and Lang.

Perse, T. L., Greist, J., Jefferson, J., Rosenfeld, R., Dar, R. (1987). Fluvoxamine treatment of obsessive compulsive disorder, *American Journal of Psychiatry, 144:*12, 1543–1548.

---

job interview, and with the anxiety felt when in unfamiliar territory, where the ability to predict events is reduced. That kind of personal experience should serve to remind nurses that, in any clinical setting, providing the patient with accurate and honest information about treatment and prognosis will function as a powerful reducer of anxiety. This cannot be emphasized too strongly.

Harry: An Anxious Patient

Harry, age 43, an executive on the move up the corporate ladder, has had a myocardial infarction for the first time. He is in the hospital and no longer in physical distress. He has been told he has had a "heart attack." Anxiety is the dominant feature of his clinical state, though he does not meet the criteria for an anxiety disorder.

Harry's anxiety, reflected in his frequent checking of his pulse, worried expression, and difficulty sleeping, is understandable, and there are a number of responses that the nurse can have to his feelings. The first is to ignore them. The second is to touch him on the arm and say something like, "Don't worry, you're going to be O.K." Neither approach will reduce his anxiety: the first for obvious reasons, the second because it is unrealistic. To find the most useful approach, the nurse can ask herself, "What would I like to be told in this situation?"

For the majority of people, this would consist of recognition that they feel anxious, that their anxiety is reasonable, and an acknowledgment that although they are in some danger, their risk can be minimized. With this approach Harry would be more likely to feel able to move on to becoming an attentive and active participant in a discussion about how to distinguish physical symptoms of anxiety from those of a heart attack, and how to minimize his risk of future heart attack. One suggestion might be to enroll in the cardiac clinic's stress management program.

It is worth distinguishing between accurate information and the word that is encountered too frequently in nursing care plans—reassurance. Reassurance is usually just an unrealistic and overoptimistic prediction about future events. Not only is this insulting to the patient, it is also a very effective way of reducing the patient's confidence in the care team if and when unpredicted aversive events occur.

The nurse can help reduce anxiety in a patient by simply explaining the physical symptoms that accompany anxiety. Many individuals with anxiety are made even more anxious by their lack of understanding of the physical manifestations of the anxiety they are experiencing. Some people who have tachycardia as a result of anxiety may believe they have a serious heart disorder; others may attribute their symptoms to a wide range of horrible physical disorders, such as a brain tumor. Other anxiety sufferers may believe that anxiety symptoms are an early sign of impending "madness," usually taking their concept of madness from Hollywood portrayals that are not particularly notable for their accuracy.

The nurse caring for Harry would explain the difference between symptoms of cardiac distress and symptoms caused by anxiety. She would talk with Harry about how he should handle each of these types of symptoms and teach him how to get his symptoms of anxiety under control with relaxation training (see Chapter 25 on the ICU patient), etc. Finally the nurse would talk with Harry about what he could do to reduce his chances of a future MI, e.g., enroll in the hospital's stress management program, stop smoking, exercise regularly, etc.

It can be an immense help to people such as Harry to have a nontechnical explanation of their experiences, emphasizing the physical events that produce the symptoms and the relationship between these and thinking about possible dangers. It should also be emphasized that anxiety is not a sign of future insanity. It is worth making this point even if the individual does not raise it spontaneously because many people are too apprehensive or embarrassed to broach the subject despite being very worried about the possibility.

The presence of trusted and familiar individuals is one of the ways in which everyone copes with anxiety. The nurse should, therefore, take every opportunity to allow her anxious patient access to such people at times of particular stress.

In addition to this general approach, graded, planned, and controlled confrontation with feared situations is the approach of choice for all sufferers of situational anxiety (including most people hospitalized for examinations and treatment); a range of anxiety management strategies is available for those with generalized anxiety.

The use of anxiolytic drugs should be discouraged, and withdrawal from these agents needs to be monitored carefully because of the wide variety of symptoms produced, as well as the danger inherent in withdrawal for the patient who has been on high doses (more than 40 mg/day) for a prolonged period. In this case, treatment is discontinued by tapering doses gradually, not exceeding a ten percent reduction each day, in order to avoid grand mal seizures and associated problems (Rosenbaum, 1982).

When access to specialized help is not possible, the nurse may consider whether a monitored self-help program would be appropriate for her patient. Many, perhaps most, phobics can overcome their fears by following such programs, although they may have less value for obsessive and generalized anxiety disorders. Probably the best self-help manual is that written by Marks (1978), the efficacy of which has been tested in a clinical trial with agoraphobics (Ghosh, Marks, & Carr, 1984).

Another useful book, specifically for and about agoraphobics, is provided by Clarke and Wardman (1985). It provides both a clinician's and a patient's view of treatment as well as a number of useful treatment suggestions. People following these programs probably do better if they have access to someone who can monitor and praise their progress and make appropriate suggestions. Also, see Chapter 25, on the intensive care patient, for additional suggestions for nursing care of the anxious patient in non-psychiatric settings.

Nursing Care Plan for Harry

Nursing Diagnosis	Desired Outcome	Interventions	Rationale
1. Anxiety (about having another heart attack).	Harry's anxiety will decrease as a result of being able to differentiate symptoms of anxiety from symptoms of an MI.	Empathize with Harry's anxiety, labeling it as normal.	Interpersonal contact with the anxious patient is possible through empathy. Labeling the patient's feelings as "normal" will decrease his anxiety.
		Explain that anxiety, like all emotional states, involves a physiological response which peaks and then begins to decrease. It does not herald "going crazy."	Reducing anxiety to a physiological state makes it seem more manageable and less mystical.
		Teach Harry what he can do to get anxiety under control, e.g., relaxation training.	Teaching Harry to attend to his anxious feelings and *use* them as a trigger for conscious muscle relaxation (see Chapter 25 on the ICU patient) can provide him with predictability and control of his anxiety, two factors with the potential to decrease it.
		Explain what symptoms of cardiac distress are like, why they occur, and what Harry should do if he experiences them.	Helping Harry differentiate between anxiety and cardiac distress and teaching him how to deal with both is likely to reduce his anxiety markedly since he is not likely to die of anxiety and cardiac distress can often be effectively treated if picked up early.
		Talk with Harry about what he can do to reduce his chances of a future MI, e.g., enroll in the hospital's stress management program, stop smoking, exercise regularly, etc.	Harry's anxiety may be an excellent source of motivation to change his lifestyle so as to reduce his chances of having another heart attack.

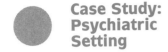

Case Study: Psychiatric Setting

Glynis, the patient with an obsessive-compulsive disorder described earlier, (p. 234) was taken off medication shortly after admission to the hospital. Withdrawal from the phenothiazines was relatively easy for Glynis and she accomplished this within a week with no adverse effects. However, benzodiazepine withdrawal proved more difficult, and her level of anxiety increased with each reduction in dosage.

At the same time, a nurse-therapist began work with her obsessions. The nurse began by touching Glynis, as Glynis felt herself to be a source of radiation contamination, and asked her to watch the therapist touch objects and then people around the ward. Initially, Glynis felt very anxious about this but, after a few sessions, found that she could tolerate it much more easily. Then the nurse-therapist asked Glynis to walk around the ward, first touching other objects and then other people without having washed beforehand. She found this very difficult but, with repeated practice, became able to do it with less and less anxiety. The nurse-therapist had discovered that contact with any object that Glynis associated with radiation would greatly increase her feelings of being contaminated, so the nurse-therapist arranged for her to receive letters from areas of the country that contained nuclear fuel stations and for her to visit laboratories where radioactive substances were used. Glynis was asked to handle the letters and the articles that had been in contact with the laboratories and then to touch objects and other people while refraining from washing. Again, anxiety was high during the first few trials but subsided as practice continued.

After fifteen sessions, Glynis was able to handle objects associated with radiation, thus increasing her feeling of being contaminated, and to touch objects such as ward furniture and other people with only a little unease (although she was occasionally tempted to handwash). Her boyfriend joined these sessions whenever possible so that he could gain an understanding of the principles involved and act as a cotherapist when the hospital staff attempted to transfer the treatment from the hospital to her home. By this time, encouraged by the progress she had made, Glynis had begun dieting and paying more attention to her personal appearance. The nurse-therapist then faced the problem of transferring the gains Glynis had made in the hospital to her home. Up to this point, Glynis had been very cooperative with treatment exercises, but she balked at the idea of contaminating her home and needed a lot of persuasion before agreeing to it. As anticipated, the first couple of sessions in her home were the most difficult but the increased anxiety soon abated and she became able to touch objects without washing first, despite feeling "contaminated." By this time, her handwashing had decreased to normal levels and she no longer asked for reassurance. Glynis continued to feel concerned about radiation for some weeks afterward and needed to carry out daily exposure exercises in order to consolidate her improvement.

Two months after her discharge, things were going well enough for Glynis to start looking for employment, although her expectations seemed rather overambitious. A month later, not having found a job, she became depressed and her symptoms resurfaced. She responded well to clomipramine, an antidepressant which has been shown to be effective in the treatment of compulsive ritualizers who are also depressed (Marks et al., 1980), and was able to tackle her obsessions largely by herself with the aid of two "booster" sessions. At a six-month followup, Glynis was once again well and had started in a job retraining program with which she was coping well. She will need to be followed up carefully over the next couple of years, however, to ensure that any reemergence of symptoms or mood disturbance is rapidly treated.

DSM-III-R Diagnosis

Axis I Obsessive Compulsive Disorder (300. 30)
Axis II none
Axis III none
Axis IV Psychosocial Stressors: 0 (inadequate information)
Axis V GAF: 0 (inadequate information)

Nursing Diagnoses

Activity Intolerance
Self-care Deficit: feeding, bathing hygiene
Social Isolation

Nursing Care Plan for Glynis

Nursing Diagnosis	Desired Outcomes	Interventions	Rationale
1. Activity intolerance: Glynis has been confined to her bed for several years, sleeping most of the day.	Glynis will resume normal activities of daily living, including self-care, social contact, school, or work.	Talk with Glynis about her goal of resuming a normal activity level, encouraging her to verbalize her feelings about doing so. Empathize with her anxiety, neither minimizing it nor overreacting to it with a lot of reassurance. Do not participate in extensive conversations about specifics of her anxiety. State clearly that you understand that this will be difficult for Glynis, but you will be available for support. State clearly that though Glynis feels anxious and is afraid, she is in a safe place; help her separate feeling afraid from being in a dangerous place.	The nurse's confidence in Glynis' ability to resume normal daily activities can help Glynis to imagine this outcome, an essential first step to achieving it. Empathy is an effective means of making interpersonal contact with the severely anxious patient. Separating feelings from reality and from behavior can help to interrupt the "paralysis" of severe anxiety.
		With Glynis, plan a daily program that will gradually increase her	Gradual desensitization is as effective as "flooding" a patient with

Nursing Diagnosis	Desired Outcomes	Interventions	Rationale
		tolerance for increased activity in spite of her anxiety. For example, during week one in the hospital, have Glynis gradually spend more time out of her room, first with maximum support, decreasing to nursing availability. Set up the plan in such a way that Glynis first spends only structured time out of her room, gradually adding unstructured time. When Glynis is allowed to be in her room, she should not be allowed to be in bed. She may get into bed to sleep only at bedtime. Glynis' activity level should at first require minimal energy expenditure, as would be the case with any type of physical exercise, such as outdoor walks.	anxiety and much less stressful. Flooding in Glynis' case would involve supportive insistence that she be up and out of her room socializing with other patients from day one of her treatment.
2. Self-care deficit: feeding, bathing, hygiene, etc.	Glynis will resume independent self-care, including nutritious meal planning, daily bathing, twice-weekly hair washing, and clothes maintenance.	Draw up a list of daily self-care activities with Glynis and talk with her about the steps required with each activity; then go through them with her. Increase expectations for unsupervised self-care on a daily basis so that Glynis is self-sufficient by the time she is eligible for discharge. Talk with Glynis about a healthy diet, identify poor eating habits, and suggest alternatives that she is likely to tolerate.	Breaking down desired outcomes into achievable steps will make Glynis' treatment task a manageable one. If she feels she must go from twelve years in bed to independent functioning, she will feel overwhelmed and give up.
3. Social isolation.	Glynis will return to the community as a fully functioning individual interested in making social contact.	Talk with Glynis about her life before her illness, using this as a springboard to suggest social involvement she will find enjoyable. Church involvement, art	Talking about each new activity with Glynis before she attempts it will give her the opportunity to "rehearse" it in her mind, beginning her

(continued on page 244)

Nursing Diagnosis	Desired Outcomes	Interventions	Rationale
		classes, volunteer work, job training, and job seeking are examples of directions she may show interest in taking.	gradual exposure to the feared event.
		Encourage Glynis to express her feelings about social involvements, including associated anxiety. Again offer empathy within a context of a reality that is not threatening. Tell Glynis that you will assist her in getting involved socially one step at a time.	Encouraging her to express her feelings about these things will give the nurse the opportunity to correct any cognitive distortions that have developed during Glynis' years of social isolation and that are increasing her anxiety about them.
		Encourage Glynis to participate in patient group activities while in the hospital. Spend at least one hour each day talking to her about her social contacts that day as well as what is ahead tomorrow.	Talking with Glynis about her experiences afterward will offer another opportunity for "exposure" to the feared events and provides a chance to positively reinforce her efforts with praise and a review of the day's accomplishments.
		Attend to Glynis' behavior in contacts with her, asking her to validate your perceptions about her responses. Encourage Glynis to talk about how she feels about spending time with you and talking with you about these things.	Glynis' interactions with the nurse provide an opportunity for the nurse to observe Glynis in social interaction first-hand and to offer support and feedback. For example, if Glynis seems anxious, the nurse can ask Glynis if she is aware of being anxious, and to try and understand where the anxiety is coming from or what is triggering it (for example, concern that the nurse will be disappointed in her if she has had a bad day). If Glynis appears calm and relaxed, the nurse can comment on this, a source of positive reinforcement for her efforts that day.

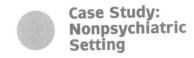

Case Study: Nonpsychiatric Setting

Geanette, a 55-year-old widow, has been admitted to the hospital with a diagnosis of probable breast cancer several days in advance of scheduled surgery to biopsy and remove the tumor. Geanette tells her nurse that she has not been hospitalized since the birth of her son 30 years earlier, and has always been fearful of hospitals, possibly because her parents (both of whom developed cancer) died in the hospital when she was twelve years old. Her husband died unexpectedly during open-heart surgery one year before. At times she is quite restless and irritable, ringing her call bell frequently. Nights are the worst so she sleeps little. She experiences hunger, but eats only small portions of her meals as she feels full after a couple of mouthfuls. Geanette's son visits her quite frequently, but she refuses to discuss her illness or its treatment and prognosis with him. She becomes very irritable when anyone tries to bring the subject up. She does complain bitterly to him about every test and procedure she undergoes. She has expressed to her primary nurse how fearful she is of the surgery and potential mastectomy, but has made no plans for her care after she goes home from the hospital. If the tumor is malignant as expected, she will undergo either chemotherapy or radiation post-operatively. While the treatment will be started in the hospital, most of it will be done on an out-patient basis. Geanette refuses to talk about either until it is a certainty, so it is not clear who will assist her in coming to the hospital for treatments, and help care for her while she recovers from her surgery and copes with the side-effects of the rest of her treatment.

DSM-III-R Diagnosis

Axis I Anxiety Disorder Not Otherwise Specified (300.00)
Axis II none known
Axis III probable breast cancer
Axis IV Psychosocial Stressors: 0 (inadequate information)
Axis V GAF: 0 (inadequate information)

Nursing Diagnoses

*Anxiety
*Fear
 Impaired Adjustment
*Potential for Isolation
 Sleep Pattern Disturbance

*A Nursing Care Plan based on these diagnoses follows.

Nursing Care Plan for Geanette

Nursing Diagnosis	Desired Outcome	Interventions	Rationale
1. Anxiety related to being in the hospital, possibly having cancer, and about to have surgery is making Geanette dysfunctional as an individual and family member.	Geanette will better manage her anxiety as demonstrated by a willingness to talk about her illness and its ramifications with the nurse and with her son.	The nurse will leave some material on breast cancer (the nurse specialist on the unit has developed a pamphlet for the patient with possible breast cancer) for Geanette to look at, offering to return later in the shift to answer any questions Geanette may have about what she reads. The nurse will attempt to engage Geanette in conversation about what is in the pamphlet, beginning with non-threatening questions/comments about it, for example: "Was the pamphlet helpful to you?" "Many patients find this pamphlet helpful to them before surgery. Did you?" "In my experience, the pamphlet doesn't answer *all* the questions patients have about going through this. Is there anything you are confused about or still have questions or concerns about?"	Before the nurse can help an anxious patient, she needs to determine where the anxiety is coming from. Misunderstanding or lack of information is often at least part of the etiology. It is important to be attuned to the patient's need to go slowly in facing anxiety. Introducing the topic, offering a resource, and giving the patient some time to get ready to talk is often more effective than just starting a discussion about feelings, especially anxiety. If the patient's anxiety increases with the first step of providing information about treatment, he is not ready to talk about his fear of death. The patient will first need time to get comfortable with talking with the nurse and to learn that it is safe to get into the anxiety he is feeling, that the nurse will understand and not be overwhelmed by it, and that she *can* help.
2. Fear of death during surgery or afterward, if surgery and followup treatment are not able to eradicate the cancer.	Geanette will put her fear of death in perspective, given her early diagnosis and treatment and continually increasing survival rates of women with breast cancer.	The nurse will assure Geanette that staff is available to her to talk about her fears or to just sit with her if that would help at times. The nurse will help Geanette face her fear of death by facing it herself and asking very directly: "Are you afraid that you are going to die?" The nurse will empathize with Geanette's understandable fears, reiterate her good prognosis, and offer to arrange for her to talk with one of the former breast cancer patient unit volunteers.	Demonstrating a willingness to talk about death and other often "unspeakable fears" conveys understanding, acceptance, and a desire to help the patient with his fears, and can give him the courage to talk about them and, eventually, to face them if necessary. Understanding that only another patient "can really understand," as well as understanding how important it is to feel *understood*, is essential to effectively supporting the anxious patient through his or her crisis.

Nursing Diagnosis	Desired Outcome	Interventions	Rationale
3. Potential for isolation.	Geanette will begin to talk with her family about her illness, and will begin to make plans with them for her care in the future.	The nurse will talk with Geanette about her need for physical and emotional support while she is ill, and how it can help her son and his wife to allow them to provide that support for her, now and throughout her recovery. With Geanette's approval, the nurse will invite the son to visit during a time when the nurse plans to talk with Geanette about what is ahead for her.	The nurse can't always help a patient with his or her anxiety as quickly and effectively as she would like to, but she *can* always help the patient not to be alone with it. Telling a "good mother" that allowing her children to take care of her is good for *them* can "give her permission" to do so.

SUMMARY

Anxiety is an experience that everyone has. There are people, objects, and situations that provoke anxious feelings in all of us. However, for some people, anxiety symptoms are intense enough to interfere with daily life; these people have anxiety disorders.

Anxiety has three major components: behavior, cognitions, and autonomic responses. An accurate assessment of anxiety takes all three into account, remembering that none of these measures differentiates between normal and pathological anxiety. The only effective criterion for pathological anxiety is interference with personal, social, or occupational functioning.

There is little evidence that psychoactive drugs, though they are widely used, are useful in treating anxiety disorders. There is no clear method of treating the anxiety states—panic disorder and generalized anxiety disorder—but some relaxation techniques and specific changes in lifestyle, such as the addition of exercise, seem to help. For the other anxiety disorders (phobias and obsessive-compulsive disorder), graded exposure is the treatment of choice.

Generalized anxiety disorder and panic disorder are different from the other disorders in that the anxiety is not produced by a situation. The other disorders are provoked by a situation or object. Post-traumatic stress disorder follows serious trauma and rarely resolves without intervention in its chronic and delayed form. Obsessive-compulsive disorder is probably the most extreme of the anxiety disorders, and it has a relationship to depression, although it is a complicated one.

In nonpsychiatric settings, the nurse may find patients who express anxiety about surgery, treatment, examinations, and so forth. The nurse can help reduce that anxiety by providing accurate information to the patient and also by explaining the physical symptoms that sometimes accompany anxiety itself.

KEY TERMS

anxiety
behavior
cognitions
autonomic responses
learning theory
neuroticism
extraversion
introversion
anxiety state
anxiety neurosis
panic disorder
generalized anxiety disorder
relaxation training
anxiety management training

stress inoculation
withdrawal
agoraphobia
safety signals
graded exposure
social phobia
social-skills training
simple phobia
systematic desensitization
guided fantasy
post-traumatic stress disorder
obsessive-compulsive disorder
response prevention

STUDY QUESTIONS

1. What are the three major components of anxiety? What is the only effective criterion for differentiating between anxious feelings and anxiety disorder?

2. Is medication indicated for the treatment of anxiety disorders? Why or why not?

3. Name the two forms of anxiety state and describe their symptoms.

4. Name the four other major anxiety disorders and describe their symptoms.

5. What is treatment by exposure and how does it work?

REFERENCES

Boyd, M. D., & Citro, K. (1988). Is your MI patient too scared to recover? *R.N.*, May, 50–54.

Clarke, J. C., & Wardman. (1985). *Agoraphobia. A clinical and personal account.* Australia: Pergamon.

Drever, J. (1952). *A dictionary of psychology.* Australia: Penguin.

Emmelkamp, P. M. G. (1982). Anxiety and fear. In Bellack, Hersen, & Kazdin (Eds.), *International handbook of behavior modification and therapy.* New York: Planum Press.

Eysenck, H. J. (1967). *The Biological Basis of Personality.* Springfield, Ill.: Charles C. Thomas.

Falloon, I. R. H., Lindley, P., McDonald, R., & Marks, I. M. (1972). Social skills training of out-patient groups. *Br. J. Psychiatry, 131,* 599–609.

Freud, S. (1919). *Collected papers 2.* London: The Hogarth Press, pp. 399–400.

Gaind, R. (1976, September). *The role of beta blockers as an adjunct in behavior therapy.* Paper presented to EABT, Greece.

Ghosh, A., Marks, I. M., & Carr, A. C. (1984). Controlled study of self-exposure treatment for phobics: Preliminary communication. *J. Royal Soc. Med., 77,* 483–489.

Goldfried, M. R. (1971). Systematic desensitization as training in self-control. *J. Consult. Clin. Psychol., 37,* 228–234.

Goldfried, M. R., & Davison, G. C. (1976). *Clinical behavior therapy.* New York: Holt, Rinehart & Winston.

Gray, J. A. (1972). *The psychology of fear and stress.* New York: McGraw-Hill.

Greden, J. F. (1974). Anxiety or caffeinism: A diagnostic dilemma. *Am. J. Psychiatry, 131,* 1089–1093.

Greden, J. F., Victor, B. S., Fontaine, P., & Lubetsky, M. (1980). Caffeine-withdrawal headache: A clinical profile. *Psychosomatics, 21,* 411–418.

Greist, J. & Jefferson, J. (1988). Anxiety disorders. In *Goldman's Review of General Psychiatry,* East Norwalk: Appleton & Lang.

Greist, J. H., Marks, I. M., & Noshirvani, H. F. Avoidance versus confrontation of fear. *Behavior Therapy, 11,* 1–14.

Hebb, D. O. (1946). *On the Nature of Fear.* Psychological Review, 53, 259–276.

Heron, K. The long road back. *New York Times Magazine,* 1988, March 6, 32–68.

Hollander, E., Liebowitz, M. R., & Gorman, J. M. (1988). Anxiety Disorders. In Talbott, Hales, & Yudofsky (Eds.), *Textbook of psychiatry.* Washington, D.C.: American Psychiatric Press, Inc.

Jacobson, E. (1938). *Progressive relaxation.* Chicago: University of Chicago Press.

Lang, P. (1978). Anxiety: Toward a psychophysiological definition. In Akiskal & Webb (Eds.), *Psychiatric diagnosis: Exploration of biological predictors.* New York: Spectrum Press.

Lang, P. J. (1977). Imagery in Therapy: an information processing analysis of fear. *Behavior Therapy, 8,* 862–886.

Lum, L. C. (1977). Breathing exercises in the treatment of hyperventilation and chronic anxiety states. *Chest, Heart & Stroke Journal, 2,* 7–11.

McCue, E. C., & McCue, P. A. (1984). Organic and hyperventilatory causes of anxiety-type symptoms. *Behavioural Psychotherapy, 12,* 308–313.

McDonald, R., Sartory, G., Grey, S. J., Cobb, J., Stern, R., & Marks, I. M. (1979). The effect of self-exposure instructions on agoraphobic outpatients. *Behav. Res. Ther., 17,* 83–85.

Maccoby, E. E. (1980). *Social development: psychological growth and the parent-child relationship.* New York: Harcourt, Brace, Jovanovich.

Marks, I. M. (1978). *Living with fear.* New York: McGraw-Hill.

Marks, I. M. (1981). *Care and cure of neuroses.* New York: Wiley.

Marks, I. M. (1982). Anxiety disorder. In J. Greist, J. Jefferson, & R. Spitzer (Eds.), *Treatment of mental disorders.* New York: Oxford University Press.

Marks, I. M. (1986). *Behavioral psychotherapy: Maudsley pocket book of clinical management.* Bristol: Wright.

Marks, I. M., & Matthews, A. M. (1979). Brief standard rating for phobic patients. *Behaviour Research and Therapy, 17,* 263–267.

Marks, I. M., Hallam, R., Connolly, J., & Philpott, R. (1977). *Nursing in behavioral psychotherapy.* London: Royal College of Nursing.

Marks, I. M., Stern, R., Mawson, D., Cobb, J., & McDonald, R. (1980). Clomipramine and exposure for obsessional compulsive rituals, 1 & 2. *Br. J. Psychiatry, 136,* 1–24.

Maxmen, Jerrold. (1986). Anxiety disorders *Essential Psychopathology.* New York: W. W. Norton & Co., p. 204.

Meichenbaum, D., & Turk, D. (1976). The cognitive-behavioral management of anxiety, anger and pain. In Davidson (Ed.), *The behavioral management of anxiety, depression and pain.* Brunner/Mazel.

Meyer, V. (1966). Modification of expectancies in cases with obsessional rituals. *Behav. Res. Ther., 4,* 273–280.

Mineka, Susan. (1987). A primate model of phobic fears. In H. Eysenck & I. Martin (Eds.) *Theoretical foundations of behavior therapy.* New York: Plenum Press.

Osgood, C. E. (1952). The nature and measurement of meaning. *Psychological Bulletin, 49,* 197–237.

Ost, L.-G. (1985). Coping techniques in the treatment of anxiety disorders: Two controlled case studies. *Behavioural Psychotherapy, 13,* 154–161.

Perse, T. L., Greist, J., Jefferson, J., Rosenfeld, R., Dar, R. (1987). Fluvoxamine treatment of obsessive-compulsive disorder. *American Journal of Psychiatry, 144,* 1543–1548.

Rachman, S. (1971). *The effects of psychotherapy.* Oxford: Pergamon.

Rachman, S. (1984). Agoraphobia—A safety-signal perspective. *Behav. Res. Ther., 22,* 59–70.

Rachman, S., Cobb, J., Gray, S., McDonald, R., Mawson, D., Sartory, G., & Stern, R. (1979). The behavioral treatment of obsessional-compulsive disorders with and without clomipramine. *Behav. Res. Ther., 17,* 467–478.

Rachman, S., Hodgson, R., & Marks, I. M. (1971). The treatment of chronic obsessional-compulsive neurosis. *Behav. Res. Ther., 9,* 237–247.

Rachman, S., Marks, I. M., & Hodgson, R. (1973). The treatment of obsessive-compulsive neurotics by modeling and flooding in vivo. *Behav. Res. Ther., 11,* 463–471.

Roper, G., Rachman, S., & Marks, I. M. (1975). Passive and participant modeling in exposure treatment of obsessive-compulsive neurotics. *Behav. Res. Ther., 13,* 271–279.

Rosenbaum, J. F., (1982). The drug treatment of anxiety. *New England Journal of Medicine, 306*(7).

Rutter, M., 1981, Stress, coping, and development: Some issues and some questions. *J. Child Psychol. Psychiat., 22:*323.

Sartory, G. (1983). Benzodiazepines and the behavioral treatment of anxiety. *Behavioural Psychotherapy, 11,* 204–217.

Seligman, M. (1971). Phobias and preparedness. *Behavior Therapy, 2,* 307–320.

Sokolov, Ye.N. (1960). Neuronal models and the orienting reflex. In M. E. B. Brazier & J. Macy, Jr. (Eds.), *The central nervous system and behavior.* New York: Foundation.

Suinn, R. M., & Richardson, F. (1971). Anxiety management training. *Behaviour Therapy, 2,* 498–510.

Suomi, S. J. (1983). Social development in rhesus monkeys: consideration of individual differences. In A. Oliverio and M. Auppella (Eds.), *Behavior of human infants.* New York: Plenum Press.

Suomi, S. J., Kraemer, G. W., Baysinger, C. M., and DeLizio, R. D., (1981). Inherited and experimental factors associated with individual differences in anxious behavior displayed by rhesus monkeys. In D. F. Klein and J. Rabkin (Eds.), *Anxiety: New research and changing concepts.* New York: Raven Press.

Thomas, A., Chess, S., & Birch, H. (1968). *Temperament and behavior disorders in children.* New York: New York, University Press.

Townsend, R. E., House, J. F., & Addario, D. (1975). A comparison of biofeedback-mediated relaxation and group therapy in the treatment of chronic anxiety. *Amer. J. Psychiat., 132,* 598–601.

Trower, P., Bryant, B., & Argyle, M. (1978). *Social skills and mental health.* London: Methuen.

Watson, J. P., Mullett, G. E., & Pillay, H. (1973). The effects of prolonged exposure to phobic situations upon agoraphobic patients treated in groups. *Behav. Res. Ther., 11,* 531–546.

Wolpe, J. (1958). *Psychotherapy and reciprocal inhibition.* Stanford, CA: Stanford University Press.

9

MOOD DISORDERS

BEV WOLFGRAM

LEARNING OBJECTIVES

After studying this chapter, the student will be able to:

- Describe and define the major mood disorders as well as the other specific mood disorders.
- Assess patients with major depression and bipolar disorder.
- Describe the psychoanalytic/ psychodynamic, behavioral/ cognitive, and genetic/ biological theories of mood disorders.
- Identify the various therapies for mood disorders.
- Identify nursing diagnoses and develop nursing care plans for patients with mood disorders.

What Are Mood or Affective Disorders?

Major mood disorders

Other specific mood disorders

Epidemiology of Mood Disorders

Gender

Age

Marital status

Social class

Life events

Personal resources

Personality characteristics

Assessment of Patients with Mood Disorders

Assessment of patients with depression

Assessment of patients with mania

Frequency, intensity, and duration of symptoms

The impact of a mood disorder on the individual

The impact of a mood disorder on the family system

Nursing Diagnoses Commonly Associated with Mood Disorders

Etiology of Mood Disorders

Psychoanalytic/psychodynamic theories

Behavioral/cognitive theories

Genetic/biological theories

Therapies for Mood Disorders

Psychoanalytic/psychodynamic therapy

Behavioral/cognitive therapies

Biological treatments (somatic therapies)

WHAT ARE MOOD OR AFFECTIVE DISORDERS?

Most people have felt "depressed," have expressed feelings of "depression," or have been described by others as being "depressed" at some time in their lives. The words "depressed" and "depression" are common expressions in our everyday conversation. It is important to note, however, that these expressions have many meanings. For some people, depression means experiencing occasional "blues" or "down times." For others, depression means an "intense, dark veil" that overshadows all aspects of their lives for extended periods. It is important to differentiate these experiences so that people in need of treatment for their depression can be identified.

People who experience *depressive symptoms* (as opposed to a depressive disorder) usually continue to function without much disruption in most aspects of their lives. The symptoms are often short-lived and the individual recovers without treatment. The normal grief that accompanies the death of a loved one is a depressive symptom that is not considered a disorder. A *depressive disorder* requiring treatment is far more intense. The affected individual experiences varying degrees of dysfunction in several areas of life. In addition, the duration of depressive symptoms far exceeds "a couple of bad days."

Mood disorders [termed "affective disorders" in DSM-III (1980)] are those that involve a disturbance in mood or affect. According to DSM-III-R the main characteristic of a mood disorder is the presence of a full or partial depressive or manic syndrome. A **syndrome** is a cluster of symptoms that a person experiences during a mood change that continues for a designated period of time. In addition to the mood change itself, the cluster of symptoms involves cognitive, motivational, physical, and behavioral changes in the individual.

DSM-III-R (1987) divides mood disorders into two diagnostic categories, bipolar disorders, characterized by one or more periods of manic or hypomanic episodes, and depressive disorders, categorized by one or more periods of depression without a history of mania. Depression and mania, however, bring with them a great variety of mood and symptom changes which vary in duration, intensity, and frequency. The DSM-III (1980) clarifies this variety by defining the major mood disorders (major depression and bipolar disorder) as those in which there is a full mood syndrome. Dysthymic disorder and cyclothymic disorder were classified as other specific mood disorders and defined as those in which there is a partial mood syndrome of at least two years' duration. Box 9–1 highlights some controversial issues in the diagnosis and treatment of mood disorders.

MAJOR MOOD DISORDERS

Major depression, also called **unipolar depression,** is characterized by sustained, intense depressive symptoms. **Bipolar disorder,** on the other hand, must include a manic episode. **Mania** is characterized as a sense of elation or euphoria. Like depression, mania varies in duration, intensity, and frequency. The assessment section of this chapter will describe in more detail the specific symptomatology of depression and mania.

OTHER SPECIFIC MOOD DISORDERS

The other specific mood disorders are **dysthymic disorder** and **cyclothymic disorder.** In both of these diagnoses the symptomatology is of insufficient intensity and duration to fulfill the diagnostic criteria for either depressive or manic episodes. The symptoms of dysthymic disorder are similar to those of the depressive syndrome. The symptoms of cyclothymic disorder are similar to those of the manic syndrome and are often referred to as **hypomania.** Again the important distinctions between dysthymia and major depression and between cyclothymia and bipolar disorder are in the severity and duration of symptomatology (American Psychiatric Association, 1980).

These diagnostic categories help differentiate the various types of mood disorders. The diagnostic criteria of each category are theory-free—they focus on the presence or absence of symptomatology rather than the reasons for the symptoms. Such diagnostic differentiation enables the clinician to distinguish those persons who are in need of treatment and can benefit from it from those individuals whose mood changes do not require treatment. In making this distinction, it is then possible for the clinician more accurately to identify and implement appropriate treatment. Also see Box 9–1.

EPIDEMIOLOGY OF MOOD DISORDERS

Mood disorders are the most common psychiatric disorders. Several studies have found that five percent of the population in the United States can be diagnosed as having a major depression at any given time and at least ten percent of the population will experience a major depression during their lifetimes. Depression is ten times more common than schizophrenia and three to five times more common than the major anxiety disorders (Griest & Jefferson, 1984). An estimated ten percent of people with depression also have manic episodes and thus are diagnosed as having bipolar mood disorder.

The incidence of mood disorders has been analyzed by many researchers to identify relationships between incidence and population subgroups. Differences in the incidence of depressive disorders among subgroups focus researchers on common characteristics of individuals who develop the disorder. These characteristics may eventually be labeled as risk factors. In turn, a knowledge of risk factors can help to understand the etiology and treatment of mood disorders. Risk factors that have so far been identified and studied include gender, age, marital status, social class, life events, personal resources, and personality characteristics. Also see Box 9–2.

GENDER

Twice as many women as men are diagnosed with unipolar or major depression. However, men are diagnosed with bipolar (manic-depression) disorder as often as women.

Weissman and Klerman (1977) believe that the prevalence of unipolar depression in women is real and not due to women seeking help more often than men. Women do not appear to experience more stressful life events or to consider life events as more stressful than do men. However, women are reported to have more intense symptoms than men. This may be a function of the different ways symptoms are expressed by women or it may be that women are more willing to express the fact that they are experiencing these symptoms. In addition, biological and psychological changes associated with postpartum and premenstrual phases are known to increase risk for depression in women (although the extent of this risk has not yet been determined). Finally, social-role expectations and conflicts as well as personality factors appear to be variables that contribute to the difference between men and women in the incidence of unipolar depression. Women in our society generally have less power and are more dependent and passive than men. These characteristics may predispose women to chronically low levels of self-esteem and little in the way of personal resources to cope with stress—conditions which may make the development of unipolar depression more likely. (See Chapter 19 on women.)

AGE

Younger people experience both unipolar and bipolar disorders more often than older people. For example, a 1981 National Institute of Mental Health study found that sixty-one percent of depressed and manic patients were younger than forty years of age. The average age of onset is different for the two disorders. Onset of unipolar disorder occurs during the middle to late thirties, with earlier occurrence in women than in men. Bipolar disorder is initially seen, on the average, during the late twenties, with an earlier age of onset for women than men (Hirschfield, 1982).

MARITAL STATUS

Unipolar depression appears to be somewhat less prevalent in married persons and in those living in an intimate relationship than in the general unmarried population. Although there are high levels of conflict reported in the marriages of bipolar patients, there appears to be no relationship between prevalence of bipolar disorder and marital status.

**Box 9–1 ●
Controversial Issues in
the Diagnosis and
Treatment of
Individuals with Mood
Disorders**

1. **Issue:** Danger to self: may include suicide attempts, suicide, or poor judgment resulting in dangerous or self-destructive behavior, for example, running through traffic.
   Questions: Who defines dangerousness: clinicians, the public, lawmakers? Should destructiveness to a person's own social role constitute "dangerousness" which calls for legal action?

2. **Issue:** Danger to others: potential or actual physical harm to family members, friends, strangers.
   Questions: Can dangerousness to others be adequately assessed when the patient is the sole provider of information? In cases where the patient has been dangerous to others, including nursing staff, should he be legally charged with criminal assault?

3. **Issue:** Refusal of treatment. This often happens when the affected individual is very depressed or considering suicide; also during hypomania and mania.
   Questions: Should a patient be allowed to sign away civil rights, i.e., sign a contract authorizing future treatment against his will? Should his behavior during previous depressive and manic episodes be accepted as evidence in present commitment hearings?

4. **Issue:** Involvement with the legal system to detain and/or treat.
   Questions: Does instituting the commitment process sabotage the therapeutic relationship between nurse and patient?

5. **Issue:** Fine line between creativity and mania.
   Questions: Does treatment of mania stifle creativity? Do we have a right to expect someone to suffer episodes of depression in order to benefit from the creativity of mania?

6. **Issue:** Given the evidence that mood disorders run in families, is there a need for genetic counseling?

   Questions: To ensure early detection, should children of parents with mood disorders be evaluated routinely for a mood disorder once the parent(s) have been diagnosed with the disorder? Should genetic counseling be routine treatment for adults?

7. **Issue:** Alcohol abuse and/or addiction as a form of self-medication.
   Questions: When is the best time to deal with the alcohol abuse—before or concurrent with treatment for the mood disorder? Can someone addicted to alcohol successfully abstain from alcohol use if the mood disorder is not treated?

8. **Issue:** Other nonprescription drugs used to self-medicate, e.g., amphetamines for depression.
   Questions: Is the use of caffeine a "legitimized" self-treatment for symptoms of decreased energy and decreased cognitive alertness? Should drug abusers be evaluated routinely for mood disorders? Are over-the-counter diet pills used as a self-treatment for the symptoms of food cravings and binge eating?

9. **Issue:** Societal stigma for being "labeled" mentally ill.
   Questions: Do the benefits of diagnosis outweigh the risk of being stigmatized, e.g., access to treatment versus the potential difficulty in running for public office?

10. **Issue:** Possible employment discrimination.
    Questions: Should employment applications and/or interviews include questions regarding treatment for a mental disorder? If so, are the rights of the person with a mood disorder infringed upon? If not, are the rights of the employer being neglected? Should patients be advised to purposely deceive the prospective employer?

Box 9—2 • Eight Questions for Future Research on Mood Disorders

1. What is the difference in impact on the individual and on the family system when the mood cycle and mood changes are unpredictable versus when they are predictable?

2. Is the adjustment that an individual with recurrent episodes of depression or manic-depression makes similar to that made by an individual with another type of chronic illness?

3. What are the effects of self-help groups for persons with depression or manic-depression? Are groups particularly useful in helping the affected individual gain an understanding of the illness in relation to his life? Do they serve as a reminder to the individual that he is different?

4. Given the higher incidence of depression in women, and given the theory of biological predisposition to depression, is depression in women a biological evolutionary adaptation to the oppression and abuse women have experienced throughout generations?

5. What would be the impact on the number of hospitalization days if a hospice-type program were developed to help family members during specific crises, e.g., depression with suicide

ideation or hypomania, in which professional intervention is required?

6. Does the practice of having a patient administer his own medication while hospitalized on an inpatient unit in any way help the affected individual to begin to take responsibility for the disorder?

7. What would be the outcome if an individual with mood disorder contracted with an inpatient unit for a particular number of hospitalization days annually? Would the number of inpatient days used by the affected individual decrease? Would there be earlier recognition of mood swings? Would the sense of failure sometimes experienced by the individual and the family when the affected individual returns to the hospital be lessened?

8. If it is true that there are specific cognitive processes that are associated with depression, could adult depression be mitigated or prevented by screening for these cognitive processes early (for example, late in high school or when there is evidence that Piaget's "formal reasoning" stage has been reached) and instituting cognitive restructuring programs at that time?

SOCIAL CLASS

Mood disorders occur in all social classes. Unipolar disorder has a higher incidence in the lower social classes than does bipolar disorder. The relationship between unipolar diagnosis and social class holds true only for dysthymia. The higher incidence of dysthymia in the lower strata of society is thought to be due to the demoralization of lower social classes; more frequent use of city, county, and state institutions versus private agencies for treatment; and poor access to those facilities due to lack of financial resources and varying degrees of social isolation (Weissman & Myers, 1978).

In the bipolar disorder, there is a direct relationship between incidence and social class (Weissman & Myers, 1978). Higher rates are seen in professional men and women and others with advanced education and social status. The increased energy, productivity, and sense of well-being that are often seen during the early stages of mania are thought to be responsible for the achievements of some of these people.

LIFE EVENTS

Both unipolar and bipolar patients experience an increase in significant life events prior to the onset of the disorder. For the person with unipolar depression, the events that take place just before the onset of the disorder are usually undesirable and out of the person's control. An exit event, such as the death of a family member or the breakup of the person's marriage or a close friendship, is an example of this. However, a cause-and-effect conclusion between these events and the onset of the disorder is not appropriate because the relationship between the event and the mood disorder cannot always be clearly established. The event may be a consequence of, the cause of, or simply coincide with the mood disorder.

PERSONAL RESOURCES

At present, no one has researched systematically the relationship between personal resources (such as intelligence or satisfying relationships) and the mood disorders. However, substantial research has been done to measure the relationship between personal resources and depressive symptoms. As a result, we know that the lack of a close confiding relationship and absence of friends is associated with the incidence of depressive symptoms; but as with life events, the loss of friendships may be a result of rather than the cause of depressive symptoms.

PERSONALITY CHARACTERISTICS

Specific personality characteristics have been found to be associated with the mood disorders. Patients with unipolar depression show higher scores than the general population on tests for introversion, neuroticism, obsessionality, dependency, and guilt. The unipolar group also shows a greater need to maintain self-esteem through approval from others than does the general population (Hirschfield & Cross, 1982).

Bipolar patients appear to score the same on these tests as the general population. When compared to the unipolar group, however, the bipolar population shows increased obsessionality and a greater need to dominate others and be aggressive.

ASSESSMENT OF PATIENTS WITH MOOD DISORDERS

The topic of assessment of patients with mood disorders is divided into five major sections. The first discusses depression, the second discusses mania, the third describes the assessment of an affected individual's symptomatology for presence, intensity, frequency, and duration of symptoms. The two final sections describe the impact of the mood disorder on the affected individual and on the individual's family.

ASSESSMENT OF PATIENTS WITH DEPRESSION

We explore five major areas in the assessment of patients with depression: mood changes, cognitive changes, motivational changes, changes in bodily functions (also called physical or vegetative changes), and behavioral changes. (See Table 9–1 for a complete list of symptoms and Table 9–2 for suggested interview questions for the assessment of depression.)

TABLE 9–1 Symptoms of major depression

MOOD
    sadness
    low self-esteem
    decreased pleasure
    decreased satisfaction
    loss of emotional attachment
    crying spells
    loss of mirth
    feeling burdened

COGNITIVE
    difficulty concentrating
    thoughts slowed down; memory loss
    difficulty making decisions
    negativism
    helplessness
    hopelessness

MOTIVATIONAL
    passivity
    paralysis of will
    escapist wishes
    suicidal ideation

PHYSICAL
    sleep disturbance
    loss of energy
    psychomotor retardation
    change in appetite
    weight loss (or gain)
    decreased sex drive
    anxiety

BEHAVIORAL
    social withdrawal
    decreased initiative
    suicide attempts
    irritability
    alcohol and drug abuse

TABLE 9–2 Suggested interview questions for assessment of depression
These questions should be addressed to both the patient and a family member or friend in order to get a more complete picture of the situation.

Individual and family history	*INDIVIDUAL:* Does the individual have a history of mood disorders? If yes, get the history of treatment. Ask what the nature of treatment was: medication, vitamins, physical activity, and so forth. Ascertain the patient's perception of the treatment, including its effectiveness. Ask whether the patient has tried using the treatment during this most recent episode. *FAMILY:* Is there a family history of mood disorder and its manifestations? Specifically, inquire about recurring episodes of depression, manic-depression, suicide, suicide attempts, alcoholism, prescription or nonprescription drug abuse, trouble with the law (a manifestation of alcoholism or of mania), spending sprees, wide fluctuations in economic status, eating disorders, and postpartum depression. *FAMILY TREATMENT:* If any family member has had a mood disorder, was he or she treated for it? Find out the nature of the treatment and its effectiveness. This data is particularly helpful in tracing the biological family history. Information about specific treatments effective for a family member may help identify a specific medication and/or treatment that will be effective for this person as well.
Mood changes	*SADNESS:* What feelings have you had lately? Have you been feeling down? Have you been feeling sad? How does this period of sadness compare to other times you've felt sad or down—is it about the same, more intense, or less intense? How have these feelings come over you—gradually or all at once? *LOW SELF-ESTEEM:* When you're feeling this way, do you like yourself? Do you find that you're feeling a greater sense of disappointment in yourself? Are there times when you like yourself? *DECREASED PLEASURE IN ACTIVITIES:* Do you find yourself feeling less satisfaction or less pleasure in some of the things that you used to do? If you still participate in them, do you experience less pleasure in the anticipation of doing these activities, during and after participating? *LESS SATISFACTION:* Do you have a sense of not being satisfied with situations that previously were satisfying? Have you had experiences in which you've accomplished something and others have praised you, yet you have felt no sense of satisfaction? *LOSS OF EMOTIONAL ATTACHMENTS:* Do you find yourself feeling disconnected from people around you? Is it hard for you to be involved emotionally with the people with whom you used to be involved? *CRYING SPELLS?* Have you wanted to cry more often lately? Have there been times you have started to cry and felt as if you couldn't stop? Have there been times when you couldn't stop crying? Do you feel as if you want to cry but can't? *LOSS OF MIRTH:* Are you someone who generally has a sense of humor, has laughed a lot and enjoyed laughter in the past? Have you noticed a change in this?
Cognitive changes	*LOSS OF CONCENTRATION AND MEMORY:* Do you find it harder to concentrate at work, in conversations, in play? Do you have difficulty tending to the task at hand or completing a task? Do you have difficulty putting thoughts together? Do you find yourself forgetting things more often? Do you feel absentminded? *DIFFICULTY WITH DECISION MAKING:* Do you find it difficult to make decisions? Have you had difficulty making decisions in the past? *NEGATIVE AND HOPELESS THOUGHTS:* Do you believe that things will be better than they are now? Do you think that bad things are going to happen to you? Do you feel you have control over what happens to you? Why do you think you feel helpless?
Motivational changes	*PASSIVITY:* Is it difficult for you to make even simple decisions? Do you feel like you don't care about anything? *PARALYSIS OF WILL:* Do you feel like you are in a state of suspended animation? Do you feel immobilized?

Escapist wishes and suicidal ideation	Do you put things off? Have you ever felt as if you wanted to end it all? Have you ever felt like hurting yourself? Have you thought of killing yourself as a way out of this? (If answer is affirmative, do suicide assessment: See Chapter 18 on Crisis.)
Physical changes	*SLEEP DISTURBANCE:* Have you noticed any change in your sleep? What is different? Do you have difficulty falling asleep and/or staying asleep? Do you wake early in the morning? Is your sleep less restful lately? Do you feel as if you want to sleep all the time? Do you find it difficult to stay awake? Has your daily sleep time increased recently?
	LOSS OF ENERGY: Have you experienced a decrease in energy available to carry out your usual activities? Do you find yourself dragging during the day or severely fatigued at the end of the day?
	PSYCHOMOTOR RETARDATION: Do you find it difficult to move around? Are you less physically active than you were previously?
	CHANGE IN APPETITE AND WEIGHT LOSS/GAIN: Have you experienced a change in your appetite? Have your eating patterns changed? Are you eating more, or less, or about the same amount? Have you lost or gained weight recently? Was the weight loss on purpose? Have you been dieting? Do you find yourself fasting or binging? Is your food intake very different from day to day? Do you feel in control of your eating? Do you crave certain foods?
	DECREASED SEX DRIVE: Has there been a change in your sex drive? Do you feel less sexy lately? Has there been a change in your sexual activity? Has your partner/spouse mentioned this? Do you find yourself going through the motions without feeling pleasure or involvement?
	ANXIETY: Do you feel anxious? Do you feel this way all the time, or does the feeling come and go? Do you have times when you experience shaking, hyperventilation, shortness of breath, palpitations, dizziness, or feelings of panic and disorientation?
	OTHER PHYSICAL SYMPTOMS: Do you have headaches? Do you have other physical changes, such as nausea, constipation, or vomiting?
Behavioral changes	*SOCIAL WITHDRAWAL AND DECREASED INITIATIVE:* Do you find that you're spending less time with your friends? Do you spend less time entertaining and being around others? Do you find that you initiate fewer social interactions? Do you respond to questions but not ask any? Do you find yourself merely making one-word responses, that is, saying just yes or no and nothing more?
	IRRITABILITY: Have you been irritable lately? Have you found yourself in more arguments or conflicts recently?
	ALCOHOL AND DRUG USE: Have you been drinking more alcohol lately? What reason do you have for doing so? What effect does it have? Do you take any prescribed medication? How much do you take on the average? What effect does it have? Do you use street drugs or nonprescription drugs on a recreational basis? How much and how often? What is the effect?

MOOD CHANGES

Sadness. Observable mood changes occur in people with depression. A person may have mild to severe feelings of sadness. Some individuals describe their mood as "a dark cloud that has settled on me" or "I'm in a black veil and can't find my way out."

Low Self-Esteem. A person with depression may develop negative feelings about self, ranging from disappointment to self-hatred. These feelings are also described as low self-esteem or low self-worth and are evidenced in such statements as "I don't deserve to be cared for" and "I don't like anything about myself."

Decreased Pleasure in Activities. A third emotional change in a person with depression is anhedonia or decreased pleasure in activities, particularly activities that the individual previously enjoyed.

**DSM-III-R
Diagnostic Criteria for
Major Depressive
Episode**

Note: A "Major Depressive Syndrome" is defined as criterion A below.

A. At least five of the following symptoms have been present during the same two-week period and represent a change from previous functioning; at least one of the symptoms is either (1) depressed mood, or (2) loss of interest or pleasure. (Do not include symptoms that are clearly due to a physical condition, mood-incongruent delusions or hallucinations, incoherence, or marked loosening of associations.)

> **1)** depressed mood (or can be irritable mood in children and adolescents) most of the day, nearly every day, as indicated either by subjective account or observation by others

> **2)** markedly diminished interest or pleasure in all, or almost all, activities most of the day, nearly every day (as indicated either by subjective account or observation by others of apathy most of the time)

> **3)** significant weight loss or weight gain when not dieting (e.g., more than 5% of body weight in a month), or decrease or increase in appetite nearly every day (in children, consider failure to make expected weight gains)

> **4)** insomnia or hypersomnia nearly every day

> **5)** psychomotor agitation or retardation nearly every day (observable by others, not merely subjective feelings of restlessness or being slowed down)

> **6)** fatigue or loss of energy nearly every day

> **7)** feelings of worthlessness or excessive or inappropriate guilt (which may be delusional) nearly every day (not merely self-reproach or guilt about being sick)

> **8)** diminished ability to think or concentrate, or indecisiveness, nearly every day (either by subjective account or as observed by others)

> **9)** recurrent thoughts of death (not just fear of dying), recurrent suicidal ideation without a specific plan, or a suicide attempt or a specific plan for committing suicide

B. **1)** It cannot be established that an organic factor initiated and maintained the disturbance

> **2)** The disturbance is not a normal reaction to the death of a loved one (Uncomplicated Bereavement)

> **Note:** Morbid preoccupation with worthlessness, suicidal ideation, marked functional impairment or psychomotor retardation, or prolonged duration suggest bereavement complicated by Major Depression.

C. At no time during the disturbance have there been delusions or hallucinations for as long as two weeks in the absence of prominent mood symptoms (i.e., before the mood symptoms developed or after they have remitted).

D. Not superimposed on Schizophrenia, Schizophreniform Disorder, Delusional Disorder, or Psychotic Disorder NOS.

Comments such as "I go to movies but I just don't enjoy them anymore," "I don't enjoy anything," and "I don't have fun" are common.

Less Satisfaction in Accomplishments. In addition to decreased pleasure in activities, the affected individual experiences less satisfaction in accomplish-

ments. For example, the individual may be unable to experience the sense of satisfaction in work that he or she formerly felt.

Loss of Emotional Attachments. The affected individual may experience a loss of emotional attachments. This detachment may range from decreasing interest in other people to alienation and/or hatred of people important in the individual's life. The person can no longer experience nurturance and intimacy in relationships. Often patients say that they feel "disconnected" from people about whom they care or used to care.

Crying Spells. Crying spells are sometimes classified as a biological/physical change; here we consider them an emotional change. The depressed person may describe constant crying or feeling the desire to cry constantly (expending a great deal of energy in not doing so). The depressed person may also describe the feeling of wanting to cry but being unable to do so.

Loss of Mirth. The loss of mirth response is another emotional change. The depressed person experiences a decreased sense of humor and laughs less frequently. People find a sense of humor helpful in keeping a perspective on life situations and find that a decreased sense of humor is accompanied by a decreased sense of perspective. The depressed person might say, "I used to be able to joke about my work, but now I can't laugh about anything."

Feeling Burdened. The depressed person often experiences a sense of being heavily burdened. This, coupled with loss of energy, produces a feeling of being overwhelmed, emotionally paralyzed, and heavily weighed down. It is difficult for the affected individual to set this feeling aside when asked to do something (such as develop or maintain a personal relationship with someone else).

COGNITIVE CHANGES

Difficulty with Concentrating and Remembering. Cognitive changes in depression involve two aspects of cognition: the process of thinking and the content of thoughts. An important change in cognitive process in the depressed individual is difficulty concentrating. The individual's thought processes slow down, as evidenced by a shorter attention span and difficulty with focusing on one topic. The affected individual may also describe feeling absentminded and having trouble with recall. Some depressed persons have described this as "the brain feeling sluggish" or "slowed down."

Difficulty with Making Decisions. The depressed person may have difficulty making decisions, feeling great frustration at an inability to make decisions previously made easily. Some people describe standing at the closet, immobilized, because they cannot decide what to wear. Or they may go to the kitchen but forget what they want when they arrive there. This difficulty may begin to interfere in all aspects of a person's life. Often it is when this symptom appears, together with difficulty in concentration, that the affected individual seeks help.

Negative and Hopeless Thoughts. When we examine the content of a depressed person's thoughts, or cognitions, we often find that the person believes that negative things are going to happen. A great deal of negativism permeates most aspects of the depressed person's life, often becoming the primary, or even the only, focus. It is difficult for the affected individual to perceive a situation as having positive as well as negative potential. For example, the person may focus on and describe only difficult and unsatisfactory aspects of work, school, or a relationship with another person.

The depressed person also feels that nothing can be done to improve a situation. The person is overwhelmed with feelings of helplessness and hopelessness, believing that circumstances are beyond his or her control and that no one can change them.

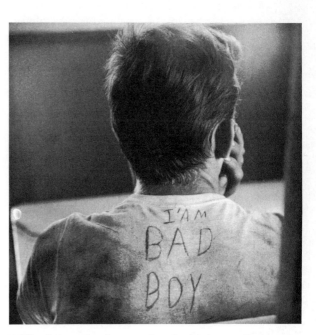

While depression is associated with low self-esteem, it is impossible to differentiate cause from effect. According to Beck (1967), cognitive symptoms of depression include a negative view of self, world, and future. At the same time, having low self-esteem, for example, due to a childhood history of physical abuse, is a potent predictor of future psychopathology.

The severity of the person's sense of loss of control or helplessness affects the individual's perception of his or her world. Comments during assessment interviews demonstrate whether the individual perceives the cause of loss of control as internal or external. If the person feels responsible, and has a negative self-concept, then he feels that the loss of control was brought upon by himself—thus circumstances cannot change because he is an awful person. "The reason things are the way they are is because I'm such a bad person," or "It's all due to me because I'm so bad things can't change and I can't get myself out of this." When an affected individual believes that outside conditions and events are in control, he is expressing a belief in external, uncontrollable causes of his suffering. Both views denote a sense of hopelessness about the future and contribute significantly to the individual's depressed mood. Distinguishing whether the individual sees causation as external or internal helps the therapist to focus intervention on changing the person's cognitions about "out there" or the self. Comments to the effect that "everything is out of my control" and "things are so bad in my life, they will never change" are common.

The sense of hopelessness experienced by the depressed person develops out of negativism and a sense of helplessness. The individual believes that the future will never be any better—things have always been bad in the past, they are bad now, and they will always be that way in the future.

In extreme depressions, **delusions** (unfounded beliefs that are rigidly held to be true, even in the face of contradictory evidence) may be present. An example of this is the affected individual who continues to believe that his job is in jeopardy even after the individual has spoken with a supervisor and has been assured that this is not the case. Also, in extreme depression, an individual may experience episodes of auditory and visual **hallucinations**. These are generally voices and sometimes images of people. Such severe cases of depression are generally referred to as **psychotic depression** because the presence of the delusions and hallucinations indicates that the individual has lost contact with reality.

MOTIVATIONAL CHANGES

Passivity. It is not uncommon for the depressed person to move from an active to a passive role in relationships, work, and the tasks of daily life. A marked shift from activity to passivity occurs most frequently in people who are *not* depressed all the time whereas those who experience *low-grade* depres-

sion all or most of the time often say that they are no more passive than usual.

It is difficult to sort out the cause and effect of a shift to passive behavior. Depressed people often prefer to be dependent, prefer to have things taken care of for them, and prefer to have decisions made by others or by external forces. These preferences correlate with the cognitive symptoms: autonomy requires energy and a sense that one is in control, that one's activities make a difference.

Paralysis of Will. A depressed person may experience paralysis of the will. The individual may be unable to summon any willpower at all, so that activities that helped lift past depressions are beyond doing. The depressed person may have previously enjoyed running, finding it a helpful weapon against depression. Now the person cannot generate enough energy to run. In fact, there may be a physical sense of immobilization.

Escapist Wishes. The depressed individual may want to withdraw or to disappear. This may take the form of procrastination of work. The ultimate escape behavior is **suicide ideation** or attempts. The person's comments may suggest that suicide is a way out of the misery, or that suicide is a way to end all the pain and suffering. These comments may convey the individual's feeling that others would be better off if he or she died. Studies of the association of depression and suicide indicate that depression was diagnosed in from thirty-five to seventy-nine percent of persons who attempted suicide (Boyer & Guthrie, 1985). The nurse should do a suicide assessment whenever dealing with a depressed individual; this assessment must be repeated at regular intervals. Chapter 18 on Crisis discusses assessment of suicide potential in greater detail. Also see Box 9–3.

PHYSICAL CHANGES

Sleep Disturbance. One of the earliest physical changes in the depressed person is disturbance in the sleep cycle. The most common disturbance is insomnia. The person has difficulty falling asleep, has difficulty staying asleep, and/or experiences early-morning awakening. In addition to reporting less sleep, the individual or his or her partner may also report very restless sleep, with tossing and turning at night. A vicious cycle can develop in which insomnia contributes to loss of energy and slowing of biological functions, which in turn intensify depressive symptomatology.

Box 9–3 ●
Determining Suicide Risk

Most mental health professionals know that some patients mask serious depression with smiles and false cheer. Not all know that even in someone who is obviously severely depressed, *improvement* in mental state sometimes heightens the risk of suicide, because the patient is no longer paralyzed by misery. It is also easy to overlook the fact that many patients who commit suicide are not suffering from severe mood disorders. Among psychiatric inpatients, most suicides are schizophrenic; in general hospitals, some suicides are in a state of delirium from alcohol or other causes. Persecutory psychoses of all kinds may culminate in suicide: some patients kill themselves to escape imaginary enemies, others in response to hallucinated commands. And even if the psychosis clears, it may be followed by suicidal despair.

In judging the danger of suicide, mental health professionals should consider the clinical history before the patient's mental state. Psychiatric inpatient departments often fail to do this adequately because they concentrate on short-term care. Many tend to treat everyone alike, working toward early discharge unless a patient is so obviously disturbed or so explicit about suicidal intentions that continued supervision is plainly necessary.

One reason for this error is that so many inpatients are now given the diagnosis of borderline personality disorder. Although such patients often threaten or attempt suicide, they are notoriously difficult to treat in mental hospitals, and ordinarily should not be kept there long. Yet misdiagnosis or incomplete diagnosis is common in these cases. Many have mood disorders (major depression or bipolar disorder) instead of, or in addition to, borderline personality. For such patients a brisk discharge after a short stay may be dangerous; at least half of all successful suicides suffer from mood disorders. The demanding, provocative behavior that seems characteristically borderline may in fact be a sign of agitated depression. Patients suffering from symptoms compatible with the diagnosis of a major depressive episode should be handled cautiously even if they are formally diagnosed as schizophrenic, alcoholic, or borderline personalities. The danger is greatest when they are deluded or hallucinating.

Source: *The Harvard Medical School Mental Health Letter,* Vol. 4 No. 7 Jan, 1988.

Some affected individuals report that, rather than having insomnia, they feel as if they could sleep continuously and often do, or at least sleep more than usual. The person with hypersomnia generally feels no more rested than the person with insomnia.

Loss of Energy. The depressed person experiences a loss of energy, is fatigued, and tires easily. "I feel like I have barely enough energy to make it through the day" and "I feel like I don't even have enough energy to get out of bed in the morning" are common statements.

Psychomotor Retardation. Another physical change in the depressed individual may be **psychomotor retardation**—the slowing down of body movement. It may be so severe that affected individuals have diffi-

culty moving from one position to another—it is a major task to move from a sitting position to a standing position or to walk to work. Some people have so much psychomotor retardation that they are catatonic—literally unable to move.

Loss of Appetite. A depressed person may have loss of appetite, may begin to eat less, and thus may experience nutritional changes. The affected individual might comment, "I've lost 10 pounds in the last two weeks and I don't know how it happened." Some depressed individuals lose their appetites but do not change their eating patterns. Comments such as, "Even though I don't feel like eating, I keep eating because I know my body needs strength," and "Since I don't feel strong and I feel fatigued, I know I have to eat," are not unusual. Some depressed persons increase their food intake and report weight gains. Food binging might occur and food cravings are common, particularly for such foods as chocolate and other sweets.

Decreased Sex Drive. The depressed person's sex drive may decrease. This symptom sometimes brings a couple into therapy, the couple presenting the problem as one person being less interested in sex than the other. An assessment must include evaluation of both individuals' sex drive, sexual responsiveness, and sexual activity. Changes in sexual responsiveness are sometimes more difficult to assess in women.

Anxiety. Some depressed persons also have a problem with anxiety. They may feel anxiety constantly, or they may have anxiety attacks and panic attacks. The depressed person may have either a general fear that something dreadful is going to happen or an exaggerated fear about a specific situation. Some people describe feeling as if something is crawling under their skin. Some are anxious about the unpredictability of the anxiety attacks, which can occur at any time. (See Chapter 8 on Anxiety Disorders for more about assessment and treatment of anxiety.)

Physical Pain. The depressed person may complain about physical pain such as headaches and muscle aches. These pains may be associated with increased muscle tension associated with anxiety.

BEHAVIORAL CHANGES

Social Withdrawal and Decreased Initiative. Depressed persons often withdraw socially, isolating themselves from others. This may take the form of less involvement in activities such as dating, entertaining, and attending social gatherings. Telephone conversations become shorter. The affected individual initiates fewer social interactions and responds only briefly to what others initiate. In conversations, the individual may respond with a single word—yes or no. Also see Box 9–4.

Irritability. Some people experience increased irritability as a behavioral manifestation of depression. This irritability arises out of the combination of negativism and sensation of being heavily burdened. It can be expressed through irritable responses to questions or statements. Irritability leads to conflict, particularly in a primary relationship. The relations of depressed people are often troubled by conflict and/or disengagement as the affected individual withdraws and the partner begins to look elsewhere for satisfaction of emotional needs. In either case the depressed person experiences less satisfaction in the relationship.

Box 9–4 • Not for Adults Only: Depression in Kids

Depression is thought of as an "adult" problem by most people, but it isn't. Children, even babies, and teenagers can also get depressed. It is true that the depressed child can look somewhat different from the depressed adult. For example, the mood change often involves irritability rather than sadness, or the child doesn't seem very childlike. He or she doesn't want to play or is "too tired" or "bored" to try.

Today's teenagers are as familiar with stress and feelings of disillusionment and self-doubt as were their counterparts in the 1960s and 1970s. Growing up, not only with "the bomb" but with the national deficit and AIDS, is more complicated than ever. Pressures to succeed, combined with the economic uncertainty of the 1980s, can intensify such feelings. Changes in the family as a result of divorce or remarriage, or trouble with grades and/or friends, add to this stress and, for some children and adolescents, result in depression.

Parents and adults who work with children and teenagers should be aware of the following warning signs of depression and, possibly, suicidality in children especially if there is a history of depression, alcoholism, or other emotional problems in his/her family. If one or more of the following symptoms appears in a child, the concerned adult should talk with him/her about it and about consulting his/her family doctor or pediatric nurse–practitioner for professional

Alcohol and Drug Abuse. The depressed individual sometimes increases consumption of alcohol for the purpose of self-medication. The alcohol may be used to decrease anxiety as well as to facilitate sleep. Alcohol use itself may become problematic and further mask the underlying depression. The same can be said for self-medication with tranquilizers such as Valium or marijuana and with stimulants such as caffeine and Dexedrine.

Other Behavioral Changes. Other behavioral changes include a sad expression, stooped posture, pacing, and wringing of hands. Also, if the patient has experienced panic attacks, he or she may avoid situations in which the panic attacks occurred. Thus phobic behavior may result from continued avoidance.

SELF-RATING QUESTIONNAIRES

Several self-rating questionnaires measure depression. One is Beck's Depression Inventory (Beck, 1971); another is the Zung Self-Rating Depression Scale (Zung, 1965). The Hamilton Rating Scale for Depression (Hamilton, 1967) was developed to quantify the severity of depression in people who have already been diagnosed as depressed. It is used in combination with the clinical interview.

Self-rating questionnaires are helpful adjuncts in assessing the presence and severity of depression.

However, the clinician should not depend too heavily on instruments that are entirely subjective, because the subjective experience of depression is highly variable. Some subjects whose self-report scores were "normal" on the Beck Depression Scale were actually severely depressed and responded dramatically to treatment (Greist & Jefferson, 1984).

ASSESSMENT OF PATIENTS WITH MANIA

MOOD CHANGES

Euphoria or Irritability. The manic mood may be one of either euphoria or increased irritability. In either case the mood has a major impact on the individual and on the family system. (See Table 9–3 for a complete list of symptoms and Table 9–4 for suggested interview questions for the assessment of mania.)

The euphoric individual experiences an increased sense of gratification, grandiosity, and heightened emotional attachment to others. There is a sense of being very important in others' lives. Others may take on greater importance in the individual's life even if he or she has never met them (this could be a "man on the street," a celebrity, a neighbor, and so on). When in a manic state, a person has a great

---

evaluation if it seems that the child may be depressed.

1. Persistent low self–esteem.

2. Negative thoughts and feelings about him or herself, the world, and the future.

3. Irritability, and/or emotional lability (cries easily), and complaints of boredom.

4. Difficulty in concentrating and/or a decline in school performance.

5. Change in eating and/or sleeping habits.

6. Loss of interest in activities he/she used to enjoy, as well as school, friends, and family.

7. Social or emotional withdrawal from friends and family and regular activities.

8. Frequent physical complaints (for example, stomachache, headache) and associated requests to stay home from school.

9. Seemingly unaffected by praise or rewards or punishment.

10. Neglect of personal appearance.

11. Aggressive or rebellious behavior or running away.

12. Drug and/or alcohol abuse.

13. Preoccupation with violence and/or death.

If it is suspected that the child is thinking of suicide, he/she should be asked directly about this. If his/her answer makes the interviewer uncomfortable, a mental health professional should be contacted immediately. (Also see Chapter 22 for more on psychopathology in children.)

Brumback, R. A., Dietz-Schmidt, S. G., & Weinberg, W. A. (1977). Depression in children referred to an educational diagnostic center: Diagnosis and treatment and analysis of criteria and literature review. *Diseases of the Nervous System, 38*(87) 529–535.

Puig-Antich, J., Chambers, W. J., & Fabrizi, M. A. (1983). The clinical assessment of current depressive episodes in children and adolescents. In Cantwell, D. P., & Carlson, G. A. (Eds.). *Affective disorders in childhood and adolescence,* Jamaica, N.Y.: Spectrum Publications, Inc.

TABLE 9–3 Symptoms of mania

Mood
  euphoria or irritability
  increased sense of gratification
  increased sense of importance (grandiosity)
  increased sense of power and influence
  decreased tolerance

Cognitive
  racing thoughts
  distractibility
  pressured speech
  impulsive decision making
  denial of problems
  delusions of grandeur
  delusions: mood-congruent or mood-incongruent
  impaired judgment

Motivational
  highly driven
  oriented toward action

Physical
  decreased sleep (insomnia)
  hyperactivity
  increased sex drive
  appetite changes
  increased energy

Behavioral
  spending sprees
  increased sexual activity
  involvement in many projects at once
  unpredictable travel
  arguments, verbal threats
  psychological, physical, sexual abuse
  alcohol and drug abuse

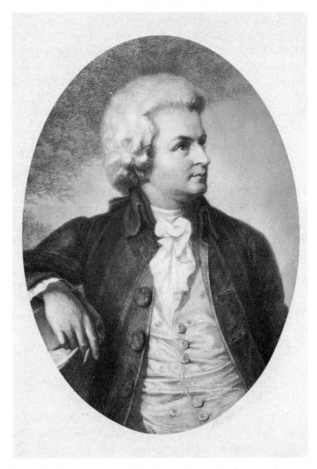

Like Mozart, many patients with manic-depressive illness are at their most creative and productive during their manic phases, as long as they do not become psychotic. For this reason, as well as unpleasant side effects, they often refuse to take their lithium, the drug most likely to control their "lows" as well as their "highs."

mirth response and a marvelous sense of humor, is very quick-witted, and experiences pleasure in nearly every activity. Grandiosity is manifested by having a sense of great power and influence and a feeling that the individual can make whatever changes the world at large might need. The individual believes that his or her view of the world is the best and the only view, and that he or she can accomplish anything. In extreme cases, the individual begins to have an even greater sense of power and influence.

The patient who is irritable also experiences grandiosity and an increased sense of importance. However, this person shows a decreased tolerance for others, is more argumentative, and is often very demanding. The individual is quick-witted but does not exhibit the sense of humor that the euphoric individual does. Like the individual experiencing a euphoric manic episode, this person has a great sense of power and influence. Comments may include, "No one else knows what they're talking about. . . . Everyone is so dumb, so boring."

COGNITIVE CHANGES

Racing Thoughts and Distractibility. As in depressed mood, cognitive changes in mania are of two types: those that involve cognitive or thinking processes and those that involve cognitive content. In the manic person, thought processes are accelerated, often described as "racing." Often thoughts come so fast that the individual cannot keep track of them. Some people have described this sensation as "a motor that runs faster and faster." A related symptom

TABLE 9–4 Suggested interview questions for assessment of mania
These questions should be directed to both the patient and a family member or
friend to get a more complete picture of the situation.

Individual and family history	*INDIVIDUAL:* Does the individual have a history of mood disorders? If yes, get the history of treatment. Ask what the nature of treatment was: medication, therapy, vitamins, physical activity, and so forth. Ascertain the patient's perception of the treatment, including its effectiveness. Ask whether the patient has tried using the treatment during this most recent episode.
	FAMILY: Is there a family history of mood disorder and its manifestations? Specifically, inquire about recurring episodes of depression, manic depression, suicide, suicide attempts, alcoholism, prescription or nonprescription drug abuse, trouble with the law (a manifestation of alcoholism or of mania), spending sprees, wide fluctuations in economic status, eating disorders, and postpartum depression.
	FAMILY TREATMENT: If any family member has had a mood disorder, was he or she treated for it? Find out the nature of the treatment and its effectiveness. This data is particularly helpful in tracing the biological family history. Information about specific treatments effective for a family member may help identify a specific medication and/or treatment that will be effective for this person as well.
Mood changes	*EUPHORIA:* Have there ever been times when you've felt really high, on top of the world, as if you were capable of doing anything? Have there been times when you've felt particularly good about all aspects of yourself? Have there been times when you've felt particularly powerful, that you could accomplish anything to which you set your mind? Have there been times when you've felt you had a special relationship with someone famous or a special relationship with a deity?
	IRRITABILITY: Have there been periods when you've been very irritable? Have there been times when you've argued with everyone constantly?
Cognitive changes	*RACING THOUGHTS AND DISTRACTIBILITY:* Have you ever felt that your thoughts were moving so fast you couldn't keep up with them or keep them straight? Do they bounce all over the place? Do you find it difficult to stay focused on one topic? Are there times when you are easily distracted?
	PRESSURED SPEECH: Have you ever felt as though you needed to talk all the time? Have you ever felt that it was difficult for your speech to keep up with your thoughts?
	IMPULSIVE DECISION MAKING: Have you ever found yourself making decisions impulsively? Have you found yourself making decisions in a way that you generally don't make decisions? Have you made purchases that you couldn't justify later on?
	DENIAL OF PROBLEMS: Has it been difficult for you to understand why family members or friends have expressed the feeling that there is something wrong with your behavior?
Motivational changes	*HIGHLY DRIVEN:* Do you feel driven to work or to accomplish things? Do you feel like you need to be doing something all the time? Is it difficult for you to sit still? Do people tell you to slow down?
Physical/biological changes	*INSOMNIA:* Have there been times when you've felt no need for sleep? How much do you sleep during those times? How rested do you feel?
	HYPERACTIVITY: Have there been times when it has been difficult for you to sit still or stay in the same place for a designated period of time? Have there been times when you paced?
	INCREASED SEX DRIVE: Are there periods when you feel an increase in your sex drive? Is there any increase in your sexual activity at those times? Do you find that you are engaging in sexual relations with people with whom you ordinarily would not?

continued

TABLE 9—4 (continued)

	APPETITE CHANGES: Have you noticed any changes in your appetite—cravings for certain foods or decrease or increase in your food intake? Have you gained or lost any weight recently?
	INCREASED ENERGY: Have there been times when you've felt you had more energy than usual? An endless amount of energy?
Behavioral manifestations	*SPENDING SPREES, INCREASED SEXUAL ACTIVITY, AND SO ON:* Do you find yourself spending more money than usual? Does it feel as though you've been buying things impulsively? Has there been increased sexual activity? Have you suddenly "taken off," traveling somewhere impulsively? Have you found yourself involved in several projects at once and leaving them before they were completed? Have you found yourself talking to almost everyone that you meet, being the "life of the party"?
	ARGUMENTS, ABUSE: Have you had increased arguments, fights, difficulty with the law? Have you physically attacked or hurt anyone? Do you find yourself speeding while driving?
	ALCOHOL AND DRUG USE: How much alcohol do you consume on a daily or weekly basis? Have you been drinking more than usual lately? Do you take any prescribed medication on a regular basis? Have you ever experimented with street drugs like marijuana or speed? Do you use any on a regular basis? (Also see Chapter 15 on Substance Abuse.)

(which some people consider to be physical) is **pressured speech.** A person with pressured speech feels the need to speak very rapidly to keep up with racing thoughts. Distractibility, which leads to difficulty in focusing attention, is common. This is related to both the acceleration of thoughts and heightened responsiveness to stimuli.

Impulsive Decision Making. Decision making is arbitrary and impulsive. A manic individual may decide to buy three cars in one day, sell one house, and buy another.

Denial of Problems. The manic person often denies problems—everything is fine, nothing is wrong. The manic individual has difficulty understanding a partner's or friend's reactions to the manic behavior and concludes that it is due to the other person's distorted view of the world.

Delusions of Grandeur. A positive self-image accompanied by a sense of optimism (as opposed to the negative expectations seen in depression) is an important cognitive manifestation in the manic person. The individual feels very powerful, capable of bringing about significant political, economic, religious, or social change. If there are problems, the manic individual blames others for them.

The manic mood is seductive to the affected individual, particularly if it is euphoric. The sense of well-being and grandiosity is exciting and much preferable to depression or euthymia (being on an even keel). Thus the person is reluctant to stop the hypomanic or manic mood before it is out of control because it feels so good.

Delusional thinking may occur in both euphoric and irritable moods. Delusions are categorized as either **mood congruent** or **mood incongruent.** Mood-congruent delusions are consistent with the themes of inflated sense of worth, power, grandiosity, and having a special relationship with a deity. A person with mood-congruent delusions may believe that he is Jesus Christ or that he is capable, alone, of solving the problem of world hunger. An example of a mood-incongruent delusion is paranoia. A person with paranoid delusions may be certain that he or she is controlled by messages on television, or that someone is inserting thoughts into his or her mind. Persons who exhibit mood-incongruent delusions may have more difficulty in treatment than those whose delusions are mood congruent. Auditory and visual hallucinations may be present in either case. The voices and images involved may convey a message of increased powerfulness or may bring messages with paranoid content.

DSM-III-R Diagnostic Criteria for Manic Episode

Note: A "Manic Syndrome" is defined as including criteria A, B, and C below. A "Hypomanic Syndrome" is defined as including criteria A and B, but not C, i.e., no marked impairment.

A. A distinct period of abnormally and persistently elevated, expansive, or irritable mood.

B. During the period of mood disturbance, at least three of the following symptoms have persisted (four if the mood is only irritable) and have been present to a significant degree:

   1) inflated self-esteem or grandiosity

   2) decreased need for sleep, e.g., feels rested after only three hours of sleep

   3) more talkative than usual or pressure to keep talking

   4) flight of ideas or subjective experience that thoughts are racing

   5) distractibility, i.e., attention too easily drawn to unimportant or irrelevant external stimuli

   6) increase in goal-directed activity (either socially, at work or school, or sexually) or psychomotor agitation

   7) excessive involvement in pleasurable activities which have a high potential for painful consequences, e.g., the person engages in unrestrained buying sprees, sexual indiscretions, or foolish business investments

C. Mood disturbance sufficiently severe to cause marked impairment in occupational functioning or in usual social activities or relationships with others, or to necessitate hospitalization to prevent harm to self or others.

D. At no time during the disturbance have there been delusions or hallucinations for as long as two weeks in the absence of prominent mood symptoms (i.e., before the mood symptoms developed or after they have remitted).

E. Not superimposed on Schizophrenia, Schizophreniform Disorder, Delusional Disorder, or Psychotic Disorder NOS.

F. It cannot be established that an organic factor initiated and maintained the disturbance. **Note:** Somatic antidepressant treatment (e.g., drugs, ECT) that apparently precipitates a mood disturbance should not be considered an etiologic organic factor.

If the individual is in the manic state during the assessment, many of these symptoms are obvious upon observation and interpersonal interaction. The truly manic person finds it difficult to sit still long enough for a thorough assessment interview.

It is very helpful to have a family member or close friend help with the assessment, because there can be tremendous disparity between how the affected individual perceives the mania and how others do. For example, one patient reported that during a period of mania, on an elevator in an elegant hotel, police suddenly entered the elevator, handcuffed him, and carried him off to jail. He had no idea why the police had done this to him. With much encouragement, eventually he added that he was verbally sex-ually abusive to women who entered the elevator. His recall of the situation was that he had been just kidding, had just wanted to have a good time, and that people had misunderstood his actions. Similarly, individuals who spend a great deal of money while manic may downplay the significance of their behavior by explaining that they need the items.

MOTIVATIONAL CHANGES. The individual experiencing mania is highly driven, at times seeming almost to be on an amphetamine-induced "high." The person acts impulsively and makes impulsive decisions. The person wants to be active and involved in everything going on. He or she strives for autonomy and independence, generally desires personal growth and self-enhancement, and wants the world to grow along at the same speed and in the same direction.

PHYSICAL/BIOLOGICAL CHANGES

Insomnia. The manic person often feels little or no need for sleep and so sleeps very little or not at all. When the individual tries to rest, the mind races so fast that it is impossible to fall asleep. If the person does fall asleep, that sleep is often not restful.

Hyperactivity. Hyperactivity—constant movement, pacing, and so forth—is a common physical manifestation of mania. It may be difficult for the person to sit still long enough to take part in the assessment interview or to order and eat a meal in a restaurant. An onlooker's impression is that the affected individual needs to be in constant motion.

Increased Sex Drive. Another physical change is increased sex drive. The individual feels an increased awareness of sexuality and often increases sexual activity. The person may seek more sexual activity with his or her spouse or lover, with friends, or even with strangers.

Appetite Changes. Appetite changes vary. Some individuals crave sweets during manic phases, others crave spicy foods; some have no food cravings at all. Some persons experience a loss of appetite. Food intake may decrease—the individual is too busy to eat and does not think much about food because he or she has plenty of energy. This person may lose weight.

Increased Energy. The manic individual feels full of an endless source of energy. The person may become involved in several projects at once, often failing to complete any of them.

BEHAVIORAL CHANGES

Spending Sprees, Increased Sexual Activity, Involvement in Many Projects, Unpredictable Travel. Behaviors commonly associated with euphoric mania include spending sprees, increased sexual activity, and extramarital affairs (sexual activity with strangers or casual acquaintances). The manic patient is likely to begin several projects at once and fail to follow any of them to completion. The individual may "take off" unpredictably, turning up almost anywhere in the world.

Arguments, Verbal Threats. Persons with irritable mania typically experience increased conflicts and arguments in all their relationships. They are likely to report and/or engage in verbal threats, insults, and other psychological abuse. They may get into difficulty with the law, be disruptive at meetings, drive irresponsibly, and, in short, enrage those around them. The irritable manic person may be physically violent toward family members as well as strangers. (See Chapter 24 on the Violent Patient.) When delusional paranoid, this individual is often both aggressive and secretive, sometimes accusing others of things that are not true.

The manic individual's impulses are nearly uncontrollable. The person's judgment may be so impaired that he or she may attempt to do things that are physically impossible, with disastrous results. For example, the individual may attempt an impossible driving maneuver in traffic or leap out a window in an effort to fly. When delusions and hallucinations (auditory and/or visual) are present, the mania is considered to be of psychotic proportions. In this situation the affected individual's judgment is severely impaired and very dangerous behavior may ensue.

Alcohol and Drug Abuse. Increased alcohol consumption and/or street or prescription drug abuse is as common in mania as in depression. Again, it is often used as self-medication and the diagnosis of mania may be difficult to make as a result.

FREQUENCY, INTENSITY, AND DURATION OF SYMPTOMS

The assessment of symptoms of depression and mania include the variables of frequency, intensity, and duration. (See Table 9–5 for suggested interview questions for the assessment of these variables.) Whether the pattern of symptom changes is predictable or unpredictable is also significant. The particular combination of variables determines the experience of the affected individual and surrounding family members. The individual whose mania occurs every September and lasts for two to three weeks is better able to plan around predicted episodes than is the individual whose manic and depressive moods occur unpredictably, or every two to three months.

When symptoms begin to occur with greater intensity or duration, previously effective interventions may become futile. When assessing an individual who has been depressed for the past month and who indicates that things are worse, it is important to clarify whether the number of symptoms has increased,

---

TABLE 9–5 Suggested interview questions for assessment of frequency, intensity, and duration of mood disorder

Frequency	Have you felt like this before? When? Are these episodes of depression/mania occurring more often than they did before?
Intensity	Is this mood becoming more severe? Are you having more symptoms as the episode continues? (After identifying specific symptoms, inquire about each: "Is your sadness/excitement becoming more intense?" "Is your sleep disturbance becoming more severe?" "Are you thinking more and more about suicide?") Over time, over different episodes of depression, has it been more difficult for you to pull yourself out of it? Over time, have the episodes become more severe, have they interfered more with how you normally live your life?
Duration	When the episodes occur, do they last as long as previous ones? Do you find it harder to pull yourself out of each succeeding depression?

---

whether the initial symptoms themselves have become more intense, or both. Is the individual becoming more dysfunctional? Is the sadness becoming more intense? Is the loss of energy more immobilizing? Is sleep now disturbed where it wasn't before? Has suicidal ideation begun?

It is essential to find out whether the patient has been depressed before, when, and whether the episodes have become more frequent or intense. Some affected individuals who at first had trouble with depression and/or mania every year or even every other year may report that they now have episodes two or three times each year. Other patients may report that the depressions have become more intense, either in severity or in the number of symptoms they experience simultaneously. As a result, their mood changes interfere more in their lives. The duration of the symptoms is important in distinguishing the individual with depressive symptoms from the individual with a depressive disorder.

SUBJECTIVE MOOD SCALE. An individual who experiences mood changes can "map out" mood swings using a subjective mood scale.

- On a scale from zero to ten (0–10), points zero to four rate the degree of depression.

- Point zero describes the *most* depressed the individual has ever been.

- Point four indicates changes in behavior and/or feelings that are cues that the individual is becoming depressed.

- Point five represents the individual's usual or normal mood.

- Points six to ten rate the degree of mania.

- Point ten describes the *most* manic the individual has ever been.

- Point six indicates changes in behavior and/or feelings that are cues that the individual is becoming manic.

An individual's cycle can be charted to show intensity, duration, and frequency of mood changes. (see Figure 9–1 for two examples.) An understanding of the pattern enables the nurse to view minor mood changes within the context of the *entire* pattern of mood changes. For example, an affected individual's sense of humor and increased productivity during hypomania can easily lead an observer to overlook the seriousness of these symptoms. This type of oversight is particularly serious if the individual's manic episodes have involved auditory and visual hallucinations and physical danger to the patient or others.

THE IMPACT OF A MOOD DISORDER ON THE INDIVIDUAL

Both the impact of the present episode and the impact of recurring mood fluctuations on the affected individual's life must be considered when doing an assessment.

The impact of a depressed mood is great. The depressed person cannot function well at work or school because of disruptions in cognitive functioning. Primary and other relationships suffer because of the affected individual's sense of isolation and failure to initiate social interaction. Intimacy is difficult. The depressed person may feel a sense of unworthiness in relationships or that he or she lacks the ability to be in a healthy relationship. The individual might consider divorce or separation from a marriage or inti-

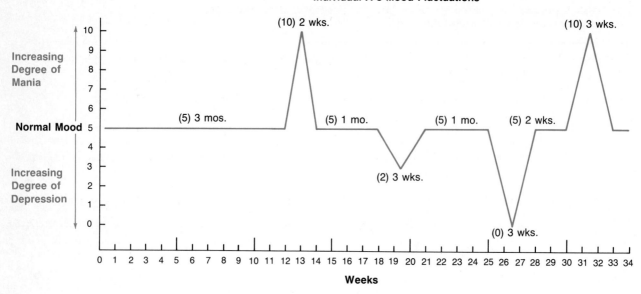

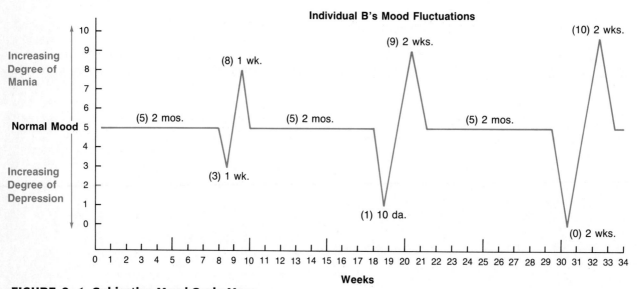

FIGURE 9–1 Subjective Mood-Scale Maps

mate relationship. If, as often happens, friends tire of trying to break through the depression, the person's sense of isolation deepens.

The manic individual also becomes dysfunctional, perhaps failing to go to work or classes. He or she may take great risks by driving recklessly, perhaps causing an automobile accident. Sometimes this individual is thought to be intoxicated and may be incarcerated without treatment.

Because of the seductiveness of the manic mood, it is difficult for the individual to set personal limits. He or she may know that a manic episode is on the way but struggle with whether or not to give it up because right then he or she is being productive and feeling really good. The person may deny what is ahead or may be willing to take the risk and take what comes. Similarly, the person who experiences episodic mania may feel that it is worth it. In both situations, the individual's family or therapist may feel differently.

Recurring mood swings leave a residual impact on the patient's life. The person may feel embarrassed or guilty if, during a manic phase, he or she engaged in sexual activity with strangers or mere acquaintances, or caused a financial burden to the family by spending the contents of a savings account. It is not uncommon for this person to become depressed after a manic episode upon recalling or hearing about extreme behavior. The affected individual may be confused, wondering "Who is the *real me?*" The patient is struggling to find his or her identity and self-image as he or she tries to define self and capabilities. He or she can lose confidence, questioning his or her ability to be in a relationship, hold a job, and/or be an effective parent. And, because the patient doesn't know whether or when the next episode will occur, or whether treatment will be effective, he or she fears losing control.

An affected individual may leave treatment during an acute phase of a mood disorder. Even though the person has learned in counseling to develop self-love, to be assertive, and to relate to others in more constructive ways, these skills may not be helpful during a mood change. The person may feel, instead, that treatment can never be helpful and that effort expended on learning and using these new skills was wasted.

THE IMPACT OF A MOOD DISORDER ON THE FAMILY SYSTEM

The family of a patient with a mood disorder feel they are losing control of the situation. They feel helpless when interventions make no difference in the affected individual or, worse, intensify the mood change. They worry that the affected person will attempt suicide or commit physical violence; they thus expend a great deal of energy fending off arguments and conflicts and avoiding situations that trigger them. Family members fear the loss of both economic and emotional stability. Can they count on the affected individual to be responsive in meeting their emotional needs? Can the spouse count on the individual to fulfill parenting responsibilities or to carry through on projects for and with the family? Family members often see the affected individual as engaging in unacceptable behaviors "on purpose," particularly those behaviors symptomatic of mania. They might view (and describe) the individual as lazy, reckless, or irresponsible. Implicit in such a point of view is the loss of respect and esteem for the affected

individual. Family members are often embarrassed about what to say to neighbors, other family members, and friends about the individual's behavior.

NURSING DIAGNOSES COMMONLY ASSOCIATED WITH MOOD DISORDERS

Assessment of the individual with a mood disorder enables the nurse to establish nursing diagnoses. Assessment of the impact of the person's mood changes on the family facilitates the formulation of nursing diagnoses for the family as well. Formulation and application of nursing diagnoses are still in the developmental stage. The North American Nursing Diagnosis Association (NANDA) has conceptualized the identification, clinical testing, and clinical application of nursing diagnoses. The following nursing diagnoses are based on nursing assessments of persons with mood disorders and are drawn primarily from nursing diagnoses developed by NANDA (Gordon, 1985).

Mood
  disturbance in self-concept (self-esteem, role performance, pleasure)
  alteration in emotional response

Cognitive changes
  sensory perceptual alterations (visual, auditory)
  alterations in thought processes

Motivational changes
  alterations in ability to initiate

Physical changes
  sleep pattern disturbance
  alterations in energy levels
  alterations in nutritional status

Behavioral changes
  alterations in parenting, actual
  impaired verbal communication
  potential for violence: self- and/or other-directed
  social isolation
  sexual dysfunction

Impact on the family system
  ineffective family coping: compromised
  ineffective family coping: disabling
  potential for violence: directed toward others
  alterations in family process

DSM-III-R Diagnostic Criteria for Cyclothymia

A. For at least two years (one year for children and adolescents), presence of numerous Hypomanic Episodes (all of the criteria for a Manic Episode, except criterion C that indicates marked impairment) and numerous periods with depressed mood or loss of interest or pleasure that did not meet criterion A of Major Depressive Episode.

B. During a two-year period (one year in children and adolescents) of the disturbance, never without hypomanic or depressive symptoms for more than two months at a time.

C. No clear evidence of a Major Depressive Episode or Manic Episode during the first two years of the disturbance (or one year in children and adolescents).

Note: After this minimum period of Cyclothymia, there may be superimposed Manic or Major Depressive Episodes, in which case the additional diagnosis of Bipolar Disorder or Bipolar Disorder NOS should be given.

D. Not superimposed on a chronic psychotic disorder, such as Schizophrenia or Delusional Disorder.

E. It cannot be established that an organic factor initiated and maintained the disturbance, e.g., repeated intoxication from drugs or alcohol.

ETIOLOGY OF MOOD DISORDERS

It is generally accepted that depression is caused by a combination of variables, including sociological, psychological, and biological. It is the way in which these variables interact that produces depression. Theories of the etiology of depression can be classified into three major categories: psychoanalytic/psychodynamic, behavioral/cognitive, and genetic/biological.

PSYCHOANALYTIC/PSYCHODYNAMIC THEORIES

Psychoanalytic theory postulates that depression is the result of a particular personality structure, one in which rage felt in reaction to threatened or real abandonment is turned inward against the self in an attempt to avoid anticipated rejection. The individual is predisposed to recurring depressions because of specific childhood experiences that shaped his or her personality structure. As an adult, he or she is sensitive to situations that are actually or symbolically similar to those childhood experiences. (The adult situations trigger feelings associated with the childhood experiences.) Although episodes of depression may be alleviated by other forms of treatment, the individual remains vulnerable to recurring episodes of depression as long as the personality structure remains unchanged.

Freud's psychoanalytic theory has become the foundation of several theories of depression. In his monograph, "Mourning and Melancholia" (Freud, [1917]1956), he described the difference between grief and depression. Freud observed that in grief the focus of loss is external; grief is directed at the lost loved one, and has no effect on self-esteem. In depression, he observed, the focus of loss (whether it involves emotional abandonment, divorce, death, and so on) is internal. This is evidenced by decreased self-esteem, internal impoverishment (lack of an inner life composed of fantasies, ideals, and so on), and self-recriminations, all of which seem to be more characteristic of the one who has been lost than of the depressed person.

INTROJECTION. Freud theorized that the self-recriminations of the depressed person involve anger directed inward as a result of **introjection** of the lost love object into the depressed person's ego. Introjection also accounts for the depressed individual's internal sense of loss and emptiness: he has, essentially, lost a part of himself.

A person who uses introjection to deal with loss probably had childhood experiences with loss. As a child, the person may have lost the mother or the mother's love. Future losses of love objects reactivate the anger persisting from the original loss. Because of introjection, this anger is turned inward and experienced as low self-esteem and possibly self-hate.

DSM-III-R Diagnostic Criteria for Dysthymia

A. Depressed mood (or can be irritable mood in children and adolescents) for most of the day, more days than not, as indicated either by subjective account or observation by others, for at least two years (one year for children and adolescents)

B. Presence, while depressed, of at least two of the following:

1) poor appetite or overeating

2) insomnia or hypersomnia

3) low energy or fatigue

4) low self-esteem

5) poor concentration or difficulty making decisions

6) feelings of hopelessness

C. During a two-year period (one year for children and adolescents) of the disturbance, never without the symptoms in A for more than two months at a time.

D. No evidence of an unequivocal Major Depressive Episode during the first two years (one year for children and adolescents) of the disturbance.

Note: There may have been a previous Major Depressive Episode, provided there was a full remission (no significant signs or symptoms for six months) before development of the Dysthymia. In addition, after these two years (one year in children or adolescents) of Dysthymia, there may be superimposed episodes of Major Depression, in which case both diagnoses are given.

E. Has never had a Manic Episode or an unequivocal Hypomanic Episode.

F. Not superimposed on a chronic psychotic disorder, such as Schizophrenia or Delusional Disorder.

G. It cannot be established that an organic factor initiated and maintained the disturbance, e.g., prolonged administration of an antihypertensive medication.

What follows is the hopelessness and helplessness of depression.

EGO-ORIENTED THEORIES. According to **ego psychology,** a theory that builds on Freud's work, a person's ego (who he is) is influenced by the drives of his id (his instinct) and by his superego (who he would like to be). The ego is also viewed as an autonomous process capable of influencing both the instinctual drives and the environment. The ego derives pleasure from experience, learning, and developing mastery. The ego's development is an evolving process of lifelong learning and maturation (Wetzel, 1984).

According to ego psychology, depression is the result of an intolerable "credibility gap" between a person's superego and ego (and the associated self-esteem). A depressed individual constantly seeks external feedback to build and maintain a satisfactory sense of self. Through others, rather than the self, a kernel of self-esteem and self-worth is maintained. When the individual realizes and/or perceives lack of support in the environment, he or she experiences overwhelming disparity. What follows is depression (Wetzel, 1984).

GRIEF AND DEPRESSION. Arieti and Bemporad (1980), two major psychiatric theorists, have expanded and refined the psychoanalytic theory of depression. They focus on the difference between grief and depression, a predisposition to depression based on early childhood experience, and the theme of loss in recurrent depression.

The difference between grief and depression for Arieti and Bemporad is that the depressed individual is incapable of having the psychological and cognitive mechanisms of normal grief. In normal grief, an individual immediately evaluates the meaning of death to him or herself, experiencing shock and then sadness. For several days or weeks, thoughts about the deceased evoke a painful sadness. The grieving individual may have difficulty believing that the loved one is really dead, but as time passes adjustment begins. The sadness begins to be eliminated, forcing reorganization of thinking and rearrangement of life so that the deceased is no longer essential to the survivor's psychological equilibrium. In time, the individual will begin to reestablish a life without the deceased (Arieti, 1977).

The depressed person is incapable of the cognitive reorganization of normal grief. The sadness of depression retards the individual's thought processes rather than forcing reorganization. The psychological mechanisms of depression appear to decrease the number of thoughts in order to decrease the amount of suffering. This slowing down of thought processes may be so intense that there is immobilization of thought and movement. The depressed person's inability to reorganize thoughts following a loss is related to his or her childhood experiences with loss (Arieti, 1962).

EARLY CHILDHOOD EXPERIENCES. Arieti and Bemporad (1978) postulate that the early childhood experiences of depressed adults involved a period of intense gratification of needs followed by withdrawal of that gratification. This withdrawal may have been caused by the birth of another child, the death or illness of a parent, or any situation involving a withdrawal of love. The child attempts to solve the dilemma in one of two ways: 1) by making himself more dependent and regressive, so that whoever takes care of him will be forced to reestablish patterns of need gratification; or 2) by attempting to live up to the expectations of whoever takes care of him, no matter how difficult it seems. Compliance and hard work become the tools by which this child tries to recapture gratification. When efforts are unsuccessful, the child believes he is at fault and tries even harder to comply. The child who chooses the first method of solving his dilemma will probably later transfer the role of mother or caretaker to others in his life. The child who tries to please those around him will carry his pattern of behavior into adult life (Arieti, 1962).

DOMINANT OTHER AND DOMINANT GOAL. Arieti (Arieti and Bemporad 1978) observes that some depressed adults tend to idealize others and need a particular primary relationship in order to function without severe depression. He has coined the term **dominant other** to describe this influential other from whom the depressed individual derives a sense of worth and well-being. The dominant other

is the symbolic representation of the caretaker who rewards self-sacrifice and hard work and punishes laziness. This relationship enables the depressed person to feel worthwhile and free from guilt and anxiety. For some individuals, the dominant other is not a person but is an organization such as a church, a business, or the military. Such dominant others provide structure, self-worth, and meaning for the depressed individual (Bemporad, 1985).

Arieti and Bemporad (1980) refer to another depressive-behavior pattern as the **dominant goal.** In this pattern, the individual pursues obsessively some unrealistic goal. This pursuit provides him with a degree of self-soothing. He becomes vulnerable to depression because the ways in which he can obtain gratification and a sense of self-esteem are so limited. His vulnerability to depression is heightened when the goal becomes unattainable.

A similarity seen in these two patterns (dominant other and dominant goal) is the associated inhibition of pleasurable activity. The individual feels he must have justification for any self-indulgence and often feels anxious and guilty when confronted with the opportunity for pleasure for its own sake. Instead, he looks for nurturance and approval by others for his participation. If he does not receive nurturance and approval, he becomes depressed (Arieti and Bemporad, 1980).

THEORY OF ATTACHMENT. John Bowlby's (1980) theory of depression includes concepts from psychoanalytic theory as well as concepts compatible with neurophysiology and developmental psychology. His view of depression is derived from his theory of attachment and bonding. An understanding of attachment theory is paramount to understanding his views on depression.

Bowlby's attachment theory facilitates our understanding of the human propensity to make strong emotional ties. **Attachment behavior** is any behavior that enables the individual to attain or retain proximity to some other differentiated and preferred individual. Attachment behavior is distinct from feeding behavior and sexual behavior and leads to the development of affectional bonds—initially between child and parent and later between adult and adult. Attachment behavior is goal corrected in that it is modified to maintain certain degrees of proximity to, or communication with, the object of attachment (Bowlby, 1980).

Attachment behavior contributes to the **attachment bond.** Attachment behaviors are active only when required. Conditions activating attachment behaviors include fatigue, unavailability or unresponsiveness of the object of attachment, and frightening experiences. Inactivation requires other conditions, such as the availability and responsiveness of the object of attachment, a familiar environment, touching, and other reassuring behavior from the significant other. Clearly there is behavior complementarity between attachment behavior and caregiving (Bowlby, 1980).

Intense emotions are aroused during formation, maintenance, disruption, and renewal of relationships involving attachment. Threatened loss arouses anxiety and actual loss results in sorrow. In addition, the threat of loss or actual loss is likely to arouse anger.

Attachment behavior becomes organized on a developmental pathway. Determinants of that pathway are the experiences an individual has had in attachment relationships during infancy, childhood, and adolescence. The pattern of emotional connections the individual makes during adult life is to a large extent determined during these three developmental phases.

Bowlby, a physician and leading psychoanalytic theorist, addresses the depressive symptoms of intense hopelessness and helplessness and feeling unwanted, unlovable, and disconnected. He believes that these symptoms are due primarily to the individual's sense of helplessness about being able to initiate and maintain affectional relationships. Such a negative belief about the self is attributed to specific experiences in the family of origin during infancy, childhood, and adolescence. Bowlby postulates that these experiences are likely to have been one or some combination of the following:

(1) Never having attained a stable and secure relationship with parents despite repeated efforts, including attempts to meet unrealistic demands and expectations. The individual develops a tendency to interpret any future loss as another failure to make or maintain a stable affectional relationship.

(2) Receiving repeated messages about how unlovable, inadequate, or incompetent he is. These messages establish his sense of self as well as a conviction that significant others are unavailable, rejecting, or punitive. Therefore, he expects others to be hostile and rejecting.

(3) Actual loss of a parent during childhood, when consequences of the loss were beyond his power to change. This confirms the belief that any effort that might be made to change the situation is doomed to failure (Bowlby, 1980).

Bowlby holds that these experiences interfere with an individual's ability to establish stable affectional relationships throughout childhood and adolescence. In the same vein, an individual who carries this deficiency into adult life is predisposed to depression.

It is clear from the discussion of these theories that loss is a central theme in psychoanalytic theory. The loss may be of a loved one, of self-esteem, of an ego ideal (what an individual aspires to be), or of attachment. It is important to note that some people have never experienced attachment or had a loved one to lose. Therefore, rather than feeling despair about what they have lost, they may despair that they will never have a stable affectional relationship.

BEHAVIORAL/COGNITIVE THEORIES

Behavioral/cognitive theories of depression are based on **social-learning theory,** which assumes that psychological functioning is best understood in terms of the interaction among the personal, behavioral, and environmental factors of a person's life. Individuals are viewed from a social-learning perspective as being capable of control over their behavior. They are not simply reactors to external influence; they are also initiators—they select, organize, and transform their environment. Depression is the interruption of established sequences of behavior that have been reinforced positively by the social environment. This reduction of positively reinforced behavior is central to the behavioral theory of depression (Hoberman & Lewinsohn, 1985).

BEHAVIORAL THEORIES OF DEPRESSION

The Reduced-Reinforcement Model. The **reduced-reinforcement model** of depression postulates that depression is a function of a low rate of response-contingent positive reinforcement. The low rate of behavioral output and **dysphoria** (unhappiness) in depression are elicited by this low rate of positive reinforcement and/or a high rate of aversive experiences. Because the low rate of positive reinforcement provides little or no rewards or satisfactions, the individual experiences dysphoria or depressed feelings. Thus there is both a causal and a maintenance relationship between reduced positive reinforcement and depression (Hoberman & Lewinsohn, 1985).

Using this model, the death of a devoted spouse of twenty-five years will provoke depression if he or she is not replaced by some other focus. The surviving spouse has lost his or her major source of positive reinforcement. The more focused on the mate, the greater the loss. The surviving spouse begins to feel that there isn't any reason to continue to do most of what he or she did (homemaking, for example). Thus she is led to inactivity (low behavioral output) and feelings of worthlessness and boredom. Inactivity can result in social isolation (an aversive experience), which removes the potential for finding new sources of positive reinforcement and maintains the depression.

Lewinsohn has proposed some etiologies for the low occurrence of positive-reinforcement interactions. One is that the individual's environment may have few positive reinforcers or may contain numerous punishing aspects. Another is that the individual lacks the skills to obtain positive reinforcers that are available or to cope effectively with aversive factors. A third is that potency of positive reinforcement may have decreased and the negative impact of aversive events may have increased (Lewinsohn, Biglan, & Zeiss, 1976).

The Depressogenic Model. Lewinsohn and his colleagues have recently proposed a model that describes the etiology and maintenance of depression. The model describes the depressogenic process and conditions most often involved in the development and maintenance of depression. A strength of the model is that it incorporates a number of the different characteristics and processes that influence depression and accounts for the heterogeneity of symptomatology observed in depressed persons (Lewinsohn et al., 1985).

The **depressogenic model** consists of seven components:

1. The first component identifies the antecedents to depression. Antecedents are those events that increase the likelihood of future depression in an individual; these include life stresses such as marital distress and work problems.

2. The second component involves the disruption of an individual's important, automatic behavior patterns (such as eating when hungry, sleeping when tired, and so on) due to the antecedents identified above. A disruption in these behavior patterns is very likely to elicit dysphoria.

3. The third component of the model recognizes the reduction of positive reinforcement in the individual's life, and/or an increase in aversive experiences. Hospitalization for any reason usually involves both. The quality of the person's interactions with environment now becomes primarily negative.

4. The fourth component is the individual's inability to reverse the process that has begun; that is, he or she cannot increase environmental positive reinforcement and resume normal behavior. As a result, self-awareness is increased but is filled with self-criticism.

5. The fifth component of the depressogenic model recognizes the individual's intensified or magnified emotions. When an individual feels responsible for an event that is producing dysphoria, and blames him or herself for failing to reverse it, then depression deepens.

6. The sixth component involves the cognitive, behavioral, emotional, and interpersonal changes that occur as the result of increasing dysphoria. These changes may help "lock" the person's increased self-awareness and dysphoria into a cycle that maintains the depressive state.

7. Finally, the seventh component of the model takes into account variations in individual factors such as gender, age, history of depression, family history of depression, and environmental factors such as an oppressive work situation, economic difficulty, and lack of social support, all of which may increase or decrease the person's vulnerability to depression. These factors may also influence all other aspects of the depressogenic process (Lewinsohn et al., 1985). For example, hospitalization for a four-year-old is likely to be more depressogenic than for a thirty-four-year-old. (See Chapter 19 on Women for one view of the influence of gender in the depressive process.)

Extinction-Trial Behavior. Observations of depressed individuals' interpersonal interactions have demonstrated that, while signs of depression elicit concern and support from others (Coine, 1976) initially, persistence of the depressed behavior may eventually elicit guilt, withdrawal, and even hostility. Hostile responses add to the individual's increasingly aversive experiences. This series of interpersonal interactions is called "extinction trial" by Arnold Lazarus (Lazarus, 1968) since motivation to continue the interpersonal relationship is gradually extinguished.

The **extinction-trial behavior** of depressed patients causes others to withdraw their support, nurturance, and attention at the very time the depressed person most wants them. For example, a depressed person may call a friend for help or advice on an upcoming job interview; the friend offers some specific suggestions. However, the depressed person keeps calling that friend for the same advice; in time, the friend becomes irritated and withdraws. If the depressed person calls his friend again to request advice about something else, the friend may be reluctant to respond because he knows that he will be asked the same thing over and over again. Ultimately, the depressed person may be unable to elicit support from others and either gives up or is unable to stop provoking people to withdraw from him.

COGNITIVE THEORIES OF DEPRESSION

Negative Cognitive-Set Theory. **Negative cognitive-set theory** (Beck, 1972) emphasizes the influence of cognitions on emotions. According to Beck, in a depressed person, the depressive affect (emotion) is secondary and the negative cognitive set is primary. The negative cognitive set involves the depressed person's negative perceptions of the self, the world, and the future, the "cognitive triad" according to Beck. These negative perceptions are responsible for the emotional, motivational, and behavioral changes in depressed patients.

The depressed person's negative perceptions of self, the world, and the future lead to an interpretation of events within a framework of self-deprecation and self-blame. Other people may challenge the depressed person's assessment of himself, but he maintains his point of view.

The negative cognitive set includes the following manifestations:

Arbitrary inference: the person draws conclusions without adequate evidence to support them.

Selective abstraction: the person draws conclusions on the basis of a single element among many possibilities.

Overgeneralization: the person makes sweeping conclusions based on a single event.

Magnification and minimization: the person makes gross errors in evaluation with little or no basis in reality (Beck, 1967).

The Learned-Helplessness Model. The **learned-helplessness model** of depression (Seligman, 1975) integrates theoretical constructs from learning theory and attribution theory. The fundamental hypothesis of the learned-helplessness model is that the individual has learned that his responses to a situation do not control the outcome(s) of that situation. He may attribute this problem to his own inadequacy, another's influence, fate, or whatever.

This model developed out of studies conducted to observe the effects of punishment on dogs. The dogs were subjected to electrical shock irrespective of their responses. The experiments produced passivity in the subjects as well as an inability to learn how to respond effectively. Seligman concluded that uncontrollability of outcomes (the outcome is unrelated to the response) can significantly debilitate an organism, resulting in motivational, cognitive, and emotional deficits (Seligman, 1975).

The motivational deficit involves a reduction in the initiation of voluntary responses. This decreased initiation is viewed as a consequence of the individual's expectation that outcomes are uncontrollable. In other words, "Why bother?" The cognitive deficit is manifested later on when the individual tries to learn that responses *can* and *do* produce a particular outcome, although previous learning indicated otherwise. It is difficult to learn, in general, that outcomes can be controlled. The emotional deficit refers to the depression, which is another consequence of learning that outcomes are uncontrollable (Abramson & Seligman, 1978). (See Chapter 25 on the ICU Patient for more on learned helplessness.)

Attribution Theory. According to **attribution theory,** after the individual has learned that he is helpless he attributes his helplessness to various factors. These attributions are along three dimensions: internal-external, stable-unstable, and global-specific. Internal attribution involves the person's belief that the outcome of a situation is the result of some internal flaw in himself. For example, the person might say, "I failed the test because I'm stupid." Note that, although he blames the outcome of the situation on himself, he does not feel in control of the situation; being "stupid" is something he cannot change. External attribution involves the belief that the outcome of a situation is as likely to happen to others as to him due to external factors. For example, he might say, "The teacher wrote a tricky test and everyone had difficulty." Internal attribution is more likely to result in decreased self-esteem (Abramson & Seligman, 1978).

The stable-unstable dimension of the attribution refers to the longevity of the "causative" factor. Stable factors are recurrent and long-lived; unstable factors are short-lived and intermittent. For example, attributing failure on an exam to "lack of ability" is considered a stable, while attributing it to "lack of effort" is an unstable factor (Abramson & Seligman, 1978).

The global-specific dimension addresses how easily the causative factor can be generalized. A global factor affects a wide variety of outcomes and suggests that the helplessness will occur across situations. Specific factors imply helplessness only in the situation that resulted originally in the learned helplessness. Attributing failure on a mathematics exam to "lack of intelligence" is global, whereas attributing it to "lack of mathematical ability" is specific (Abramson & Seligman, 1978).

Application of this model to depression helps to clarify our understanding of cognitions and behaviors of depressed individuals. Studies indicate that depressed students are more likely to attribute failure to internal factors than are nondepressed students. Studies of depressed persons' attributions for success and failure have found that they often make internal, global, and stable attributions for failure and tend to make external, specific, and somewhat less stable attributions for success (Abramson & Seligman, 1978). Common statements about failure and success are: "I failed the exam because I'm stupid" (internal, global, stable) and "I passed the exam because it was easy" (external, specific, less stable).

The propensity to attribute failure to internal factors results in decreased self-esteem. Thus the depressed person emerges from this learned-helplessness process with deficits in four areas: motivational, cognitive, emotional, and self-esteem.

The intensity of these deficits depends on how certain the individual is that the outcomes of situations are uncontrollable. In addition, the importance to the individual of a desired outcome to a situation influences the intensity of the decreased self-esteem and emotional deficit. This model predicts that depression results when a person believes that an outcome he desires is improbable—or that an undesirable outcome is probable—and that whatever he does to influence it, he will have no effect on the outcome (Abramson & Seligman, 1978).

GENETIC/BIOLOGICAL THEORIES

GENETIC THEORY. The nature versus nurture (genetics versus environment) controversy about likely etiology inevitably surfaces in any discussion of the etiology of a psychiatric disorder. It has received attention because of reports of evidence for a genetic and biological basis of major depression and manic-depression.

According to genetic theory, people in the same family are more likely to have major depression than are random individuals in the general population. The closer the biological relationship, the greater the probability will be that if one family member has major depression, other members will, too. In other words, while two cousins may have major depression, the probability of a brother and sister or parent and child having it is greater. The increased probability reaches its maximum with identical twins and bipolar disorder. If one twin has bipolar disorder the probability that the other will have it is between fifty and eighty percent (Wender & Klein, 1981).

Studies have also found that relatives of people with major depression are more likely to develop mild depression (dysthymia) than random individuals in the general population. However, these relatives may have fewer and less noticeable depressive symptoms than the relatives with major depression and are less likely to be treated (Wender & Klein, 1981).

Studies of adoption cases have been used to distinguish between the effects of nature and nurture in individuals with mood disorders. In Belgium, researchers have studied the biological and adoptive parents of adults with bipolar mood disorder (Mendlewicz & Rainer, 1977). The biological and adoptive parents were compared to each other and to the biological parents of adults with polio and the biological and adoptive parents of normals. The researchers concluded that the biological parents of the adopted adults with manic-depressive illness had as high an incidence of major depression (unipolar) as the biological parents who raised their own children, many of whom developed manic-depressive illness as adults. The adoptive parents of the adult manic-depressives had no greater incidence of psychiatric disorders than did the biological parents of the adult polio patients or the adoptive parents of the normal adoptees (Mendlewicz & Rainer, 1977).

Cadoret (1978) arrived at similar results. He also concluded that adoptees with affectively ill biological parents had a higher incidence of depression than did adoptees with normal biological parents or adoptees whose biological parents had other psychiatric disorders.

Family and genetic studies support the distinction between bipolar and unipolar illness. They indicate that the incidence of mood disorders among first-degree relatives of individuals who have bipolar disorder is twice that occurring in relatives of individuals with unipolar disorder (Cadoret, Winocur, & Clayton, 1970).

BIOLOGICAL THEORY: BIOGENIC-AMINE THEORY. The **biogenic-amine theory** of depression suggests that the etiology of major depression is underactivity of nerve cells whose neurotransmitters are the biogenic amines (such as serotonin and norepinephrine). This theory evolved from research on essential hypertension. When some patients with hypertension were treated with the drug reserpine, they became severely depressed. Experimental work with animals found that reserpine depleted the brain of three chemicals belonging to the monoamine (biogenic-amine) family. It was tentatively concluded that the biogenic amines are associated with mood. A deficiency of these amines produces depression and an excess produces a state of excitement or mania (Wender & Klein, 1981).

The biogenic-amine theory is supported by the action of antidepressant drugs, which increase the availability of certain biogenic amines (neurotransmitters) at critical receptor sites in the brain. The biogenic amines are involved in the transmission of nerve impulses in the brain and other parts of the central nervous system. Two of these neurotransmitters, norepinephrine and serotonin, have received special attention in the study of depressive illness. The following are variations on the biogenic-amine hypothesis:

> (1) The catecholamine theory hypothesizes that norepinephrine depletion causes depression. The catecholamine brain system is associated with positive action, pleasant circumstances, and arousal.
>
> (2) The indolamine theory hypothesizes that serotonin depletion causes depression. This brain system is associated with sleep, unpleasant or painful circumstances, and decreased responsiveness.
>
> (3) The permissive theory hypothesizes that depletion of both norepinephrine and serotonin causes depression.
>
> (4) The two disease theory hypothesizes that: (a) norepinephrine depletion coupled with a normal level of serotonin causes depression, and (b) serotonin depletion with a normal level of norepinephrine causes depression. This new emphasis is less on individual neurotransmitters and more on interdependent relationships (Wetzel, 1984, pp. 243–244).

The biogenic-amine hypotheses are controversial because findings have been inconsistent. In addition, present technology allows the neurotransmitters to be measured only indirectly. The inductive logic that is used as a result of that indirect method results in hypotheses, not necessarily explanations. For example, although it is known that antidepressant drugs that increase the output of norepinephrine alleviate depressive symptomatology, it does not necessarily follow that replacing norepinephrine will alleviate depression or that depression is a norepinephrine deficiency. More research is needed. This issue will be taken up again in the section on antidepressant medications, on pages 285–288.

BIOLOGICAL TESTS FOR DEPRESSION. Interest in understanding the mood disorders from a biological basis is increasing. As a result, laboratory tests are being developed and studied to determine the effectiveness of biological measurements in diagnosing mood disorders.

Dexamethasone-Suppression Test (DST). The **dexamethasone-suppression test (DST)** has become the most widely used biological test for diagnosis of a psychiatric disorder. Under normal conditions, the administration of dexamethasone, a potent synthetic steroid, completely suppresses the production and release of cortisol from the adrenal gland. However, in many depressed patients there is only a partial suppression or an early recovery (escape) from suppression of cortisol output (Sternberg, 1984).

The standard method for the DST is to administer 1 mg of dexamethasone orally at 11 P.M. or midnight and then determine the plasma cortisol concentrations at 4 P.M. and 11 P.M. the following day. If postdexamethasone plasma cortisol concentration is 5 μg per dl or greater, the test is considered positive because there has been a failure to suppress cortisol (Carroll et al., 1981). Studies have suggested that, on the average, forty-five percent of patients with major depression produce an abnormal DST. Thus the DST may be useful in diagnosing major depression or a variant of affective illness, such as atypical depression. A negative DST result is not as valuable diagnostically because more than fifty percent of patients with major depression show normal cortisol suppression (Sternberg, 1984).

Thyrotropin-Releasing Hormone Test (TRH). Use of the **thyrotropin-releasing hormone (TRH)** in the diagnosis of depression developed during a study of TRH in the treatment of depression. Researchers found that there is a smaller amount of thyroid-stimulating hormone (TSH) released after TRH infusion in depressed patients than in control subjects (Prange et al., 1972).

To administer the TRH, the nurse gives the patient 500 μg of TRH by intravenous push over thirty seconds, following an overnight fast. An in-dwelling intravenous catheter is used to draw a baseline blood sample (pre-TRH infusion) and then additional samples are taken at fifteen-minute intervals for ninety minutes after the TRH infusion. A TSH level of less than 5 or 7 μg per ml and greater than fifteen is considered abnormal (Prange et al., 1972). A blunted TSH response to TRH infusion is found in twenty-five to sixty-five percent of patients with major depression. Abnormal TRH test results are relatively independent of DST nonsuppression. Thus the use of both tests may increase the identification of depression (Sternberg, 1984).

Other Laboratory Tests. Some other laboratory tests have not been fully proven to be useful in diagnosing depression; these include the growth-hormone–stimulation test and the measurement of platelet-serotonin transport and platelet-imipramine binding, all of which are biological correlates of mood disorder. Research on these correlates is in its infancy and so, as yet, what produces the relationship between these factors and mood disorders is not known. Growth-hormone release has been found to be lower in depressed patients than in control subjects following insulin-induced hypoglycemia or ingestion of the drug clonidine. Preliminary research indicates that the speed of platelet-serotonin transport is decreased in unipolar and bipolar depression but is normal during manic phases. Research has also indicated that the number of imipramine-binding sites (imipramine being one of the tricyclic antidepressant drugs) on the platelets of depressed patients is fewer than in controls. Imipramine has been associated with serotonin transport (Sternberg, 1984).

THERAPIES FOR MOOD DISORDERS

Although the physician may be the one to administer procedures and order tests and medications, the nurse always knows and understands what is happening. A nurse's role may vary from one clinical setting to another, but she always knows the meaning of a procedure, the outcome of a test, and the therapeutic and side effects of medications.

PSYCHOANALYTIC/PSYCHODYNAMIC THERAPY

Psychoanalytic/psychodynamic therapy is designed to restructure the personality pattern of a depressed individual so that future episodes of depression are prevented and the person's everyday functioning and well-being are improved. Therapy is based on the theory that the preexisting personality structure predisposes the individual to depression when he or she experiences a loss. The personality structure requiring change affects interpersonal relationships, the means of obtaining self-esteem, and the basic view of the self.

STAGES OF THERAPY. The process of psychoanalytic/psychodynamic therapy for depression can be broken into four stages: engagement, initial, working-through, and termination. Each stage involves therapeutic tasks or goals. Transition between stages is not abrupt; it often consists of overlapping therapeutic tasks and processes.

The Engagement Stage. During the **engagement stage,** the therapist establishes rapport with the patient, expresses a genuine interest in helping, is open and honest regarding her limitations, and offers clarity about certain issues, such as availability and charges. The therapist also conveys to the patient that ultimately he has the power to help himself and that she will help him mobilize that power through confrontation and interpretation. The patient often seeks therapy during or following a loss and focuses primarily on his depressive symptoms and sadness. It is important that the therapist not accept the patient's assessment of himself as helpless, inadequate, or overwhelmed. If she does, she quickly develops a pattern that supports the patient's regression and interpersonal stance of helplessness and dependency. The therapist is active and empathic in directing the patient to focus on feelings and on trying to better understand himself (Bemporad, 1976).

The Initial Stage. The **initial stage** of psychoanalytic/psychodynamic therapy sets a foundation for the work of personality reorganization. During this stage, the therapist attends to the transference relationship that develops. The therapist also relates the patient's particular life situation(s) to his specific personality organization. The therapist also attempts to connect the precipitating events of the depression to the patient's maladaptive ways of achieving and maintaining a sense of self-worth (Bemporad, 1985).

The development of transference in the therapeutic relationship is paramount to the psychoanalytic therapy process. **Transference** is an unconscious process wherein the patient projects the characteristics of a loved one (possibly, a loved one who has been lost) onto the therapist, initiating and reacting to the therapist as if she were that person. He may demonstrate resistance to therapy, request premature termination of therapy, or sink into more severe depression as a result. It is crucial that the therapist recognize the transference phenomenon as it develops and deal with it within the context of therapy. Transference can be a powerful tool—it brings the depressed person's actual interpersonal and internalized struggles into the therapeutic relationship where they can be reexperienced in a safe context and be examined. (See Chapter 5 on Assessment.)

Relating particular life situations to specific personality organization requires that the patient recall and describe childhood experiences. Recall is facilitated through dream interpretation, memory exploration, and the transference phenomena. During this reconstruction of the patient's early life, the therapist encourages him to identify and appreciate the forces that led him to adopt certain defenses, ways of relating, and means of achieving and maintaining self-esteem. This process also enables the patient to identify valuable and gratifying aspects of his personality that have been suppressed and/or repressed to maintain self-esteem (Bemporad, 1985).

The Working-Through Stage. The **working-through stage** is the process by which the patient relinquishes his depressive and other maladaptive modes of behavior. This stage is characterized by frequent advances, stalemates, and regressions. Although the patient begins to see that his behavior and psychological defenses are dysfunctional or pathological, they continue to provide him with some sense of security, predictability, and gratification. His resistance is usually based on the unconscious fear that his life will be completely empty or chaotic without the pathological but familiar structure on which his life is based. The depressed patient's basic struggle often consists of giving up his excessive reliance on external sources for self-esteem, and trying new ways of obtaining gratification and meaning (Bemporad, 1976).

As therapy progresses, the patient's interpersonal relationships assume a new form. For example, the patient openly expresses his feelings of anger as well as spontaneous enjoyment. He also relinquishes his role as the inferior in the "dominant other" pattern and achieves a more realistic view of how others can fulfill his needs. Self-esteem becomes internalized. This enables the patient to see others as more than simple bestowers of praise or rewards. He begins to perceive other people as struggling with the difficulties of life and relationships that he does, and as individuals who are influenced by childhood experiences similar to his. The therapist encourages the patient to understand that significant others in his past were influenced by their own childhood experiences and, as a result, had their own problems. This understanding of the past increases the patient's ability to be empathic to other people and not to revert to his dysfunctional ways of relating to them and himself (Bemporad, 1985).

The Termination Stage. The **termination stage** of therapy is designed to bring closure to the therapeutic relationship. This may involve review of the therapy with the patient, including whether the patient has achieved his goals, his feelings regarding his behavioral changes, and his plans for the future. It is very important to deal with the patient's feelings about separation from the therapist. Successful termination of therapy is crucial because it provides an experience for dealing with separation and loss in a new and constructive way.

The psychoanalytic/psychodynamic approach is not limited to patients and therapists in a psychiatric setting. Depressed patients in nonpsychiatric settings may benefit from nursing care based in part on the psychoanalytic/psychodynamic treatment model; however, referral to a psychotherapist should be considered in certain cases. For example, a 34-year-old woman on a general internal-medicine unit for regulation of her diabetes mellitus is withdrawn, tearful, and expresses intense sadness. She states that the diabetes became unmanageable following her separation from her husband three months ago after ten years of marriage. She says that loss has always been difficult for her and feels she has suffered more than her share of losses. Her father was killed in a car accident when she was five; her paternal uncle, who was active in her parenting following her father's death, died of a heart attack when she was fifteen; and her mother died three years ago. She wonders whether there is some way to deal with the present loss that would be less disruptive to her life.

In this situation, which involves chronic as well as current loss, psychoanalytic/psychotherapy may be the best approach to treatment. The nurse can discuss with the patient the goals and process of psychoanalytic/psychodynamic psychotherapy and recommend two or three psychotherapists in her geographical area. She can also encourage the patient to focus on and talk with her about the feelings related to her losses and respond with empathy and support.

BEHAVIORAL/COGNITIVE THERAPIES

BEHAVIORAL THERAPY. Behavioral therapies are based on the theory that depression is maintained by reinforcement of depressed behavior and inadequate reinforcement of nondepressed behavior. Behavioral therapies, then, increase positive reinforcement for nondepressed behavior and teach the individual how to elicit positive reinforcement from other people. This is accomplished through the process of **contingency management,** in which reinforcement for depressed behavior is withdrawn and positive reinforcement for nondepressed behavior is substituted. The nurse identifies effective reinforcement for each patient, and then observes the patient's response, making modifications in the reinforcement program as appropriate.

Three behavioral therapies used in the treatment of depression are discussed here: social-skills training, assertiveness training, and reality therapy. The principles of the behavior therapies particularly lend themselves to use by the nurse working with the depressed patient, whatever the setting, on becoming an active participant in his treatment (medical or psychiatric).

Social-Skills Training. **Social-skills training** is designed to increase the depressed individual's social interactions by strengthening his social skills. Techniques focus on increasing the frequency of positive social interaction through positive reinforcement. Social interactions are broken down into steps, and the individual is encouraged to increase his social interaction one step at a time. Reestablishing social contact, for instance, can be broken down into 1) calling a friend and inviting him to do something that involves minimal interaction (like attending a movie); 2) having lunch with the same friend; and 3) planning further social interaction with him or someone else. The nurse positively reinforces the patient's successful social-interaction activity and focuses discussion on how that success can be carried over to other social interactions.

When planning to use this treatment mode, the nurse considers the following basic interventions:

Establish a baseline for a desired activity, say walking outdoors, that includes its frequency, degree of pleasure for the patient, and duration.

Establish a contract in which the patient and nurse decide together on a plan of action as well as mutual and separate responsibilities and expectations. The contract between the 34-year-old diabetic woman described earlier and her nurse might include: talking about feelings instead of keeping them to herself, exercising regularly, and making at least one social contact per day. The contract would also specify the steps toward these goals in behavioral terms as exemplified above, the reward for the achievement of each step, and negative consequences for engaging in undesirable behavior (such as avoiding all social

contact for a period of time). Rewards can consist of self-nurturing of various kinds; consequences can be physical exercise or financial contributions to a charity of the individual's choice.

Offer substitute behavior for dysfunctional behavior, such as walking instead of sleeping when morale is low.

Provide continuous reinforcement for the successful behavior, with plans to increase the period of time that elapses between the behavior and the reinforcer.

Plan increased social interaction around activities that are already of interest to the patient; for example, an individual with a special interest in movies would take someone to the movies.

The principles and techniques of social-skills training are applicable to patients both in psychiatric and nonpsychiatric settings. For example, it would not be unusual for a young man with a spinal-cord injury to become quite depressed and become increasingly socially withdrawn. During his rehabilitation process, his primary nurse might plan an activity that gradually increases his experience with positive social interaction. The activity would be one of special interest to the patient as well as have the potential for success. The nurse would provide acknowledgment and praise for the patient's attempts and accomplishments. A therapeutic alliance between nurse and patient is important to the success of any such behavioral program. Trust and openness in the relationship enhance the patient's ability to recognize how he sabotages his success.

Assertiveness Training. **Assertiveness training** can be an effective therapy for depressed persons who tend to be nonassertive and lack communication skills, often a result of feeling inadequate. Nonassertiveness can also be related to fear of vulnerability and a sense of loss of control over situations. Assertiveness training can increase the affected individual's sense of control over himself and his self-confidence, and reduce his sense of vulnerability.

The first step in teaching assertive behavior to the depressed person is to help him distinguish between nonassertive, assertive, and aggressive behavior. Nonassertive behavior is not standing up for one's rights in order to avoid conflict and to please others. The nonassertive individual seems to be passive and deferential to other people, without self-respect. Aggressive behavior involves standing up for oneself at the expense of others. The aggressive individual exhibits domineering, coercive, and abusive behavior. Assertive behavior is standing up for one's rights without violating others' rights. Assertive expression is direct, honest, and straightforward.

Nonassertiveness may also be manipulative. That is, the nonassertive individual may work indirectly to obtain what he needs. Ironically, the manipulative behavior often originates in the individual's sense of powerlessness in a situation, while the behavior is controlling the situation in a subtle and underhanded manner. Such interactions are successful temporarily but ultimately reinforce the person's sense of powerlessness and guilt.

Assertiveness training is most often done in a group, but it can be carried out on an individual basis as well. Assertive behavior can be taught to depressed individuals by using a variety of behavioral techniques, such as positive reinforcement, modeling, role playing, and role reversal. With positive reinforcement, for example, the group leader and members compliment, or reinforce, an individual when he demonstrates assertive behavior. With modeling, the individual may design or "model" his behavior on the behavior of others in the group on someone in another setting, such as a television character whose behavior is identified as assertive in specific situations. In role playing, the individual practices assertive behavior that he plans to carry out in life situations. The group leader and members take on the role of other persons in a specific life situation. In role reversal the depressed person must demonstrate nonassertive behavior while group members demonstrate assertive behavior. This provides an opportunity for the individual to observe the interaction from the stance of nonassertiveness (Smith, 1975).

Several phenomena may occur as the depressed person begins to learn assertive behavior. The individual may manifest behavior that is more aggressive than assertive. It is thought that, once given permission to express himself, the depressed person acts aggressively because he has not yet had sufficient experience in learning and integrating assertive behavior. The depressed individual's family may complain of the disruption they experience. As the depressed person becomes more assertive and assumes greater responsibility for his behavior, the family will be able to reduce its responsibility for the depressed member. In addition, the depressed person's sense of vulnerability is decreased because he has learned how to express his needs and wants.

Assertiveness training can be a useful intervention in both psychiatric and nonpsychiatric settings.

A woman admitted to an orthopedic unit may be feeling very depressed and overwhelmed by her temporary incapacitation due to a broken leg. She expresses concern about taking care of her two preschool children but is reluctant to ask her husband and extended family for assistance. The nurse can role play with the patient how best to express her needs and requests to her husband and family. The nurse then seeks followup information regarding the success of the interaction, helps the patient plan further assertive interaction if necessary, and praises her for her accomplishment. The nurse can also encourage the patient to use her newly acquired assertive skills while still a patient with the nursing, medical, and physical-therapy staff rather than, for example, "not bothering" the doctor and nurse with questions, requests, and so on.

Reality Therapy. Reality therapy, developed by William Glasser (1975), is based on the principle that a person is responsible for his own behavior. Reality therapy is intended to help change the depressed person's self-image from one associated with passivity, dependency, and helplessness to one that embraces activity, independence, and power. It is based on the premise that the depressed person is in control of the depression. Therapists who adhere to this framework refer to the affected individual's behavior as "to depress" rather than "to be depressed." The therapeutic process is intended to help the individual identify behavior that depresses him, to plan strategies to change this behavior, and to continually assess progress. As with other therapies, rapport between the patient and the therapist is essential.

The first step in reality therapy is to clarify what the patient "wants" and to restate these desires as goals to be achieved when the patient is not depressed. The nurse encourages the patient to focus on his depressed behavior as it relates to the established goals. The nurse might ask, "Why are you depressing yourself now? What might you do differently?" The nurse and patient discuss the conflicts between the patient's goals and his depressing behaviors in order to help the patient better define the problem.

Patient and nurse together develop a plan and establish a specific contract to change behavior that is identified as not helpful. The plan is constantly modified and improved. The behavioristic rationale for continuous modification is that when changes in an individual's behavior do not occur according to the plan, the failure is the plan's rather than the patient's. The patient is not criticized, nor are excuses permitted or accepted. The nurse continues to convey a hopeful attitude to the patient by continuing to work on and improve previous plans (Glasser, 1975).

Reality-therapy techniques can be applied in both psychiatric and nonpsychiatric settings. For example, a patient attempting to learn care of his ostomy may express feeling depressed because he continues to fail to do it adequately. The nurse intervenes to assist him in identifying the behavior that interferes with his learning and success. Such behavior, if continued, serves to depress the patient because it represents failure. Alternative behavior is identified that is likely to increase the potential for the patient's mastering his ostomy care. If the patient does not achieve success, the nurse encourages him to identify how the alternative behavior might be further modified.

COGNITIVE THERAPY. The primary treatment technique based on cognitive therapy is called **cognitive restructuring.** The therapist encourages the depressed person to identify his errors in thinking, to associate these errors with his depressed feelings, and to replace his negative cognitions with thoughts that enhance his self-image and represent reality more accurately. Therapeutic techniques based on cognitive theory include role rehearsal, assertiveness training with role playing, recording automatic thoughts, identifying underlying assumptions or predictions in thought patterns, and modifying "should" messages.

As in other therapies, the therapeutic relationship in cognitive therapy is extremely important. The therapist is empathic as well as objective. The therapist attempts to think as the patient thinks, and to gain an understanding of the patient's emotional and cognitive responses—in short, to view the world through the patient's eyes. Objectivity and a logical approach to situations under discussion as well as to the patient's thought processes are required of the nurse. A balance between empathy and objectivity is crucial. Objectivity is requisite for identification of the patient's cognitions. Empathy allows the nurse to recognize the patient's tendency to overpersonalize interactions and helps her frame discussion in terms that help the patient not feel criticized or attacked.

The initial phase of cognitive restructuring focuses on situations in which the patient becomes depressed. He is encouraged to identify the "automatic thoughts," such as "I never get anything right," that he experiences in these situations.

The therapist then relates the patient's negative cognitions to his feelings of depression. Thought processes associated with these negative thoughts are examined to exemplify illogical and invalid connections that the patient may be making. For example, a young woman feels that her fiancé's moodiness and recent angry outbursts are evidence that he really doesn't love or want to marry her. In fact, his feelings may have nothing or little to do with her. Other logical errors include arbitrary inference, overgeneralization, overpersonalization, magnification, and minimization. Another common illogical connection is the "if-then" pattern. In this pattern, the patient's thought process could be like the following: "*If* my husband would rather go out with the guys than stay home with me, *then* he doesn't love me, and the reason for this is that I am not lovable." The patient is asked to keep track of her cognitions (thoughts) as well as what triggers them. Patient and therapist together examine the content and process of the patient's cognitions.

Replacement of negative cognitions and restructuring of thought processes into more logical ones can be achieved in a variety of ways. The affected individual might keep a log of his depressed feelings, thoughts associated with those feelings, the logical processes used to draw conclusions, and the positive thoughts and logic that are successful in interrupting negative thought processes.

The therapist identifies cognitions consistent with learned helplessness and challenges them. The therapist then teaches the patient to substitute thoughts of power for thoughts of powerlessness and helplessness. The therapist may also teach problem-solving skills, which can enable the individual to develop a sense of mastery over his environment. Identifying the problem and breaking it down into manageable parts helps the patient focus on specifics, which in turn enables him to identify solutions. In the example above, the problem is the woman's turmoil about her husband's behavior which she interprets as evidence that he doesn't love her. The problem can be broken down into his behavior and all its possible meanings, and her feelings about it which seem unmanageable. Specificity and reduction of a problem to parts reduce the patient's sense of being overwhelmed. After the patient has mastered a situation previously viewed as out of control, the therapist can refer to that success as the patient tackles other problems.

As mentioned in the discussion of learned helplessness, the depressed person generally attributes his failures to internal, stable, and global factors. Cognitive restructuring is directed at changing his invalid attributions in the direction of external, unstable, and specific factors. Cognitive change is required if the depressed person is to feel involved in his success. Attribution of success to internal, stable, and global factors increases the individual's self-esteem and self-confidence (Abramson & Seligman, 1978).

The depressed person's expectation that the outcome of a situation is uncontrollable is an important cognition that requires change. The depressed person's cognitive restructuring is directed toward changing his expectation from that of uncontrollability to controllability. His actual behavioral responses may require some training, but first the patient must believe that his behavior can influence or control the outcome.

The effectiveness of cognitive therapy has been studied primarily with nonpsychotic, unipolar depressed persons. Cognitive therapy has been found to be as effective as antidepressant-medication therapy in mild to moderate depression. However, the effectiveness of antidepressant medication and cognitive therapy in combination is greater than the effectiveness of either treatment alone, particularly in severe depression (Rush et al., 1982).

Although cognitive therapy is effective in symptom reduction, it is important to remember that symptom reduction is not the only objective. Cognitive therapy is also intended to help prevent future depression by changing the patient's automatic negative thought processes. The approach may be especially beneficial for depressed patients who, as a result of other illnesses, cannot take antidepressant medication (Rush, 1983).

Cognitive therapy can be extremely useful in rehabilitation of cardiac patients. For example, a woman executive referred for rehabilitation following a myocardial infarction expresses feeling hopeless about her future. She believes that she will never again be able to function effectively as an executive, will become economically dependent on others, and will have to give up all physical activity. The nurse encourages her to examine the basis of her assumptions and asks questions that direct her to examine her thought processes: "Are there other directions your life may take? Is there anything in the rehabilitation process that may help you prevent those outcomes?" The patient and nurse examine how the patient's cognitive processing results in her feeling sad, hopeless, and out of control of future events. The nurse makes suggestions about how such thought processes can be interrupted. For example, "When you are feeling depressed, say 'Stop what am I thinking' and question whether you are assuming that there is only one possible outcome or alternative."

BIOLOGICAL TREATMENTS (SOMATIC THERAPIES)

ANTIDEPRESSANT MEDICATIONS. The tricyclic antidepressants, the newer second-generation antidepressants, and monoamine oxidase inhibitors are the major medications used in the treatment of depression. The purpose of these medications is to alleviate the symptoms associated with depression, and make it possible for the patient *not* to feel depressed. They are not mood stimulants.

TRICYCLIC AND SECOND-GENERATION ANTIDEPRESSANTS.

The **tricyclic antidepressants** are called tricyclic because their chemical form includes three-ring structures. Imipramine, the first of the antidepressants to be used in the treatment of clinical depression, was introduced in 1958 and development of other tricyclics quickly followed. Recently, antidepressant medications with different chemical structures have been developed. One, maprotiline, has a four-ring structure and is referred to as a tetracyclic. These newer medications are called second-generation antidepressants. Other second-generation antidepressants include amoxapine, trazadone and fluoxetine.

In general, the tricyclic antidepressants show a high level of effectiveness in alleviating depressive symptomatology. Various studies report that sixty to ninety-five percent of depressed persons experience a remission of symptoms when treated with these drugs. Researchers continue to attempt to predict individual response to the tricyclics on the basis of particular patient characteristics, symptomatology, onset of symptoms, and biological markers like an elevated DST (Noll, Davis, & DeLeon-Jones, 1985).

Studies have evaluated the effectiveness of the **second-generation antidepressants** as compared to "standard," that is, tricyclic treatment. Initial reports indicate that the newer drugs may have an earlier onset of action. However, these results have not been replicated, and none of the second-generation drugs has been shown superior to imipramine or amitriptyline, another commonly used tricyclic antidepressant, in relieving symptoms of depression. An important advantage of the second-generation group is the decreased incidence of anticholinergic and cardiovascular effects as compared to the tricyclics; however, they have other adverse effects (Rudorfer, Golden, & Potter, 1984). See Tables 9–6 and 9–7 for the type, incidence, and rating of side effects of the tricyclic and second-generation antidepressants.

TABLE 9–6 Side effects of tricyclic and second-generation antidepressants

Tricyclic Antidepressants

Type of side effect	Description
Anticholinergic	Dry mouth Blurred vision Urinary retention Constipation Sweating Increased intraocular pressure
Cardiovascular	Orthostatic hypotension Tachycardia Palpitations
Other	Restlessness and/or agitation Insomnia Skin rash Mild tremors Weight gain or loss Agranulocytosis (rare)

Second-Generation Antidepressants*

Drug	Side Effect
Amoxapine	Parkinson-like extrapyramidal symptoms Akithisia Akinesia Increased serum prolactin and galactorrhea Tardive dyskinesia Impotence Inhibition of ejaculation Painful ejaculation In women, inability to reach orgasm
Trazadone	Psychosis Cardiac arrhythmia Prolonged and painful penile or clitoral erection Confusional state (including ataxia, fatigue, inability to think clearly, drowsiness)
Maprotilene	Seizures
Fluoxetine	Nausea Nervousness Headache Insomnia

*As a group, these medications produce fewer anticholinergic and cardiovascular side effects than the tricyclics.

Source: From Noll, K. M., Davis, J. M., and DeLeon-Jones, F. (1985). Medication and somatic therapies in the treatment of depression. In E. E. Beckham and W. R. Leber (Eds.), *Handbook of depression*. Homewood, IL: Dorsey Press. Fluoxetine information from The Medical Letter on Drugs and Therapeutics, 30: 45, 1988.

Mechanisms of Action of the Antidepressants. For a long time, it was thought that antidepressants selectively enhanced neurotransmitter activity in the brain. The tricyclics were thought to block neuronal reuptake of the monoamine neurotransmitters nor-epinephrine and serotonin, while monoamine oxidase inhibitors acted by decreasing the rate of breakdown of the neurotransmitters. This theory, however, failed to account for all therapeutic effects of the drugs when used with clinically depressed patients.

TABLE 9—7 Tricyclic and second-generation antidepressants, dose, side effects rating

Agent		Usual Daily Starting Dose* (mg)	Usual Effective Daily Dose* (mg)	Relative Sedative Effects	Relative Anticholinergic Effects	Relative Hypotensive Effects
Generic name	Trade name					
Tricyclic antidepressants						
Amitriptyline	Endep Elavil Amitid	75	150–300	High	High	More
Desipramine	Norpramine Pertofrane	50	100–300	Low	Low	More
Doxepin	Adapin Sinequan	75	75–300	High	Medium	More
Imipramine	Janimine Sk-Pramine Tofranil	75	150–300	Medium	Medium	More
Nortriptyline	Aventyl Pamelor	50	50–100	Low	Medium	Less
Protriptyline	Vivactil	15	15–60 (divided into 4–5 doses)	Low	High	More
Trimipramine	Surmontil	75	50–200	High	Medium	More
Second-Generation Antidepressants						
Amoxapine	Asendin	50 tid	150–400	Medium	Low	Less
Trazadone	Desyrel	50 tid	150–400	High	Low	Less
Maprotilene	Ludiomil	75	125–225	Medium	Low	Less
Fluoxetine	Prozac	20 A.M.	20–40			

*Lower doses (often one-third to one-half of the usual dose) are used with older patients.
Source: Adapted from Griest, J. H., and Jefferson, J. W. (1984). *Depression and its treatment*. Washington, D.C.: American Psychiatric Press, p. 45. Fluoxetine information from The Medical Letter on Drugs and Therapeutics, 30: 46, 1988.

Some studies have attempted to identify the mechanisms of the antidepressant action. Reuptake blockage of neurotransmitters occurs almost immediately after administration of the tricyclic antidepressant, and observation has confirmed that there is usually some relief of symptoms during the first week of treatment. Full remission of depressive symptoms, however, requires three weeks or more, leading to rejection of reuptake blockage as the single explanation for the therapeutic effect. Other studies are evaluating the drugs' effects on receptors and receptor sites rather than on the amount or location of the neurotransmitters themselves (Noll, Davis, & De-Leon-Jones, 1985).

MONOAMINE OXIDASE INHIBITORS (MAOIs). The **monoamine oxidase inhibitors (MAOIs)** were first studied and used as antituberculars. They received attention as antidepressants when it was noted that they relieved depressive symptomatology. It was also noted, however, that some patients receiving this type of medication who ingested foods high in the amino acid tyramine developed hypertensive crisis, sometimes to the extent that they suffered intracranial bleeding and death. Thus initial use of MAOIs in the treatment of depression was quite conservative, and doses were probably too small to be effective. This cautious approach no doubt contributed to the early impression that MAOIs were less effective than tricyclics (Noll, Davis, & DeLeon-Jones, 1985).

Recently, the use of MAOIs for treatment of depression has become more common. Some depressed patients who have not responded to other treatments respond well to MAOIs. The affected individuals who are most likely to respond to MAOIs are those experiencing atypical depression (or depressive disorder not otherwise specified, according to DSM-III-R), for example, emotional responses to loss that are prolonged or pathological in degree. These people generally have not responded to tricyclics or electroconvulsive therapy, another biological treatment which will be discussed later, and so had

been regarded as having "characterological" depression, a type thought to be nonresponsive to biochemical treatment (Noll, Davis, & DeLeon, 1985).

The range of side effects from MAOIs is similar to that of the tricyclics, with one important addition: hypertensive crisis. The MAOI medications inhibit oxidase, the enzyme that breaks down monoamines in many parts of the body, including the intestine. Because of this, more monoamines than usual may be absorbed by the intestine, among them tryamine, a monoamine that affects blood pressure. Extreme elevations in blood pressure may occur, precipitating intracranial bleeding that can lead to stroke or death. For this reason, foods that contain large amounts of tyramine must be avoided (see Table 9–8).

LITHIUM. **Lithium** has become increasingly popular in the United States since it was approved by the Food and Drug Administration in the early 1970s for use in treating and preventing mania. Lithium has also been found effective in treatment of some

---

TABLE 9—8 Monoamine oxidase inhibitors (MAOIs)

Generic Name	Trade Name	Daily Dose*
Phenelzine	Nardil	60–90 mg
Tranylcypromine	Parnate	20–60 mg

Side effects for both drugs	Foods to avoid**
Similar to tricyclic antidepressants	Aged cheese in any form
Hypertensive crisis	Yogurt
flushing	Liver
sweating	Broad bean pods
weakness	Pickled, fermented, smoked, or aged meat, fish, or poultry
headache	Caffeine in large amounts
ringing in the ears	Chocolate in large amounts
pounding heartbeat	Alcohol, especially Chianti wines
shortness of breath and chest pain	

*Generally taken in divided doses.
**Most psychiatric units have a patient-education handout that is more detailed and includes medications to avoid.
Source: Noll, K. M., Davis, J. M., and DeLeon-Jones, F. (1985). Medication and somatic therapies in the treatment of depression. In E. E. Beckham and W. R. Leber (Eds.), *Handbook of depression*. Homewood, IL: Dorsey Press.

depressions and cyclothymia (Jefferson, Griest, & Ackerman, 1983).

Lithium has become well-established as the drug of choice for maintenance therapy of bipolar mood disorder. Approximately seventy to eighty percent of persons with bipolar disorder respond to lithium, though there is variation in the degree and type of response. Some affected individuals experience no further episodes of mania and depression. Others experience varying degrees of decreased length and/or severity of both moods. A third response is the suppression of manic episodes but little or no effect on depressive symptoms. A subgroup of the above consists of persons who experience intolerable side effects from the lithium (such as hand tremors, gastrointestinal symptoms, and acne) (Wender & Klein, 1981). Alternative treatments are being pursued for the twenty to thirty percent of nonresponders. One is carbamazepine (CBZ, Tegretol), which will be discussed later.

In some cases, there is recurrence of depressive and/or manic episodes despite maintenance of a therapeutic blood level of lithium (level associated with remission of symptoms). In these situations, supplemental medication is used to help alleviate the symptoms. Neuroleptics (antipsychotic medication) such as thiothixene (Navane), thioridazine (Mellaril), and chlorpromazine (Thorazine) are administered during manic episodes. Depressive episodes may be treated by adding antidepressant medications such as amitriptyline (Elavil), imipramine (Tofranil), and doxepin (Adapin).

The rate at which lithium is absorbed by the digestive tract varies among individuals; thus measurement of the concentration of lithium in blood plasma has become the accepted method of monitoring the amount of lithium in the biological system. The goal of treatment with lithium is maintenance of the patient's plasma lithium level in the therapeutic range of 0.8–1.2 mEq/L. The dose is individualized through medication trial and monitored for blood level, therapeutic response, and signs of toxicity. When the blood level is below 0.8 mEq/L, generally there is no therapeutic response, and if the level is above 1.2 mEq/L, there may be toxic effects. There is a large variation in response among individuals. Some patients experience alleviation of symptoms at a plasma level on the lower end of the therapeutic range, while others require a higher level of lithium for therapeutic effects (Wender & Klein, 1981).

Mechanism of Action of Lithium. The chemical properties of lithium make it unique as a psychotropic medication, one used in the treatment of psychopathology. Lithium is the simplest solid element (atomic number three). It shares characteristics with calcium, magnesium, potassium, and sodium. It is not protein bound, has no metabolites, is absorbed from the gastrointestinal tract, and is excreted by the kidneys (Jefferson, Griest, & Ackerman, 1983).

Lithium's effectiveness in treating mood disorders has generated research designed to understand how the drug relieves symptoms of depression and mania and protects patients from both. Because of lithium's chemical simplicity as a single atom in ionized form, there was hope that understanding its mechanism of action would lead to understanding the ultimate cause of the mood disorders. However, after thirty-five years of lithium use and study, there is still no specific answer. Recent research and understanding of lithium run parallel to the increase in understanding of the brain and its function.

The changes that lithium brings about in the central nervous system are similar to those brought about by other treatments for mood disorders. Changes that have been observed include changes in serotonin, acetylcholinesterase, and cholinergic function; and effects on catecholamines, peptide neurotransmitters, sleep, and changes in and effects on circadian rhythms of neurotransmitters and receptors. However, the present level of understanding does not account for all of the symptomatology of mood disorders on the basis of any of these changes. It is thought that future research will reveal that several mechanisms of action and etiologies interact to result in the various combinations of symptoms seen in the mood disorders (Noll, Davis, & DeLeon-Jones, 1985).

As with any medication, it is important to observe the patient carefully for side and toxic effects (see Table 9–9). Instructions to the lithium user and his or her family help ensure safe use of the medication. When lithium is administered within the correct dosage range, when followup is conscientious, and when the individual and the family members are aware of toxic effects and have a plan of action to follow should they appear, lithium is a safe medication. The nurse may choose to use a flow sheet (Table 9–10) to monitor the dose, blood level, effectiveness, side effects, and laboratory values of the individual receiving lithium therapy.

TABLE 9–9 Lithium carbonate

Dose **900–1,500 mg/day, in divided doses,** **maintenance**	Starting dose for acute mania is 600 mg three times a day. Dose must be carefully determined for each individual.
Blood level **0.8–1.2 mEq/L**	Level is carefully determined for each individual.

Side effects	Benign diabetes insipidus reaction
	    increased thirst, increased urinary output
	    in some severe cases, resulting in electrolyte imbalance
	
	Hand tremors (usually fine tremors)
	
	Precipitation and exacerbation of acne
	
	EKG changes (flattening or inversion of T waves)
	
	Decrease in thyroid hormone levels
	
	Gastrointestinal symptoms (mild)
	    common during early treatment and intermittently thereafter
	    more severe or persistent symptoms are associated with impending
	    toxicity
	
	Renal abnormalities
	    reported damage to the concentrating ability of the kidneys; however,
	    no evidence of the kidney's primary ability to excrete waste products
	    is impaired
	
	    occurrence of chronic renal failure in clients receiving lithium is no
	    higher than rate in general population
	
	Weight gain (more likely in persons with previous weight problems)

Toxic effects **(arranged from most to least common)**	Abdominal pain Loss of appetite Nausea Vomiting Diarrhea Gross tremor Uneven gait Slurred speech Muscle twitching Feelings of weakness Feelings of giddiness "Ill"-gray appearance Seizures

CARBAMAZEPINE (CPZ, TEGRETOL). Though lithium salts have been the primary medical treatment for persons with manic depression since the 1970s, some persons unfortunately do not respond to lithium during acute episodes (Goodwin & Zis, 1979). Nearly thirty percent of those who respond to acute treatment relapse during maintenance treatment (Prien, Caffey, & Klett, 1973). Many of those who do not respond to lithium experience four or more mood changes per year and are thus considered "rapid cyclers" (Lerer, 1985). In addition, some persons cannot tolerate the side effects of lithium treatment. Therefore, alternative medical treatments are being explored. One alternative is **carbamazepine** (Tegretol), which has been found to be effective for acute and prophylactic treatment of manic depression

Monitoring

Pretreatment

1. Baseline renal function testing: desirable extent of testing controversial—varies from serum creatinine to 24-hour urine creatinine clearance, urinalysis, and testing renal concentrating ability
2. Thyroid function tests: TSH serum level a sensitive indicator of hypothyroidism
3. Additional laboratory tests when indicated, e.g., serum electrolytes, chemistry panel, EKG, hemogram, EEG

During Treatment

1. Serum lithium levels
   a. during initial treatment every 5–7 days
   b. during establishment of maintenance once every two weeks, then once a month, then every three months
   c. whenever there is a dosage adjustment and/or signs of toxicity
   d. blood sample is drawn 12 hours *after* the last dose and *before* the first daily dose is taken
2. Renal function
   Annual serum creatinine clearance unless symptoms indicate more extensive followup or if symptoms of renal dysfunction occur
3. Thyroid function
   Annual unless symptoms of thyroid dysfunction occur
4. Signs of toxicity
   After blood levels are stabilized they tend to remain stable except in certain circumstances:
   a. large variations in sodium intake: increase in sodium decreases lithium blood levels while decreased sodium increases lithium blood levels which may cause toxicity
   b. illness with flu-like symptoms (vomiting and diarrhea) may produce an increase in lithium blood levels due to sodium loss, which can cause toxicity (more vomiting and diarrhea) which in turn exacerbates toxicity

Source: Adapted from Jefferson, J. W., Griest, J. H., and Ackerman, D. L. (1983) *Lithium encyclopedia for clinical practice*. Washington, D.C.: American Psychiatric Press. Noll, K. M., Davis, J. M., and DeLeon-Jones, F. (1985) Medication and somatic therapies in the treatment of depression. In E. E. Beckham and W. R. Leber (Eds.), *Handbook of Depression*. Homewood, IL: Dorsey Press; and Wender, P. H., & Klein, D. F. (1981). *Mind, mood and medicine*. New York: New American.

(Ballenger & Post, 1985). Because there is more experience with lithium, however, it is usually tried first.

Medication Classification of Carbamazepine and Mechanism of Action. Carbamazepine is an anticonvulsant medication that has been effective in the treatment of temporal lobe neurological disorders.

Initial interest in the psychotropic properties of CBZ arose out of clinical reports that the medication relieved some of the psychiatric symptoms observed in persons with temporal lobe disorders (Lerer, 1985).

It is speculated that CBZ acts on the limbic system. Seizures originating in the limbic areas are more readily suppressed by CBZ than are cortical seizures. CBZ acts as an anticonvulsant by preventing exces-

TABLE 9–10 Lithium flow sheet

A flow sheet may be used to monitor the dose, blood level, effectiveness, side effects, and laboratory values of the individual receiving lithium therapy. Some individuals and family members have found the following flow sheet helpful.

Date	Dose	Blood Level	Mood Value (0–10)	GI	Tremor	Thyroid	Renal	Other

sive discharges by pathologic neurons and by preventing normal neurons from firing after being triggered by pathological discharges (Varga, 1984). See Table 9–11 for doses, blood level, side effects, toxic effects, and monitoring of patients on carbamazepine treatment.

ELECTROCONVULSIVE THERAPY (ECT). Following Cerletti's discovery in 1937 of the therapeutic benefit of seizures induced by electric currents passing through the brain (Cerletti, 1956), **electroconvulsive therapy (ECT)** was used for a number of years in a variety of clinical situations. Sometimes the treatment was quite terrifying for patients, as neither anesthesia nor a muscle-relaxant medication was administered to ameliorate the violence of the seizures. In addition, patients often experienced acute amnesia with slow memory return and sometimes experienced residual memory loss many years after treatment. In view of this, it is not surprising that ECT soon became an unpopular form of treatment for depression. Recently, however, ECT has begun to gain recognition as an acceptable and effective treatment for depression. Electroconvulsive therapy as it is now performed is dramatically different from the ECT of the past. Patients are anesthetized before and during treatment. Muscle-relaxant medications are administered to prevent injury to bones and muscles. Oxygen therapy permits oxygen loading of the blood before the seizure is induced to decrease the possibility of brain injury from seizure anoxia. Recent research has indicated that ECT is nearly as effective if current is passed through only the dominant brain hemisphere as when current is passed through both hemispheres. Individuals treated with this type of ECT have extremely few complaints of memory loss. Patients recovering from unilaterally induced seizures are as alert and in contact with their pasts as are persons awakening from brief general anesthesia.

As with any treatment process, the nurse or other mental-health professional who recommends ECT must cultivate the patient's trust and confidence. Depressed patients with severe biological and emotional symptoms are the primary candidates for ECT. The nurse informs the patient about the nature of ECT and its expected outcome. Informed consent procedure requires that the physician also review the treatment with the patient. A complete medical history and routine laboratory screening tests are obtained during the pretreatment evaluation. Particular attention is paid to the patient's bone structure and his capacity to metabolize the muscle-relaxant drug succinylcholine (Anectine) rapidly, as slow metabolism of the drug will produce an apneic period after the treatment (Fink, 1979).

ECT treatments are usually administered in the morning. Standard anesthesia precautions are observed. The patient is permitted to have nothing by mouth from 10 P.M. of the preceding evening to decrease the risk of aspiration. An anticholinergic medication is recommended to reduce secretions of the mouth and digestive tract. The anticholinergic also mitigates the cardiac response to vagal stimulation, which occurs during the seizure. A small dose of amybarbital or a benzodiazepine may be administered to the anxious patient. It should be kept in mind, however, that these drugs are likely to elevate the seizure threshold and thus make it harder to induce a seizure (Fink, 1979).

The machines that deliver the electric shock are designed to keep the application of current within safe and therapeutic limits. The goal is to use the least amount of current possible to produce a therapeutic seizure, that is, a seizure that is safe (that does not cause brain damage) and that has the fewest undesirable aftereffects. It is important that the nurse monitor whether or not a seizure has occurred. For example, when a muscle relaxant is used, the patient

TABLE 9–11 Carbamazepine

Dose
400 mg–2,000 mg daily

Blood level
6–10 nanograms/ml

Side effects*	Dizziness
	Fatigue
	Diplopia
	Drowsiness
	Clumsiness
	Nausea (rare)
	Vomiting (rare)
Adverse and toxic effects	Dermatologic reactions (minor to severe)**
	nonspecific rashes
	urticaria
	exfoliative dermatitis
	toxic epidermal necrolysis
	Hematologic reactions
	transient decreases in white blood cell count***
	thrombocytopenia: mild to moderate (rare)
	anemia: mild to moderate (rare)
	agranulocytosis: serious, generally occurs within first two months
	aplastic anemia: rare, can be rapidly fatal, generally occurs within first year
Hematologic monitoring	Baseline complete blood count, platelet count, creatinine, and liver function tests
	CBC followup: every two weeks for two months, then every three weeks
	Observe for signs of bone-marrow suppression: infection, fever, pallor, weakness, petechiae. Client is instructed to contact physician immediately, discontinue medication, and have CBC drawn if signs appear.

*Some of the side effects can be minimized by initiating therapy at lower doses and gradually increasing to the therapeutic dose.

**Dermatological reactions may be early signs of serious toxicity. When a skin rash is accompanied by chills, fever, arthralgia, myalgia, lymphadenopathy, and eosinophila, toxicity is present.

***Counts as low as 3,000/cc^3 are common and do not appear to be dose-related or a sign of impending agranulocytosis or aplastic anemia

Source: Massachusetts General Hospital (1985). Carbamazepine (Tegretol) for manic-depressive illness: An update. *Biological Therapies in Psychiatry, 6,* 21–24.

may manifest a response delay or the treatment may fail altogether. On the other hand, a seizure in a paralyzed patient may be "missed." The most reliable method of monitoring ECT effects is to monitor the patient's brain activity with an EEG (Fink, 1979).

Cardiac and respiratory monitors are also used. Through this type of monitoring, the staff will know if an adequate seizure has been produced and, therefore, if the treatment has been effectively administered.

Maintenance of an adequate airway and ventilation are essential during the treatment. Anesthesia and oxygen equipment and emergency medications must be available, as must a physician skilled in emergency resuscitation. An anesthesiologist may not be required if the person administering anesthesia has had special training in the use of the rapid and light anesthesia used in ECT. Forced ventilation with oxygen as soon as anesthesia is induced is recommended (Fink, 1979).

The effectiveness of ECT has been studied primarily as it compares to other treatments. There are methodological problems in studying ECT, due to variations in procedure, particularly variations in induction and monitoring of the seizures. Despite these methodological problems, the evidence warrants the conclusion that ECT is an effective treatment for major depression. In addition, ECT is more effective than pharmacological treatments, particularly when the depression is severe, includes delusional thinking (Scovern & Kilmann, 1980), and when it is chronic (a type of depression that has not responded to drug treatment or psychotherapy).

RESPONSIBILITIES OF THE NURSE IN A PSYCHIATRIC SETTING

It is essential that the nurse understand the nature and treatment of mood disorders in order to work effectively with patients who have them. The nurse's specific responsibilities include patient and family education about mood disorders and their treatment, monitoring the effectiveness of medication as well as its side effects, ongoing assessment of symptoms, and helping the patient and his family cope with the effects of what may be a chronic illness.

PATIENT AND FAMILY EDUCATION

The nurse has a major role in educating the patient and his family about the patient's specific manifestations of the mood disorder. The nurse explains the patient's cycle (pattern of mood changes) with emphasis on the predictability or unpredictability of the changes. The nurse also emphasizes that the purpose of medication is to stabilize the patient's moods and that if one medication fails to do so, or if its side effects outweigh therapeutic effects, other medications can be tried.

MONITORING MEDICATION

In helping to evaluate the effectiveness of the medication a patient is taking, the nurse observes whether the patient's mood is stabilizing and his symptoms are reduced. The nurse identifies any side effects and teaches both the patient and his family how to do so as well. When lithium is part of a patient's treatment, it is important for the nurse to make sure that the patient's blood lithium level is within therapeutic limits. If the patient shows any signs of toxicity with lithium or any other medication, the nurse, patient, or family should not administer another dose and should inform the physician of the situation.

It is important to discuss with the patient how he feels about taking the prescribed medication and to assess whether he understands the place the drug has in the treatment of his mood disorder. Asking the patient how he views taking the medication will help the nurse assess whether the patient has faced the fact that he has a psychiatric disorder in need of treatment. If he has not accepted this, he may not take the medication.

The nurse checks for orthostatic hypotension when major tranquilizers and antidepressants are being used. This process involves taking a blood pressure and pulse while the patient is seated and again sixty seconds after the patient stands. Naturally, the nurse also observes the patient for dizziness and faintness at this time. The nurse instructs the patient and family regarding how to assess orthostatic changes and what to do if they occur.

Monitoring the patient's sleep pattern is one way to assess the effectiveness of the medication. It may also be helpful to teach the patient with insomnia behavioral techniques to get to sleep. One strategy is to encourage the patient to count backward from 300 sequentially. The individual experiencing a manic mood may have a "p.r.n." medication, such as Xanax (alprazolam) or Ativan (lorazepam), both antianxiety agents sometimes prescribed for sleep which the nurse can offer when appropriate.

Close monitoring of nutritional status is essential with patients whose depression involves loss of appetite. Patients taking an MAOI must learn and observe the requisite dietary restrictions. Patients treated with lithium must maintain a stable salt intake and consult the physician before altering it. The nurse can help the patient and his family learn and implement dietary changes by asking about usual eating habits and pointing out where change will be necessary. A nutritionist or dietician can also be consulted.

MAINTAINING ONGOING ASSESSMENT OF SYMPTOMS

The nurse must engage in ongoing assessment for suicide risk in all patients with mood disorders. With patients who report active suicidal ideation this will include regular observation, being alert for sharp objects or medications in the patient's possession, and possibly making a no-suicide contract with the patient on a shift-to-shift or day-to-day basis. (Also see Chapter 18 on Crisis.) Nursing responsibilities also include helping the individual to identify other means of dealing with feelings and life situations.

It is often the nurse who arranges for decreased environmental stimulation for the patient who presents in a manic mood. It may be necessary to take precautions to ensure the safety of other patients as well as that of the affected individual. This might mean temporary use of the "quiet room" (isolation room) on the psychiatric unit. When a patient oversteps the bounds of acceptable behavior, firmness and directness are essential, particularly in the case of a manic individual who presents with behaviors indicative of his loss of control. The individual experiencing a manic episode may not know that he is out of control. It is essential that he know that someone in the environment will take charge when necessary.

Maintaining a therapeutic, professional stance with an individual experiencing a manic episode is difficult but essential. The nurse addresses both the content and the process of manic behavior. Individuals experiencing mania can be extremely persuasive. The nurse must be careful not to lose perspective on the manic process, which includes distractibility, intensity, and sense of righteousness on the part of the patient. The patient can be convincing in his sense of power and can leave the nurse with a distorted view of how things are or could be. This particularly applies to a hypomanic patient. Hypomania can be "contagious," particularly if the hypomanic mood is one of euphoria. One can also get caught up in arguing with a patient experiencing an irritable manic or hypomanic mood. The nurse must remember that there is no way to win an argument with a person who is manic because he will keep escalating the argument or will maneuver the topic into a different area to regain control. It is impossible to convince an individual experiencing a manic episode that he is "wrong," or to "reason" with him.

The nurse can help the manic individual, particularly between manic episodes, to deal with feelings of shame and guilt related to things he has done while manic. He may have had sexual relations with someone he wishes he had not, broken the law, or harmed someone psychologically, socially, or physically. For some affected individuals, the feeling of shame and guilt is so severe that they become depressed and even suicidal, feeling that suicide is one sure way to protect themselves and others from their disorder.

With the range of mood changes (depressive and manic) possible, it is crucial that the nurse understand a patient's symptomatology within the context of his entire mood-cycle pattern. As has been mentioned, hypomania can appear to be delightful but can be the beginning of a nightmare for the affected individual and his family. The same applies to early symptoms of a depressed mood. Mild withdrawal and a little sadness can be the beginning of a process that may lead to more severe symptomatology, suicide attempts, and even death. The mood disorders have the potential to be life threatening and the nurse keeps this in mind when designing interventions.

WORKING WITH THE FAMILY

The nurse works with the patient and his family to help identify specific behavioral or emotional changes that indicate he is "cycling." For example, the patient may realize that a change in sleep pattern is one of the early signs of a mood change for him. At the first point of change, the individual should contact his therapist since the mood change may suggest that a change in medication is warranted.

The nurse works with the family to help them recognize the point in mania at which the affected individual is out of control. At this point, it is no longer productive to tell him to "get it together." It is time to take charge. When the patient is between manic episodes, the nurse can help him and his family recognize behaviors that indicate loss of control. The patient and family can then together identify these specific unacceptable behaviors and make clear plans for action when they occur.

The nurse discusses with the family how the mood disorder affects various aspects of family life. For example, there may be an increased incidence of argument and conflicts during the patient's mood-change episodes. The nurse can help the family develop the ability to distinguish whether a given conflict has interpersonal etiology or is a symptom of the disorder. During family conferences, information about the nature of the stress at home can be elicited. The nurse can then work with the family to help them learn how to problem solve and share responsibility for problems that occur.

The nurse can help the patient's family avoid blaming him for his behavior and focus on his responsibility for dealing with it and how, together, to prevent it from controlling his life and theirs. Though family members should not take on the responsibility of ensuring that the patient takes his medication, they should know when it is necessary for them to take charge.

The nurse can also assist the family in understanding that, for many people, a mood disorder is chronic and requires reexamination of individual and family expectations and goals and the time frame for achieving them. Self-help groups for individuals with mood disorders and their families, including children, may be useful. If none are available, the nurse may want to establish one in the community. (Also see Chapter 21 on Families.)

RESPONSIBILITIES OF THE NURSE IN A NONPSYCHIATRIC SETTING

Application of knowledge about mood disorders in a nonpsychiatric setting is not only beneficial to patient care but also a major nursing responsibility. Patients in nonpsychiatric settings may manifest depressive symptomatology at any time in the course of treatment for an illness. Anticipation, assessment, and treatment of the symptomatology are integral to nursing practice in any setting.

Persons at risk for developing a mood disorder and those presently experiencing a mood disorder are, like the general public, in need of a variety of health-care services. Those not at risk for developing a mood disorder may also manifest depressive symptoms as a reaction to a physical illness, the impact of the illness and its treatment on the family, associated disruption in their own lives, and the health-care setting environment. These patients, however, may be more likely to respond to the therapeutic interventions of the staff in the nonpsychiatric setting, without clinical psychiatric consultation. Some patients, however, may require psychiatric treatment in addition to the therapeutic approaches utilized by the nursing staff.

Anticipation of depression in a patient requires the nurse to identify variables in the treatment setting and the illness process that could contribute to its development. Uncontrollability of the outcome of treatment, decreased positive reinforcement, attribut-

ing treatment failure to self, life stressors, and disruption of autonomous behaviors can all contribute to the development of depression in a patient.

A physical illness or trauma is a life stressor that disrupts not only the routine behavior of the patient but that of his family as well. There may be economic, social, and personal loss. The treatment setting disrupts the patient's and family's routine behavior and results in a sense of dependency on medical and nursing staff. The hospital setting also represents loss of privacy, of intimacy with loved ones, and of control of the immediate environment.

The nurse's responsibility consists of identifying how these variables are manifested in a specific treatment setting. Policies, procedures, physical environment, staff-patient relationships, and availability of the nurse are the components of the patient's world wherein a depression-producing environment can develop. The nurse has a responsibility to be sensitive to the patient's vulnerability and, as far as she is able, to prevent the development of a situation conducive to depression.

ASSESSING DEPRESSIVE SYMPTOMATOLOGY

The nurse assesses depressive symptomatology in her patients. She obtains information from the clinical interview, family and friends of the patient, observation, and colleagues' observations. (Also see Chapter 5 on Assessment.) Further psychiatric assessment may be necessary, and the nurse initiates and facilitates consultation with psychiatric clinicians. She also assesses the family's support system and, when indicated, facilitates the development of an extended family and/or social-support system. The family is directed to hospital or community resources that can help them improve their problem-solving skills and master the threatening situation.

THERAPEUTIC INTERVENTIONS

Therapeutic interventions instituted by the nurse may include providing for direct positive reinforcement of nondepressed behavior, redirecting negative thoughts through cognitive restructuring, and focusing on outcomes that are controllable. The illness may have both controllable and uncontrollable aspects and processes. The nurse assists the patient in identifying the controllable processes that he is capable of mastering. The treatment process itself may also consist of controllable and uncontrollable processes and outcomes that will increase the patient's sense of mastery over the situation. (Also see Chapter 25 on the ICU patient.)

The depressed patient in a nonpsychiatric setting may require treatment by a psychiatric clinician. This treatment may include medication as well as a particular therapy modality (such as psychotherapy, cognitive restructuring, or assertiveness training). The nurse coordinates the psychiatric and nonpsychiatric treatment and provides feedback to the psychiatric clinican(s) regarding the patient's condition. When a psychiatric medication is used, the nurse evaluates its effectiveness, observes for side effects, and teaches the patient and his family about the medication.

CHALLENGING THE MYTHS ABOUT MOOD DISORDERS

Another important nursing responsibility is challenging the myths about mood disorders. Patients with mood disorders experience real physical illnesses and symptomatology, and their credibility regarding these should not be questioned because of their mood disorder. It may be necessary for the nurse to advocate for this patient when it appears that physical symptomatology is being minimized or is regarded solely as a manifestation of the mood disorder. The nurse needs to question her own beliefs and values regarding patients with mood disorders and must identify how these values operate in her practice. Once the nurse has committed herself to this self-examination she invites her colleagues to join her in

that process. Occasional regular consultation between nursing staff and mental-health clinicians may be helpful in planning comprehensive patient care.

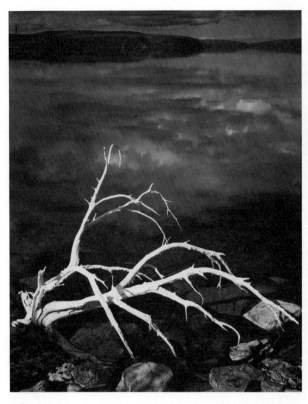

Why me?
("White Branches, Mono Lake, California, 1950" photograph by Ansel Adams.)

**Case Study:
Nonpsychiatric
Setting**

Mary is a 44-year-old woman who had a mastectomy due to breast cancer four months ago. Because of two positive lymph nodes, she is being treated for one year with adjunct chemotherapy in an ambulatory setting. Mary has been informed that the chemotherapy is not necessarily a cure and that she has a higher than average risk of having a primary lesion in her other breast.

Mary expresses feelings of frustration and discouragement with the chemotherapy because of the side effects and the uncertainty of its outcome. Side effects have included intermittent nausea, weight loss, and hair thinning. Mary has tried all kinds of medications and eating strategies to control the nausea, with varying success. She increases her food intake when she feels better in order to compensate for the weight loss. Additionally, for two to three days during each monthly chemotherapy cycle, she feels particularly anorexic and exhausted. During these times it is difficult for her to go to work and to maintain her previous level of excellent functioning as a nursing supervisor. As a result of her difficulty functioning at work, her staff is expressing dissatisfaction with her performance and are seeking out others for decision making. Mary's supervisors have also expressed concern regarding her apparent inability to manage her nursing unit consistently in an efficient and effective manner. Recently she was asked to consider temporary reassignment to a position with little or no management responsibility.

Mary wonders whether she should go through the entire chemotherapy treatment process, particularly given that there is no guarantee regarding its outcome. She wonders whether the difficulties caused by the treatment are worth it. She appears despondent as she discusses this dilemma and expresses how difficult it is to "hold it together from one day to the next." She denies feeling suicidal but wishes this all would end.

Mary describes feelings of sadness fluctuating with a sense of emotional numbness. These feelings are almost always present and on occasion include bouts of uncontrollable crying. During the past two months her sleep has been consistently disrupted in that she has difficulty falling asleep, sleeps restlessly, and frequently awakens during the night.

Mary's socialization has markedly decreased since her surgery and chemotherapy. Prior to her illness, Mary regularly attended dinner parties, the theater, and movies. She played on a summer softball team and a winter basketball team and also played racquetball on a regular basis. She dated frequently and was sexually active. Mary reports that she has not participated in any of the above activities since her surgery and chemotherapy. She attributes most of her nonparticipation to recovery from surgery, decreased energy, fatigue, and fear of rejection. She also expresses concern that her friends will "give up on me because I'm not much fun to be with."

Mary defines her family as a committed and intimate network of five friends. The six of them have known each other for seven years and the relationships are described as nurturing and supportive. However, she states that this family is expressing increased frustration with her social withdrawal and feels helpless in knowing what to do.

Mary's family of origin consists of three siblings (twin sister and two brothers) and parents in their early seventies. The family of origin is not geographically close but maintains phone contact a couple of times per month. The relationships are described as somewhat supportive but emotionally distant. Mary's twin sister has become quite unavailable since Mary's illness. Mary attributes this to her sister's fear that she too will develop breast cancer. The emotional distance is very painful for Mary since she has always considered her sister as her closest family tie.

DSM-III-R Diagnosis

Axis I: Major depression, single episode, severe, without psychotic features (296.23)
Axis II: Unknown
Axis III: Breast cancer
Axis IV: Psycho-social stressors: 0 (inadequate information)
Axis V: GAF: 0 (inadequate information)

Nursing Diagnoses

Disturbance in self-concept; body image, role performance
Sleep-pattern disturbance
Ineffective family coping (compromised): sister, friends
Social isolation
Powerlessness

Nursing Care Plan for Mary

Nursing Diagnosis	Desired Outcomes	Interventions	Rationale
1. Disturbance in self-concept: body image, role performance	Integration of physical changes in appearance and body image: integration of performance changes that are necessary as a result of illness and/or treatment; acceptance of reestablished role in workplace	Discuss mastectomy and its impact on Mary's body image	This involves identification of previous body image and its meaning to the patient; specific identification of loss; assistance with grieving; identification of meaning of mastectomy to Mary's sense of wholeness (sexual, psychological, physical).
		Connect Mary with other women who have had a mastectomy (as in Reach for Recovery).	These patients are likely to have also experienced unpleasant side effects (hair loss, nausea, fatigue) from chemotherapy, and can offer Mary a sense of understanding missing in the professional who has never been a cancer patient.
		Discuss chemotherapy and its impact on Mary's work performance.	Focusing on specific changes in Mary's performance and her perceptions of her ability to reachieve that level of performance post-treatment can begin to make what has been an overwhelming problem manageable. Helping Mary develop problem-solving strategies for the present discrepancy in performance can help her reestablish a sense of being in control. Identifying work-related losses and assisting with associated grieving can help her define and integrate a new role.
		Consider psychiatric consultation or refer Mary for continued counseling to achieve the above outcome if necessary.	The clinic nurse may not have the time or inclination to do such extensive counseling at the time of outpatient chemotherapy appointments. (Another alternative would be to work with clinic and program administration to develop a position for a nurse who would be available solely for counseling with cancer patients.)

Nursing Diagnosis	Desired Outcomes	Interventions	Rationale
2. Sleep pattern disturbance	Alleviation of difficulty falling asleep and alleviation of early awakening	Teach Mary techniques that interrupt thinking or worrying, such as counting backwards from 300. Teach relaxation techniques and/or self-hypnosis. Consult with Mary's physician for an evaluation of need for antidepressant medication.	If behavioral techniques along with above-described counseling are not effective treatments for a sleep pattern disturbance, antidepressant medication might be indicated.
3. Ineffective family coping (compromised): sister, friends	Interaction with sister and friends that enhances emotional connectedness and functioning in the context of life-threatening illness	Assist Mary in identifying interactions with her sister that invite emotional engagement: expressing to her sister how the emotional distance feels (loss), expressing understanding of her sister's fear, identifying various modes of interaction for expression (letters, cards, direct contact, phone calls), expressing to her sister what she specifically needs from her now, inviting her sister to visit, inviting her sister to join her for a clinic visit.	Emotional contact between Mary and her sister is a potential source of empathy and support for both.
		Assist Mary in identifying interactions with friends that are complementary to their initiation for connectedness and social involvement: contract to participate in at least one weekly activity, identify how friends can express their caring, write down the ideas, encourage Mary to share ideas with friends.	Reconnecting Mary to her friends (her social system), if there has been an emotional break, is as essential to their coping as it is to hers.
		Encourage Mary to invite her sister and friends for a conference to focus on how they can be helpful as well as identify what they need from Mary. Refer Mary to continued counseling to achieve the above, if necessary.	

Nursing Diagnosis	Desired Outcomes	Interventions	Rationale
4. Social isolation	Satisfying social relationships and activities; resumption of social activities	Engage Mary in planning process for resuming social activities; assist in identifying the obstacles to participate in former activities such as dating (fear of rejection) and theater (fatigue, nausea); select an activity at which Mary can succeed; elicit help from friends in carrying out this activity.	Specific problem-solving of obstacles increases Mary's chances of succeeding as well as her sense of mastery and power in the situation.
		Engage in agreement to increase gradually social activities; plan around days when sick from chemotherapy; plan activities in advance (change if necessary); write down plans.	Agreements facilitate the collaborative nature of the therapeutic relationship between Mary and the nurse. Increases the likelihood for joint future problem-solving and "fine-tuning" the plans.
		Consult with Mary's physician about the need for psychiatric evaluation to consider treatment with antidepressant medication if her social isolation continues.	Duration and severity of symptomatology are significantly disruptive to her capacity to function effectively. Mary's biological system needs the biological assistance to help Mary to cope and to adapt.
5. Powerlessness	Experiencing a sense of power regarding direction and quality of life	Discuss Mary's sense of powerlessness in relation to her illness: focus on her feelings about cancer and the unpredictability of its outcome; assist Mary in identifying her values, behaviors, and/or activities that would be indicative of *quality* life for her; encourage her to share this with her family.	Lack of predictability and controllability can result in learned-helplessness symptomatology. Increasing either or both, especially in regard to her illness and its treatment, can prevent and/or effectively treat such symptoms, including depression.
		Discuss Mary's sense of powerlessness in relation to treatment; identify how health-care system enhances or inhibits her sense of power in treatment; advocate for her; assist her in being assertive to staff; identify degree to which side effects can be controlled; identify what is controllable and what is not.	

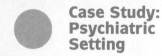

**Case Study:
Psychiatric
Setting**

Fran is a 42-year-old single parent and a successful lawyer in private practice. She has a 14-year-old son whose father, her first husband, lives out of state. Fran's second ex-husband also lives in another state. There is a history of bipolar mood disorder in Fran's family and her mother committed suicide when Fran was fourteen.

Fran has been encouraged to seek counseling by her friends because of her increasing depression and talk about suicide. Although Fran is reluctant to seek treatment, fearing stigmatization, she recognizes that her feeling of wanting to hurt herself is becoming stronger and is beginning to feel out of control. She agrees to a psychiatric evaluation and then states that her preference is to deal with her problems on an outpatient basis.

Fran describes herself as depressed and feels that her depression is beginning to interfere with her life socially and professionally. A primary symptom is sleep disturbance. Fran describes taking from two to three hours to get to sleep, then awakening after three to four hours. She feels extremely tired when she wakes up and has difficulty getting out of bed. She also reports a decrease in energy, saying that it is very difficult for her to get through the day because of fatigue. Fran's interest in being around people has decreased, and she has become socially withdrawn. She says that it is very difficult for her to put forth the energy required to interact with friends. Additional symptoms include her decreased pleasure in dining out and attending concerts—in fact she has decreased motivation and enthusiasm for most of the activities she previously enjoyed. Her professional law practice has been disrupted because she has difficulty concentrating and focusing on her work for any period of time. She also finds it difficult to make decisions about cases, despite having had experience with the legal issues.

Fran expresses concern that her depression will become as intense as her mother's had been during the separation and divorce from Fran's father. When her mother sought treatment, she was hospitalized. Despite hospitalization, she got no relief from the symptoms she experienced (the same ones Fran is experiencing now)—an increased appetite with binging and weight gain, night sweats, and suicidal thoughts.

Fran reports that she has struggled with depression much of her life. She remembers her late teens as being an especially difficult time for her. She remembers feeling depressed because she was "extremely unattractive." She made a suicide attempt at the age of sixteen by overdosing with aspirin, following a breakup initiated by her boyfriend.

Fran describes college as a relatively good time in her life. She married for the first time a year after graduation. She describes her ex-husband, a high-school teacher, as a very nice, bright, passive man. Their sexual relationship was not good and she began feeling attracted to other men. After being married for six years she became sexually involved with a divorced friend, a criminal lawyer, who later became her second husband. She got involved with him because she found him exciting. They lived together for two years, married, and together raised her son from her first marriage. She finished her law degree and began practicing with a law firm. After four years of marriage, her husband left her and disappeared. She discovered that he had moved to another state with a woman with whom he had been having an affair.

During her second marriage, Fran experienced recurring depressions and binging behavior. Following her second separation she became more depressed and self-medicated with alcohol. While drinking helped her insomnia, it did not alleviate her depression, which increased along with her sense of loss of control.

Fran reports that at times she feels extremely productive. During these times she feels very energetic and becomes active in other lawyers' cases as well as her own. She describes feeling "wonderful"; she feels very powerful and feels that she can accomplish anything. During these periods, she becomes more socially active by having several parties and attending others. She occasionally invites strangers to her home and has at times impulsively flown to various parts of the country. During these times her legal cases are either put on hold or dealt with by her law partners. As a result her law partners have indicated an interest in dissolving their partnership with her.

During these times of elation, Fran has very little need for sleep and sleeps only two or three hours per night. She feels extremely attractive and acts on her increased sense of sexuality. While recounting some of her experiences, she expresses embarrassment and guilt about her behavior. She has also apparently created some financial hardship for herself by spending a great deal of money during these episodes. Fran also seems to have experienced auditory hallucinations during her "high" times. She describes seeing and hearing angels who encourage her to join them. These experiences are very frightening.

Fran remembers that her father experienced marked mood swings, including highs similar to what Fran experienced. In addition, she describes him as being depressed most of the time when he was not "high." Her father was never treated for these mood swings. He died a year ago of cancer. Fran does not know her paternal grandparents and her father was their only child.

Fran's mother is described as a nondisclosing parent who often told Fran to "snap out of being down" when Fran was depressed. At times she became extremely irritable and was verbally abusive. At other times she was very withdrawn and punished Fran with silence by staying in her room for as long as three days. Her mother was extremely overweight, experienced food binging, craved sugar, and often appeared very unhappy and very tired.

Fran's parents' relationship was a stormy one and they separated several times. Fran wishes her parents had divorced sooner so that she would not have had to deal with their conflicts as a young child.

Fran describes her brother (her only sibling) as very unhappy and irritable. He seems to be burdened by everything in life and often tells Fran that he "exists" from day to day.

As Fran describes her family, she expresses both sadness and anger about their past relationships with one another and with her. She is able to identify some parallels between her parents' relationship and her own marriages. At present, she wonders if she can ever feel better about herself since she is so much like her parents. She expresses sadness about how disconnected her family members were from each other, as well as the emotional isolation she has always felt. She feels isolated emotionally from everyone at this point, including her son, and has concluded that she would be better off dead. Because of her emotional emptiness and continuing struggle with her depression, she has become preoccupied with thoughts of death and suicide.

DSM-III-R Diagnosis

Axis I: Bipolar disorder, depressed, severe, without psychotic features (296.53)
Axis II: Unknown
Axis III: Unknown
Axis IV: Psychosocial stressors: 0 (inadequate information)
Axis V: GAF: 0 (inadequate information)

Nursing Diagnoses

Disturbance in self-concept: low self-esteem
Alterations in thought processes
Alteration in nutritional status
Sleep-pattern disturbance
Self-destructive thoughts/behaviors
Social isolation
Ineffective family coping

Nursing Care Plan for Fran

Nursing Diagnosis	Desired Outcomes	Interventions	Rationale
1. Disturbance in self-concept: low self-esteem	Increased self esteem; better-balanced view of self with respect to attributes; clear perception of attributes that enhance achievement of life goals and attributes that inhibit achievement of these goals	Assess timing of interventions: involves assessing depressive symptomatology to ascertain whether Fran is at a point where she can benefit from interventions. Symptoms of depression may be interfering so much that further immobilization, rather than decrease of symptomatology, may occur.	Appropriately timed cognitive-behavioral therapy techniques can help interrupt Fran's negative thoughts about herself and her situation, the first step on her journey to overcoming her mood disorder.
		Cognitive restructuring: focus on the messages to the self that reinforce negativism; identify and reinforce thoughts and feelings that are nurturing and self-enhancing to Fran.	
		Encourage Fran to continue therapy following discharge from the hospital to continue work in this area.	
		Refrain from making statements to Fran that oversimplify the task of feeling better about herself, for example: "Tomorrow is another day."	Cognitive therapy must be done in an empathic context to be effective.

Nursing Diagnosis	Desired Outcomes	Interventions	Rationale
2. Alterations in thought processes: (1) difficulty with decision making and concentration. (2) Sensory-perceptual alterations: visual and/or auditory hallucinations (during mania).	Ability to make decisions; ability to stay focused.	Identify Fran's symptoms as part of the depressive syndrome. Involve her in projects that do not require long periods of attention. Express understanding of her frustration.	Empathizing with Fran's feelings of frustration and anxiety while helping her to manage them, through labeling them as treatable symptoms of her illness, setting up *experiences* of treatment success, and not being overwhelmed by them herself, are the means to help a patient who is depressed begin again to feel in control of her life.
	Absence/alleviation of visual and/or auditory hallucinations (if manic).	If manic, identify the nature of the hallucinations, e.g., voices calling her to her death, angels burning her. Stimulate as many senses as possible to keep Fran focused on reality. For example, have her keep her eyes open and look at you; remind her of her location; give clear statements that you will not let the voices/images harm her or let her follow through on the messages; let her know that you are there to protect and help her. Caring forms of touching may help ground Fran in reality, such as holding her hand while staying with her until she begins to feel safe.	Assisting Fran to maintain some contact with reality can decrease the risk of self-harm and also her fear.
3. Alteration in nutritional status	Weight within normal range	Monitor intake and weight. Encourage Fran to eat; to have smaller portions of food or snacks between meals. If on an MAOI, provide food low in tyramine; teach Fran specifics of MAOI diet and its rationale. Monitor symptoms of appetite changes as part of evaluation of effectiveness of medication.	Attention to Fran's physiological as well as psychological needs is important to maximize her functioning, including her active cooperation with her treatment. Appetite changes may reflect her progress or lack of it; they may also be a side effect of antidepressant medication.

Nursing Diagnosis	Desired Outcomes	Interventions	Rationale
4. Sleep-pattern disturbance	Alleviation of difficulty falling asleep and early awakening without feeling rested	Decrease stimuli that may keep Fran awake. Provide as many familiar surroundings as possible in the hospital setting, such as Fran's own pillow, own clothing. Teach behavioral techniques that can interrupt thinking or worrying at bedtime such as counting backward from 300, and getting *up* when not successful at falling asleep within 10–15 minutes, then trying again to go to sleep when tiredness is again felt.	Improvement in sleeping is often an early therapeutic effect of antidepressant medication. If this is not the case, behavioral techniques which promote the association of bed with sleep (rather than other activities, including *not* sleeping) can be very helpful in the treatment of a sleep disturbance.
5. Self-destructive thoughts/behaviors	Absence of self-destructive thoughts/ behaviors.	Determine presence of suicidal ideation, plan, access to plan, and Fran's willingness to seek help if ideation or impulses feel out of control. If Fran is capable of entering into a no-suicide contract, establish such a contract on a shift-by-shift or 24-hour basis, whichever is more appropriate. If Fran is incapable of entering into a no-suicide contract, institute suicide precautions (see Chapter 18). Help Fran to identify other options for dealing with her feelings. Help her to identify consequences of suicide for family members and friends.	While the non-psychotic suicidal patient cannot promise to not have suicidal feelings, she can promise *not to act* on those feelings. Separating suicidal thoughts and feelings from suicidal behavior can help Fran feel less out of control.
6. Social isolation	Satisfying social relationships	With a severely withdrawn patient, the nurse may initiate social contact.	Social contacts are an important source of positive reinforcement in Fran's life. The depressed patient needs

Nursing Diagnosis	Desired Outcomes	Interventions	Rationale
		Plan other social contacts with Fran. Social-skills training and assertiveness training may be used, but these interventions must be timed considering the presence and degree of other symptomatology.	to make social contact, despite the lack of any desire to do so. This is a case in which a change in feelings is likely to follow a change in behavior rather than vice versa.
7. Ineffective family coping	Family's coping styles enhance rather than inhibit functioning of the family unit.	Teach the family signs and symptoms of depression and mania as well as the theories regarding its etiology. Teach the family the purpose and side effects of the medication(s). Help the family recognize early signs of depression and mania and to identify resources to utilize at that time. Help the family learn an interactional style that results in less conflict and disconnectedness. This includes recognizing when Fran's mood change and its effect on interactions occurs, verbalizing the feeling of wanting to stay connected, and planning ways to do that together. Help the family identify oppressing, demeaning, and belittling messages that continue to reinforce the affected individual's low self-esteem and sense of powerlessness. Give examples of messages that are more affirming and nurturing. Help the family recognize messages that escalate or ignore the mania. Give examples of messages that are firm, directive, and caring.	The family can be a rich source of social, psychological, and physical support to the depressed patient both in the hospital and after discharge if they understand the nature and treatment of mood disorders and are helped to appreciate their potential for being a part of the treatment process and significantly helping their affected family member.

SUMMARY

Mood disorders are those that involve primarily a disturbance in mood or affect. According to DSM-III-R the main characteristic of a mood disorder is the presence of a full or partial depressive or manic syndrome. The major mood disorders are major depression (also called unipolar depression) and bi-polar disorder which includes a manic episode. The other specific mood disorders are dysthymic disorder and cyclothymic disorder. Although similar to the major mood disorders, they are different in the severity and duration of symptoms. Mood disorders have an impact on both the patient and his family. They affect an individual's quality of life, productivity in society, and the psychological well-being of his family.

Patients with mood disorders are assessed in terms of their mood changes, cognitive changes, physiological changes, and behavioral changes.

There are three main theories regarding the etiology of mood disorders: psychoanalytic/psychodynamic, cognitive/behavioral, and genetic/biologial. Psychoanalytic theory, based primarily on Freud's work, postulates that depression is the result of a particular personality structure. The behavioral theories are based on social-learning theory, which assumes that psychological functioning is best understood in terms of the interaction among the personal, behavioral, and environmental factors of a person's life. According to genetic theory, people in the same family are more likely to have major depression (or other mood disorders) than are random individuals in the general population. Biological theory suggests that the etiology of major depression is underactivity of nerve cells whose neurotransmitters are the biogenic amines.

Therapies for mood disorders are based on psychoanalytic, behavioral, and biological treatments. Psychoanalytic therapy is designed to restructure the personality patterns of the affected individual. Behavioral therapies are based on the theory that depression is maintained by reinforcement of depressed behavior and inadequate reinforcement of non-depressed behavior. Biological therapy involves the use of various antidepressant medications to alleviate symptoms. Lithium has become well-established as the drug of choice for maintenance therapy of bipolar mood disorder. Electoconvulsive therapy can be an effective treatment for depression, especially in the case of a depression that has been resistant to medication and psychotherapy.

The nurse who cares for a patient with a mood disorder in a psychiatric setting plays a role in educating the patient and his family about the illness, monitors the effects of medication, monitors an ongoing assessment of the patient's symptoms, and works with the treatment team as well as the patient's family in the attempt to understand and effectively treat his mood disorder. The nurse who cares for a patient with a mood disorder in a nonpsychiatric setting assesses depressive symptomatology, makes therapeutic interventions, initiates psychiatric consultations, and challenges myths about mood disorders.

KEY TERMS

mood disorders
syndrome
major depression
unipolar depression
bipolar disorder
mania
dysthymic disorder
cyclothymic disorder
hypomania
delusions
hallucinations
psychotic depression
suicide ideation
psychomotor retardation
pressured speech
mood-congruent delusions
mood-incongruent delusions
psychoanalytic theory
introjection
ego psychology
dominant other
dominant goal
attachment behavior
attachment bond
social-learning theory
reduced reinforcement model
dysphoria
depressogenic model
extinction-trial behavior

negative cognitive-set theory
learned-helplessness model
attribution theory
biogenic-amine theory
dexamethasone-suppression test (DST)
thyrotropin-releasing hormone (TRH)
psychoanalytic/psychodynamic therapy
engagement stage
initial stage
transference
working-through stage
termination stage
behavioral therapy
contingency management
social-skills training
assertiveness training
reality therapy
cognitive restructuring
tricyclic antidepressants
second-generation antidepressants
monoamine oxidase inhibitors (MAOIs)
lithium
carbamazepine
electroconvulsive therapy (ECT)

STUDY QUESTIONS

1. Name and describe the clinical symptoms of depression and manic-depression.

2. Name and describe the five major areas of assessment of patients with depression.

3. Name and describe the five major areas of assessment of patients with mania.

4. Name and describe briefly the three major theories of mood disorders.

5. Name and describe briefly the three major types of treatments of mood disorders.

REFERENCES

Abramson, L. Y., & Seligman, M. E. P. (1978). Learned helplessness in humans: critique and reformulation. *Journal of Abnormal Psychology, 87,* 49–74.

American Psychiatric Association (1980). *Diagnostic and statistical manual of mental disorders, third edition.* Washington, D.C.: American Psychiatric Association.

American Psychiatric Association (1987). *Diagnostic and statistical manual of mental disorders, third edition, revised.* Washington, D.C.: American Psychiatric Association.

Arieti, S. (1962). The psychotherapeutic approach to depression. *American Journal of Psychotherapy, 16,* 397–406.

Arieti, S. (1977). Psychotherapy of severe depression. *American Journal of Psychiatry, 134,* 864–8.

Arieti, S., & Bemporad, J. R. (1978). *Severe and mild depression: The psychotherapeutic approach.* New York: Basic Books.

Arieti, S., & Bemporad, J. R. (1980). Psychological organization of depression. *American Journal of Psychiatry, 137,* 1360–5.

Ballenger, J. C., & Post, R. M. (1985). Carbamazepine in manic-depressive illness: A new treatment. *American Journal of Psychiatry, 137,* 782–90.

Beck, A. T. (1967). *Depression.* Philadelphia: University of Pennsylvania Press.

Beck, A. T. (1972). *Depression: Cause and treatment.* Philadelphia: University of Pennsylvania Press.

Beck, A. T., Rush, A. J., Shaw, B. F., & Emery, G. (1979). *Cognitive therapy of depression.* New York: Guilford Press.

Bemporad, J. R. (1976). Psychotherapy of the depressive character. *Journal of the American Academy of Psychoanalysis, 4,* 347–72.

Bemporad, J. R. (1985). Long-term analytic treatment of depression. In E. E. Beckham & W. R. Leber (Eds.), *Handbook of depression.* Homewood, Illinois: Dorsey Press.

Bowlby, J. (1980) *Loss: Attachment and loss.* Vol. 3. New York: Basic Books.

Boyer, J. L., & Guthrie, L. (1985). Assessment and treatment of the suicidal patient. In E. E. Beckham & W. R. Leber (Eds.), *Handbook of depression.* Homewood, Illinois: Dorsey Press, 606–33.

Cadoret, R. J. (1978). Evidence for genetic inheritance primary affective disorder in adoptees. *The American Journal of Psychiatry, 135,* 463–66.

Cadoret, R. J., Winocur, G., & Clayton, P. (1970). Family history studies, VII: Manic-depressive disease versus depressive disease. *British Journal of Psychiatry, 116,* 625–35.

Carroll, B. J., Feinberg, M., Greden, F., et al. (1981). A specific laboratory test for the diagnosis of melancholia. *Archives of General Psychiatry, 38,* 15–22.

Cerletti, U. (1956). Electroshock therapy. In F. Marti-Ibanez et al. (Eds.), *The great physiodynamic therapies in psychiatry.* New York: Hoeber-Harper.

Coine, J. C. (1976). Toward an interaction description of depression. *Psychiatry, 39,* 28–40.

DiMascio, A., Weissman, M., Prusoff, B., et al. (1979). Differential symptom reduction by drugs and psychotherapy in acute depression. *Archives of General Psychiatry, 36,* 1450–6.

Ferster, C.B. (1973, October). A functional analysis of depression. *American Psychologist,* 857–70.

Fink, M. (1979). *Convulsive therapy: Theory and practice.* New York: Raven Press.

Freud, S. ([1917], 1956). Mourning and melancholia. In *Collected papers.* Vol. 4. London: Hogarth Press.

Gambrill, E. D. (1977). *Behavior modification: Handbook of assessment, intervention and evaluation.* San Francisco: Josey-Bass.

Glasser, W. (1975). *Reality therapy: A new approach to psychiatry.* New York: Harper & Row.

Goodwin, F. K., & Zis, A. P. (1979). Lithium in the treatment of mania. *Archives of General Psychiatry, 36,* 840–6.

Gordon, M. (1985). *Manual of nursing diagnosis 1984–85.* New York: McGraw-Hill.

Griest, J. H., & Jefferson, J. W. (1984). *Depression and its treatment: Help for the nation's number one mental health problem.* Washington, D.C.: American Psychiatric Press.

Hamilton, M. (1967). A rating scale for depression. *British Journal of Social and Clinical Psychology, 6,* 278–96.

Hirschfield, R. M. A., & Cross, C. K. (1982). Epidemiology of affective disorders. *Archives of General Psychiatry, 39,* 35–46.

Hoberman, H. M., & Lewinsohn, P. M. (1985). The behavioral treatment of depression. In E. E. Beckham & W. R. Leber (Eds.), *Handbook of depression.* Homewood, Illinois: Dorsey Press.

Jacobson, E. (1971). *Depression: Comparative studies of normal, neurotic, and psychotic conditions.* New York: International Universities Press.

Jefferson, J. W., Griest, J. H., & Ackerman, D. L. (1983). *Lithium encyclopedia for clinical practice.* Washington, D.C.: American Psychiatric Press.

Lazarus, A. (1968, February). Learning theory and treatment of depression. *Behavioral Research Therapy,* 80–9.

Lerer, B. (1985). Alternative therapies for bipolar disorder. *Journal of Clinical Psychiatry, 46,* 309–16.

Lewinsohn, P. M. (1975). The behavioral study and treatment of depression. In M. Hensen (Ed.), *Progress in Behavioral Modification.* New York: Academic Press.

Lewinsohn, P. M., Biglan, T., & Zeiss, A. (1976). Behavioral treatment of depression. In P. Davidson (Ed.), *Behavioral management of anxiety, depression, and pain.* New York: L Brunner/Mazel.

Lewinsohn, P. M., Hoberman, H. M., Teri, L., & Hautzinger, M. (1985). An integrative theory of depression. In S. Reiss & R. Bootzin (Eds.), *Theoretical issues in behavior therapy*. New York: Academic Press.

Lindemann, E. (1960). Psychosocial factors as stressor agents. In J. Tanner (Ed.), *Stress and psychiatric disorders*. Oxford: Blackwell.

Massachusetts General Hospital (1985). Carbamazepine (Tegretol) for manic-depressive illness: An update. *Biological Therapies in Psychiatry, 6*, 21–24.

Mendlewicz, J., & Rainer, J. D. (1977). Adoption study supporting genetic transmission in manic-depressive illness. *Nature, 268*, 327–9.

Noll, K. M., Davis, J. M., & DeLeon-Jones, F. (1985). Medication and somatic therapies in the treatment of depression. In E. E. Beckham & W. R. Leber (Eds.), *Handbook of depression*. Homewood, Illinois: Dorsey Press.

Prange, A. J., Wilson, I. C., Lara, P. D., et al (1972). Effects of thyrotropin-releasing hormone in depression. *Lancet, 2*, 999–1002.

Prien, R. F., Caffey, E. M., & Klett, C. J. (1973). Prophylactic efficacy of lithium carbonate in manic-depressive illness: Report of the Veteran's Administration and National Institute of Mental Health collaborative study group. *Archives of General Psychiatry, 28*, 337–41.

Rudorfer, M. V., Golden, R. N., & Potter, W. Z. (1984). Second-generation antidepressants. *Psychiatric Clinics of North America, 3*, 519–34.

Rush, A. J. (1983). Cognitive therapy of depression: Rationale, techniques, and efficacy. *Psychiatric Clinics of North America, 6*, 105–27.

Rush, A. J., Beck, A. T., Kovacks, M., et al. (1982). Differential effects of cognitive therapy and pharmacotherapy on hopelessness and self concept. *American Journal of Psychiatry, 1390*, 862–66.

Scovern, E. W., & Kilmann, P. R. (1980). Status of electroconvulsive therapy: Review of the outcome literature. *Psychological Bulletin, 87*, 260–303.

Seligman, M. P. (1975). *Helplessness*. San Francisco: W. H. Freeman.

Smith, M. (1975). *When I say no, I feel guilty*. New York: Dial Press.

Sternberg, D. E. (1984). Biologic tests in psychiatry. *Psychiatric Clinics of North America, 7*, 639–50.

Varga, E. (1984). Tegretol in affective disorders. *Carrier Foundation Letter, 94*, 1–3.

Weissman, M. M., & Klerman, G. L. (1977). Sex differences and the epidemiology of depression. *Archives of General Psychiatry, 34*, 98–111.

Weissman, M. M., & Myers, J. K. (1978). Affective disorders in a U.S. urban community: The use of research diagnostic criteria in an epidemiological survey. *Archives of General Psychiatry, 35*, 1304–11.

Wender, P. H., & Klein, D. F. (1981). *Mind, mood, and medicine*. New York: New American Library.

Wetzel, J. W. (1984). *Clinical handbook of depression*. New York: Gardner Press.

Zung, W. K. (1965). A self-rating depression scale. *Archives of General Psychiatry, 12*, 63–70.

10

SCHIZOPHRENIA

FAYE GARY

INTRODUCTION

Schizophrenia is a devastating mental illness estimated to affect about 1 percent of the general population (Maxmen, 1986). It is actually a group of several disorders that strike at an early age and are chronic in nature, with periods of acute episodes. The resulting costs on the affected individual, the schizophrenic's family, and society in general are enormous. Schizophrenia's causes are unclear, prevention difficult, and treatment inadequate. In recent years, however, the outlook for schizophrenic patients has greatly improved. The antipsychotic drugs currently in use, though limited in their ability to control all symptoms of schizophrenia, can relieve the worst symptoms associated with the illness. In addition, new information about family and environmental factors related to schizophrenia has helped the patient and family cope with the disease. Ongoing research into the genetic and neurochemical bases of schizophrenia promises hope for more effective treatment measures in the future.

Though schizophrenia is primarily a **thought disorder** as opposed to a **mood disorder,** individuals with schizophrenia exhibit a wide variety of symptoms including withdrawal, difficulty concentrating, unintelligible communications, bizarre and unusual behavior, and disturbances in reality testing. Frequently there is a history of unusual behaviors documented since early childhood; some children will have autistic-like uncommunicative behaviors, with limited emotional attachments; still others display behavioral problems and learning disabilities. On the other hand, some children who later become schizo-

phrenic will lead "normal lives" until their first schizophrenic episode in late adolescence or early adulthood.

The disorder is so complex that symptoms might arise without any identifiable contributing causes. In other instances, schizophrenia may be precipitated by a wide variety of stressors, such as death of a family member or loved one, the loss of a job, substance use and/or abuse, an accident, a move to a new culture or neighborhood, or a threat to body image (Harvard Medical School Mental Health Letter, 1986).

In spite of the devastation this disease can cause, society has not yet provided the type of resources, both human and material, that are needed for comprehensive treatment (Bassuk & Gerson, 1978).

This chapter will focus on the characteristics of schizophrenia, theories about etiology and treatment, related nursing diagnoses and interventions, and rehabilitation strategies. Because of the chronic nature of schizophrenia, this chapter also addresses issues regarding deinstitutionalization and homelessness among schizophrenic persons.

HISTORICAL DESCRIPTIONS OF SCHIZOPHRENIA

The symptoms and behaviors of schizophrenia were reported as early as 1400 B.C. in Sanskrit writings. Persons with schizophrenia were described as poorly groomed, walking around without clothing, without memory, and exhibiting disturbed psychomotor activity (Kaplan & Sadock, 1985). The care provided for those individuals labeled as "mad" was and still is determined by the social, economic, religious, and societal ideology of a particular period and culture (Bassuk & Gerson, 1978). For hundreds of years, schizophrenics were considered criminals and frequently were housed in jails or other institutions designed for those possessed by devils or their evil spirits.

In the early 1900s the German psychiatrist Emil Kraepelin (1919) made two important distinctions in the description of this disorder. In observing patients with dementia, he noticed that some patients' symptoms, e.g., delusions, began at a relatively early age, while in other patients, the deterioration did not begin until later in life. He used the term "dementia praecox" to describe the illness afflicting the first group. The dementia of patients whose onset of cognitive impairment begins relatively late in life is now referred to as Alzheimer's disease (Black, Yates, & Andreason, 1988). Kraepelin also distinguished between those patients who were chronically afflicted with dementia and those with mood disorders who suffered bouts of emotional instability but who did not appear to worsen over time. The Swiss psychiatrist Eugen Bleuler built on Kraepelin's observations of dementia and coined the term "schizophrenia" referring to the splitting off or dissociation of parts of the self. He observed that the patient experiences separation of integrated functioning that blends thoughts and feelings. Bleuler (1950) described four key characteristics of schizophrenia, the 4 A's—ambivalence, disturbance in association, disturbance in affect, and autism that are used to this day to help in the diagnosis of schizophrenia (Tsuang, Faraone, & Day, 1988):

Affective disturbances can include depression, anxiety and/or flat emotional responses to situations that require more dramatic responses.

Ambivalence exhibits itself through extreme, contradictory emotions and thoughts about a person or object.

Autism is characterized by a drastic withdrawal from reality and little interest in human relationships.

Looseness of association is revealed by bizarre, illogical verbalization that often contains a message to be "decoded," but is hard to follow and seems to make no sense. This symptom is unique to schizophrenia.

Schneider (1959) made the point that a number of symptoms are necessary for the diagnosis of schizophrenia. He developed a system referred to as the "Schneiderian First and Second-Rank Symptoms." According to Schneider, a patient who is in a schizophrenic episode will exhibit some of the symptoms in each category:[1]

First-Rank Symptoms:

Voices speaking personal thoughts out loud (thought broadcasting)

Hearing voices discussing him (auditory hallucinations)

Hearing voices describing his behavior and comments upon his thoughts and activities

Command hallucinations (auditory hallucinations directing the patient, often, to do self-harm or to hurt someone else)

Delusions

Somatic Passivity (psychomotor retardation)

Thoughts being placed into his mind (thought insertion)

Thoughts and experiences being controlled by external forces

Second-Rank Symptoms

Perplexity

Depression

Euphoric states

The International Pilot Study of Schizophrenia (WHO, 1975) provides yet another classification of schizophrenia. Conducted under the auspices of the World Health Organization, this study looked at diagnostic criteria for schizophrenia in industrialized and developing countries. Participating countries included Nigeria, England, the Soviet Union, Taiwan, the United States, Czechoslovakia, Denmark, India, and Columbia. The study produced a list of behaviors specific to the diagnosis of schizophrenia that were common to the countries. These included restricted affect, poor insight, hearing one's thoughts spoken aloud, absence of early waking, poor rapport, lack of elation, widespread delusions, incoherent speech, unreliable information given, bizarre delusions, and nihilistic delusions. This study also revealed that schizophrenic patients in developing countries tended to have a much better chance of coping with their illness than those patients in highly industrialized nations.

---

[1]Schizophrenics almost never experience visual hallucinations, more common in the organic psychoses. (See Chapter 11 on Organic Mental Disorders.)

DSM-III-R Diagnostic Criteria for Schizophrenia

A. Presence of characteristic psychotic symptoms in the active phase: either (1), (2), or (3) for at least one week (unless the symptoms are successfully treated):

    (1) two of the following:

        (a) delusions

        (b) prominent hallucinations (throughout the day for several days or several times a week for several weeks, each hallucinatory experience not being limited to a few brief moments)

        (c) incoherence or marked loosening of associations

        (d) catatonic behavior

        (e) flat or grossly inappropriate affect

    (2) bizarre delusions (i.e., involving a phenomenon that the person's culture would regard as totally implausible, e.g., thought broadcasting, being controlled by a dead person)

    (3) prominent hallucinations [as defined in (1)(b) above] of a voice with content having no apparent relation to depression or elation, or a voice keeping up a running commentary on the person's behavior or thoughts, or two more voices conversing with each other

B. During the course of the disturbance, functioning in such areas as work, social relations, and self-care is markedly below the highest level achieved before onset of the disturbance (or, when the onset is in childhood or adolescence, failure to achieve expected level of social development).

C. Schizoaffective disorder and mood disorder with psychotic features have been ruled out, i.e., if a major depressive or manic syndrome has ever been present during an active phase of the disturbance, the total duration of all episodes of a mood syndrome has been brief relative to the total duration of the active and residual phases of the disturbance.

D. Continuous signs of the disturbance for at least six months. The six-month period must include an active phase (of at least one week, or less if symptoms have been successfully treated) during which there were psychotic symptoms characteristic of schizophrenia (symptoms in A), with or without a prodromal or residual phase, as defined below.

Prodromal phase: A clear deterioration in functioning before the active phase of the disturbance that is not due to a disturbance in mood or to a psychoactive substance use disorder and that involves at least two of the symptoms listed below.

CURRENT DIAGNOSTIC CLASSIFICATION OF SCHIZOPHRENIA

Today, the DSM-III-R provides the most commonly used criteria for the diagnosis of schizophrenia. The DSM-III-R description represents a combination of contributions from past theories and current research. Many of the symptoms described by Bleuler and Schneider are included in the list of defining symptoms. Kraepelin's distinction of chronicity and gradual deterioration is also included.

Criteria developed in the 1970s and 1980s at Washington University in St. Louis helped to increase reliability of the diagnosis and to narrow its focus (Black, Yates, & Andreason, 1988). The most important distinction arising from this work is that an individual with all other symptoms, but whose illness has not lasted for at least six months, is given the diagnosis of Schizophreniform Disorder, a classification outside the category of Schizophrenic Disorders (Black, Yates, & Andreason, 1988). It is thought that the absence of long-term progression of the characteristics of schizophrenia may signal a greater

Residual phase: Following the active phase of the disturbance, persistence of at least two of the symptoms noted below, these not being due to a disturbance in mood or to a psychoactive substance use disorder.

Prodromal or residual symptoms:

(1) marked social isolation or withdrawal

(2) marked impairment in role functioning as wage-earner, student, or homemaker

(3) markedly peculiar behavior (e.g., collecting garbage, talking to self in public, hoarding food)

(4) marked impairment in personal hygiene and grooming

(5) blunted or inappropriate affect

(6) digressive, vague, overelaborate, or circumstantial speech, or poverty of speech, or poverty of content of speech

(7) odd beliefs or magical thinking, influencing behavior and inconsistent with cultural norms, e.g., superstitiousness, belief in clairvoyance, telepathy, "sixth sense," "others can feel my feelings," overvalued ideas, ideas of reference

(8) unusual perceptual experiences, e.g., recurrent illusions, sensing the presence of a force or person not actually present

(9) marked lack of initiative, interests, or energy

Examples: Six months of prodromal symptoms with one week of symptoms from A; no prodromal symptoms with six months of symptoms from A; no prodromal symptoms with one week of symptoms from A and six months of residual symptoms.

E. It cannot be established that an organic factor initiated and maintained the disturbance.

F. If there is a history of autistic disorder, the additional diagnosis of schizophrenia is made only if prominent delusions or hallucinations are also present.

tendency toward acute onset and resolution and a greater chance of recovery to previous levels of functioning. The clinical picture of Schizophreniform Disorder is otherwise similar to that of Schizophrenia except that Schizophreniform Disorder is more often characterized by emotional turmoil, fear, confusion, and especially vivid hallucinations (APA, 1987). The distinction between these two diagnoses, however, may be crucial to management of the patient. Schizophrenia is a stigmatizing disease, and diagnosis must be very carefully determined by exclusion of possible organic causes (including tumors and substance abuse); symptoms are then differentiated from affective disorder, dissociative disorder, and personality disorder.

TYPES OF SCHIZOPHRENIA

The DSM III-R (1987) has specified five types of schizophrenic disorders: **catatonic type, disorganized type, paranoid type, residual type,** and **undifferentiated type.** This diagnostic system requires that mental health professionals make judgment calls about the overall functioning of the patient (Tsuang,

**DSM-III-R
Diagnostic Criteria for
295.2x Catatonic Type**

A type of schizophrenia in which the clinical picture is dominated by any of the following:

(1) catatonic stupor (marked decrease in reactivity to the environment and/or reduction in spontaneous movements and activity) or mutism

(2) catatonic negativism (an apparently motiveless resistance to all instructions or attempts to be moved)

(3) catatonic rigidity (maintenance of a rigid posture against efforts to be moved)

(4) catatonic excitement (excited motor activity, apparently purposeless and not influenced by external stimuli)

(5) catatonic posturing (voluntary assumption of inappropriate or bizarre postures)

Faraone, & Day, 1988). The criteria by which clinical judgments are made follow.

CATATONIC TYPE SCHIZOPHRENIA

Catatonic schizophrenia is characterized by bizarre motor behavior in which the patient is either in a stupor or a state of excitement (Kaplan & Sadock, 1985). When the patient is in a stupor, he may exhibit stiff muscle tone, muteness, echopraxia, childlike obedience to directions, and disorganization of the personality (Kolb & Brodie, 1982). Other behaviors include preoccupation with self, little interest and participation in the external environment, and emotional impoverishment, with a characteristic avoidance of eye contact.

When in a catatonic stupor, the patient needs direct care and continuous observation for assistance in the activities of daily living, such as eating, toileting, grooming, and hygiene.

The patient may move from stupor to catatonic excitability. Excitability is accompanied by some psychomotor activity that is unrelated to external stimuli. This phase of the illness also involves restlessness, bizarre and pressured speech, hallucinations, grimaces, feelings of anger, hostility and rage. The patient may become self-destructive or aggressive (Schultz & Kilgalen, 1969). In addition, the patient does not maintain good hygiene and may require assistance with activities of daily living.

Dwayne: A Catatonic Schizophrenic

Dwayne was a 25-year-old student at a community college and an office manager in a small insurance company. He was brought to the emergency room of a large teaching hospital by his fiancée. He lay on a stretcher in a very still manner and resisted all attempts by the nurses and physicians to be moved. His eyes remained closed. According to Dwayne's fiancée, he had become increasingly "weird" in the past six months. His physical appearance had deteriorated; he seemed preoccupied and would not talk. At times, he refused to eat, to attend classes at the community college, or to go to work. Instead, he would remain in bed for long periods of time and stare. His fiancée became frightened when he began to lose weight and had several episodes during which he shouted obscenities. Then, he would return to his previous state of staring, remaining mute, and lying "lifeless-like" in bed.

DISORGANIZED TYPE (HEBEPHRENIC) SCHIZOPHRENIA

Disorganized or hebephrenic schizophrenia usually begins in adolescence. The individual regresses to very primitive behavior, with minimal ability to execute the activities of daily living. The patient tends to be withdrawn and reclusive; his eating habits are sloppy, and he may use neologisms (his own "made-up" words for things) and experience hallucinations. In addition, the patient may often giggle or be silly inappropriately. All or some of these behaviors may continue for years.

Rather than having well-developed delusional systems, patients with disorganized type schizophrenia tend to be as fragmented and disorganized in

DSM-III-R Diagnostic Criteria for 295.1x Disorganized Type

A type of schizophrenia in which the following criteria are met:

A. Incoherence, marked loosening of associations, or grossly disorganized behavior.

B. Flat or grossly inappropriate affect.

C. Does not meet the criteria for catatonic type.

their thinking as in the rest of their behaviors. The nurse might experience difficulty relating to the patient because of severe thought disorganization, withdrawal, and social isolation. The patient does not connect with events that are occurring in the patient's external world. For example, the patient might exhibit continuous silliness and giggling which seems uncontrollable and permeates all interpersonal relationships. Regression occurs at a fairly rapid rate and does not easily lend itself to immediate intervention. The patient loses his capacity to attend to such basic personal activities as toileting, and is likely to become autistic and unapproachable by others. Disintegration of personality and ego functions is perhaps in its most extreme form in this type of schizophrenia (Kolb & Brodie, 1982). The onset of illness usually occurs during adolescence and early adulthood. Diagnoses of disorganized schizophrenia have been made, however, as early as age 9 or 10 (Spotnitz, 1976).

Pam: A Patient with Disorganized Type Schizophrenia

Pam was an 18-year-old woman who was admitted to the hospital because of withdrawn behaviors and a lack of interest in participating in family and peer activities of daily living. Her mother reported that Pam's physical appearance had become disheveled. She seldom combed her hair or brushed her teeth. Her mother complained that Pam had begun laughing loudly when she was alone in her bedroom, and seemed to have been participating in a conversation with some of her schoolmates although no one else was with her and she wasn't on the telephone. During the admitting interview, Pam's mother reported that Pam interrupted other people's conversations, ate in a hurried and sloppy manner, and stayed away from the house for long hours, reporting upon return that she had been in the National Geographic Forest. The mother stated that Pam had been a very obedient child, quiet, nice, and a model student, until recently. No precipitating event could be identified; however, there was a history of schizophrenia in Pam's maternal grandmother.

PARANOID TYPE SCHIZOPHRENIA

The paranoid schizophrenic can best be described as a person with an intellectual psychosis, an all-consuming delusional system, who uses projection as a pathological mode of defense (Freud, 1895 in Frosch, 1983). Freud hypothesized that people develop paranoia about things which they cannot tolerate within themselves, provided that a predisposition exists for the use of projection (Freud, 1895 in Frosch, 1983, p. 28). The use of projection alleviates anxiety and inner tensions by placing the problem on others. Hence, the ego is somewhat protected from dealing with the intolerable, at least until the defense of projection fails him and the repressed anxiety begins to "leak out."

Because of the tension and suspicion that he experiences, even when well-defended against his own inner experience, the patient may be subject to outbursts and fits of rage with little provocation (Kolb & Brodie, 1982). Nothing seems to comfort the paranoid patient. Because of the nature of the illness, the paranoid patient can sometimes be dangerous to himself and/or others. Deterioration is usually slower than with other types of schizophrenia.

Jim: A Patient with Paranoid Schizophrenia

Jim, a 45-year-old veteran who was once a fighter pilot, was hospitalized for "suspicious behavior." His paranoid ideas started to develop at the time the American embassy staff was being held hostage in Iran. Jim entered the hospital unit dressed in fatigue

**DSM-III-R
Diagnostic Criteria for
295.3x Paranoid Type**

A type of schizophrenia in which there are:

A. Preoccupation with one or more systematized delusions or with frequent auditory hallucinations related to a single theme.

B. *None* of the following: incoherence, marked loosening of associations, flat or grossly inappropriate affect, catatonic behavior, grossly disorganized behavior.

Specify stable type if criteria A and B have been met during all past and present active phases of the illness.

boots and a camouflage suit and carried a supply of foods and medicine. He refused to talk to the staff because of his "secret clearance papers." He kept his back to the wall, looked around the unit in a very suspicious manner, and refused food. He had difficulty sleeping because he felt that his body would be invaded at "that opportune time." These invasions would be in the form of laser beams shot from another country through an elaborate satellite mechanism that was brought in by a complex computer system. Moreover, this same satellite would transfer laser type messages back to a coordinating station and produce images of the patient to the enemy that was looking for him to execute his death sentence.

UNDIFFERENTIATED TYPE SCHIZOPHRENIA

Undifferentiated schizophrenia is characterized by a variety of prominent psychiatric symptoms such as delusions, hallucinations, incoherence, and grossly disorganized behaviors.

Mac: A Patient with Undifferentiated Schizophrenia

Mac was a 30-year-old man who exhibited bizarre delusions: He believed that his daily medications were transmitted from his body to his dead mother. He also heard voices that commanded him to speak or not to speak. At times, he needed assistance with hygiene and dressing, and on occasion, required supervision of his nutritional intake. He was withdrawn and did not socialize with others. After his numerous failed attempts at living in the community, Mac's family requested that he remain in the hospital where he had been a long-term patient. Mac eventually resided in a group home located on the grounds of a state hospital.

RESIDUAL TYPE SCHIZOPHRENIA

Residual type schizophrenia suggests that the prominent symptoms of the illness have abated. Inappropriate or flat affect behavior and illogical or magical

**DSM-III-R
Diagnostic Criteria for
295.9x
Undifferentiated Type**

A type of schizophrenia in which there are:

A. Prominent delusions, hallucinations, incoherence, or grossly disorganized behavior.

B. Does not meet the criteria for paranoid, catatonic, or disorganized type.

DSM-III-R Diagnostic Criteria for 295.6x Residual Type

A type of schizophrenia in which there are:

A. Absence of prominent delusions, hallucinations, incoherence, or grossly disorganized behavior.

B. Continuing evidence of the disturbance, as indicated by two or more of the residual symptoms listed in criterion D of schizophrenia (see p. 314).

---

thinking may persist, however. Hallucinations and delusions may be present. This disorder is either chronic or subacute.

Jose: A Patient with Residual Type Schizophrenia

Jose, a hotel employee who worked in the laundry room, reported to work regularly each day. In "his corner," he folded towels and sheets in a slow and methodical fashion; he ate alone, talked to himself, and responded to questions from others in a monotone. At times, his conversations became difficult to follow: ". . . Horses are beautiful. They sometimes fly . . . they are larger than pigs. Pigs have guns. Horses don't."

EPIDEMIOLOGY

It is difficult to determine epidemiological characteristics of schizophrenia because of deficiencies in diagnostic procedures, case identification, and data regarding onset. It has been determined, however, that among age groups 15 years and older, schizophrenia occurs at a rate of 0.30 to 1.20 per 1000 population; each year, roughly 200,000 new cases are reported in the United States, while around 2 million new cases are reported throughout the world. Nearly .025 to .05 percent of the total population will be diagnosed with schizophrenia and will receive treatment within the year of their initial diagnosis; two thirds of these individuals will need hospitalization (Kaplan & Sadock, 1988).

GENDER

Schizophrenia is about equally prevalent among men and women, although women tend to have a slightly better prognosis than men. The illness may occur at a later age in women than in men.

AGE

The onset of schizophrenia is most likely to occur between the ages of 15 and 25 for men, and ages 25 to 35 for women (Kaplan & Sadock, 1988). In middle class patients, however, onset of schizophrenia tends to be higher among patients between the ages of 35 to 44 years (Goodman et al., 1983; Gregory & Smeltzer, 1983).

MARITAL STATUS

The schizophrenic patient is usually unmarried, divorced, or widowed.

SOCIOECONOMIC CLASS

Some researchers have found that there is a relationship between schizophrenia and socioeconomic status, with a prevalence among lower socioeconomic groups (Hollingshead & Redlich, 1958; Dowhrenwend, 1975; Warheit, Bell & Schwab, 1977). Determining socioeconomic status, however, involves measuring income, occupation, and education—all of which might be greatly affected by the schizophrenic's inability to function in daily life (Goodman et al., 1983). More important, it is not clear why this relationship between lower socioeconomic status and schizophrenia exists. Some have hypothesized that schizophrenic individuals tend to "drift" or migrate to the center of a city and join other "fringe livers" or "street people" because their illness prevents them from holding down jobs and maintaining relationships (Dunham, 1965). Others attribute the correlation of schizophrenia and lower socioeconomic status to the stresses of poverty and crowding associated with living in central urban areas; i.e., it is thought that such a living situation can produce schizophrenia in vulnerable individuals (Gregory and Smeltzer, 1983). Much additional research is needed in this area (Tsuang, Faraone, & Day, 1988).

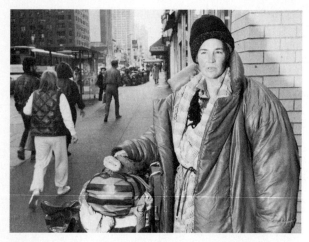

It has been hypothesized that because schizophrenic individuals are unable to maintain employment or other significant relationships, they become "street dwellers," or one of the many homeless.

ASSESSMENT OF SCHIZOPHRENIA

RATING SCALES

A complete patient assessment is a prerequisite for effective and efficient treatment of schizophrenia. Rating scales which cover degree of psychopathology, family environment, and social competence are essential areas for the nurse to consider (Curran, Faraone, & Dow, 1985; Tsuang, Faraone, & Day, 1988).

SEVERITY OF PSYCHOPATHOLOGY. The assessment of psychopathology is done in order to verify the diagnosis, reconsider prognosis, and oversee the progression of the disorder. Tools that are useful for the assessment of pathology include the psychiatric interview (see Chapter 5, Assessment) and a scale that targets the severity of symptoms such as the Brief Psychiatric Rating Scale (BPRS) which can be administered at the beginning and end of hospitalization, and on an outpatient basis at about every three months (Curran, Faraone, & Dow, 1985). (See Figure 10–1.)

FAMILY ENVIRONMENT. Much evidence exists to support the idea that patients who live in families with a high level of expressed emotions (EE) are more likely to experience an exacerbation of symptoms than are patients who live in families where there is low expressed emotion (Curran, Faraone, & Dow, 1985; Hooley, 1986; Brown, Carstairs, & Topping, 1958). Expressed emotion can be assessed

using the Camberwell Family Interview (CFI) in which a relative of the patient is interviewed. Scoring for this instrument, however, is difficult, making the tool limited for everyday use. Nonetheless, the general underpinnings of the CFI can be used by the clinician for the assessment of family function. The nurse should be familiar with the problem of overinvolvement of relatives with patients and should interview families in a manner that allows the members to express their criticisms of the patient. These general guidelines can be adapted to each unique clinical situation.

SOCIAL COMPETENCE. Social competence can best be determined by observing the patient in his own environment. Although this option is frequently unrealistic, the nurse can observe the patient on the psychiatric unit and record behavioral data in a systematic way. The Simulated Social Interaction Test (SSIT) (Curran, 1982) can also be used to assess social competence. It provides the clinician with a range of eight situations that the patient is likely to experience with some difficulty. (See Figure 10–2.)

The Social Adjustment Scale-11 (SAS-11) was designed specifically for schizophrenic patients. Fifty-two questions address work, interpersonal relationships, sexual adjustment, romantic involvement, family role/functions, leisure activity, and personal well-being (Schooler, Hogarty, & Weissman, 1977).

CHARACTERISTICS AND SYMPTOMATOLOGY

The nurse who assesses the schizophrenic patient in order to formulate nursing diagnoses and plan and deliver appropriate care will find a wide variety of symptoms and behaviors. The patient may exhibit disturbances in mood, cognition (including thought form and content), perception, physiological functioning, interpersonal skills and functioning, self-perception, volition, and motor ability. Following is a description of some of these behaviors, with a summary provided in Table 10–1 on pages 324–325.

MOOD CHANGES. The schizophrenic patient experiences increasing anxieties, tensions, and irritations. There is a tendency toward withdrawal and an aloofness about important issues and concerns. There is no ambition or interest in anything; spontaneity is lost. The patient will find reasons to isolate himself from people and will manifest no interest in his environment. Confused and alone, the patient will become increasingly unable to harmonize and balance emotions. Values that previously reigned may no

1. Somatic Concern	Degree of concern over present bodily health. Rate the degree to which physical health is perceived as a problem by the patient, whether complaints have a realistic basis or not.	1
2. Anxiety	Worry, fear, or over-concern for present or future. Rate solely on the basis of verbal report of patient's own subjective experiences. Do not infer anxiety from physical signs or from neurotic defense mechanisms.	2
3. Emotional Withdrawal	Deficiency in relating to the interviewer and to the interviewer situation. Rate only the degree to which the patient gives the impression of failing to be in emotional contact with other people in the interview situation.	3
4. Conceptual Disorganization	Degree to which the thought processes are confused, disconnected or disorganized. Rate on the basis of integration of the verbal products of the patient; do not rate on the basis of patient's subjective impression of his own level of functioning.	4
5. Guilt Feelings	Over-concern or remorse for past behavior. Rate on the basis of the patient's subjective experiences of guilt as evidenced by verbal report with appropriate affect; do not infer guilt feelings from depression, anxiety or neurotic defenses.	5
6. Tension	Physical and motor manifestations of tension, ''nervousness,'' and heightened activation level. Tension should be rated solely on the basis of physical signs and motor behavior and not on the basis of subjective experiences of tension reported by the patient.	6
7. Mannerisms and Posturing	Unusual and unnatural motor behavior, the type of motor behavior which causes certain mental patients to stand out in a crowd of normal people. Rate only abnormality of movements; do not rate simple heightened motor activity here.	7
8. Grandiosity	Exaggerated self-opinion, conviction of unusual ability or powers. Rate only on the basis of patient's statements about himself or self-in-relation-to-others, not on the basis of his demeanor in the interview situation.	8
9. Depressive Mood	Despondency in mood, sadness. Rate only degree of despondency; do not rate on the basis of inferences concerning depression based upon general retardation and somatic complaints.	9
10. Hostility	Animosity, contempt, belligerence, disdain for other people outside the interview situation. Rate solely on the basis of the verbal report of feelings and actions of the patient toward others; do not infer hostility from neurotic defenses, anxiety or somatic complaints. *Rate attitude toward interviewer under "uncooperativeness"*.	10
11. Suspiciousness	Belief *delusional or otherwise* that others have now, or have had in the past, malicious or discriminatory intent toward the patient. On the basis of verbal report, rate only those suspicions which are currently held whether they concern past or present circumstances.	11
12. Hallucinatory Behavior	Perceptions without normal external stimulus correspondence. Rate only those experiences which are reported to have occurred within the last week and which are described as distinctly different from the thought and imagery processes of normal people.	12
13. Motor Retardation	Reduction in energy level evidenced in slowed movements. Rate on the basis of observed behavior of the patient only; do not rate on basis of patient's subjective impression of own energy level.	13
14. Uncooperativeness	Evidence of resistance, unfriendliness, resentment, and lack of readiness to cooperate with the interviewer. Rate only on the basis of the patient's attitude and responses to the interviewer and the interview situation; do not rate on basis of reported resentment or uncooperativeness outside the interview situation.	14
15. Unusual Thought Content	Unusual, odd, strange, or bizarre thought content. Rate here the degree of unusualness, not the degree of disorganization of thought processes.	
16. Blunted Affect	Reduced emotional tone, apparent lack of normal feeling or involvement.	16
17. Excitement	Heightened emotional tone, agitation, increased reactivity.	17
18. Disorientation	Confusion or lack of proper association for person, place or time.	18

FIGURE 10–1 Brief Psychiatric Rating Scale Brief Psychiatric Rating Scale used for evaluation of the schizophrenic patient. For each of the 18 symptom areas, the interviewer marks the scale according to the degree of presence of that symptom, from "not present" to "extremely severe."

Source: Overall, J. E., & Gorham, D. R. (1962). The brief psychiatric rating scale. *Psychological reports, 10,* 799–812.

1. **Disapproval or criticism**
   Narrator: You are at work, and one of your bosses has just finished inspecting one of the jobs that you have completed. He says to you —
   Confederate: That's a pretty sloppy job. I think you could have done better.

2. **Social assertiveness or visibility**
   Narrator: Let's suppose you respond to an ad in the newspaper and go for a job interview. As the interview goes on, the interviewer says —
   Confederate: What makes you think that you're a good person for the job?

3. **Confrontation and anger expression**
   Narrator: For the past two weeks you have been saving your money to go out to dinner. Now you are at the restaurant with some friends. You order a very rare steak. The waitress brings a steak to the table that is so well done it is burnt and tastes awful. After you have a few bites, the waitress comes over and says —
   Confederate: Are you enjoying your steak?

4. **Heterosexual contact**
   Narrator: You are at a party, and you notice a woman has been watching you all evening. Later, she walks up to you and says —
   Confederate: Hi, my name is Jean.

5. **Interpersonal warmth**
   Narrator: You are seated in a very quiet restaurant with your date. She has been looking depressed all evening. You ask her what's wrong, and she says —
   Confederate: I'm really down. Everything seems to be turning out badly.

6. **Conflict with or rejection by parent or relative**
   Narrator: One of your close relatives has come to visit you. Although you enjoy him, tonight he is dominating the conversation and is very critical and rejecting of you. At one point in the conversation, your relative says —
   Confederate: The way you are running your life is a disgrace.

7. **Interpersonal loss**
   Narrator: You have had an argument with a close friend. She says to you —
   Confederate: I don't want to talk about it anymore. I'm leaving.

8. **Receiving compliments**
   Narrator: You just helped one of your neighbors move several large pieces of furniture. He is very grateful for your help. He says to you —
   Confederate: Thanks a million. Not many people would have given me a hand. You're a really good friend.

FIGURE 10–2 The Simulated Social Interaction Test

longer be adhered to, and social graces are compromised (Kolb & Brodie, 1982). The schizophrenic person may also display what appears to be a rehearsal of emotions before expressing them: words come out stilted, pressured, and disconnected. The incongruous nature of thought and affect, the impoverished cognitive and emotional expressions, and the retarded psychomotor activities constitute behavior that demonstrates components of the patient's so-called "split personality" (Gregory & Smeltzer, 1983; Frosch, 1983; Kolb & Brodie, 1982; Bleuler, 1950; Gordon, 1982).

Blunted Affect. The schizophrenic patient often presents with a blunted, flat affect. The patient's expression is emotionless.

> Upon observing the U.S. Challenger shuttle disintegrate into fire and smoke, a schizophrenic patient sat quietly and commented to the nurse, without any concern, warmth, excitement, or regard for the astronauts, "It's gone now."

Anhedonia. Anhedonia is another symptom associated with schizophrenia. The schizophrenic patient presents a state of continuous apathy. Nothing seems to make him happy. The patient will not be able to experience pleasure from any activity. It should be noted that this may also be characteristic of the depressed patient.

Mutism and Stupor. Some schizophrenic patients will not talk with the nurses; however, that should not prevent them from talking to him. In addition, the nurse observes for variation in facial expressions, body posture, and leg and foot movement. The facial expression may be blank (as in catatonic reactions), or it may display deep depression or melancholy.

Delusions. Sometimes the patient feels as if the world is changing right before his eyes, with no explanation for the change. This state may last for several days or weeks; it can occur as the patient approaches the development of a definite delusional belief system (Leff & Isaacs, 1981).

> My family looks strange to me . . . I hardly recognize them any more . . . The earth has rejected me . . . I am a part of another universe that I don't understand.

Aloofness. The patient presents an image of one not concerned about anything or anyone. When possible, he will select situations void of interpersonal contacts.

I would rather be at home alone, in my room, with my radio, than attending the company party tomorrow.

COGNITIVE CHANGES. Cognitive changes are obvious in the schizophrenic patient's disturbed communication. The patient gradually loses the ability to present a logical, relevant series of thoughts. Instead, the disturbed thought process results in fragmented, illogical, and loosely associated elements. The patient's thoughts may have meaning to the patient, but because he uses highly personal metaphors, similes, or eccentric expressions, it is difficult for others to understand him. He uses symbolism in a highly personal manner, thus obstructing effective communication with others. Bizarre thought connections, highly personal symbolism, disregard for cause/effect relationships, and creation of personal phraseologies are just some of the forms this expression takes (Sullivan, 1962; Kolb & Brodie, 1982). Here is an example of disturbed thought process from a patient whose career in biomedical sciences was interrupted by schizophrenia:

My tubes are tied to the test tubes that are connected to the inner tubes. The sunlight, the solar computer, and by remote control my insides are microwaved for the formal meeting that will occur at sunlight—no sundark. My fate rests in the hands of the unicorn from the forest of the unicorn . . . who enter, infect, and evaporate away . . . leaving me in salt and vinegar, to evaporate into atmospheric nothingness.

Loss of Concentration. The schizophrenic loses the ability to concentrate and focus on ideas, people, or objects in the environment. The nurse might incorrectly assume that the patient is intellectually impaired. Rather, his interests and concerns are selective and not necessarily the same as the nurse's, so the patient tunes her out and lets his mind wander.

"John, can you share with us your activities of last week?" No response. Instead: slow, disjointed, comment: "Share . . . activities . . ."

An appropriate comment and one likely to be successful in getting the patient's attention, would be: "You don't seem to be with us today in group, John. Maybe the group could help if something is bothering you."

Passive Attention. Passive attention allows the patient a degree of contact with reality by means of practical, though detached, routines devoid of concentration and intellectual content or response to challenge.

John may not engage in conversation but will respond to medication call and basic activities of daily living.

Disturbances in Thought Form. In *loosening of associations* the patient presents ideas which shift from one subject to another in an oblique manner. In its most severe form, speech will be incoherent.

The house burned last night, but I didn't . . . I was hot and there was hot sex . . . six of one and half a dozen of another . . . sox are hot, though. Maybe it will rain.

Overinclusiveness and tangential thought refer to the patient's inclusion of an enormous amount of irrelevant material within the normal flow of thought.

I was walking my dog last night when I noticed the new growth on the trees. . . . My readings had focused on the bark, but that is directly related to the species. There are 1000 types of oak trees. The origin of this oak is in Alaska. Alaska was once owned by Russia. Russia is a communist country where one finds few citizens walking dogs.

Neologism is the patient's coining of new words and phrases usually incomprehensible to others.

A schizophrenic patient was very angry with a judge because of his statements during a commitment hearing and commented, "I am going to sue that judge because of hibockery and mosologious behavior."

In the distracting thought form referred to as *thought blocking,* the patient experiences internal intrusions that block his flow of speech. Usually he can, after a pause, resume normal thought and speech. The frequency and duration of thought blocking will vary according to acuity level. That is, it is likely to be most intense during an acute psychotic episode.

I will present my information to the . . . (pause) er, er . . . group therapy members . . . tomorrow, . . . next week . . . er . . . .

Other disturbed thought forms include clanging, echolalia, impoverished thought, and concrete thinking.

Clanging is the patient's rhyming of words within sentences, in which rhyming seems more important to the patient than the sentence content.

The tree has a tap root . . . Watch my toot . . . and fix my flute.

Echolalia involves the patient's repeating of words and phrases in a rhythmic fashion with little concern about effective communication.

TABLE 10–1 Characteristics of schizophrenia

Behavior	Definition/Description
Cognitive Disturbances	
Thought Form	
Loosening of association	Thoughts expressed are inexact, diffuse, and without central themes, as in tangential speech
Overinclusiveness	Numerous details, descriptions; unfocused speech
Tangential thought	Enormous and confusing amount of irrelevant details included in speech; loosely related thoughts or associations
Neologisms	Made-up words that have meaning only to the patient
Clanging	Words rhyme, but content is incomprehensible
Echolalia	Repetition of the speech of another person
Impoverished thought	Restricted concepts, ideas, constructs
Concrete thinking	Loss of ability to abstract
Blocking	Inhibited flow of thought and speech
Thought Content	
Delusions of grandeur	False beliefs of extreme wealth, exceptional powers, or special missions
Delusions of reference (self-referential ideation)	Individual claims personal ownership of communication and events that have nothing to do with him
Paranoid delusions	False belief that forces, individuals, family, groups, and so forth, have targeted the individual for hostile and destructive purposes
Mood Disturbances	
Blunted affect	Emotionless and flat expression; voice flat and monotonous
Anhedonia	No pleasure in experience
Autism	Without communicative speech
Aloofness	Detached; uninvolved; indifferent
Motor Disturbances	
Stupor	Blank facial expression; may look like acute organic brain syndrome in which patient goes back and forth between delirium and stupor
Peculiar mannerism	Peculiar; odd behavior such as grimacing
Catatonic type	Rigid and fixed posture
Spontaneity	Uninhibited, often purposeless activity, or, complete loss of spontaneity

Interviewer: Mrs. Brown, what brings you to the hospital?

Mrs. Brown: Mrs. Brown, what brings you to . . . the hospital?

Impoverished thought is a condition in which the patient talks but communicates little.

The nurse asked Mrs. Brown about a recent visit with her daughter. Mrs. Brown replied, "My daughter is my daughter. She was born . . . some years ago, and she visited me."

With excessively *concrete thinking,* the patient possesses intellectual capabilities but loses the ability to engage in abstract thought.

Interviewer: Mrs. K, what brings you to the hospital?

Mrs. K: My LTD.

Disturbances in Thought Content. *Disturbances* in the thought content of the schizophrenic patient are exhibited in the patient's *delusions:* false beliefs that

Perceptual Disturbances	
Hallucinations	
Auditory	Hears voices outside himself that do not exist, feels that voices within him can be heard by others.
Visual	Sees things that do not exist in the environment
Olfactory	Smells odors that are not in the environment
Tactile	Feels sensations that are not produced by anything in reality
Somatic	Thinks that parts of body are altered, diseased, changed in location and/or structure
Illusion	Misinterpretation of visual images that are in the environment
Motivational Changes	Appears "worn out"; lacks energy and initiative
Physical Disturbances	
Autonomic nervous system changes	Cold and slightly discolored hands and feet; blotchy skin; dilated pupils; moist hands; mild tachycardia; grimaces; odd movements referred to as "waxy flexibility" and "schizophrenic float"; shuffling gait; tick-like movements; highly developed rituals (usually associated with the chronically ill)
Weight flexibility	Early phase: gains weight; later phase: loses weight
Illness	Malnutrition, tuberculosis, and other communicable diseases occur as a result of poor living conditions and limited resources for the deinstitutionalized chronically mentally ill.
Interpersonal Disturbances	
Social withdrawal and social isolation	Limited contact with family and friends; reclusive; increased time spent asleep.
Increased sleep	Facilitates isolation
Highly personal use of language	Results in disturbed, and so decreased, interpersonal contacts
Limited interest in environment	Detached; aloof
Difficulty with intimacy	Limited, if any, emotional attachments
Psychological discomfort	Uncomfortable in presence of others; clings, intrudes, is withdrawn, and so forth
Lack of social graces	Diminished use of commonly acceptable etiquette within a particular reference group
Disturbances in Sense of Self	Confusion about one's identity; blurred ego boundaries
Disturbances in Volition	Limited goal-directed behaviors; impairment in occupation, recreation, and interpersonal relations

in the acute phase of schizophrenia may be disorganized and nonsystematic.

> My brain is connected to a remote control that dictates to the Pentagon chiefs and birds that can't fly.

Delusions may sometimes be highly organized, systematic, and manifested as *fixed* false beliefs.

> When a student nurse was interviewing a patient, he told her that his arm was broken. . . . X rays were made, and it was learned that there was no

fracture. The patient continued to believe, however, that his arm was broken and made a sling for it. The nurse and other personnel could not change the patient's belief.

Delusions of grandeur may include thoughts about extreme wealth, exceptional powers, or special missions.

> I own the world . . . I can ignite the space shuttle Challenger . . . I control food for the hungry all over the world.

With *delusions of reference* the patient interprets and assigns personal ownership to communications (written, verbal, or nonverbal) that have no relevance to him.

> A young man hospitalized for his first psychotic episode read an article in a newspaper about someone who had the same birthday as his and concluded that person was his twin brother. His mission in life became centered on finding him.

A patient with *paranoid delusion* feels that some force—person, family, group, or organization—has targeted him for destructive reasons. In reality, there is usually no basis for this belief; however, to the patient it is real and extremely frightening and anxiety provoking. It can also lead to violent behavior on the patient's part if he feels "attack" of some kind is imminent and he must protect himself.

> The electric camera in the church records my prayers and thoughts. . . . My wife put poison in my coffee.

Of course, the nurse must assess the apparent paranoid delusion for a "kernel of truth." For example, a woman in her initial interview complained that she was being watched by someone. The staff followed through with questions about this belief to the patient's family and learned that the family had hired a private detective to follow her and report back to them.

A patient with *nihilistic delusions* believes that a part of his body, family, group, or the world is destroyed or is about to be.

> My liver is being removed . . . I am turning purple . . . Tomorrow at 7 AM the world will go poof! The end.

PERCEPTUAL CHANGES. The most frequent type of perceptual disturbance is hallucinations. Hallucinations are of four types: auditory, visual, olfactory, and tactile. Auditory hallucinations are the most common type. A patient hears voices: the voices often have conversations with each other, give commands or directions, or are broadcast aloud. When the patient first experiences these voices, they are frightening and may seem unreal, but later the voices become a characteristic part of the patient's experience.

> A tape recorder is in my mind, and it beeps out my comments to every question you ask me.

Visual hallucinations, most commonly associated with organic psychosis, occasionally trouble the patient with a functional disorder. They are images that occur in the patient's mind or that derive from the outside. They require no external stimuli and can be fleeting experiences or mental pictures manifested continuously for weeks, even years.

> Look, my fingers are turning into knives!

Olfactory hallucinations are relatively rare but include those experiences in which the patient smells an odor that does not exist in the external environment.

> I smell smoke under your arm.

Tactile hallucinations include those experiences in which the patient feels something on his skin or body part (often bugs) not substantiated by reality. They are uncommon and usually associated with organic psychosis.

> Nurse, there are ants crawling all over me!

Another form of perceptual disturbance is the illusion. This type of disturbance involves a misinterpretation of a stimulus in the environment. For example, a patient with illusions might look at a curtain moving in the wind and decide that a spirit is entering his room through the window.

MOTIVATIONAL CHANGES. The schizophrenic manifests such a variety of symptoms that at times he may appear "worn out" from the illness. He can become afraid to take action for fear of fatal consequences. Since his reality-testing apparatus is faulty, the patient may seek refuge from interpersonal situations, delay making decisions, and even become disinterested in his external environment. Conversely, the patient, on other occasions, might express feelings of rage, murder, or suicide. These uncontrollable thoughts are easily converted to action because of the lack of internal boundaries and the ability to control impulses and drives. An awesome degree of ambivalence may be displayed during which the patient switches from love to hate, from gentleness to gauche expressions, from excitement and investment in a person or idea to complete disengagement.

PHYSICAL CHANGES. Physical changes also occur in schizophrenic patients. Autonomic nervous system symptoms include cold or slightly discolored hands and feet, and blotchy skin. During the acute phase of schizophrenia, the patient may present with dilated pupils, moist palms, and mild tachycardia (Kaplan & Sadock, 1985). The catatonic patient, of course, presents the most drastic physical involvement because of his long period of immobility. The patient's weight is likely to fluctuate. During the early phase of the disease, the patient will lose weight, but during the latter stages of the disease, he is likely to gain weight. The fluctuations are frequently related to antipsychotic drug therapy.

Other physical or psychomotor activity changes in the chronically mentally ill vary in duration and intensity and may include grimaces, shuffling gait, tic-like movements, or highly developed rituals.

Patients who are chronically mentally ill are candidates for malnutrition as well as tuberculosis and other communicable diseases. With improved living conditions in hospitals and in home- or community-based programs for the mentally ill, however, these conditions can be ameliorated and controlled.

With the exception of the subgroup of schizophrenic patients who manifest excitement, most schizophrenic patients experience little difficulty sleeping. In many instances, their retarded psychomotor activity, depressed mood, and isolation and alienation from social contacts tend to facilitate sleep.

The deinstitutionalization movement, which has involved an increasing number of patients being discharged to the home or community, has exposed many patients to harsh or unhealthy living conditions (Bassuk & Gerson, 1978). About 25 percent of the homeless in the United States have been found to be psychiatric patients (Lamb, 1984).

INTERPERSONAL DISTURBANCES. Many bizarre and inappropriate behaviors are observed in the schizophrenic patient. These include rude or inappropriate behavior, mutilation of body parts, disturbed motor behavior, social withdrawal, and suicide attempts. *Mutilation of body parts* may involve banging the head against the wall or floor or burning the tips of the fingers while smoking cigarettes. *Rude or socially inappropriate behavior* involves violation of social norms that commonly govern behavior in the presence of others. For example, the patient might pick his nose, cough over others, or pass gas and laugh.

> Bob would enter the family home, sit in the living room with other family members, pass gas, and say "Air pollution, air pollution."

The schizophrenic patient experiences many incongruous feelings, ideas, and thoughts which may result in suicide attempts resulting from his inability to negotiate the variety of conflicts he is experiencing. Ambivalent feelings will appear in dramatic shifts from love to hate and can lead to cryptic and labyrinthine suicidal behaviors (Kolb & Brodie, 1982; Pao, 1979).

> A 60-year-old man, admitted to a hospital with a diagnosis of schizophrenia, had cooperated with the staff in his treatment. Within two months, the patient showed marked improvement, and discharge plans were made for the patient's daughter to take him home. The morning of the planned discharge the patient went into the bathroom, removed the window screen, and jumped from the sixth-floor window to his death. The nurse found a note from the patient to his daughter which simply stated, "Love you!"

The schizophrenic patient is at risk for suicide during the acute phase of the illness. It should be remembered that this is in direct contrast to the depressed patient, who is more susceptible to suicide in the latter phases of the illness (See Chapter 9 on mood disorders). Also, schizophrenics are at risk for attempting suicide during periods of transition (that is, upon entering the hospital, upon entering or coming out of a psychosis, or upon discharge) (Rosenbaum & Beebe, 1975).

Social withdrawal is a common behavior in the schizophrenic. The patient will seek those environments where he can be alone and will remain disconnected from the emotion and concerns of others. Increased sleeping, autistic thought, the use of highly personal language, and the incongruity of feelings, thoughts, and impulses exacerbate this kind of withdrawal. Gradually, the patient ceases contact with friends and associates. Communication is strained and tinged with indifference or irritability. The patient will have a passive attitude, with little spontaneity or interest in events in the environment.

DISTURBANCES IN MOTOR FUNCTIONING. *Disturbed motor functioning* may consist of catatonic-type behaviors of rigid posture and no interaction with the environment. The patient may select a body posture and remain in that position for long periods of time (days, weeks, or months), resisting all attempts to reposition or move him. Catatonic behavior with excitability includes rigid and fixed posture with brief periods of excitement when the patient may become irritable and highly excitable.

NURSING DIAGNOSES RELATED TO SCHIZOPHRENIA

A history and assessment of the patient's mental status enables the nurse to establish nursing diagnoses that aid in planning, implementing, and evaluating care. The following nursing diagnoses are those that are most likely to be established by the nurse caring for a schizophrenic patient. Related interventions are discussed in a later section of this chapter.

Anxiety

Altered thought processes

Self-esteem disturbance

Personal identity disturbance

Body image disturbance

Sensory perceptual alterations: Visual, auditory, gustatory, tactile, olfactory

Impaired verbal communication

Ineffective individual coping

Family coping: potential for growth

Ineffective family coping: compromised, leading to disabling

Altered family processes

Potential for violence (self-directed or directed at others)

Social isolation

Impaired social interaction

Powerlessness

Self-care deficit (feeding, bathing/hygiene, dressing/grooming, or toileting)

Altered health maintenance

Sleep pattern disturbance

Activity intolerance

Noncompliance (difficulties with initiation and followthrough)

Spiritual distress

THEORIES OF SCHIZOPHRENIA
PSYCHOANALYTIC OR PSYCHODYNAMIC THEORY

The psychoanalytic model of human behavior focuses on intrapsychic conflict, interpersonal relationships, and environmental influences (Arieti, 1974; Wing, 1978). The psychodynamic model of schizophrenia is based on the concept of psychic determinism, which purports that human behavior at any point is related to events that have occurred in the past, during key developmental stages (which may now be out of conscious awareness). If developmental conflicts and traumatic events are not made conscious and mastered the individual will continue to repeat them in unhealthy or maladaptive behaviors without any awareness of their powerful connections to psychological pain and unhappiness (Karasu, 1977).

Arieti (1974) divides the developmental period into three major time frames: childhood (birth to six years), puberty (six to twelve years), and adolescence-to-adulthood (twelve to eighteen or twenty years). According to psychoanalytic theorists, the child who does not master the developmental tasks of these stages may be at risk for developing psychopathology including schizophrenia.

CHILDHOOD. Disturbances in the mother-child relationship during childhood are thought to provide the foundation for the development of schizophrenia. Fromm-Reichman (1950) used the term "schizophrenogenic mother" to indicate that some mothers, by failing to transmit adequate emotional warmth, trust, and support, could produce a disturbed child. A child needs to develop trust and a feeling of security (Erikson, 1968; Arieti, 1974); this development is hampered by a mother who is overly anxious, insecure, and inadequate in her role as mother (Sullivan, 1953; Reynolds, 1980). Spitz (1965) and Dunn (1977) have pointed out that prolonged separation of mother and child can also have a devastating effect upon the child and his development.

The father of the schizophrenic is discussed less often by clinicians and theoreticians. Lidz (1960; 1968), however, contends that fathers of schizophrenics are generally weak and ineffective in their parental roles. Schizophrenics tend to perceive their fathers as insecure, and this impression manifests itself in the patient's low self-esteem.

PUBERTY. During late childhood and puberty (six to twelve years of age), the child is increasingly engaged in school and other activities and is away from home for a good part of each day. Through outside activities, the child is exposed to numerous and diverse cultural, religious, and ethical standards, and behavior that is unfamiliar to him.

During this phase of development, the child must learn to tolerate ambiguity, obscure communications, diversity of opinions, different levels of significance in interpersonal relations, and so forth. It is, for example, important for the child to develop a working knowledge of intimate relationships, such as those with family members, versus acquaintance (less intimate) relationships with friends and other relatives. During this period, three emotions are thought by some to predominate in children who are later diagnosed as schizophrenic: 1) anxiety, 2) anger, and 3) withdrawal (Arieti, 1974).

ADOLESCENCE TO ADULTHOOD. The adolescent-to-adulthood phase of development (twelve to twenty years of age) is considered the most turbulent by many psychoanalytic theorists because of the demands placed on the individual to come to terms with so many issues in a brief time period. Cross-cultural studies have indicated that these demands are culturally determined, and that not all cultures approach development of their young in the same fashion (Mead, 1953).

The adolescent-to-adulthood phase tests the fitness of the individual that was developed during the two earlier phases. It is during this phase that demands are placed on the person for academic and job performance, for development and maintenance of relationships with the opposite sex, and for the refining and internalization of values and codes of moral and social conduct and religious beliefs. Many people in this age group are also pressured to make choices about a career.

If an individual has failed to develop adequately during the previous two stages, he may begin in this stage (if not before) to manifest negative or pathological behavior. A poor developmental history, for example, due to neglect-abuse, or trauma, may produce a person with a poor or ill-defined self-image or identity. In addition, the individual may be unclear and/or confused about his sexual identity, his sense of competence, and society's expectations of him. Instead of a confident attitude and mature behavior, extreme fluctuations of mood and attitude may be observed, along with a variety of behaviors that seem to have no consistent pattern (Erikson, 1963; Arieti, 1974; Spitz, 1965; Nicholi, 1988). Erik Erikson, in particular, saw the growth process as one involving biological, psychodynamic, sociocultural, cognitive and interpersonal growth and development on other levels. (See Chapter 5 on Assessment.)

All this confusion tends to contaminate other phases of the growth process that normally occur during this period, resulting in interpersonal deficits and poor conflict management (Sullivan, 1953; Fromm-Reichman, 1950; Fagan, 1974; Dunn, 1977). As crises occur and are inadequately resolved, the individual may again and again experience psychological defeats. This has the cumulative effect of damaging an already weak personality structure.

BEHAVIORAL THEORY

Although behaviorists have in the past proposed theories to explain the development of schizophrenia, few behavioral theorists currently view schizophrenia as a completely environmentally caused illness. Many, however, do see the benefits of behavioral therapy in helping the schizophrenic individual.

One of the few behavioral theories viewing schizophrenia as a learned maladaptive behavior was developed by Ullmann and Krasner (1975). They proposed that schizophrenia may be caused by the lack, over a period of time, of adequate positive and growth-producing environmental reinforcements. As a result of this the schizophrenic person learns not to attend to the same stimuli that others respond to and is left, then, with his own internal stimuli such as fantasies, daydreams, preoccupations, and other irrelevant stimuli that do not facilitate the development of healthy interpersonal relationships and adaptive behaviors (Mears & Gatchel, 1979).

The stigma associated with aberrant and maladaptive behaviors tends to provoke negative responses from others in the environment, causing the individual to withdraw, retreat, and seek refuge in the behaviors most familiar to him, which are by this time bizarre and pathological. When this occurs, a cyclical process is observed: 1) there is a lack of positive reinforcement in the environment; 2) the patient tends to respond to internally generated cues (bizarre and pathological); 3) behaviors manifested by the patient are observed by others as weird, crazy, and bizarre, which causes them to withdraw from the schizophrenic; 4) the schizophrenic patient escalates responses with heightened internal processes that are even more bizarre. The longer this process goes on, the more reversals the patient experiences. Eventually these symptoms can become an integral part of the patient's repertoire of behaviors, and may be extremely difficult to change (Mears & Gatchell, 1979; Ullman & Krasner, 1975; Bandura, 1969). Although this theory may no longer stand up to the results of studies demonstrating a biological basis for schizophrenia, it does provide some direction for behavioral treatment measures (Kaplan & Sadock, 1988).

BIOLOGICAL THEORIES

GENETIC THEORIES. Schizophrenia is a complex disorder and cannot be accounted for by just one theory. There is evidence, however, that a genetic component does exist in the transmission of schizophrenia. Family studies have shown that the frequency of occurrence of schizophrenia is about 46 percent among children with two schizophrenic parents, about 10 percent with a first degree relative (parent, sibling, or child) afflicted with the illness, and about 3 percent with an affected second degree relative (uncle, aunt, nephew, niece) (Gottesman & Shields, 1972). Family studies, while confirming the strong familial nature of the illness, do not provide conclusions about whether the illness is genetically or environmentally caused (see Table 10–2).

The most powerful studies in demonstrating the genetic predisposition to the development of schizophrenia have been twin and adoption studies. Identical (monozygotic) twins have the same genetic make-up, and the comparison of the development of schizophrenic twins raised together and apart provides a way of directly testing the genetic and environmental theories of the causes of schizophrenia. Twin studies have shown a significantly high concordance rate among identical twins of 45.6 percent, while the concordance rate among fraternal twins (twins who do not have the same genetic make-up) is 12.7 percent. In other words, in monozygotic twins where one twin suffers from schizophrenia, there is a 45.6 percent chance that the other twin will also be affected regardless of whether they are raised together or apart. This percentage goes down to 12.7 percent in fraternal twins, who do not have the same genetic make-up (Tsuang & Vandermey, 1980; Gottesman & Shields, 1972; Wing, 1978; Kety et al., 1978; Maxmen, 1986).

In a classic adoption study (Heston, 1966), grown children of schizophrenic mothers who had been raised by someone other than their natural mothers were compared to adopted children born to non-schizophrenic mothers. Heston found a 16.6 percent risk of the development of schizophrenia in the children of schizophrenic mothers, while none of the control adoptees had schizophrenia. These twin and adoption studies have demonstrated that genetic predisposition, and not environment, is powerfully associated with the development of schizophrenia, virtually putting an end to the concept of the "schizophrenic mother" (see Table 10–2).

BIOCHEMICAL THEORIES. Although the relationship between biochemical processes and schizophrenia is not fully understood, researchers continue to investigate the association.

TABLE 10–2 Risk for relatives of a schizophrenic

Schizophrenic Patient	Person at Risk	Percent of Risk
General population	Everybody	0.8–1.0
Father	Each child	1.8
Mother	Each child	10–16
Both parents	Each child	25–46
Child	Each parent	5
One sibling	Each sibling	8–10
Second-degree relative	Another second-degree relative	2–3
Monozygotic twin	Other monozygotic twin	40–50
Dizygotic twin	Other dizygotic twin	12–15
Adoptive parents (schizophrenic)	Adoptee with "normal" biological parents	4.8
Biological parents (schizophrenic)	Adoptee reared by "normal" adoptive parents	19.7

Source: Maxmen, J. (1986). *Essential psychopathology.* New York: W. W. Norton Co, p. 152.

There are two predominant hypotheses related to biochemical aspects of schizophrenia: 1) schizophrenia is the result of hyperactivity of dopaminergic pathways in the brain; and 2) the symptoms that accompany schizophrenia are indicative of some type of abnormal brain function in which catecholamines and/or indoleamines are not properly metabolized. This brain dysfunction is thought to play a role in producing an abundance of endogenous psychotogens. Schizophrenia is thought to develop when there is an imbalance between two or more neuroregulators, chemical compounds in the brain that act like chemical transmitters or modulators (Losonczy, Davidson, & Davis, 1987).

The predominant hypotheses have led to the investigation of several other possible etiologic pathways. These include the dopamine (DA) hypothesis, the monoamine oxidase (MAO) hypothesis, the transmethylation hypothesis, and the auto-immune hypothesis (Gregory & Smeltzer, 1983; DeLisi, 1987; Losonczy, Davidson, & Davis, 1987).

Dopamine Hypothesis. The dopamine hypothesis suggests that behaviors manifested in schizophrenics are specifically related to an excess of dopamine activity in the limbic system. This hypothesis was constructed after the introduction of phenothiazines, the first antipsychotic drugs. Researchers and clinicians observed that these drugs produced extrapyramidal side effects much like the symptoms observed in patients with Parkinson's disease (constant movement of the mouth, tremor of the hands and legs, and constant movement of the head and neck). They deduced that since Parkinson's disease is a result of a deficiency of dopamine in the substantia nigra (part of the midbrain that controls rigidity or involuntary movements in the body), schizophrenia may be the result of excess dopamine in the central nervous system. It follows, then, that the therapeutic effects of the phenothiazines in the treatment of schizophrenia may be due to their dopamine-receptor blocking activity.

In 1962, Carlsson proposed that schizophrenia may be linked to an excess of dopamine (DA) (Carlsson & Lindquist, 1963). It was further suggested that drugs such as the phenothiazines (Thorazine) and the butyrophenones (Haldol) that block postsynaptic DA activity should be classified as antipsychotic agents or neuroleptics (Tamminga & Gerlach, 1987). The phenothiazines are labeled antipsychotic rather than antischizophrenic. This is because these drugs ameliorate the blatant psychotic symptoms, characteristic of any functional psychosis, not just schizophre-

nia, and can be useful in the treatment of some organic psychoses as well. Since it has not been determined that schizophrenia is caused by an excess of dopamine, researchers continue to investigate the relationship between genetic make-up, stress, environment, and family dynamics in the development of schizophrenia. The dopamine hypothesis, however, remains the most important biochemical theory of schizophrenia today (Losonczy, Davidson, & Davis, 1987).

Transmethylation Hypothesis. Although seriously questioned in recent years, the transmethylation hypothesis suggests that there is an oversupply of methylated metabolites such as dimethoxyphenylethylamine (DMPEA). DMPEA has been isolated in the urine of schizophrenic patients (Gregory & Smeltzer, 1983). Since the methylated metabolites like DMPEA so closely resemble the molecular structure of hallucinogens such as mescaline or lysergic acid diethylamide (LSD), it has been hypothesized that the psychotic phenomena observed in schizophrenia could be explained by the presence of endogenous hallucinogens (Van Kammen & Gelernter, 1987). DMPEA is also clinically significant because of its association with catatonic-type behaviors produced in laboratory animals (Gregory & Smeltzer, 1983).

Monoamine Oxidase Hypothesis. The monoamine oxidase (MAO) enzyme is important because it oxidizes amines such as serotonin and the catecholamines. Thus, MAO inhibitors act as energizers for the psyche (Baldessarini & Cole, 1988). The MAO hypothesis regarding the etiology of schizophrenia suggests that the blood platelets of schizophrenic patients have a significant decrease in the level of MAO activity compared to the platelets of non-schizophrenics (Wyatt et al., 1980; Meltzer, 1987). At present, findings are inconclusive. MAO activity has a genetic base but is influenced by diet, hormonal activity, age, and ingestion of certain classes of drugs such as the MAO-inhibitors, a class of antidepressants.

Autoimmune Hypothesis. The autoimmune hypothesis is another speculative biochemical theory regarding the etiology of schizophrenia. It holds that there may be an abundance of antibodies that accumulate in the nucleus accumbena septi in the limbic system of the schizophrenic. Much work needs to be done to substantiate this hypothesis and provide relevant clinical application.

In summary, the biochemical theories, though not fully substantiated, offer another theoretical framework within which to explore the causes and treatment of schizophrenia.

NEUROANATOMY THEORIES. Biomedical technology, such as computed tomography (CT), and magnetic resonance imaging (MRI), has made it possible for researchers and clinicians to examine more carefully changes in the brain structure of schizophrenic patients. According to Weinberger, Wagner, and Wyatt (1983), clinicians and researchers have for quite some time suspected that the brains of schizophrenic patients might be structurally different from the brains of non-schizophrenics.

Four abnormalities of the brain structure have been identified: enlargement of the lateral cerebral ventricles; a markedly smaller frontal lobe; atrophy of portions of the cerebellum; and abnormal asymmetries in the cerebral hemisphere (Meltzer, 1987; Weinberger, Wagner, & Wyatt, 1983). The first three abnormalities indicate tissue degeneration in the brain (Meltzer, 1987). The enlarged ventricles that occur as a result of cerebral atrophy could be a consequence of two things: 1) the disease process itself; or 2) the result of the confinement, and medications that are associated with the treatment of the disease (Maxmen, 1986). The fourth abnormality is associated with cognitive disorders (autism and dyslexia) (Weinberger, Wagner, & Wyatt, 1983).

The results of brain studies of schizophrenics have potential for future understanding and suggest, by interpretation, that schizophrenia is not one consolidated disease but rather an assorted grouping of aberrations that influence pathological behavior (Weinberger, Wagner, & Wyatt, 1983).

It is clear that new biomedical technologies are enhancing the possibilities of studying anatomic structures of the brain, as well as brain biochemistry, and the biological bases of psychiatric disorders will be vigorously explored in future years (Garber et al., 1988).

INFORMATION PROCESSING THEORY. There are two basic methods associated with processing cognitive information: automatic and conscious. The automatic processes occur without intention; they may or may not lead to awareness, and may or may not interfere with other information processing activity.

Conscious (controlled) information processes are thought to be serial, slow, and less effectual than automatic information processing. The conscious and deliberate focus on task hinders the person's overall functioning. Schizophrenia is thought to be associ-

ated with difficulties in controlled, serial processing. Additional research is needed to further elucidate the differences between automatic and conscious information processing in schizophrenia (Liberman et al., 1984).

THERAPIES FOR TREATING SCHIZOPHRENIA
PSYCHODYNAMIC THERAPY

Psychoanalysts once believed that the schizophrenic patient could not benefit from psychoanalytic methods because of their difficulties with communication and the maintenance of satisfactory interpersonal relationships. Fromm-Reichman (1950), Sullivan (1953), Searles (1967), and others, however, have attempted to treat schizophrenic patients using the psychoanalytic method based on regression in the service of the ego, transference, countertransference, and changing intrapsychic structure (Greerson, 1967; Schultz, 1985).

The primary focus of the psychoanalytic method involves the patient's development of basic trust (Sullivan, 1953; Erikson, 1963; Fromm-Reichman, 1950). Only after the patient has developed trust in the therapist can he begin to reach out into the world and develop satisfying relationships with others. Psychoanalytic therapy with schizophrenic patients focuses on improving interpersonal relationships and socialization skills, and is action-oriented (Liberman, 1985; Schultz, 1985).

Most people agree, however, that psychotherapy is not constructive in the treatment of schizophrenia unless used in conjunction with other forms of therapy such as pharmacotherapy. Nonetheless, the nurse should recognize that a solid therapeutic alliance is essential for other types of treatment to be effective (Tsuang, Faraone, & Day, 1988). (See Chapter 7 on the Nurse as Therapist.)

There are five basic forms of psychoanalytic psychotherapy used with schizophrenia: individual, group, family, milieu, and therapeutic community.

INDIVIDUAL THERAPY. In individual therapy, the therapist is concerned with: 1) the development of trust; 2) identifying feelings and conflicts associated with dysfunction and helping the patient find words to talk about them; 3) recognizing and therapeutically managing regression, transference, countertransference, and feelings such as intense anger; 4) the exploration of significant past life-events, life

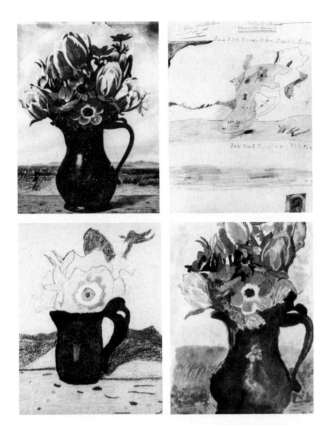

A patient diagnosed with paranoid schizophrenia was asked to copy the picture in the upper left-hand corner of these illustrations. At first, the patient was unable to comply but did finally complete the upper right-hand drawing. After a year of psychoanalytic therapy, the patient's altered perceptions appear to be much improved, and he was able to do the drawing at the bottom right.

stressors, failed expectations, and conflicts and resolutions; and 5) synthesizing data and determining patterns of behaviors, as well as antecedents to behaviors (Fromm-Reichman, 1950; Searles, 1967; Bellak et al., 1973).

GROUP THERAPY. With the therapist, patients explore problems in daily living in a group setting by utilizing each other's experiences, thoughts, and feelings. Group therapy can help schizophrenic patients develop socialization and interpersonal skills (Yalom, 1985).

FAMILY THERAPY. Family therapy within a psychoanalytic framework centers on intrapsychic forces and conflicts within the family of the schizophrenic patient which affect him by increasing or decreasing his psychotic symptomatology. A major theoretical component of this therapy is psychic determinism, which holds that all behavior is internally moti-

vated—one's emotional life is the result of specific causes, whether known or unknown, and is not just the result of chance (Jones, 1980). In family therapy, the schizophrenic patient is never seen by himself but rather with the spouse or parents and in many cases the siblings as well. Niell and Kniskern (1982) have described this family unit as a " 'people salad,' each member confined in a network of interlocking relationships." (p. 232). The goal of family psychotherapy is for the family group to begin to make an effort to break up interlocking defenses and patterns that prevent growth of the individual members (Niell & Kniskern, 1982).

MILIEU THERAPY. The goal of milieu therapy is the development of an environment that is structured, free of excessive stimuli, designed to allow the patient to assimilate stimuli at his own rate, and in an environment that the patient feels is physically and psychologically safe (McReynolds, 1960; Van Putten & May, 1976).

THERAPEUTIC COMMUNITY. In a therapeutic community, patients and staff collaborate in therapeutic activities. This approach clearly moves the patient from the status of a helpless, passive recipient, to an active participant in his own treatment process.

BEHAVIORAL THERAPY

In behavioral therapy, the schizophrenic patient is viewed as one who has responded to a combination of reinforcement, lack of reinforcement, and aversive experiences that have facilitated the development and maintenance of schizophrenic behaviors such as social withdrawal, poor interpersonal relations, regressive behavior, and hallucinations (Karasu, 1977; Nathan & Harris, 1987; Kazdin & Bootzin, 1972; Paul & Lentz, 1977).

The nurse who uses behavioral therapy shapes, extinguishes, and accelerates/decelerates behaviors through systematically applying reinforcers such as tokens which can be exchanged for privileges or mildly aversive consequences such as withdrawal of privileges like smoking (Karasu, 1977).

Behavioral therapy addresses four priority areas of treatment of the schizophrenic patient: resocialization (self-care and social skills); specific role performance, for example, in daily living; reduction of intensity and frequency of bizarre behaviors (hallucinations, delusions, inappropriate or flat affect; and the identification and mobilization of support services in the community (Paul, 1969; Flanagan, 1978).

Ayllon and Michaels (1959) published a landmark study of the psychiatric nurse's use of behavioral therapy with hospitalized psychiatric patients. In this study, nurses used positive reinforcement (systematic increase of attention) when the patient engaged in desirable behaviors, and delivery of negative or mildly aversive consequences (systematic withdrawal of attention) when the patient engaged in undesirable behaviors, such as psychotic conversations. Since this study, behavioral therapy has been used successfully in the treatment of schizophrenic and other psychotic patients in the hospital and community.

SOCIAL LEARNING PROGRAMS. Social learning programs provide another way of helping the patient take more responsibility for his own behavior. Using principles such as social skills training and token economies, these programs, like the study cited above, use the mental health staff as reinforcing agents to help patients develop more socially acceptable behavior.

SOCIAL SKILLS TRAINING. Social skills training emphasizes the acquisition and improvement of specific social skills, often focusing on conversational skills. In one social skills training program described by Curran, Faraone, and Dow (1985), small groups of stabilized patients were given lessons on each skill, homework, opportunities for practice and role playing, videotaping, and feedback from participants and therapists. Lessons stressed interpersonal skills such as starting a conversation, speaking, listening, receiving criticism, self-disclosure, and handling specific problems such as apologies and "saving face."

TOKEN ECONOMY METHOD. The token economy method is another type of positive reinforcement useful in treating schizophrenic patients. The patient is given the responsibility of earning tokens through acquired desirable behaviors (Ayllon & Haughton, 1962; Liberman, 1985). This system provides a systematic method of rewarding and accelerating the development of desirable and adaptive behaviors. For example, if the nurse has targeted the reduction of bizarre behaviors, the following treatment plan might be used.

Goal: The patient will engage in conversations with staff that are free of delusional content and bizarre behaviors, for three minutes; five minutes; seven minutes; and so forth.

Patient's behaviors: Talking about delusions; inappropriate or bizarre behavior.

Staff responses: Ignore delusional talk; engage in rational discussions with patient. Do not engage in conversation with patient when his discussion has delusional content.

Token Schedule: Reward (reinforce) patient with tokens when his conversation with staff is free of delusions for three minutes (10 tokens); five minutes (20 tokens); seven minutes (30 tokens); and so forth. The tokens will be exchanged for walks with staff (20 tokens); trips with other patients and staff to recreational sites outside the hospital (30 tokens); toilet articles, cigarettes, candy, and so forth.

The nurse must be aware of the fact that modifying a patient's behaviors by using a token economy system within an institutional setting is relatively easy; complexities arise, however, when the nurse seeks to generalize these changes to a home and/or community setting (Kazdin & Bootzin, 1972). She also needs to understand that the patient may still be engaging in delusional thinking or hearing "voices" but has learned not to talk about these things. This raises some ethical issues: Who is the treatment for? What will the patient experience during behavior modification? The patient may decrease social isolation by appearing more normal, but this may not be what the patient most needs or wants. In the process, he may be left alone to deal with frightening delusions and hallucinations.

Paul and Lentz (1977) undertook a six year study comparing social learning and milieu programs for inpatient schizophrenics. They reported a striking decrease in symptomatic behaviors as well as earlier releases from the hospital among those patients who were treated in a social learning program when compared to patients in milieu therapy and those who received traditional hospital treatments (control group). Figure 10–3 illustrates their findings. There were 28 chronic schizophrenic patients in each treatment group, matched for age, sex, socioeconomic level, symptomatology, and duration of hospitalization (Carson, Butcher, & Coleman, 1988). The results showed that patients receiving either milieu or social learning therapy had significant improvement in overall functioning compared to the hospitalized patients. The social learning program, however, clearly provided the most impressive results.

FAMILY THERAPY. Behavioral theory based family therapy can also be useful in the treatment of the schizophrenic patient and family. Unlike psychoanalytically based family therapy which sees the entire family unit as dysfunctional, behavioral family therapy sees the family only as an important source of

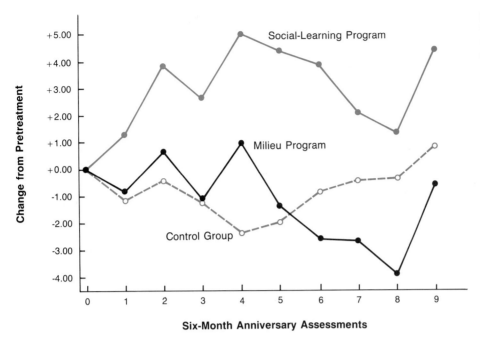

FIGURE 10–3 Social Learning Versus Milieu Programs for Inpatient Schizophrenics When inpatients in three types of behavioral treatment programs were compared at six month intervals, those in the social-learning program showed remarkable increases in overall functioning, while patients in the control and milieu groups showed slight changes in functioning.

Source: Paul, G. L., & Lentz, R. J. (1977). *Psychosocial treatment of chronic mental patients: Milieu versus social learning programs.* Cambridge: Harvard University Press, p. 374.

support for the patient. Curran, Faraone and Graves (1986) advise that family therapy for schizophrenics has three foci: education, communication, and problem solving. The educational component addresses methods by which the family's guilt, shame, and self blame about the patient's illness can be reduced. Content of family therapy sessions should include information on what is known about the biological bases of schizophrenia, and discussion of the fact that the patient's behaviors are outside his control as well as discussion of the effect of environmental stressors on the patient. Communication skills emphasized include active listening, giving and accepting feedback about one's behavior in a useful fashion, and discussing feelings.

It has been found that improving the family's problem-solving skills will help to reduce stress and anxiety within the family. Several basic steps are recommended to families: 1) define the problem; 2) generate as many solutions as possible; 3) thoroughly evaluate each potential solution; 4) seek the best alternative and evaluate it; 5) implement the selected alternative and 6) evaluate the outcome (Curran, Faraone, & Graves, 1986; Tsuang, Faraone, & Day, 1988).

BIOLOGICAL (SOMATIC) THERAPIES

Over the years, numerous somatic or biological therapies have been employed for the treatment of

schizophrenia. Among them are electroshock, insulin coma, psychosurgery, megavitamin therapy, and hydrotherapy. Most of these have been abandoned in favor of the use of antipsychotic medication, which, along with the interpersonal therapies, is the primary mode of treatment of schizophrenia today.

ELECTROSHOCK THERAPY. Little evidence currently exists to support the use of electroshock therapy in schizophrenic patients (Kalinowsky & Hoch, 1973). Electroshock therapy, also called electroconvulsive therapy or ECT, is used primarily to treat mood disorders. It may be used in the acute phase of schizophrenia or when the schizophrenic patient does not respond to pharmacotherapy. Electroconvulsive therapy can produce elevated intracranial pressure and should not be used with patients with any intracranial lesion.

Complications of electroshock therapy include: 1) memory impairment that can last from a few days to several months; 2) fractures and dislocations, (now quite rare, since a muscle relaxant is used during the therapy); and 3) bradycardia that can be prolonged (Kolb & Brodie, 1982). (See Chapter 9 on Mood Disorders for more on ECT.)

INSULIN COMA THERAPY. Similarly, there is little evidence to support the use of insulin coma therapy in the treatment of schizophrenia (Kalinowsky &

Hoch, 1973). Previous justifications included the belief that nerve cells became overactive and oversensitive to normal stimuli in the schizophrenic patient's environment. Treatment, it was theorized, would decrease the level of activity in nerve cells by neutralizing the neurological excitant, a type of hormone. The schizophrenic was thought to have injured young intracellular pathways, e.g., at birth or due to head injury, after which older nerve pathways were reactivated. Insulin therapy supposedly reversed this process (Kalinowsky & Hoch, 1973). Clinical observations indicated that sleep tended to improve the overall mental state of patients. Introduced by Sakal in 1933, insulin coma therapy was a fairly widespread practice until the 1970s. Currently, however, insulin coma therapy is not used, primarily because of the treatment's associated risks.

PSYCHOSURGERY. Prefrontal lobotomy, a surgical procedure in which part of the frontal lobe of the brain is surgically "disconnected" from the remainder of the brain, produces an emotionless, "bland" affect (and a decrease in drive). This treatment is based on the assumption that the prefrontal area is the location of emotions. Again, efficacy has not been adequately demonstrated, and numerous associated ethical and legal issues have been debated. The rationale for employing psychosurgery in the treatment of functional psychosis was to reduce the amount of the schizophrenic's "self-involvement" (Millon, 1973; Gregory & Smeltzer, 1983). The Nobel Prize in medicine was awarded to Moniz for his work in psychosurgery (Kolb & Brodie, 1982). More recently, however, safer and more effective psychosurgical procedures have been developed, though their use remains experimental.

MEGAVITAMIN THERAPY. This type of therapy utilizes large amounts of vitamins; it is thought that vitamins, especially niacin, will control schizophrenic-type symptoms. There is no empirical evidence whatsoever to support this assumption, and this treatment modality is seldom employed.

HYDROTHERAPY. Hydrotherapy includes whirlpool baths, showers, and alternating chilling and warming techniques to calm aggressive and disturbed patients. These means were widely used until fairly recently. Today, many people use variations of these methods, such as sauna and Jacuzzi, for simple relaxation.

PSYCHOPHARMACOLOGIC THERAPIES

The successful introduction of psychopharmacologic agents for the treatment of schizophrenia has made many of the biological therapies obsolete. The antipsychotics, or neuroleptics, have been used in the treatment of schizophrenia for over 30 years. While there are many types of neuroleptic drugs, all are pharmacologically equivalent in their primary therapeutic action and have demonstrated superiority to placebo in drug trials (Black, Yates, & Andreason, 1988). Antipsychotic medications can control symptoms that would otherwise be present (maintenance), and can prevent the unpredictable exacerbation of psychotic symptoms (prophylaxis). The regular use of low dose medication modifies psychotic symptoms and facilitates the therapeutic effects of higher doses in the presence of florid psychotic symptoms.

Neuroleptic drugs are classified as either low-potency or high-potency. The lower potency neuroleptics are associated with autonomic side effects such as dry mouth, constipation, urinary retention, and postural hypotension as well as sedation. The extrapyramidal side effects of these agents are less severe than those of the high-potency drugs. The high-potency drugs produce fewer autonomic side effects, but more significant extrapyramidal effects such as tremors, shuffling gait, motor retardation, and drooling. The main classes of neuroleptics are the phenothiazines, the butyrophenones, the thioxanthenes, the dibenzoxazepines, and the dihydroindolones.

METHODS OF ACTION. Antipsychotic drugs are believed to work through a series of blocking type actions that occur in various sections of the brain, causing the blocking of dopamine and neurotransmitter receptors (Gelenberg, 1984; 1987). This view corresponds with the theory that schizophrenic psychosis results from an excess of dopamine or abnormal activity of certain dopamine receptors (Black, Yates, & Andreason, 1988, p. 773). Several dopamine pathways affected by the neuroleptics have been identified in the brain. It is hypothesized that the mesolimbic dopamine pathway is involved in the antipsychotic efficacy of neuroleptics; the nigrostriatal dopamine pathway is thought to be involved with extrapyramidal (central nervous system) side effects. The mesocortical pathway is implicated in the sedative action of these drugs; and the hypothalmic-hypophyseal and incertohypothalmic pathways are responsible for the neuroendocrine side effects (Swonger & Matejski, 1988, p. 257).

SELECTION OF SPECIFIC DRUG. The neuroleptics as a group are very similar in therapeutic benefit and vary most according to side effects (see Table 10–3). While the range of possible side effects is similar from drug to drug, the frequency and severity with which the various side effects occur differ significantly, making this one important criterion for drug selection for the individual client. Side effects may be complicated by interactions with a symptom of the psychosis itself or by interaction with other medical problems or drugs sensitivities of the patient. Drug choice, therefore, is made with goals of maximizing desired therapeutic effects while minimizing the potential unwanted side effects of the drug (Swonger & Matejski, 1988). Some specific guidelines for antipsychotic drug selection are summarized below:

TABLE 10–3 Side effects of various neuroleptics

Drug	Early Side Effects				Continuing		
	Anticholinergic	Sedation	Orthostatic hypotension	Blood cell disorders	Lowered seizure threshold	Hypothalamic	Extrapyramidal
Phenothiazines, aliphatic							
Chlorpromazine (Thorazine)	+ +	+ + +	+ + +	+ +	+ + +	+ +	+ +
Promazine (Sparine)	+ + +	+ +	+ +	+ +	+ + +	+ +	+ +
Triflupromazine (Vesprin)	+ + +	+ + +	+ +	+ +	+ + +	+ +	+ +
Phenothiazines, piperidine							
Thioridazine (Mellaril)	+ + +	+ + +	+ + +	+	+	+ +	+
Mesoridazine (Serentil)	+ +	+ + +	+ +	+	+	+ +	+
Piperacetazine (Quide)	+ +	+ +	+ +	+	+	+ +	+ +
Phenothiazines, piperazine							
Prochlorperazine (Compazine)	+	+ +	+	+ +	+	+ +	+ + +
Perphenazine (Trilafon)	+ +	+	+	+ +	+	+ +	+ + +
Fluphenazine (Permitil, Prolixin)	+	+	+	+ +	+	+ +	+ + +
Trifluoperazine (Stelazine)	+	+	+	+ +	+	+ +	+ + +
Acetophenazine (Tindal)	+ +	+ +	+	+ +	+	+ +	+ + +
Carphenazine (Proketazine)	+	+ +	+	+ +	+	+ +	+ + +
Butyrophenone							
Haloperidol (Haldol)	0	+	+	+	+ +	+ + +	+ + +
Thioxanthenes							
Chlorprothixene (Taractan)	+ +	+ + +	+ + +	+ +	+ + +	+ +	+ +
Thiothixene (Navane)	+	+	+	+ +	+ +	+ +	+ + +
Dihydroindolone							
Molindone (Lidone, Moban)	+ +	+ +	+	+	0/ +	+	+ +
Dibenzoxazepine							
Loxapine (Daxolin, Loxitane)	+	+ +	+	+ +	+ +	+	+ + +
Dibenzodiazepines							
Clozapine (experimental)	+ + +	+ +	+ + +	+ +	+	0/ +	0
Benzamides							
Sulpiride	+	0/ +	+	0/ +		+ +	+

Source: Adapted from Swonger, A., & Matejski, M. (1988). *Nursing pharmacology.* Glenview, IL: Scott, Foresman and Company, p. 266.

1. It is important to review the patient's medical history and, if an effective drug has been used previously, to continue using that agent.

2. If florid psychotic symptoms occur while the patient is on a particular low-dosage maintenance drug, the dosage of that particular medication should be increased and the patient observed closely to see if the symptoms subside.

3. If the patient exhibits adverse side effects such as acute dystonia or oculogyric crisis, the drug should be discontinued.

4. If the patient has not taken a particular drug and the clinician wishes to prescribe it, family members' previous experiences and perceptions about the drug should be elicited and used as a factor in determining whether to prescribe the antipsychotic drug.

5. When all else fails, the clinician should use her clinical experiences and knowledge about drugs and their therapeutic and adverse side effects in selecting a drug for her patient.

Other factors that are considered in drug selection are dosage requirements (see Table 10–4), price, mode of administration, and planned duration of therapy (long- or short-term).

TABLE 10–4 Equivalent dose and daily oral adult dosage range for commonly used neuroleptics

Generic Name Drug	Trade Name	Equivalent Dose[a]	Adult Daily Oral Dosage Range (mg)
Phenothiazines, aliphatic			
Chlorpromazine	(Thorazine)	100	30–1,000
Promazine	(Sparine)	200	40–1,000
Trifluoromazine	(Vesprin)	25	60–150
Phenothiazines, piperidine			
Thioridazine	(Mellaril)	100	150–800
Mesoridazine	(Serentil)	50	30–400
Piperacetazine	(Quide)	10	20–160
Phenothiazines, piperazine			
Prochlorperazine	(Compazine)	15	15–150
Perphenazine	(Trilafon)	10	12–64
Fluphenazine	(Permitil, Prolixin)	2	0.5–20
Trifluoperazine	(Stelazine)	5	2–40
Acetophenazine	(Tindal)	20	60–120
Carphenazine	(Proketazine)	25	25–400
Butyrophenone			
Haloperidol	(Haldol)	2	1–15
Thioxanthenes			
Chlorprothixene	(Taractan)	100	75–600
Thiothixene	(Navane)	5	6–60
Dihydroindolone			
Molindone	(Lidone, Moban)	10	15–225
Dibenzoxazepine			
Loxapine	(Daxolin, Loxitane)	10	20–250

*Dose equivalent to 100 mg of chlorpromazine.
Source: Adapted from Swonger, A., & Matejski, M. (1988). *Nursing pharmacology*. Glenview, IL: Scott, Foresman and Co., p. 265.

ADVERSE EFFECTS OF ANTIPSYCHOTIC DRUGS. As stated earlier, the adverse effects of antipsychotic drugs are severe enough to require extreme caution when prescribing and evaluating the efficacy of any one particular drug. Most adverse effects, with the possible exception of tardive dyskinesia, can be reversed by lowering the dosage or switching to a new drug. Generally, low and high potency medications have different adverse side effects (see Table 10–5). Psychotropic drugs are generally not prescribed for the pregnant or lactating woman owing to possible toxic effects on the fetus or infant.

Extrapyramidal Effects. Considered the most serious side effects of neuroleptic therapy, and thought to be caused by the blocking of post-synaptic dopamine receptors, extrapyramidal side effects include acute dystonia, akathesia, Parkinson's syndrome, and tardive dyskinesia. A discussion of each syndrome is presented below.

Acute Dystonia. Acute dystonic reactions, more likely to occur if the patient is on high-potency neuroleptics, include facial grimacing or muscle spasms involving the tongue, face, neck, and back. They are most likely to develop within the first five days of treatment (Swonger & Matejski, 1988). These reactions, though uncomfortable and anxiety provoking for the patient and family, are seldom dangerous or life threatening. Initial treatment for dystonia usually consists of intravenous parenteral drugs, such as benzodiazepine, (diazepam/Valium), diphenhydramine (Benadryl), and caffeine (injectable type). Once acute symptoms subside, the patient is placed on oral preparation of one of these drugs.

Parkinson's Syndrome. The greatest risk for the development of Parkinson's syndrome, often called pseudoparkinsonism, is between 5 and 30 days after initiating treatment (Swonger & Matejski, 1988). This syndrome is characterized by muscle tremor, rigidity, shuffling gait, drooling, and looseness of arm movements. The examiner should look for muscle tremor in the hands ("pill-rolling" appearance), wrists, elbows, head, palate, and all other body parts. Rigidity is demonstrated by resistance to passive motion and a slowness of an extremity to return to position after it has been raised. The patient may turn his body as if it were one solid structure. An examiner would also notice that the patient takes small, rapid steps with a stooped posture.

The nurse should be especially aware of Parkinson's syndrome at the beginning of drug therapy if the patient is receiving high-potency drugs. (The Rabbit syndrome—rapid tremor of the mouth and jaw—can occur later in drug treatment.) A decrease in the antipsychotic dosage or the administration of a less potent antipsychotic medication is the usual approach to the management of this syndrome. Debate continues as to whether drugs such as Cogentin and Benadryl should be prescribed prophylactically, to prevent the development of extrapyramidal side effects, or whether the extrapyramidal symptoms should be treated as they develop.

TABLE 10–5 Spectrum of adverse effects caused by antipsychotic drugs

Low-potency	High-potency
Fewer extrapyramidal reactions (especially Thorazine)	More frequent extrapyramidal reactions
More sedation, postural hypotension	Less sedation, postural hypotension
Decreases seizure threshold, alters electrocardiogram (especially Thorazine)	Less effect on the seizure threshold, cardiovascular toxicity
Skin pigmentation and photosensitivity	Fewer anticholinergic effects
Occasional cases of cholestatic jaundice	Occasional cases of neuroleptic malignant syndrome (irreversible tardive dyskinesia including diminished cognitive capacity)
Rare cases of agranulocytosis	

Source: Adapted from Gelenberg, A. (1984). Psychosis. In E. Bassuk, S. Schoonover, & A. Gelenberg (Eds.). *The practitioner's guide to psychoactive drugs,* 2nd ed. New York: Plenum, p. 125.

Tardive Dyskinesia. Tardive dyskinesia is usually a late-occurring and persistent side effect of neuroleptic therapy. It first appears as gnarling, curling, or twisting movements of the tongue (Swonger & Matejski, 1988). Tardive dyskinesia can also involve abnormal movements of the head, neck, and extremities. Affecting from 15 percent to 45 percent of the patients on neuroleptics, tardive dyskinesia is particularly troublesome because there are so few treatment options and because they may persist and even become irreversible (Swonger & Matejski, 1988). Little is known about why some patients develop tardive dyskinesia and others do not.

Treatment of tardive dyskinesia begins with prevention. Antipsychotic medication should be prescribed only when absolutely necessary and in the lowest possible dosage for the shortest period of time. The patient should be thoroughly evaluated for abnormal movements before beginning any antipsychotic medication and evaluated every six months after (Silver & Yudofsky, 1988). An examination procedure is summarized in Table 10–6. In addition, the nurse should continuously observe the patient for any early signs of tardive dyskinesia. She must be familiar with the abnormal movements that are likely to develop and report these findings immediately to the physician. Acute facial and/or tongue dystonia is an indication for stat IM Benadryl, 25–50 mg, to prevent compromise of the airway. A standing medical order should be written to cover this emergency nursing intervention so time isn't wasted obtaining an order during the emergency when the patient's anxiety is likely to increase rapidly and worsen the situation.

When antipsychotic medication is indicated, the patient and his family (or advocate) should be presented with all pertinent information about its side effects. The physician, nurse, patient, family, and appropriate others should weigh the benefits and risks associated with the patient's antipsychotic drug therapy. If observed movements become problematic, the clinician might consider giving the patient benzodiazepine (Valium), clonazepam (Clonopin), baclofen (Lioreasal), or propranalol (Inderal).

Recently, more attention has been given by mental health care providers, attorneys, and patient advocates to the risks of tardive dyskinesia. The lip-smacking, chewing, puckering of lips, tongue protrusion, and wormlike movement of the tongue during the early stages of the symptoms can range from minimal to severe and can interfere with the patient's activities of daily living (eating, dressing, communicating). In the most severe forms, these symptoms can (though rarely) affect swallowing and breathing. Because of the severity of these problems, the clinician will always try to inform the patient and family about

---

TABLE 10–6 Examination procedure for tardive dyskinesia

Either before or after completing the examination procedure, unobstrusively observe the patient at rest (e.g., in waiting room). The chair to be used in this examination should be a hard, firm one without arms.

Examination procedure

1. Ask patient whether there is anything in his or her mouth (gum, candy, etc.) and if there is, to remove it.

2. Ask patient about the *current* condition of his or her teeth. Ask patient if he or she wears dentures. Do teeth or dentures bother patient *now*?

3. Ask patient whether he or she notices any movements in mouth, face, hands, or feet. If yes, ask to describe and to what extent they *currently* bother patient or interfere with his or her activities.

4. Have patient sit in chair with hands on knees, legs slightly apart, and feet flat on floor. (Look at entire body for movements while patient is in this position.)

5. Ask patient to sit with hands hanging unsupported. If male, between legs, if female and wearing a dress, hanging over knees. (Observe hands and other body areas.)

6. Ask patient to open mouth. (Observe tongue at rest within mouth.) Do this twice.

7. Ask patient to protrude tongue. (Observe abnormalities of tongue movement.) Do this twice.

8. Ask patient to tap thumb, with each finger, as rapidly as possible for 10 to 15 seconds; separately with right hand, then with left hand. (Observe facial and leg movements.)

9. Flex and extend patient's left and right arms (one at a time). (Note any rigidity.)

10. Ask patient to stand up. (Observe in profile. Observe all body areas again, hips included.)

11. Ask patient to extend both arms outstretched in front with palms down. (Observe trunk, legs, and mouth.)

12. Have patient walk a few paces, turn, and walk back to chair. (Observe hands and gait.) Do this twice.

From the Abnormal Involuntary Movement Scales (AIMS) from Department of Health, Education, and Welfare, Public Health Service, Alcohol, Drug Abuse, and Mental Health Administration, National Institute of Mental Health. Also from Silver & Yudofsky (1988).

the risks of antipsychotic medications, though informed consent may be difficult to obtain from the acutely psychotic patient. It is recommended that the family be educated about antipsychotic drug therapy and their consent obtained. The patient is then gradually educated about psychosis and its treatment, and informed consent obtained from him to continue drug treatment as soon as the most florid psychotic symptoms subside (Silver & Yudofsky, 1988).

Anticholinergic Side Effects. Anticholinergic side effects may be caused either by the antipsychotic medication itself or by an anticholinergic drug used to treat extrapyramidal side effects (Rifkin & Siris, 1987). Generally, antipsychotic drugs with the most extreme anticholinergic properties produce fewer extrapyramidal side effects; there is also evidence, however, that the most potent anticholinergic drugs may have a negative effect on antipsychotic potency (Swonger & Matejski, 1988). Anticholinergic side effects usually occur within the first few weeks of treatment.

Anticholinergic side effects fall into two major categories, peripheral (or autonomic) nervous system and central nervous system. Common peripheral side effects include dry mouth, blurred vision, decreased gastric motility, urinary retention, and drying of bronchial secretions. Central side effects include memory problems, confusion, and loss of concentration.

Treatment of anticholinergic side effects consists of using the least amount of drug necessary to control psychiatric symptomatology and treating the side effects. Table 10–7 summarizes peripheral side effects with associated nursing diagnoses and suggested nursing interventions for prevention and management. If side effects become more acute, the prescribing clinician should consider another antipsychotic drug with less anticholinergic activity.

The use of an anticholinergic antiparkinson agent along with an anticholinergic antipsychotic drug (such as thioridazine [Mellaril]) can cause drug toxicity. The nurse should be alert to signs of confusion, disorientation, and possible agitation; enlarged pupils; dry mucous membranes; flushed skin; tachycardia and diminished bowel sounds.

Physostigmine, given intravenously (1–2 mg) can provide therapeutic and diagnostic assistance in toxicity. First, it will reverse the untoward symptoms,

TABLE 10–7 Nursing diagnoses and interventions for anticholinergic side effects

Side Effect	Nursing Diagnosis	Nursing Intervention
Decreased salivation	Alteration in comfort	Offer gum and lozenges for dry mouth.
	Potential for infection (dental caries)	Encourage good oral hygiene.
Decreased bronchial secretions	Ineffective airway clearance	Educate about coughing to clear bronchial passages. Encourage high fluid intake.
Decreased sweating	Hyperthermia	Educate about importance of maintaining normal body temperature through proper dress for the environment.
Difficulty urinating	Altered pattern of urinary elimination	Offer water frequently and educate about importance of maintaining high fluid intake.
Decreased gastric motility	Constipation	Offer patient a stool softener or natural laxative. Educate about importance of fiber and fluid intake.
Increased pupil size	Sensory perceptual alteration: visual	Advise patient to protect eyes from exposure to sunlight with sunglasses; schedule periodic visual exams.
Confusion, loss of memory	Altered thought processes	Warn patient not to drive alone, in unfamiliar places, or at night, or operate dangerous equipment.

and second, it will reverse the peripheral and central nervous system symptoms that accompany toxicity related to anticholinergic drugs.

When physostigmine is administered, it should be given slowly; cardiac monitoring is essential, as is the nurse's readiness for cardio-respiratory resuscitation. The benefits versus complications of administering the drug should be carefully considered. Extreme caution should be taken when the patient has cardiovascular involvement.

Effects on the Cardiovascular System. Antipsychotic drugs can cause orthostatic hypotension. Hypotension occurs most frequently among patients who are receiving low potency drugs, such as chlorpromazine (Thorazine), and has a greater chance of occurring when administered parenterally. Because of this possible side effect, special caution should be taken when administering neuroleptics to elderly people. Elastic stockings may help to reduce hypotension by preventing blood from pooling in the extremities. The nurse should monitor blood pressure and instruct the patient to rise slowly from a sitting or lying position. If symptoms do not subside, the clinician may administer intravenous fluids to increase the blood volume. Other agents used to bring about the desired clinical effect are metaraminol (Aramine) and norepinephrine (Levophed). These drugs should be used with extreme caution.

Neuroleptics have been found to produce cardiac effects that show up on the electrocardiogram (Kaplan & Sadock, 1988). Lesions in the heart tissues of patients who received antipsychotic drugs have also been attributed to antipsychotic medications. Low-potency drugs, such as thioridazine (Mellaril), appear to be cardiotoxic.

It is important for the nurse to be aware that antipsychotic drugs can cause cardiac arrhythmias when used in overdoses and can be treated with antiarrhythmic agents such as lidocaine (Xylocaine). Sudden deaths reported to occur among patients who receive antipsychotic drugs (see page 343) might be attributed to ventricular arrhythmias.

Effects on Vision. Mydriasis (dilation of pupils) makes the patient sensitive to light. The patient might complain of blurred vision. Antipsychotic drug usage may cause pigment deposition in lens, cornea, conjunctiva, and retina. The nurse should advise the patient who is on long term antipsychotic therapy about this possibility and schedule annual ophthalmologic examinations.

Effects on Skin. Allergic reactions to the antipsychotic drugs can vary from mild to severe. The nurse should observe the patient for erythematous, itchy sensations likely to appear around the neck, face, and trunk. Though this condition is rarely considered life threatening, the nurse should report any suspicious signs and symptoms. Frequently this condition is treated with steroids (topical). In cases where the patient has cutaneous reactions, the clinician should consider using another family of antipsychotic medication.

Hormonal, Sexual, and Hypothalmic Reactions. Antipsychotic drugs can cause galactorrhea (excessive or spontaneous flow of milk), decreased frequency and/or flow of menstruation, decreased libido, and pituitary enlargement. It is recommended that women who receive long-term antipsychotic drugs have regular breast examinations (owing to the possibility of prolactin-sensitive tumors).

Testosterone levels tend to be lower in males who receive antipsychotic medications and may have a negative effect on libido. The neuroleptics may interfere with sexual functioning in that they frequently cause delayed or retrograde ejaculation. Patients who experience retrograde ejaculation report orgasm with no accompanying emission but do have a foamy-appearing urination. The clinician in these situations should consider changing the patient to high-potency antipsychotic drugs.

Chlorpromazine, in particular, interferes with glucose tolerance and insulin release when used with the pre-diabetic patient.

The patient might also experience an increase in appetite with an accompanying increase in weight. If this occurs, the clinician should consider changing medication to high potency agents. The nurse should also assist the patient with diet and exercises. These side effects, while not life-threatening, are extremely troubling to the patient, and the nurse should pay special attention to the diagnosis and management of hormonal and sexual side effects, working closely with the patient.

Hepatic Effects. Low-potency drugs can rarely produce cholestatic jaundice that is accompanied by fevers, chills, nausea, malaise, and pruritus. If this occurs, the medication should be discontinued, and the physician should consider a high-potency drug.

Hematalogic Effects. Low-potency antipsychotic drugs can cause some toxicity to bone marrow. Leukopenia (a drop in the number of white blood cells, especially granulocytes) can occur suddenly, but rarely does a patient develop agranulocytosis (Swonger & Matejski, 1988). The nurse must watch for signs of possible infection, immediately reporting information about a patient's sore throat, fevers, malaise, or other signs of respiratory infection. If infection is suspected, a complete blood count should be ordered and appropriate action taken.

Effects on Pregnancy and Lactation. The antipsychotic drugs are not teratogenic; however, they can cross the placenta and come in contact with the fetus. Newborns have been observed to show neuroleptic withdrawal symptoms. Extreme caution should be used in treating a pregnant or lactating woman with antipsychotic medications as these drugs can be found in the milk of lactating mothers.

Sedative Effects. The nurse needs to know that low-potency drugs (that is, chlorpromazine, thioridazine, and chlorprothixene) are sedatives. This information is useful when determining the most desired time for sedation (that is, if night sedation is desired, give drug at bedtime).

Withdrawal Reactions. Antipsychotic drugs are seldom used for recreational purposes. They are not addictive and are non-habit forming. When these drugs are stopped suddenly, however, rebound reactions, such as nausea and vomiting and sleep disturbances occur; cholinergic reactions to the drugs include increased salivation and diarrhea.

Overdose. The ingestion of antipsychotic drugs seldom causes death. In the case of overdose, gastric lavage should be done. These drugs have an antiemetic effect; therefore, inducing vomiting is difficult.

Effects on Seizure Threshold. The low-potency drugs lower the patient's seizure threshold. The nurse should assess for a history of seizures; alcohol or drug withdrawal also tends to lower the patient's seizure threshold. The phenothiazines in particular are contraindicated for patients undergoing alcohol withdrawal because of the increased likelihood of seizures.

Sudden Death. Approximately 30 years ago, numerous reports appeared in the literature that suggested a relationship between antipsychotic drugs and incidences of sudden death. No definitive relationship has ever been established, however. Suspicion has led the American Psychiatric Association Task Force on Sudden Death (1988) to establish four criteria for the diagnosis of sudden death: death occurs within 24 hours after the onset of untoward reactions; the patient is healthy with no preexisting illness and is receiving the standard recommended dosage of antipsychotic drug; the autopsy shows no obvious cause of death; and all medical data will be available for analysis.

Kelly, Fay, and Laverty (1963) suggest that some individuals are more highly susceptible to the effects of antipsychotic medications than others. Although there is insufficient data to support the hypothesis that neuroleptics cause sudden death, it does seem appropriate that periodic EKGs be performed on those patients receiving antipsychotic drugs who have prior histories of repolarization problems or other cardiac dysfunctions. The use of lower doses of a drug is considered to be the best prophylactic treatment against sudden death among schizophrenic patients.

LONG-TERM ANTIPSYCHOTIC THERAPY. The objective of long-term therapy with schizophrenic patients is to minimize the possibility that deterioration and the more severe symptoms associated with the disorder will reoccur. Schizophrenic patients who stop taking their medications, or are placed on a placebo, will have a 60–80 percent chance of experiencing florid psychotic symptoms again within the period of one year. Over the course of a year or two, a very small percentage of these patients will not have relapsed because they do not need long-term drug therapy. It is extremely difficult, however, for the nurse and physician to detect which patients will and will not need long-term drug therapy (Gelenberg, 1984; 1987).

Instead of *drug holidays* (when a patient's medications are withheld for a certain period of time; also known as *drug vacation*), Gelenberg (1984) and others recommend that the drug be tapered to the lowest most effective maintenance dosage for the patient. Since schizophrenic patients are vulnerable to various types of stress (familial, interpersonal upheavals), their needs for antipsychotic medications varies and they should be periodically assessed for a need for more or less medication. The assessment should include general health status, neurological, psychological, and psychosocial functioning.

Depot Medications. Depot medications, such as fluphenazine enanthate (Prolixin enanthate) and fluphenazine decanoate (Prolixin decanoatel), are long acting. These drugs help control florid symptoms and are especially useful when maintenance therapy, over a long period of time, is indicated. This group of drugs also assists in increasing compliance among patients who have a history of being unreliable about taking their medications.

These medications are given to the patient by injection; the first several days following the injection, it is likely that the patient will have some side effects from the drug. The goal, however, is to stabilize the patient and keep him as symptom-free as possible with a minimum dose of the drug. Usually, injections are given to the patient every one to six weeks (Munkvad, Fog, & Kristjansen, 1976; Gregory & Smeltzer, 1983).

Tardive dyskinesia remains a problem with this type of therapy; this condition is one of the major complex side effects that might occur in long-term drug therapy for the schizophrenic patient. Because it has a late onset, is serious, and can be irreversible, the clinician, patient, and family members should always discuss the benefits, complications, and risks of neuroleptic therapy before any drugs are prescribed (Crane, 1972; Kety, 1978a).

SCHIZOPHRENICS AND THEIR FAMILIES

IMPACT OF THE FAMILY ON THE PATIENT

Research has shown that family interactions play a significant role in determining the outcome of a patient's schizophrenia. Brown, Carstairs, and Topping (1958) pioneered the theory of expressed emotions (EE) among relatives of the mentally ill. They developed the categories of emotions listed below (Hooley, 1986; Vaughn, 1986; Brown, Carstairs, & Topping, 1958):

Criticism: Remarks made by relatives about the ill member, with content and voice tones that are negative

Hostility: Pervasive negative feelings, and critical remarks about the patient, such as "He is strange," or "She is crazy and stupid," rather than comments on the patient's behavior

Emotional Overinvolvement: Inflated and overstated emotional response to the patient's illness, and overprotectiveness of the patient

Warmth: Relatives' tonal changes that indicate positive thoughts and feelings about the patient

Positive Regard: Relatives express praise or appreciation of the patient

The latter two categories (warmth and positive remarks) have not received much attention in the literature. More in-depth investigation of these two components will assist professionals in better understanding why some patients have longer successful tenure in the community (Hooley, 1986) (see Table 10–8).

According to this construct, the patient's relatives, and not the patient, determine the degree of expressed emotions (EE) that occur in a family. As

TABLE 10–8 Characteristics of relatives of schizophrenics with high EE and low EE

High Expressed Emotions	Low Expressed Emotions
Little effort to understand patient.	Attend to ill family member.
Little empathy.	Sensitive to ill member and his requests for privacy and autonomy.
Critical of bizarre behaviors.	View patient's illness as genuine, and have lower expectations of the patient.
Patient's behaviors are perceived as a personal affront to relatives.	Manifest empathy and strive to understand the patient's suffering.
Strong disapproval of patient and use of emotionally charged words such as revolting, crazy, and so forth.	Accepting of bizarre behaviors; tolerant.
Poor problem-solving skills.	Dissatisfaction with patient is muted or not openly expressed.
Limited ability to adapt to ill family member's disorder.	Better problem-solving skills.
Relatives are significant source of tension, conflicts, and frustration in the family.	Adaptable; uses trial-and-error approach to dealing with patient.
	Calm and self-contained reactions to patient's bizarre behaviors.

Source: Adapted from Vaughn, C. E. (1986). Patterns of emotional response in the families of schizophrenic patients. In M. Goldstein, I. Hand, & K. Hahlweg, *Treatment of schizophrenia, family assessment and intervention.* New York: Springer-Verlag, pp. 97–106.

might be expected, there are markedly different family reactions to mentally ill family members (Vaughn, 1986; Hooley, 1986).

Vaughn and Leff (1976) looked at relapse rates for patients who returned to high and low EE homes as a function of medication compliance and degree of patient-relative contact. They found that patients who experienced more than 35 hours of face-to-face contact with critical, hostile, and over-involved (high EE) families were more likely to suffer a relapse. Patients who were not taking antipsychotic medications were at extreme risk for relapse, while patients who were taking antipsychotic medication had about a 50/50 chance of relapse. Patients who returned to low EE families and who received antipsychotic medications had the lowest relapse rates, followed by patients in low EE families who were not receiving antipsychotic drugs (Vaughn & Leff, 1976; Hooley, 1986). While this study does not provide definitive clinical findings about the differences between high EE and low EE families and their effect on the schizophrenic patient, it does point out that EE is an important line of ongoing inquiry that could yield significant data of use to the patient and his relatives, as well as to mental health care providers.

IMPACT OF THE PATIENT ON THE FAMILY

Just as the schizophrenic is directly affected by his family, so the family is directly affected by the schizophrenic. Family members must provide for treatment (the costs of which can be astronomical) and adapt their feelings and needs to the demands and needs of the ill family member. The financial and emotional costs can be overwhelming. In addition the family has to deal with the stigma that is associated with having a mentally ill member. Some patients, because of a regressed or incapacitated state do not separate easily from the family, though they are often forced to do so. In some cases, the family is the only resource for the patient; thus, their association continues even though it can be deleterious both to the patient and to the family. Families who live with a chronically ill member tend to feel "tied down" and trapped. They have little social life. The lost hopes and dreams of parents of a schizophrenic son or daughter result in frustration and conflict (Willis, 1982; Levine, 1983).

Family members may have to grapple with several issues at one time, including the diagnosis of illness in the family member and other family members' perceptions of how they may have participated in the development of the illness. Moreover, family members need to be alert continuously to how the ill member's behavior affects each family member, as well as the family's functioning as a whole (Caplan, 1974; Askren, 1987).

In times of crisis, the family and others can be of tremendous help or hindrance to the patient and to the family unit as a whole. During these periods, the integrity of the entire family structure should be considered. The nurse needs to assess continuously for the potential "breakup" of the family because of stress associated with the ill member. If she detects a "split," she should confront the family with her observation and work with them in deciding what to do about it. Parents may feel that the situation requires more mental and physical energy and financial support than they can handle. Respite care, that is, removal of the patient from the home for short periods of time, will offer the family and patient a reprieve from each other. This method is more desirable than complete removal of the patient from the family and community because of the appearance of florid psychotic symptoms (Caplan, 1974). Within the family structure, members might observe that the patient sleeps too much, or not enough, or eats too much, or not enough. The patient might have little motivation and be unable to manage his money and other activities of daily living. Yet, he might refuse therapeutic medication, making the statement that the treatment is "no good"; at the same time he may be prone to taking street drugs that exacerbate symptoms. Such are the frustrations of living with a schizophrenic family member, and the reason they need an available support system (such as the county mental health center crisis intervention team) and a family therapist.

The schizophrenic patient's thought form and content make the patient even more vulnerable to mishandling by society. Jobs are frequently lost or never attained; relationships with friends are strained; financial difficulties may occur. If the disease progresses, the patient will become more withdrawn, regressive, and dependent on family and others. The process is one that he does not understand and cannot control (Bassuk & Lamb, 1986).

Encounters with the police and the court system are an ever-present fear among many families with a schizophrenic member. Families have to endure occasional violence perpetrated against the self (patient) and themselves. Those who provide care for their schizophrenic family member have identified the following behaviors as most distressing: aggression, withdrawal, social inappropriateness, unpredictability, irrational beliefs, talking to self, poor hygiene, and not assisting with household tasks (Holden & LeWine, 1982; Askren, 1987). In addition to these struggles, family members may also experience difficulty communicating with health professionals (Askren, 1987). In fact, many families have cared for the ill member for years without ever having known the diagnosis and probable outcome of the illness (Holden & LeWine, 1982).

Organizations such as Families and Friends of the Adult Mentally Ill (FFAMI) and the National Alliance for the Mentally Ill (NAMI) have been created for the purpose of helping families cope with the mentally ill through support and education (see Box 10–1). The National Schizophrenic Fellowship (NSF) publishes a newsletter that discusses the needs of the ill member and his family. Its major aim is to provide information and education about schizophrenia to the patient and his family.

THE TREATMENT SETTING

In recent years, the advancement in the use of antipsychotic drug therapy, along with a focus on community mental health care, have drastically changed the "tradition" of institutionalization for schizophrenic patients. The current goals in mental health care include keeping the patient in the community when at all possible. Hospitalization is used for crisis stabilization and the treatment of florid psychotic symptomotology. The long-term aim of treatment during hospitalization is to return the patient to the community (and the county mental health care system) as quickly as possible. The average stay in hospitals ranges from 10 to 42 days, depending upon the patient's responsiveness to treatment and the type of institution.

As a consequence of community-based care, the mental health care delivery system is in the process of change. At outpatient rehabilitation service centers, hospitals are now linked directly to other community agencies with the objective of providing continuity of care for the schizophrenic patient (Bassuk & Lamb, 1986; Bassuk & Gerson, 1978).

DEINSTITUTIONALIZATION AND CHRONIC MENTAL ILLNESS

Deinstitutionalization began during the early 1960s and is based on the principle that patients can receive more humane and therapeutic care in the community than in mental hospitals (Greenblatt, 1977; Lamb, 1980). This principle, along with the development and use of antipsychotic medications that provide control of psychotic symptoms (Davis, et al., 1980; NIMH, 1986) served as the impetus for the development of the nation's county mental health care centers.

Several other factors hastened the deinstitutionalization process. The mentally ill who were living in the community became eligible for financial assistance (known as Supplemental Security Income). This money was intended to provide the patient with resources to purchase food, shelter, and other necessities (Lamb, 1980; Lamb, 1984). In addition, federal legislation provided funds for the construction and staffing of community mental health centers throughout the United States.

These initiatives provided resources for professionals to treat the mentally ill within the community. With these resources in place and through the work of professionals concerned about the rights of the mentally ill, commitment laws throughout the nation changed. At the same time, family groups and concerned citizens began to vocalize their concerns about the mentally ill: inhumane treatment, involun-

Box 10–1 ● Helping Families Cope

The National Alliance for the Mentally Ill was formed in 1979 by families of the mentally ill. Its purpose is to work toward the improvement of mental health care delivery to the chronically mentally ill. This organization advocates for increased funding for research, training, and public education regarding mental illness and more effective public policies that address attitudinal and behavioral change among members of the general population. They also form pressure groups to monitor access to and quality of mental health services rendered to the chronically mentally ill.

tary commitment, and long-term hospitalization (Greenblatt, 1977; Lamb, 1980; Lamb, 1984).

The impact of these developments can be understood by examining these data: in 1955, there were approximately 559,000 patients in public mental institutions; in 1984 there were about 132,000 (Lamb, 1984) (see Fig. 10–4).

The chronically mentally ill, many of whom have been diagnosed as schizophrenic, make up a highly dependent and needy portion of our population. With deinstitutionalization, the chronically mentally ill have, in some cases, fallen through the cracks of our mental health care system.

Five characteristics of the chronically mentally ill patient have been described by Kuchnel, DeRisi, Liberman, and Mosk (1983, p. 248):

1) Vulnerability to stress: minimal to moderate stress can produce pathology.

2) Deficits in coping skills: deficient in performing activities of daily living to include financial and meal management, personal hygiene, and so forth.

3) Dependency: their helplessness demands support and care from family and friends, public agents and agencies.

4) Difficulties with interpersonal relationships: individual has problems with developing and maintaining relationships; he tends to withdraw, so experiences isolation, alienation, and loneliness.

5) Difficulty with working in competitive job market: the individual has problems in finding and/or maintaining a job.

Wing (1978) posits that schizophrenia in particular is accompanied by or followed with social disablements. He suggests two groups of intrinsic impairments: the syndrome of negative traits (which include apathy, retarded thoughts and movement, lack of motivation and drive, social withdrawal, underactivity, hallucinations, and delusions), and impairment of inner language (patient uses "unusual associations;" confusion, incoherence, and vagueness are pervasive).

The description of these impairments helps to highlight a variety of the needs of the chronically mentally ill (Kuchnel, DeRisi, Liberman, & Mosk, 1983; Wing, 1978). The chronically mentally ill experience major problems with money management, transportation, compliance with medication instructions, meal preparation, and articulating their needs for other basic services (Lamb, 1984; Reynolds, 1980).

Schizophrenics and other chronically mentally ill in the community are frequently without basic services, living impoverished lives (Lamb, 1984), void

of services that were available in state hospitals and other institutions (Talbott, 1977; Lamb, 1984; Bassuk and Lamb, 1986).

Today, the population of mental hospitals has been reduced by two-thirds. That achievement is offset, however, by huge increases in the rate of admissions to those hospitals (signifying a high turnover of patients after short periods of hospitalization), and in the number of discharged but severely and chronically disturbed patients consigned to bleak lives in nursing homes, single room occupancy hotels, and skid-row rooming houses (Bassuk & Gerson, 1978, p. 46).

PROBLEMS WITH DEINSTITUTIONALIZATION. The deinstitutionalization movement in the United States has raised serious concerns about inhumane treatment of the mentally ill in and out of institutions, their deplorable living conditions, and failure of the attempt to mainstream mentally ill patients into society. Although the problem is complex, several contributing factors have been identified:

1. Major gaps in the existing network of community service (Bassuk, 1986);

2. Inability of mental health professionals to recognize the various types of chronic and long-term patients, and their diverse physical and psychological needs;

3. Variability in each patient's capacity to be successfully rehabilitated (differences in ego strength, motivation, family support, and capacity to manage stress); and

4. Overzealous goals for patients sometimes encouraged by professionals without the patient's support that therefore yield failure (Morrisey, 1967; Mosher & Keith, 1980; Lamb, 1984; Bassuk, 1986).

Lipton and Sabatini (1984) point to two basic flaws in the deinstitutionalization process. First, there was a deficit in the conceptualization of deinstitutionalization. Emphasis was placed on the biomedical model of treatment of schizophrenia, which emphasizes its chronicity and deteriorating course. Too little attention was given to the role of psychosocial variables (withdrawal, dependence, and isolation) and their effects on the course of the illness. Second, there was a flaw in the implementation of deinstitutionalization, in that needed community services were poorly conceptualized and seldom readily available for the mentally ill who reentered the community (Bassuk & Lamb, 1986).

Homelessness. As a result, deinstitutionalization has led to homelessness, high recidivism rates, and a

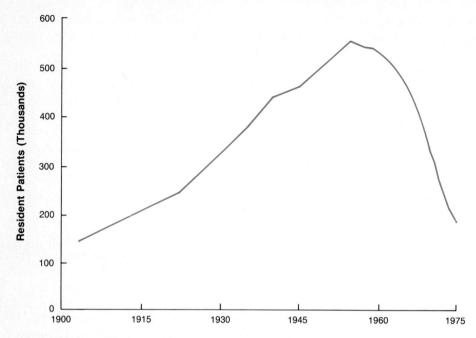

A. Inpatient population of state and county mental hospitals rose steadily from the turn of the century until 1955; since then it has decreased sharply. These data do not include private or Federal hospitals, whose population has held fairly constant at between 50,000 and 75,000.

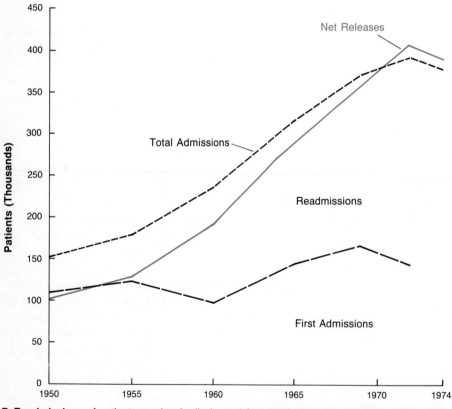

B. Readmissions of patients previously discharged from institutions have exceeded first admissions since 1960; in 1972 they accounted for 64 percent of admissions. Rise in net releases (discharges minus returns from long-term leaves) reflects shorter periods of hospitalization.

FIGURE 10—4 Patterns of Admission to State Hospitals

low quality of life for the chronically mentally ill in this country. The homeless mentally ill (many of whom are schizophrenic) "enter the health care system as stigmatized patients . . . they lack an address, cash in one's pocket, a friend—homeless persons lack dignity, respect, and, more important, an identity. As individuals without status in society, they are less recognizable. Without the health care system they are almost invisible" (Bassuk & Lauriat, 1984, p. 310).

The Alcohol, Drug Abuse, and Mental Health Administration (ADAMA) of the U.S. Public Health Service has estimated that there are approximately 2,000,000 homeless people in the United States. Clearly, state mental hospital personnel and community mental health personnel have not effectively coordinated programs and services for this population (Bachrach, 1984; Talbot & Lamb, 1984; Bassuk & Lamb, 1986). (See Box 10–2.)

A report of The American Psychiatric Association Task Force on the Homeless Mentally Ill (Lamb, 1984) has made recommendations that address psychiatric care for these individuals. An outline of these recommendations follows: 1) meet the individual's basic needs (food and shelter); 2) provide a range of step-wise, supervised housing; 3) provide accessible and effective psychiatric treatment and rehabilitation programs; 4) provide medical treatment and crisis intervention programs; 5) assist society in the development of a sense of responsibility for the chronically mentally ill; 6) make changes in the legal and administrative programs that impact upon community care for the chronically mentally ill; 7) improve coordination between funding resources and program implementation; 8) educate professionals and paraprofessionals to provide services for the chronically mentally ill; 9) provide social services; 10) provide hospitalization for the patients who do not respond to outpatient treatment; 11) research epidemiological factors and causes, and explore treatment methods for the chronically mentally ill; and 12) provide additional financial resources for the development of long-term solutions for the homeless mentally ill.

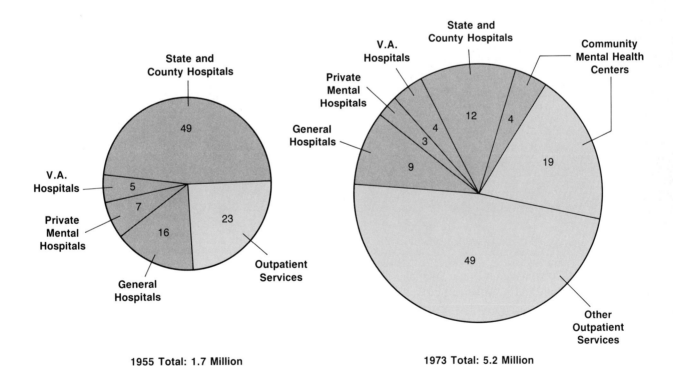

1955 Total: 1.7 Million

1973 Total: 5.2 Million

C. **Shift to outpatient services** is illustrated by the two pie charts. The numbers give the percent of total episodes accounted for in 1955 and 1973 by various facilities offering either inpatient (gray) or outpatient (color) services. The community mental health centers that have been established since 1963 account for much of the outpatient increase, but other outpatient facilities have also expanded.

Box 10–2 ● First-Hand Lesson

Although I was aware of our country's growing problem of homeless people and that many street dwellers suffer from psychiatric illnesses, the plight of these persons did not seem real until recently when I intervened on behalf of a homeless person.

While vacationing in a beautiful resort city in Florida, a friend and I visited a popular restaurant and outdoor bar located in the downtown area. As we sat outdoors, waiting for other friends to arrive, we admired the reflections of the lights on the nearby water and the majestic fountains in the park, around which couples walked hand in hand. There were horse-drawn carriages circling the edge of the park, and the people strolling around were dressed lavishly for a Saturday night on the town.

As we watched the pleasant scene before us, we noticed a large plastic garbage bag on a bench in the center of the neatly groomed park lawn near us. We assumed that the abandoned garbage bag contained cans or other trash. However, as numerous people walked past, occasionally scowling and glancing at the bag, it became apparent to us that the bag was moving. We asked one of the passersby about the contents of the bag and learned that a woman was sitting inside the well-sealed bag, flicking a lighter. She had intimated to passersby that those outside her bag were "dead" and that the outside air was unsafe to breathe.

A well-meaning young man, slightly inebriated, prodded the woman to remove the bag for her own safety; she threatened him with a sharp object, and he finally left her alone. We felt obligated to do something to help this poor creature who apparently was delusional and hallucinating to the point of being potentially harmful to herself and others. We summoned two passing police officers and suggested that she be placed in protective custody under Florida's Baker Act (for involuntary psychiatric placement). The officers gently and carefully took the woman into custody and transported her to the local crisis unit.

Later we learned from the police that the woman had a history of involuntary psychiatric hospitalizations. She was typically stabilized on medications and released after the three-day holding period, only to neglect her medications and repeat the cycle again and again.

This first-hand lesson emphasized to me the glaring need for follow-up psychiatric care for the homeless population of our country. We see so many homeless people in our streets and many times consider their psychotic behavior a normal consequence of their plight. In some ways, the woman's perception may have been correct; many of us have truly become "dead" to the needs of the homeless.

The deinstitutionalization of the mentally ill has not been a total failure. Its implementation, however, was faulty in many respects (Bassuk & Lamb, 1986). It has provided alternative living arrangements for thousands of patients who are able to adapt to community living. The focus here, however, is on the population of patients who have not been able to adapt to the community, and whose needs nurses, physicians, and other mental health professionals have not been able to meet (Bassuk & Lamb, 1986).

Nurses can play a major role in improving services to the chronically mentally ill, especially those who have, for one reason or another, not been able to adapt well to community living. Krauss (1989) has exhorted nurses to participate in the shaping and planning of new systems of care for this population. She feels that of all mental health professionals, nurses are the best prepared to focus on "comprehensiveness, continuity, and care" which she describes as the watchwords of the deinstitutionalization movement.

Evelyn: A Homeless, Chronic, Paranoid Schizophrenic

Evelyn Moutz was a 29-year-old woman who resided in large state hospitals in New York for approximately eight years. During that time she was diagnosed as a chronic paranoid schizophrenic. She was discharged on four occasions, but had short tenure in the community, during which time she lived either on the street or in shelters. Hence, she was regularly rehospitalized for periods of time ranging from a few weeks to months.

In anticipation of discharge for the fifth time, the nurse, social worker, and psychiatrist at the midtown shelter sought to make things different for Evelyn with regard to her adjustment to the community. The team began to plan with Evelyn about one month before her actual discharge date.

The team provided Evelyn with information about schizophrenia, and how the disease affected her. She and the nurse discussed medications and the necessity to comply with a schedule for taking the neuroleptic drugs. The side effects were discussed with Evelyn, as well as the therapeutic benefits. Evelyn had a history of refusing or hiding medications.

The nurse and Evelyn visited the community and located a suitable group home for Evelyn, in an area of the city with which she felt somewhat familiar. The nurse and social worker helped Evelyn complete forms for supplemental income entitlements and health care benefits. Evelyn and the nurse toured the neighborhood and located the stores, a church, laundry, and restaurant that Evelyn could use on a regular basis. Evelyn gradually became more familiar with the area, and was discharged to the group home.

At the group home, Evelyn met other nurses and social workers who helped her become involved in social skills training. She was later referred to vocational rehabilitation where she received funds for transportation, books, and other expenses associated with training. She studied basic electronics with the hope of getting a job assembling portable radios.

Twice weekly, Evelyn participated in supportive group therapy at the group home. There she and other patients discussed their difficulties, fears, failures, and successes. Social skills training at the group home involved learning how to eat at a table with others, dress appropriately, and other social graces.

Despite her progress, Evelyn eventually began to complain of tension headaches, she showed lack of interest in returning to her vocational training classes, and she wanted to stop participating in group therapy. During individual counseling, the nurse became aware that Evelyn had stopped taking her medicine. In fact, she had been flushing the medication down the toilet for more than a week. The nurse and

Evelyn discussed this problem with the psychiatrist and the three of them determined that Evelyn should be placed on a low dose of Prolixin that would be given to her weekly by injection. Evelyn felt frightened because she would be receiving injections but she realized the advantage of not having to struggle with her ambivalence about the medication each morning and night.

The nurse and Evelyn returned to the school where Evelyn received her training. With the nurse's support, Evelyn was able to ask for a chance to complete all assignments that were outstanding. Evelyn remained in school and completed her assignments. After graduation, Evelyn was interested in employment but was terrified of the responsibility it entailed. She and the nurse, with the assistance of a social worker affiliated with the group home, located a radio assembly business where technicians were needed. Before her interview, Evelyn role played the interview with the social worker. Then the nurse and Evelyn went together to the job interview. Evelyn discussed, in a candid fashion, her previous work history. The nurse provided additional information when appropriate. Evelyn was hired.

Evelyn worked, lived in the group home, and participated in group therapy sessions twice weekly. She began, however, to seem quite stressed and tired at times. Apparently, Evelyn had begun to think that a co-worker was "watching" her. She became frightened and feared that she would be fired. The nurse observed other behavior changes as well. Evelyn seemed to be withdrawn in group therapy, wasn't sleeping well, and had lost some weight. She suggested that Evelyn might benefit from individual counseling until the stress of her job and associated responsibilities had subsided. Evelyn agreed to meet with her twice a week.

By the time Evelyn had been working for six months, she had learned to manage a personal checking account. She stated that she wanted to move into her own apartment but did not feel that the community was safe. She was afraid of drugs on the streets and being mugged. The nurse and social worker offered to help Evelyn to deal with these realities. Evelyn also began to be interested in locating her family who lived in another state (mother, father, and five sisters), with whom she had lost contact. The nurse and Evelyn discussed how they might go about doing this.

REHABILITATION OF THE SCHIZOPHRENIC PATIENT

Rehabilitation of the patient with schizophrenia begins after psychotic symptoms have subsided. If some symptoms persist, rehabilitation should proceed anyway, based on the patient's capacity to respond to interventions by nurses and other professionals.

Psychiatric rehabilitation is founded on the philosophy that "disabled people need skills and support to function in the living, learning, and working environments of their choice" (Anthony & Nemec, 1984, p. 382). The goals of psychiatric rehabilitation are attained through two significant interventions: 1) assisting the patient to develop the type of skills he needs to function in his environment; and 2) providing the environmental resources, both physical and human, that are needed to maintain and/or strengthen the patient's current status of functioning.

Psychiatric rehabilitation represents components from two major disciplines, physical medicine and principles of psychotherapy (Anthony & Nemec, 1984). The nurse, because of her orientation to the biological and psychosocial aspects of health care, should be uniquely able to provide rehabilitative care to the psychiatric patient.

Skills training is an integral part of psychiatric rehabilitation. Skills programs are grounded in social learning theory and include such activities as role playing, shaping of behaviors, coaching, and strengthening problem-solving skills. The skills can be taught in individual, group, family, and milieu therapies. Vocational training is also an important aspect of this approach (Anthony & Nemec, 1984; Anthony & Liberman, 1986). When patients have been discharged from the hospital, case management is an important component of the treatment process, providing a way to coordinate all aspects of the patient's rehabilitation needs (see Box 10–3).

PSYCHOSOCIAL SKILL CENTERS. *Psychosocial skill centers* are mental health self-help clubs located in cities throughout the country. They were initiated by patients and nonprofessionals to provide aid and support to mentally ill patients by assisting them with life's problems through an emphasis on reality factors in the here-and-now. These programs focus on providing shelter and employment opportunities, enhancement of role performance, improvement of interpersonal relationship skills, and greater efficiency in managing stress (Anthony & Liberman, 1986).

COMMUNITY SUPPORT PROGRAMS. *Community support programs* (CSP) are designed to provide services to chronically mentally ill adults who are severely impaired and experience major problems in activities of daily living. These include few and poor interpersonal relationships, housing problems, un-

employment, and social skills deficits. These adults, however, do not need the long-term, 24-hour-a-day care that has traditionally been provided by hospitals and other types of residential facilities. Community support programs are composed of individuals who provide service to the chronically mentally ill by assisting them with activities of daily living while residing in the community (NIMH, 1982).

OUTREACH PROGRAMS. An *outreach program* is a program that facilitates and provides for treatment for the homeless and chronically mentally ill. To be effective, *outreach programs* must approach the needs of the chronically and homeless mentally ill in a nontraditional fashion. These programs send professional and nonprofessional workers into the streets, subways, bus stations, parks, vacant lots, shelters, soup kitchens, and everywhere else the mentally ill exist. The "point of contact" is where the patient happens to be. The team approach is essential for access to patients, as well as assistance in connecting them to the variety of services that they need. Trust between the patient and mental health worker must first be established and maintained. Only after there is true and mutual respect can the outreach worker and patient begin to develop lines of communication and discuss the patient's needs and possible ways of meeting them (Levine, Lezak, & Goldman, 1986).

The outreach worker typically gets involved in assisting the patient with basic human needs: assisting with the procurement of psychiatric and other health care services; arranging for hospitalization when necessary; providing for case management and follow-up; and separating from the patient and fostering his/her independence when the time comes (Axelrod & Toff, 1987).

RESPONSIBILITIES OF THE NURSE IN A PSYCHIATRIC SETTING

The nurse has a myriad of responsibilities related to the care of the patient with schizophrenia in a psychiatric setting. The acute phase of treatment frequently requires hospitalization or admission to a crisis stabilization facility. During this phase of the illness, positive symptoms of schizophrenia, such as hallucinations, delusions, ideas of reference, and agitation are treated and psychosocial and vocational deficiencies are assessed (Crow, 1980a&b; Kane, 1987). Negative symptoms associated with the dis-

Box 10–3 ● Case Management and the Schizophrenic Patient

Case management has been a valuable method for providing treatment to both physically and mentally ill patients, and it is an essential component of the rehabilitation process. Case management is a process designed to coordinate and provide continuity of care to an individual by assigning major responsibility for that care to one professional (Levine & Fleming, 1984; Ridgway, Spaniol, & Zipple, 1986).

Basic components of case management for any type of patient are (Levine & Fleming, 1984):

1. *Patient identification and outreach.* Identify patients to be served through outreach activities.

2. *Patient assessment.* Strengths, weaknesses, potential for independent living, and value system are evaluated.

3. *Service planning.* Based on assessment data with goals and objectives clearly identified.

4. *Linkage with requisite services.* Creative, formal, and informal ways of providing service to the patient.

5. *Monitoring of service delivery.* Professional's and patient's perceptions of care are reviewed, and the appropriateness and effectiveness of services is evaluated.

6. *Patient advocacy.* Assertive efforts are used to secure services for the patient. Case managers, psychiatrists, nurses, and paraprofessionals might provide service to street people, individuals in shelters, or group homes. They might also provide crisis intervention, health care services, assistance with money management, drug monitoring, and assistance with other activities of daily living.

According to the American Nurses' Association (June, 1988, p. 1). "Case management is a system of health assessment, planning, service procurement/delivery/coordination, and monitoring, through which multiple service needs of patients are met. Case management optimizes the patient's self-care capability, promotes efficient use of resources, and stimulates the creation of new services as they are needed across the continuum of health care. The goals of case management are provisions of quality care, enhancement of the patient's quality of life, and cost containment."

Case management has been implemented to circumvent the many problems associated with system bureaucracy and solve continuity of care problems when providing services to the diverse and mobile chronically mentally ill population (Bachrach, 1984; Intagliata, 1982).

---

order, such as withdrawal, isolation, apathy, and ambivalence, if evident, must also be addressed.

The nurse should first focus on the safety of the patient (and/or staff). External controls, such as space allocation, should be considered. The nurse is often responsible for evaluating the patient's acuity level and determining if the doctor's orders regarding where to house the patient are appropriate. For example, can the patient be managed on an open (unlocked) unit (Albiez-Gibbons, 1986)?

If the patient requires seclusion and restraint, the setting must have proper ventilation, a level of stimulation that the patient can manage, and be assessed for potential to activate the patient's psychotic symptoms (for example, delusions, hallucinations, and/or illusions).

The patient's ambivalence regarding treatment and staff is likely to be intense. On the one hand, the patient recognizes and will state that he needs treatment; on the other, he might become uncooperative and request immediate discharge minutes later (Tucker, Ferrell, & Price, 1984).

The nurse is responsible for observing carefully and recording the patient's behaviors. It can be reassuring to the patient and his family to know that the nurse and the physician will be working together with the patient and his family members. Hospitalization or residential treatment always involves loss of control for the patient and his family to some extent. This can be frightening and anxiety provoking to both. Knowing who is in charge, and that they are approachable can help.

ASSESSMENT OF THE PATIENT'S DELUSIONS

The nurse, regardless of the practice setting, should know how to evaluate thoughts and behaviors that she suspects to be delusional. Several dimensions of the patient's delusions can be evaluated: persistence, complexity, bizarreness, behavioral impact, and the degree of doubt (Andreasen, 1986). Briefly, persistence can be gauged by determining the frequency with which the patient is engrossed in the delusional thought and/or actions; complexity is decided by the magnitude to which the patient's false belief content is connected, is cohesive, consistent, and has central focus; bizarreness of the delusion is determined by the degree of credibility the nurse assigns to the patient's thoughts and actions; behavioral impact is determined by assessing the extent to which the patient acts on his false thoughts and beliefs; and the degree of doubt is determined by the extent to which the patient actually believes/or doubts his false thoughts and beliefs. The nurse will observe that some patients might question their delusions while others present their thoughts with majestic assurance and conviction.

The nurse must always evaluate the patient's delusional beliefs and behaviors within the context of his cultural or religious orientation and experiences.

ASSISTING THE PATIENT IN REALITY TESTING

The schizophrenic patient is likely to have difficulty with reality testing, that is, the ability to evaluate the external world objectively and differentiate it from the internal world. His environment should be designed to facilitate interactions and interpersonal relationships within the context of his cultural experiences as well as his clinical acuity level. The nurse should explain rules, roles, routines, and expectations in the psychiatric unit at the patient's level of comprehension. Also, determinations should be made about the demands and composition of the current inpatient milieu and the patient's ability to handle them. The staff must be aware, however, that the patient might experience their concerns as their judgment that he is not able to function without their assistance. In such instances, the patient can fall into or get stuck in "sick role behavior" that impedes his treatment (Beebe, 1975).

The nurse can assist the patient with reality testing in the following ways. First, she can help him distinguish where specific stimuli and sensations originate. Are they within the person or in the environment? That is, the nurse might say, "the voice you heard telling you to stand next to the wall is coming from your head, and is not a command from someone in the room" (it originates from within). Second, the nurse must try to determine what might be causing the sensations. Then, she can help the patient with his understanding about what might be causing these stimuli and sensations. Discussions about the stimuli and sensations (voices, bodily sensations, or illusions) as they relate to the patient's conflicts and frustrations can help the patient cope with them. Third, the nurse should try to find the purpose and significance of the sensations, and verify this with the patient. This step can be referred to as the interpretation of meaning of the sensation. An incorrect interpretation can influence the patient's behavior. These incorrect interpretations may provide the basis for paranoia or suspiciousness. The patient may act on these and display pathological behaviors that are associated with them. The final step involves searching for the appropriate response to the stimuli and sensations (Balint, 1942). If the nurse understands these four features of reality testing, she can develop systematic nursing interventions that help the patient improve his ability to differentiate reality from his psychotic beliefs and experiences.

The nurse can also support the patient in improving his memory, aid in his identification of feelings and thoughts, assist the patient in learning how to anticipate certain events and consequences, and help the patient with problems with concentration, focusing, and attention to tasks (Schafer, 1968; Bellak et al., 1973). Moreover, the nurse can facilitate the patient's ability to more accurately perceive, interpret, and gauge the feelings and moods of others in a manner that is free of distortions and anxieties (Modell, 1968; Bellak et al., 1973). Accurate reality testing improves judgment functions for the schizophrenic patient. Reality therapy methods can be employed to assist the patient in recognizing that reality does indeed exist and that he will need to learn to meet his needs within that context (Glasser, 1965).

MANAGING DRUG THERAPY

In recent years, much inpatient treatment of schizophrenia has focused on the use of neuroleptic drugs. There is a small group of patients, however, who do not benefit from drug treatment. Since the patient's drug responses are influenced by biological, environmental, and interpersonal factors, it is understandable that all patients do not have the same response to neuroleptics.

The nurse's knowledge about antipsychotic medications and characteristic symptomatology of schizophrenia, along with her clinical observations of the patient, becomes vital to the patient's treatment. She must make clinical inferences, plan and implement treatment strategies, record data on the patient's records, and become an active participant in the clinical discussion where the patient's treatment options and dispositions are determined. Too, she must serve as an advocate for the patient and family.

During the patient's inpatient treatment, the physician considers the selection of neuroleptic drugs, their recommended dosage and side effects, and attempts to choose the medication most likely to help an individual patient. Inpatient treatment, hopefully, is brief; its objective is finding an effective dose of neuroleptic medication and the development of a thorough after-care plan which includes community based psychosocial treatment (Schooler & Carpenter, 1983; Kane, 1987).

SHORT- AND LONG-TERM GOALS. The short-term goal in administration of neuroleptics is reduction of the intensity of psychotic behavior. Control of the psychotic disorder is the goal of the long-range therapeutic plan. The nurse, physician, and other members of the treatment team need to grapple with such questions as: 1) Is it likely that the patient's symptoms will subside completely or only abate in intensity? 2) What is the drug of choice and why? 3) What are the anticipated side effects? 4) What should the dosage of medication be? 5) What is the mode of administration? 6) What is the frequency of administration? 7) What is the likely duration of treatment? 8) What are the current and potential compliance issues that will need to be considered (Todd, 1981; Donaldson, Gelenberg, & Baldessarini, 1983)? Here, too, the nurse is responsible for documenting the therapeutic effects of the drug used, its side effects, and the patient's general reactions to it.

COMPLIANCE ISSUES IN DRUG THERAPY. The nurse must pay particular attention to compliance behaviors of the patient and family. Drug noncompliance is one of the most common causes of relapse and rehospitalization in the schizophrenic patient (Kaplan & Sadock, 1988).

The nurse discusses with the patient and family members issues such as:

1. The benefits to the patient, the family, and others

2. The *therapeutic* effects of the drug

3. The risks associated with the chosen drug

4. Possible side effects, such as extrapyramidal symptoms and tardive dyskinesia, and what will be done to prevent them

5. The recommended schedule for administering the drug

6. Those signs and symptoms that should be brought to the attention of the nurse or physician (nausea, vomiting, diarrhea, increased blurred vision, stiffness, and tremors)

7. Information about the person or agency to contact regarding (a) questions about the drug, (b) need for consultation, (c) what constitutes a need for emergency care (or hospitalization), and/or (d) who to call or where to go for support

8. Fears that neuroleptic medications may cause sedation or death (this will not occur unless an enormous amount is ingested)

9. Fears that neuroleptic medication is addictive (it is not)

10. What to expect from the patient; coping methods that family members might utilize if the patient's psychotic symptoms recur

11. Psychiatric rehabilitation programs such as Community Support Programs (CSP) and skill centers. Also, the nurse should inform family about community support groups for themselves, such as the National Alliance for the Mentally Ill (NAMI)

12. Goals of treatment and anticipated outcome.

MONITORING PATIENTS ON NEUROLEPTIC DRUGS. There can be severe side effects associated with neuroleptic therapy. The nurse must observe for extrapyramidal and autonomic side effects, and record these in the patient's chart as well as bring them to the attention of the physician and other team members (see pages 339–341 and Table 10–7 for the discussion of extrapyramidal and anticholinergic side effects and related nursing measures).

MANAGEMENT OF OVERDOSE. Neuroleptic drugs are seldom lethal when taken in overdose. The nurse, however, should be alert for drowsiness and the possibility of coma as well as signs of twitching, dystonic movements, tardive dyskinesia, convulsions, tachycardia, hypotension, or confusion. Extrapyramidal side effects may be treated or prevented with anti-Parkinson agents such as benztropene (Cogentin), trihexyphenidyl (Artane), or diphenhydramine (Benadryl), given either orally or intramuscularly.

MANAGING THE SUICIDAL OR HOMICIDAL PATIENT

The risk of suicide among schizophrenic patients continues to be a major problem. It can occur at any time and in any setting during the course of the illness, although it is thought to occur most often during the first 10 years of illness. Depression, which is considered to be an important risk factor for potential suicide, must be assessed on a regular basis (Drake & Cotton, 1986). Depression is likely to occur once the patient understands his illness and its projected long-term course, which is likely to involve exacerbations of acute symptoms, multiple hospitalizations, and gradual deterioration (Seeman & McGee, 1982).

Alleback et al (1986) caution that a history of previous suicidal attempts is one of the best predictors of suicide. Yet there are schizophrenic patients who make attempts without any previous history of suicidal behaviors.

Among chronic schizophrenics, feelings of hopelessness, including negative expectations about the future, may increase the risk of suicide. Drake and Cotton (1986) report that when depression, but not hopelessness, is present, the risk of suicide is diminished.

Isolation, alienation, difficulties with maintaining satisfying interpersonal relationships, interruptions with employment, and conflicts with family members make it extremely difficult for the schizophrenic to lead a purposeful and worthwhile life (Dingman & McGlashon, 1986). Thus the patient begins to feel worthless, which is another factor that increases the risk of suicide. Johns, Stanley, & Stanley (1986) tested the following risk factors as predictors of suicide among schizophrenic patients:

—age and sex (young male schizophrenics at greatest risk)

—first 10 years of illness

—chronicity with exacerbation and remission of psychotic symptoms

—numerous hospitalizations

—recently discharged from the hospital

—clinical depression

—feelings of hopelessness

—negative attitude about treatment

Nyman and Johnsson (1986) have identified several groupings of behaviors that the nurse might take as warnings about the schizophrenic patient's potential self-destruction. They include self-destructive acts without suicidal intent (scratching, cutting); suicidal "planning" (purchasing weapons, saving pills and razor blades); suicidal talk (content focusing on hopelessness and misery); aggression (fits, rage, tantrums); and fantasies with aggressive content (pleasure derived from pain, fear, and anguish).

The role of neuroleptics in schizophrenic suicide is controversial. At one time, it was thought that antipsychotic drugs (especially depot, long-acting type) increased depression and therefore the risk of suicide among schizophrenics (DeAlarcon & Carney, 1969). More recent research has not corroborated this (Johns, Stanley, & Stanley, 1986). It appears that antipsychotic drugs neither prevent nor precipitate suicide.

Given the ambivalence of the schizophrenic patient and his distorted reality testing, the nurse should assess the patient for suicidality at regular intervals. This is accompanied by observing the patient's behaviors (verbal and nonverbal) and being alert for suicidal ideation and the potential for acting on it. Then she and the rest of the treatment team learn, along with the family, the appropriate interventions. Sometimes the schizophrenic patient's withdrawal, isolation, and alienation from others is so profound that life becomes overwhelming and a decision is made to leave it all, to commit suicide (Drake et al., 1984; Nyman & Johnsson, 1986).

If the patient believes that another person is there for him and genuinely and unconditionally cares about him, he may be more apt to "hold on" and go on living. The hope of ever mastering the inner conflicts and frustrations will be sustained (Meerloo, 1962).

If the patient is truly suicidal, a staff person, preferably his primary nurse, should be with him at all times. If indicated, the patient may need to be placed in a secluded area, with personnel constantly in attendance. As a last resort to ensure safety, suicidal patients are placed in four-point restraints.

The homicidal patient also needs special attention, because of the possibility of injury to other patients or staff in the hospital. Medications may be used to assist in the control of aggressive behavior. Isolation and separation from others might also be necessary. The patient should not be on an open ward unless there are adequate security and personnel to handle an attempted escape or an attempted act of violence against the self or others (Sclar, 1981; Salamon, 1976) (see also Chapter 24, Psychiatric Mental Health Nursing with the Violent Patient).

MONITORING THE PATIENT FOR PHYSICAL HEALTH PROBLEMS

The nurse is responsible for monitoring the schizophrenic patient's physical health. Frequently, schizophrenic patients have neglected their physical health through poor nutrition, limited access to adequate health care, poor housing, and noncompliance with prescribed medication regimens. Hospital admission procedures should include, in addition to the psychiatric assessment, a physical examination, X-ray, and routine blood work. The patient may require additional tests to detect the presence of sexually transmitted diseases.

Pregnancy tests for all women of child-bearing age should be considered. Further intervention depends upon the patient's history and mental status, and the results of these examinations.

Based on her observations and assessments of the patient, the nurse might need to request dietary consultation for help in assisting the patient in maintaining near normal weight or in providing foods high in fiber and bulk, and large amounts of water and juices to treat constipation.

MONITORING PATIENT-PATIENT AND PATIENT-STAFF RELATIONSHIPS

The nurse has the responsibility to observe subgroupings and "falling in love" behaviors among patients and sometimes between staff members and patients in a variety of settings. She should be sensitive to the patient's often faulty perceptions of interpersonal relationships, ambivalence, the tendency to isolate himself, and regression. The nurse must also be sensitive to the patients' developing unhealthy and mutually exploitive, destructive relationships, and intervenes, for example, by meeting together with the parties involved and confronting their self- and other-destructive behavior. This may need to be done several times

and/or with the help of the patients' therapists or staff physician.

ADVOCATING FOR THE PATIENT

In addition to the responsibilities discussed above, the nurse is responsible for protecting the patient's rights. Most states have codes of patient's rights that might be required by law to be posted in patient areas (in hospitals, in clinics, and so forth) (see Chapter 27).

The nurse assists in determining the assets and liabilities of the patient's family system. Frequently, the patient will have conflicts, delusions, suspicions, and numerous anxieties about specific family members. The nurse assesses these beliefs in the family context via a home visit or family session in the hospital or clinic and helps the patient and his family cope with both the reality of their situation and the patient's psychotic thinking.

Patient (and family) should be actively involved from the beginning of nursing care planning. Some facilities require the involvement of an appointed advocate for the patient or the hospital ethics committee (see Chapter 28) when:

1. The patient is too psychotic to participate.

2. Family members are not readily available to assist in planning care.

3. Treatment regimens involve a controversial or potentially controversial procedure/therapy.

COUNTERTRANSFERENCE

As the nurse performs her many different functions in the psychiatric setting, she needs to be aware of her fears, prejudices, provocative behaviors, limitations, motivations, knowledge deficiencies, and emotional sensitivity that different types of patients touch off or stir up in her. She must also recognize the varieties of cultural differences among patient populations and their unique needs (see Chapter 6). She must be cognizant of the many types of pathological and coping behaviors that a variety of patients exhibit and her internal reactions (as well as behavior) to these patients. At times, the nurse will need in-depth supervision and support. If support does not come automatically, she should be assertive enough to ask for supervision by the nurse specialist, staff psychiatrist or psychologist, or the patient's therapist in order to provide optimal nursing care.

Box 10—4 ● The Outcome of Schizophrenia

Frederick L. and Catherine S. are clients at a community mental health center. Mr. L., 27, now lives in a shelter for the homeless; he has had episodes of schizophrenia and alcohol abuse for ten years. Ms. S. is 32 and lives in a board-and-care home on Social Security disability payments. She has had episodes of schizophrenia for seven years and can do only occasional volunteer work. Mr. L. often fails to follow his treatment plan and take the medications prescribed for him. His clinician sees him as a dull, colorless person who will always live on the fringes of society. Ms. S.'s flamboyance and escapades have so exasperated the people caring for her that she has been diagnosed as a borderline personality.

The professionals who treat these patients doubt that they will recover or even significantly improve; they hope only for stabilization and maintenance. Yet recent long-term studies show improvement even in some schizophrenic patients who seem to be hopelessly ill. Why does clinical experience apparently contradict this research? The answer has many implications for the understanding of schizophrenia, the care of schizophrenic patients, and the training of professionals who treat them.

Clinicians see a stream of chronically ill patients who need more than antipsychotic drugs and psychosocial treatment; their lives are in total disarray. They need food, clothing, shelter, and treatment for physical illnesses. They often require help in obtaining a source of income and dealing with personal and legal problems. Many clinicians find that their caseloads are too large and their training is insufficient to deal with these patients. The paperwork is burdensome. There is no payment for extra time spent on ancillary activities. Clinicians often feel overwhelmed, and find it hard to believe that these patients could even improve, much less recover.

But the vision of clinicians is obscured by the atmosphere of constant crisis and seeming hopelessness. They are so busy that they rarely have time to think about patients they are no longer seeing. They often assume that these patients are in someone else's care or living in decrepit hotels. Recovered patients hardly ever call their former therapists and say "Hi, this is Joe. I just wanted you to know that I finally got my life together, married Jane, and found a decent job. Thanks for all the help you gave me." Working without such feedback creates a persistent bias in clinical perspective.

Over Fifty Percent Improve

The earliest studies gave a discouraging impression of the long-term out-

MANAGING THE PATIENT WITH POSITIVE HIV STATUS

PATIENT CARE. The American Psychiatric Association (1988) has developed a policy for the management of AIDS on inpatient psychiatric units. The policy states that a patient should receive the necessary psychiatric treatment, regardless of his HIV status and serologic status; he should be informed that he will be or has been tested and of the results of the test; all inpatients should be perceived as having the potential for receiving or transmitting the HIV infection or other infections; and if an infected patient engages or threatens to engage in behaviors that put

others at risk, the physician has the responsibility to take the least restrictive but effective action (educate, counsel, isolate, and/or restrain the patient) to control these behaviors.

CONFIDENTIALITY. If a patient with positive HIV status is hospitalized, whether or not to discuss the patient's HIV status with other staff is a decision made by the physician. After discussing the situation with the patient, the physician may determine that disclosure is necessary for treatment; if the patient's behavior is such that other patients and staff on the unit are at risk, and control of these behaviors is dif-

come in schizophrenia, because they included only hospitalized patients. For a more accurate picture, researchers should follow the lives of patients both in and out of treatment. In the last two decades there have been five such studies, including more than 1300 subjects. Every study has shown that half or more of people hospitalized for chronic schizophrenia recover or significantly improve over a period of 20 years or more. . . .

. . . [C]linicians should reconsider their pessimism about the long-term prognosis of schizophrenia. Patients often recover the capacity to care for themselves and participate in society. Symptoms, both positive (such as delusions and hallucinations) and negative (such as apathy or withdrawal) often subside. Clinicians should avoid suggesting to patients that they will never recover, will deteriorate, or will have to take antipsychotic drugs for the rest of their lives. That betrays hope and discourages self-healing. Instead, mental health professionals could show through their words, actions, and attitudes that recovery is possible; patients are more likely to improve if they believe they can.

We should also reconsider the practice of describing schizophrenia as if it had only two forms; acute, with a rapid resolution, and chronic, with continual recurrence and gradual deterioration. Most patients would be better described by an intermediate term. The existing systems for diagnosing schizophrenia are not very useful in predicting long-term outcome: more attention might be paid to the differences among people who are labeled schizophrenic. Some researchers have proposed substituting "person with prolonged psychiatric illness" for "schizophrenic patient." Furthermore, the time spent in treatment is only part of the lives of these people. It would make sense to think of treatment as "walking along part of the path" with them. That clinical perspective would encourage patients to clarify who they are, what they want to do, and when they want to do it. It would relieve the pressure for rapid improvement and allow both patients and clinicians to cope more realistically with fluctuating symptoms.

Outcome Unpredictable

Many patients, of course, do not improve. Some succumb to a particularly severe form of the illness. Others receive inadequate treatment or lack opportunities for returning to society. Still others are prevented from changing their lives by the side effects of medications, the stigmatizing label of mental illness, personality disorders, or the demoralizing effects of prolonged institutionalization. But no one can know in advance which patients will improve and which will not. We and other researchers have recorded history after history of patients who, after years of sitting in the day room of a hospital watching television, get on their feet and make new lives for themselves—as much to their own as to their therapists' surprise. Mental health care could be reorganized to provide long-term options in the light of these variations.

Under the present system most clinicians, families, and patients are already resigned to low expectations by the time the symptoms of the illness begin to lift. Recovery would be more likely if mental health programs treated all patients as if they might recover. Legislators should be urged to enact long-range budgets: 15- to 20-year instead of 2- to 5-year plans. Bright young mental health professionals should be encouraged to work with these difficult but surprisingly rewarding patients. And we should develop research strategies to determine which treatments are best for which patients in the various phases of prolonged psychiatric illness.

Source: Harding, C. (1988). *Harvard Medical School Mental Health Letter*. May 1988, Vol. 4 No. 11. Reprinted with permission.

---

ficult, then disclosure of a patient's HIV infectious status is appropriate. This must be done with sensitivity and caution. (See Box 18–1.)

DISCHARGE. When the patient is clinically ready for a psychiatric discharge from the unit, but is perceived to possibly place others in the community at risk, the staff should not retain the patient as a form of quarantine or prevention. Educating the patient about his disease and the risks it poses for others is appropriate. The nurse should make sure that the patient has had an appropriate level of counseling to effect a behavioral change. If his behaviors do not change, the nurse will then need to decide the appropriate course to take when there is conflict between two fundamental principles: the individual's right to privacy and the responsibility of health professionals to warn those that they suspect or know are in danger (Martin, 1988) (see Chapter 28).

DISCHARGE PLANNING

As the nurse and other psychiatric personnel plan for the patient's discharge to the community, the nurse should assess for social competence by determining the patient's social support and social adjustment

(Curran, Faraone, & Dow, 1985) (see Chapter 5, on assessment). The nurse will need to have information about the following: the size of the patient's social network; the extent of the linkage and connectedness of the persons in the network; the length of time that people have been in the network; the average amount of contact the patient has with the network; the extent to which the patient enjoys and is comfortable with the network members; the sense of openness and straightforwardness with which problems can be discussed by patient and network members; and the extent to which the network members are helpful (Curran, Faraone, & Dow, 1985). The astute nurse can use these data when preparing the patient for discharge by constructing specific nursing interventions and outcome criteria for increasing the patient's access to or involvement in his social network, e.g., regular family therapy, referral to group therapy for the chronically mentally ill, AA, Alanon, etc., to be added to the patient's ongoing nursing care plan.

While the effects of schizophrenia may be devastating, much evidence exists to support the belief that schizophrenia may not necessarily resign a person to the back wards of a mental health hospital or a life fraught with constant relapses. Throughout the period of care, and finally, in discharge planning, nurses can be instrumental in promoting the individuality of each patient by seeing that person as an individual with unique symptoms and needs—and always capable of recovery (see Box 10–4).

FUTURE DIRECTIONS IN THE CARE OF SCHIZOPHRENIC PATIENTS AND THEIR FAMILIES

BIOLOGICAL AND GENETIC RESEARCH

New technologies in the area of molecular genetics and brain imaging are likely to provide a better understanding of the pathophysiology, etiology, and treatment possibilities for schizophrenia in the future. Advances in biomedical technology have made it possible to study the gross structure and function of the brains of schizophrenic and nonschizophrenic patients. Examples include positron emission tomography (PET) which measures the flow of glucose in the brain and computer axial tomography (CAT) which has made it possible to study the structure of the ventricles of the brain (Buchsbaum & Haier, 1987). Electroencephalogram (EEG) technology will provide clinicians and researchers with data regarding brain electroactivity mapping (BEAM) which measures delta and theta activity of the brain (Tsuang, Faraone, & Day, 1988).

Much recent research has focused on the study of neurotransmitters: serotonin, norepinephrine, dopamine, and GABA. An understanding of the functions of these neurotransmitters (especially dopamine) is thought to be critical to the improvement of antipsychotic drugs and other somatic therapies for the treatment of schizophrenia.

"Season of birth" studies are designed to determine if schizophrenics are more likely to be born during the time of year (winter months) when infections (bacterial and viral) are present. The role of infection in the etiology of schizophrenia needs further exploration.

PSYCHOSOCIAL STUDIES

Family studies, especially the study of Expressed Emotion (EE) levels in the families of schizophrenics and its association with relapse, continues to be an area of great interest to researchers, with much potential for clinical application (Hooley, 1986).

Studies that examine the role of deprivation, distress, poverty, and other sociocultural stressors are also needed for a more in-depth understanding of schizophrenia. It remains unclear as to whether poverty is a cause or consequence of schizophrenia (Tsuang, Faraone, & Day, 1988; Warheit & Scharb, 1977). Studies of psychosocial treatment and rehabilitation cover four major areas: psychosocial factors associated with the etiology, history, and outcome of schizophrenia; the creation of effective treatment and rehabilitation programs utilizing this framework; process and outcome studies of specific treatment programs; and combined treatment approaches. These types of studies will provide valuable information about the effectiveness of community based programs, and methods that can be employed to increase the patient's tenure in the community (National Institute of Mental Health Research Highlights, 1986).

ROLE OF THE PROFESSIONAL NURSE

Aiken (1987) has presented several strategies that the nurse may use to improve the type of assistance currently provided to the mentally ill. She proposes: 1) consolidating authority and accountability in fiscal management of clinical programs; 2) rooting authority in local government where local officials can manage broad-based programs; 3) developing new service settings to include group homes, foster homes, mobile clinics, and the streets (Mechanic, 1986; Aiken, 1987); 4) creating outreach programs, much like the public-health nursing model where nurses meet the patient in the home, in the streets, and on the job; 5) reforming financial methods of reimbursement; 6) attracting professionals to public-sector careers (essential, but difficult); and 7) joining the national public debate about homelessness and the chronically mentally ill (Aiken, 1987).

Similarly, Crosby (1987) has communicated that care, not cure, is an important factor in treatment of the chronically mentally ill; that treatment in a community with adequate resources for the chronically mentally ill is desirable and preferable to long-term care in institutions. In addition, the focus on care, if accepted by professionals, should assist the nurse in emerging as a key player in the delivery of service to the chronically mentally ill.

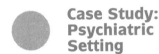

Case Study: Psychiatric Setting

Demographic Data

Name: Carrie Davis
Age: 17 years
Geographic: 5151 Parkside Drive, Houston, TX
Ethnicity: Caucasian
Religious Preference: Protestant
Referring Agency: Parents (in the Emergency Room)
Occupation: College Student

Presenting Problem

At the time of her admission in the emergency room, Carrie was mute and nonresponsive to all inquiries from the treatment staff. She presented with a rigid body posture. Prior to this time, Carrie had been an active athlete and an outstanding student in her academic courses.

History of Problem

Carrie's parents reported their perceptions of the current problem. Recently, Carrie had told her parents that she was pregnant and that she and her fiancé were planning to be married. Her parents were devastated; they demanded that she have an abortion. Carrie did not want to have an abortion and pleaded with her parents to allow her to keep the baby.

Carrie's parents were outraged and felt that their image in the community would be tarnished. Furthermore, they felt Carrie's image at school and in the community would also be tarnished. Carrie's father stated, "I have plans for her to study law and join me in my transcontinental shipping business. I won't let these plans go up in smoke."

Carrie's parents arranged the abortion and proceeded with it against her will. The parents had thought that the "crisis" was over. However, shortly thereafter, the parents observed that Carrie was losing weight, refusing food, grimacing, crying frequently, and becoming increasingly withdrawn. They also commented that Carrie appeared "totally indifferent toward everything and everyone. It was as if Carrie had no feelings." These behaviors had gone on for about seven months and had increased in intensity during the two weeks prior to Carrie's hospital admission. Carrie's mother observed that her body had become stiff and rigid and that she would remain in one position for hours, even days. Carrie appeared to be oblivious to any discomfort or pain that might be induced from remaining in one position.

Over a period of days, Carrie's behaviors increased in intensity: she stared at the ceiling in her room, did not engage in personal hygiene, and became mute. Her parents were extremely frightened and sought immediate help from a psychiatrist. The psychiatrist recommended inpatient treatment and proceeded to make the necessary arrangements to hospitalize Carrie.

Psychiatric History

Schizotypal personality disorder in paternal grandmother.

Family History

Carrie's mother and father had no history of psychiatric illness. They both described themselves as hardworking and dedicated to their business and family. Carrie's mother described herself as being a bit compulsive; Carrie's father described himself as being demanding and having high expectations of himself and others.

Mrs. Davis described her own father as exacting, hard working, and success oriented. She described her mother as an "excellent mother": gentle, dutiful, superb cook, counselor, and friend. Mr. Davis's father was dead, and he provided no additional information about him. He seemed embarrassed as he described his mother as "a little odd" and not very involved with him. She never had friends and the other kids called her a witch, as she always dressed in black and was never friendly like the other mothers. He mumbled that "today she is the local 'bag lady.'"

There were three other children in the family: three sons who were college graduates and working in their father's business in different parts of the world. The three sons were married and had their own families. No history of mental illness was reported.

Social History

Mr. and Mrs. Davis reported that Carrie had a normal and uneventful childhood. She was an obedient child, worked hard in school, and received excellent grades.

Education

In high school, Carrie was popular and high achieving. She planned to attend college and major in engineering, as her three brothers and her father had. A very attractive young woman, Carrie had an active social life, and worked hard at meeting all of her academic and family responsibilities.

Support

Mrs. Davis commented that Carrie had one close friend and many other school acquaintances. She also had a special teacher who has served as her mentor. Her fiancé was one important component of her support system.

Physical History

Normal physical development. Currently, Carrie's mouth was dry, she was underweight (105 pounds; 5'7"), and there was redness at pressure points.

Drug Use

Mrs. Davis felt that Carrie had probably tried marijuana and cocaine at some point in her life, but she had no evidence of regular use.

Mental Status

Appearance: disheveled, mute, wearing wrinkled clothes, hair uncombed, eyes cast downward.

Sensorium: unresponsive to positive or mildly aversive external stimuli.

Mood: mute.

Motoric Behavior: rigid, stiff body (no movements observed).

Thought Content and Thought Process: unable to assess.

Medication: no known prescription medications.

Potential for Violence: could not be assessed at this time; no history of violent behavior.

Summary

Carrie Davis is a 17-year-old, who was brought to the emergency room by her parents. She had recently had an abortion and was disheveled, unkempt, and staring downward. She presented a rigid body posture and was mute.

The Five Axes

Axis I: Schizophrenia, Catatonic Type (295.2x)*
Axis II: No diagnosis
Axis III: a) Dry mouth; skin red at pressure points; b) not eating; dehydrated; c) severely underweight; d) poor bowel/bladder control
Axis IV: Psychosocial Stressors-4-Severe: a) pregnancy and abortion; and b) separation from boyfriend
Axis V: Current GAF: 12; Past GAF: 86

Nursing Diagnoses

** 1) Alteration in health maintenance
** 2) Impaired verbal communication
** 3) Ineffective individual coping
   4) Ineffective family coping
   5) Potential improved skin integrity
   6) Disturbance in self-concept
   7) Altered patterns of urinary elimination related to change in lifestyle
   8) Self-Care Deficit: feeding, bathing/hygiene, toileting, dressing/grooming
   9) Altered nutrition: less than body requirements
  10) Potential for violence related to inability to control behavior
  11) Grieving
  12) Alteration in bowel elimination related to change in lifestyle

*Note: Because the psychotic symptomatology reported by Carrie's parents has been going on for more than 6 months, Carrie is given a diagnosis of Catatonic Schizophrenia. If the symptoms were present for less than 6 months, Carrie would have been given a diagnosis of Schizophreniform Disorder (295.40).

**Nursing diagnoses developed in care plan that follows.

Nursing Care Plan for Carrie

Nursing Diagnosis	Desired Outcomes	Interventions	Rationale
1. Alteration in health maintenance.	Carrie will increase food and fluid intake to 1200 calories per day.	Offer 1200 calorie diet, fluids, etc., and monitor and record patient's intake of food and fluids; observe behaviors. Offer nutritious liquids and foods in small quantities; offer food that does not require much activity/energy to consume (easily chewed, attractive color, and aroma).	Improved nutrition is essential to full physical and mental recovery.
	Carrie will resume normal elimination habits.	Monitor and record elimination patterns and activities.	Constipation is likely because of immobility, limited intake, and if patient is taking phenothiazines.
		Offer 60-100 cc's juice and other fluids every hour.	Fluids help to prevent dehydration and constipation.
		Offer stool softener.	
		Assess need for parenteral fluids, e.g., if patient refuses oral fluids.	
	Carrie's body will become less stiff and rigid.	Apply passive range of motion exercise to arms and legs. Explain to Carrie why this is being done. Nurse may comment, "Feel free to help me with your care, Carrie. I think you will be able to exercise yourself again, soon!"	Passive exercise prevents contractions, additional stiffness, and provides a method of "communication" with patient.
	Carrie will have adequate circulation and skin integrity maintained.	Turn Carrie approximately every four hours, and utilize a schedule such as: back to right side; right side to left side; left side to back; and so forth.	Prevents pneumonia and decubiti; increases opportunities for communication; promotes comfort and increases environmental stimulation for Carrie.
		Massage pressure areas such as hips, back, and all bony prominences.	

Nursing Diagnosis	Desired Outcomes	Interventions	Rationale
		Use footboard to prevent foot drop and sliding.	
		Explain the procedures to Carrie and invite her to help whenever she feels she can.	
2. Impaired verbal communication.	Carrie will demonstrate improved communication as evidenced by increased verbalization of needs, frustrations, conflicts, and anger.	Introduce self to patient.	Carrie needs to know who the nurse is; what to expect from her; the general plan of care; how long the nurse will care for her.
		Continually observe and record patient's attempts to communicate.	A baseline set of data is essential for purposes of discerning change; the nurse then records psychological regression or progress, physical deterioration or improvement.
		Assess (by observation, history, and mental status examination) the patient's behaviors, attitudes, problems (especially the abortion), needs, and patterns of coping. Then, express expectations to Carrie. Once Carrie begins to respond, suggesting that family problems be dealt with in family therapy before discharge is likely to reduce her ambivalence about getting well.	In order to recover, Carrie needs to feel understood, and needs to feel hopeful about the future.
		Inform the patient how long the nurse will provide the physical, therapeutic, and interpersonal care, and explain that the nature of the relationship will end when she is able to care for herself.	A genuine, honest, matter-of-fact approach is beneficial. It also communicates the nurse's expectation to Carrie that she will return to a higher level of functioning, and return to the community.
		Provide immediate feedback for positive behaviors; be consistent with Carrie; and state expectations clearly.	Be cautious about making secondary gains so gratifying that Carrie becomes too comfortable, and loses motivation to become self-sufficient and independent.

Nursing Diagnosis	Desired Outcomes	Interventions	Rationale
		Communicate that you understand the specific problems that precipitated this hospitalization.	To provide therapeutic care, the nurse needs to be aware of initial conflict and precipitating events.
		Determine a schedule for social activities; explain this schedule to patient. Tell her that expectations are that she go to OT, for example, and at least observe until she feels comfortable enough to participate.	Development of trust is facilitated by follow-through with promises and scheduled activities.
		Determine how much of your presence Carrie can tolerate. Plan contact with Carrie around your findings.	Controlling interactions with Carrie will prevent undue anxiety, frustrations, and conflicts.
		Discuss with Carrie expectations of her behavioral change and commitment to her toward achieving that objective.	This conveys to the patient that the nurse thinks she has the capacity to improve, and that the nurse is committed to helping her become well again.
		Observe for pattern of eye movement—partially closed/open. Observe for clutching of fist, biting or grinding teeth, sucking and spitting behaviors (regressive and infantile behaviors), and record all such behaviors. Note kinesics: "What might this body posture mean?"	Detailed observations of subtle behavior changes are essential. The behavioral clues are limited; therefore, plan of care is often based upon limited data.
3. Ineffective individual coping.	Carrie will verbalize thoughts and feelings associated with her current illness and begin to seek alternative methods of dealing with current problems.	Remove patient from "hub of activities" if environment appears too stimulating. Be careful not to overwhelm Carrie by persistently talking about things that make her anxious (parents or her abortion).	Catatonic excitement is a possibility and can be dangerous to Carrie and others in the environment. Other patients in the environment might become extremely frightened and develop feelings of anxiety or hopelessness about their own illnesses.

Nursing Diagnosis	Desired Outcomes	Interventions	Rationale
		Empathize with Carrie's anxiety and how it interferes with her functioning.	An explanation will clarify situations; assist in orienting the patient to reality; encourage communication; engage the patient's thoughts; provide a model for "talking" about feelings; enhance trust.
		Spend a designated amount of time with the patient. Touch Carrie, being sensitive to her comfort level. Convey concern, interest in, and commitment to a different method of communicating (talking about feelings).	Physical presence reassures patient; provides base for reality testing; touch for some patients is effective method of communication; nurse should determine if and when appropriate.

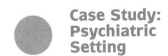

Case Study: Psychiatric Setting

Demographic Data

Name: James (Jimmy) Wilder
Age: 31 years
Address: 1010 Fremount Street, Chicago, IL
Ethnicity: Irish
Religious Preference: None Stated
Referring Agency: Wife and self
Occupation: Professor, Computer Science

Presenting Problem

James, who prefers to be called Jimmy, states that he has begun to isolate himself from colleagues at work and family at home. His productivity at work is slowly deteriorating; he is argumentative and suspicious that his friends and family are planning to harm him. He also states that he recently was a candidate for an important University award, but was not chosen. He thinks that his colleagues sabotaged him. His wife, Mary Wilder, states that Jimmy has lost about twenty pounds in the last two months.

He has, for the past seven months, accused his wife of thirteen years of having an affair with the man next door, and insisted that the entire house be illuminated at night, lest his wife's lover enter the house and "spend time with her."

Jimmy also reported that faces, but not heads, would yell obscene comments at him and threaten to send laser beams through his body if he had sex with his wife. According to Jimmy's wife, he has become increasingly demanding and argumentative. (At 3:00 A.M. recently Jimmy tried to kill his wife. Jimmy agreed to go to the hospital if his wife would also agree to treatment, too; she did.)

At the time of hospitalization, Jimmy stated that he was suspicious about his food, his wife's fidelity, and his neighbors. He believed that laser beams were destroying his body, and the faces with voices, but no heads, had begun to scream louder and louder. The voices also commented on his behaviors as they occurred. Mrs. Wilder commented that Jimmy was having difficulty resting and complained of swelling in his legs. He was frightened, nervous, anxious, and angry. In an effort to deal with these feelings, Jimmy created an elaborate computer within himself which was designed to store and protect information in his brain.

History of Problem

Jimmy is a dedicated professor of computer science. He worked hard to finance his graduate education. In the pursuit of becoming a professor, he worked about sixteen hours each day for several years. He has been successful in producing patents of software he has developed, publishing, and attracting excellent students to his program.

Mary Wilder reported that Jimmy began to show suspicious behaviors about seven months ago when several things seemed to happen all at once: his father died of a heart attack; his department chairman gave him only a fair annual performance rating; and he was not selected for the prestigious University Scholars Award. Jimmy felt that the recipient of the award was not as productive and scholarly as he. Jimmy began to complain to his wife and colleagues that "they are out to stop me."

On occasion, Jimmy would refuse to eat and would yell, "Woman, you are trying to kill me . . . Woman, you are trying to poison me!" He cursed, slammed doors, and entered data into his home computer until the early morning.

He lost a lot of rest because he would watch to see if the neighbor would enter the home to be with his wife. Mrs. Wilder reported that Jimmy seldom mentions the computer that he thinks is in his brain. He does, however, think that his "personal computer" is the one inside his brain, and he would remark, ". . . The best kind to have, you know!"

Psychiatric History

Jimmy does have a history of being somewhat eccentric; he is a loner, is secretive, and easily becomes upset when someone disagrees with him about computers. Mary Wilder reported that when Jimmy was a doctoral student, he thought that his professor was trying to steal his ideas for publication. Jimmy received crisis counseling at the University's student mental health service during the time that he was writing his dissertation.

Family History

Jimmy's father (at age 63) died of a heart attack less than a year ago. He was a property appraiser in a large real estate company in Chicago. Jimmy remembers his father as a driven man, exacting, demanding, and sometimes rejecting. Jimmy's mother (age 64) is alive and works as a secretary in an alcohol rehabilitation center. Mary Wilder reported that Jimmy's mother is a recovering alcoholic, but Jimmy did not corroborate that impression. He has one sister who is a missionary in Central America. They communicate several times each year via mail. Jimmy has twin daughters, Marcia and Molly (age 7). Mary Wilder states that he is fond of "the girls," but makes it clear to them that he does not tolerate noise, questions, and challenges.

Social History

Jimmy states that his mother was kind, but spacey, while his father was always working and demanding. He feels that he had a decent childhood, and enjoyed many creature comforts.

Jimmy was an average student in high school, but began to excel when in college. He received a scholarship for graduate and doctoral studies. Mary Wilder indicates that he is dedicated to his work, and spends long hours at the University, but shows little interest in social contacts.

Supports

Jimmy's mother and wife are his supports. Colleagues at work are potential supports.

Substance Abuse

Mary Wilder states that Jimmy used amphetamines, marijuana, and cocaine during his student days. She is not aware of recent drug use. He does drink bourbon late at night, however, "after the girls go to bed."

Health History

Occasional headaches; treated with aspirin, Tylenol.

Mental Status

Appearance: In pajamas. Composed, articulate, and cautious in speech.
Sensorium: Oriented to time, place, and person; intact memory and recall.
Emotion: Controlled and angry-sounding.
Mood: Fearful and suspicious; hesitant to talk.
Speech: Normal, matter-of-fact type fashion. Slow and monotonous.
Motoric: He is sitting in chair, with legs crossed and arms folded across his chest.
Thought Content: Coherent, but delusional; hallucinations.
Thought Process: Presents thoughts in an organized, controlled, and pressured fashion.
Medications: No prescription medications.
Potential for Violence: Yes. Assess for feelings of anger. Determine a history of violent behavior—any other instances besides attacking his wife? Take necessary precautions.

Summary

This 31-year-old man has a 7-month history of being suspicious about his wife, neighbor, and colleagues at work. He has recently experienced sleep disturbance and has refused to eat because he fears food is poisoned. Jimmy also thinks that he has a personal computer in his head that stores information about patents and research. Jimmy has been successfully employed at the University for eleven years.

DSM-III-R Diagnosis

Axis I: Paranoid Schizophrenia (295.30)
Axis II: Diagnosis deferred.
Axis III: Cramps in legs, and irritation on tongue. Weight loss of approximately 20 pounds in the last two months.
Axis IV: Psychosocial Stressor: 3—Moderate
Axis V: Current GAF: 27, Past GAF: 80

Nursing Diagnoses

*Altered thought processes
Impaired verbal communication
Potential for violence
Altered family processes
Ineffective family coping
Ineffective individual coping
Altered health maintenance
Self-esteem disturbance
Sleep pattern disturbance
Social isolation
Anxiety
*Altered nutrition: less than body requirements

*Nursing diagnosis developed in care plan that follows.

Nursing Care Plan for Jimmy

Nursing Diagnosis	Desired Outcomes	Interventions	Rationale
1. Altered thought processes.	Jimmy will have decreased delusional thinking as evidenced by his ability to discuss anxieties, disappointments, conflicts, and interpersonal difficulties with his wife, neighbors, and colleagues.	Encourage ventilation but do not cross-examine Jimmy; do not become argumentative. Explain all ward routines to Jimmy; provide an orientation to the unit.	Information will assist Jimmy in predicting events and outcomes. Assists in forestalling suspicions.
		Be honest and genuine in all communications. Don't say anything you aren't sure about, e.g., when Jimmy can go home.	Facilitates trust, openness, and encourages the disclosure of honest/genuine expressions from Jimmy.
		Provide positive feedback when Jimmy successfully engages in a reality-oriented activity.	Genuine and positive feedback enhances self-esteem.

Nursing Diagnosis	Desired Outcomes	Interventions	Rationale
	Decreased anxiety, fears, and increased psychological comfort.	Acknowledge the delusions as "real to Jimmy"; then, discuss other methods of approaching problems such as talking about his anxieties.	Demonstrates empathy for Jimmy; enhances trust; encourages communication.
		Do not challenge Jimmy's delusions. Accept them as real to him.	Argument mitigates against trust, increases anxiety, and reinforces Jimmy's notion that his reality is not understood.
		Select an area in Jimmy's experiences that has been free of delusional content and interact with him around it.	The healthy component of the personality needs to be a) identified, b) nurtured, and c) used to connect the patient with reality.
		Do not joke or make mocking and cryptic comments about Jimmy's delusions and other maladaptive behaviors.	His feelings and thoughts are real to him, and cause him anguish and emotional pain. Respect Jimmy and develop a therapeutic alliance with him.
		Restrain any use of sarcasm or wit.	This type of behavior will erode the development of trust, increase anxiety and fears, and provoke hostile behaviors.
		When trust has been established and nurse is comfortable with patient, present more realistic aspects of a situation/event to Jimmy, for example, his not winning the award, and discuss them with him.	Alternative method of viewing the situation/event might be the beginning of self-examination for Jimmy. It must take place within a trusting and non-threatening environment.
		Discuss the delusional content with regard to specific problems experienced and verbalized by patient.	An examination of the delusional content and its connection to real problems can yield an understanding about a) outcome of situation, b) responses from others in the situation, and c) an exploration with patient about how he might handle things differently.

Nursing Diagnosis	Desired Outcomes	Interventions	Rationale
	Jimmy will learn ways of handling anxiety, fear, and low self-esteem that are free of delusions.	Facilitate the expression of anger, guilt, and frustration through ventilation and other forms of expressions (sublimation).	Ventilation of anger/frustration will help relieve the patient of anxiety and tension. Provides nurse with greater understanding of her patient's conflicts.
2. Altered nutrition: less than body requirements.	Jimmy will experience a decrease in suspicions and delusions about food being poisoned and achieve desired body weight.	Provide group eating situations. Use paper plates and cups. Staff members might eat with Jimmy. Provide food in ready-to-serve containers. When possible, encourage Jimmy to assist in preparation and serving of food. Encourage Jimmy to select his own food.	Eating in group might allay thoughts about food being poisoned.
		When possible, establish a comfortable and familiar pattern of eating for Jimmy.	Increases psychological comfort; reinforces a familiar behavior that can be used in recreating additional healthy behaviors.
		Do not threaten Jimmy with intravenous fluids or gastric feedings when food is refused.	Explain, discuss food/delusions, but refrain from stating, "The surgeon will insert a tube in your veins if you don't eat." Such comments might be viewed as hostile, and provoke violent behavior in self-defense.

SUMMARY

Schizophrenia is a functional psychosis characterized by delusions, hallucinations, incoherence, catatonic behavior, inappropriate affect, and chronicity. There are five types of schizophrenia described by the DSM-III-R: catatonic, disorganized type (hebephrenic), paranoid, undifferentiated, and residual.

It has been thought that fewer than 10 percent of patients who experience their first schizophrenic episode will recover completely, however, recent research indicates that the outlook is much brighter. As many as two-thirds have been found to be recovered upon 30-year follow-up. The onset of schizophrenia usually takes place between the ages of 15 and 24, and the illness is equally prevalent among men and women.

The psychodynamic theory of schizophrenia posits that disturbances in the mother-child relationship when the child is between birth and six years of age may provide the foundation for schizophrenia. If an individual does not successfully pass through the various stages of psychosexual development, he may begin to manifest pathological behavior. Most behavioral theories related to schizophrenia focus not on the causes of the disorder, but on principles from behavioral theory that may be used to change the psychotic behavior itself. Biological theories of schizophrenia include genetic theories, biochemical theories, and anatomic theories related to brain hemisphere functioning.

The psychoanalytic approach to treating schizophrenia includes individual therapy, group therapy, milieu therapy, and therapeutic community. Behavioral therapy focuses on resocialization, role performance, reduction of intensity and frequency of bizarre behaviors, and enhancement of support systems in the community. Former biological therapies included malarial therapy, electroshock therapy, psychosurgery, insulin coma therapy, and hydrotherapy. Psychopharmacological therapies include the neuroleptic drugs often given as depot medications.

The family can have great impact on the schizophrenic patient. Five categories of expressed emotions identify the attitude that family members have toward the patient: 1) criticism, 2) hostility, 3) emotional overinvolvement, 4) warmth, and 5) positive remarks. The schizophrenic's illness has great impact on the family as well. The family is responsible for the patient's care, including its cost. The family may feel "tied down" and have little social life as a result. Their dreams and aspirations for the ill family member create frustration in themselves and the patient. There are organizations designed to help the family cope with schizophrenia, for example, the National Alliance for the Mentally Ill.

The treatment setting has changed over the years; many patients are now deinstitutionalized and, unfortunately, homeless. Thus it is now more difficult for mental-health care professionals to reach and treat them. Outpatient services include psychosocial skill centers, community support services, and outreach programs.

The nurse is responsible for helping the patient improve reality testing, monitoring the patient's response to medication, assessing for suicide risk, and monitoring the patient for physical health problems. She may be responsible for case management in the outpatient setting; she is a major source of support for the chronically mentally ill patient and his family.

KEY TERMS

schizophrenia
  catatonic type
  disorganized type
  paranoid type
  undifferentiated type
  residual type
reality testing
schizophreniform disorder
dopamine hypothesis

computed tomography
antipsychotic medications
neuroleptics
high-potency medications
low-potency medications
extrapyramidal side effects

tardive dyskinesia
Parkinson's syndrome
dystonias
anticholinergic side effects
depot medications

Expressed Emotions (EE)
deinstitutionalization
chronic mental illness
homelessness
case management

STUDY QUESTIONS

1. Name and describe the major characteristics of the five types of schizophrenia.

2. What kind of impact can the family have on the schizophrenic patient?

3. Describe briefly the positive and negative aspects of pharmacotherapy with schizophrenic patients.

4. Compare and contrast the theoretical bases of behavioral and psychoanalytic therapy in treating schizophrenia.

5. How has deinstitutionalization affected the chronically mentally ill?

REFERENCES

Aiken, L. (1987). Unmet needs of the chronically mentally ill: Will nursing respond? *Image: Journal of Nursing Scholarship, 19*(3), 121–125.

Alleback, P., Varla, A., Kristjansson, E., & Wistedt, B. (1986). Risk factors for suicide among patients with schizophrenia. *Acta Psychiatr. Scand., 74,* 414–419.

Alleback, P., Varla, A., & Wistedt, B. (1987). Suicide and violent death among patients with schizophrenia. *Acta Psychiatr. Scand., 74,* 43–49.

Albiez-Gibbons, A. (1986). Mental health acuity system: the measure of nursing practice. *Journal of Psychosocial Nursing and Mental Health Services, 24*(7), 16–20.

American Nurses Association (June, 1988). *Nursing case management.* Kansas City, MO: American Nurses Association, 1.

American Psychiatric Association (1987). *Diagnostic and statistical manual of mental disorders,* 3rd ed. Washington, D.C.

American Psychiatric Association (1988). AIDS Policy: Inpatient psychiatric units. *The American Journal of Psychiatry, 145*(41), 542.

Andreason, N. C. (1986). Comprehensive assessment of symptoms and history. Unpublished manuscript cited in Tsuang. Faraone, and Day (1988), Schizophrenic disorders. In A. Nicholi (Ed.). *The new Harvard guide to psychiatry.* Cambridge, MA: The Belknap Press of Harvard University Press.

Anthony, W., & Liberman, P. (1986). The practice of psychiatric rehabilitation: Historical, conceptual, and research base. *Schizophrenia Bulletin, 12*(4), 542–559.

Anthony, W. A., & Nemec, P. B. (1984). Psychiatric rehabilitation. In A. S. Bellack (Ed.) *Schizophrenia: Treatment, management, and rehabilitation.* New York: Grune and Stratton, Inc., 375–414.

Arieti, S. (1974). *Interpretation of schizophrenia,* 2nd ed. New York: Basic Books.

Askren, D. (1987). Family caring for chronic schizophrenic members: An ethnographic study. Unpublished masters thesis, University of Florida, Gainesville, Florida.

Axelrod, S., & Toff, G. (1987). Outreach services for homeless, mentally ill people. *Proceedings of the first of four knowledge development meetings on issues affecting homeless mentally ill people.* Washington, D.C.: The Intergovernmental Health Policy Project, George Washington University, NIMH Contract Number 278–86–0006 (ES).

Ayllon, T., & Haughton, E. (1962). Control of the behavior of schizophrenic patients by food. *Journal of Experimental Analysis of Behavior, 5,* 343–352.

Ayllon, T., & Michaels, J. (1959). The psychiatric nurse as a behavior engineer. *Journal of Experimental Analysis of Behavior, 2,* 323–334.

Bachrach, L. (1984). The homeless mentally ill and mental health services: An analytical review of the literature. In H. R. Lamb (Ed.), *The homeless mentally ill: A task force report of the American Psychiatric Association.* Washington, D.C.: American Psychiatric Association.

Bachrach, L. L., & Lamb, H. R. (1982). Conceptual issues in the evaluation of the deinstitutionalization movement. In G. J. Stahler & W. R. Tash (Eds.), *Innovative approaches to mental health evaluation.* New York: Academic Press.

Baier, M. (1987). Case management with the chronically mentally ill. *Journal of Psychosocial Nursing and Mental Health Services, 25*(6), 17–20, 33, 35.

Baldessarini, R. J., and Cole, J. O. (1988). Chemotherapy. In A. M. Nicholi, Jr. (Ed.), *The new Harvard guide to psychiatry.* Cambridge, Massachusetts: Belknap Press of Harvard University Press, pp. 481–533.

Balint, M. (1942). Contributions to reality testing. *British Journal of Medical Psychology, 19,* 201–214.

Bandura, A. (1969). *Principles of behavior modification.* New York: Holt, Rinehart, & Winston.

Bassuk, E. (Ed.) (1986). Concluding comments. In E. Bassuk & H. R. Lamb (Eds.), *The mental health needs of homeless persons.* San Francisco: Jossey-Bass.

Bassuk, E., & Gerson, S. (1978). Deinstitutionalization and mental health services. *Scientific American, 238*(2), 46–53.

Bassuk, E., & Lamb, H. R. (1986). Homelessness and the implementation of deinstitutionalization. In E. Bassuk & H. R. Lamb (Eds.), *The mental health needs of homeless persons.* San Francisco: Jossey-Bass.

Bassuk, E., & Lauriat, A. (1984). The politics of homelessness. In H. R. Lamb (Ed.). *The homeless mentally ill: A task force report of the American Psychiatric Association.* Washington, D.C.: The American Psychiatric Association, p. 310.

Beebe, J. (1975). Acute inpatient intervention. In C. P. Rosenbaum & J. Beebe (Eds.), *Psychiatric treatment—Crisis/clinic/consultation.* New York: McGraw-Hill.

Bellak, L. (1958). The schizophrenic syndrome: a further elaboration of the unified theory of schizophrenia. In L. Bellak, & P. K. Benedict (Eds.), *Schizophrenia: A review of the syndrome.* New York: Logan Press.

Bellak, L., Hurvick, M., & Gediman, H. (1973). *Ego functions in schizophrenics, neurotics, and normals.* New York: John Wiley and Sons.

Black, D. W., Yates, W. R., & Andreason, N. C. (1988). Schizophrenia, schizophreniform disorder, and delusional disorders. In J. A. Talbott, R. E. Hales, & S. C. Yudofsky (Eds.), *Textbook of psychiatry.* Washington, D.C.: The American Psychiatric Press, pp. 357–402.

Bleuler, E. (1950). *Dementia praecox—the group of schizophrenias.* Translated by J. Zinkin, New York: International University Press.

Brown, G. W., Carstairs, G. M., & Topping, G. W. (1958). The post hospital adjustment of chronic mental patients. *The Lancet, 2,* 685–689.

Buchsbaum, M., & Haier, R. (1987). Functional and anatomical brain imaging: impact on schizophrenia research. *Schizophrenia bulletin. 13,* 1, 115–132.

Crane, G. E. (1972). Prevention and management of tardive dyskinesia. *American Journal of Psychiatry, 129*(4), 446–467.

Caplan, G. (1974). *Support systems and community mental health.* New York: Behavioral Publications.

Carlsson, A. & Lindquist, M. (1963). Effect of chlorotpromazine or haloperidol on the formation of 3-methoxytyramine and normetanephrine in mouse brain. *Acta Pharmacologica et Toxicologica, 20,* 140.

Carson, R., Butcher, J., & Coleman, J. (1988). *Abnormal psychology and modern life.* Glenview, IL: Scott, Foresman/Little, Brown.

Casey, D. (1987). Tardive dyskinesia. In H. Y. Meltzer (Ed.), *Psychopharmacology: The third generation of progress.* New York: Raven Press, 1411–1419.

Coler, M. (1984). I am nursing diagnosis . . . color me DSM-III green: a comparative analysis of nursing diagnoses and diagnostic categories of the Diagnostic and Statistical Manual III of the American Psychiatric Association. In M. Kim, G. McFarland, & A. McLanes (Eds.), *Classification of nursing and diagnoses: Proceedings of the fifth national conference.* New York: C. V. Mosby, pp. 313–324.

Curran, J. P., Faraone, S. V., & Graves, D. (1986). Behavioral family therapy in an acute inpatient setting. In I. A. Falloon (Ed.), *Handbook of behavioral family therapy.* New York: Guilford.

Crosby, R. (1987). Community care of the chronically mentally ill. *Journal of Psychosocial Nursing and Mental Health Services, 25*(1) 33–37, 43, 45.

Crow, T. J. (1980a). Discussion of positive and negative schizophrenic symptoms and the role of dopamine. *British Journal of Psychiatry, 137,* 383–386.

Crow, T. J. (1980b). Molecular pathology of schizophrenia: More than one disease process? *British Medical Journal,* Jan. 12(6207), 66–68.

Curran, J. (1982). A procedure for the assessment of social skills: The simulated social interaction test. In J. P. Curran & P. M. Monti (Eds.), *Social skills training: A practical handbook for assessment and treatment.* New York: Guilford Press. 348–372.

Curran, J., Faraone, S., & Dow, G. (1985). Inpatient treatment of schizophrenia and other psychotic disorders.

In Hersen, M. (Ed.), *Practice of inpatient behavior therapy: A clinical guide.* New York: Grune and Stratton.

Davis, J. M., Schaffer, C. B., Killian, G. A., Kuard, C., & Chan, C. (1980). Important issues in the drug treatment of schizophrenia. *Schizophrenia Bulletin, 6,* 70–87.

DeAlarcon, R., & Carney, M. W. (1969). Severe depressive mood changes following slow release intramuscular fluphenazine injection. *British Journal of Psychiatry, 3,* 564–567.

DeLisi, L. (1987). Viral and immune hypothesis for schizophrenia. In H. Y. Meltzer (Ed.), *Psychopharmacology: The third generation of progress.* New York: Raven Press. 765–771.

DeVane, C. L., & Tingle, D. (1988). Psychiatric disorders. In J. C. Delafuente and R. B. Stewart (Eds.), *Therapeutics in the elderly.* Baltimore, MD: Williams and Wilkins.

Dingman, C., & McGlashan, T. H. (1986). Discriminating characteristics of suicide. *Acta Psychiatr. Scand., 74,* 91–97.

Donaldson, S., Gelenberg, A., & Baldessarini, R. (1983). The pharmacologic treatment of schizophrenia. A progress report. *Schizophrenia Bulletin, 9*(4), 504–527.

Dowhrenwend, B. P. (1975). Sociocultural and social-psychological factors in the genesis of mental disorders. *Journal of Health and Social Behaviors, 16,* 365–392.

Drake, R., & Cotton, P. (1986). Depression, hopelessness and suicide in chronic schizophrenia. *British Journal of Psychiatry, 148,* 554–559.

Drake, R. E., Gates, C., Cotton, P. G., & Whitaker, A. (1984). Suicide among schizophrenics. Who is at risk? *Journal of Nervous Mental Disorders, 172,* 613–617.

Dunham, H. (1965). *Community and schizophrenia: An epidemiological analysis.* Detroit: Wayne State University Press.

Dunn, J. (1977). *Distress and comfort.* Cambridge: Harvard University Press.

Erikson, E. (1963). *Childhood and society.* New York: W. W. Norton Co., p. 273.

Erikson, E. (1968). *Identity: Youth and crisis.* New York: W. W. Norton.

Fagan, C. (1974). Aspects of therapeutic intervention with adolescents. In C. Fagan (ed.), *Readings in child and adolescent psychiatric nursing.* St. Louis: C. V. Mosby.

Flanagan, S. (1978). Behavioral treatment of psychosis. In R. Liberman (Ed.), *Symposium on Behavior Therapy in Psychiatry,* in the *Psychiatric Clinics of North America.* Philadelphia: W. B. Saunders.

Freud, S. (1949). *An outline of psychoanalysis.* Translated by James Strachey. New York: W. W. Norton.

Fromm-Reichman, F. (1950). *Principles of intensive psychotherapy.* Chicago: University of Chicago Press.

Frosch, J. (1983). *The psychotic process.* New York: International Universities Press.

Garber, H. J., Weilburg, J. B., Budnanno, F., Manschreck, T., & New, P. F. J. (1988). *American Journal of Psychiatry, 145*(2), 165–171.

Gelenberg, A. J. (1987). Antipsychotic drugs: Current issues. Syllabus for psychopharmacology course sponsored by the Massachusetts General Hospital and the Harvard Medical School Department of Continuing Education. Boston: October 16–18, 1987.

Gelenberg, A. J. (1984). Psychoses. In E. L. Bassuk, S. C. Schoonover, & H. J. Gelenberg (Eds.), *The practitioner's guide to psychoactive drugs.* New York: Plenum. 167–203.

Glasser, W. (1965). *Reality therapy.* New York: Harper and Row.

Goodman, A., Siegel, C., Craig, T., & Lin S. (1983). The relationship between socioeconomic class and prevalence of schizophrenia, alcoholism, and affective disorders treated by inpatient care in a suburban area. *American Journal of Psychiatry, 140,* 166–170.

Gordon, V. (1982). *Schneiderian first rank symptoms: A distribution profile.* Unpublished master's thesis, University of Florida, Gainesville, Florida.

Gottesman, I., & Shields, J. (1972). *Schizophrenia and genetics: A training study vantage point.* New York: Academic Press.

Gregory, I., & Smeltzer, D. G. (1983). *Psychiatry: Essentials of clinical practice.* Boston: Little, Brown.

Greenblatt, M. (1977). The third revolution defined: It is sociopolitical. *Psychiatric Annals, 7,* 506–509.

Greerson, R. R. (1967). *The technique and practice of psychoanalysis.* New York: International Universities Press.

Harvard Medical School Mental Health Letter (1986). 2, 12, 1–4.

Holden, D., & LeWine, R. (1982). How families evaluate mental health professionals, resources, and effects of illness. *Schizophrenia Bulletin, 8*(4), 626–633.

Hollingshead, A. B., & Redlich, F. C. (1958). *Social class and mental illness.* New York: John Wiley and Sons.

Hooley, J. M. (1986). An introduction to EE measurement and research. In M. Goldstein, I. Hand, K. Hahlweg (Eds.), *Treatment of schizophrenia, family assessment and intervention.* New York: Springer-Verlag.

Intagliata, J. (1982). Improving the quality of community care for the chronically mentally disabled: The role of case management. *Schizophrenia Bulletin, 8,* 655–674.

Johns, C. A., Stanley, M., & Stanley, B. (1986). Suicide in schizophrenia. *Annals of New York Academy of Science, 487,* 294–300.

Kalinowski, L. & Hoch, P. (1973). Theories of somatic treatment. In T. Millon (Ed.), *Theories of psychopathology and personality.* Philadelphia: W. B. Saunders.

Kane, J. M. (1987). Treatment of schizophrenia. *Schizophrenia Bulletin, 13*(1), 133–156.

Kaplan, J., & Sadock, B. (1985). *Modern synopsis of/comprehensive textbook of psychiatry IV,* 4th ed. Baltimore, MD: Williams and Wilkins.

Kaplan, J., & Sadock, B. (1988). *Synopsis of psychiatry: Behavioral sciences clinical psychiatry,* 5th ed. Baltimore, MD: Williams and Wilkins.

Karasu, R. (1977). Psychotherapies: An overview. *The American Journal of Psychiatry, 134,* 8.

Kazdin, A. E., & Bootzin, R. R. (1972). The token economy: An evaluative review. *Journal of Applied Behavior Analysis, 5*(3), 343–372.

Kelly, H. G., Fay, J. E., & Laverty, S. G. (1963). Thioridazine hydrochloride (mellaril): Its effect on the electrocardiogram and a report of two fatalities with electrocardiographic abnormalities. *Canadian Medical Association Journal, 89,* 546–554.

Kety, S., Rosenthal, D., Wender, P. H., & Schulsinger, F. (1978). The biologic and adoptive families of adopted individuals who became schizophrenic: Prevalence of mental illness and other characteristics. In L. C. Wynne, R. L. Cromwell, and S. Matthysse (Eds.). *The nature of schizophrenia: New approaches to research*. New York, NY: Wiley, pp. 25–37.

Kety, S. (1978). Strategies of basic research. In M. Lipton, A. DiMascio, & K. Killan (Eds.), *Psychopharmacology, a generation of progress*. New York: Raven Press.

Kim, Mi Ja, McFarland, G., & McLane, A. (1984). *Classification of nursing diagnosis: Proceedings of the fifth national conference*. St. Louis: The C. V. Mosby Co.

Kolb, L., & Brodie, H. K. (1982). *Modern clinical psychiatry*, 10th ed. Philadelphia: W. B. Saunders.

Kraepelin, E. (1919). *Dementia praecox and paraphrenia*. Edinburgh: E. S. Livingston.

Krauss, J. B. (1989). The three Cs and the chronically mentally ill. *Archives of Psychiatric Nursing*, 111 (2). April, 59–60.

Kuchnel, T. G., DeRisi, W. J., Liberman, R. P., & Mosk, M. D. (1983). Treatment strategies that promote deinstitutionalization of chronic mental patients. In W. P. Christian, G. T. Hannah, & T. J. Glahn (Eds.), *Deinstitutionalization: Strategies for effective transition of clients to the community*. New York: Plenum Press. 246–265.

Lamb, H. R. (1980). Board and care for home wanderers. *Archives of General Psychiatry*, 37, 135–137.

Lamb, H. R. (1984). Deinstitutionalization and the homeless mentally ill. In H. R. Lamb (Ed.), *The homeless mentally ill: A task force report of the American Psychiatric Association*. Washington, D.C.: The American Psychiatric Association.

Leff, J., & Isaacs, A. (1981). *Psychiatric examination in clinical practice*. Oxford: Blackwell Scientific Publications.

Levine, I. S. (1983). Homelessness: Its implications for mental health policy and practice. Presented at the *Annual Meeting of the American Psychological Association*, Anaheim, CA, August 30, 1983.

Levine, I. S., Lezak, A. D., & Goldman, H. H. (1986). Community support systems for the homeless mentally ill. *New Directions in Mental Health Services*. June (30), 27–42.

Levinson, D., & Simpson, G. (1987). Serious nonextrapyramidal adverse effects of neuroleptics: Sudden death, agranulocytosis and hepatotoxicity. In H. Y. Meltzer (Ed.), *Psychopharmacology: The third generation of progress*. New York: Raven Press, pp. 1431–1436.

Liberman, R. P., Marshall, B. D., Marder, S. R., Dawson, M. E., Neuchterlein, K. H., & Doane, J. A. (1984). The nature and problem of schizophrenia. In A. S. Bellack (Ed.), *Schizophrenia: Treatment, management, and rehabilitation*. New York: Grune and Stratton, Inc.

Lidz, T. (1968). Family organization and personality structure. In N. Bell & E. Vogel (Eds.), *A modern introduction to the family*, revised. New York: Free Press.

Lidz, T. (1960). Schizophrenia, human integration and the role of the family. In D. Jackson (Ed.), *The etiology of schizophrenia*. New York: Basic Books.

Lipton, F., & Sabatini, A. (1984). Constructing support systems for homeless chronic patients. In H. R. Lamb (Ed.), *The homeless mentally ill: A task force report of the American Psychiatric Association*. Washington, DC: American Psychiatric Association.

Losonczy, M., Davidson, M., & Davis, K. (1987). The dopamine hypothesis of schizophrenia. In H. Y. Meltzer (Ed.), *Psychopharmacology: The third generation of progress*. New York: Raven Press. 715–726.

Martin, D. (1988). *Personal communication*. Senior staff specialist, American Nurses' Association. Kansas City, Mo.

Maxmen, J. (1986). *Essential psychopathology*. New York: W. W. Norton, Co. 152.

McBride, K., & Mulcare, R. (1986). Peripheral vascular disease in the homeless. In P. Brickner, L. Scharer, B. Conanan, A. Elvy, & M. Savarese (Eds.), *Health care of homeless people*. New York: Springer Co.

McReynolds, P. (1960). Anxiety, perception, and schizophrenia. In D. D. Jackson (Ed.), *The etiology of schizophrenia*. New York: Basic Books, pp. 248–292.

Mead, M. (1953). *Coming of age in Samoa*. New York: Modern Library.

Mears, F., & Gatchel, R. (1979). *Fundamentals of abnormal psychology*. Chicago: Rand McNally.

Mechanic, D. (1986). The challenge of chronic mental illness: A retrospective and prospective view. *Hospital and Community Psychiatry*, 37(9), 891–896.

Meerloo, J. A. M. (1962). *Suicide and mass suicide*. New York: Grune and Stratton.

Meltzer, H. Y. (1987). Biological studies in schizophrenia. *Schizophrenia Bulletin*, 13(1), 77–111.

Millon, T. (1973). *Theories of psychopathology and personality*. Philadelphia: W. B. Saunders.

Modell, A. (1968). *Object love and reality*. New York: International Universities.

Morrisey, J. (1967). The case for family care of the mentally ill. *Community mental health journal, monograph N. 2*. New York: Behavioral Publications. 7–59.

Mosher, L., & Keith S. (1980). Psychosocial treatment: Individual, group, family and community approaches. Special Report *Schizophrenia Bulletin*. Department of Health and Human Services Publication No. (ADM) 81–1064. Superintendent of Documents, U.S. Government Printing Office, Washington, D.C.

Munkvad, I., Fog, R., & Kristjansen. (1976). The drug approach to therapy, long-term treatment of schizophrenia. In D. Kemali, G. Bartholini, & D. Richter (Eds.), *Schizophrenia Today*. New York: Pergamon Press.

Nathan, P., & Harris, S. (1987). *Psychopathology and society*. New York: McGraw-Hill.

National Institute of Mental Health. (1982). A network of caring: The community support program of the National Institute of Mental Health. ADM–81–1063. Washington, D.C.: National Institute of Mental Health.

National Institute of Mental Health. (1986). Schizophrenic disorders. *Research highlights, 1986—Extramural research*. Rockville, MD: National Institute of Mental Health. 1–12.

Neill, J. R., & Kniskern, D. P. (Eds.) (1982). *From psyche to system: The evolving therapy of Carl Whitaker*. New York: Guilford Press.

Nicholi, A. M. (1988). The adolescent. In A. M. Nicholi (Ed.), *The new Harvard guide to psychiatry*. Cambridge: Belknap Press of Harvard University. 637–664.

North American Nursing Diagnosis Association. (1986).

Classification of nursing diagnosis. St. Louis: C. V. Mosby.

Nyman, A., & Johnsson, H. (1986). Patterns of self-destructive behavior. *Schizophrenia Acta Psychiatr. Scand., 73,* 252–262.

Overall, J. E., & Gorham, D. R. (1962). The brief psychiatric rating scale. *Psychological Reports, 10,* 799–812.

Pao, P. (1979). *Schizophrenic disorders*. New York: International Universities Press.

Paul, G. L. (1969). Chronic mental patient: Current status—Future directions. *Psychological Bulletin, 77,* 81–94.

Paul, G. L., & Lentz, R. J. (1977). *Psychosocial treatment of chronic mental patients: Milieu vs. social learning programs*. Cambridge: Harvard University Press.

Peplau, H. (1952). *Interpersonal relations in nursing*. New York: Putnam's Sons.

Pepper, B., Kirshner, M. C., & Rijglewicz, H. (1981). The young adult chronic patient: Overview of a population. *Hospital and Community Psychiatry, 32,* 463–469.

Pothier, P. (1987). The issue of prevention in psychiatric nursing. *Archives of Psychiatric Nursing, 1*(3), 143–144.

Reynolds, E. (1980). Activities of daily living: A needs assessment of chronic schizophrenics. Unpublished master's thesis. University of Florida, Gainesville, Florida.

Ridgway, P., Spaniol, L., & Zipple, H. (1986). Case management services for persons who are homeless and mentally ill: Report from an NIMH workshop, The Center for Psychiatric Rehabilitation, Sargent College of Allied Health Professions, Boston University.

Rifkin, A., & Siris, S. (1987). Drug treatment of acute schizophrenia. In H. Y. Meltzer (Ed.), *Psychopharmacology: The third generation of progress*. New York: Raven Press. 1095–1102.

Rosenbaum, C. P., & Beebe, J. (1975). *Psychiatric treatment—Crisis/clinic/consultation*. New York: McGraw-Hill.

Salamon, I. (1976). Violence and aggressive behavior. In R. A. Glick, et al. (Eds.), *Psychiatric emergencies*. New York: Grune and Stratton, p. 113.

Schafer, R. (1968). *Aspects of internalization*. New York: International Universities.

Schneider, K. (1959). *Clinical psychopathology*, 5th rev. ed. M. W. Hamilton, Translator. New York: Grune and Stratton (originally published, 1958).

Schooler, N., & Carpenter, W. (1983). New drug treatment strategies in schizophrenia. In W. Carpenter & N. Schooler (Eds.), *New directions in drug treatment for schizophrenia*. Reprinted from *Schizophrenia bulletin*. U.S. Department of Health and Human Services. Rockville, MD: National Institute of Mental Health.

Schultz, C. G. (1985). Schizophrenia: Individual psychotherapy. In H. I. Kaplan & B. J. Sadock (Eds.), *Comprehensive textbook of psychiatry/IV, Vol. I*, 4th ed. Baltimore, MD: Williams and Wilkins, pp. 734–746.

Schultz, C. G., & Kilgalen, R. K. (1969). *Case studies in schizophrenia*. New York: Basic Books, Inc.

Schultz, J., & Dark, S. (1986). *Manual of psychiatric nursing care plans*. Boston: Little, Brown.

Sclar, B. (1981). Psychiatric emergencies. In A. W. Burgess (Ed.), *Psychiatric nursing in the hospital and the community*, 3rd ed. Englewood Cliffs, NJ: Prentice-Hall, Inc., pp. 471–487.

Searles, H. (1967). The schizophrenic individual's experience of his world. *Psychiatry, 30,* 119–131.

Seeman, M., & McGee, H. (1982). Treating depression in schizophrenic patients. *American Journal of Psychotherapy, 36,* 14–22.

Seltzer, B. (1988). Organic mental disorders. In A. M. Nicholi, Jr. (Ed.), *The new Harvard guide to psychiatry*. Cambridge, Massachusetts: Belknap Press of Harvard University Press, pp. 358–386.

Silver, J. M. & Yudofsky, S. C. (1988). Psychopharmacology and electroconvulsive therapy. In J. A. Talbott, R. E. Hales, & S. C. Yudofsky (Eds.), *Textbook of psychiatry*. Washington, D.C.: American Psychiatric Press.

Spitz, R. (1965). *The first year of life*. New York: International Universities Press.

Sullivan H. S. (1953). *Interpersonal theory of psychiatry*, (Ed.) Perry and Garvel. New York: W. W. Norton and Co.

Sullivan, H. S. (1962). *Schizophrenia as a human process*. New York: W. W. Norton.

Swonger, A., & Matejski, M. (1988). *Nursing pharmacology*. Glenview, IL: Scott, Foresman/Little Brown College Division.

Talbott, J. A. (1977). Deinstitutionalization: Avoiding the disasters of the past. *Hospital and Community Psychiatry, 30*(9), 621–624.

Talbott, J. A., & Lamb, H. R. (1984). Summary and Recommendations. In H. R. Lamb (Ed.), *The homeless mentally ill, A task force report of the American Psychiatric Association*. Washington, DC: American Psychiatric Association.

Tamminga, C., & Gerlach, J. (1987). New neuroleptics and experimental antipsychotics in schizophrenia. In H. Y. Meltzer (Ed.), *Psychopharmacology: The third generation of progress*. New York: Raven Press, pp. 1129–1140.

Taube, C. A. & Barrett, S. A. (1985). Mental health, United States. Rockville, MD: National Institute of Mental Health.

Todd, B. (1981). Reasons people don't take their medicine. *R.N., 19,* 54–57.

Tsuang, M., Faraone, S., & Day, M. (1988). Schizophrenic disorders. In A. Nicholi (Ed.), *The new Harvard guide to psychiatry*. Cambridge: The Belknap Press of Harvard University Press.

Tsuang, M., & Vandermey, R. (1980). *Genes and the mind—Inheritance of mental illness*. Oxford: Oxford University Press.

Tucker, G. J., Ferrell, R. B., & Price, T. R. P. (1984). The hospital treatment of schizophrenia. In A. S. Bellack (Ed.), *Schizophrenia: Treatment, management, and rehabilitation*. New York: Grune and Stratton, Inc., pp. 175–191.

Ullmann, L. P., & Krasner, L. (1975). *A psychological approach to abnormal behavior*, 2nd ed. Englewood Cliffs, New Jersey: Prentice-Hall.

Van Kammen, D. P., & Gelernter, J. (1987). Biochemical instability in schizophrenia I: The norepinephrine system. In H. Y. Meltzer (Ed.), *Psychopharmacology: The third generation of progress*. New York: Raven Press, pp. 745–751.

Van Kammen, D. P., & Gelernter, J. (1987). Biochemical instability in schizophrenia II: The serotonin and gamma-aminobutyric acid systems. In H. Y. Meltzer

(Ed.), *Psychopharmacology: The third generation of progress*. New York: Raven Press, pp. 753–758.

VanPutten, T. V., & May, P. (1976). Milieu therapy of the schizophrenics. In L. West & D. Finn (Eds.), *Treatment of schizophrenia: Progress and prospects*. New York: Grune and Stratton.

Vaughn, C. E. (1986). Patterns of emotional response in families of schizophrenic patients. In M. Goldstein, I. Hand, & K. Hahlweg (Eds.), *Treatment of schizophrenia: Family assessment and intervention*. New York, NY: Springer-Verlag, pp. 97–106.

Vaughn, C. E., & Leff, J. P. (1976). The influence of family and social factors in the course of psychiatric illness: A comparison of schizophrenia and depressed neurotic patients. *British Journal of Psychiatry, 129*, 125–137.

Warheit, G. J., Bell, R. A., & Schwab, J. J. (1977). *Needs assessment approaches: Concepts and methods*. Rockville, MD: National Institue of Mental Health.

Weinberger, D., Wagner, R., & Wyatt, R. (1983). Neuro-pathological studies of schizophrenia: a selective review. *Schizophrenia Bulletin, 9*(2), 193–212.

Willis, M. J. (1982). The impact of schizophrenia on families: One mother's point of view. *Schizophrenia Bulletin, 8*(4), 617–620.

Wing, J. K. (1978). *Reasoning about madness*. Oxford: Oxford University Press.

World Health Organization. (1975). *Report of the international pilot study of schizophrenia, Vol I.: Results of the initial evaluation phase, Geneva, 1973*. Geneva: World Health Organization.

World Health Organization. (1979). *Schizophrenia: An international follow-up study*. New York: John Wiley and Sons.

Wyatt, R. J., Potkin, S. G., Bridge, T. P., Phelps, B. H., & Wise, D. C. (1980). Monoamine oxidase in schizophrenia: An overview. *Schizophrenia Bulletin, 6*, 199–207.

Yalom, I. (1985). *The theory and practice of group psychotherapy*. New York: Basic Books.

11

ORGANIC MENTAL DISORDERS

JONATHAN T. STEWART

LEARNING OBJECTIVES

After studying this chapter, the student will be able to:

- Define delirium and dementia and describe the difference between the two.
- Describe the primary and secondary symptoms of delirium and dementia.
- Name and describe the major organic mental disorders.
- Discuss the etiologies of the major organic mental disorders.
- Develop teaching plans for families of patients with organic mental disorders which focus on helping them deal with their own emotions.
- Establish nursing diagnoses and develop appropriate nursing care plans for patients with organic mental disorders.

INTRODUCTION

Chapter 7 on mood disorders and Chapter 10 on schizophrenia include mental disorders to which there is no known specific pathophysiology. They are thus referred to as "functional" illnesses. In contrast, there is a large group of mental illnesses with very well-described pathophysiologies, and these are referred to as the **organic mental disorders,** or **organic brain syndromes.** The hallmark of an organic mental disorder is that the associated mental changes are caused by a specific lesion in the central nervous system. This lesion may be structural or chemical.

Patients with organic mental disorders have problems with the intellectual functions such as comprehension, calculation, general knowledge, abstract reasoning, and memory, and language, referred to as a group as **cognitive functions.** They are also sometimes referred to as **higher cortical functions** because they are carried out by the cerebral cortex. (In contrast, functional psychoses are rarely associated with any deficits in intellectual functioning.)

The nurse confronts the health care needs of patients with organic disorders with knowledge about the biological, psychological, and social needs of this population and their families. She provides expert health care in a variety of settings; consults with families regarding comprehensive health care; serves as an advocate for the individual and family; and assists in the promulgation of policy for the elderly and others with organic mental disorders (Abdellah, 1981; Hagerty, 1984; Robinson, 1986).

Robinson (1986) suggests that nurses who care for patients with long-term disabilities, such as organic mental disorders, will need to expand their roles and learn how to become effective case managers; intervene in crisis situations in the home and community; and be proficient in the assessment and management of behavioral, psychological, and physical problems that the patient experiences.

Organic disorders can be found in any age group. The elderly, however, require special attention. The elderly are the fastest growing segment of the population in the United States. It has been estimated that by the year 2030, persons over the age of 65 will comprise approximately 17 to 20 percent of the total U.S. population (Abdellah, 1981). Although the elderly have been portrayed as a homogeneous population, there is evidence that the older adult communities represent a multiplicity of psychosocial, developmental, and interpersonal experiences.

This chapter details a variety of organic mental disorders that the nurse may encounter in patients for whom she might provide nursing care.

The organic mental disorders fall roughly in two categories: acute (referred to as **delirium** or **encephalopathy**) and chronic (referred to as **dementia**). This distinction is important because it has implications for prognosis, treatment, and nursing management.

Organic mental disorders are sometimes referred to as **senility,** which is a misnomer. However, the adjective **senile** is correctly used to refer to an illness occurring in the senium, which means only that the patient's age is greater than sixty years. Thus physicians may refer to "senile cataracts" or "senile changes of the esophagus" without any reference to mental changes.

As a group, the organic mental disorders are perhaps the most devastating illnesses. Acute organic brain syndromes are terribly frightening for family members to witness because they cause behavioral changes in the patient that range from embarrassing to life-threatening. The confusion associated with an acute organic brain syndrome may lead to extreme degrees of combativeness or to dangerously impaired

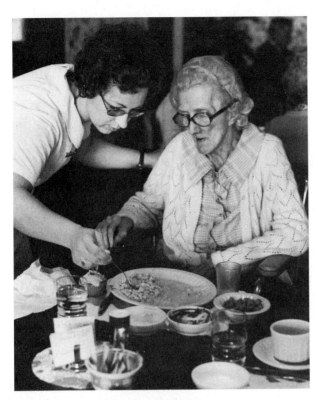

By 2030, elderly persons will comprise approximately one-fifth of the total population in the United States.

judgment. Also in some cases the central nervous system dysfunction may progress to severe morbidity such as aspiration pneumonia or even death. For the family of a patient with a chronic organic mental disorder, the loved one gradually deteriorates to the point of institutionalization and ultimately death.

The differential diagnosis of organic mental disorders includes a wide variety of diseases. There are many different organic mental disorders that may present with the same symptoms but with completely different medical treatments and prognoses. Fortunately, nursing management is fairly similar for most dementias and many deliria. However, this diversity dictates that differential diagnosis is essential in any patient with an organic mental disorder. To diagnose a patient with an organic mental disorder is similar to diagnosing a patient with a "fever"; such diagnoses merely describe symptoms rather than reflecting specific treatable illnesses. In this chapter, the most common forms of organic mental disorders will be discussed in terms of etiology, prevalence, behavior, treatment, and nursing care.

DESCRIPTION OF DELIRIUM AND DEMENTIA

Although the two broad classes of organic mental disorders—acute and chronic—present differently, most deliria are similar in terms of symptomatology, as are most dementias. This underscores the importance of differential diagnosis. (See Box 11–1.)

Table 11–1 highlights the important differences between a delirium and a dementia; however, these distinctions are not as definite in reality as the table might indicate.

An organic mental disorder may evolve over a course of hours (an electrolyte disturbance), days (hepatic encephalopathy), weeks (Wernicke-Korsakoff syndrome), months (hypothyroidism), or years (Alzheimer's disease). The important principle is that the more acute the evolution of an organic mental disorder, the more similar will its presentation be to a classic delirium, and the more chronic, the more similar to a classic dementia.

The acute nature of a delirium makes its presentation quite dramatic, both to family and professionals. The patient will appear obviously sick to family members, manifesting a dramatic change in behavior and abilities as described below. As such, patients with symptoms of acute deliria will always require immediate medical attention.

In contrast, dementias are typically quite insidious and progress slowly. As a result, the diagnosis is obvious only in retrospect, often after several years of cognitive problems. It is common for the family of a patient presenting with Alzheimer's disease to report that the first symptoms appeared as much as four to five years previously. This delay in seeking medical attention may represent denial on the part of the family or the mistaken notion that such changes are normal consequences of aging.

TABLE 11–1 Delirium vs. dementia

Delirium (Encephalopathy)	Dementia
Acute	Chronic
Obviously "sick"	Insidious—obvious in retrospect
Clouded sensorium	Clear sensorium
Confusion	Denial
Often reversible	Often progressive, irreversible

Box 11–1 ● A Loss of Judgment

Neurology and psychology, curiously, though they talk of everything else, almost never talk of 'judgment'—and yet it is precisely the downfall of judgment . . . which constitutes the essence of so many neuropsychological disorders. Judgment and identity may be casualties—but neuropsychology never speaks of them.

And yet, whether in a philosophic sense (Kant's sense), or an empirical and evolutionary sense, judgment is the most important faculty we have. An animal, or a man, may get on very well without 'abstract attitude' but will speedily perish if deprived of judgment. Judgment must be the *first* faculty of higher life or mind—yet it is ignored, or misinterpreted, by classical (computational) neurology. And if we wonder how such an absurdity can arise, we find it in the assumptions, or the evolution, of neurology itself. For classical neurology (like

classical physics) has always been mechanical—from Hughlings Jackson's mechanical analogies to the computer analogies of today.

Of course, the brain is a machine and a computer—everything in classical neurology is correct. But our mental processes, which constitute our being and life, are not just abstract and mechanical, but personal as well—and as such, involve not just classifying and categorizing, but continual judging and feeling also. If this is missing, we become computer-like. . . . And by the same token, if we delete feeling and judging, the personal, from the cognitive sciences, we reduce them to something . . . defective—and we reduce our apprehension of the concrete and real.

From Sacks, Oliver (1987). *The Man who Mistook His Wife for a Hat and Other Clinical Tales.* New York: Harper and Row, pp. 19–20.

The main characteristic of delirium is the **clouded sensorium.** Delirious patients appear confused or bewildered. They are profoundly inattentive and are therefore unable to carry on a conversation or perhaps even answer simple questions. Their attention may shift rapidly from one person or object to another. They misunderstand or misperceive things; this is often frightening to them. These misperceptions may manifest themselves as actual visual illusions or hallucinations (an illusion is a misperception of a sensory stimulus, whereas a hallucination is the perception of a sensory stimulus when there is actually nothing there). Finally, although delirious patients may be unable to give a coherent history, there is usually some evidence that they realize something is wrong with them.

In contrast, patients with dementia are described as having a **clear sensorium.** Although they may misperceive things, they will not usually appear bewildered; their attention span and ability to carry on a conversation are relatively good. As a result, these patients, especially in early stages, do not look "sick." It is common for someone to take a complete medical history from a demented patient and subsequently to

discover, to much surprise, that the patient is quite disoriented, with numerous deficits in cognitive functioning.

Patients with dementia often engage in some degree of **denial.** They are genuinely unaware that there is anything wrong. They will steadfastly deny any problem with memory, for example, and will subsequently confabulate (that is, fabricate answers) or otherwise try to cover up a deficit. They may become quite irritable when any deficit is brought to their attention. Often this denial is quite effective in covering up the illness, giving credence to the idea that the patient is not really "sick."

As a rule, most deliria are reversible with medical treatment, usually dictating a good prognosis. In contrast, most dementing illnesses are progressive and irreversible. Despite this fact, however, skilled nursing management can lead to an improved quality of life.

The following case examples highlight some of the major clinical features of delirium and dementia. The reader should notice that more extensive case studies about selected disorders appear at the end of the chapter.

Mr. Anderson: A Victim of Hepatic Encephalopathy (Delirium)

Mr. Anderson was a 42-year-old man with a long history of chronic alcoholism. He was brought to the hospital by his family after an uncontrollable tantrum in which he smashed a lamp on the floor. The family reported that Mr. Anderson had appeared quite confused for forty-eight hours prior to admission. They stated that he could not carry on a conversation and was at times incoherent. He would occasionally appear to see things on the walls and had screamed "Get it out of here!" as he smashed the lamp. On examination, Mr. Anderson mumbled unintelligibly. He occasionally appeared frightened and constantly shifted his gaze from person to person and place to place in the examining room. Subsequently, the diagnosis of hepatic encephalopathy was made by a neurologist on the basis of elevated liver enzymes. Mr. Anderson responded well to treatment with intravenous fluids and lactulose. Within several days Mr. Anderson's condition cleared, and he stated that he felt "back to normal." He was discharged to his family after ten days of hospitalization, and they reported that he was entirely back to normal at that point.

Mrs. Borelli: A Patient with Alzheimer's Disease (Dementia)

Mrs. Borelli was a 67-year-old woman who was, somewhat reluctantly, taken to her family physician by her daughter, who stated that Mrs. Borelli had been having trouble with her memory. The daughter reported that during the previous six months Mrs. Borelli had had more and more trouble remembering her grandchildren's names. Two days prior to their visit, Mrs. Borelli had forgotten to turn off the stove after cooking something and caused a small fire. Her daughter stated that, in retrospect, she had noted problems with her mother's memory for perhaps two or three years. Originally, these were trivial matters, such as misplacing things or forgetting appointments, but the problem had gradually become more serious. Mrs. Borelli denied any problems, stating that she came in "just to get a checkup." She specifically denied any problems with memory. She was quite pleasant with the nurse and gave a fairly good past medical and personal history, exhibiting no problems at all in attending to the interview. When asked about her living situation during the previous five years, the patient gave a coherent history. However, subsequent discussion with the daughter revealed that numerous details were confused or incorrect. When asked about her memory, Mrs. Borelli denied any problems. When specifically tested, she initially resisted, stating rather angrily, "I told you that there is nothing wrong with my mind." Later, when the examiner asked Mrs. Borelli to repeat three things that he had asked her to remember, she stated, quite angrily, "I didn't bother to remember your stupid things because I don't feel like playing children's games." Mrs. Borelli was subsequently diagnosed as suffering from Alzheimer's disease. Her memory and other cognitive functions continued to deteriorate over the next three years to the point that her daughter could no longer care for her at home, and she was eventually admitted to a nursing home, where she died of aspiration pneumonia six years after the initial visit.

PRIMARY SYMPTOMS OF DEMENTIA AND DELIRIUM

Aside from the above-mentioned differences between delirium and dementia, the symptoms of virtually all organic mental disorders are often similar. It is useful to think of symptoms as either primary or secondary. **Primary symptoms** are the actual cognitive symptoms of an organic mental disorder and are the true essence of the illness. **Secondary symptoms** are adaptive (or maladaptive) responses. Secondary symptoms are far more variable from patient to patient, and even from situation to situation, than are primary symptoms.

Primary symptoms consist of the patient's actual intellectual deficits as well as the difficulties encountered (getting lost, for example) as a direct result. The severity of these primary symptoms mirrors the severity of the organic mental disorder itself. This is not necessarily the case with secondary symptoms. In addition, the nature of primary symptoms may be characteristic of the specific diagnosis. For example, patients with Wernicke-Korsakoff syndrome tend to have more severe memory difficulties, whereas patients with normal pressure hydrocephalus may have more difficulties with bowel and bladder control. Finally, primary symptoms tend to be responsive only to definitive treatment of the organic mental disorder and be less responsive than secondary symptoms to environmental manipulation.

ORIENTATION

Orientation is perhaps the most commonly used barometer of a patient's cognitive functioning. **Orientation** refers to the patient's awareness of time, place, and situation. A person is said to be oriented to time if he can state the approximate time of day (within ninety minutes), the day of the week, the date, month, and year. It should be remembered, however, that orientation to time is subject to many confounding factors. For example, the exact date has far less significance for a self-employed farmer than it does for a bank teller. Furthermore, hospitalized or nursing-home patients, even if not organically impaired, may have an especially difficult time keeping track of the date. Patients in intensive care units may also have a great deal of difficulty keeping track of the time of day and even day versus night, since medications, nursing care, and so forth may be evenly spaced throughout a twenty-four-hour period.

Orientation to place refers to the patient's ability to identify his building and city. This requires much less awareness than time and date and is usually not subject to the same confounding variables as time.

Orientation to situation refers to the patient's awareness that he is in a hospital or clinic and being interviewed and cared for by the nurse. Further details, such as the nurse's or hospital's name, may not be important here, as many normal people have a hard time remembering them.

Orientation is actually a fairly complex function, requiring attention, memory, and intuitive sense of time. It may serve as a convenient longitudinal measure of a given patient's cognitive functioning. However, it must be borne in mind that some organically impaired individuals will remain oriented. Also, it is not at all uncommon to see perfectly healthy people manifest a degree of disorientation to date or time if they are not commonly attuned to date or time (Snyder, 1983).

Typically, as a demented patient deteriorates, he or she first loses track of time and date, followed by place, and finally situation. If the organic process is reversible, orientation returns in the opposite sequence: situation first, followed by place, and finally time (Snyder, 1983).

Mr. Crenshaw: A Patient with Pyelonephritis (Delirium)

Mr. Crenshaw was a 49-year-old man with a history of multi-infarct dementia. He was forty-seven when admitted to the hospital for an evaluation. At that time he could identify correctly the hospital, the city, and the fact that his primary nurse was interviewing him. When asked the date, his answer was incorrect by approximately three months. Following his admission, Mr. Crenshaw deteriorated fairly rapidly. Two days following his admission, he stated that he thought the year was 1958. He was still aware of the city but felt that he was in an apartment house. Within three more days, Mr. Crenshaw would no longer attempt to identify the date or year. He was unaware of the city he was in; he thought that his primary nurse was his wife, and that she was making sexual advances toward him. Eventually, Mr. Crenshaw's rapid deterioration was explained by a urinary tract infection with pyelonephritis. With appropriate antibiotic therapy, he again became oriented to place and situation but still was unable to report the date with an accuracy greater than three months.

MEMORY

Most, but not all, organic mental disorders result in impairment of memory. In this sense, memory refers to the ability to learn new things, such as where the hospitalized patient's room is or the reason for hospitalization. Typically, long-term memory in the organically impaired patient is spared; patients usually have no difficulty remembering their youth or other past events. As a general rule, the more chronic the organic brain syndrome, the more long-term memory will be impaired. For example, a patient who has been delirious for forty-eight hours will probably, if interviewable, exhibit good memory of events up to perhaps three days prior to admission, while a patient with a five-year history of dementia will have very poor recall for events over the past six years or more. Notice that this loss of memory usually precedes the onset of the organic brain syndrome by a relatively brief period of time; this is known as **retrograde amnesia.** In the case of delirium, memory function will return as the delirium itself resolves. However, since memory function was impaired during the period of delirium, the patient will not have registered any new memories during the illness. This explains why delirious patients will often not remember anything about their illness or hospitalization. This distinction between retaining old memories and registering new ones is a very important one. Families may be surprised that with early dementia a demented patient will have markedly impaired recent memory but completely intact memory for the past ("She remembers high school as if it were yesterday, but she can't remember what she had for breakfast").

As memory impairment progresses, the names of people who are important to the patient are forgotten, such as grandchildren and close friends or business associates. At this stage, it is common for the patient to have difficulty remembering entire events rather than simply details. The patient may begin to make dangerous mistakes, such as forgetting to turn off the stove or the bath water. Patients with this degree of memory impairment normally need close supervision for their own safety.

Mrs. D'Angelo: A Patient with Alzheimer's Disease (Dementia)

Mrs. D'Angelo was an 87-year-old woman who had had difficulty keeping appointments and remembering people's names for several years. Two years prior to her admission, she had forgotten to close her front door when she went out to shop, and her house was robbed. Her son and daughter-in-law then encouraged her to move in with them. Her memory continued to worsen; she forgot her daughter-in-law's name with increasing frequency. On two occasions, Mrs. D'Angelo decided to take a bath but subsequently forgot that she had turned on the water. One of these occasions resulted in extensive damage to her son's home. Her condition continued to deteriorate, and she eventually became incontinent. This, coupled with occasional episodes of combativeness, prompted the family to admit her to the hospital for evaluation. A diagnosis of Alzheimer's disease was made, and a program of education for her family was begun. This, combined with antipsychotic medication and referral to a geriatric day treatment program, ultimately enabled Mrs. D'Angelo to return to her son's home.

LANGUAGE FUNCTION

Some organically impaired patients may have difficulties with **language function.** Typically, this behavior begins as a problem with word finding. The patient has difficulty thinking of the names for things, first more infrequently named objects and eventually simpler objects. In the early stages, the patient will describe himself as "having words on the tip of my tongue." He will describe objects rather than naming them, for example, asking for "the stuff in the bottle that you put on your hamburger" rather than "ketchup." This type of naming difficulty is known as **anomia,** and it is a form of **aphasia.** In some patients, primarily patients with Alzheimer's disease, language difficulties may progress to include difficulty in understanding speech as well as difficulty in naming things. As the disease progresses, the patient may have difficulty understanding the simplest of statements. During this phase, the patient is still quite verbal, although his speech at times may not make any sense. The patient himself cannot understand what he is saying.

At this stage the patient may make mistakes with specific words: for example, calling a pencil a "pencip," or calling a cat a "fat." These types of errors are known as **paraphasic** errors. In many of the progressive dementias, such as Alzheimer's disease, this phase may eventually progress to a phase in which the patient begins to lose spontaneous speech and hence becomes more and more mute.

Mr. Ellsworth: A Patient with Alzheimer's Disease (Dementia)

Mr. Ellsworth was a 62-year-old man with a diagnosis of Alzheimer's disease. His family reported that he was having a great deal of difficulty speaking. They stated that he would occasionally become irritable when he could not remember words. He would become angry when he asked his family for "the stuff you put on your steak," and they were not aware that he was asking for salt. This difficulty progressed, and within two years Mr. Ellsworth, although quite talkative, was very difficult to understand. The family felt that Mr. Ellsworth was unable to understand anything at this point, but they were eventually taught that he could follow very simple commands, such as "come here" or "stand up."

VISUOSPATIAL ORIENTATION

Some patients with organic mental disorders have difficulties with what is referred to as **visuospatial orientation.** This means that they have difficulty finding their way around and remembering how they got to a new place. This problem may initially manifest itself as increasing difficulty finding one's way around in unfamiliar places. This, like orientation, is somewhat individual, as many unimpaired individuals have a good deal of difficulty in strange buildings or cities. Most important, then, is whether the patient is having more difficulty than usual. This sort of problem may progress to the point where the patient will get lost in increasingly familiar surroundings.

One dangerous symptom that may arise from a combination of memory problems and visualspatial problems is wandering. Many moderately to severely organically impaired patients will wander, either from home or from the hospital ward. This is an especially difficult problem when it occurs at night, as there is usually less nursing supervision at that time.

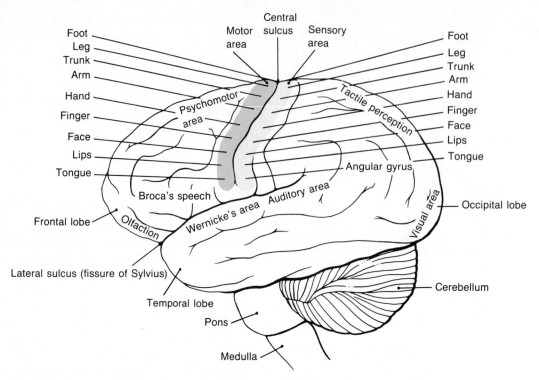

FIGURE 11–1 Topographic Organization of the Brain

Source: Bullock, B., & Rosendahl, P. (1988). *Pathophysiology: Adaptation and alterations in function*, 2nd ed. Glenview, IL: Scott, Foresman/Little, Brown.

Mrs. Farnham: A Case of Pick's Disease (Dementia)

Mrs. Farnham was a 58-year-old woman with a diagnosis of Pick's disease. Throughout their married life, Mrs. Farnham and her husband had enjoyed traveling by car. Mr. Farnham drove while Mrs. Farnham read maps and "navigated." For the past three years, Mrs. Farnham has had increasing difficulty in reading maps and identifying landmarks, at times resulting in the couple becoming lost in unfamiliar cities. Mr. Farnham finally sought hospitalization for his wife when she went out to go shopping one morning and got lost; she was eventually brought home by the police.

During the hospitalization, the diagnosis of Pick's disease was made. Mrs. Farnham returned home, but her condition deteriorated over the next four years. In addition to memory and orientation difficulties, she began to wander outside the house unsupervised. Finally, Mrs. Farnham disappeared one evening and was not found for twenty-four hours. She was found to have fallen over a retaining wall approximately six blocks away, resulting in a fractured hip. Mrs. Farnham was subsequently hospitalized and transferred to a nursing home following hip surgery.

Mr. Gerraghty: A Patient with a Brain Tumor (Dementia)

Mr. Gerraghty was a 37-year-old attorney who, six months prior to hospitalization, began to have difficulty getting dressed. He sometimes put his shirt on inside out or his pants on backward. In spite of this, his work remained as good as ever. He experienced no difficulties with his memory or with his functioning in court. Several weeks prior to his admission, Mr. Gerraghty was called to another city to meet with colleagues. Although he had made this trip several times before, he became lost on the way, having to call for directions twice. Concerned with this sudden change, Mr. Gerraghty made an appointment with his family physician. Since his presentation seemed rather unusual in the absence of other cognitive difficulties, the physician referred Mr. Gerraghty to a neurologist who subsequently hospitalized him. During the hospitalization, a cranial CT scan was performed, which revealed a calcified meningioma pressing on the right parietal lobe. This was excised surgically, and Mr. Gerraghty's recovery was normal. He eventually returned to work, approximately eight weeks post-op, and he has not had any problems since.

FRONTAL LOBE SYMPTOMS

Most organic mental disorders are accompanied by at least some **frontal symptoms,** or symptoms related to dysfunction of the frontal lobes of the brain. These symptoms are difficult to characterize because they may resemble functional psychiatric illnesses such as depression or some personality disorders. Frontal symptoms include difficulties with judgment and reasoning, social sense, personal hygiene, motivation, and emotional regulation. Unlike most functional psychiatric illnesses, bowel and/or bladder control may also be impaired. (See Figure 11–1.)

REASON AND JUDGMENT. The patient with frontal-lobe dysfunction is impaired in the ability to reason or to solve problems. However, this does not relate to memory or other difficulties per se. The patient has difficulty planning and anticipating consequences of his actions. For example, the patient may have a great deal of difficulty playing a simple game of cards because of his inability to develop a strategy and to anticipate the consequences of his play. He will have trouble making appropriate plans for the family finances, such as budgeting or anticipating the need for insurance. Such difficulties with judgment can sometimes be mistaken for disinterest and apathy, or even depression. These types of impairments in reasoning and judgment are especially noticeable in a person who is involved in a profession.

LOSS OF SOCIAL SENSE. Along with loss of reasoning comes a characteristic loss of social sense. The patient with frontal lobe impairment will gradually lose his social grace and intuitive sense of politeness. This may appear initially as inappropriate familiarity with people and progress to greater degrees of tactlessness, such as telling obscene jokes to strangers. The patient may eventually experience even more profound losses of social sense, such as eating with his hands or urinating in public. Again, this may be mistaken for a functional psychiatric illness.

LOSS OF PERSONAL HYGIENE. Another feature of frontal-lobe impairment is the loss of personal hygiene. Just as people have an intuitive sense of tact and social grace, they also have an intuitive sense of cleanliness. This is gradually lost in the frontally impaired patient. He may fail to see the need for showering, sometimes for days or weeks at a time, and be quite resistant when this activity is suggested to him. He may not see any need to shave, comb his hair, or change his clothing daily. As mentioned below, in-continence often is a feature of frontal-lobe impairment: at that late stage, the frontally impaired patient will normally not see the need to clean himself after having an episode of incontinence.

INERTIA. The patient with frontal-lobe impairment experiences an increase in **inertia.** Inertia is the property by which an object, if set in motion, continues in the same way, and if at rest is difficult to get moving. A patient experiencing inertia, once having begun a task, such as brushing his teeth or walking, may have trouble stopping. He may continue to shave the same side of his face repeatedly or write the same words over and over again when drafting a letter. This inability to inhibit repetitive behaviors is known as **perseveration.** More characteristically, the patient may remain at rest and be quite resistant to beginning any new tasks. Frontally impaired patients are frequently comfortable spending days and weeks at a time in bed without doing anything. They may be extremely resistant to getting out of bed to participate in activities, or even to allow themselves to be moved in order to perform routine nursing care. When less impaired, the patient appears unmotivated or stubborn.

EMOTIONAL LABILITY. The patient with frontal-lobe impairment will frequently exhibit an extremely labile mood. He will cry suddenly and easily at things that are only mildly sad, laugh excessively at jokes, and become surprisingly angered at minimal frustrations. These affects typically disappear just as suddenly as they begin. The most severe cases are referred to as **emotional incontinence** and are typically due to a neurological condition known as **pseudobulbar palsy,** which results from frontal lobe impairment or damage. When not labile, this patient's affect may be described as shallow.

INCONTINENCE. People with moderate to severe frontal lobe impairment usually have problems with bowel or bladder control. If noted very early, some patients will report that the urge to urinate comes very quickly and overwhelmingly. These patients learn to hurry to the bathroom as soon as they feel the need. This eventually progresses to frank urinary incontinence, which occurs with increasing frequency. As the patient becomes more impaired, fecal incontinence occurs as well. By this time, the patient's social sense and sense of personal hygiene are usually also impaired and he remains unconcerned with his incontinence (Konstantinides, 1986; Walsh, Persons, & Wieck, 1987; Brown, 1986). This behavior is especially difficult for the family, which is invariably convinced that the loved one is very depressed, becoming psychotic, or, unfortunately, just being lazy and difficult. A good awareness of the nature of this symptomatology is essential in counseling families of these patients.

Mr. Han: A Patient with Normal Pressure Hydrocephalus (Dementia)

Mr. Han was a 48-year-old man who was well until two years prior to his hospitalization. At that time Mr. Han's wife reported personality changes, which she originally attributed to a "midlife crisis," and eventually to depression. Initially, Mrs. Han was concerned that her husband had begun to behave differently in social situations. He would occasionally greet guests in his home wearing an undershirt and boxer shorts, and his wife would have to encourage him to change. Eventually, he began to refuse to change, and on several occasions he made comments to visitors that Mrs. Han felt were quite rude. Soon after this, Mr. Han was fired from his job as a grocery store manager. This was attributed by his employer to his increasingly casual interactions with customers, for example, telling an obscene joke to an elderly woman who had asked him where in the store she could find a loaf of bread. During the next year, Mr. Han had increasingly neglected his personal hygiene. He wore the same undershirt and shorts every day and physically resisted his wife's efforts to replace them with clean clothing. He refused to bathe and spent increasing periods of time in bed, eventually becoming bedridden. At the same time, although he would cry quite easily, Mr. Han denied any problems with sleeping, appetite, or sadness. He would invariably tell his wife, "I just don't feel like doing anything right now." Mr. Han was initially seen by a psychiatrist who prescribed antidepressant medication, which was ineffective. Finally, Mr. Han became incontinent of urine and began to have difficulties walking. Mrs. Han took him to see a neurologist, who admitted him to the hospital. A workup at that time revealed a diagnosis of dementia due to normal pressure hydrocephalus. Mr. Han was subsequently referred to a neurosurgeon who inserted a ventriculoperitoneal shunt. Mr. Han's post-op recovery was smooth and he returned home in three weeks. One year following surgery, a community nurse stated that Mr. Han was no longer incontinent and was spending a major portion of the day working around the house. He was much more conscious of his personal hygiene, although his wife still needed to help him select clothing in the morning. His judgment was still somewhat impaired, and he did not return to work.

SECONDARY SYMPTOMS

The primary symptoms of organic mental disorders described above represent symptoms that arise directly from the patient's intellectual disabilities. The ways in which a patient adapts to these deficits, as well as the maladaptive coping mechanisms that may arise, are quite individual. These may be thought of as the secondary symptoms of an organic mental disorder.

In contrast to primary symptoms, secondary symptoms are quite variable. Whereas the pattern of primary, cognitive symptoms may offer some differential-diagnostic assistance, the pattern of a patient's secondary symptoms reflects individual personality and immediate adaptation to the environment rather than diagnosis. For example, any organic mental disorder may be accompanied by a greater or lesser degree of denial or the presence or absence of psychosis. In addition, while the severity of primary symptoms correlates with the severity of the organic mental disorder itself, the severity of secondary symptoms does not necessarily correlate. Secondary symptoms are usually far more responsive to treatment and management than are primary symptoms, regardless of the underlying pathology.

The organically impaired individual is faced with the difficult task of trying to understand a complicated environment with ever-decreasing cognitive abilities. Obviously he or she cannot correct a cognitive disability, so the only logical strategy that remains is to try to simplify the environment. This is the primary coping mechanism that the organically impaired patient uses. Simplification of the environment involves decreasing the number of changes and unexpected surprises—this is done by rigidly trying to maintain the status quo in the environment. Thus the demented patient manifests progressively increasing **rigidity,** insisting that things always be done in the way to which he is accustomed. He may become upset if dinner is not served at the usual time or in the usual place, or if there are guests in the house. In the hospital, he may become quite upset with a change in his primary nurse, complaining that the new nurse "doesn't do things right." This rigid stance, as grouchy as it may seem, is to be encouraged, since it helps the patient cope with a difficult environment by simplifying it to an acceptable level.

Likewise, many organically impaired patients develop **obsessive-compulsive behaviors** in order to ensure that they are adequately taking care of themselves. A mildly impaired patient may check the door at night five or six times to be sure that he has locked

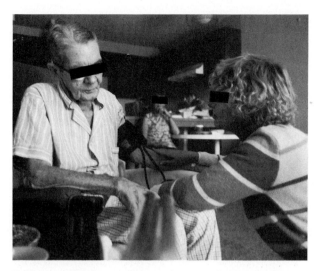

Patients with dementia may become increasingly agitated if things are not done according to their accustomed routine.

it. These are quite good coping strategies and should be encouraged. Encouraging a mildly demented patient to write down obsessively in an appointment book everything he needs to do may extend his ability to function independently by months or even years. Similarly, the nurse or physician may suggest that the patient weekly sort his medications into a compartmentalized pill box, in order to ensure that he neither misses nor repeats doses.

Mr. Isaacs: A Victim of Moderately Advanced Alzheimer's Disease (Dementia)

Mr. Isaacs was a 79-year-old man with moderately advanced Alzheimer's disease. He had been living in a nursing home for three years. One day, several new patients were admitted, necessitating moving Mr. Isaacs to a new room. At first, Mr. Isaacs was angry about the move and protested, to no avail. During the first few days after the move, Mr. Isaacs became quite confused and increasingly disoriented. He repeatedly went in to the wrong room and became enraged when he thought another patient was in his bed. He had difficulty finding his clothing and personal effects, which had been moved to the new room, and repeatedly accused staff members of stealing his clothing. After five days, arrangements were made to return Mr. Isaacs to his original room. This was accomplished quickly, and within a matter of hours all of the above problems had been resolved.

The patient's denial of illness is characteristic of dementia. A person's loss of intellectual functioning represents a far more serious attack on the concept of self than the loss of an arm or even of eyesight. Fortunately, virtually all demented patients exhibit a greater or lesser degree of denial. Far from disguising the problems for social reasons, the demented patient is actually unaware of his or her cognitive difficulties, at least on most levels. When interviewed, he or she will defend this denial by changing the subject, fabricating responses to questions that he or she cannot answer (known as **confabulation**), or by becoming irritable and refusing to answer. The last response may become quite maladaptive; when asked if he is aware of the date, the patient may stand up and state angrily, "I don't have to answer any of your stupid questions." He may then leave the room or even the hospital. Some patients will go as far as walking away from anyone who attempts to talk to them for fear of being unable to respond appropriately. This irritability, coupled with an attempt to flee from the difficult situation, is known as a **catastrophic reaction.**

Mrs. Jimenez: A Patient with Dementia Paralytica

Mrs. Jimenez was a 52-year-old woman with a two-year history of neurosyphilis and memory deficit. She was known to cope with this memory deficit by confabulating. She had been living in a foster care home and had been brought to see her family physician for a fever and productive cough. When her doctor asked about her home situation, she offered a detailed explanation of her penthouse apartment and her job as the director of a television show. When asked to recall three objects that she had been asked to remember, she initially changed the subject, preferring to talk about the "more important" subject of dealing with actors and their agents. When the doctor became somewhat more insistent, Mrs. Jimenez confidently named three completely different objects and then proceeded to discuss further her television career.

Although the secondary, adaptive symptoms that a patient manifests have very little to do with the underlying diagnosis, they do reflect the patient's personality and responses to the environment. For example, a previously obsessive-compulsive person may experience less difficulty with secondary symptoms than most because obsessive-compulsive organization of the environment (writing notes and schedules) will be second nature to him. A patient with a long his-

DSM-III-R Diagnostic Criteria for Delirium

A. Reduced ability to maintain attention to external stimuli (e.g., questions must be repeated because attention wanders) and to appropriately shift attention to new external stimuli (e.g., perseverates answer to a previous question).

B. Disorganized thinking, as indicated by rambling, irrelevant, or incoherent speech.

C. At least two of the following:

1) reduced level of consciousness, e.g., difficulty keeping awake during examination

2) perceptual disturbances: misinterpretations, illusions, or hallucinations

3) disturbance of sleep-wake cycle with insomnia or daytime sleepiness

4) increased or decreased psychomotor activity

5) disorientation to time, place, or person

6) memory impairment, e.g., inability to learn new material, such as the names of several unrelated objects after five minutes, or to remember past events, such as history of current episode of illness

D. Clinical features develop over a short period of time (usually hours to days) and tend to fluctuate over the course of a day.

E. Either (1) or (2):

1) evidence from the history, physical examination, or laboratory tests of a specific organic factor (or factors) judged to be etiologically related to the disturbance

2) in the absence of such evidence, an etiologic organic factor can be presumed if the disturbance cannot be accounted for by any nonorganic mental disorder, e.g., Manic Episode accounting for agitation and sleep disturbance.

---

tory of responding angrily toward others may be relatively more irritable than most. A person who tended to avoid finding fault with himself may use more denial and confabulation than others and be more prone to catastrophic reactions if confronted. A patient in an unfamiliar environment, such as a hospital, or in a very demanding environment, such as a big city or a shopping mall, may require more adaptive behaviors than a patient who is in a more familiar environment, such as at home.

Of course, the above mechanisms, while adaptive, may progress in severity to become maladaptive. For example, a person's rigidity may progress to the point where he cannot tolerate any environmental changes at all, such as a custodian sweeping the floor in his room or a change in medication. Likewise, denial may progress to catastrophic reactions that are so frequent or severe as to prevent effective nursing care. This progression to maladaptive symptomatology occurs when the primary, cognitive symptoms become too overwhelming to compensate for, or when they evolve too quickly to compensate for, as in the case of delirium.

PSYCHOTIC SYMPTOMS AND ORGANIC MENTAL DISORDERS

The classic example of maladaptive behavior in an organic mental disorder is the onset of **psychosis.** Psychosis occurs when, as a result of cognitive disabilities, the patient can no longer understand his environment. He begins to develop an incorrect concept of what is happening and how to deal with it. In contrast to psychotic symptoms associated with functional psychoses, psychotic symptoms associated with organic mental disorders include visual illusions, hallucinations, and simple nonbizarre delusions. Psychotic symptoms arising from organic mental disorders are quite frightening to the patient and should be brought to medical attention as soon as possible. Fortunately, these problems are treatable through environmental manipulation, such as the reduction of irritating stimuli, and/or the administration of antipsychotic medications, such as haloperidol (Haldol) and thioridazine (Mellaril).

The organically impaired patient often responds to the misperceived environment with fear. For example, he may be unable to identify his primary

DSM-III-R Diagnostic Criteria for Dementia

A. Demonstrable evidence of impairment in short- and long-term memory. Impairment in short-term memory (inability to learn new information) may be indicated by inability to remember three objects after five minutes. Long-term memory impairment (inability to remember information that was known in the past) may be indicated by inability to remember past personal information (e.g., what happened yesterday, birthplace, occupation) or facts of common knowledge (e.g., past presidents, well-known dates).

B. At least one of the following:

1) impairment in abstract thinking, as indicated by inability to find similarities and differences between related words, difficulty in defining words and concepts, and other similar tasks

2) impaired judgment, as indicated by inability to make reasonable plans to deal with interpersonal, family, and job-related problems and issues

3) other disturbances of higher cortical function, such as aphasia (disorder of language), apraxia (inability to carry out motor activities despite intact comprehension and motor function), agnosia (failure to recognize or identify objects despite intact sensory function), and "constructional difficulty" (e.g., inability to copy three-dimensional figures, assemble blocks, or arrange sticks in specific designs)

4) personality change, i.e., alteration or accentuation or premorbid traits

C. The disturbance in A and B significantly interferes with work or usual social activities or relationships with others.

D. Not occurring exclusively during the course of Delirium.

E. Either (1) or (2):

1) there is evidence from the history, physical examination, or laboratory tests of a specific organic factor (or factors) judged to be etiologically related to the disturbance

2) in the absence of such evidence, an etiologic organic factor can be presumed if the disturbance cannot be accounted for by any nonorganic mental disorder, e.g., Major Depression accounting for cognitive impairment

Criteria for severity of Dementia:

Mild: Although work or social activities are significantly impaired, the capacity for independent living remains, with adequate personal hygiene and relatively intact judgment.

Moderate: Independent living is hazardous, and some degree of supervision is necessary.

Severe: Activities of daily living are so impaired that continual supervision is required, e.g., unable to maintain minimal personal hygiene; largely incoherent or mute.

---

nurse and fear that this "stranger" in his room is there to harm him.

Mrs. Lewiston: A Patient with Alzheimer's Disease (Dementia)

Mrs. Lewiston was a 92-year-old woman with a ten-year history of Alzheimer's disease. She had lived in a nursing home for eight years. Mrs. Lewiston had trouble remembering the names of her grandchildren. When her eldest grandson came to visit, she failed to recognize him. When he identified himself by name, she said that she didn't have a grandson by that name. When he corrected her, she became quite irritated, accused him of trying to swindle her out of her money, and tried to slap him.

An organically impaired patient may also experience illusions or hallucinations. The most common is a visual illusion; for example, the patient may misperceive a piece of furniture as an animal or a person, or misperceive a medication tablet as an insect. Such illusions can be quite frightening to the patient; they are somewhat common in visually impaired patients and in patients with deliria but can occur in any organic mental disorder.

Mr. Monroe: A Patient with Multi-Infarct Dementia

Mr. Monroe was a 54-year-old man with a five-year history of multi-infarct dementia. He also suffered from mild cataracts. Recently he was admitted to a general hospital for prostate surgery. During his first evening of hospitalization, his nurse, Suzanne, heard Mr. Monroe screaming. When Suzanne went to his room, he demanded that she "get that dog out of my house." Mr. Monroe was pointing to a chair in the corner of the room. Suzanne turned on a light in the room, explaining that the chair did indeed look somewhat like a dog in the dark, and that "lots of people make that kind of mistake." She then left a night light on in the room. Mr. Monroe had no further visual illusions during the hospitalization.

Finally, organically impaired patients may experience the phenomenon known as **sundowning.** Recall that organically impaired patients seek a simple, easily understood environment. If such an environment is provided, they will frequently compensate for their cognitive disabilities quite well. However, it can be difficult to provide an easily understood environment at night. For example, it is difficult for the patient to orient himself visually in the dark. There may be fewer people available in the unit or at home to help orient the patient at night. Finally, there are few orienting cues for the patient at night, such as meals or other specific, time-related activities. As a result, many demented patients function quite well during the day but become more confused and disoriented, and occasionally even psychotic, at night. This change is known as sundowning.

Mr. Noonan: A Patient with Alcoholic Dementia

Mr. Noonan was a 52-year-old man with a five-year history of alcoholic dementia. He had recently become abstinent from alcohol and was living with his brother and sister-in-law. During the day Mr. Noonan stayed fairly active, tending a garden and helping his sister-in-law with housework. However, in recent months he had been waking between 3 and 5 A.M. and wandering through the house. On one occasion, he inadvertently got into bed with his young nephew, who was quite frightened by the experience. On another occasion he wandered out of the house, only to be brought back by the police at 4:30 A.M. At that time, he stated that he was "going to work."

SENILE DEMENTIA, ALZHEIMER'S TYPE

EPIDEMIOLOGY

Currently, three percent of Americans over age 65 and more than nine percent of Americans over age 75 suffer from severe organic brain syndromes (Kramer et al., 1985). Schneck, Reisberg, and Ferris (1982) report that more than four million Americans currently suffer from a moderate to severe dementia, including 58 percent of the one million Americans living in nursing homes. This, coupled with the steadily increasing percentage of people living past age 65, has lead Plum to refer to dementia as "an approaching epidemic" (Plum, 1979). It is difficult to say whether our current health care delivery system will be able to handle this ever-increasing load. Certainly, though, every health care provider must be well-versed in the management of these complex illnesses.

Alzheimer's disease is by far the most prevalent type of dementia, accounting for between 50 and 70 percent of all dementias. The actual prevalence rate for Alzheimer's disease is not entirely clear but is probably around six percent of the population over age 65 (Kay, Bergman, & Foster, et al., 1970). Alzheimer's disease occurs frequently in men and women of all races and socioeconomic groups. The prevalence of Alzheimer's disease gradually increases from age 50 on, plateauing around age 90.

The diagnosis of Alzheimer's disease is usually subsumed under the heading of senile dementia, Alzheimer's type (SDAT) (or **primary degenerative dementia** in DSM-III-R). This is because Alzheimer's disease remains a purely clinical diagnosis; definitive laboratory evidence of Alzheimer's disease is not yet available (at least short of brain biopsy). Thus, strictly speaking, the diagnosis is never completely confirmed until an autopsy is performed. The term SDAT is used because only 98 percent of such patients suffer from Alzheimer's disease, the remaining two percent suffering from the much rarer Pick's disease.

ASSESSMENT OF ALZHEIMER'S DISEASE

Alzheimer's disease has a slow, insidious onset with a very gradual but steady deterioration, usually over five to ten years. Patients typically manifest a variety of primary and secondary symptoms, with no single groups of symptoms predominating. (See Box 11–2.)

Reisberg and his associates (Schneck, Reisberg, & Ferris, 1982; Reisberg, Ferris, DeLeon, & Crook, 1982; Reisberg, 1985) have roughly divided the stages of Alzheimer's disease into three phases: the **forgetfulness phase,** the **confusional phase,** and the **dementia phase.**

In the forgetfulness phase, the patient remains functional, although he or she may occasionally forget the names of people or very specific details about day-to-day experiences. While he or she may experience some difficulties at work, these are not readily apparent to the employer. During this phase the patient will frequently be aware of, and concerned with, memory difficulty. This awareness will often facilitate attempts to adapt to the problem by simplifying the work schedule, maintaining an appointment book, writing lists of things to do, and so forth. While the patient's difficulties are evident to himself, and possibly his spouse, they are not readily apparent to the clinician.

It has recently been shown that about 95 percent of the patients in this forgetfulness phase have a benign longitudinal course at a four-year followup. In other words, while this forgetfulness phase may represent the earlier evidence of dementia, it may not progress further, and hence would indicate a diagnosis of **benign senescent forgetfulness,** a mild, nonprogressive cognitive dysfunction.

In the confusional phase, the patient becomes more objectively dysfunctional, and this is evident to the people around him or her. Performance at work may deteriorate, possibly necessitating forced or early retirement. Likewise, the patient will be increasingly unable to handle responsibilities at home, such as financial planning, preparing meals, or house repairs and maintenance. Travel becomes increasingly difficult, as the patient is unable to adapt to unfamiliar environments. The patient will exhibit more frequent memory loss and will have problems with orientation, perhaps having difficulty finding the way in unfamiliar or partially familiar environments. There may be some problems with word finding, but speech is still fluent. At this point, the patient loses the awareness of memory deficit, and denial becomes more evident. Apart from this, the patient may still appear surprisingly intact to the casual observer. Usually there are no maladaptive symptoms such as psychosis or catastrophic reactions.

In the dementia phase, the patient is obviously quite dysfunctional, even to the casual observer. At this stage, he is incapable of surviving without at least some assistance. He will require assistance with bathing, dressing, and grooming and may also require supervision to prevent wandering off or serious mishaps, such as leaving the stove turned on. He is quite disoriented and may occasionally forget the names of his children or even his spouse. His memory deficit may become so severe as to prevent him from finishing anything that he has started because of an inability to remember what he was doing. During the more advanced part of the dementia phase, more serious language deficits may be noted, such as comprehension problems and, ultimately, mutism. The patient will also begin to manifest incontinence. During the very latest stages of the dementia phase, neurological signs, contractures, and aspiration are noted. The latter is the most common cause of death in these patients.

Far from having a benign course, patients with Alzheimer's disease have three to four times the mortality rates of age-matched controls (Kay, Bergman, & Foster, 1970). Like most other dementing illnesses, Alzheimer's disease is progressive, ultimately resulting in the patient's inability to compensate for

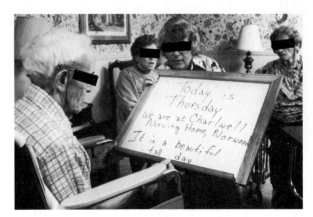

Alzheimer's disease progresses through three phases: forgetfulness phase, confusional phase, and dementia phase. During the more advanced part of the dementia phase, severe language deficits are evident, such as comprehension problems.

Box 11–2 ● Another Name for Madness

In the autumn of 1979, my mother killed the cats. We had seven; one morning, she grabbed four, took them to the vet and had them put to sleep. She said she didn't want to feed them anymore. It occurred to me that she might be going mad.

A few months later, she disappeared. When she returned, after four days, she had no idea where she had been. By now, she, too, knew that something was wrong. Over the next two years, she was subjected to periodic memory tests and physical examinations by a battery of general practitioners, gynecologists, neurologists and other physicians. Day by day, she became more disoriented. She would seem surprised at her surroundings, as if she had just appeared there. She stopped cooking, and had difficulty remembering the simplest things.

Finally, in September 1981, the neurologist who by then was in charge of the case, told my sister, Margaret, what he had suspected for some time: My mother had Alzheimer's disease.

I had heard of Alzheimer's, but I knew little about it. I didn't know that Dr. Lewis Thomas, the science writer and chancellor of the Memorial Sloan-Kettering Cancer Center, has called it "the disease of the century," because, "of all the health problems in the 20th century, this one is the worst."

I didn't know that it ravages the brain so severely that today it is believed to be this country's fourth leading killer. I didn't know that two million American adults are afflicted with it. I didn't know that what looked to me like madness is, in fact, an organic brain disorder which begins with forgetfulness and causes a progressive—and relentless—loss of intellectual and physical functioning. I didn't know that it is irreversible, incurable and virtually untreatable. I didn't know that the doctors would be unable to tell me what causes the disease. I didn't know that I would soon begin to wonder, every time I forgot someone's first name or misplaced my keys, whether the disease could be passed from one generation to the next.

Today, my mother can no longer drive a car. She cannot be left alone. Until my sister locked the phones several months ago, she called the operator or friends many times each morning to ask what day it was. Now she just asks whoever is at the house.

She frequently looks disheveled. Until she recently began to take sedation, she would hallucinate that the television or the toaster was in flames. She repeats the same few questions and stories over and over again, unable to remember that she has just done so a few moments before.

My mother, a college graduate who used to say television "rots the mind," now spends most of her days watching it—literally watching, for she rarely turns on the sound—and smoking cigarettes. When I visit her on Sundays now, I always find her watching one of those disco dance shows. She stares at it and smokes. Until last fall, she had gone 13 years without a cigarette. She cannot remember how much she smokes—and so, she smokes about four and a half packs a day. It is one of the few things she still remembers how to do.

My mother is 54 years old. She has been a widow for almost five years. Soon, within several years, her brain will forget not only what day it is but how to perform what for most people are automatic functions: how to eat, how to walk—in short, how to live.

Source: Marion Roach, *The New York Times Magazine,* January 16, 1983, pp. 22–31. Reprinted with permission.

environmental stresses and intercurrent illnesses. Aspiration pneumonia is the most common cause of death. The sequelae of Alzheimer's disease account for 100,000 to 120,000 deaths annually in the United States, making it the fourth most prevalent cause of death (Katzman, 1976). In spite of this, the diagnosis is only rarely listed on death certificates, with death being typically attributed to pneumonia or cardiorespiratory arrest; physicians seem to think more of the intercurrent illness than the dementia in these cases.

Perhaps the most useful rating instrument for patients with Alzheimer's disease from a nursing standpoint is Reisberg's Global Deterioration Scale (Reisberg, Ferris, & DeLeon, 1982). This scale essentially parallels the description above of the course of Alzheimer's disease and is equally useful in the assessment of other dementias as well. Other rating instruments include Pfeiffer's Short Portable Mental Status Questionnaire (Pfeiffer, 1975) and Folstein's Mini-Mental State Test (Folstein, Folstein, & McHugh, 1975). These are brief, easily administered tests that yield a dementia "score" based on the severity of cognitive impairment.

Dementia can be the most devastating illness that a person may experience. Organic brain syndromes causing behavioral changes that range from embarrassing to life-threatening are terribly frightening for family members to witness. The confusion associated with any organic brain syndrome may lead to extreme degrees of combativeness or to dangerously impaired judgment. To watch a formerly productive loved one gradually and unceasingly deteriorate to the point of requiring institutionalization and ultimately death is one of the most difficult crises that any family faces. (Family issues related to dementia are discussed in more detail on pages 403–415.)

THEORIES OF ETIOLOGY

Prior to the mid-nineteenth century, dementia was not generally recognized as an illness; it was frequently thought of as possession by evil spirits. In 1838, Esquirol first recognized "demence senile" as an illness. Toward the end of the nineteenth century, Kraepelin noted a form of "insanity" that was frequently accompanied by grossly apparent changes in the brain. Finally during the beginning of the twentieth century, Alzheimer discovered the characteristic histopathological changes of Alzheimer's disease, **senile plaques** and **neurofibrillary tangles.** Alzheimer believed that the illness was caused by changes in the arterioles and subsequent ischemia. This was the pre-

dominant point of view until as late as the mid-1960s, at which time Corsellis and Evans proved that patients with Alzheimer's disease have no more atherosclerotic brain disease than age-matched normal controls. At that point it became apparent that Alzheimer's disease was indeed a primary degenerative illness of the central nervous system (Schneck, Reisberg, & Ferris, 1982).

Pathophysiologically, Alzheimer's disease is characterized by a degeneration of neurons in the cortex of the brain. Some actual cortical atrophy may be noted both on CT scan and at autopsy, but this is quite variable. As the neurons degenerate, tangles of abnormal neurofilaments may form in the cell bodies. These are known as neurofibrillary tangles and are quite characteristic of Alzheimer's disease, although they do occur in other illnesses. Abnormal neuronal material may also accumulate around an amyloid core, producing a senile plaque, or neuritic plaque. These are also characteristic of, but not diagnostic of, Alzheimer's disease. Finally, recent research has shown that patients with Alzheimer's disease have a consistent decrease in activity of the neurotransmitter substance acetylcholine. While the significance of this is not clear, much research is currently underway to determine whether patients can benefit from medications that increase acetylcholine activity (Schneck, Reisberg, & Ferris, 1982).

The etiology of Alzheimer's disease remains quite mysterious. It is possible that it is actually a group of diseases with a common pathology. Patients with Down's syndrome invariably develop Alzheimer's disease in the fourth or fifth decade of life; this has suggested the possibility of a genetic component of Alzheimer's disease, perhaps transmitted on the twenty-first chromosome, the chromosome associated with Down's syndrome. The brains of patients with Alzheimer's disease show a high concentration of aluminum in some studies, and Alzheimer's-type changes can be induced in a cell culture by adding aluminum—suggesting a possible toxic etiology. There has also been a great deal of research into the possibility that Alzheimer's disease may be caused by an infectious agent, although this seems doubtful at this time (Schneck, Reisberg, & Ferris, 1982).

TREATMENT OF ALZHEIMER'S DISEASE

Currently, there is no definitive treatment for Alzheimer's disease. While the patient's ability to function can be maximized and any maladaptive secondary symptoms can be managed, no treatment will arrest or reverse the neuronal degeneration or primary symptoms, and deterioration is inevitable. However, research into etiology and treatment, some of it quite promising, continues at a vigorous pace.

Although definitive treatment is not available, there are many interventions that may be quite helpful in the management of Alzheimer's disease and other dementias. These are discussed in the section on "Therapies for Organic Mental Disorders," pages 403–415. (See Box 11–3.)

MULTI-INFARCT DEMENTIA
EPIDEMIOLOGY

Less than ten years in the wake of the discovery that Alzheimer's disease was not related to atherosclerosis, Hachinski and his associates began to describe **multi-infarct dementia** (MID) (Hachinski, Lassen, & Marshall, 1974). In contrast to primary degenerative dementia, multi-infarct dementia is a disease of the blood vessels rather than the neurons and thus is related to atherosclerotic brain disease.

As previously mentioned, perhaps 50 to 70 percent of all dementia is of the Alzheimer's type. The vast majority of the remaining dementias are multi-infarct dementias. While quite frequently difficult to distinguish from Alzheimer's disease, multi-infarct dementia usually exhibits several distinct characteristic features, as described on pages 397–398.

Multi-infarct dementia is predominant among men, which may parallel the increased incidence of atherosclerotic diseases in general in men. It occurs most frequently between the ages of 40 and 60, declining after age 60. This is in contrast to Alzheimer's disease, the incidence of which rises steadily with increasing age, at least to age 90. In contrast to Alzheimer's disease, several illnesses predict increased risk for development of multi-infarct dementia, including hypertension, strokes, diabetes mellitus, and other atherosclerotic diseases. Cigarette smoking may also be a risk factor.

ASSESSMENT OF MULTI-INFARCT DEMENTIA

The clinical course of multi-infarct dementia has been described by some authors as a "step-wise deterioration." In contrast to the steadily deteriorating course

---

Box 11–3 ● Families' Responses to Alzheimer's disease

Families with members that develop Alzheimer's disease may go through a five stage reaction process.

Stage One

The family might recognize some changes in the ill member's behaviors, but react with comments like, "It is due to aging." Such comments may indicate the family's denial and a wish for the ill family member to be well and healthy. Families might fail to recognize gross disturbances and maladaptive behaviors. This denial serves several purposes including: coping against the dread and fear of loss of the individual's previous state of functioning, delaying such a painful experience, and, therefore, delaying comprehensive treatment for the ill member and support and guidance for the entire family. In fact, some families may deny the illness to the extent that they have to be helped by professionals before they are willing to seek help for the ill family member.

Stage Two

When the deterioration of the family member can no longer be denied, the family may become over-involved with its ill member. Such behavior as sacrificing personal life, and neglecting social relationships and individual freedom, becomes the norm. Yet, the family must realistically assess the ill member's ability to care for himself and manage his finances and other affairs. The nurse should recall that family reactions to the ill member are also based on culturally determined factors. Knowledge about the cultural folkways and mores of a particular ethnic group need to be considered, as well as the wishes and desire

of primary degenerative dementia, the course of multi-infarct dementia is characterized by periods of abrupt and rapid deterioration, alternating with more or less long plateaus and even transient improvements. It has been postulated that these abrupt "steps" may represent the occurrence of the lacunar infarcts, tiny thrombotic strokes that are characteristic of the illness. This "step-wise deterioration" is not always readily apparent to the clinician but can frequently be described by a spouse or close relative.

Unlike Alzheimer's disease, multi-infarct dementia tends to be accompanied by relatively more damage to the frontal lobes, at least early in the illness. Thus patients may present with more frontal symptoms than those with Alzheimer's disease—personality changes, emotional lability, and loss of personal hygiene—early in the course of their illnesses. Such changes are typically seen much later in the course of Alzheimer's disease. In addition, as would be expected, the patient with multi-infarct dementia may become incontinent sooner than the patient with primary degenerative dementia.

The differentiation of multi-infarct dementia from primary degenerative dementia is made chiefly by history. However, patients with multi-infarct de-mentia will frequently have minor neurological signs, such as reflex asymmetry or gait changes, early in the course of their illness, and this can help with differential diagnosis as well. Finally, the cranial computerized axial tomography (CT) scan of a patient with multi-infarct dementia will often reveal numerous lacunar infarcts. Magnetic resonance imaging (MRI) and positron emission tomography (PET) scans are also helpful in making the diagnosis.

The same rating instruments used for Alzheimer's disease may be used for assessment of multi-infarct dementia (or any other dementia for that matter). In addition, Hachinski and his associates have developed a rating scale, the Hachinski Ischemia Scoring System, that helps differentiate multi-infarct dementia from SDAT (Hachinski, Lassen, & Marshall, 1974).

THEORIES OF ETIOLOGY

Pathophysiologically, multi-infarct dementia is characterized by numerous small thrombotic strokes, mostly in very small vessels. The strokes, when they occur, are typically too small to produce any clinical symptoms. As more and more of these strokes accrue over a period of years, however, clinical deficits be-

---

of the patient (when possible) and individual family members.

and must be recognized and effectively dealt with.

made, tension, anger, and guilt are likely to surface.

Stage Three

Family members are likely to be angry. This occurs because of the physical and psychological burden associated with care of the ill member; the array of behavior problems that the ill member manifests; and the family's sense of having been abandoned by the afunctional ill member. Frequently, feelings of anger are directed toward the nurse and other health care professionals whose very function is to assist and serve the ill member and his or her family. In such circumstances, the professional must assist the family in dealing with their feelings of anger and rage. Transference and countertransference issues might surface among family and staff,

Stage Four

When anger begins to subside, guilt may surface, sometimes associated with family members' subconsciously wanting the ill member to die. Family members may also feel guilt because they delayed treatment by not having provided more immediate care for the ill member. The nurse and other health professionals should learn to recognize the guilt and effectively assist the family to work toward resolution of these feelings. Family counseling may be indicated when families are confronted with difficult decisions. When different family members, and (in some instances) the patient, disagree with the decisions other family members have

Stage Five

If family members understand the disease process and the myriad of behaviors that the ill member can evidence, they will be more likely to accept the disease that affects the loved one. Resources within the family and in the community can be implemented to assist the family in coping with the burdens associated with care of the ill member.

Source: Adapted from Tusink, J. P., and Mahler, S. (1984). Helping families cope with Alzheimer's disease. *Hospital and Community Psychiatry, 35*(2) 152–156.

come evident. These very small strokes are referred to as **lacunar infarcts** and may often be seen on a cranial CT scan as very small radiolucent "holes." These small lacunar infarcts may often be punctuated by several larger, clinically apparent strokes.

The most important clinical differences between multi-infarct dementia and primary degenerative dementia are summarized in Table 11–2.

TREATMENT OF MULTI-INFARCT DEMENTIA

Management of the patient with multi-infarct dementia is essentially the same as that for the patient with Alzheimer's disease. However, since these patients tend to have more problems with social sense and personality change, family education becomes especially important. It may be difficult for family members to conceive of such changes as being due to a physical illness. Although there is no definitive treatment for multi-infarct dementia, some authors believe that its progression may be retarded somewhat by vigorously controlling hypertension, if it is present (Merritt, 1979).

WERNICKE-KORSAKOFF SYNDROME AND ALCOHOLIC DEMENTIA
EPIDEMIOLOGY

Alcohol abuse is one of the major preventable health problems in the world today. The Surgeon General

Heckler's Report estimates that as many as ten percent of all Americans are alcoholics (U.S. Department of Health, Education, & Welfare, 1979; Secretary's Task Force on Black and Minority Health, 1985). In addition to the psychosocial, hepatic, and other health problems associated with alcoholism, it should be remembered that alcohol is also a potent neurotoxin. Chronic alcohol abuse leads to a number of neurological dysfunctions, including peripheral neuropathy, cerebellar degeneration, and a number of organic mental disorders. Of the latter, the two most important for this discussion are **Wernicke-Korsakoff syndrome** and **alcoholic dementia.**

Wernicke-Korsakoff syndrome is a subacute delirium that typically occurs in advanced alcoholism; it seems to be directly related to a deficiency of thiamine (vitamin B_1). This deficiency leads to a dysfunction of the structures responsible for memory.

Wernicke-Korsakoff syndrome has been rarely seen in recent years, possibly because so many foods are currently enriched with B vitamins. Thus the illness will be seen primarily in relatively malnourished alcoholics.

ASSESSMENT OF WERNICKE-KORSAKOFF SYNDROME AND ALCOHOLIC DEMENTIA

Clinically, Wernicke-Korsakoff syndrome is divided into two parts: Wernicke's encephalopathy and Korsakoff's psychosis. These two syndromes usually occur together. Wernicke's encephalopathy is characterized by gaze palsies and ataxia. The gaze palsies may also be associated with diplopia. Korsakoff's psy-

TABLE 11–2 Primary degenerative dementia vs. multi-infarct dementia

	Primary Degenerative Dementia	**Multi-Infarct Dementia**
Epidemiology	Men and women affected equally	More common in men
	Incidence increases until age 90	Peak incidence age 40–60
	No relationship to previous illness	High correlation with hypertension, stroke
Clinical Course	Steady deterioration	Stepwise deterioration
	Personality changes late	Personality changes early
	Incontinence late	Incontinence early
Dementia Workup	Neurological signs late	Neurological signs earlier
	CT scan normal (may be atrophy)	Lacunar infarcts, strokes on CT scan

chosis refers to a subacute delirium, much like any other delirium, but associated with an unusually extensive degree of memory impairment. Patients will frequently be unable to remember things for more than a matter of seconds.

In addition to Wernicke-Korsakoff syndrome, there is a relatively poorly defined dementia associated with alcohol abuse, known simply as alcoholic dementia. The pathophysiology of alcoholic dementia is poorly understood, but may relate to irreversible toxic damage to the cortex, primarily the temporal lobes. Other researchers believe that alcoholic dementia is a chronic form of Wernicke-Korsakoff syndrome, but the relationship between these two illnesses is not at all clear (Cutting, 1978).

Alcoholic dementia closely resembles primary degenerative dementia, although memory deficits are usually much more prominent in the former. A history of alcoholism is probably the most important differential-diagnostic clue.

TREATMENT OF WERNICKE-KORSAKOFF SYNDROME AND ALCOHOLIC DEMENTIA

Wernicke-Korsakoff syndrome responds rapidly to treatment with parenteral thiamine. Typically, gaze palsies will resolve within a matter of hours of treatment and memory deficits within days. Subsequent to acute treatment, of course, a plan must be developed to aid the patient in maintaining sobriety.

Thiamine is involved in the metabolism of glucose. Quite often an alcoholic will be admitted to a hospital in a dehydrated condition. If rehydrated with intravenous fluids that contain glucose, the result may be a relative deficiency of thiamine, precipitating an acute Wernicke-Korsakoff syndrome. Typically, this problem is avoided by adding vitamins to the intravenous fluid.

In the case of alcoholic dementia, there is no definitive treatment. These patients do not respond to thiamine; management is essentially the same as for a patient with primary degenerative dementia. However, the progression of alcoholic dementia can be arrested or at least slowed by abstinence from alcohol. Therefore, the nursing care plan must provide some mechanism to enforce such abstinence (Bennett, Mowery, & Fort, 1960; Guthrie & Elliott, 1980; O'Leary, Radford, Chaney, et al., 1977; Page & Linden, 1974; Cummings & Benson, 1983). (Also see Chapter 15 on substance abuse.)

NORMAL PRESSURE HYDROCEPHALUS
EPIDEMIOLOGY

Normal pressure hydrocephalus has only been recently described as a type of dementia. It is caused by decreased reabsorption of cerebrospinal fluid, which gradually leads to the enlargement of the lateral ventricles of the brain. Approximately two-thirds of patients with normal pressure hydrocephalus have had some physical problem, usually meningitis, head trauma, or a subarachnoid hemorrhage, that may impede the flow of cerebral spinal fluid. Normal pressure hydrocephalus affects men and women equally, and usually begins prior to age 65. It is probably responsible for two to three percent of all dementias.

ASSESSMENT OF NORMAL PRESSURE HYDROCEPHALUS

Clinically, normal pressure hydrocephalus is characterized by a triad of symptoms: dementia, incontinence, and gait problems. The dementia associated with normal pressure hydrocephalus is quite similar to that of any other dementia, although there may be more frontal symptoms, such as lability and personality change. The dementia also progresses somewhat more rapidly than primary degenerative dementia. Incontinence, first of urine and then of feces, tends to occur early in the course of normal pressure hydrocephalus. Gait problems are somewhat variable but most frequently are characterized by difficulties with automaticity of gait or with turning or stepping over objects.

The presence of this triad of symptoms is quite characteristic of normal pressure hydrocephalus and will usually warrant further investigation. Diagnosis is established by a cranial CT scan, which will reveal dilated lateral ventricles.

TREATMENT OF NORMAL PRESSURE HYDROCEPHALUS

Many patients with normal pressure hydrocephalus improve either partially or completely with the placement of a ventriculoperitoneal shunt, a neurosurgical procedure designed to relieve pressure by draining excess CSF into the peritoneum. This is not a benign procedure; it is associated in adults with a fairly high degree of mortality and failure, and patients are very carefully selected. If the shunting procedure is successful, the progression of the illness will be at least arrested and in many cases reversed. Management of the inoperable patient or the patient who has failed to respond to the shunting procedure is essentially the same as management of any other dementia.

THE METABOLIC ENCEPHALOPATHIES

A number of systemic illnesses may be accompanied by mental-status changes, often involving organic mental disorders. Since most of these conditions, hyponatremia for example, tend to occur quite acutely, the typical picture is that of a delirium or encephalopathy; thus these conditions are usually referred to as **metabolic encephalopathies.** However, there are important exceptions to this generalization. Hypothyroidism, for example, tends to evolve quite slowly and insidiously, leading to the clinical picture of a dementia. Thus, in spite of the use of the term metabolic encephalopathy, it should be remembered that, as with all other organic mental disorders, the more acute the onset, the more the illness will resemble a delirium, and the more chronic, the more it will resemble a dementia.

Many of these metabolic encephalopathies are associated with systemic illnesses, such as peptic ulcer disease and renal failure. Hence they are seen quite commonly in general hospitals. They are also somewhat more common in the elderly, who tend to have multiple systemic illnesses. It is therefore especially important to be aware of these illnesses in the elderly population; not all organically impaired older patients have Alzheimer's disease.

Electrolyte abnormalities consistently produce a variety of delirious conditions. Increases or decreases in sodium, potassium, or calcium levels are the most common electrolyte abnormalities. There may be distinguishing features, such as lethargy or seizures, depending on whether a given electrolyte is abnormally high or low, but the presence of delirium is universal. Treatment consists of correction of the electrolyte disturbance.

Uremia as a result of renal failure is often associated with a typical delirium; this usually occurs only when the uremia is severe. Some authors feel that this uremic encephalopathy is rather unusual in an otherwise healthy patient unless the urea nitrogen is over 100 to 120 mg/dl. Treatment consists of dialysis or other definitive treatment for the uremia itself (Merritt, 1979).

Hepatic encephalopathy is a condition seen in patients with severe liver disease, most commonly alcoholics. The pathophysiology of this illness is not clear, but it probably involves the liver's inability to detoxify nitrogenous waste products. Clinically, the patient manifests a fairly classical delirium, evolving over a period of several days to weeks, eventually progressing to coma. Currently, there is no definitive laboratory test to confirm the presence of hepatic encephalopathy. Treatment involves restriction of nitrogen intake via a protein-restricted diet and the administration of lactulose, which prevents absorption of the nitrogenous materials. The underlying hepatic condition is also treated, if possible.

Hypothyroidism, and to a lesser extent **hyperthyroidism,** may both cause a relatively chronic dementia. These are especially important diagnoses to be aware of—they are frequently overlooked and often lead to an inaccurate diagnosis of Alzheimer's disease. Furthermore, hypothyroidism will frequently present with depressive symptoms, and hyperthyroidism will present with anxiety symptoms, further complicating the diagnosis. The symptoms of dementia in hypothyroidism are strikingly similar to those of primary degenerative dementia. However, other stigmata of hypothyroidism, such as weight gain, cold intolerance, and hair and skin changes, will usually be present as well. Patients with hyperthyroidism will also exhibit dementia, but again, other signs will be present, such as heat intolerance, tachycardia, and tremor. Both illnesses are usually completely curable with appropriate treatment of the underlying thyroid condition.

Vitamin B$_{12}$ deficiency may also cause a chronic organic brain syndrome. It is most frequently seen in patients with gastrointestinal conditions (such as pernicious anemia), with various malabsorption syndromes, and less often with malnourishment. In addition to exhibiting dementia, the patients may have both motor and sensory deficits due to an associated spinal-cord condition known as *subacute combined degeneration of the cord.* The diagnosis is confirmed by a decreased serum B$_{12}$ level, and the illness is readily treatable with B$_{12}$ injections.

There are numerous **iatrogenic** causes of organic brain syndromes. These may occur in any patient but are far more common in the elderly, who have difficulty metabolizing and eliminating medications. Elderly patients with underlying dementias or with mild cognitive dysfunctions (see "Benign Senescent Forgetfulness," below) are probably at greatly increased risk for iatrogenic organic brain syndromes. The most common agent to produce such cognitive impairments are anticholinergic medications, sedatives, and steroids. The most commonly used anticholinergic drugs are atropine, many of the antidepressants, antihistamines, and over-the-counter sleeping pills. Sedative hypnotics are quite frequently prescribed, and occasionally a mildly demented, rigid, obsessive-compulsive patient will erroneously be prescribed a minor tranquilizer such as diazepam (Valium), only leading to further decompensation and perhaps even psychosis. Steroids are not prescribed quite as frequently as anticholinergics and sedatives, but quite frequently cause a delirium or mood disturbance. Diagnosis involves taking a thorough medication history, paying especially close attention to the patient's use of over-the-counter medications or medications prescribed by several different physicians. Treatment consists of removing the offending agent.

Sedative-hypnotic withdrawal syndrome consistently produces a severe delirium and is extremely common. Alcohol-withdrawal syndrome is the most common of these, but barbiturate and benzodiazepine withdrawal are also quite common. (Narcotic withdrawal does not typically produce a delirium.) The patient with this syndrome will present with an agitated delirium, often accompanied by visual hallucinations, tachycardia, hypertension, tremor, and possibly seizures. (See Chapter 15 on substance abuse.) These illnesses, if left untreated, are life-threatening; patients often die in status epilepticus or from circulatory collapse. Diagnosis is established through a thorough history, frequently involving the patient's family and friends. Response to treatment is excellent, involving gradual detoxification with a similar substance and correction of any metabolic derangements that may occur. Chlordiazepoxide (Librium) is most commonly used for alcohol and benzodiazepine withdrawal and phenobarbital for barbiturate withdrawal. Thiamine is also given in the case of alcohol withdrawal, to prevent the development of Wernicke-Korsakoff syndrome.

OTHER CAUSES OF ORGANIC MENTAL DISORDERS

As recently as fifty years ago, prior to the era of antibiotics, syphilis was a true epidemic in this country. In the late stages of the illness the central nervous system is affected in a variety of ways, including **dementia paralytica**, which at one time accounted for as many as twenty percent of psychiatric hospitalizations in this country. Advanced syphilis is relatively rare now, but there are occasional cases. Onset of dementia paralytica usually occurs several decades after the initial infection. It is characterized by a rapidly progressive dementia, leading inevitably to death in three to five years if left untreated. Classically, patients tend to present with personality changes (possibly due to frontal-lobe involvement) and poor personal hygiene as well as grandiose delusions. Treatment consists of high-dose penicillin therapy, typically given intravenously.

Many neurodegenerative diseases (notably Huntington's disease, Wilson's disease, and sometimes advanced Parkinson's disease) are associated with a progressive dementia. Treatment and prognosis depend on the nature of the underlying illness.

There are many less frequent causes of organic mental disorders, including AIDS and other central nervous system infections (bacterial, viral, and fungal), tumors, trauma, post-anoxia damage, collagen-vascular diseases, and heavy metal intoxications. Medical treatment for these disorders is quite variable, while nursing care is similar to that for other organic mental disorders.

PSEUDODEMENTIA

Chapter 9 on mood disorders discusses the broad range of symptoms present in the depressed patient. Depressed patients may suffer from vegetative symptoms, such as sleep and appetite disturbances, as well as symptoms such as anhedonia and hopelessness. In addition to these, the elderly depressed patient may also suffer from cognitive symptoms.

It was believed for many years that the earliest symptoms of dementia were depressive symptoms, supposedly because the patient retained some degree of insight into what was happening to him. Thus when a patient presented with both depressive and cognitive symptoms, it was quite common for him to be diagnosed with an early dementia. In recent years, however, it has been learned that, while a dementia may occasionally masquerade as a depression, it is far more common for a depression to masquerade as a dementia. The latter condition has been termed **pseudodementia** (Kiloh, 1961; Wells, 1979).

Pseudodementia is not an organic mental disorder at all; it is probably best thought of as one of an entire array of depressive symptoms. It is extremely important to be aware of this diagnosis—the patient with a pseudodementia may appear quite similar to a truly demented patient, but be completely curable. Table 11–3 summarizes the important differences between pseudodementia and a true dementia.

TABLE 11–3 Dementia vs. Pseudodementia

Dementia	Pseudodementia
Insidious onset, slow progression	Abrupt onset, rapid progression
Usually no history of depression	Usually positive history of depression
Does not appear depressed	Appears depressed
Denies cognitive problems	Complains of cognitive problems, may feel guilty about them
Confabulates or gives approximate answers	Gives "don't know" answers

Typically, a pseudodementia has an abrupt onset and rapid progression from normal to noticeably demented in a matter of weeks or a very few months. This occurs in marked contrast to other dementias, in which the onset takes place over a period of years and is usually noticed only in retrospect. While some dementias and deliria do present this rapidly, the possibility of a pseudodementia should always be considered.

As mentioned above, patients with a pseudodementia typically appear depressed. They usually complain of other depressive symptoms such as hopelessness, sleep and appetite disturbances, and guilt, and quite frequently have a past history of depression as well. In contrast, a truly demented patient may be somewhat emotionally labile but will only very rarely appear depressed.

Finally, the patient with a pseudodementia lacks the characteristic denial noted in truly demented patients. When asked about cognitive problems, the patient with a pseudodementia usually admits to these, often complaining bitterly about them. Furthermore, he may exhibit some degree of associated guilt, for example, feeling that his memory loss is a terrible burden on his family. When actually tested, the pseudodemented patient will often give many "I don't know" responses to questions, whereas the truly demented patient will either change the subject, confabulate, or give an approximate answer.

Pseudodementia responds quite well to treatment. Since it may be thought of as a depressive symptom, appropriate treatment is the same as the appropriate treatment for the underlying depression, be it a major depression, a dysthymic disorder, or an adjustment reaction. Treatment may thus include tri-cyclic or other antidepressants, electroconvulsive treatments, individual psychotherapy, family therapy, appropriate interventions by a nurse, or, in the case of an adjustment reaction, perhaps simply time.

SENSORY DEPRIVATION

While it does not cause a true organic brain syndrome, **sensory deprivation** may lead to confusion, disorientation, and even hallucinations. This has been referred to as a sensory-deprivation psychosis, or ICU psychosis, since it occurs frequently in intensive care units.

When completely sensory deprived, most normal people have a great deal of difficulty with orientation and may eventually experience auditory and visual hallucinations. Complete sensory deprivation is rather unusual, but partial deprivation occurs fairly often. For example, the patient in an intensive care unit may have nothing to look at but the ceiling and nothing to listen to but the sound of the heart monitor; such a situation is quite disorienting. The patient may have even fewer orienting clues; for example, he may be receiving tube feedings on a 24-hour basis, which eliminates mealtimes. Or there may be no window in his room, thus preventing the awareness of day or night. The nursing staff may rotate shifts so that there are no consistent personnel on any given shift. The patient will almost certainly be disoriented and may appear somewhat confused. The severe medical problems that lead to placement in the ICU also may lead to organic brain syndromes.

Patients with severely impaired vision or hearing also suffer from a degree of sensory deprivation. While they may learn to adapt quite well, they may become quite easily confused, sometimes even to the point of developing delusions. This is far more common in people who have been blind or deaf for only a brief period of time and in people who are otherwise impaired cognitively.

Patients who are already demented or who have benign senescent forgetfulness are especially vulnerable if they become sensory deprived. These patients may become disoriented or agitated quite rapidly if appropriate steps are not taken. Patients with these disorders will find it even more difficult to adapt to losses in their vision or hearing. In general, the more cognitively impaired a patient is, the less sensory deprivation he or she can tolerate. On the other hand, such impaired patients may also have difficulty dealing with sensory overstimulation, as discussed on page 408.

Once identified, treatment of sensory deprivation involves providing the patient with as much visual and auditory stimulation as possible (without overstimulation). Orienting cues, such as clocks and windows, should be provided if possible. Since the avoidance of sensory deprivation is an important part of the treatment of any organic brain syndrome, further treatment strategies will be discussed in the section on treatment on pages 403–415.

BENIGN SENESCENT FORGETFULNESS

One of the greatest challenges of geriatic health care is to distinguish that which is normal for age from that which is pathological. This difficulty leads many clinicians to conclude erroneously that many treatable diseases, such as arthritis and erectile dysfunction, are "normal for old age." Likewise, some clinicians and many lay people consider dementia "normal for old age" and fail to appreciate the need for further diagnosis. The nurse should keep in mind that all organic mental disorders are pathological and dictate diagnosis and treatment. However, one form of cognitive deterioration does represent a normal consequence of aging. This is known as **benign senescent forgetfulness** and was first described by Kral (1962). It is important to distinguish this entity from a true dementia, as the prognosis is quite different.

Benign senescent forgetfulness is characterized by a mild cognitive deficit, mostly involving memory function. The patient maintains insight about his problem, freely discusses his memory problems, and compensates successfully by keeping lists, appointment books, and so forth. In other words, the clinical picture is identical to the forgetfulness phase of a dementia.

The primary distinguishing feature of benign senescent forgetfulness is its nonprogressive course. When followed longitudinally, the memory dysfunction does not progress, nor does the patient lose insight. This longitudinal history, plus a thorough medical workup, is essential for establishing the diagnosis of benign senescent forgetfulness.

Since the course of benign senescent forgetfulness is nonprogressive, patients are not subject to the increased physical morbidity or mortality noted in primary degenerative dementia. However, while benign senescent forgetfulness does not render the patient dysfunctional, it may render him vulnerable to decompensation. Probaby the most important causes of such decompensation are sensory deprivation, iatrogenic problems, and intercurrent illnesses.

Once the presence of benign senescent forgetfulness is established, no definitive treatment is necessary. The patients may benefit from frank discussion of ways to adapt to memory difficulties (such as the use of appointment books). It is especially important to impress on patients and their families that their difficulties do not represent a dementia and will not progress; most patients are somewhat fearful that their condition will deteriorate. Finally, the patients and their families should be made aware of the potential for decompensation. They should be advised that such decompensation is an indicator that something physical is wrong and that they should seek prompt medical attention.

THERAPIES FOR ORGANIC MENTAL DISORDERS
ENVIRONMENTAL APPROACHES

Although some organic mental disorders are curable with appropriate medical treatment, most require long-term management, the major responsibility for which lies with the nurse or primary caregiver.

Once the nurse understands a few basic principles, the environmental management of the organically impaired patient can be extremely rewarding, often resulting in a surprising degree of symptomatic improvement. Treatment of most organically impaired patients involves primarily day-to-day management and manipulation of the environment. The nurse is probably in the best position to work with the patient to maximize his ability to function, thus reaping the greatest rewards from being with the patient. Even following discharge from the hospital or nursing home, the nurse may help the patient to bring these improvements home with him by educating his family members or other caretakers (Snyder, 1983).

Table 11–4 outlines the basic principles for caring for the organically impaired patient. The nurse should be familiar with these principles and be prepared to teach them to family members who will be caring for the patient.

GOALS. Prior to developing any care plan, it is essential for the nurse to develop realistically attainable goals for the patient. For the delirious patient the goals may involve complete remission of the delerium; far more modest goals will be set for most demented patients. Because the primary symptoms in a demented patient will not improve to a great extent,

---

TABLE 11–4 Treating the patient with an organic mental disorder

---

Set realistic goals

Provide a consistent, easily understood environment (reality orientation)

 Provide orienting cues to time—clocks, calendars, windows

 Provide orienting cues to place—signs on doors, maps

 Leave dim light on at night

 Do not allow patient to stare at ceiling for prolonged periods

 Encourage the availability of familiar objects, people, and activities—familiar routines, personal effects, family visits

 Develop a consistent routine—provide the patient with a schedule

 Avoid changes in the routine—room changes, changes in primary nurse, schedule changes (if changes are anticipated, prepare the patient in advance)

 Simplify the sequence of the patient's activities of daily living—try a checklist

 Simplify your own speech patterns:

  Use simple, subject-verb-object structure

  Avoid using pronouns

  Always identify yourself initially

  Stand in plain view of patient

  Maintain good eye contact

  If the patient does not understand, repeat exactly

---

the nurse sets goals that involve the secondary symptoms instead. Some patients may be expected to perform virtually all of their activities of daily living independently, while others may be expected to do little more than to cooperate with toileting and bathing. The determination of appropriate treatment goals can frequently be quite difficult; experience is usually the best teacher. If the nurse sets goals too low, the patient will be deprived of the opportunity to make maximum use of his or her abilities, leading to more rapid intellectual deterioration as well as demoralization. On the other hand, if the nurse sets goals too high, it results in frustration for the patient and disappointment for the family.

As treatment goals are developed, it is important to bear in mind that the demented patient's condition will usually deteriorate; therefore, the nurse must anticipate a gradual modification of goals. It can be quite disheartening for both the nurse and the

patient's family to see progressively less demanding goals first met and then lost. This is to be expected, however, and the nurse should think of treatment goals as being limited time-wise and revise them based on a periodic review of the nursing care plan. Thus a goal may be written as "will dress independently of any assistance until next care plan review," rather than simply "will dress independently of any assistance." If the nurse formulates treatment goals in this way, the expected progression of disability is reflected as a progression of the disease process itself, rather than as a failure on the part of the nurse or patient (Snyder, 1983).

ENVIRONMENTAL MANIPULATION. As previously mentioned, rigidity and obsessive-compulsive behavior are important adaptive mechanisms used by the organically impaired patient. Far from being pathological, these mechanisms are attempts to simplify the environment. Herein lies an essential principle in the care of patients with organic mental disorders: *Make the environment simple for the patient to understand.* Situations which are difficult to understand or which are ambiguous, such as schedule changes and unannounced trips, should be kept to a minimum. Everything should be explained to the patient repeatedly in a very simple, straightforward manner. Likewise, the environment should contain redundancy; in other words, there should be several ways for patients to orient themselves to where their rooms are or what time of day it is (Snyder, 1983; Steele, Lucas, & Tune, 1982; Trockman, 1978).

The most important technique for maintaining orientation is **reality orientation.** Reality orientation involves the nurse repeatedly reminding patients of the date, the time, where they are, what is happening around them, and any important upcoming events. This is not as easy as it sounds, however. If this information is simply stated, it may remind some patients of their disability and they may take offense, sometimes quite emphatically. Thus it may be difficult to present this information while at the same time conveying the appropriate degree of respect for the patient. Often the best solution is to work the orienting material into a casual conversation. For example, the nurse may say, "Since it is Tuesday, your doctor will be making rounds later this afternoon," or "We usually give medicines at 7:00 A.M. here at the County Hospital." Often such reality orientation can be quite subtle, and the nurse may wonder if it has been effective if the patient does not acknowledge it. The organically impaired patient listens attentively for such information, however, and the technique is quite effective. The important principle is to make the information available without implying to the patient that it is necessary.

Sensory deprivation is the greatest enemy of organically impaired patients because it robs them of orienting cues and promotes misperceptions. One important strategy to combat this is to provide a light in the patient's room at night. This should be bright enough so that the patient can figure out where he or she is and not misperceive objects in the room. However, it should not be bright enough to give the appearance of daytime. This nightlight is the primary treatment for the sundowning syndrome, described previously.

The demented patient may be kept in bed for prolonged periods of time because of illness, or because of resistance to getting out of bed. This is quite common in a hospital setting, and is surprisingly common in nursing homes and even at home. This is an extremely sensory-depriving situation and should be avoided as much as possible. Instead, a patient should be seated in a dayroom or hallway, or even outdoors, to provide adequate sensory stimulation. If the patient is ambulatory, he or she may be encouraged to take walks in areas in which he is not likely to become lost. If the patient must remain in bed, then sensory stimulation, such as a view, pictures, and personal effects, will help him or her remain oriented. The organically impaired patient at bedrest needs more human contact and reality orientation than the mentally normal patient. The nurse should expect to spend far more time with this patient, although family members, volunteers, and even other patients may also help to provide the necessary contact.

A familiar environment is obviously easier to cope with than a new, unfamiliar one. Thus an organically impaired patient will function best at home and have the greatest difficulties in a hospital or a new nursing home. The demented patient should be kept at home for as long as possible. However, circumstances eventually necessitate the patient leaving home, either temporarily or permanently, and the presence of familiar objects and people in the unfamiliar environment will aid in this transition.

Most people are accustomed to a specific daily routine. They may prefer to shower before or after breakfast, or to watch television at specific times during the day. By their very nature, hospitals and nursing homes tend to change these routines. However, the organically impaired patient will fare much better if as much of his or her usual routine as possible can be maintained. This usually does not significantly inconvenience anyone, and a seemingly insignificant change in "routine procedures" may help the patient a great deal. The nurse should actively seek such information by asking the patient about his or her normal routine, then working to conform to these patterns as much as possible. When it is not possible to conform, the nurse should repeatedly explain the new routine to the patient to help him learn it, at the same time acknowledging that it is indeed different from his usual routine. She may say, "I know that you are used to bathing in the evenings, but here at the County Hospital, patients bathe at 8:00 A.M., right after breakfast." She repeats this statement daily until it becomes a part of the patient's new routine. At the same time, the nurse is acknowledging that this is a new routine to learn and implying that any difficulties in getting used to the new routine are normal and to be expected. Allowing this degree of denial is far more adaptive than disruptive.

In addition to trying to maintain a familiar routine, the presence of familiar objects may be quite reassuring to the organically impaired patient. Personal effects, mementos, and photographs are especially useful and should be well within the patient's view. Besides providing a somewhat more familiar, less frightening environment, these personal articles may also serve as starting points for conversations with the patient (Davidhizar, Gunder, & Wehlage, 1978; King, 1982).

Family members provide the most familiar presence for the organically impaired patient. For the organically impaired patient living in an increasingly confusing world, the consistent presence of known and trusted family members is invaluable. This is doubly important when circumstances necessitate removal of the patient from his home. Cultural attitudes toward this vary greatly. In many Eastern societies, for example, advancing age is highly revered and respected, and families naturally care for their elders who become demented. Many highly industrialized societies such as the United States, however, respect instead youth and productivity with a tendency to avoid the elderly or demented patient (Butler, 1979). This may lead family members to become quite reluctant to visit their organically impaired relative. In spite of this, continued family involvement with the organically impaired patient must be encouraged. This may be quite simple or virtually impossible and may at times require the involvement of the nurse, the physician, the social worker, the psychologist, or any number of other health care professionals (Cobe, 1985).

As previously mentioned, a consistent routine is essential in the treatment of the organically impaired patient. Once this routine is established, it should be followed as consistently as possible. In addition, it is helpful to provide the patient with a schedule. This should be easily read and understood, and should reflect the patient's daily activities. This can be as effective at home as in a hospital or nursing home.

Any change in the patient's routine is to be avoided. For example, demented patients will invariably have a great deal of difficulty if their room is changed, whether at home or in an institution. Besides having difficulty finding their room, patients may become more disoriented and even psychotic following a room change. This may even apply to bed changes in the same room. Thus, if room reassignments become necessary, organically impaired patients should have high priority for keeping the same room, even if they are considered quite stable medically.

Likewise, personnel changes can be quite difficult for these patients. The patient's primary nurse should not change, if at all possible, nor should the physical therapist, recreational therapist, physician, and so on. This is obviously much more difficult in an acute hospital setting.

Of course, some changes in the routine are inevitable. These may include visits to the doctor, relatives coming for a weekend, a surgical procedure, transfer to a new ward, or a variety of other things. When these changes are anticipated, it is important to prepare the patient well in advance. This becomes a modification of the usual reality-orientation technique. The patient will be frequently reminded of the upcoming change for several days prior to its taking place. Often the patient will be reminded as much as four or five times a day for an entire week. The patient's feelings about the upcoming change should also be explored. Once the change does take place, it should be repeatedly acknowledged as a change from the usual routine. Of course, it is not always possible to anticipate changes and prepare the patient in advance, and in those cases the patient will require a great deal more reassurance and reality orientation following the change.

Organically impaired patients usually have difficulty with carrying out a sequence of tasks. For example, a patient may try to shave before plugging in an electric razor. The nurse can simplify any sequential tasks that the patient will be performing by eliminating unnecessary steps. For example, if a male patient shaves himself, his razor can be left plugged in, and he may not need to use aftershave. The patient's clothing may be laid out for him in the morning, eliminating his need to make a decision about what

to wear. Clothing itself can be made simpler for such patients: Velcro fasteners are easier to handle than shoelaces, and pullover shirts are easier than shirts with buttons. In general, the patient's room can be arranged to eliminate complicated sequences of tasks. This arrangement may involve a degree of apparent disarray, such as leaving the patient's razor and toothbrush next to the sink rather than in the medicine chest, but it will enable the patient to remain maximally independent with his activities of daily living (Snyder, 1983).

The nurse can also provide the patient with a checklist to help with complicated tasks. For example, a list of personal hygiene tasks to perform every morning or a list of steps involved in heating a prepared meal can help the patient complete these tasks alone. Such checklists can be specific or general, much like a list of chores, depending on the patient's level of cognitive impairment. This is actually just an extension of the appointment book system (Snyder, 1983).

Many organically impaired patients have some difficulty with language function. Even if not truly aphasic, patients may have a problem with complex sentence structures. Very long or complicated sentences also require a certain degree of memory to comprehend fully. Bartol (1979) has developed a number of excellent suggestions to help enhance the patient's comprehension. For example, the nurse can make an effort to use very simple sentence structure, that is, subject–verb–object. The patient is apt to misunderstand more complicated sentences and sentences involving many small connector words. Also, it may be difficult for the organically impaired patient to follow the use of pronouns. Although at first a bit awkward, avoiding the use of pronouns may dramatically increase comprehension. Questions should be simply put and answerable with "yes" or "no" if possible.

When speaking with such impaired patients, it is important for the nurse to identify herself initially, even if she has only been gone for a matter of minutes. While speaking, the nurse should stand in plain view and maintain good eye contact. This will help to maintain the patient's attention and will also provide the patient with valuable nonverbal communication. Finally, if the patient does not seem to understand, the nurse may repeat a question or statement verbatim as many times as it takes for the patient to understand. This provides the patient with additional opportunities to understand what is being said; such repetition does not usually irritate the patient (See Table 11–5) (Bartol, 1979).

TABLE 11–5 Guidelines for nurse-patient communication in dementia

I. Verbal
  A. Speech construction
    1. Short words.
    2. Simple sentences (not compound or complex).
    3. No pronouns; only nouns.
    4. Begin each conversation (particularly at night) by identifying yourself and calling the person by name.
  B. Speech style
    1. Speak slowly.
    2. Say individual words clearly.
    3. If you increase your speech volume, *lower* the tone; raise the volume only for deafness, not because you do not get a response you understand.
    4. If you ask a question, wait for a response.
    5. Ask only one question at a time.
    6. If you repeat a question, repeat it exactly.
    7. Utilize self-included humor whenever possible.

II. Nonverbal (facial motion, torso position, upper extremity gestures)
  A. General
    1. Convince yourself that your nonverbal style can be felt all the way across the room and by several people, not just by the patient or staff person you are addressing.
    2. Make sure that every verbal communication is delivered with proper nonverbal gestures.
  B. Specific
    1. Stand in front (or directly in the line of vision) of the person.
    2. Maintain eye contact.
    3. Move slowly.
    4. If the person starts or continues to walk while you are talking to him, do not try to stop him as your first move. Instead keep moving along in front of him and persevere.
    5. Use overemphasis and exaggerated facial expression to emphasize your point, particularly if vision or hearing is impaired.

III. General Guidelines
  A. Listen actively. If you don't understand, say you don't understand and ask for a repetition of the statement. If this request precipitates a catastrophic reaction, offer your best guess. If you receive a "no," try another guess. Continue until resolution.
  B. Assume there is capability for insight. If someone refuses to join an event she normally engages in, assume she has become sad, angry, frustrated, embarrassed, or anxious about her condition. Your first job is to check to see if that is so—not just to ask, "Are you okay?" or some such ritualistic question.
  C. Chart all phrases and nonverbal techniques utilized that consistently "get through" for a particular person and a particular situation. Use one another's techniques. Compare notes on successes and failures.
  D. When encouraging participation in activities, regulate your exuberance according to the following criteria: If you push the patient beyond a certain point you may precipitate a catastrophic reaction, and you must have planned your time and energy so that you can now treat the reaction with verbal and nonverbal techniques.
  E. When possible, utilize an observer to watch your exchange, make suggestions, and perhaps trade off with you. If you have not really "gotten anywhere" in 5 minutes or less, you will probably do better to leave and either return in 5 minutes or have a colleague try.
  F. If you say you are going to do something, *do it*. If you forget, find the person and apologize. Assuming that the person has forgotten the episode insults both your intelligence and his.
  G. If you need to stop a patient–patient interchange, do it firmly and quickly, get the participants out of each other's territory, wait 5 minutes, and then return and explain to each one why you acted as you did. Use factual explanations, not guilt induction.

Source: Bartol, M. A. Nonverbal communication in patients with Alzheimer's Disease. *J. Geront. Nurs.* 5:21–31, 1979. Page 23. Reprinted by permission.

COGNITIVE STIMULATION. Another major principle in the treatment of the organically impaired patient is to maintain adequate cognitive stimulation. In poorly managed institutional settings, the demented patient has very little stimulation, if any. There may be little recreational activity, the daily routine being essentially limited to meals and personal hygiene. In the face of this lack of stimulation, patients may deteriorate intellectually quite rapidly. Furthermore, such deterioration, coupled with the inevitable sensory deprivation, may lead to an increased incidence of psychotic symptoms. An appropriate environment for the organically impaired patient will provide a good deal of intellectual stimulation.

It is extremely important to maximize reasonable expectations of the patient. The hospital staff should encourage the patient to remain as independent as possible. Often, it is much faster and more convenient for the nurse to assist the patient with tasks, but the patient will fare better if he can be allowed to handle as much as he can on his own. If a patient who can dress himself independently is assisted daily, he will soon be unable to dress without assistance. Of course, as the patient's condition deteriorates, he will inevitably require increasing amounts of assistance. The principle here is not to prevent such inevitable decline but to retard it and to maximize the patient's abilities at any given time (Cowdry, 1968).

The optimum environment for the demented patient will provide an appropriate degree of stimulating activities. These may include various social and recreational activities as well as groups. Current events groups and reminiscing groups (see below) are especially useful. Patients should also be encouraged to continue involvement with hobbies, and may, in fact, develop new hobbies in an optimal setting. Patients may also benefit from occasional changes in the environment. For some patients this may involve a limited degree of travel, usually day trips, and for others brief outings to restaurants or shopping centers, or walks outdoors. Television and movies may also provide a degree of intellectual stimulation, but these are best used in moderation because they provide minimal opportunity for social interaction.

In general, the best type of intellectual stimulation for the demented patient is interpersonal contact. Therapy and other types of groups provide this type of contact quite well, as do churches and social organizations such as the Knights of Columbus or the American Legion. Many patients are uncomfortable in large groups, however, and may need some encouragement to join. Another solution is to provide socialization on a smaller scale, such as family visits and involvement of volunteers. Many communities have a form of "foster grandparent" program in which children or adolescents regularly visit older or demented patients. These programs are generally quite helpful.

Reminiscing therapy is a relatively new innovation in the care of the aging or demented patient (King, 1982) and may be executed individually or within a group. Reminiscing therapy encourages the patient to discuss his past experiences. Sometimes

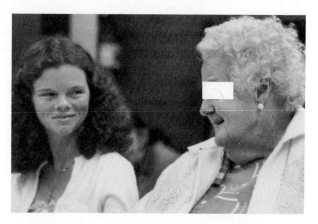

The best type of intellectual stimulation for a demented person is interpersonal contact. One example of interpersonal contact is the "foster-grandparent" program, designed to encourage contact between children/adolescents and elderly/demented persons on a routine basis.

personal effects or photographs may serve as starting points for discussion. Any health care professional can easily master this technique. Many people have the mistaken notion that the demented patient "lives in the past," and that this is harmful. Actually, the process of positive life review is essential to the aging process; it is a great source of self-esteem. In addition, it will be remembered that the demented patient will normally have intact memory for the past. People enjoy sharing their experiences with other people, and reminiscing therapy may provide tremendous interpersonal success and satisfaction for even the most demented patient (King, 1982).

It is essential to monitor the patient closely for signs that intellectual stimulation has been excessive. This may manifest itself as irritability, refusal to participate in activities, or even catastrophic reactions or psychosis. Experience is an excellent teacher in gauging just how much stimulation is adequate and how much is excessive for a particular patient (Trockman, 1978).

Above all, it is essential to remember which of a patient's symptoms are adaptive and which are maladaptive. The nurse should not attempt to decrease a demented patient's rigidity or compulsivity, as these are important adaptive coping mechanisms. Frequently, people accuse a demented patient of being "too set in his ways," and attempt to remedy the situation by bombarding the patient with changes in the usual routine. Of course, this results first in a great deal of irritability, followed by decompensation and catastrophic reactions. Contrary to what many people believe, it is essential to encourage the patient to *remain* set in his ways, or even to become *more* set in his ways.

Likewise, a certain degree of denial is normal in all dementing conditions and is probably adaptive. This may account for the fact that demented patients do not generally become severely depressed. The nurse learns not to confront this denial, no matter how overwhelming, unless it is actually dangerous to the patient. For example, a patient who insists that he is going to enroll in law school as soon as he leaves the nursing home need not be confronted unless he is about to walk out of the nursing home to enroll or to send money for tuition. Nor does the nurse "humor" the patient by discussing the law school curriculum with him. It is usually best to sidestep such comments. If denial does become dangerous, it is still preferable to confront the patient in an indirect, face-saving way. For example, rather than saying, "You can't go to law school because you are too sick," the nurse may say, "I know you're looking forward to going to law school, but you really shouldn't go today because your family will be coming to see you." This type of indirect confrontation works most of the time. (For an outline describing appropriate cognitive stimulation, see Table 11–6.)

FAMILY EDUCATION

The organically impaired patient and his or her family have profound effects on each other (Robins, Mace, & Lucas, 1982). Family members care for demented patients far more often than nurses: Contrary to popular belief, the majority of demented patients are cared for in the home by family members. Thus the family usually represents the greatest single resource available for caring for the organically impaired patient. Even in a nursing home setting, the family may provide a great deal of care to the patient through their interactions as well as through actual physical care such as feeding, dressing, and so on (Pitt, 1982).

The emotional and physical burden of caring for a demented family member can be overwhelming. There have been numerous reports of depression in the spouses of demented patients, and one recent study indicated that as many as 87 percent of family members caring for a demented relative reported problems such as chronic fatigue, anger, and depression (Robins, Mace, & Lucas, 1982). Caring for the demented patient involves constant vigilance, day and night, and physically difficult work (Robins, Mace, & Lucas, 1982; Snyder, 1983). Unlike nurses, family

TABLE 11–6 Nursing measures for enhancing cognitive stimulation

Encourage patient to function as independently as possible

Provide stimulating activities—groups, recreational activities, hobbies, some limited travel

Provide as much interpersonal contact as possible

Consider reminiscing therapy

Closely monitor patient to avoid inadvertent overstimulation

Do not discourage rigidity and obsessive-compulsive behavior

Do not confront denial, unless actually dangerous to the patient

Be alert to the possibility of intercurrent illnesses

Provide education and support for family members

members have not been trained in dressing, bathing, and transferring patients. Also, the family, unlike the nurse, works 24 hours each day.

As difficult as the physical burden may be, the emotional burden of such care is far more overwhelming. Family members may become depressed, almost as a form of chronic grieving, over the patient's gradual and inevitable decline. They will become frustrated as, in spite of their best efforts, the patient gradually loses abilities. They may experience guilt, feeling that their care is not good enough. Or, more commonly, they may feel angry about being burdened with this monumental task and guilty about their anger. This anger may also be displaced on other family members, on health care providers, or even on the patient himself. When the anger is displaced on the patient, it usually manifests itself as feelings that the patient is not really sick or not trying hard enough. Comments such as, "He can dress himself if he wants to," are quite indicative of such feelings. This type of comment may also indicate denial of an otherwise devastating reality (Pitt, 1982).

On the other hand, families may overindulge the patient as a result of their guilt. This may take the form of intellectual understimulation, which leads to further decline. More important, overindulgence can literally exhaust the family, leading to further anger or less effective care for the patient. Sometimes a family member will quit his or her job to care for the patient, resulting in insurmountable financial difficulties (Pitt, 1982).

Usually emotions are very strong and unstable in such a difficult situation. Families may be ambivalent about important decisions such as financial guardianship and nursing home placement and may have a great deal of difficulty in deciding (Hogstel, 1981). Family members may also be bitterly divided about decisions.

Superimposed upon all of these problems, there is, invariably, a tremendous fear of the unknown. Family members are concerned about what will happen to the patient, whether they will be able to care for him, and what will happen if they are not able. As a result, in attempts to master these fears, they may alternately cling to false hopes and prematurely view the patient as terminal (Eisdorfer, Cohen, & Veith, 1980).

The nurse or other health care professional can do a great deal to remedy these problems by working with the family. Family education will help allay fears, making the family feel more in control. It will help them anticipate problems before they arise and develop rational solutions that will be in the patient's best interest. By helping the family to see the situation more realistically, guilt and frustration may be alleviated. The family will also learn new ways to perform routine care and new sources of assistance, thus decreasing their burden. Above all, this education may help promote a better relationship between the patient and his family, temporarily or permanently forestalling the need for nursing home placement or other placement outside the home (Steele, Lucas, & Tune, 1982).

The nurse who works with the family of a demented patient should quickly identify who the patient's primary caregiver will be. While all family members will be involved in the educational process, the nurse will concentrate on developing the closest alliance with this primary caregiver. The nurse should at all times be viewed as supportive and available, and should be quite frank, open, and willing to discuss the patient's disease and its prognosis. At the same time, the nurse should focus more on the patient's remaining abilities than his progressing disabilities, so as not to imply utter hopelessness. She also focuses on the family's emotional reaction to their situation, remaining constantly alert for signs of emotional difficulties that may be maladaptive for family members or dangerous to the patient. She may refer serious difficulties to a psychiatric nurse clinical specialist, psychiatrist, psychologist, or family therapist (Hogstel, 1981). The primary focus of the nurse is to assist the family in a practical way with decisions and difficult situations (Hogstel, 1981).

The nurse begins with a frank discussion of the nature of the patient's illness. The family should know what the nature of the illness is, what to expect, and, perhaps more important, what not to expect. The patient's current abilities and disabilities should be discussed as well as a general idea of what will happen with these disabilities over time. The nurse discusses openly any specific problems that the family will face, but not so far in advance that the patient is made to seem worse than he actually is. If the patient is exhibiting behavioral problems, such as frontal lobe or psychotic symptoms, the nurse discusses these in detail with the family. These are often extremely difficult for a family to understand, and such discussion will prevent them from seeing the patient's behavior as purposeful or "bad."

It is often difficult to determine appropriate goals and demands for the patient. This is even more difficult for inexperienced and emotionally involved family members than it is for a skilled nurse. Therefore, a great deal of family education will involve very specific discussion of appropriate goals for the patient. These, of course, will be gradually modified. At the same time, the primary caregiver may be taught a variety of specific nursing skills. The extent of this will be based on the amount of time and skill that the caregiver has as well as other family resources (Taylor & Ballenger, 1980).

Most important, the primary caregiver must learn all of the management strategies for providing a consistent environment and appropriate cognitive stimulation, as described in the previous section on "Environmental Approaches." These are not intuitively obvious to the lay person and are perhaps more important to convey than any other nursing skill. This should be approached quite practically, with specific suggestions in mind. These suggestions should be tailored individually to the patient's home environment and the family situation. Often, home visits may be helpful in facilitating this.

The nurse may also refer the family to appropriate agencies for assistance. In many cities, geriatric day-treatment programs and other programs for demented patients are available through churches or the community mental health system. These are quite useful, providing both intellectual stimulation for the patient and free time for the family. As the family's resources are increasingly tapped, the family may be referred to sources of financial support, such as the Social Security system, or to housekeeping or meal-preparation services. Sources of assistance for patients with specific disabilities, such as blindness or paralysis, should not be overlooked. Finally, the nurse may refer the family to one of the many support groups available for families of demented patients, so that family members can obtain more emotional support. These groups are usually run by other family members of demented patients who are extremely supportive and knowledgeable about available resources.

As the patient's condition deteriorates, and demands on the family and the need for skilled nursing care increase, the nurse will discuss with the family the possibility of placing the patient in a nursing home. Usually the family has already considered this and has general feelings and ideas about it. It is usually a good idea to discuss nursing home placement in advance, before the need becomes urgent. Specific criteria that the family will use for nursing home placement, as well as the selection of a nursing home and the financial and logistical arrangements, should be discussed openly (Hogstel, 1981).

The demented patient functions best at home as a result of the familiar environment and the presence of family. Quite often, however, the patient will reach a point at which he or she can no longer be cared for at home. At this point, the family may begin to seriously consider nursing home placement. Besides skilled nursing care, the nursing home will provide a safe environment and twenty-four-hour supervision for the patient, things that are quite difficult to provide at home. The ideal nursing home will also provide the appropriate degree of cognitive stimulation for the patient as well as a constant, understandable environment.

Every family has a different set of unspoken criteria for seeking nursing home placement. These criteria vary tremendously from family to family and reflect, among other things, the amount of physical and emotional burden that the family can tolerate. These criteria are very much culturally determined but are also influenced by other obvious factors, such as the number of family members available to help, the financial situation, the patient's symptoms and medical needs, and even the physical layout of the home. It is helpful to think of the family as having a sort of "nursing home threshold" which, if exceeded, will incite the family to seek placement.

The family's "threshold" must be respected at all times. While it is important to discuss nursing home placement, it is equally important not to attempt to coerce a family into or out of seeking placement. If the family is coerced into premature nursing home placement, a tremendous amount of guilt and ill feelings may result. Talking a family out of nursing home placement may have even more serious consequences; typically, the family feels even more burdened, feeling

that the clinician cannot be relied upon as a source of support. Family members may begin to feel a great deal of anger and frustration, which may be displaced onto the patient. Any discussion of the family's thoughts about nursing home placement must be conducted with the patient's best interests in mind, remembering always that the maintenance of a good family support system is very much in the patient's best interest (Reichel, 1978).

Quite often, families seek nursing home placement on an emergency basis. This usually results from the occurrence of an especially dangerous or disturbing behavior, such as incontinence, wandering away from home, or accidentally starting a fire. Such an emergency situation is, of course, undesirable, as it deprives the family of valuable time to discuss nursing home placement with each other, make financial arrangements, and find the ideal nursing home. Sometimes these situations are unavoidable, but quite often they can be anticipated and dealt with well in advance. This underscores the importance of family education (Hogstel, 1981).

As nursing home placement becomes a consideration, other alternatives should be explored. Quite often, the patient will not require any extraordinary level of care, but the family will gradually become exhausted. In these cases, providing a break in the family's unending responsibility may prove to be an effective option. Other family members should be considered as resources, either for several hours during the day or for several weeks or months once or twice a year. If this is not an option, some nursing homes provide **respite programs** in which patients are admitted for a few weeks, several times per year. Such periods of respite allow family members to regain their strength. Family members are encouraged to take vacations and spend time relaxing and caring for themselves.

Most communities have some form of geriatric day-treatment program, either through churches, the local community mental health center, or organizations such as the Older Americans Council. These programs have the dual benefits of providing the proper degree of cognitive stimulation while supervising the patient for several hours per day, thus allowing the primary caregiver valuable respite time, both for other duties and for relaxation. Although they do not provide the same degree of stimulation, often a variety of other resources available in the community can provide several hours a day of supervision for the patient.

Besides respite, families attempting to care for a demented patient at home will usually need a variety of other services. Besides caring for the demented patient, the family has the added burden of having to assume those responsibilities that the patient himself can no longer meet. Thus, housekeeping, shopping, financial planning, and home-repair services may be helpful to the family. The family will often be in need of financial assistance as well, due to medical costs and loss of income (both the patient's and often the primary caregiver's). A social worker may make these types of referrals. The patient may also be in need of some degree of skilled nursing care. In these cases a visiting nurse can often be provided, either through the local health department or a private agency.

If it becomes evident that the patient will need to be placed outside of the home, then a number of less restrictive alternatives may be considered. One such alternative is a supervised apartment, which typically provides meals, laundry, and housekeeping services, as well as scheduled activities. Supervised apartments may have nurses available 24 hours per day, as well as physician coverage. In some facilities, nurses make rounds daily and dispense medications. Another option to be considered is foster care. Larger foster homes are well staffed, with good supervision twenty-four hours per day. They may also provide some assistance with personal care, as well as meals and housekeeping. However, they do not provide skilled nursing care.

Once the family has decided on nursing home placement, several other tasks remain, perhaps the most difficult of which is informing the patient. This responsibility lies with the family, although the nurse or other clinician may be invaluable in providing support and guidance. Patients frequently resist nursing home placement, but this often relates more to fear of a major change in the environment than to fear of the nursing home itself. Therefore, several weeks of advanced preparation and perhaps visits to the proposed nursing home may be helpful. In addition, numerous other arrangements need to be made prior to nursing home placement. These include selection of a nursing home (one close enough to family members to allow frequent visits), financial arrangements, and a variety of legal arrangements. The nurse, along with the social worker (if there is one involved), may be of great help with many of these arrangements.

Above all, it should be remembered that the decision to seek nursing home placement is a difficult one, associated with a great deal of guilt and ambivalence on the part of the family. Once the decision is made, it must be consistently and wholeheartedly supported. It is essential for family members to feel that they have done the right thing for the patient,

and this must be reinforced. At this difficult time a trusting, nonjudgmental relationship with the nurse may be the greatest asset that the family has.

In conclusion, while it is not actually psychotherapy, this process of family education may afford dramatic results for the families of patients suffering from organic mental disorders. At the same time, it can significantly improve the patient's quality of life by offering him a stronger and more knowledgeable support system.

SOMATIC ISSUES

THE MEDICAL WORKUP. The medical workup (which is almost identical for the delirious or demented patient) is usually performed by a neurologist, a psychiatrist, or an experienced primary care physician. The workup may be performed on an outpatient basis, although it is somewhat more convenient to admit the patient to the hospital for a brief period of time. The workup consists of a thorough medical history, usually given both by the patient and by family members. The history will also include a complete review of the patient's current medications including over-the-counter medications. This is followed by a complete physical examination, with extra attention given to the neurological examination and an examination of cognitive functions. The latter consists of simple tests for orientation, memory, language function, and so forth. Appropriate lab work includes a complete blood count, assessments of serum glucose, electrolytes, liver enzymes, urea nitrogen, and creatinine, as well as vitamin B_{12} and folic acid levels, tests for thyroid dysfunction and collagen-vascular diseases, and a test for syphilis. Other appropriate tests may include a cranial CT or MRI scan, a lumbar puncture, an electroencephalogram, and possibly referral to a psychologist for detailed neuropsychological testing (Sabin, Vitag, & Mark, 1982). This entire workup is relatively inexpensive and noninvasive and will ultimately lead to a specific diagnosis and treatment plan.

MEDICAL COMPLICATIONS. Like anyone else, patients with organic mental disorders are apt to become ill from time to time. The likelihood of this is, of course, increased in the very old or profoundly demented patient and poses a number of special problems. Because demented patients often do not receive adequate attention, intercurrent illnesses may be overlooked. Their complaints may be glossed over as merely a product of their dementia or may not be treated aggressively enough because the patient is perceived as "hopeless." In addition, health care professionals may undertreat the elderly patient because they feel that his illness is "normal for age" (Butler, 1975).

An even more important problem is the fact that organically impaired patients have a great deal of difficulty in reporting or localizing symptoms. In addition to the obvious difficulties in presenting a coherent history, patients may be physiologically unable to localize pain or describe its quality. They may also have difficulty in reporting more subjective symptoms, such as malaise, dizziness, or fatigue. As a further complication to diagnosis, elderly patients may not develop a febrile response to infections. For example, a younger patient with pneumococcal pneumonia may complain of acute onset of malaise, chills, rigors, a productive cough, and dyspnea, and would certainly be febrile. An elderly patient with Alzheimer's disease, however, may be afebrile and virtually asymptomatic, exhibiting only a sudden exacerbation of his dementia. The diagnosis will be made only on the basis of physical examination and chest x-ray (Goodstein, 1985).

Intercurrent medical illnesses represent the most common cause of decompensation in organically impaired patients. This decompensation will usually, but not always, be sudden, and certainly out of character for the patient's usual mental status. This is so common that any abrupt change in mental status in a demented patient should be considered as undiagnosed medical illness until proven otherwise. Such mental status changes should be brought to the physician's attention as soon as possible (Taylor et al., 1983).

Probably the most common intercurrent illnesses that present this way are urinary tract infections and pneumonia. In the severely impaired patient, the latter is often a result of aspiration, and recurrences must be prevented. Other infectious processes, such as cellulitis or sinusitis, or more serious infections such as peritonitis, will also cause decompensation. In addition, virtually any condition associated with severe pain, such as an acute abdomen, kidney stone, or broken hip, can cause decompensation. Finally, exacerbation or progression of any serious illness, such as congestive heart failure, diabetes, or cancer, can lead to the same problems. It should also be borne in mind that the demented patient is not immune to the various causes of delirium, such as electrolyte problems, uremia, and vitamin B_{12} deficiency.

Intercurrent illnesses may lead to a degree of sensory deprivation, also leading to decompensation. Most obvious are illnesses that lead to impairments of vision or hearing. However, any illness that results in decreased ambulation or mobility will also cause a degree of sensory deprivation. Thus a fractured hip may cause serious problems, as may a stroke or leg ulcer. Treatment involves correction of hearing, visual, and mobility problems, such as with a hearing aid, cataract extraction, or physical therapy, but also adaptation of the environment. For example, large-print or talking books may be provided for the visually impaired patient. People can be encouraged to enunciate clearly for the hearing impaired patient, or he can be taught to lip read. In the case of the patient who has lost his ability to ambulate, prolonged periods of bedrest should be discouraged if medically possible, and he should be taught from an early point to use a wheelchair, walker, handrails, or whatever else is appropriate. Of course, an effort should also be made to make the patient's environment more wheelchair- or walker-accessible.

Decompensation may be due to iatrogenic problems (discussed previously). Both patients with benign senescent forgetfulness and patients with true organic mental disorders are quite susceptible to these problems. Treatment, of course, involves reduction or removal of the problems (Butler, 1975).

Organically impaired patients are not immune to functional psychiatric problems, either new or preexisting. This may present an extremely complicated picture, as a functional illness may exacerbate organic deficits, and a dementia may impair the patient's ability to report subjective symptoms. These difficult situations are discussed further in Chapter 23 on psychiatric mental health nursing with the elderly.

PSYCHOSIS. Psychosis may occur in an organically impaired patient who is unable to adapt to his or her cognitive disability. Psychosis may be a result of increased stress from the environment, such as a disruption of the patient's routine, or from a rapid loss of cognitive function, either as a result of a medical illness or in the case of a rapidly progressive delirium. The psychotic symptoms consist of (usually visual) hallucinations, or more commonly illusions, and delusions. They may vary in severity from casual statements to major concerns that the patient will be quite upset about, even to the point of taking dangerous action. For example, a patient may state casually to the nurse that his roommate stole his socks, or he may report this quite angrily, accuse his roommate, attempt to notify the hospital administrator, or strike his roommate. Thus psychosis may represent an entire spectrum of severity, from nondestructive mechanisms to serious and even life-threatening problems (Taylor & Ballenger, 1980).

The presence of psychosis always demands immediate attention. The psychotic patient is upset and frightened, and his distress must be alleviated. Furthermore, the psychosis is extremely distressing to family members and other patients, and at times the patient may present a real danger to them. The abrupt onset of psychotic symptoms in an organically impaired patient is always a foreboding sign in need of immediate intervention. Such acute decompensation can never be ignored, as it will prove to be due to a medical illness or some other serious problem (Taylor et al., 1983).

Some organically impaired patients chronically exhibit psychotic symptoms. Once established, these symptoms no longer demand a complete medical workup unless they suddenly increase in severity. However, appropriate management will minimize the severity of the psychotic symptoms, as well as the difficulties that they may cause.

When psychosis does occur, the first step is to rule out any treatable cause, such as a medical illness or an iatrogenic problem. Major psychological stresses, sensory deprivation, or sudden changes in the patient's routine should also be ruled out. Once ruled out, the patient's environment and care plan should be reassessed, ensuring that they are optimal. Afterwards an increase in reality orientation, maximal consistency with the patient's usual routine, and either an increase or decrease in cognitive stimulation (experience will dictate which) will quite often improve or resolve the psychosis (Trockman, 1978).

If the strategies above prove ineffective, further interventions are necessary. In the case of psychotic symptoms that are mild and neither disturbing nor dangerous to the patient, gentle, indirect confrontation may prove effective, as long as the patient is allowed to save face. For example, the patient who accuses his roommate of stealing his socks may be assured that the socks will eventually turn up and that it isn't worth wasting his time. Likewise, a patient who speaks of leaving a nursing home to manage his staff can be asked to stay because the other patients enjoy his company. In the case of a patient who is hallucinating, the nurse may say, "Your eyes are playing tricks on you," quickly adding that "Lots of people make that same mistake."

If such face-saving confrontation is ineffective, or in the case of more serious or dangerous psychotic symptoms, neuroleptic medication is extremely effec-

tive. However, medication should be used only when the strategies above have proven ineffective. Admittedly, the use of medication is far simpler than any of the above suggestions, but nonpharmacologic management is usually far more beneficial to the patient.

PSYCHOPHARMACOLOGY. Neuroleptic, or antipsychotic, medication decreases the patient's behavioral and emotional responses to psychotic symptoms. In the case of psychoses associated with organic mental disorders, these medications will often resolve the psychotic symptoms completely. Usually, though, the patient will maintain a degree of face-saving denial, for example, stating that even though his socks were stolen, he has more important things to do with his time than to pursue it. Neuroleptic medications may be used either routinely or on a p.r.n. basis, depending on the nature and chronicity of the psychosis. They are usually titrated to the minimum effective dosage for resolving the dangerous behavior and rendering the patient amenable to reality orientation (Taylor et al., 1983).

Several different neuroleptic medications are available for this purpose but haloperidol (Haldol) and thioridazine (Mellaril) are the most common. Dosages are extremely low in comparison to those used for functional psychoses. For example, a typical dosage of haloperidol for a 70-year-old patient with Alzheimer's disease might be between 0.5 mg and 6 mg per day, compared to 15 to 40 mg per day for a young schizophrenic. All neuroleptics may be given either in divided doses or once a day, usually at bedtime. Table 11–7 lists some common neuroleptic agents used for the management of psychosis in the organically impaired patient.

All neuroleptics may oversedate. In addition, low-potency agents, such as thioridazine, may cause anticholinergic problems such as dry mouth, blurred vision, constipation, and urinary retention, as well as postural hypotension. The latter is especially common with chlorpromazine (Thorazine) and may even cause the patient to fall. High-potency agents, such as haloperidol, are relatively devoid of these side effects, causing instead Parkinsonian symptoms such as slowness, rigidity, and tremor. These high-potency agents may also cause a peculiar sort of motor restlessness known as *akathisia.* They may also occasionally cause acute muscle spasms known as *dystonic reactions,* although this is far more common in younger patients who are receiving neuroleptics. All these side effects of high-potency neuroleptics may be reversed with anticholinergic agents such as benztropine (Cogentin), trihexyphenidyl (Artane), or diphenhydr-

TABLE 11–7 Common neuroleptic medications for psychosis in organically impaired patients

Generic Name	Trade Names	Typical Doses mg/day
Haloperidol	Haldol	$\frac{1}{2}$–6
Fluphenazine	Prolixin, Permitil	$\frac{1}{2}$–6
Trifluoperazine	Stelazine	1–10
Thiothixene	Navane	1–10
Perphenazine	Trilafon	2–16
Loxapine	Loxitane	10–50
Chlorpromazine	Thorazine, others	10–150
Thioridazine	Mellaril	10–150

Note:
High-potency agents (toward top of table) cause more Parkinsonian side effects.

Low-potency agents (toward bottom of table) cause more sedation and anticholinergic side effects.

amine (Benadryl). However, these agents cause even more anticholinergic problems than the low-potency neuroleptics.

When neuroleptic medication is used, it is important to remember that its effect is only to alleviate the psychotic symptoms that have occurred; it will not improve the primary, cognitive symptoms of the organic mental disorder. Often family members have this mistaken impression, as they do not distinguish primary from secondary symptoms. Again, neuroleptics will often merely correct the emotional and behavioral reactions to the psychosis rather than completely resolving the psychosis itself. This is an appropriate goal for most patients.

RESTRAINTS. Due to their inherent sensory-depriving effects, restraints should be used only in an emergency situation in which serious harm will result if the patient's behavior is not controlled immediately. In these cases, restraints should be used only until adequate control is achieved through the use of medications and correction of the underlying cause of the acute decompensation. If the patient is restrained, it should be in a quiet, well-lighted room, and the nurse should provide vigorous reality orientation as frequently as possible. Is should also be repeatedly reinforced to the patient that he has not done anything wrong and that he is not being punished. He should be told that the restraints are temporary measures to prevent his harming himself. In these situations, restraints are far preferable to the use of a seclusion room where a confused, organically impaired patient might easily harm himself.

NURSE'S RESPONSIBILITIES IN NONPSYCHIATRIC AND PSYCHIATRIC SETTINGS

The nurse needs to be knowledgeable about a variety of organic disorders. They can be observed in almost any setting (intensive care units, nursing homes, medical/surgical wards, private homes, public health agencies, and so forth).

The nurse might find her services a welcome component of the total treatment process in any of these settings. For example, she might find herself as the conduit of information to the physician about the patient's behavioral patterns and syndromes. Her observational skills and twenty-four-hour contact with the patient provide many opportunities for gathering patient data and constructing nursing diagnoses and plans for nursing care.

The family, regardless of the setting, will need to be involved in health care planning for its ill member. Furthermore, support to family members, as they become involved with the health care system, is an essential part of the nurse's professional responsibility. It consists of educating and clarifying the prescribed treatment for the patient. Reassuring the patient and family is also an important activity.

Patients with organic brain syndromes are very challenging to the nurse. The survival rates of these patients can range from one to twenty-five years after onset of illness; there is always uncertainty about longevity and prognosis (Wells, 1977). This variable alone can be very perplexing to patients, families, and nurses.

In the event the patient needs psychiatric care, family members will need to understand clearly the rationale for treatment (inpatient and outpatient) and be guided and supported as they attempt to arrange for care. On the other hand, if the patient is already under the care of a health professional, then the professional must make every effort to involve the family in the plans for institutional care, as well as care in a variety of other settings.

Professional organizations for the purpose of supporting families with ill members can be of tremendous therapeutic value. For example, Alzheimer's family support groups and family support groups for patients with epileptic disorders are active in communities through the nation.

Finally, the nurse can play a vital role in primary prevention of irreversible organic brain disorders. She can also facilitate treatment of a functional illness in the demented patient. In fact, the nurse might be the first health care professional to observe early disturbances in mood, intellect, physiology, and motivation. She must be knowledgeable about organic disorders in order to discern the symptoms associated with them as well as symptoms of other, possibly coexistant, problems.

PROVIDING CARE FOR PHYSICAL NEEDS

There are several different types of organic brain syndrome. While their etiologies are different, and diagnostic and medical treatment might vary, the nursing care is fairly consistent and includes the following:

- The nurse is familiar with all drugs prescribed for the patient, their side effects, therapeutic benefits, and the typical responses to the effects of these drugs.
- A "baseline" understanding of the patient's dietary habits is established. This type of information assists the nurse in determining any changes in the patient's eating habits that might indicate either increased pathology or a patient's adaptation to further his own deterioration.
- The nurse's assessment skills are extremely useful as these patients will require continuous monitoring of physical condition. The patient's ability to communicate clearly and intelligently is limited.
- The nurse monitors the patient for blood pressure fluctuations as a side effect of neuroleptic and antidepressant drugs.
- The nurse also monitors the patient's intake of adequate fluids and nutrition. Suspicions, delusions, hallucinations, and so forth, along with physical limitations, may interact to forestall adequate nutrition.
- Physical hygiene and personal care (toileting, showering, and so on) are frequently neglected. This type of neglect can cause patients, family, and even staff to view the patient as repulsive. Withdrawal from the patient is a common consequence. In fact, depending on acuity level, the patient may require monitoring of some or all activities of daily living.

- The differences between delirium (acute onset) and dementia (insidious) should be clearly understood by the nursing staff. The nurse must, when assessing the patient, determine whether the presenting symptoms are an advancement of the present illness or if the symptoms represent a more acute onset of physical problems.
- The nurse monitors the patient's tolerance for on-unit and off-unit programs. The patient's condition may fluctuate due to the physical environment or psychological changes, so the nurse determines what the differential variables are and manipulates them when possible.
- The milieu is the nurse's responsibility. It should be arranged to enhance the patient's functioning. A unit that is well-lighted, has a comfortable temperature, and is considered "safe" is a basic custodial requirement.
- Occasionally the patient will need to be placed in restraints (two and four-point types) for self-protection. The entire staff should be aware of nursing protocol for restraint usage. Those assisting the nurse must be observed for undue roughness and the nursing personnel's responses to patient's resistance. Once the patient is restrained, the nurse observes him frequently (every 15 minutes) and releases one, then two, of the points as soon as the patient can tolerate it. In fact, when possible, the nurse remains with the patient and assists in 1) control of anxiety, 2) reality testing, and 3) orientation and relaxation. As soon as it is therapeutically possible, the nurse removes the restraints. She explains to the patient and staff the reason for using the restraints.

PSYCHIATRIC CARE OF PATIENT

Orientation to time, place, and date will perhaps be continuously distorted for many dementia patients. This never-ending behavior can be very anxiety producing for the nurse. She will need to discuss her fears, anxieties, and resentments about the patient's clinical state. Supervision by knowledgeable nurses and other professionals can be extremely helpful. Over time, supervision can assist in the enhancement of quality nursing care. When dealing with demented patients, the nurse must remember the following points.

- When providing care, the nurse speaks calmly and distinctly to the patient. Her sentences are short and directive.
- She provides and encourages opportunities for the patient to discuss past events in his life. The

nurse might hear about the same events over and over; however, reminiscing therapy encourages interpersonal relationships, assists in intellectually stimulating the patient, and enhances the patient's self-esteem.

ASSISTANCE WITH FAMILY

Organic disorders can be extremely troublesome for families. The slow and insidious onset, as well as the acute onset, is frustrating and baffling to loved ones. Family members might deny that the ill member is expressing maladaptive behaviors. The nurse is in a unique position to:

- Explain the illness to the family. The nurse might consider drawing simple diagrams or providing written information about the illness.
- Teach the family about medications prescribed for the patient: their therapeutic effects and side effects (short and long-term).
- Discuss the inpatient routine (ward schedule) with family members. For example: 7:30 A.M., breakfast; 9–11 A.M., bathing, dressing, and so on; 1–9 P.M., visitors. If the family understands the routine, this aids in two ways: 1) it facilitates their psychological comfort and "demystifies" the treatment process; and 2) it enhances cooperation with health care professionals.
- Teach the family methods of more effectively communicating with the patient. Conversely, the nurse might learn from the family how better to communicate with the patient. At any rate, the family and nurse ought to take advantage of every opportunity to communicate.
- Describe the total treatment plan, its goals and objectives, to enlighten and educate the family. This is especially necessary as patients are frequently cared for by family and other types of community-based programs.
- Inform the family members of agencies in the community that can provide assistance (financial, physical care, emotional support, respite care). This is extremely important as plans for discharge are being made.
- Support the family members who are involved with the patient. Professionals who treat and care for patients with organic problems can unintentionally force family members into an untenable situation: 1) the family is told to accept the loss of its previously functioning member; 2) at the same time, they are asked to remain in constant contact and encourage the highest level of functioning possible for the patient.

Case Study: Nonpsychiatric Setting

Demographic Data

Name:	Mr. James Munroe
Age:	58 years
Geographic:	Rocky Mount, North Carolina
Ethnicity:	Caucasian
Religious Preference:	Lutheran
Referring Agency:	Family Physician
Education:	Community College Graduate
Occupation:	U.S. Postal Service, Mail Carrier

Mr. James Munroe is a 58-year-old white man, who is employed as a postal mail carrier. He is married and the father of two adult daughters. He has come to the hospital for prostate surgery.

Patient's Perception of Problem

"I feel okay most of the time. My knees and legs hurt. My blood pressure is high. Medication helps. I am having surgery and I'm going to get out of here as soon as I can!"

History of Problem

Mr. Munroe is known to his colleagues and neighbors as a diligent and committed worker. About five years ago, Mr. Monroe began to complain to his wife that, on occasion, he felt weak in his knees—like his knees could no longer hold his body—but he continued working. Sporadically, he complained to his wife about his right leg feeling extremely weak. He could no longer complete his mail delivery route in the designated time. Gradually, Mr. Munroe was slower and slower with his mail delivery.

After several days of his complaining, Mrs. Thelma Munroe took her husband for a routine physical examination. The examination revealed he had high blood pressure (162/120). He was given an antihypertensive drug (Hydrochlorothiazide 50 mg q a.m.) for treatment of high blood pressure. No other intervention was done at this time. Mr. Munroe has also suffered from cataracts for several years, although he had little difficulty with them.

Mr. Munroe continued his employment at the post office. His wife remained very concerned about his overall health, but did not know what else to do. At times, she observed that, "My James seems strange and says things that are out of the ordinary." He had begun to neglect his personal hygiene and would refuse to shave, take his medication, and so forth for several days at a time.

Colleagues at the post office began to complain that Mr. Munroe seemed "spaced out" and not interested in what was going on in his environment. He would become confused and was observed trying to open another worker's locker. Others had observed that Mr. Munroe was not thinking on the job and reported him to their superiors.

Concurrently, Mr. Munroe's superiors had begun to receive complaints from the patrons on his postal route that he had "acted unprofessionally" toward the women in the neighborhood. Although he looked healthy and continued to report to work on time, his superiors found it necessary to remove him from his duties.

Mr. Munroe continued to act weird, and seemed to be attracted to the young women in the neighborhood. His behavior disturbed Mrs. Munroe, but Mr. Munroe refused to discuss these concerns with her.

Psychiatric History

No history of previous psychiatric problems.

Family History

Mr. Munroe's father lived until age 90; his mother recently died of a cerebrovascular accident (CVA). Mr. Munroe had two brothers. One brother was killed in the Korean War; the other brother is a Certified Public Accountant, and has no known mental or physical problems.

Social History

Mr. Munroe has always taken pride in being able to provide financial support for his wife and two daughters. He is perceived by his wife as "a good husband and devoted father." Mr. Munroe completed high school. During his high school years, he won several trophies for outstanding performance in sports, including football and soccer.

Mr. Munroe married his wife at age 23. They have had an active role in the community: Boy Scouts and Girl Scouts, Little League football, and numerous church and civic functions. During the years their two daughters were in college, Mr. Munroe worked two jobs. He felt physically strained and mentally tense during these years. "Somehow," he said, "I had to get those girls through college." He was diagnosed as having mild hypertension, but felt the condition was related to working two jobs. The hypertension subsided after Mr. Munroe quit his second job.

He denied ever smoking. He would drink 2–3 cans of beer when watching his favorite sports on television.

Health History

A history of hypertension and cataracts for several years. Currently scheduled for prostate surgery.

Current Mental Status

General Appearance: Unshaven, somewhat disheveled; quiet, but tense.
Sensorium: Coherent responses to nurse's questions about time, place, and person. On one occasion during the interview, patient burped aloud. (Wife was embarrassed.)
Emotions: Mr. Munroe was cooperative and relaxed during the first part (10 minutes) of the interview, but became irritable and uncooperative during the latter.
Mood: Showed a range of sadness to moderate elation.
Speech: Unable to respond to specific questions about recent activities. Speech appeared pressured at times.
Motor Behavior: Sat still. On occasion appeared disinterested in nurse's questions, looking away from nurse and focusing on different objects in the room.
Thought Content: Coherent (when elected to be cooperative). Some recent memory impairment.
Thought Process: Distracted, periods of silence; appeared disinterested in interview.

Medication

Hydrochlorothiazide 50 mg every morning for hypertension.

Violence Potential

No history of violence. Observe patient.

Summary

Mr. Munroe is a 58-year-old disabled mail carrier who is being admitted to the hospital for prostate surgery. He has a history of hypertension; recently, he has had difficulty completing his responsibilities as a mail carrier.

Mr. Munroe was admitted to a general hospital for prostate surgery. During the first evening of hospitalization, the nurse heard Mr. Munroe screaming. When she went to his room, he demanded that she "get that dog out of my house." Mr. Munroe was pointing to a chair in the corner of the room. The nurse turned on a light in the room, explaining that the chair did indeed look somewhat like a dog in the dark and that "sometimes people make that kind of mistake." She then left a night light on in the room. Mr. Munroe had no further problems during hospitalization.

Mr. Munroe's nurse suggested a neurology consultation, and after a neuropsychological evaluation, a diagnosis of multi-infarct dementia was made.

DSM-III-R Diagnosis

Axis I Multi-Infarct Dementia (290.4x)
Axis II No diagnosis made
Axis III Hypertension
Axis IV Psychosocial stressors: Physical illness diagnosed; surgery planned for prostate problems; severity: 3 moderate.
Axis V Current GAF: 31—40; Highest GAF in past year, 80

Nursing Diagnoses

Dressing/grooming, self-care deficit
Sensory perceptual alterations (visual, kinesthetic)
Ineffective individual coping

Nursing Care Plan for Mr. Munroe

Nursing Diagnosis	Desired Outcomes	Interventions	Rationale
1. Dressing/grooming, self-care deficit.	Mr. Munroe will attain the highest possible level of functioning and return to the least restrictive environment.	Provide a schedule for bathing, shaving, and medications, and explain all procedures to Mr. Munroe.	A regular schedule will reduce anxiety, provide predictability, and encourage independence through self-care.
		Encourage Mr. Munroe to participate in as many self-care activities as he is able to handle.	Encourages Mr. Munroe's independence and autonomy.
		When appropriate, engage Mrs. Munroe in her husband's care.	An excellent opportunity for (a) nurse to demonstrate nursing care technique to Mrs. Munroe; (b) Mrs. Munroe to share her knowledge about Mr. Munroe with nurse; (c) nurse to do health teaching.
		Provide an environment that is quiet and free of unnecessary distraction. At night, keep a light on in his room.	The patient might be annoyed and distracted by objects in the environment. Alleviates anxiety and disturbance.
		Ask Mr. Munroe about his bedtime routine at home. Also, get information from Mrs. Munroe about his sleeping habits and preferences.	Provides nurse with important information that will assist in planning care during hospitalizations. Information can also be used in a diagnostic sense: compare data received from Mr. Munroe with data from his wife. Inconsistencies

Nursing Diagnosis	Desired Outcomes	Interventions	Rationale
			in information can assist the nurse in making determinations about Mr. Munroe's cognitive functions, reality testing, memory, self-care capabilities, and so forth.
		Provide activity and stimulation during the day.	Activity is an important component of self-care. It stimulates intellectual functioning; increases opportunities for social participation; and enhances patient's sense of competence and autonomy.
		Allow sufficient time for Mr. Munroe to bathe, shave, dress, take medications, and so forth. The nurse should lay out clothes and shaving apparatus for him. Provide mechanical aids such as Velcro closures or dressing stick, if needed. Also, the nurse should explain to Mr. Munroe in clear and concise statements just what she expects him to accomplish.	These types of actions will assist Mr. Munroe in learning or relearning some adaptive behaviors. Mastery at this level will increase his sense of achievement and competence.
2. Sensory perceptual alterations (visual, kinesthetic).	Mr. Munroe will demonstrate an improvement in his contact with reality, and assume his highest possible level of self-care.	Encourage Mr. Munroe to remain active on unit (walk), and be out of bed as much as possible.	These types of activities stimulate interest in the environment; promote desired physical functioning; increase interest in self-care; and enhance possibilities for social and interpersonal interactions.
		Provide a safe environment for Mr. Munroe by checking him frequently throughout the night; providing a light for his room at night; removing all unnecessary objects or furniture from his room. Example: explain to Mr. Munroe that a dog is not in the room, but do not argue with him. Remain with him until fears have subsided.	Mr. Munroe is likely to misinterpret common objects in his environment at night. A light will assist him in identifying these objects, and decrease his fears and anxieties that are associated with misinterpretation.

Nursing Diagnosis	Desired Outcomes	Interventions	Rationale
		Discuss with Mr. and Mrs. Munroe the physical design of their bedroom at home. Assist them in arranging the bedroom furniture/objects in a fashion that will enhance Mr. Munroe's reality testing and self-care activities.	The physical environment should be safe, attractive, and enhancing for the patient (and Mrs. Munroe). Moreover, this is an excellent opportunity to provide health teaching for Mr. and Mrs. Munroe about Mr. Munroe's health care when he is at home recuperating from surgery.
		Assist Mr. and Mrs. Munroe in determining the degree to which they will need assistance with activities of daily living at home, and the availability of caregivers to provide assistance.	Family routine needs to be considered; amount of time the caregivers will have to assist the patient should be discussed. Required care during the night should be given special consideration. The amount of care/supervision required upon return home is not always known. Mr. and Mrs. Munroe would be provided with follow up care/supervision to assist in the enhancement of self-care activities and optimal contact with reality.
		When communicating with Mr. Munroe, be sure to be specific and direct. Do not use body gyrations, non-verbal communications, and so forth.	Misperceptions and misinterpretations are likely to occur. They will probably intensify at night.
		Discuss with Mr. Munroe (and Mrs. Munroe) the reasons he has been hopitalized. Explain the anticipated activities associated with surgery, such as: (a) administration of intravenous fluids and medications; (b) personnel, dressed in blue/green with head, feet, and mouth covered, etc.; (c) pre-operative and post-operative care, and so forth.	Mr. Munroe is likely to be more cooperative if informed about all procedures and techniques. He will be less fearful and anxious, and more likely to participate in self-care activities.

Nursing Diagnosis	Desired Outcomes	Interventions	Rationale
3. Ineffective individual coping.	Mr. Munroe will develop effective methods of problem solving and decision making that facilitate his optimal level of functioning.	Encourage Mr. Munroe to discuss activities in his life that he once felt good about, but can no longer adequately perform, such as bathing, dressing, and participating in social and civic activities.	The determination of Mr. Munroe's strengths and desires will be useful in realistically planning future care. Activities that he formerly enjoyed can be designed in such a manner to allow Mr. Munroe's participation; a more limited role in participation of activities might be an adaptive alternative to no participation.
		Help Mr. Munroe develop a daily schedule that includes activities that he enjoys such as walking the block in the neighborhood, or attending a Boy Scout meeting in the community.	These activities are designed to utilize the patient's strengths. They will assist in enhancing interests in interpersonal relationships, autonomy, and self-care.
		Assist Mr. and Mrs. Munroe in mobilizing a support system of friends and relatives who care about them, and who will (can) understand Mr. Munroe's physical and mental condition.	Support systems can offer opportunities for ventilation, empathy, information sharing, and emotional nurturance to Mr. and Mrs. Munroe. Also, a support system will limit feelings of isolation and alienation.
		Instruct Mr. and Mrs. Munroe about how to participate in self-relaxation activities such as deep breathing and stretching exercises.	A method of tension release; assists in exercising certain muscles; a time of reflection and quiet; and so forth.

Case Study: Psychiatric Setting

Demographic Data

Name: Benjamin Isaacs
Age: 73 years
Geography: Miami, Florida
Religion: Jewish
Education: Masters degree, Education Administration, University of Miami
Occupation: Retired High School Principal

Patient's Perception of Problem

"My neighbors are stealing my money and food! You need to have them put in jail! Don't leave me here. Take me home!"

Mrs. Isaacs stated that her husband has become more difficult to manage. Recently (last month) he began to display behaviors such as roaming through the house at night looking for the dean's office, accusing his wife of stealing his money, and occasionally becoming combative, threatening to assault the man next door because he too was stealing Mr. Isaacs' money and food. Mrs. Isaacs stated, "I had to do something quickly when early one morning, Benjamin got out of bed and attempted to rearrange the electrical wiring in the house in preparation for an important pep rally to be held in the gym."

History of Problem

During his earlier years, Benjamin Isaacs was known as a dynamic and committed high school principal. He was principal at one of the city's largest and most prestigious high schools. His intellectual acuity, values, and desire to teach students self-discipline were qualities that made him the envy of many professionals.

Mr. Isaacs retired approximately two years earlier than planned because of beginning memory problems and other deterioration of intellectual abilities. For example, Mr. Isaacs had begun experiencing difficulty when presiding over faculty meetings at which issues were presented that involved complex and emotionally charged content. He would respond to these situations by telling inappropriate ethnic jokes and making light of the importance of items presented during the meetings.

His activities in the community ended rather abruptly. His speech became a source of embarrassment for him and his wife. Mrs. Isaacs reported observing her husband's language usage deteriorate to a stage where sentences were long, with extensive verbage: there was vagueness with increasing difficulty in recognizing and naming objects.

Gradually, Mr. Isaacs became less effective in his communications. Similarly, he tended to withdraw, preferring to remain at home. He was described as being sporadically "irritable and cross" with increasing frequency.

Psychiatric History

Benjamin Isaacs has no history of psychiatric illness. According to his wife, he has always worked hard and taken pride in his school and the community.

Family History

Benjamin's father was a prominent neurosurgeon who practiced in New York City. He died at the age of 56 as a result of an auto accident. Benjamin's mother, age 98, is in a nursing home in North Miami. She has a 30-year history of dementia.

Benjamin has one sister who is a practicing attorney in Illinois. She lives with her husband and two sons. Benjamin and his sister have, through the years, enjoyed a close and gratifying relationship with each other. Mr. and Mrs. Isaacs have no children.

Social History

Mrs. Isaacs reported that Benjamin grew up in New York City. His mother and father stressed excellence and achievement. He tended to be methodical in his approach to tasks. Benjamin was a hard worker and an outstanding student. He was always fond of children and youth. At an early age, he decided to become a high school principal, and to be the "best in the business." He and his sister made a contract with each other some years ago that the two of them would always stick by each other, no matter what their fate.

Benjamin likes to swim and play golf. In fact, he frequently swam in the high school pool. His golf playing buddies were prominent community leaders, members from the synagogue, and other school officials.

Health History

Occasional leg pain that is associated with an old injury sustained several years ago while swimming in the high school pool.

Tylox prn for occasional leg pain.

Current Mental Status

General Appearance: Neatly dressed in sports shirt, sneakers, and slacks. As the nurse began the interview, he sat quietly in his chair and looked out of the window.

Sensorium: Not able to provide coherent responses to nurse's questions about time, place, and person. Judgment is impaired; memory of present events, poor; memory of past events, questionable (patient did not respond to nurse's queries).

Emotions: Looking around room, eyes occasionally fixed on an object in room; little eye contact with nurse; seems blank, vacant.

Mood: Shallow affect; seems to be off in his own world.

Speech: Barely audible, mispronounces names of common objects in the environment.

Motor Behavior: Tends to walk with caution; movements are deliberate and slow.

Thought Content: Incoherent at times; distracted easily; poor judgment and memory.

Thought process: Incoherent thought process. Slow, nonresponsive to nurse's queries; disorganized and pressured.

Summary

Mr. Benjamin Isaacs is a 73-year-old man with a diagnosis of Alzheimer's disease, moderate, who has been placed in a nursing home because his wife could no longer provide care and supervision for him in their home. He has been assigned to a room of his liking, and is becoming familiar with his surroundings. Personal items and selected pieces of furniture from his home were placed in his room at the nursing home. His wife visits him every day.

DSM-III-R Axes

Axis I - Primary degenerative dementia of the Alzheimer type (290.00)

Axis II - No diagnosis made

Axis III - Left leg injury

Axis IV - Psychosocial stressors: dementia diagnosed; severity: 3

Axis V - Current GAF: 16

Highest GAF Past Year: 21

Nursing Diagnoses

*Impaired verbal communication
*Bathing/hygiene, dressing/grooming: self-care deficit
*Anxiety
 Alteration in health maintenance
 Powerlessness
 Role performance disturbance
 Self-esteem disturbance
*Social isolation
 Altered thought processes

*Nursing diagnoses developed in care plan that follows.

Nursing Care Plan for Mr. Isaacs

Nursing Diagnosis	Desired Outcomes	Interventions	Rationale
1. Impaired verbal communication.	Mr. Benjamin Isaacs will demonstrate improved communication by effectively expressing his thoughts and feelings to staff and family with a minimum of frustrations.	Communicate in a straight forward and honest manner.	It is important not to overwhelm this patient with information, especially if it is ambiguous.
		Orient Mr. Isaacs to his environment; be sure that he is in a safe environment where he can be easily observed. Explain to Mr. Isaacs where he is and why he is there.	Information enhances cooperation, orients him to place, person, and time, enhances feelings of security and comfort.
		Encourage conversation but do not cross-examine Mr. Isaacs even if his comments are blatantly conflictual.	Cross-examination heightens suspicions/anxiety and will provoke anger, distrust, confusion, disorientation, and so forth.
		Provide opportunities for Mr. Isaacs to reminisce. Follow train of thought and determine, when possible, interests and strengths.	The nurse can utilize content from reminiscent talk to structure interpersonal dialogue and selected activities that might be free of confusion, irritability, and anxiety.

Nursing Diagnosis	Desired Outcomes	Interventions	Rationale
		Encourage visits from Mrs. Isaacs and Mr. Isaacs' sister (and her family) who live in Illinois. Also, encourage Mrs. Isaacs to invite friends and former associates in the community to visit him. Do not overstimulate or overwhelm him.	The family and other familiar people can assist in (a) enhancing interpersonal relationships; (b) increasing opportunity for reality testing; (c) facilitating social interactions; (d) decreasing withdrawal and feelings of powerlessness.
		Introduce self: "My name is _____; I am the nurse who will be assisting you with your care." State date, name of place, time, and so forth when conversing with Mr. Isaacs.	Assists in alleviating anxiety and embarrassment; he might not recognize nurse, nor familiar objects in the environment.
		Each day, assign the same nurse to supervise and participate in Mr. Isaac's care.	Builds trust; increases socialization, reality testing, and so forth.
		Encourage Mr. Isaacs to express his thoughts and feelings in the best manner that he can; observe for the most effective method of communication and share with other personnel and his wife.	Continuous observation and assessment will provide data for planning, and assist nurse in implementing methods that enhance effective communication.
		Observe and monitor the effect that patient's behavior has on you and other personnel.	Discuss the impact of patient's behavior in staff meetings and supervisory sessions. Always be alert for possible transference issues. Monitor self and other persons for feelings of hopelessness, fear, anger, anxiety, psychological discomfort, and so forth.
		Speak on an adult level, but make sentences simple, brief, and in appropriate tone, with accompanying eye contact.	Enhances respect, trust, and appropriate adult-adult communication. Eliminates frustration and anger associated with impaired verbal expression.

Nursing Diagnosis	Desired Outcomes	Interventions	Rationale
2. Anxiety.	Mr. Isaacs will experience a decrease in feelings of anxiety and an enhancement of psychological comfort.	Determine the proximity of physical closeness that tends to forestall/alleviate the patient's anxiety. Determine if and when verbalizations are important.	Aloneness with faulty reality testing can be extremely anxiety provoking. It increases confusion, irritability, and impaired thought processes.
		The nurse must become familiar with her own anxieties regarding the patient's clinical state through consultation or supervision on a regular basis.	An anxious nurse will increase patient's anxiety. The patient needs to know that the nurse can contol the situation when he cannot.
		Encourage relaxation activities such as retreating to a quiet room, or walking on hospital grounds. Mrs. Isaacs should be offered the option of walking with her husband on the grounds.	Provides method of self-control, independence (though limited), and enhances self-esteem. Provides privacy and alone-time for Mr. and Mrs. Isaacs.
		Help the patient identify possible sources of anxiety.	If the nurse and patient can identify anxiety-producing situations, then specific action can be instituted to allay and alleviate the anxiety. The patient and nurse can also seek alternatives to the situations.
		Encourage routines and a structured approach to all activities, such as dressing, mealtime, bedtime, socialization skills, medication time, arrangement of furniture in the room, and the structure of the environment.	The patient will be able to function better and longer if his environment is simple and undisturbed. His frustration and anxieties will decrease.
3. Social Isolation.	Mr. Isaacs will increase his social and interpersonal activities within the nursing home.	Interact on a one-to-one basis. Gradually progress toward small group, then larger group interactions.	A gradual approach minimizes fears, anxieties, and threats, and encourages success.
		Intervene when the patient separates himself from others on the unit.	Frequent and prolonged separation can increase opportunities for delusions, hallucinations, and increases social isolation and withdrawal.

Nursing Diagnosis	Desired Outcomes	Interventions	Rationale
		Speak in a matter-of-fact fashion but in a kind and sincere voice.	A matter-of-fact voice increases the conveyance of the importance of the message. A kind and sensitive voice provides comfort and a sense of security.
		Always tell Mr. Isaacs your name and how long you will be with him. Also, tell him the date, time, and place. Explain all activities and procedures before they begin.	This is part of reality testing. It enhances trust and security, and diminishes the need to deny memory problems that cause embarrassment for the patient.
		Physical presence is important. Remain with Mr. Isaacs but do not force conversations.	Physical presence with silence is very useful for the patient *but* difficult for the nurse to endure. The nurse must learn to be comfortable with silence.
		Monitor non-verbal behaviors and cues. These messages will probably be subtle, but highly meaningful to the patient.	The subtle and detailed movements such as (a) eye movement, (b) shoulder positioning, (c) head movement, (d) eye contact, and (e) arm and hand movement can be the only expressive behaviors manifested. Study these behaviors and make interpretations within the context of the situation and your knowledge of the patient.
4. Bathing/hygiene self-care deficit.	Mr. Isaacs will have adequate nutritional/fluid intake; he will also have adequate bowel and bladder elimination.	Remain with the patient during meals. Monitor nutritional intake.	Promotes reality orientation and enhances socialization.
		Talk with the patient about memories, positively reinforcing him for sharing them.	Enhances socialization and reality orientation, and stimulates a desire to have satisfying interpersonal relationships.
		Monitor bowel/bladder evacuation.	Constipation can occur because of limited activity; decreased food intake; and general feeling of hopelessness.

Nursing Diagnosis	Desired Outcomes	Interventions	Rationale
		Arrange furniture and artifacts in room in an attractive but simple manner. Leave in that order.	Enhances sense of security; provides a more functional environment.
		Put patient's personal items in same place every day. Encourage structured and methodical behaviors.	Facilitates the patient's reality testing; provides a sense of security; increases mastery and competence in dressing and other self-care behaviors.
		Continuously assess the patient's level of tolerance for stimulation; his capacity for self-care; his capacity to tolerate numbers of people. Be careful about expectations for the patient.	The appropriate amount of stimuli will enhance feelings of security and self-confidence. People can be stimulating or anxiety-provoking.

SUMMARY

Organic mental disorders make up the largest group of mental illnesses with very well-described pathophysiologies. The hallmark of an organic mental disorder is that the associated mental changes are caused by a specific lesion, either structural or chemical, in the central nervous system. Patients with organic mental disorders have trouble with intellectual functions such as memory and language.

Organic mental disorders fall into two categories: delirium and dementia. Delirium is acute, with rapid onset; dementia is chronic, with slow onset. The main characteristic of delirium is clouded sensorium—the patient appears sick or bewildered. The demented patient, on the other hand, does not appear to be bewildered. The demented patient often engages in denial and is genuinely unaware that anything is wrong mentally.

Dementia and delirium produce primary and secondary symptoms. Primary symptoms are the actual cognitive symptoms of organic mental disorder; secondary symptoms are adaptive or maladaptive responses. Primary symptoms include difficulty with orientation (to time, place, and situation), memory, language function, visuospatial orientation, and frontal-lobe symptoms. Secondary symptoms include behaviors such as rigidity, obsessive-compulsive syndrome, confabulation, catastrophic reactions, psychosis, and sundowning.

DSM-III-R divides organic mental disorders into two subsections. One includes primary degenerative dementia (including Alzheimer's disease, multi-infarct dementia, and substance-induced disorders). The other subsection includes all other organic mental disorders. Alzheimer's disease, the most prevalent of all dementias, can be roughly divided into three phases: the forgetfulness phase, the confusional phase, and the dementia phase. Some patients never progress beyond the forgetfulness phase, thus obtaining a diagnosis of benign senescent forgetfulness. Other dementias include multi-infarct dementia, Wernicke-Korsakoff syndrome, alcoholic dementia, normal pressure hydrocephalus, neurosyphilis, Parkinson's disease, and Huntington's disease. Pseudodementia, a depressive symptom, may mimic dementia.

There are a number of systemic illnesses that may be associated with organic mental disorders. These conditions are called metabolic encephalopathies, and include electrolyte abnormalities, uremia, hepatic encephalopathy, hypothyroidism and hyperthyroidism, vitamin B$_{12}$ deficiency, and sedative-hypnotic withdrawal syndrome all of which can have iatrogenic causes.

Many organic mental disorders are curable with appropriate medical treatment, but responsibility for management of the patient lies with the nurse. The nurse develops realistic goals: for the delirious patient, complete remission of symptoms; for the demented patient, reduction of secondary symptoms (the primary symptoms do not improve much, if at all). The goals are reviewed periodically and adjusted to the patient's capabilities as the illness progresses or arrests. The nurse also manipulates the patient's environment so that it is familiar and understandable; she also watches to make sure that neither sensory deprivation nor sensory overload occurs.

Finally, the nurse works with the patient's family to help them deal with their own emotions and set goals for the patient. She may also be instrumental in helping them decide whether or not to place the patient in a care facility outside the home, such as a nursing home.

KEY TERMS

organic mental disorders

organic brain syndromes

cognitive functions

higher cortical functions

delirium

encephalopathy

senility

clouded sensorium

clear sensorium

denial

primary symptoms

secondary symptoms

orientation

retrograde amnesia

language function

anomia

aphasia

paraphasic

visuospatial orientation

frontal symptoms

inertia

perseveration

emotional incontinence

pseudobulbar palsy

rigidity

obsessive-compulsive behaviors

confabulation

catastrophic reaction

psychosis

sundowning

Alzheimer's disease

primary degenerative dementia (PDD)

forgetfulness phase

confusional phase

dementia phase

senile plaques

neurofibrillary tangles

multi-infarct dementia (MID)

lacunar infarcts

Wernicke-Korsakoff syndrome

alcoholic dementia

normal pressure hydrocephalus

metabolic encephalopathies

electrolyte abnormalities

uremia

hepatic encephalopathy

hypothyroidism

hyperthyroidism

vitamin B$_{12}$ deficiency

iatrogenic

dementia paralytica

pseudodementia

sensory deprivation

benign senescent forgetfulness

reality orientation

reminiscing therapy

respite programs

sedative-hypnotic withdrawal syndrome

STUDY QUESTIONS

1. Define organic mental disorders. How are they different from functional psychoses and mood disorders?

2. Define delirium and dementia. What is the difference between the two?

3. Define primary symptoms and secondary symptoms of organic mental disorders. Name three of each.

4. Name and describe four organic mental disorders.

5. How can a nurse help the family of a patient with an organic mental disorder?

REFERENCES

Abdellah, F. G. (1981). Nursing care of the aged in the United States of America. *Journal of Gerontological Nursing, 7,* 657.

Adams, R. D., Fisher, C. M., Hakim, S., Ojemann, R. G., & Sweet, W. H. (1965). Symptomatic hydrocephalus with "normal" cerebrospinal-fluid pressure. *N. Eng. J. Med., 273,* 117–126.

American Psychiatric Association, Committee on Nomenclature and Statistics. (1987). *Diagnostic and statistical manual of mental disorders 3rd ed., revised.* Washington: American Psychiatric Association, pp. 97–163.

Bartol, M. A., (1979). Nonverbal communication in patients with Alzheimer's disease. *J. Gerontol. Nurs., 5*(4), 21–31.

Bennett, A. E., Mowery, G. L., & Fort, J. T. (1960). Brain damage from chronic alcoholism: The diagnosis of intermediate stage of alcoholic brain disease. *American Journal of Psychiatry, 116,* 705–711.

Birren, J. E., & Sloane, R. B. (1980). *Handbook of mental health and aging.* Englewood Cliffs, N.J.: Prentice-Hall.

Brown, P. (1986). The nursing process for clients with gastrointestinal system dysfunction. In C. Kneisl and S.

Ames (Eds.), *Adult health nursing—A biopsychosocial approach*. Menlo Park: Addison-Wesley.

Butler, R. N. (1975). Psychiatry and the elderly: An overview. *Am. J. Psychiatry, 132,* 893–900.

Butters, N., & Miliotis, P. (1985). Amnesic disorders. In K. M. Heilman & E. Valenstein, *Clinical neuropsychology* (2nd Ed.). New York: Oxford University Press, pp. 403–449.

Cassell, C. K., & Jameton, A. L. (1981). Dementia in the elderly: An analysis of medical responsibility. *Ann. Intern. Med., 94,* 802–807.

Cobe, G. M. (1985). The family of the aged: Issues in treatment. *Psychiatr. Ann., 15,* 343–347.

Cowdry, E. V. (1968). *The care of the geriatric patient.* St. Louis: C. V. Mosby Co.

Cummings, J. L., & Benson, O. F. (1983). *Dementia: A clinical approach.* Boston: Butterworths, p. 44.

Cuttings, J. (1978). The relationship between Korsakov's syndrome and "alcoholic dementia." *Br. J. Psychiatry, 132,* 240–251.

Damasic, A. R. (1985). The frontal lobes. In K. M. Heilman & E. Valenstein, *Clinical neuropsychology* (2nd Ed.). New York: Oxford University Press, pp. 339–375.

Davidhizar, R., Gunder, E., & Wehlage, D. (1978). Recognizing and caring for the delirious patient. *J. Psychiatr. Nurs., 16*(5), 38–41.

Eisdorfer, C., Cohen, D., & Veith, R. (1980). *The psychopathology of aging.* Kalamazoo, Mich.: The Upjohn Company, pp. 20–21.

Folstein, M. F., Folstein, S. E., & McHugh, P. R. (1975). "Mini-mental state": A practical method for grading the cognitive state of patients for the clinician. *J. Psychiatr. Res., 12,* 189–198.

Gibson, J. (1988). *We kept her at home.* Unpublished manuscript, 1309 Raa Avenue, Tallahassee, FL.

Goodstein, R. K. (1985). Common clinical problems in the elderly: Camouflaged by ageism and atypical presentation. *Psychiatr. Ann., 15,* 299–312.

Guthrie, A., & Elliott, W. A. (1980). The nature and reversibility of cerebral impairment in alcoholism. *Journal of the Study of Alcoholism, 41,* 147–155.

Hachinski, V. C., Lassen, N. A., & Marshall, J. (1974). Multi-infarct dementia. *Lancet, 1,* 207–210.

Hagerty, B. K. (1984). Assessing organic mental disturbances. In *Psychiatric-mental health assessment.* B. K. Hagerty (ed.). St. Louis: Mosby.

Hogstel, M. O. (1981). *Nursing care of the older adult.* New York: John Wiley & Sons.

Joynt, R. J., & Shoelson, I. (1985). Dementia. In D. M. Heilman & E. Valenstein, *Clinical Neuropsychology* (2nd ed.) New York: Oxford University Press.

Katzman, R. (1976). The prevalence and malignancy of Alzheimer's disease: A major killer. *Arch. Neurol., 33,* 217–218.

Kay, D. W. K., Beamish, P., & Roth, M. (1964). Old age mental disorders in Newcastle upon Tyne. *Br. J. Psychiatry, 110,* 146–148.

Kay, D. W. K., Bergmann, K., Foster, E. M., McKechnic, A. A., & Roth, M. (1970). Mental illness and hospital usage in the elderly: A random sample followed up. *Compr. Psychiatry, 11,* 26–35.

Kiloh, L. G. (1961). Pseudo-dementia. *Acta Psychiatr. Scand., 37,* 336–351.

King, K. S. (1982). Reminiscing psychotherapy with aging people. *JPNMHS, 20*(2), 21–25.

Konstantinides, N. (1986). The gastrointestinal system in health and illness. In C. Kneisl and S. Ames (Eds.), *Adult health nursing—A biopsychosocial approach.* Menlo Park: Addison-Wesley.

Kral, V. A. (1962). Senescent forgetfulness: Benign and malignant. *Can. Med. Assoc. J., 86,* 257–260.

Kramer, M., German, P. S., & Anthony, J. C. et al. (1985). Patterns of mental disorders among the elderly residents of eastern Baltimore. *J. Am. Ger. Soc., 33,* 236–245.

McHugh, P. R., & Folstein, M. F. (1985). Organic mental disorders. In R. Michaels, J. O. Cavenard, & H. K. H. Brodie, et al. *Psychiatry,* v. 1. Philadelphia: J. B. Lippincott Co.

Merritt, H. H. (1979). *A textbook of neurology,* 6th Ed. Philadelphia: Lea & Febiger.

O'Leary, M. R., Radford, L. M., Chaney. E. F., & Schau, E. J. (1977). Assessment of cognitive recovery in alcoholics by use of the trail-making test. *Journal of Clinical Psychology, 33,* 579–582.

Page, R. D., & Linden, J. D. (1974). "Reversible" organic brain syndrome in alcoholics. *Journal of the Study of Alcoholism, 35,* 98–107.

Pfeiffer, E. (1975). A Short Portable Mental Status Questionnaire for the assessment of organic brain deficit in elderly patients. *J. Am. Geriatrics. Soc., 23,* 433.

Pitt, B. (1982). *Psychogeriatrics: An introduction to the psychiatry of old age.* Edinburgh: Churchill Livingstone.

Plum, F. (1979). Dementia: An approaching epidemic. *Nature, 279,* 372–373.

Reichel, W. (1978). *The geriatric patient.* New York: H. P. Publishing Co., pp. 185–186.

Reisberg, B. (1985). Alzheimer's disease update. *Psychiatric Annals, 15,* 319–322.

Reisberg, B. (1986). Dementia: A systematic approach to identifying reversible causes. *Geriatrics, 41*(4) pp. 30–46.

Reisberg, B., & Ferris, S. H. (1982). Diagnosis and assessment of the older patient. *Hosp. & Comm. Psychiatry, 33,* 104–110.

Reisberg, B., Ferris, S. H., DeLeon, M. J., & Crook, T. (1982). The global deterioration scale for assessment of primary degenerative dementia. *Am. J. Psychiatry, 139,* 1136–1139.

Report on the secretary's task force on black and minority health, vol. 1 (1985). Washington, D.C.: U.S. Department of Health and Human Services.

Robins, P. V., Mace, N. L., & Lucas, M. J. (1982). The impact of dementia on the family. *JAMA, 248,* 333–335.

Robinson, L. (1986). *The future of psychiatric/mental health nursing in nursing clinics of North America*, E. A. Rankin (ed.). Philadelphia: W. B. Sanders.

Sabin, T. D., Vitag, A. J., & Mark, V. H. (1982). Are nursing home diagnosis and treatment inadequate? *JAMA, 248*, 321–322.

Salzman, C. (1982). Basic principles of psychotropic drug prescription for the elderly. *Hosp. & Comm. Psychiatry, 33*, 133–135.

Schneck, M. K., Reisberg, B., & Ferris, S. H. (1982). An overview of current concepts of Alzheimer's disease. *Am. J. Psychiatry, 139*, 165–173.

Snyder, M. (1983). *A guide to neurological and neurosurgical nursing*. New York: John Wiley & Sons.

Steele, C., Lucas, M. J., & Tune, L. E. (1982). An approach to the management of dementia syndromes. *Johns Hopkins Med. J., 151*, 362–368.

Stipe, J. G. (1967). *The development of physical theories*. New York: McGraw-Hill Book Co., p. 49.

Stuart, G. W., & Sundeen, S. J. (1983). *Principles and practice of psychiatric nursing*. St. Louis: C. V. Mosby Co.

Taylor, J. W., & Ballenger, S. (1980). *Neurological dysfunctions and nursing intervention*. New York: McGraw-Hill.

Taylor, R. B., Buckingham, J. L. Donatelle, E. P., Jacott, W. E., & Rosen, M. G. (1983). *Family medicine: Principles and practice* (2nd ed.). New York: Springer-Verlag.

Tomlinson, B. E., Blessed, G., & Roth, M. (1970). Observations on the brains of demented old people. *J. Neurol. Sci., 11*, 205–242.

Trockman, G. (1978). Care for the confused or delirious patient. *Am. J. Nurs., 78*, 1495–1499.

U. S. Department of Health, Education and Welfare, Public Health Service (1979). *Healthy people: The surgeon general's report on health promotion and disease prevention*. Washington D.C.: U.S. Department of Health, Education and Welfare, Public Health Service, DHEW (PHS) Publication No. 79-55071

Walsh, J., Persons, C., & Wieck, L. (1987). *Manual of home health care nursing*. Philadelphia: J. B. Lippincott.

Wells, C. E. (1977). Dementia: Definition and description. In C. E. Wells (ed.) *Dementia* Ed. 2. Philadelphia: F. A. Davis Co.

Wells, C. E. (1979). Pseudodementia. *Am. J. Psychiatry, 136*, 895–900.

Wisniewskitt, M., Coblentz, J. M., & Terry, R. D. (1972). Pick's disease: A clinical and ultrastructural study. *Arch. Neurol., 26*, 97–108.

12

PERSONALITY DISORDERS

CHARLES HODULIK

LEARNING OBJECTIVES

After studying this chapter, the student will be able to:

- Identify the role of defense mechanisms in personality disorders.
- Identify and describe manifestations of the three major subgroups of personality disorders.
- Identify and describe the specific personality disorders.
- Assess patients for personality disorders.
- Plan and participate in practical management of patients with personality disorders in the general health-care setting.
- Make nursing diagnoses and propose nursing care plans for patients with personality disorders.

DESCRIPTION OF PERSONALITY DISORDERS

Personality disorders are among the most common of psychiatric disorders and are the most difficult to treat. Unlike depression, anxiety disorders, neuroses, and adjustment disorders, personality disorders are chronic, unremitting, and more subtly debilitating. Patients with personality disorders are often blamed for their problems and described by others in pejorative terms. They often frustrate and alienate the professionals who try to help them. Frequently neglected, these patients are a major challenge to mental health professionals. Patients with personality disorders need understanding and empathy but often drive away those who attempt to understand them.

In this chapter we describe personality disorders specifically for the nurse generalist. Her goal is not to engage in psychotherapy designed to treat the disorders and correct the underlying character pathology; her goal is to design and manage the nursing care of these patients so that they do not inadvertently undermine their health care. The discussion focuses on the patient with borderline personality disorder because that disorder is likely to be the most difficult to deal with in the health care setting. The nurse who not only can identify the borderline patient and modify nursing care to specifically meet her needs, but who can also empathize with this patient's struggle despite the practical problems it creates for nursing care, should be able to intelligently and sensitively manage patients with the gamut of personality disorders briefly described in this chapter.

MANIFESTATIONS OF PERSONALITY DISORDERS

Most personality disorders best manifest themselves in affected individuals' troubled relationships with other people. The nurse who understands the various personality traits or disorders is best able to elicit maximum cooperation from the patient. Without this understanding, reasonable approaches to these patients may cause major difficulties. An approach that works with one personality type may not work with another. What may be helpful in motivating one personality type may provoke anger and a refusal to cooperate in another.

DSM-III-R has defined the personality disorder as a deeply ingrained, inflexible, maladaptive pattern of relating to, perceiving, and thinking about the environment and the self that is of sufficient severity to cause either significant impairment in adaptive functioning or personal distress. Patients with these disorders generally do not assume responsibility for their lives and feelings; rather, they tend to blame others.

Patients with personality disorders lack sufficient coping mechanisms to adapt successfully to the stresses and problems of everyday life. Debilitating anxiety and psychosis usually are not present. Problems are related to a more general difficulty in working and loving.

Patients with personality disorders frequently and rigidly use defense mechanisms. According to psychoanalytic theory, **defense mechanisms** are psychological maneuvers that provide us with defenses against unpleasant impulsive feelings or memories. The psychologically healthy person uses defense mechanisms flexibly to control the intensity of impulses, feelings, and memories. If the defense mechanisms are used rigidly and frequently enough to cause interpersonal difficulties, subjective distress, or a disruption in functioning, the diagnosis of a personality disorder may be justified. For example, the patient with a compulsive personality disorder rigidly uses lists, schedules, orderliness, cleanliness, and punctuality to control feelings. While compulsive traits are useful for memorization, becoming organized, and accomplishing tasks, rigid use of this defense mechanism does not allow warmth, love, tolerance, or spontaneity to enter interpersonal relationships.

Conversely, the patient with a diagnosis of histrionic personality disorder represses (forgets) details, facts, memories, schedules, and other information required for successful functioning. The patient focuses exclusively on dramatics, flattery, attention seeking, and successful rivalry to maintain good feelings about him or herself. Pathology is manifested by an inability to function well without flattery and attention from others.

The rigid use of the defense mechanism called **projection** is central to the diagnosis of paranoid personality disorder. Via projection, unpleasant impulses and fantasized internal motives are attributed to (projected onto) another, making others appear dangerous and not to be trusted. Rigid use of this defense mechanism results in obvious interpersonal difficulties. Although a detailed presentation of defense mechanisms is not possible in this chapter, Nemiah (1961) provides an excellent overview of this topic.

A difficulty frequently encountered in the Axis II diagnosis of personality disorder occurs when a patient meets the criteria for several personality disorders. At present, DSM-III-R does not provide a system for organizing personality disorders. It does not provide a structure for comparing one personality disorder diagnosis to another in terms of etiology, severity of pathology, or any other comparative model. There is no mechanism for separating traits and behaviors from psychopathology. This makes DSM-III-R, Axis II, differential diagnosis complicated. Mental health professionals often disagree in diagnosing personality disorders (Mellsop et al., 1982). An improved method of organization may improve diagnostic agreement.

Vaillant and Perry (1980) describe three personality-disorder clusters based on the concepts of Eysenck (1956). This classification system is useful because it provides a higher organizing concept for subgrouping the personality disorders. However, it does not take into account some recent information from studies of the patient with borderline personality disorder (Kernberg, 1984). The classification system of personality disorders presented here uses the concepts of personal identity, interpersonal relationships, defense mechanisms, and Axis V highest level of functioning. (See Table 12–1 for a complete list of defense mechanisms.)

Personality disorders can be divided into three subgroups, based on the patient's self-perception and personal identity, quality of interpersonal relationships, expression of affect, and use of defense mechanisms. These three subgroups are 1) confused thinking and social withdrawal; 2) borderline personality organization; and 3) cohesive personality (see Table 12–2).

CONFUSED THINKING AND SOCIAL WITHDRAWAL

Prior to DSM-III, the most disturbed of the **confused thinking and socially withdrawn** patients were thought to be schizophrenic. These patients tend to be isolated emotionally from other people. They may display strange behavior (bizarre dress, inappropriate social behavior, and so on) that reinforces their isolation. Aloof and avoidant of others, they withdraw emotionally into themselves during times of stress. These patients function poorly in society and are occasionally hospitalized (as a result of extreme personal neglect, substance abuse, or behavior dangerous to self or others). The highest functioning members of this group, the individuals with avoidant personality disorder, are capable of closer

relationships but often continue to suffer in isolation, fearing rejection. The schizoid patient seems to have accepted loneliness as a way of life; the schizotypal patient often appears too chaotic and disturbed to be close to others.

BORDERLINE PERSONALITY ORGANIZATION

Patients with **borderline personality organization** exhibit a lack of a cohesive and well-integrated sense of self (Kernberg, 1984). Unlike the socially withdrawn and confused patients who cope by using autistic fantasy and protective confusion, patients with borderline personality organization are more likely to become overwhelmed by powerful feelings of anger and anxiety.

The term borderline personality organization implies a broader and more general concept than the specific diagnosis of **borderline personality disorder**. Borderline personality disorder is one of the three personality disorders within the borderline personality organization group.

DEFENSE MECHANISMS. Patients with borderline personality organization use the developmentally primitive defense mechanisms of splitting and denial. These pathological defense mechanisms protect them from experiencing unpleasant aspects of themselves but do not allow the development of a more stable

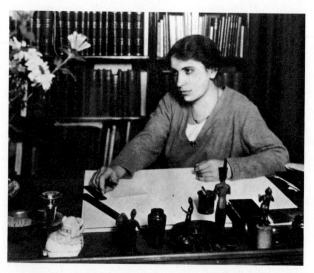

Anna Freud, the daughter of a genius, elaborated on her father's theory of defense mechanisms. She is also known for her application of psychoanalytic theory in the treatment of children.

TABLE 12—1 Defense mechanisms*

Acting-out is the direct expression of impulses without any apparent reflection, guilt, or regard for negative consequences. (Whereas "acting-*up*" is a lay term for any misbehavior, acting-*out* is a misbehavior that is a response to, and a way of coping with, stress or conflict.) After breaking up with his girlfriend, a teenager acts-out by impulsively overdosing. [Immature]

Altruism is involved when the person dedicates himself to the needs of others, partly to fulfill his own needs. [Mature]

Denial is the lack of awareness of *external* realities that would be too painful to acknowledge. It differs from repression (see below), which is a "denial" of *internal* reality. Denial operates when a woman says, "I'm sure this lump on my breast doesn't mean anything." Denial may be temporarily adaptive. [Narcissistic]

Devaluation occurs when the person demeans another or himself by the attribution of exaggerated negative qualities to either. By constantly ridiculing his competence, a patient devalues a therapist to avoid facing her sexual feelings toward him. [Immature]

Displacement is the discharge of pent-up emotions, usually anger, onto objects, animals, or people perceived as less dangerous than those which originally induced the emotions. Kicking the dog. [Neurotic]

Fantasy is the excessive retreat into daydreams and imagination to escape realistic problems or to avoid conflicts. Also called "autistic fantasy" or "schizoid fantasy." [Immature]

Humor is involved when the person uses irony, paradox, or absurdity to reduce what otherwise might be unbearable tension or fear. Hawkeye Pierce in "M*A*S*H." [Mature]

Idealization is used when the person unduly praises another or himself by exaggerating virtues. "Better" to idealize a spouse than to see the jerk for what he is and be a very lonely divorcée. [Immature]

Identification is the unconscious modeling of another's attributes. It differs from role modeling or imitation, which are conscious processes. Identification is used to increase one's sense of self-worth, to cope with (possible) separation or loss, or to minimize helplessness, as with "identification with the aggressor," as seen in concentration-camp prisoners who assumed the mannerisms of their Nazi guards. [Immature]

Intellectualization involves the overuse of abstract thinking which, unlike rationalization (see below), is only self-serving in aiming to reduce psychic discomfort. Alcoholics use intellectualization when they quibble over the definition of alcoholism as a way of avoiding their problem drinking. [Neurotic]

Introjection is the incorporation of other people's values, standards, or traits to prevent conflicts with, or threats from, these people. Introjection may also serve to retain a lost loved one, as when people adopted John Kennedy's accent after his death. [Immature]

Isolation of affect is the compartmentalization of painful emotions from their events. It involves the experience or recollection of an emotionally traumatic situation, without the anxiety customarily or originally associated with it. A soldier may kill without experiencing—that is, by isolating—the terror or guilt he would otherwise feel. [Neurotic]

Projection is the unconscious rejection of unacceptable thoughts, traits, or wishes by ascribing them to others. [Narcissistic when delusional; immature otherwise]

Rationalization is the self-serving use of plausible reasons to justify actions caused by repressed, unacceptable emotions or ideas. Psychotherapist: "I charge a lot so therapy will be meaningful to the patient." [Neurotic]

Reaction formation is preventing the expression or the experience of unacceptable desires by developing or exaggerating opposite attitudes and behaviors. "The lady doth protest too much." [Neurotic]

Regression is retreat under stress to earlier or more immature patterns of behavior and gratification. On hearing terrible news, an adult begins sucking his thumb. [Immature]

Repression is the exclusion from awareness of distressing internal feelings, impulses, ideas, or wishes. Repression is unconscious, suppression (see below) is conscious. A man is unaware that he resents his more successful wife. [Neurotic]

Somatization is reaction to psychologically stressful situations by an excessive preoccupation with physical symptoms. [Immature]

Splitting is involved when the person views himself or others as all good or all bad, as opposed to being a balance of positive and negative attributes. In splitting, the person frequently alternates between idealization and devaluation. [Immature]

Sublimation is the gratification of a repressed instinct or unacceptable feeling by socially acceptable means. Better a surgeon than a sadist. [Mature]

Suppression is the conscious and deliberate avoidance of disturbing matters: Scarlett O'Hara: "I'll think about it tomorrow." [Mature]

Source: Adapted from Maxmen, J. S. (1986). *Essential Psychopathology*. New York: W. W. Norton.

TABLE 12—2 Three subgroups of personality disorders

Description	Sense of Self	DSM-III-R Diagnoses	Defense Mechanisms	Axis V Highest Level of Functioning
Confused thinking Socially withdrawn	Vague and confused	Avoidant Paranoid Schizoid Schizotypal	Fantasy Projection Confusion Withdrawal Isolation of affect	Poor
Borderline personality organization	Fragmented	Narcissistic Borderline Antisocial	Acting out Splitting Projective identification	Poor
Cohesive personality	Consistent and cohesive	Histrionic Compulsive Passive-aggressive Dependent	Repression Reaction formulation Intellectualization Undoing	Fair to good

and secure sense of self that remains stable when the environment changes.

Everyone has good and bad characteristics, strengths and weaknesses. The healthy person is able to integrate these characteristics into a cohesive and stable self that is acceptable to him and to society. Out of this cohesiveness comes a stable sense of goals, values, direction, moral standards, cultural and societal responsibility, and secure sexual orientation. Healthy people are able to tolerate external stress and difficulty without emotionally decompensating, that is, being overwhelmed and becoming dysfunctional.

Splitting. **Splitting** is the pathological defense mechanism that tries to contain the anxiety generated by emotional decompensation or **fragmentation.*** If formation of a cohesive self-perception is not possible, partial grouping provides at least some, although structurally weak, organization. Perceptions of self and others are often split into categories of all good and all bad. Patients who use splitting are unable to describe themselves and others in more than brief, confusing, or stereotypic terms. For example, these patients, when asked to describe others, can describe

*Fragmentation in the extreme involves disintegration anxiety in which it is not physical extinction that is feared, but the loss of humanness and the ascendancy of a nonhuman or inorganic environment (Kohut, 1984).

physical traits, roles, and judgments, but can provide little sense of personality. A patient may state, "My mother was tall, with blue eyes. She worked as a housewife. She was good. My father was a farmer. He was angry and scared me. My mother protected me from him." Patients who use splitting depend heavily on their perceptions of good and bad. They are unable to deal with themselves and others as whole people, seeing only discrete characteristics.

Denial. In the example above, the patient perceives her mother as having all the good attributes of both a father and a mother, while she perceives her father as having all the bad attributes. **Denial** simply describes the ability not to see (deny) the existence of the good traits of the father and the less good traits of the mother. Another illustration of denial is seen in the chronic alcoholic who is jaundiced and suffering from severe liver failure but who denies the existence of a drinking problem.

Splitting and denial are weak and often ineffective defenses. They usually do not contain the anxiety that surfaces unpredictably in the vulnerable individuals who use them. For example, early in an interview a patient described his mother as beautiful, energetic, and liked by everyone. Later, he described her as angry, violent, abusive, and demanding. When confronted by these two different perceptions of the same person, the patient became very upset and began to cry. He was unconsciously using splitting to protect himself from a clear but disturbing perception of a confusing mother.

People with borderline personality organization are not able to integrate all aspects of themselves into a cohesive self. They remain fragmented, that is, they experience themselves as sometimes grandiose and powerful and other times as inadequate and vulnerable, rather than as somewhere in between. The nature of the fragmentation determines the specific personality-disorder diagnosis.

THREE TYPES OF BORDERLINE PERSONALITY ORGANIZATION

Borderline Personality Disorder. Patients with *borderline personality disorder* exhibit the least successful mastery of fragmentation. These patients desperately require other people to give them a sense of definition as parents, children, lovers, friends, or employees. Because of splitting, their relationships are unstable and full of conflict, thereby producing secondary problems (such as difficulty functioning) and intense symptoms (such as feelings of abandonment or suicidality) when the relationships deteriorate.

Narcissistic Personality Disorder. Patients who suffer from **narcissism** have achieved a slightly more successful adaptation. They have been able to bring together their positive traits, perceptions, and talents into a somewhat stable sense of self, which remains intact except during severe distress. These patients, however, are unable to relate to their own shortcomings and feelings of loss and sadness and are unable to empathize with others who have such feelings.

Antisocial Personality Disorder. Patients with **antisocial personality disorder** avoid the anxiety and unpleasant emotions associated with fragmentation by acting out their conflicts with society. They do not assume responsibility for their actions and do not trust others. Their value system often consists of attitudes such as, "If it feels good, do it. If you want it, take it. If others get hurt, too bad. Others would do the same if they had the opportunity."

COHESIVE PERSONALITY

Patients with **cohesive personality** have a more developed and realistic sense of self. They think clearly, have a sense of who they are, and have meaningful interpersonal relationships. These patients function better than those in the other two subgroups, but they make rigid use of higher level defense mechanisms, such as repression and compulsive behavior. There is some question about the validity of this subgroup of personality disorders: many of the criteria for cohesive personality are only exaggerations of traits present in many people considered to be healthy.

Comparison of Borderline to Cohesive Personality. The assessment of a cohesive personality is difficult. The patient with a cohesive personality is able to separate the self from external events. Although mood and self-esteem may be affected by external events, the basic sense of self is constant. Patients with a cohesive sense of self are able to tolerate being alone. They are not tormented by disjointed, antagonistic, and seemingly unintegratable fragments of themselves. Unlike borderline patients, patients with cohesive personality disorders have the ability to sustain long-term friendships and develop a work history. Patients with a cohesive sense of self are also able to give accurate and complete descriptions of themselves and others. They are able to respond to requests such as, "Tell me about yourself," and "How would you describe yourself as a person?" While these are not easy questions, patients with cohesive personalities are able to respond with a description of themselves that includes values, feelings, preferences, a sense of right or wrong, a moral code that defines good and bad, and an integrated sense of sexuality. The fragmented patient is usually only able to describe portions of the self that seem to change in different situations.

Borderline patients describe significant others as stick people, without human features. As a result, the listener is unable to generate an image of the person described. A borderline patient may describe his or her parents in all good or all bad terms, or inconsistently. For example, early in an interview, an individual may describe his mother as abusive, violent, and demanding. Later he may refer to her as beautiful and loving. When confronted with these inconsistencies, he is likely to experience anxiety and confusion and possibly acknowledge that he is unable to retain a consistent mental picture of his mother.

Other patients who have problems with a stable sense of self include those suffering from an organic brain syndrome. They cannot grasp a concept so subtle and abstract as sense of self. For similar reasons, this is also not possible for patients of limited intelligence. Others, such as anxious or depressed patients, who have a relatively stable sense of self, may be too preoccupied, lethargic, or not motivated enough to struggle with personal questions during an interview. With them, assessment of sense of self must be done over time with continued development of the therapeutic relationship.

ASSESSMENT OF PERSONALITY DISORDERS

Many patients display symptoms of personality disorders when they are hospitalized. It is important for the nurse to obtain sufficient history to be able to place the present behavior of the patient in context. The hospital setting often precipitates regression and feelings of dependency in patients; thus symptoms of personality disorder tend to be more prominent at times of hospitalization. The personality disorder is less obvious at times of less stress when there is less of a need for defensive activity. Patients in the hospital may also develop personality disorder symptoms secondary to their medical problems.

Conversely, some patients appear emotionally healthier while hospitalized. Extremely dependent or borderline patients (when not threatened with discharge) may be more comfortable on a unit, where the role of patient is clear. At discharge, they may appear much more upset and demanding. Their fear of loss and anxiety related to their need for structure and clear expectations is expressed through anger. Understanding that such patients are expressing manifestations of their personality disorders allows for planning of required outpatient structure such as visiting-nurse services, family support, or psychiatric followup.

When the nurse has obtained sufficient history and data to determine that the maladaptive personality pattern of the patient is chronic and well-established, the diagnosis of personality disorder can be made. Since dependency is a feature of most personality disorders, it is important to differentiate the diagnosis of dependent personality from dependent features of the more serious and difficult-to-treat (and deal with) personality disorders and borderline personality organization.

The existence of an overwhelming primary psychiatric diagnosis such as schizophrenia, mood disorder, or anxiety disorder severely complicates Axis II diagnosis. Often the major disruptive symptoms of the Axis I diagnosis must be controlled before the underlying personality becomes evident. In schizophrenia, however, the degree of personality disorganization is chronic and severe. An Axis II personality-disorder diagnosis is usually not possible in patients with schizophrenia because of the disorganization present and the confusion about sense of self.

BORDERLINE PERSONALITY DISORDER

It is probably more difficult to work with the individual with borderline personality disorder than with any other patient. Despite the best efforts of knowledgeable and experienced clinicians, these patients (usually women) are often dysfunctional and present with serious problems, such as suicidality. (See Chapter 18 on crisis for more on suicide assessment.) In addition, the nurse or therapist is likely to be blamed by the patient for the consequences of her destructive behavior. Worse, an appropriate approach to a borderline patient at one time may result in disastrous effects at another. The anger and self-destructiveness of these patients make them extremely difficult to deal with. In short, these patients are taxing even for the most highly trained professional. To work with them in the health care system requires highly coordinated teamwork by all involved. A failure in coordination (perhaps as a result of the patient's "splitting") may sabotage the treatment.

Borderline patients usually manifest their pathology through intensely overinvolved, self-serving relationships with other people. For the borderline patient, the only thing worse than having one of these relationships is *not* having one. When deprived of a relationship with a significant other because of death, separation, divorce, abandonment, or rejection, the most flagrant of the DSM-III-R symptoms (such as temper displays, affective instability, or self-destructive behavior) are likely to become manifest. Also see Box 12–1.

Although everyone requires others for warmth, love, and support in order to be happy, borderline patients require others for their very existence. Other people are required because borderline patients lack a cohesive sense of self. They are not able to integrate feeling happy at one time and sad at another, loving at one time and hating at another, and strong at one time and weak at another. People who are secure in their sense of self can accept broad ranges of behavior, thoughts, and feelings within themselves as consistent with a flexible personality. Borderline patients do not possess such flexibility and are unable to achieve a realistic sense of self.

ETIOLOGY OF BORDERLINE PERSONALITY DISORDER. Hypotheses regarding the etiology of borderline personality disorder involve biological,

Box 12–1 ● At the Movies

Fatal Attraction, one of the most successful movies of 1987, dubbed "the AIDS movie" because it argues that sex can be lifethreatening (*People,* October 26, 1987, p. 89), is thought by some mental health professionals to be a vivid portrait of borderline personality disorder at its most destructive (University of Wisconsin Department of Child Psychiatry Journal Club, November 1987). In the movie, actress Glenn Close portrays Alex, a "tragic, bewildering mix of sexuality and rage" (*People,* October 26, 1987, p. 89). According to *People* reporters, one psychiatrist has pointed out that the Close character's pathology includes a weak sense of identity, a tendency to become obsessed with an idealized love object, and very low self-esteem. These and other borderline traits, e.g., a sense of worthlessness (sometimes expressed as "emptiness") and the in-

ability to contain affect and impulses, can result in self as well as other directed violence as depicted in *Fatal Attraction.* (Of course, borderline personality disorder isn't the only DSM-III-R diagnosis associated with violence. See Chapter 24, *The Violent Patient.*)

Interestingly, according to *People,* test audiences voted down the movie's original ending in which Alex slits her own throat, framing her lover to be convicted of her "murder." In the final version of the film, the one released to the public, *Alex* gets it in the end. The test audience reportedly felt avenged in viewing it, and gave their "approval," a good example of how much negative countertransference can be stirred up by an individual (or a woman?) with borderline personality disorder.

Source: *People,* October 26, 1987.

psychological, and sociological factors. Some knowledge and expertise is required in all of these areas in order to develop the understanding required to work well with the borderline patient. Another organizing concept in attempts to better understand these patients is their inner struggle with accumulated rage.

Biological Factors. Biological factors play a significant role in borderline pathology. One hypothesis is that the borderline patient is genetically predisposed to a higher than normal level of aggression and rage, making her more difficult to care for as a child and relate to as an adult (Kernberg, 1984). This is disputed by theorists who acknowledge the borderline patient's pathological anger but who feel that it is impossible to tell whether it is the cause or effect of the psychopathology (Wolberg, 1982). (Also see Box 12–2.)

The borderline and mood disorders share biological markers, that is, biological signs of disorder. Two of these are the **dexamethasone-suppression test** and the **REM latency test.** The dexamethasone-suppression test evaluates the integrity of a hypothalamic pituitary adrenal-cortical axis. Both patients with borderline personality disorder and those with

mood disorders have abnormalities in this system. The REM (rapid eye movement) latency test measures the time between falling asleep and the onset of REM sleep. Again, patients with borderline and mood disorders show similar abnormalities on this measure (Akiskal, 1981). These data have led to the hypothesis that borderline personality disorder is not a valid concept but is only a variant of mood disorders. This appears to be an oversimplification—most patients who meet the criteria for borderline personality disorder do not satisfactorily respond to treatment for mood disorders (such as tricyclic antidepressant medication). Also many patients with borderline personality disorder do not suffer from clinical depression. Nevertheless, medications used to treat symptoms of mood disorders may be helpful to some patients with borderline personality disorder. (See Chapter 9 on mood disorders for more on biological markers and antidepressant medication.)

Psychological Factors. The borderline concept was developed initially in psychoanalytic literature to describe patients who appeared healthy enough to benefit from psychoanalysis, but who began to decompensate, or fragment, and become transiently

Box 12–2 • Genetics and Personality

Results of behavioral genetics research are beginning to seriously challenge the conventional wisdom about the importance of childhood environment to developing personalities. Behavioral geneticists are finding that genes account for about 50% of the variance in personality type (or 50% of the range found in a study population). Similarly, studies of identical twins reared together and reared apart indicate that genetic influences on personality development predominate. The result is the same for the development of altruism and aggressiveness, personality traits which are commonly thought to be the result of parent modeling or parenting style.

The longest running prospective study of genetic influences on personality and behavior, initiated by the late Ronald Wilson of the University of Louisville in the 1950s, has shown that "behavioral development is guided by a genetic strategy analogous to that for biological development" (Holdon, 1987, p. 600). In fact, according to researchers working on this project and others, "the common environment seems to have a negligible role in creating personality similarities among family members" (p. 600). The most explicit statement about all of this is credited to Harvard sociobiologist E. O. Wilson: "The behavioral genes . . . probably influence the ranges of the form and intensity of emotional responses, the thresholds of arousals, the readiness to learn certain stimuli as opposed to others, and the pattern of sensitivity to additional environmental factors that point cultural evolution in one direction as opposed to another" (p. 601).

Source: Holdon, Constance. (1987) The genetics of personality. *Science*, 237, 7 August, p. 598–601.

psychotic during the unstructured psychoanalytic treatment process. The search for reasons for the large discrepancy between the apparent health of these patients and their potential to become psychotic in stressful situations has produced a large and sophisticated psychoanalytic literature. Margaret Mahler's (1971) theory regarding psychological birth is an example. According to Mahler, babies are born autistic (unable to interact significantly with others); they then begin to fuse with the mother until they become psychologically symbiotic. During the symbiotic phase, the baby perceives no separation or difference between himself and his mother. This phase peaks when the infant is six to eight months old. After this, the child begins to separate and become an individual distinct from his mother. This phase is called *separation-individuation*. It is a difficult time for both child and mother. Some theorists feel that it is most difficult for a female child because she must separate from the same-sex parent, and our culture is tolerant of (even supportive of) close mother-daughter ties. Boys, on the other hand, from preschool through adolescence are encouraged by the world to be strong and autonomous.

A toddler will only be able to separate if he or she is convinced that mother will be there when he

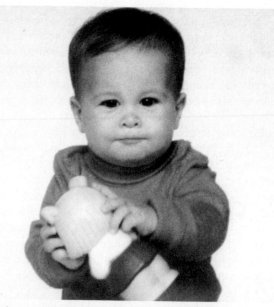

At about 8 months of age, according to Margaret Mahler, a psychoanalytic theorist of the object-relations school, the infant begins the most important work of his or her life: "psychological birth" through the process of separation and individuation from his or her mother, a previously symbiotic partner, to become a person in his or her own right.

**DSM-III-R
Diagnostic Criteria for
Borderline Personality
Disorder**

A pervasive pattern of instability of mood, interpersonal relationships, and self-image, beginning by early adulthood and present in a variety of contexts, as indicated by at least *five* of the following:

1) a pattern of unstable and intense interpersonal relationships characterized by alternating between extremes of overidealization and devaluation

2) impulsiveness in at least two areas that is potentially self-damaging, e.g., spending, sex, substance use, shoplifting, reckless driving, binge eating (Do not include suicidal or self-mutilating behavior covered in [5].)

3) affective instability: marked shifts from baseline mood to depression, irritability, or anxiety, usually lasting a few hours and only rarely more than a few days

4) inappropriate, intense anger or lack of control of anger, e.g., frequent displays of temper, constant anger, recurrent physical fights

5) recurrent suicidal threats, gestures, or behavior, or self-mutilating behavior

6) marked and persistent identity disturbance manifested by uncertainty about at least two of the following: self-image, sexual orientation, long-term goals or career choice, type of friends desired, preferred values

7) chronic feelings of emptiness or boredom

8) frantic efforts to avoid real or imagined abandonment (Do not include suicidal or self-mutilating behavior covered in [5].)

---

or she wants to be close. That is, the mother must continue to be perfectly available. Since imperfection is intolerable to the toddler, and mothers are not perfect, a defense is needed against fear of abandonment—specifically, the defense of splitting. Splitting allows the child to deny the existence of the bad (imperfect) parts of the mother and thus feel safe enough to separate and begin to become a distinct individual. If all goes well, the toddler eventually is able to tolerate the fear of separation and to perceive and accept all parts of the mother, the self, and others.

Developmentally, the borderline patient, usually female, has not successfully worked through this normal separation-individuation process. It is thought by psychoanalytic theorists (Kernberg, 1984; Masterson, 1975) that as a toddler, the borderline patient was not able to make the transition from an infant fused symbiotically with her mother to a child with the ability to separate and become autonomous without significant fear and anxiety. Because of this developmental arrest, the borderline patient has not developed the appropriate mental apparatus to control impulses and powerful affects. The individual with borderline personality disorder is therefore unable to develop an accurate self-perception and understanding of the nature of the relationship between herself and others. The inability to be alone, chronic feelings

of emptiness or boredom, and identity disturbance are the manifestations of this arrest in development.

Daniel Stern, a psychiatrist and researcher like Mahler, takes a different view of the psychological development of borderline personality disorder. In his research on the "observed infant" (1985, p. 13), he has focused on the development of self from infancy as well as the role of "attunement" (p. 138) or affect-matching in early relationships. Stern, like Kernberg, theorizes that affect has a major role in psychological development and that affect attunement between mother and infant is essential to the development of the sense of subjective self between the ages of nine and 15 months. This attunement involves more than a mother's empathy for her child, according to Stern. A form of affective transaction, it involves one person's reflection of the inner state of another, in order to be with him.

In contrast to Mahler, Stern holds that sense-of-self first emerges in the first two months of life, develops its "core" which consists of four self-invariants: agency, coherence, affectivity, and continuity, between the ages of two and six months; becomes intersubjective between seven and 15 months; and evolves into the verbal sense of self between 18 and 30 months. The self that evolves may be the true self if that is what the mother has attuned to. However, if intersubjective sharing involves selective attunement (based on the mother's affective state rather than the infant's), misattunement, or nonattunement, the true self is disavowed and a false self develops. Like Kohut (1977), a psychoanalyst who developed the theory of self-psychology (see Chapter 2 on theoretical models of psychopathology), Stern describes pathology due to deficits in interpersonal reality, not conflict, and focuses on attachment rather than separation in his attempt to explain the development of character disorders such as borderline personality disorder. Even in discussing rapprochement, Stern emphasizes the resetting of the *attachment* balance that occurs, rather than the autonomy and separation that is its context. He states: "For Mahler (and Kernberg) connectedness implies a failure in differentiation; for us, success in psychic functioning" (Stern, 1985, p. 241). For Stern (and Kohut) togetherness is the essential state of human existence.

Sociological Factors. Borderline patients have interpersonal relationships that are significantly impaired. By definition, it is difficult for borderline patients to have supportive, caring, and helpful friends who are willing to be available to them during times of stress and crisis. Borderline patients tend to burn out their support systems, leaving themselves isolated during times of greatest difficulty. Although cause and effect are difficult to sort out, these patients often have severely strained relationships with their families. Biologically oriented theorists argue that the borderline patient's genetically determined symptomatology leads to significant stress in his or her family and the development of family pathology (Kernberg, 1984). Family theorists argue that pathology within the family is the cause of the borderline patient's psychopathology (Wolberg, 1982). They argue that there is often a lack of appropriate generational boundaries. For example, role reversal frequently exists between the parents and the child.

In psychologically healthy families, the parents are responsible for providing structure, support, and guidance for the children. Parents are also responsible for taking care of the children, disciplining them, and providing intangibles such as comfort, warmth, and affection, as well as setting appropriate limits. When a child is out of control in an inappropriate or dangerous way, it is the role of the parent to help contain and protect the child until he or she regains control. In many families of borderline patients, the children are often charged with providing gratification, pleasure, and a sense of accomplishment for the parent. When the child is upset or needy, the parents become frustrated because the child is making them

appear to be bad parents as a result of his "bad" behavior. This cycle escalates into rage and destructiveness and is likely to be repeated in the next generation. That is, the child of an individual with borderline personality disorder is likely to develop the disorder also. Many theorists feel that this is the result of heredity *and* this type of environment.

The ultimate example of the child who is responsible for caring for the needs of the adult is in the case of incest. Many clinicians find a high incidence of incest in borderline patients, leading to the hypothesis that incest is the cause of the borderline personality disorder (Hodulik, unpublished manuscript). Although it has been reported that the mothers of borderline individuals are often borderline themselves (Masterson, 1975), recent research has not supported this (Gunderson, 1984). More often, the parents are found to be needy and often not emotionally available to the child. There is no consistent or predominant psychiatric disorder in the parents of individuals with borderline personality disorder, although the incidence of depression is higher than among normals (Gunderson & England, 1981).

TREATMENT FOR BORDERLINE PERSONALITY DISORDER. Although in this chapter we focus on managing patients within their personality pathology rather than providing psychotherapeutic treatment designed to change the personality, our distinction is not so clear in the case of the individual with borderline personality disorder. These patients perceive themselves as victims, not taking responsibility for their problems or the potential solutions to them. They blame others extensively for their problems and often feel justified in self-destructive behavior. As a result, borderline patients generate increasing amounts of anger and frustration, which they blame on others, while feeling increasingly less responsible for themselves and their behavior. This situation can become volatile and dangerous. Both practical management of these patients when they are hospitalized and ongoing psychotherapy should attempt to manage the borderline patient in the same way. The patient should be encouraged to try harder to take more responsibility for herself. She needs to receive a consistent message from her therapist, family, and all important people who work with her—nurses, clergy, teachers, and nonpsychiatric physicians—that she has the ability to keep herself alive and safe during stressful times. She will also need reinforcement that there is growth, strength, and stability to be gained by merely surviving. When this is not possible or enough to help the patient contain the very painful feelings which she acts out in self-destruction, psychiatric hospitalization is usually recommended. Also see Box 12–3.

At the time of hospitalization, if not before, the patient must be assessed carefully for the presence of any additional Axis I disorders. It is consistent with DSM-III-R for a patient with borderline personality disorder to have an additional Axis I diagnosis of a mood, anxiety, substance abuse, or other disorder. Although medication cannot "cure" a personality disorder, antidepressant, antianxiety, and/or antipsychotic medication may help to control symptoms of agitation, insomnia, depression, dissociation, and poor impulse control (Hodulik, 1984).

In order to begin psychotherapy with a borderline patient, the therapist must have a commitment from the patient to stop the destructive behavior that provides a distraction from painful emotions. The patient is unlikely to make this commitment unless she is in a relationship with a secure and competent therapist.

PRACTICAL MANAGEMENT OF PATIENTS WITH BORDERLINE PERSONALITY DISORDER

1. The nurse does not necessarily agree with the patient's perceptions of events or other people.

2. The nurse does not take sides in the patient's disputes with other people.

3. The nurse does not attempt to rescue the patient from the consequences of her actions.

4. The nurse does not try to solve problems the patient is capable of solving herself. This would only undermine her competence and ability to solve problems.

5. The nurse does not get caught up in the patient's "splitting" and remains a member of a coordinated and well-led treatment team.

6. The nurse only tries approaches that are consistent with the approaches of other treatment-team members.

7. The nurse obtains ongoing consultation from a competent advisor or peer when dealing with the patient.

8. The nurse is not ashamed of her frustrations or negative feelings toward the borderline patient. She talks about this openly with other members of the treatment team in order to resolve her feelings.

9. The nurse does not attempt to compensate for a therapist or physician who appears not to be doing a good job of treating the borderline patient. If she is concerned about this, she should talk with the therapist or physician directly. She may obtain significant information that the patient did not tell her.

The management of patients with borderline personality disorder is filled with frustrations, and progress is slow. But with practice the nurse can master the skills to work with these patients, and be of significant help to them in their struggles.

Mary: A Patient with Borderline Personality Disorder

Mary was a 21-year-old woman who first sought treatment after an ingestion of pills following a fight with her boyfriend. Although Mary experienced feelings of anger and anxiety that escalated after her boyfriend threatened to leave her, she did not make clear her exact reasons for the overdose. She claimed not to remember a logical train of thought. Immediately after taking the overdose, she began thinking more coherently and called the rescue squad to transport her to the hospital. She agreed to admission to the psychiatric unit.

Mary's mental status revealed anxiety and a guarded manner of interaction. She was quite withdrawn initially and minimized the seriousness of her overdose. When questioned in depth about herself and her problems, she was either vague and uninterested or resentful and angry that people were asking these questions. She blamed the hospital staff for causing problems for her and making her feel bad.

When Mary's boyfriend called and expressed interest in her, she insisted she was ready to leave. Her admitting psychiatrist discharged her uneasily and made an outpatient appointment that she did not keep. Mary quickly returned to a relatively high level of functioning. With her relationship restored, she felt more secure and able to use her energy and high level of intelligence.

Mary's boyfriend felt guilty and was accepting the blame for Mary's suicide attempt (as a result of her defense of projective identification).* In only a short period of time, he felt controlled and defensive around Mary. (This is a common feeling among people who work with or have relationships with borderline patients.) Although he felt compelled to stay, the fights related to control and unreasonable demands left Mary's boyfriend feeling angry and frustrated. The tension rose.

When Mary began experiencing insomnia and increased agitation, she asked her personal physician

*Projective identification is a primitive form of projection, characterized by 1) the tendency to continue to experience the impulse that is simultaneously being projected onto the other person, 2) fear of the other person under the influence of that projected impulse, and 3) the need to control the other person under the influence of this mechanism (Kernberg, 1984).

Box 12–3 ● Marilyn

Certainly, the grown-up Norma Jeane continued to neglect herself, just as she had been neglected as a child. She could not break the pattern. Alone, without the public pressure of being Marilyn, she sometimes wouldn't bother to bathe, or wash her hair, or change out of an old bathrobe. She could ignore runs in her stockings, or menstrual stains on her skirt. When the mist of drugs took over, some of this carelessness overlapped into her public life. Singer Eddie Fisher, who was then married to Elizabeth Taylor, remembers Marilyn after her separation from Arthur Miller, at a party at a Nevada gambling casino where Frank Sinatra was performing. "Elizabeth and I sat in the audience," he recalled, "with Dean and Jeanne Martin and Marilyn Monroe, who was having an affair with Sinatra, to watch his act. But all eyes were on Marilyn as she swayed back and forth to the music and pounded her hands on the stage, her breasts falling out of her low-cut dress. She was so beautiful and so drunk." A few months later, a

guest at Peter Lawford's beach house, where Marilyn was often a guest during the last two years of her life, described her sad figure "half doped a lot of the time," oblivious to the spreading bloodstain on her white pants as she lounged on cushions or walked aimlessly on the beach.

The woman who feared most of all becoming a joke, being used or victimized, was succumbing to her greatest fear. Only Norma Jeane would have known the cruel distance between the nightmare of the nonperson she believed herself to be and the dream of the public Marilyn—and that distance was diminishing. She felt "unimportant and insignificant," her last psychiatrist, Dr. Ralph Greenson, explained. "The main mechanism she used to bring some feeling of stability and significance to her life was the attractiveness of her body."

Whenever the public artifice failed and the private Norma Jeane seemed to be her only fate again—when another man she looked to for fathering had abandoned her, when

---

to prescribe medication to help her relax. Unaware of her personality disorder, he prescribed an antianxiety medication that decreased her impulse control. As a result, Mary acted on her self-destructive impulses and overdosed with the medication. She was admitted to the intensive care unit for monitoring. The consulting psychiatrist found Mary again minimizing her irresponsible behavior and the seriousness of her overdose. She was angry when asked questions that confronted inconsistencies in her story. At times other than questioning, she adopted a chameleonlike willingness to comply with procedures and requests.

Although the consulting psychiatrist recommended psychiatric hospitalization for Mary, she refused. Mary claimed that all she needed was a better attitude, and she planned to work on this. The situation worsened considerably when Mary's boyfriend announced he could not handle her anymore and that he was ending the relationship.

Mary threatened to leave the unit against medical advice. The psychiatrist knew that since she would probably deny suicidal intent if asked by legal authorities, it was unlikely she could be forced legally to re-

ceive treatment. (See Chapter 27 on legal issues and Chapter 28 on ethics for more on involuntary detention and treatment.)

The nurses became increasingly worried that Mary would act out her anger in a physically destructive manner. She would explode into rages when the nursing staff tried to make her accept routine vital-sign checks and other procedures she had previously easily tolerated. The nurses were concerned that restraints might become necessary. (Also see Chapter 24 on the violent patient.)

The attending physician was also upset by Mary's behavior. He was angry that the psychiatrist could not make her go to the psychiatric unit, and that the nurses were frequently calling him with questions about Mary's care. The whole system was becoming paralyzed with feelings of anger and anxiety.

The hospital staff and physicians had taken on the problems of the borderline patient (projective identification again). The head nurse, attending physician, and consulting psychiatrist met to clarify roles and responsibilities, to set up approaches to the patient's demanding, angry behavior, and to discuss

she was criticized or blamed, when she had failed to have a child or otherwise bring reality to her public persona—then depression and hopelessness took over. Marilyn said she had attempted suicide twice before she was nineteen. When she was twenty-four, Natasha Lytess saved her a third time. There were three near-deaths during her marriage to Arthur Miller, and at least two more close calls before the final act.

She was still beautiful and a good actress to the end. The costume tests and outtakes from the unfinished *Something's Got to Give* show a luminescence and magic that her imitators can't capture. Studio executives of that film knew she had just been saved from self-induced death by overdose, accidental or not, but, as one explained callously, "If she'd had a heart attack we'd never get insurance for the production. We don't have that problem. Medically, she's perfectly fit."

And indeed she did appear miraculously free of the usual physical symptoms of addiction. Greenson concluded that, "Although she resembled an addict, she did not seem to be the usual addict." When she oc-

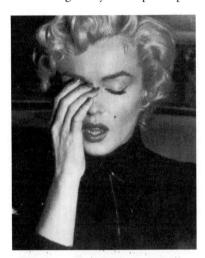

After being disappointed again and again by the men in her life who she hoped would not think of her only as a sex-object, and after eight suicide attempts between the ages of 19 and 36, Marilyn took a fatal overdose of drugs and alcohol and died as she lived, alone.

casionally gave up drugs, she apparently did not experience withdrawal. Lee Strasberg, who had taken her into his family in New York, said he tried to help her sleep without pills by giving her the nurturing she had missed as a child. "She wanted to be held," he explained. "Not to be made love to but just to be supported, because when she'd taken the pills they'd somehow react on her so that she would want more. We wouldn't give them to her. That's why she got in the habit of coming over and staying over. I'd hold her a little and she'd go to sleep."

But no one can reach back into the past. Only we can love and accept that child in ourselves, and so have the strength to change the pattern.

Perhaps Marilyn could not have achieved that. Perhaps she had been abandoned too early. But she lived in a time when her body was far more rewarded than the spirit inside. Her body became her prison.

Source: Steinem, Gloria, *Marilyn.* (New York: Henry Holt and Company), 1986) pp. 152–154. Used by permission.

what could or could not be done legally. With everyone in agreement about a consistent approach, Mary's behavior became more reasonable. When she began to feel more in control, Mary was willing to begin outpatient psychotherapy with the consulting psychiatrist. She was able to transfer her dependency from her boyfriend to her psychiatrist, an important first step in achieving responsible independence, the major goal of psychotherapy.

NURSING CARE PLAN. The only background information Mary's primary nurse, Beth, had about Mary was "second overdose in a month"; both overdoses related to conflict with her boyfriend. After two shifts of caring for her, Beth also learned that Mary was emotionally labile but denied having any emotional problems except for anxiety when she felt that her boyfriend wanted to end their relationship. She also denied the seriousness of her two suicide attempts. Beth was aware of feeling angry at Mary

but felt that this might be because she reminded her of her younger sister, whom she had always considered a "spoiled brat."

The combination of Mary's history and a brief exposure to her emotional instability and the intensity of her anger was enough for Beth to hypothesize a possible diagnosis of borderline personality disorder, which the consulting psychiatrist confirmed. She reasoned that, though Mary's problems needed to be dealt with in psychotherapy, there were things she could do to help Mary regain emotional equilibrium. Beth could set limits in the context of empathy for the emotional experience Mary was having. The following is the start of the nursing care plan Beth developed for Mary while Mary was hospitalized in the ICU.

NARCISSISTIC PERSONALITY DISORDER

Narcissistic people are not good patients. Life is very hard for them when they are sick or injured. They

Nursing Care Plan for Mary

Nursing Diagnosis	Desired Outcome	Interventions	Rationale
1. Anxiety	Mary will verbalize, rather than act out, and cope effectively with anxiety regarding loss of a primary relationship.	Encourage Mary to explore and express her feelings about her boyfriend and their relationship, previous relationships, and her need for a primary relationship.	Helping Mary identify her needs, expectations, and anxieties, and helping her see patterns, take responsibility for problems, and find behavioral alternatives to avoid them in the future will help Mary reestablish a sense of being in control of her life (a sense of self) and less vulnerable to external threat.
2. Ineffective individual coping	same	Help Mary relate her anger to her anxiety about being left and help her see how angry behavior (not feelings) alienates people. Explore with her ways to express anger without being self-destructive or sabotaging valued relationships.	Helping the patient with borderline personality disorder separate feelings from behavior allows the nurse to acknowledge and empathize with the patient's very intense affect without condoning or encouraging self-destructive behavior.
3. Potential for injury (potential for self-directed violence)	Mary will make and keep a no-suicide contract. She will not act on suicidal feelings but contact her therapist or support person about them.	Label suicide as an unacceptable alternative, acknowledging Mary's power to kill herself despite hospitals, psychiatrists, etc., and offering to help her avoid its tragic (for her) irreversible outcome.	Taking Mary's suicidality seriously and acknowledging her power is likely to decrease her need to act out her self-destructive feelings.
		Differentiate suicidal feelings from suicidal behavior.	Mary can't control her feelings but she can control her behavior.
		Offer the nursing staff's help in controlling Mary's suicidal impulses while she is in the unit. Renew a no-suicide contract (see Chapter 18) every shift.	The increased opportunity to have her feelings understood or at least acknowledged by nursing staff will decrease Mary's tendency to act those feelings out. A no-suicide contract is one way to acknowledge the intensity of Mary's feelings while helping her contain them.

DSM-III-R Diagnostic Criteria for Narcissistic Personality Disorder

A pervasive pattern of grandiosity (in fantasy or behavior), lack of empathy, and hypersensitivity to the evaluation of others, beginning by early adulthood and present in a variety of contexts, as indicated by at least *five* of the following:

1) reacts to criticism with feelings of rage, shame, or humiliation (even if not expressed)

2) is interpersonally exploitative: takes advantage of others to achieve his or her own ends

3) has a grandiose sense of self-importance, e.g., exaggerates achievements and talents, expects to be noticed as "special" without appropriate achievement

4) believes that his or her problems are unique and can be understood only by other special people

5) is preoccupied with fantasies of unlimited success, power, brilliance, beauty, or ideal love

6) has a sense of entitlement: unreasonable expectation of especially favorable treatment, e.g., assumes that he or she does not have to wait in line when others must do so

7) requires constant attention and admiration, e.g., keeps fishing for compliments

8) lack of empathy: inability to recognize and experience how others feel, e.g., annoyance and surprise when a friend who is seriously ill cancels a date

9) is preoccupied with feelings of envy

become demanding, angry, and easily offended. Since they feel entitled to special treatment, receiving care that is only as good as everyone else's is not good enough for them.

Like borderline and antisocial patients, narcissistic patients lack the ability to perceive themselves and others accurately. They only acknowledge their good, strong, positive, and virtuous characteristics. However, fantasies of power, conquest, fame, and success are often not powerful enough to ward off feelings of failure and worthlessness. Since pain, illness, suffering, and depression do not easily fit into these patients' systems of belief, they are difficult to work with when they are sick.

There is no empirical evidence of either a biological or genetic factor in this disorder. One theory suggests that these patients may not have been valued or shown affection to as children for themselves, but only for what they could do (Wolberg, 1982). Theorists hypothesize that the parents of these patients needed their children to be special or talented in order to maintain their own self-esteem.

Norman: A Patient with Narcissistic Personality Disorder

Norman considered himself an important man. He dressed well, acted confident and self-assured, and possessed an attitude of entitlement. The nursing staff noticed, at first with amusement, later with irritation, that his doctor treated him as a special patient who did not have to follow the usual rules on the unit.

The amusement changed to irritation when the nursing staff was asked to check Norman's surgical wound twice as often as usually required. Norman did not seem to appreciate how difficult it was to make time for the extra dressing change, as he was rarely in his room when the nurse needed to begin it, and he expressed no thanks for his special care.

When confronted about the impact of his special treatment, Norman exploded with a list of criticisms about the operation of the unit and quality of care. He very perceptively identified several areas of dispute concerning the operation of the unit. The staff quickly polarized and began fighting about unit policies. Part

DSM-III-R Diagnostic Criteria for Antisocial Personality Disorder

A. Current age at least 18.

B. Evidence of Conduct Disorder with onset before age 15, as indicated by a history of *three* or more of the following:

    1) was often truant

    2) ran away from home overnight at least twice while living in parental or parental surrogate home (or once without returning)

    3) often initiated physical fights

    4) used a weapon in more than one fight

    5) forced someone into sexual activity with him or her

    6) was physically cruel to animals

    7) was physically cruel to other people

    8) deliberately destroyed others' property (other than by fire-setting)

    9) deliberately engaged in fire-setting

    10) often lied (other than to avoid physical or sexual abuse)

    11) has stolen without confrontation of a victim on more than one occasion (including forgery)

    12) has stolen with confrontation of a victim (e.g., mugging, purse-snatching, extortion, armed robbery)

C. A pattern of irresponsible and antisocial behavior since the age of 15, as indicated by at least *four* of the following:

    1) is unable to sustain consistent work behavior, as indicated by any of the following (including similar behavior in academic settings if the person is a student):

        (*a*) significant unemployment for six months or more within five years when expected to work and work was available

        (*b*) repeated absences from work unexplained by illness in self or family

        (*c*) abandonment of several jobs without realistic plans for others

    2) fails to conform to social norms with respect to lawful behavior, as indicated by repeatedly performing antisocial acts that are grounds for arrest (whether arrested or not), e.g., destroying property, harassing others, stealing, pursuing an illegal occupation

---

of the staff became even more attentive to Norman's concerns, increasing his irritation at those who were less attentive.

Psychiatric consultation was obtained. Somewhat surprisingly, Norman reacted very positively to the psychiatrist and was much easier to manage. The psychiatrist was able to focus on the difficulty for Norman of being in a situation that he could not control. When the nursing staff was encouraged to focus on his pain and his difficulty remaining immobile, he became less demanding and seemed to require only slightly more than routine care. The nursing staff was able to assign coverage to him so that the nurses who could legitimately feel some concern and positive feelings toward him worked with him. Those who could find no empathy or positive feelings for Norman did not work with him.

When it was realized that Norman's style was based on his personality and that his sense of entitlement was only a way of compensating for deep feelings of insecurity and fear of rejection, the nursing staff found it easier to feel concern for Norman. Their concern was the key ingredient in reducing behaviors that only escalated when confronted.

PRACTICAL MANAGEMENT OF PATIENTS WITH NARCISSISTIC PERSONALITY DISORDER. It is natural to react negatively to the narcissistic patient, but the most useful approach is to respond positively to his sense of entitlement. It is helpful to focus either on his positive traits (his tolerance of pain or the hospital routine's unpredictabil-

3) is irritable and aggressive, as indicated by repeated physical fights or assaults (not required by one's job or to defend someone or oneself), including spouse- or child-beating

4) repeatedly fails to honor financial obligations, as indicated by defaulting on debts or failing to provide child support or support for other dependents on a regular basis

5) fails to plan ahead, or is impulsive, as indicated by one or both of the following:
(*a*) traveling from place to place without a prearranged job or clear goal for the period of travel or clear idea about when the travel will terminate
(*b*) lack of a fixed address for a month or more

6) has no regard for the truth, as indicated by repeated lying, use of aliases, or "conning" others for personal profit or pleasure

7) is reckless regarding his or her own or others' personal safety, as indicated by driving while intoxicated, or recurrent speeding

8) if a parent or guardian, lacks ability to function as a responsible parent, as indicated by one or more of the following:
(*a*) malnutrition of child
(*b*) child's illness resulting from lack of minimal hygiene
(*c*) failure to obtain medical care for a seriously ill child
(*d*) child's dependence on neighbors or nonresident relatives for food or shelter
(*e*) failure to arrange for a caretaker for young child when parent is away from home
(*f*) repeated squandering, on personal items, of money required for household necessities

9) has never sustained a totally monogamous relationship for more than one year

10) lacks remorse (feels justified in having hurt, mistreated, or stolen from another)

D. Occurrence of antisocial behavior not exclusively during the course of Schizophrenia or Manic Episodes.

ity) or on his feelings of pain, loss, and rejection. Being critical of his behavior is likely only to make him more demanding and difficult. If the patient views the nurse as an empathic person, he will be more likely to reconstitute his defenses and feel less needy. If the nurse relates to his special, talented, and impressive qualities, the patient will be more likely to feel positive toward the nurse and also be less demanding and more reasonable. Responses such as, "I would like to have more time to spend with you," and "It must be difficult to be in so much pain," are more successful than "I'm too busy to spend any more time with you; I have other patients to take care of." The nurse's response must be genuine to be effective. Even the most competent and confident nurse is likely to have trouble dealing with this pa-

tient. She should obtain psychiatric consultation and direction if possible. If not possible, she at least should discuss her approach to the patient with a peer. She needs to remember that narcissistic patients are masters at dividing staff against each other.

ANTISOCIAL PERSONALITY DISORDER
The DSM-III-R diagnostic criteria for patients with antisocial personality disorder include illegal, delinquent, and disruptive behavior. Psychodynamically, these patients suffer from an inability to trust. Unlike paranoid patients, who are suspicious and often feel that others are out to get them, antisocial individuals believe that it is dangerous to depend on other people since all people are considered unreliable. Anti-

social patients feel that it is fair to take advantage of others; they assume that others would behave in the same way toward them.

Like the patient with borderline personality disorder, the antisocial patient does not see himself realistically. He seems, however, to have a better defense against anxiety than the borderline patient. The antisocial patient has adopted a lifestyle that values immediate pleasure rather than delayed gratification and long-term success. He does not consider school or a long-term work commitment with a system of promotions to be worth the effort. Antisocial individuals frequently come in conflict with the law because they see no value in laws or rules.

Antisocial personality disorder is one of the most studied scientifically of the personality disorders. There is strong support for a biological or genetic factor in this disorder. An individual's chances of developing an antisocial personality disorder are higher if he comes from a family with an antisocial biological parent, even if that individual was adopted at birth and raised by other, nonantisocial parents. Also, subtle neurologic abnormalities in children are correlated with the development of antisocial personality disorder in adults (Robins, 1966).

___

Jason: A Patient with Antisocial Personality Disorder

Jason, a 19-year-old patient, was admitted to a medical unit because of increasing lethargy and confusion, possibly related to poor glucose regulation. Jason was diagnosed as having diabetes mellitus at age 14, and was initially difficult to regulate due to his lies about his intake, physical fighting with peers, and tendency to stay out all night. With group home placement and counseling Jason's behavior improved and his diabetes was effectively regulated. Regulation had become difficult again recently for unknown reasons.

Although the nursing staff initially felt empathic toward Jason and admired his tough independent style, attitudes changed as Jason did not improve and seemed to become more angry and demanding. Nurses who insisted on supervising his insulin injections felt intimidated by his angry behavior but noted improvement in his condition. When the pattern of improvement after supervised insulin injection was noticed, the treatment plan was changed to require nursing staff supervision. This resulted in rapid improvement in symptoms but an increase in demanding and manipulative behavior.

Only when limits were set (required supervision) did the underlying reason for hospitalization become clear. Jason was being evicted from his apartment and knew that he could live in a hospital if he appeared sick.

___

PRACTICAL MANAGEMENT OF PATIENTS WITH ANTISOCIAL PERSONALITY DISORDER. Patients with antisocial personality disorder do not seek long-term success. They seek immediate gratification and pleasure. The only reason an antisocial person does not do something enjoyable is his fear of punishment. Thus it is useful to be clear about expectations and the consequences of failing to meet them. Stressing to these patients that a treatment or procedure is in their long-term best interest will have little effect. A matter-of-fact, straightforward approach and statement of expectations is more useful. In the case of Jason, the nurse appropriately insisted on supervision of his self-administered insulin injection rather than allowing him age-appropriate independence. Giving the antisocial patient control is often not in his best interest. The nurse must expect that these patients will refuse to do things, only to agree later, in an attempt to maintain control. The nurse, as a health care professional, is usually not trusted by these patients.

HISTRIONIC PERSONALITY DISORDER

Histrionic personality disorder has had a controversial history. The term "hysteria" has been associated with flamboyant behavior, migrating uteruses, conversion disorder, and society's version of stereotyped femininity (for example, the "dumb blond"). In DSM-III, the term histrionic replaced hysterical in order to avoid this controversial past.

Early psychiatric literature makes reference to "good hysterics" and "bad hysterics." Bad hysterics are angry, impulsive, destructive, and sometimes suicidal individuals. They are dependent on others for their personal identity, their basic sense of self. According to DSM-III these bad hysterics would be better diagnosed as having borderline personality disorder. Good hysterics are flamboyant, attention seeking, dramatic, and dependent on attention from the opposite sex for a sense of well-being. It is important to differentiate the purpose of attention seeking in the two patients. The bad hysteric (borderline) requires attention to maintain a basic sense of self. The good hysteric requires attention only for mood support. The loss of a significant interpersonal relationship may precipitate rage, anger, confusion, psychosis, desperation, and self-destructive behavior in

DSM-III-R Diagnostic Criteria for Histrionic Personality Disorder

A pervasive pattern of excessive emotionality and attention seeking, beginning by early adulthood and present in a variety of contexts, as indicated by at least *four* of the following:

1) constantly seeks or demands reassurance, approval, or praise

2) is inappropriately sexually seductive in appearance or behavior

3) is overly concerned with physical attractiveness

4) expresses emotion with inappropriate exaggeration, e.g., embraces casual acquaintances with excessive ardor, uncontrollable sobbing on minor sentimental occasions, has temper tantrums

5) is uncomfortable in situations in which he or she is not the center of attention

6) displays rapidly shifting and shallow expression of emotions

7) is self-centered, actions being directed toward obtaining immediate satisfaction; has no tolerance for the frustration of delayed gratification

8) has a style of speech that is excessively impressionistic and lacking in detail, e.g., when asked to describe mother, can be no more specific than, "She was a beautiful person."

---

the bad hysteric (borderline). This loss will produce dysphoric mood without psychotic symptoms in the good hysteric. The DSM-III-R diagnosis of histrionic personality disorder describes the good hysteric.

Helen: A Patient with Histrionic Personality Disorder

Helen held court in her hospital room. Her walls were covered with pictures of herself and friends, and she dressed as though she was on a cruise rather than in a hospital. She paid more attention to who was visiting her than to her medical recovery. She always fixed her hair and put on make-up before her attending physician visited in the morning, but remained in her sexy lingerie.

Helen got along well and was cooperative with the nurses who paid attention to her and were empathic regarding her problem of finding a good catering service that would deliver to the hospital. She was irritable and demanding toward the nurses who seemed to her to be more interested in rules and details than in her desires, for example, her wish to be allowed to sleep until 10 A.M., and to have visitors after visiting hours.

PRACTICAL MANAGEMENT OF PATIENTS WITH HISTRIONIC PERSONALITY DISORDER. Patients with histrionic personality disorder generally are highly functioning. They are successful socially and at work. It is important to remember that as long as these patients receive attention, flattery, and admiration, they are happy, cooperative, and infrequently request psychiatric treatment. They rarely are admitted to psychiatric inpatient units. These patients seek treatment for depression, often with atypical symptoms of increased sleep, anxiety, and somatic complaints when significant or romantic relationships end. This type of depression has been

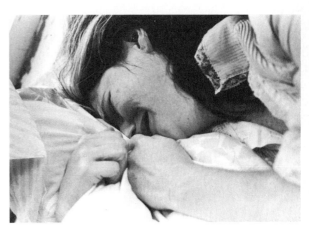

The "bad hysteric" or borderline individual requires attention from others to maintain a basic sense of self. A break up with a boyfriend (of one month) can be a crisis and precipitate suicidal ideation and behavior. She usually says afterwards that she didn't want to die—instead she just wanted her boyfriend to know how badly she felt.

referred to as *hysteroid dysphoria* or *rejection-sensitive depression*. The DSM-III-R diagnosis would be depressive disorder not otherwise specified. These patients often respond well to one class of antidepressant medication, monoamine oxidase inhibitors, and poorly to electroconvulsive treatment. (See Chapter 9 on mood disorders for more on treatment with MAO inhibitors.)

COMPULSIVE PERSONALITY DISORDER

In contrast to the dramatic, flamboyant, affectively charged histrionic is the patient with **compulsive personality disorder.** These patients avoid feelings and intimacy by rigid adherence to rules, order, and organization. They are tidy, well-organized, and punctual. Issues of power, money, cleanliness, and order are important to them. Although in some ways they are dutiful and diligent workers and patients, they often emotionally decompensate when they become ill and are unable to control their lives. Although they are usually stoic in suffering, they may become unreasonable when overwhelmed.

These patients struggle with issues of control and mastery that normally have been resolved in children by ages two to four. In the toddler stage, children attempt to gain control over their bowels and bladder. Harsh and demanding parenting at this time and around other developmental milestones according to psychoanalytic theory (Hartman and Kris, 1946), may predispose children to feel intense shame when out of control, and, so, to develop compulsive personality traits. Although this disorder tends to run in families, biological and developmental factors have not been clearly separated.

PRACTICAL MANAGEMENT OF PATIENTS WITH COMPULSIVE PERSONALITY DISORDER. It is important for the nurse to assist this patient to gain control of as much of his treatment as is safely possible. He will become less anxious and more reasonable when in control. The nurse should give this patient choices whenever possible and include him in treatment planning. Being casual, informal, or mellow may not be appreciated; the patient is likely to feel insecure with staff who do not pay strict atten-

---

DSM-III-R Diagnostic Criteria for Obsessive Compulsive Personality Disorder

A pervasive pattern of perfectionism and inflexibility, beginning by early adulthood and present in a variety of contexts, as indicated by at least *five* of the following:

1) perfectionism that interferes with task completion, e.g., inability to complete a project because own overly strict standards are not met

2) preoccupation with details, rules, lists, order, organization, or schedules to the extent that the major point of the activity is lost

3) unreasonable insistence that others submit to exactly his or her way of doing things, **or** unreasonable reluctance to allow others to do things because of the conviction that they will not do them correctly

4) excessive devotion to work and productivity to the exclusion of leisure activities and friendships (not accounted for by obvious economic necessity)

5) indecisiveness: decision making is either avoided, postponed, or protracted, e.g., the person cannot get assignments done on time because of ruminating about priorities (do not include if indecisiveness is due to excessive need for advice or reassurance from others)

6) overconscientiousness, scrupulousness, and inflexibility about matters of morality, ethics, or values (not accounted for by cultural or religious identification)

7) restricted expression of affection

8) lack of generosity in giving time, money, or gifts when no personal gain is likely to result

9) inability to discard worn-out or worthless objects even when they have no sentimental value

tion to detail and who thus do not seem professional to him.

DEPENDENT PERSONALITY DISORDER

Patients with **dependent personality disorder** function relatively well as long as there are dominant or forceful significant others providing direction. Although there is little empirical data providing validity for this diagnosis, the concept seems widely accepted and understood, possibly because dependency is a concept common to many disorders. Since dependency is also an element of psychologically healthy people, pathology is possibly only a matter of degree.

People who suffer from dependent personality disorder go to great lengths and submit to extreme abuse in order to stay in relationships. They become symptomatic when the cost of staying in the relationship becomes too much for them to bear or when the source of dependency gratification is lost. Two of the best examples are the person who cannot function after the death of a spouse and the partner of an abusive alcoholic who finds another equally abusive relationship to enter into upon leaving the first.

There are no known biological factors in this disorder. Dependent people seem to feel that the world is dangerous and that they must always rely on the direction of others whom they trust not to abandon them. They do not trust their own ability to make decisions, feeling that others have better ideas.

PRACTICAL MANAGEMENT OF PATIENTS WITH DEPENDENT PERSONALITY DISORDER. Patients with dependent personality disorder usually follow directions well. The nurse need not be afraid to appear directive or authoritarian. These patients are usually more comfortable being directed than having to make choices. As long as the goal is not personality change, giving advice may be the easiest way to manage these patients. However, whenever possible, the nurse should emphasize that the patient is the one in the best position to make certain decisions about his case. If the goal were personality change through psychoanalytic psychotherapy, the therapist would be more likely to refuse to give advice and focus on the patient's feelings of frustration and perceived incompetence. This approach is usually not productive for management of practical problems, but in order not to encourage increased regression, it is important for the nurse to encourage a dependent patient gradually to do as much as possible for himself.

PASSIVE-AGGRESSIVE PERSONALITY DISORDER

Patients with **passive-aggressive personality disorder** are angry people who seem to be unaware of their angry feelings and do not understand the impact or power of their behavior. Although superficially courteous, polite, and agreeable, their actions

---

DSM-III-R Diagnostic Criteria for Dependent Personality Disorder

A pervasive pattern of dependent and submissive behavior, beginning by early adulthood and present in a variety of contexts, as indicated by at least *five* of the following:

1) is unable to make everyday decisions without an excessive amount of advice or reassurance from others

2) allows others to make most of his or her important decisions, e.g., where to live, what job to take

3) agrees with people even when he or she believes they are wrong, because of fear of being rejected

4) has difficulty initiating projects or doing things on his or her own

5) volunteers to do things that are unpleasant or demeaning in order to get other people to like him or her

6) feels uncomfortable or helpless when alone, or goes to great lengths to avoid being alone

7) feels devastated or helpless when close relationships end

8) is frequently preoccupied with fears of being abandoned

9) is easily hurt by criticism or disapproval

DSM-III-R
Diagnostic Criteria for
Passive-Aggressive
Personality Disorder

A pervasive pattern of passive resistance to demands for adequate social and occupational performance, beginning by early adulthood and present in a variety of contexts, as indicated by at least *five* of the following:

1) procrastinates, i.e., puts off things that need to be done so that deadlines are not met

2) becomes sulky, irritable, or argumentative when asked to do something he or she does not want to do

3) seems to work deliberately slowly or to do a bad job on tasks that he or she really does not want to do

4) protests, without justification, that others make unreasonable demands on him or her

5) avoids obligations by claiming to have "forgotten"

6) believes that he or she is doing a much better job than others think he or she is doing

7) resents useful suggestions from others concerning how he or she could be more productive

8) obstructs the efforts of others by failing to do his or her share of the work

9) unreasonably criticizes or scorns people in positions of authority

(or lack of actions) betray a rigid demand to control and dominate. They procrastinate, dawdle, and fail to meet deadlines for projects if deadlines are imposed by others. They seem to feel that they should not have to be accountable for their actions and they often feel misunderstood. They usually make excuses for not doing things. Predictably, they are very difficult patients.

Like dependent personality disorder, passive-aggressive personality disorder is a widely held concept that has had little scientific validation as a disorder. The behavior pattern associated with it is common in other diagnoses and in people considered normal. No scientific studies clearly support a biological or family inheritance pattern.

PRACTICAL MANAGEMENT OF PATIENTS WITH PASSIVE-AGGRESSIVE PERSONALITY DISORDER. It is important for the nurse to stay out of power struggles with these patients. They do much better when they feel that they are in control. It is also important for the nurse to remain sensitive to these patients' wishes, especially when they are unclear or passive. Instead of dictating to this patient the type of treatment he is to receive, the nurse can be creative in offering alternatives, even if the patient eventually chooses all of them. The nurse frequently inquires if plans for care or treatment meet the patient's approval. He is likely to be cooperative as long as he does not feel disrespected.

PARANOID PERSONALITY DISORDER

The distinguishing characteristic of patients with **paranoid personality disorder** is inalterable suspicion of others. They are usually unable to acknowledge and accept their own negative and angry feelings toward others. Instead, they project, or attribute these feelings to those around them. Because of this projection, during times of danger or stress they find it difficult to trust people, since anyone might be out to hurt them, use them, or take advantage of them. Paranoid people are more likely to be successful in careers in which vigilance and secrecy are important. Unlike the paranoid-schizophrenic patient, these patients do not lose contact with reality. They are not delusional about their perceptions; they are just guarded and suspicious.

Before the development of the concept of schizotypal personality disorder, attempts were made to link paranoid patients to schizophrenics. After extensive study, no good evidence has been found supporting genetic transmission of this disorder; however, there is some evidence for increased incidence in families with a schizophrenic member.

**DSM-III-R
Diagnostic Criteria for
Paranoid Personality
Disorder**

A. A pervasive and unwarranted tendency, beginning by early adulthood and present in a variety of contexts, to interpret the actions of people as deliberately demeaning or threatening, as indicated by at least *four* of the following:

1) expects, without sufficient basis, to be exploited or harmed by others

2) questions, without justification, the loyalty or trustworthiness of friends or associates

3) reads hidden demeaning or threatening meanings into benign remarks or events, e.g., suspects that a neighbor put out trash early to annoy him

4) bears grudges or is unforgiving of insults or slights

5) is reluctant to confide in others because of unwarranted fear that the information will be used against him or her

6) is easily slighted and quick to react with anger or to counterattack

7) questions, without justification, fidelity of spouse or sexual partner

B. Occurrence not exclusively during the course of Schizophrenia or a Delusional Disorder.

PRACTICAL MANAGEMENT OF PATIENTS WITH PARANOID PERSONALITY DISORDER. The nurse should deal with this patient as she would a paranoid-schizophrenic patient (see Chapter 8). The only difference is degree of disturbance, with the personality disorder patient more responsive to nursing interventions than the psychotic one (who additionally needs medication).

It is important for the nurse to respect these patients' needs for interpersonal distance by being more "professional" than friendly and more matter of fact than warm. The nurse can explain what needs to be done and why, in a straightforward and candid manner. She should avoid becoming defensive when challenged or accused of something by these patients. Humor does not work well with these patients, since it may threaten them with a level of candor and intimacy that increases defensiveness.

SCHIZOTYPAL PERSONALITY DISORDER

Schizotypal personality disorder was new to DSM-III. Prior to DSM-III, many schizotypal patients would have been diagnosed as schizophrenic. DSM-III-R criteria require that clearly psychotic features (hallucinations or delusions) be present in order to make the diagnosis of schizophrenia.

Schizotypal patients are severely disturbed individuals. They display strange behavior such as bizarre speech or beliefs, poor social skills, and strained and distant interpersonal relationships. The most disturbed of this population closely resemble schizo-phrenic patients, the only difference being the absence of frank psychosis. Better functioning or healthier schizotypal individuals are eccentric and remain interpersonally distant.

The schizotypal diagnosis was developed to describe the healthier end of the schizophrenic spectrum. Predictably, this disorder is more common in biological relatives of people with schizophrenia. Because the category is relatively new, little else is known about it.

PRACTICAL MANAGEMENT OF PATIENTS WITH SCHIZOTYPAL PERSONALITY DISORDER. Although it is clear that psychotic-schizophrenic patients are usually significantly helped by antipsychotic medication, the data are not as clear for patients with schizotypal personality disorder. Some of these patients are being helped by low doses of antipsychotics such as Navane (thiothixene) or Mellaril (thioridazine hydrochloride).

Since patients with schizotypal personality disorder tend to misinterpret and personalize what is going on around them as well as have poor coping skills, they are easily overwhelmed by difficult situations, such as hospitalization for serious illness or surgery. When stressed, they tend to withdraw autistically into their fantasies and ignore aspects of the outside world. For this reason, they cannot be expected to make important decisions quickly and may need to be approached several times about the same issue. They may only be able to attend to the problem and the nurse when the level of stress is reduced.

**DSM-III-R
Diagnostic Criteria for
Schizotypal
Personality Disorder**

A. A pervasive pattern of deficits in interpersonal relatedness and peculiarities of ideation, appearance, and behavior, beginning by early adulthood and present in a variety of contexts, as indicated by at least *five* of the following:

1) ideas of reference (excluding delusions of reference)

2) excessive social anxiety, e.g., extreme discomfort in social situations involving unfamiliar people

3) odd beliefs or magical thinking, influencing behavior and inconsistent with subcultural norms, e.g., superstitiousness, belief in clairvoyance, telepathy, or "sixth sense," "others can feel my feelings" (in children and adolescents, bizarre fantasies or preoccupations)

4) unusual perceptual experiences, e.g., illusions, sensing the presence of a force or person not actually present (e.g., "I felt as if my dead mother were in the room with me")

5) odd or eccentric behavior or appearance, e.g., unkempt, unusual mannerisms, talks to self

6) no close friends or confidants (or only one) other than first-degree relatives

7) odd speech (without loosening of associations or incoherence), e.g., speech that is impoverished, digressive, vague, or inappropriately abstract

8) inappropriate or constricted affect, e.g., silly, aloof, rarely reciprocates gestures or facial expressions, such as smiles or nods

9) suspiciousness or paranoid ideation

B. Occurrence not exclusively during the course of Schizophrenia or a Pervasive Developmental Disorder.

Understanding and accepting the limitations of these patients is likely to reduce the stress they are experiencing. Since these patients are likely to relate unusually well to some staff while shunning all others, the nurse needs to keep this in mind when making out patient assignments. Stress reduction, not personality change, should be a goal of the nursing care plan for this patient.

Schizoid patients are *not* schizophrenic. Although both populations may have significantly impaired relationships, schizoid patients maintain a firm grip on reality. Their major problem is their inability to relate warmly to other people. They are often reclusive and live with parents or in isolation. Although they do occasionally marry, the marriage relationship usually remains distant and without emotional intensity. They seem to have little need for human contact or comfort. This deficiency is compensated for by an active fantasy life.

The diagnostic criteria for schizoid personality disorder are designed to separate this disorder from the more disturbed schizophrenic and schizotypal patients. There have been no good studies describing genetic or biological features. This disorder has been difficult to study since these patients infrequently request treatment.

PRACTICAL MANAGEMENT OF PATIENTS WITH SCHIZOID PERSONALITY DISORDER. Schizoid individuals seldom create management problems when they are ill since they are not usually emotionally stormy, demanding, or impulsive. Instead they tend to be withdrawn, polite, and controlled, and as long as their need for privacy and emotional distance is reasonably respected, equilibrium will be maintained. If the nurse attempts to get emotionally close to these patients or to push them to express their feelings, they will only retreat further into social isolation.

Patients with schizoid and **avoidant personality disorders** have much in common since both experience significant difficulty in establishing relationships.

DSM-III-R Diagnostic Criteria for Schizoid Personality Disorder

A. A pervasive pattern of indifference to social relationships and a restricted range of emotional experience and expression, beginning by early adulthood and present in a variety of contexts, as indicated by at least *four* of the following:

1) neither desires nor enjoys close relationships, including being part of a family

2) almost always chooses solitary activities

3) rarely, if ever, claims or appears to experience strong emotions, such as anger and joy

4) indicates little if any desire to have sexual experiences with another person (age being taken into account)

5) is indifferent to the praise and criticism of others

6) has no close friends or confidants (or only one) other than first-degree relatives

7) displays constricted affect, e.g., is aloof, cold, rarely reciprocates gestures or facial expressions, such as smiles or nods

B. Occurrence not exclusively during the course of Schizophrenia or a Delusional Disorder.

Schizoid individuals eventually give up, but the avoidant patient continues to acknowledge suffering because of loneliness. Avoidant patients will form relationships with others, but only if they feel reasonably sure that they will not be rejected. Loss and rejection are so painful to these patients that they choose isolation rather than exposing themselves to risk. This diagnosis was new to DSM-III. There are no known familial or other biological features.

PRACTICAL MANAGEMENT OF PATIENTS WITH AVOIDANT PERSONALITY DISORDER. Patients with avoidant personality disorder have some ability to trust and invest in relationships but do not handle surprises well, for example, a last-minute change in plans for surgery. The nurse should let this type of patient know when she will be available or unavailable. He may need explanations about rotating shifts and why staff are at times unavailable

DSM-III-R Diagnostic Criteria for Avoidant Personality Disorder

A pervasive pattern of social discomfort, fear of negative evaluation, and timidity, beginning by early adulthood and present in a variety of contexts, as indicated by at least *four* of the following:

1) is easily hurt by criticism or disapproval

2) has no close friends or confidants (or only one) other than first-degree relatives

3) is unwilling to get involved with people unless certain of being liked

4) avoids social or occupational activities that involve significant interpersonal contact, e.g., refuses a promotion that will increase social demands

5) is reticent in social situations because of a fear of saying something inappropriate or foolish, or of being unable to answer a question

6) fears being embarrassed by blushing, crying, or showing signs of anxiety in front of other people

7) exaggerates the potential difficulties, physical dangers, or risks involved in doing something ordinary but outside his or her usual routine, e.g., may cancel social plans because she anticipates being exhausted by the effort of getting there

to him. In the case of the avoidant patient whose progress is slow, he can move forward if he feels secure that a trusted other person is committed to remaining with him through the experience. There is usually little difficulty working with these patients on medical and surgical units.

NURSING CARE FOR PATIENTS WITH PERSONALITY DISORDERS

Although in this chapter we described practical approaches for managing patients with personality disorders, the techniques will not serve as substitutes for competence, concern, respect for patients, and professionalism. In addition, everyone has a personality style, and it is important for the nurse to know what impact her own personality has on patients. Warmth and friendliness can facilitate interacting with a histrionic patient but frighten a schizotypal or paranoid patient. Attention to protocol and detail may impress the compulsive patient but leave the narcissistic patient feeling unloved. Strength and the ability to set limits may be helpful with antisocial and dependent patients but will offend the narcissistic patient and enhance the pathology of the passive-aggressive patient. In working with any of these individuals, understanding oneself is as important as understanding the patient.

Such understanding is required for the development of **empathy.** Empathy is the ability to put oneself emotionally in someone else's place—to be able to feel what another person feels. To feel accepted while feeling emotionally and intellectually understood is therapeutic as well as reassuring for the patient. Without this understanding, the nurse will have little protection from the anger and frustration that some of these patients evoke. If the nurse's reaction to the patient results in a lack of empathy, he is likely to feel more stressed, and the symptoms of his disorder will intensify. The nurse's attitude that the patient can handle the problem with her support can be extremely helpful.

The ability to understand intellectually why a patient with a personality disorder is behaving self-destructively, or in such a way as to undermine his care, can help the nurse remain empathically involved while maintaining objectivity and professionalism. When the nurse's own problems interfere, supervi-

sion or consultation can help her to understand the situation, get support for her efforts, and take the best course of action.

A good supervisor can help the nurse clarify her clinical assessment of a situation, her theoretical reason for choosing a particular course of action, and her personal reactions. If supervision is done in an atmosphere of concern and respect, it will leave the nurse with a sense of security and confidence that she is doing all that she can for her patient. Such reassurance is needed for her own well-being and professional self-esteem, both of which are essential to doing good work with personality-disorder patients.

SUMMARY

Personality disorders are among the most common of psychiatric disorders and the most difficult to treat. Personality disorders are chronic and unremitting and may be debilitating. In addition, other psychiatric disorders, such as mood disorders, may be present and thus will complicate the issue. DSM-III has defined personality disorder as a deeply ingrained, inflexible maladaptive sense of self and the environment that is of sufficient severity to cause either significant impairment in adaptive functioning or subjective distress.

There are three major subgroups of personality disorders: confused thinking and socially withdrawn, borderline personality organizaton, and cohesive personality. Patients with personality disorders frequently and rigidly use defense mechanisms, including projection, splitting, and denial.

Practical management, rather than therapy designed to change personality, is the treatment of choice for health care patients with personality disorders. However, in some cases, the use of psychotropic medication can be helpful. The nurse needs to develop empathy toward patients with personality disorders while remaining objective and professional. Accurate assessment of the patient's personality type or personality disorder, if one is present, is important, since the approach that helps one type of patient may harm another. For example, the nurse's strength and ability to set limits may help the antisocial patient but will enhance the pathology of the passive-aggressive patient.

It must be kept in mind that personality disorders are difficult for the experienced mental health professional to diagnose, often requiring a period of time with the patient in psychotherapy to be determined. The nurse generalist can appropriately hypothesize about a patient's possible personality disorder and implement a trial of nursing intervention based on the principles put forth in this chapter. If things go well or improve, she is probably on the right track. If they don't, or worsen, she should try again and, possibly, obtain psychiatric consultation.

KEY TERMS

personality disorder

defense mechanism

projection

confused thinking and social withdrawal

borderline personality organization

splitting

fragmentation

denial

narcissism

antisocial personality disorder

cohesive personality

dexamethasone suppression test

REM latency test

histrionic personality disorder

compulsive personality disorder

dependent personality disorder

passive-aggressive personality disorder

paranoid personality disorder

schizotypal personality disorder

avoidant personality disorder

empathy

STUDY QUESTIONS

1. Why are personality disorders so difficult to diagnose and treat?

2. Name three major defense mechanisms used by patients with personality disorders. What role do the mechanisms play in personality disorders?

3. Name and describe the three major subgroups of personality disorders.

4. Name and describe five other personality disorders.

5. Why is practical management, rather than therapy designed to change personality, the treatment of choice for patients with personality disorders?

REFERENCES

Akiskal, H. (1981). Sub-affective disorders, disthymic, cyclothymic and bipolar II disorders in the borderline realm. *Psychiatr Clin North Am, 4,* 25–46.

American Psychiatric Association (1980). *Diagnostic and statistical manual of mental disorders.* Third Edition. Washington, D.C.: American Psychiatric Press, Inc.

American Psychiatric Association (1987). *Diagnostic and statistical manual of mental disorders.* Third Edition, Revised. Washington, D.C.: American Psychiatric Press.

Eysenck, H. J. (1956). The inheritance of extroversion-introversion. *Acta Psychol (Amst), 12,* 95.

Frosch, J. P. (Ed.) (1983). *Current perspectives on personality disorders.* Washington, D.C.: American Psychiatric Press.

Gunderson, J. (1984). *Borderline personality disorder.* Washington, D.C.: American Psychiatric Press, Inc.

Gunderson, J., & England, D. (1981). Characterizing the families of borderlines. *Psychiatr Clin North Am, 4,* 159–168.

Hartman, H., and Kris, E. (1946). Comments on the Formation of Psychic Structure, in Eissler, R. S., et al. (Eds), *The Psychoanalytic study of the child,* vol. 2, 11–38, New York: International Universities Press.

Hodulik, C. (1984). *Psychiatry knowledge and skills assessment program.* Washington, D.C.: American Psychiatric Press.

Hodulik, C. Borderline personality disorder and incest. (unpublished manuscript).

Kernberg, O. (1967). Borderline personality organization. *J Am Psychoanal Assoc, 15,* 641–685.

Kernberg, O. (1984). *Severe personality disorders.* Binghampton, NY: Vail-Ballou Press, p. 16.

Kohut, Heiny. (1977). *The restoration of the self.* New York: International Universities Press.

Kohut, H. (1984). *How does analysis cure?* Chicago: University of Chicago Press, p. 18.

Mahler, M. (1971). A study of the separation-individuation process and its possible application to borderline phenomena in the psychoanalytic situation. *Psychoanalytic Study Child, 26,* 403–424.

Masterson, J., & Rinsley, D. (1975). The borderline syndrome: The role of the mother in the genesis and psychic structure of the borderline personality. *Int J Psychoanal, 56,* 163–177.

Mellsop, G., Varghese, J. F., et al. (1982, October). The reliability of Axis II of DSM-III. *Am J Psychiatry, 139,* 10.

Millon, T. (1981). *Disorders of personality. DSM-III, Axis II.* New York: John Wiley & Sons.

Nemiah, J. (1961). *Foundations of psychopathology.* New York: Oxford University Press.

Robins, L. N. (1966). *Deviant children grown up.* Baltimore: Williams and Wilkins.

Stern, David. (1985). *The interpersonal world of the infant.* New York: Basic Books.

Vaillant, G. E., & Perry, J. C. (1980). *Personality disorders.* Friedman, Kaplan, & Saddock, ch. 22.

Wolberg, A. (1982). *Psychoanalytic psychotherapy of the borderline patient.* New York: Thieme-Stratton, Inc.

13

PSYCHOPHYSIOLOGICAL DISORDERS

LINDA J. BAKER

LEARNING OBJECTIVES

After studying this chapter, the student will be able to:

- Define and differentiate between psychosomatic (or psychophysiological) and somatoform disorders.
- Identify and describe the three etiological models of psychosomatic disorders.
- Identify assessment criteria and develop nursing care plans for patients with psychosomatic disorders.
- Define and describe somatoform disorder.
- Describe the four types of somatoform disorders.
- Identify assessment criteria and develop nursing care plans for patients with somatoform disorders.

INTRODUCTION

Health practitioners have long recognized that psychological and social variables play a role in the development and course of physical illness. People interact continuously with their environment and with other people. A realistic view of health and disease must therefore attend to environmental and psychological factors and must not treat individuals simply as diseased organ systems or upset metabolic processes. In this chapter we will examine psychological conditions that present as physical illness or complaints of physical distress. We focus on the relationship among personality factors, life situations, and illness.

Psychiatric diagnoses in which patients have physical complaints and demonstrable tissue damage or impairment are called **psychosomatic** or **psychophysiological disorders.** These will be discussed in the next section. Later in this chapter another group of conditions will be discussed in which there are physical complaints and apparent physical distress, but with little or no evidence of tissue damage or impairment. These are called **somatoform disorders** because the symptoms *suggest* somatic impairment, although no physical evidence of impairment is detectable.

In general, individuals who suffer from these types of conditions do not seek help from a mental health or psychiatric clinic. Rather they seek help and

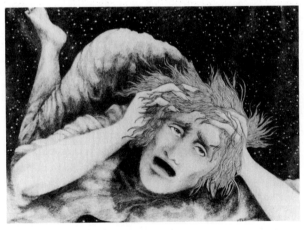

When caring for the person with stress-related illness, it is extremely important for the nurse to recognize and treat the physical symptoms and their emotional by-products before exploring the possible role of psychological factors. In this illustration entitled "Matter, Energy, Space and Time" the artist, Jane Kley, portrays her feelings of helplessness, weightlessness, and overall agony during a migraine attack.

relief for their physical symptoms from doctors and nurses in a general medical setting. So unless there is a request for psychiatric consultation, the nurse often plays a critical role in the assessment, treatment, and management of such patients. Often these patients do not make a connection between their physical symptoms and their emotional or life stress problems. Some, however, seem to sense intuitively that although they are in physical distress, the real source of their problems may be emotional.

Although it may be tempting for the nurse and other health practitioners to try to separate the organic from the functional or the physical from the psychological, it is an impossible and fruitless task to pursue this mind-body dichotomy. The approach taken in this chapter accepts the inseparability of the mind and the body, and attempts to examine ways in which psychological factors may be affecting the individual's health and/or perception of health, and the way in which distress and disease are communicated to the practitioner.

PSYCHOLOGICAL FACTORS AFFECTING PHYSICAL CONDITION

Nowhere in the study of psychology or psychopathology does the issue of mind-body come into focus more clearly than in the DSM-III-R classification of psychological factors affecting physical condition (American Psychiatric Association, 1987). Other terms used for these types of disorders are psychophysiological or psychosomatic. (The latter, from Greek, literally means the intersection of mind or soul [psyche] and body [soma].) In psychophysiological disorders or psychosomatic illness, psychological and environmental factors play a role in the initiation, maintenance, or exacerbation of a disease or symptom.

Psychosomatic disorders occur in a wide variety of physiological systems, including gastrointestinal (such as gastric and duodenal ulcer, ulcerative colitis, or irritable bowel syndrome), cardiovascular (such as hypertension, angina pectoris, acute myocardial infarction, or migraine headache), respiratory (such as asthma or hyperventilation), skin (such as psoriasis, urticaria or acne), and musculoskeletal (such as tension headache or rheumatoid arthritis). The immune system may be involved, making an individual more prone to infectious diseases. If it is the endocrine system that is "vulnerable," the individual may develop diabetes or thyroid disease. The above are all exam-

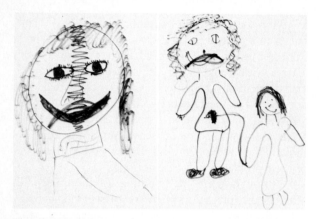

These drawings by a 12-year-old girl suffering from migraines depict the pain she endures. At times, she feels as though her stomach is being punched and she has to vomit, while at other times she only experiences nausea.

ples of diseases that are commonly thought of as psychosomatic. Psychological factors may also play a role in other diseases or conditions in which a single symptom is present (such as vomiting or frequent micturition).

The presence of demonstrable organic pathology or pathophysiological process distinguishes psychosomatic disorders from somatoform disorders. A person with hypertension does have high blood pressure. The asthmatic experiences labored breathing and gasping as a result of constriction in the bronchial airways. The person suffering from a peptic ulcer or ulcerative colitis has a lesion that requires medical treatment. However, it is the relationship between emotions and physical illness that makes psychosomatic disorders a controversial subject in medical science. How does a life experience, and an individual's emotional reaction to the experience, translate to damage to an organ system? How can health professionals understand the chain of events that start from a life event and its emotional concomitants and progress to physiological changes that lead to disease? A great deal of research has explored this important question and a number of theories have been proposed. We will discuss three of these theories in the next section.

ETIOLOGY

PSYCHOANALYTIC MODEL. The psychoanalytic or psychodynamic model of psychosomatic illness, first discussed by Freud as "hysteria," proposes that the individual dissociates unacceptable feelings about important events and people from consciousness and displaces them onto the body. Freud called this "that mysterious leap from the mental to the physical" (Freud, 1938, p. 229). The bodily symptoms function to keep the anxiety stemming from intrapsychic conflicts from reaching consciousness.

During the 1940s and 1950s Franz Alexander (1950, 1968) and his colleagues studied clinically a variety of psychosomatic diseases including bronchial asthma, rheumatoid arthritis, ulcerative colitis, essential hypertension, neurodermatitis, duodenal peptic ulcer, and thyrotoxicosis. Alexander's theory, largely based on psychoanalytic sessions with patients, includes several basic assumptions: 1) there are certain constitutional (genetic) factors that may make an individual more likely to experience a certain type of disease; 2) there are personality factors or central or "nuclear conflicts" that are specific to a particular disease; and 3) events in the life of the individual may arouse these conflicts, which then stimulate onset or exacerbation of disease. According to Alexander, all three factors, a genetic-organ vulnerability, a specific underlying psychodynamic conflict, and a precipitating life event, interact to produce the disease. For example, the hypothesized specific nuclear conflict associated with hypertension is the individual's constant struggle against expressing angry, hostile feelings for fear of losing the affection of others. It has been theorized that the asthmatic individual has conflicts about independence, experiencing excessive unresolved dependency on the mother, and a wish to be encompassed or protected by her.

Grace and Graham (1952) proposed another "specificity" theory. This theory, initially supported by statements made by patients in therapeutic interviews and later supported by research evidence (Graham, 1972), states that each different psychosomatic disease is associated with a "specific attitude" expressed by the individual (see Table 13–1). An *attitude* was defined as a statement consisting of what the person feels is happening to him or her, and what he or she wishes to do about it. For example, the individual with a migraine headache felt something had to be achieved and then relaxed after his effort. The person with urticaria felt he was "taking a beating" and was helpless to do anything about it. Like Alexander's theory, Graham's theory holds that life events are critical in stimulating these specific attitudes and are related to the onset or exacerbation of disease.

BEHAVIORAL MODEL. The behavioral model of psychosomatic illness starts with the premise that illness is the result of a failed attempt to cope ade-

TABLE 13–1 Attitudes associated with psychosomatic illness

Illness	Specific Attitude	Patient Statements
Urticaria (hives)	Takes a beating and helpless to do anything about it.	"My husband pushes me around and walks all over me, but what can I do?"
Eczema	Intruded upon and helpless to deal with the associated frustration.	"I want to make my mother understand that I need to do it myself, but I can't." "I feel terribly frustrated."
Asthma and rhinitis	Abandoned or wanting to shut out a person or situation.	"I feel he's left me out in the cold." "I want to build a wall between him and me."
Duodenal ulcer	Deprived of one's due and desire for revenge.	"He hurt me and I don't deserve it so I want to hurt him." "I want to get back at him."
Migraine headache	Unable to relax until something is achieved or gets done.	"I can't relax until I get it done." "I had a million things to do before lunch."
Hypertension	Threatened with harm and needing to be ready for anything.	"Nobody is ever going to beat me; I'm ready for anything."
Constipation	Grimly perseverant though it seems that nothing good can come from the situation.	"This marriage is never going to be any better but I can't leave."

Source: Grace, W. J., & Graham, D. T. (1952). Relationship of specific attitudes and emotions to certain bodily disease. *Psychosomatic Medicine, 14,* 243–251. And Graham, D. T. (1972). Psychosomatic medicine. In N. Greenfield & R. Sternback (Eds.), *Handbook of psychophysiology.* New York: Holt, Rinehart & Winston.

quately with stressful life events. Therefore, it is important for an individual to be able to identify particular stresses and demands in his or her life and to learn more adaptive responses to these situations. Learning more adaptive responses includes changing overt behavior (such as learning to say "no" when already overcommitted) and also modifying emotional or psychological reactions to stressors that may be contributing to illness.

Psychologists Holmes and Rahe (1967) developed a list of stressful life events called the Social Readjustment Rating Scale, or the Life-Change Scale. The scale was developed by having individuals rate certain life events according to how stressful they were thought to be. These events were then ranked, ordered, and assigned a numerical value (for example, death of a spouse = 100, divorce = 73, retirement = 45, change in residence = 20). This scale was then used in studying the medical histories of other individuals. The researchers found that as the life-change score increased, the probability of illness increased. In other words, the more life events an individual experiences (within a certain time frame), the more likely he or she is to become ill. (See Table 13–2.)

The most serious life event on the Holmes and Rahe scale, death of a spouse, was studied by Parkes, a British investigator, and his colleagues (1969). Widowers, aged 55 or older, were followed for nine years after the deaths of their wives. Of 4,486 widowers, 213 died within the first six months after their spouses had died. This was 40 percent higher than the statistically predicted rate. But after the first year, the widowers' mortality rate did not differ from that of the general male population. Thus the period of bereavement may be a time of greater risk for physical illness (see Box 13–1).

BIOMEDICAL MODEL. The biomedical model of psychosomatic illness incorporates the **diathesis-stress** concept—a diathesis (a weakness or physical predisposition), when coupled with stress, triggers illness. This is also sometimes called the **specific-organ vulnerability** hypothesis. It proposes that when an individual is under stress, the weakest link in the chain, or the most vulnerable organ, is affected. There is evidence that such organ vulnerability may be inherited (McConnell, 1966). For example, an ulcer is a lesion in the stomach or duodenum lining. Normally, small breaks in this mucous lining

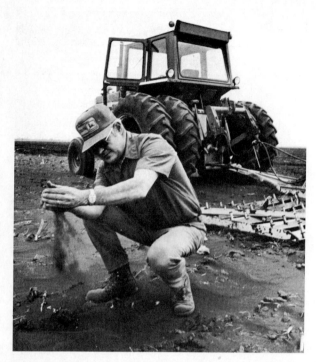

The Family Farm—as American as you can get. Rural life today, however, along with farming, is not what it used to be. Stressors as wide-ranging as long hours to handling dangerous equipment to drought or even worse, bankruptcy, lead to the highest incidences of depression and suicide in the rural areas of the country.

repair themselves quite easily and no ulcer will form. If, however, there is a diathesis (such as an oversecretion of acid or pepsin, a particularly weak mucous lining, or a lining that regenerates very slowly), then an ulcer is more likely to develop. Any of the three diatheses mentioned, which may be genetically inherited, can make a person more prone to ulcers.

Unlike the specificity theories discussed above, other biomedical models postulate that there is a general stress reaction that is similar for all individuals. Hans Selye (1956) developed a theory describing the **general adaptation syndrome,** in which the same series of physiological events is produced whenever an individual is stressed. Stressors, both psychological and physical (for example, extreme cold), activate the autonomic nervous system, stimulate hormonal secretions from the pituitary and adrenal glands, bring about biochemical changes, and alter the brain's level of electrical activity. The triphasic pattern of physiological response includes: 1) an alarm reaction that is an initial acute phase of lowered resistance, immediately following exposure to a stressor (for example,

body aches and chills); 2) resistance, which is a stage of heightened resistance when the body is trying to counteract the stressor (for example, fever and inflammation); and 3) exhaustion, during which there is a collapse of adaptive responses (for example, sepsis). If the stressor continues, illness, and in some cases death, may follow (Selye, 1956; 1976).

In summary, models of psychosomatic illness focus on three factors that appear to be important in the development of disease: 1) genetic factors (such as specific-organ vulnerability, 2) personality factors (such as psychological conflicts or specific attitudes), and 3) life events. Whether specific personality factors and life events are associated with specific diseases or whether disease is an overall reaction to general levels of stress is a matter for further research. However, the nurse's responsibility includes attending to the specific life events and personality factors that characterize a specific patient and his or her physical disorder. Such an individualized approach is more likely to bring about both insight and relief from distress.

CLINICAL PICTURE

Since psychosomatic disorders occur across such a broad range of physiological systems (gastrointestinal, cardiac, respiratory, and so on), it is difficult to present a typical clinical picture. The onset and course of illness will vary as a function of the type of physical condition. Patients with asthma will present quite differently from those with irritable bowel syndrome, and those with irritable bowel syndrome will differ markedly from patients who suffer from migraine headaches. Patients with different physical conditions will describe their distress and discomfort differently. There will be differences in the onset of symptoms and the course of illness that enable a clinician to formulate a diagnosis for each different physical condition. However, the common thread that joins these seemingly disparate "physical" diagnoses lies in the psychological factors that contribute to the disease.

The DSM-III-R category for psychosomatic disorders acknowledges that the symptoms reflect real changes in the body and that psychological factors are involved. In a sense, nearly all bodily illnesses to which humans are subject may be affected by psychological factors. However, the category of psychological factors affecting physical condition draws attention to those disorders that are most commonly thought of by mental health professionals as being influenced by psychological factors. Which disorders

TABLE 13–2 The stress of adjusting to change

Events	Scale of Impact
Death of a spouse	100
Divorce	73
Marital separation	65
Jail term	63
Death of close family member	63
Personal injury or illness	53
Marriage	50
Fired at work	47
Marital reconciliation	45
Retirement	45
Change in health of family member	44
Pregnancy	40
Sex difficulties	39
Gain of new family member	39
Business readjustment	38
Change in financial state	38
Death of close friend	37
Change to different line of work	36
Change in number of arguments with spouse	35
Mortgage over $10,000	31
Foreclosure of mortgage or loan	30
Change in responsibilities at work	29
Son or daughter leaving home	29
Trouble with in-laws	29
Outstanding personal achievement	28
Wife begins or stops work	26
Begin or end school	26
Change in living conditions	25
Revision of personal habits	24
Trouble with boss	23
Change in work hours or conditions	20
Change in residence	20
Change in schools	20
Change in recreation	19
Change in church activities	19
Change in social activities	18
Mortgage or loan less than $10,000	17
Change in sleeping habits	16
Change in number of family get-togethers	15
Change in eating habits	15
Vacation	13
Christmas	12
Minor violations of the law	11

Source: Adapted from: Holmes, T. H., and Masuda, M. (1972). Psychosomatic syndrome. *Psychology Today*, April.

should and should not be classified under this category will be discussed using case examples.

Charles: A Victim of Migraine Headaches

Charles, a 45-year-old independent businessman, suffered from migraine headaches off and on for twenty-five years. During some periods, he would have several headaches a month, but then he would go for many months without having a headache at all. He could usually tell when he was about to have a headache because he experienced an "aura." His eyes became very sensitive to light, flashes of light appeared to cross his field of vision, there was a ringing in his ears, and he felt nauseated. The headache itself was a throbbing, intense pain that lasted for several hours. Usually the pain occurred on the left side of his head, although sometimes it was on the right or in front.

Charles remembered that his first headache occurred after he graduated from college, a few months after starting his first job. His headaches seemed to occur during periods of inactivity, such as weekends and vacations, and often followed a particularly busy time. The last headache occurred following the completion of a business deal he had been working on for several weeks. "I just had to get the job done," he explained. "There were a million things to do, and I really put in overtime those last few days."

Charles's case satisfies the DSM-III-R criteria. His migraine headaches have a known pathophysiological process, and psychologically meaningful events appear to be associated with the onset of a headache and its accompanying symptoms. The types of life events that are associated with migraine headaches are not necessarily the serious events found on the Holmes and Rahe (1967) Life-Change Scale,

Box 13–1 ● Dangers of Bereavement

According to a review of records in Finland from 1972 through 1976, widows and widowers have an increased death rate in the first five years after bereavement. Among 95,000 widowed persons, the rate of death from all causes was 6.5 percent higher than expected for their age and sex. The rate of death from natural causes was three percent higher and the rate of violent death 93 percent higher. The suicide rate was 242 percent higher than expected and the rate of traffic deaths 153 percent higher.

The death rate rose most in the first weeks and months. Mortality from natural causes doubled in the first week for both men and women. Among women, the rate returned to average by the end of the first month, and among men over 65, it returned to average by the sixth month; but widowers under 65 had a natural death rate 50 percent higher than expected even in the third year. Men had more than doubled mortality from heart disease in the first week, and nearly doubled mortality from strokes in the first month. In men under 65, the rate of deaths from stroke quadrupled during the first month. In women, the rate of death from heart disease more than

tripled in the first week. Cancer deaths rose 25 percent among men in the first month and 60 percent among women in the first week, but did not increase after that.

Violent death was also most common in the first month; for example, suicides increased 17 times among widowers and 4.5 times among widows. After that, the rate of violent deaths gradually fell, but the excess remained substantial, especially among those under 65.

The authors suggest that emotional distress precipitates heart attacks in the first months of widowhood, and stress combined with sleeplessness may cause psychotic reactions that lead to suicide. Impaired immune functioning might also account for some of the deaths. The effects of bereavement may last longer in men under 65 partly because after the death of a wife they eat poorly, smoke, and drink more, and reduce their physical activity.

Jaakko Kaprio, Markku Koskenvuo, and Heli Rita. Mortality after bereavement: a prospective study of 95,647 widowed persons. *American Journal of Public Health, 77:*283–287 (March 1987).

Source: *The Harvard Medical School Mental Health Letter.* (1987) 4(5), p. 7.

(death of a spouse or divorce). They appear to be more or less everyday events, but ones that have a very important impact on the particular individual and, therefore, are important in assessment and treatment. A complete DSM-III-R diagnosis is as follows:

AXIS I 316.00 Psychological Factors Affecting Physical Condition

AXIS II None known

AXIS III Migraine Headaches

AXIS IV Psychosocial stressors: Change in work schedule. Severity: 3—Mild

AXIS V Highest level of functioning past year: 90

Carol: A Victim of Nausea

Carol was a 24-year-old woman who complained of nausea and vomiting. She had recently started a new job in which she was required to give lectures to various civic groups. She feared failure, became anxious, felt nauseated, and often vomited before one of these presentations. Eventually, she became nauseated if she even thought about giving a talk, which interfered with her preparation of material for her lectures. She recognized that her fears were unreasonable and she usually managed to give her talk but found that her physical symptoms were becoming debilitating.

DSM-III-R Diagnostic Criteria for Psychosomatic Disorders (Psychological Factors Affecting Physical Condition)

A. Psychologically meaningful environmental stimuli are temporally related to the initiation or exacerbation of a specific physical condition or disorder.

B. The physical condition has either demonstrable organic pathology (such as rheumatoid arthritis) or a known pathophysiological process (such as migraine headache, vomiting).

C. The condition does not meet the criteria for a somatoform disorder.

In Carol's case, a psychologically meaningful stimulus, public speaking, is associated with a single physiological symptom, vomiting. Therefore, a diagnosis of psychological factors affecting physical condition is appropriate. However, it is also true that an additional diagnosis of social phobia (see Chapter 8 on anxiety disorders) may be correct. The complete DSM-III-R diagnosis would then be:

AXIS I   316.00 Psychological Factors Affecting Physical Condition
         300.23 Social Phobia, Public Speaking Anxiety

AXIS II None known

AXIS III Nausea, vomiting

AXIS IV Psychosocial Stressors: New career
         Severity: 3—Moderate

AXIS V   Highest level of functioning past year: 70

John: A Victim of Chest Pain

John was a 54-year-old man who suffered severe, crushing substernal chest pain off and on for about four hours before coming into the hospital. He was admitted, and EKG and enzyme criteria substantiated a diagnosis of myocardial infarction. His recovery and rehabilitation went well and he returned to work in six weeks.

John was married and had three children, one still living at home. He was a successful executive in a large insurance corporation where he had started as a salesman twenty-nine years before. Prior to his heart attack, John was under tremendous pressure at work and had been working late hours and weekends. He had also suffered a severe financial loss in a business deal with his son-in-law. His youngest son had been arrested for shoplifting, and family life was fraught with tension and arguments. Once John returned home, he had episodes of angina several times a week, which he alleviated with nitroglycerin tablets. These episodes tended to occur when he overexerted himself physically or when he became involved in one of the family arguments.

In John's case, it seems quite clear that psychological factors were involved in John's heart attack, and, subsequently, in his episodes of angina. Therefore, a diagnosis of psychological factors affecting physical condition is appropriate. John experienced a number of significant events found on the Life-Change Scale (Holmes & Rahe, 1967) that may have contributed to his heart attack. Personality factors may also have been involved. That is, John could probably be labeled a "Type A" individual, one who is hard driving, competitive, and time urgent. This type of individual is more than twice as likely to suffer a heart attack as is an easygoing, "Type B" personality type (Rosenman et. al., 1975). (Also see Chapter 20 on men for more on "Type A" personality.)

In addition to John's own psychological history, his medical and family history revealed a hereditary factor. Both his father and grandfather died of heart disease. John smoked one and one-half packs of cigarettes a day, had a history of hypertension, and had abnormally high levels of serum cholesterol. This illustrates that other factors are quite often involved in the development of disease and that these factors must be considered in the process of developing a treatment plan. John was treated for his hypertension and elevated serum cholesterol with medication and diet. He was also advised to quit smoking. *Psychosomatic* does not necessarily mean *psychogenic*. In other words, psychological factors may contribute to a disease process or development of a symptom, but may not be the sole or major factors involved. Most diseases or physical conditions may be thought of as having multifactorial etiologies. The complete DSM-III-R diagnosis in this case would be as follows:

AXIS I   316.00 Psychological Factors Affecting Physical Condition

AXIS II   None known

AXIS III Myocardial infarction
          Angina Pectoris
          Hypertension

AXIS IV   Psychosocial stressors: Change in work level, change in financial status, problems with family members, legal problems with son.
          Severity: 4—Severe

AXIS V   Highest level of functioning past year: 80

Louise: A Victim of Palpitations, Dizziness, and Dyspnea

Louise was a 44-year-old woman who went to her family doctor reporting peculiar "spells" that had left her feeling anxious and frightened that something was seriously wrong with her. She described these spells as starting quite suddenly, when she felt slightly dizzy and had a sensation that things going on around her weren't "real." Her breathing became difficult, as though she couldn't catch her breath, and she felt her heart pounding. She felt sweaty and shaky. During the last episode she experienced a tingling feeling in her hands and her face.

The first of these episodes occurred about a month before her visit to the doctor. Two weeks prior to the episode, she had placed her aging mother in a nursing home after many weeks of family discussions and soul searching. She felt that the responsibility for making this decision and caring for her mother was thrust upon her by other family members. She reported being preoccupied with her decision during subsequent weeks, feeling guilty and wondering if she had done the right thing. She wondered whether the "spells" she had been having were related to the family problems that had been bothering her for several months.

In Louise's case, it is likely that her physical symptoms are related to the family stress she described and therefore fit the criteria for a DSM-III-R diagnosis of psychological factors affecting physical condition. However, this particular cluster of symptoms also fits the DSM-III-R diagnosis of panic dis-

order (see Chapter 8 on anxiety disorders). Thus a more specific and accurate diagnosis would be panic disorder, even though, technically, the episodes are physical symptoms that are affected by psychological factors. The complete diagnosis would be:

AXIS I   300.01 Panic Disorder

AXIS II   None known

AXIS III Palpitations, dizziness, dyspnea

AXIS IV   Psychosocial stressors: illness of mother
          Severity: 3—Moderate

AXIS V   Highest level of functioning past year: 90

Dan: A Victim of Chest Pain and Dyspnea

Dan, a 19-year-old college student, complained of wheezing, labored breathing, and chest constriction whenever he went jogging or played basketball outdoors. This was particularly likely to happen on a cold day. Dan's difficulty in breathing usually started ten to fifteen minutes after he started to exercise, and continued for thirty minutes to an hour after he stopped. Dan reported no other times when he experienced these difficulties.

When asked about how he was doing in general, this patient did not report any recent or chronic stress; he described a satisfying primary relationship and supportive family. He talked about school and his major in political science with enthusiasm. There seemed to be no psychologically stressful events correlated with his breathing problems. A diagnosis of asthma may be made, but there is no evidence that psychological factors are affecting Dan's illness. Therefore, a diagnosis of psychological factors affecting physical condition is not appropriate.

NURSING DIAGNOSES FOR PSYCHOLOGICAL FACTORS AFFECTING PHYSICAL CONDITION

As with the DSM-III-R diagnoses, the nursing diagnoses for psychological factors affecting physical condition include both the organic pathology or pathophysiological process and the psychological or emotional factors. For example, as in Charles's case (migraine headache), the nursing diagnoses would include 1) pain, 2) sensory-perceptual alteration (visual), and 3) ineffective individual coping. The nursing diagnoses for Carol (phobia and nausea) would include 1) anxiety and 2) ineffective individual coping (fear). In John's case (chest pain) the nursing diagnoses would include 1) potential activity intolerance, 2) pain, 3) ineffective family coping (disabling), and 4) ineffective individual coping. Louise's case (panic disorder) would include 1) ineffective breathing pattern, 2) anxiety, 3) fear, 4) anticipatory grieving, and 5) alteration in family process. It is important to identify and treat both the presenting "medical" complaint and the psychological factors which may be contributing to them.

NURSING INTERVENTIONS

Nurses working in inpatient or outpatient settings are responsible for teaching psychosomatic patients about pain management, especially nonpharmacological techniques. For example, a cold compress may be soothing for migraine pain and could allow a migraine sufferer to get by with less narcotic medication.

Teaching about the pharmacological and nonpharmacological management of anxiety is also important. In Carol and Louise's cases, the nurse can explore with each patient her fears and anxieties, and whence they come. She can teach the patient that anxiety is best dealt with through exposure, not avoidance. Referral for behavioral or psychoanalytic psychotherapy may be indicated. If so, the nurse can tell the patient what to expect and how therapy can help.

Nurses working with Charles and Louise can point out sources of illness-associated stress at work and in the family. Encouraging the migraine sufferer to learn to say "no" and to arrange for breaks during the work day, as well as exercise and adequate rest and nutrition, may lead to fewer attacks. Planning with John how to decrease the number of cardiac risk factors in his life (caffeine intake, poor nutrition, lack of exercise, smoking, and so on) as well as teaching him about the potential health benefits of family therapy is his primary nurse's responsibility, and something she is in a good position to do if she has established an effective therapeutic relationship with him during his stay in the coronary care unit. (See Box 13–2.)

ASSESSMENT

The most important part of the assessment of psychological factors affecting physical condition is the interview. Usually the physician will conduct a physical exam and order any laboratory tests that are indicated. The physician will formulate a preliminary diagnosis of the physical part of the disorder (for example, asthma, ulcerative colitis). If any information about the patient's psychosocial history, current life situation, or emotional status is lacking in the data collected by the physician, the nurse conducts an interview directed at assessing these issues. The key diagnostic issue is whether or not psychologically meaningful environmental stimuli are temporally related to the onset or exacerbation of the symptom.

DIFFICULTIES IN ASSESSMENT. Three things make an interview aimed at assessing the importance of psychological factors difficult. First, patients often do not make a connection between their physical symptoms and emotional or life-stress problems. Almost by definition, these patients dissociate feelings about significant life events from conscious awareness and transform them into bodily symptoms. Therefore, these patients have difficulty making mind-body connections. Some patients, however, do sense that the source of their problems may be emotional. To encourage such thinking, the nurse may ask such questions as, "Have you ever noticed that when you are upset, your symptoms get worse?" "Do you ever feel that events in your life affect your asthma?" "What events in your life seem to make your stomach pain worse?" "You say you felt worse on Tuesday morning. Let's look at what happened on Monday."

A second factor making it difficult to take a psychosocial history and explore possible precipitating life events is that patients may interpret the questions above as accusations. They may think that the nurse is implying, "It's all in your head." The word *psychosomatic* has come to have a pejorative meaning to many people; it is often thought to imply that the pain and the symptoms of psychosomatic illness are not real. This attitude comes from an assumption that mind and body are two separate and distinct entities, and symptoms can be categorized as stemming from problems only in one *or* the other. A brief explanation about how stress affects the body may make the patient more receptive to ideas about mind-body connections. Because in the past few years the media have legitimized the concept of stress and its relationship to illness, many patients will now be more willing to accept this interpretation of their symptoms.

A third factor that makes interviewing difficult is that many of these patients have great trouble recognizing and verbally expressing feelings. This lack of ability to verbalize emotions has been labeled **alexithymia,** which means "without words for mood"

Box 13–2 • Stress Management for Nurses

Stress affects different people in different ways. Some people may be more susceptible to stress-related illness than others, and researchers in this area have been exploring the personality traits that may help a person cope with stress and maintain mental wellness. Nursing is a profession considered high on the stress scale, and many nurses consider job burnout a major threat. Recently nurse researchers have become interested in determining how to cultivate those qualities which would help a person avoid job burnout. Rich and Rich (1987) discovered that "hardiness" may be related to the avoidance of staff burnout: "By conceptualizing crises as challenges rather than as threats and by adopting a 'can do' attitude in the work situation, hardy nurses may not experience their job as being as stressful as do nonhardy nurses." The following guidelines developed by Paula Tedesco-Carreras (1988) are aimed at helping nurses (and others) realize that they are responsible for their own physical and mental well-being and can work to manage stress on an individual level:

1. Develop a self-care philosophy. Take responsibility for your own physical and mental wellbeing; be at-tentive to your needs—they are important!

2. Get to know yourself. Clarify your own personal philosophies, values, and goals; become aware of your reactions to certain stressors and the feelings that are evoked; notice behaviors that you would like to change.

3. Avoid being self-critical. Many people feel that they should be able to handle any situation and any demands placed upon them, then they feel badly about themselves for not being able to meet unrealistic (usually self-imposed) expectations! Lachman suggests four methods for decreasing what she calls negative self-talk.

a. Steadily increasing your belief that you can control your emotional responses, not external events.

b. Increasing your wisdom about the difference between what you can control and what you cannot.

c. Knowing, perhaps redefining, and living according to your values.

d. Setting time aside each day to do planning for your day, as well as your life.

(Sifneos, 1973). If asked about emotions associated with a significant life event, the alexithymic patient typically either does not understand the question, is bewildered by the notion of feelings, or continues to describe inner responses in terms of physical symptoms. This inability to report feelings is not attributed to resistance or denial on the part of the patient, but rather to a lack of experience with the emotional self.

ASSESSMENT FOR DEPRESSION. In addition to assessing the impact of psychological factors on the patient's illness, the nurse also assesses the psychosomatic patient for possible depression. This is because an underlying depression can be, and often is, masked by a presentation of physical complaints (Lesse, 1967). Even when the patient does not report a mood disturbance, an evaluation of the vegetative signs of depression (appetite loss, sleep distur-bance, fatigue, sexual difficulties, and so on) can assist in making a diagnosis of depression, which warrants a psychiatric consultation regarding the potential usefulness of antidepressant medication and/or psychotherapy. (See Chapter 9 on mood disorders for more on the assessment and treatment of depression.)

The outcome of a psychological or psychosocial assessment interview should be a complete psychosocial history, preliminary DSM-III-R diagnosis, and nursing diagnoses, which can be entered in the patient's chart. The written assessment includes the history and current status of the presenting problem; past psychiatric history and treatment; current family, occupational, and social information; genetic or relevant medical information; developmental, childhood, and family history; information on appearance and behavior; information on affect and mood; and possible psychological factors contributing to the pre-

4. Build social support systems. Make a habit to talk about your feelings with peers, co-workers, family, and friends. Commiserating with those who share similar values and goals is mutually supportive. Somehow, things do not feel so bad knowing "we are all in this together."

5. Learn to communicate clearly and precisely in a non-aggressive manner. Learn to feel comfortable saying the word "no!" when possible, especially when it is in the interest of lowering your own personal stress.

6. Pay attention to nutrition. Eat well-balanced meals at regular intervals; take time to eat lunch away from a stressful environment; avoid excessive fats, salt, sugar, and caffeine. Include fresh fruits and vegetables and fiber in your diet. Maintain your ideal weight.

7. Exercise. It is necessary for muscular, skeletal, and cardiovascular fitness, a wonderful way to relieve tension, clear your head, and "get the crazies out." Aerobic exercise done properly three to four times per week promotes relaxation and a general feeling of well-being.

8. Get sufficient rest and sleep. They are necessary for their restorative and reparative powers. The amount of sleep each person needs is an individual matter. Especially when normal biorhythms are interrupted (during shift work or pulling an all-nighter), it is important to find creative ways of obtaining undisturbed periods of rest and sleep.

9. Relax, take breaks, or change your activity for a short time; learn deep-breathing, progressive relaxation, and visualization exercises. Give yourself the time and permission to participate in an enjoyable hobby or activity on a regular basis. Learn to meditate.

10. Manage time. Learn to set priorities and organize; when possible, allow more time than necessary to complete a task so as not to feel rushed. When possible, disregard the clock.

11. Become aware. No matter the origin, the beliefs and philosophies a person holds can be a source of solace during stressful times. Our spirituality can give us strength to confront the difficult moral and ethical dilemmas we must face in the nursing profession. "The beliefs that emerge from our spiritual sense give hope in times of crises, provide a perspective for the day-to-day struggles of living, and offer guidance to our lives. Our beliefs contribute to our notion of what can be done to handle stress."

12. Cultivate humor. Laughter is an activity that can often break tense moments; learn to laugh at yourself.

13. Avoid addictive substances. Following the prescriptions for maintaining mental wellness is not always easy. We sometimes desire quick and easy solutions for relieving stress and "fixers" are readily available to us. Reliance on the use of alcohol, prescription and over-the-counter drugs, illegal substances, and nicotine for the management of stress may lead to addictive problems.

Source: Tedeso-Carreras, P. NSNA/ Imprint, Feb/Mar 1988, p. 39.

---

senting symptoms. If specific assessment instruments are used, such as the Holmes and Rahe Life-Change Scale or the Beck Depression Inventory, the results are also included in the written assessment.

TREATMENT

In today's health care settings, the first type of treatment attempted for many psychosomatic disorders is some form of pharmacological intervention. A variety of medications alleviate or reduce many of the physical symptoms (for example, cimetidine for ulcers, ergotamine and certain psychotropic medications* for migraine headache, theophylline for asthma). However, this by no means reduces the necessity for attention to psychological factors that may be contributing to the physical symptoms. Most medications have side effects, and long-term use of most drugs carries some risk. Treatment aimed at the psychological aspects of the disease may reduce the need for medication as well as prevent relapse in the future.

The first step in the treatment of patients with psychosomatic disorders is the development of a warm, supportive, working relationship with one of the health care professionals (such as the nurse) involved in the case. If the patient suspects that psychological factors are critical in his or her disease, then these issues may be directly addressed early in treatment. Sometimes the patient may prefer to be referred to a psychotherapist, because of a previous therapy experience, the nurse's style (sometimes nurse and patient, like therapist and patient, just

*Many migraine sufferers obtain relief from the disorder after a few days or weeks of treatment with one of the antidepressants (selection depends on therapeutic response and patient's tolerance of side effects; any or all may be tried), or lithium despite not having a diagnosis of mood disorder (Couch & Hassanein, 1979; Kimble, Williams, & Agras, 1975).

don't "click"), or the type of issues involved. If, however, the patient is unaware of, or unwilling to consider, psychological factors, it is best to wait until a stable relationship with one of the treating professionals, based on symptom management, is established. At that point, or soon after, the patient may be able to discuss some of the stressful problems in his or her life without feeling defensive.

The relationship that develops, for example, between the patient and the nurse forms the basis of treatment. The nurse's understanding and validation of the patient's view of the situation, including his or her symptoms, is vital. Confrontation with psychological issues, deep interpretations of the "meaning" of symptoms, and directives are likely to be counterproductive. Empathy and listening with a sympathetic ear are more likely to bring important issues out in the open. The patient's gradually increasing comfort in discussing feelings and life events with the physician or nurse is, in itself, therapeutic. Practical suggestions, problem solving, support, and encouraging the expression of feelings are the main elements of treatment.

Some patients may respond well to keeping a diary of their symptoms. The patient can track a symptom and any significant events or emotions that might be related to its onset and development. Together, the patient and, perhaps, the nurse can work to discover whether the symptoms seem to follow any pattern, or if a specific type of event seems to be a precipitating factor.

Insight-oriented, or psychodynamic, psychotherapy may be indicated for patients who are verbally expressive and interested in exploring how psychological factors may be influencing their health. In this case, the nurse can make a referral to a mental health professional who has interest and expertise in treating psychosomatic disorders. Many patients, however, will not be appropriate for insight-oriented psychotherapy. For some, such as the alexithymic patient, such anxiety-provoking psychotherapies may even make the symptoms worse (Sifneos, 1975).

SOMATOFORM DISORDERS

Somatoform disorders fall into four distinct diagnostic groups: **somatization disorder, conversion disorder, somatoform pain disorder,** and **hypochondriasis.** Four distinct features characterize this group of disorders: 1) a loss of or an alteration in physical functioning; 2) the symptoms not being explained by a known physiological mechanism; 3) evidence that psychological factors have precipitated the problem; and 4) the symptoms not being under voluntary control of the patient.

Ford (1983) describes somatization as a process by which the patient uses his or her body for psychological purposes (**primary gain**) or for personal gain (**secondary gain**). Psychological purposes, or primary gain, often serve a conflict-resolving function and include 1) conversion of unpleasant or conflicting emotions into a physical symptom (for example, preoccupation with bowel dysfunction in place of experiencing underlying depression); 2) use of a symptom to communicate symbolically an idea or emotion (for example, a paralysis symbolizing a feeling of helplessness); and 3) alleviation of guilt through suffering (for example, chronic pain beginning after the death of a person whom the patient regarded ambivalently). Personal or secondary gain includes 1) the ability to manipulate interpersonal relationships; 2) release from duties or responsibilities; 3) financial gain (such as disability compensation); and 4) attention or sympathy from others. Secondary gain is not found exclusively in the somatoform disorders; it may also be observed in cases of organic disease.

Traditionally, these disorders have been difficult to diagnose and treat. Like patients who have psychosomatic disorders, these individuals are generally seen in general medical settings rather than psychiatric ones. However, unlike complaints related to psychosomatic disorders, somatoform complaints cannot be confirmed by medical examination or laboratory procedures, although the symptoms persist.

As medical examinations fail to find causes for the symptoms, the nurse and physician begin to consider the possibility of psychological factors. At this point, if the nurse or physician suggests a psychiatric consultation or refers the patient to a psychotherapist, the patient may feel misunderstood and mistreated. He or she may be convinced that the illness is physical and therefore continue to seek medical solutions. Rather than accept a psychiatric diagnosis, this patient is likely to seek medical help elsewhere, "doctor shopping" until finding one who will provide a medical explanation for the symptoms. For these reasons, health providers often find these patients very difficult to treat. They have long, complicated medical histories that include many frustrated attempts at treatment. Often physicians and nurses ultimately respond to these patients with anger, frustration, and derision. They label these patients "crocks," "chronic complainers," or "thick-chart patients"; and they may refer to the medical history, or positive review of systems as an "organ recital."

Somatoform disorders can be confused, sometimes tragically, with 1) undiagnosed physical illness; 2) psychosomatic disorders; 3) malingering; and 4) factitious disorder. Unlike psychosomatic disorders, there is no known pathophysiological process for somatoform disorder. However, the two are alike in that the symptoms presented in both disorders are not under the voluntary control of the patient. A patient with **malingering** voluntarily produces false or grossly exaggerated physical symptoms. This patient uses symptoms in an attempt at manipulation to gain some recognizable goal, such as avoiding military conscription or a particular type of work. A patient with **factitious disorder with physical symptoms** presents with physical symptoms to such a degree that he or she is able to obtain and sustain multiple hospitalizations and even surgery. The physical signs of illness are voluntarily produced through physiological tampering, for example, ingesting or injecting a bacterially contaminated substance, in the hope of gaining medical attention and assuming the role of patient. This disorder is also known as **Munchausen syndrome.**

SOMATIZATION DISORDER

Somatization disorder, once known as hysteria, is characterized by multiple somatic complaints that are recurrent or chronic. It can involve a variety of physiological systems (cardiovascular, gastrointestinal, gynecological, and so on). It is often referred to as **Briquet's syndrome,** after the French physician who first described it in 1859. The disorder usually begins before the age of 30 and has a chronic, fluctuating course. It rarely occurs in men. Patients with a diagnosis of somatization disorder may also have a history of conversion symptoms and/or be diagnosed as histrionic personality (Kimble, Williams, & Agras, 1975). There is also evidence of an association with sociopathy. Delinquency from school, repeated fighting, running away from home, a poor work record, a poor marital history, sexual promiscuity, heavy drinking, and trouble with the police are found in the histories of many hysterics (Goodwin & Guze, 1979). (See Chapter 12 on personality disorders).

Somatization disorder, or Briquet's syndrome, is characterized by the following: 1) a complicated history of repeated medical complaints, often presented in a dramatic fashion; 2) a wide variety of symptoms, such as headaches, back pain, fainting spells, weight problems, and breathing difficulties; and 3) symptoms severe enough to have led to medication or visits to the doctor, or to have somehow interfered with the patient's life.

Marie: A Patient with Somatization Disorder

Marie was a 32-year-old woman who came to a general medical clinic seeking help for a number of problems that had been plaguing her. She presented her complaints in such a dramatic and complicated fashion that the nurse who took her medical history had a difficult time determining when the present illness began and which symptom brought her to the clinic. Marie said, "I am fatigued and tired all the time now . . . I feel dizzy and I faint a lot . . . My heart starts to beat very fast and it is so loud that I'm surprised I haven't had a stroke . . . I have been having trouble with my bowels lately . . . My menstrual cramps are so bad I practically have to go to bed for a week . . . I have been sick all my life."

Marie reported nineteen symptoms that had, over the years, resulted in three hospitalizations and visits to more than twenty doctors. She had taken a multitude of medications, including minor tranquilizers and narcotics. Extensive diagnostic procedures, including exploratory surgery six months ago, had resulted in a number of unsubstantiated diagnoses and ineffective treatments.

Marie was married to a man who was fifteen years older than she. When first married, she worked part-time as a receptionist in a local business office, but then began to feel too ill to work. Marie and her husband had no children, though he wanted them. He worked full-time as the manager of a department store, and also often shopped and cooked for the two of them, as well as helped Marie with the housework.

The case of Marie highlights some of the more prominent diagnostic features of somatization disorder. There is also a suggestion that Marie was obtaining secondary gain from her illness because she had been relieved of her adult responsibilities.

Once a diagnosis of somatization disorder has been made, treatment, or more accurately, management (as this patient is usually resistant to potentially effective psychiatric treatment) is the next step. Usually, this patient is best managed in a primary care or general medical setting. Confrontation about whether a symptom is real or not will prove fruitless. This patient is likely to resent and reject even a psychiatric consultation. Someone like Marie might desert the physician or nurse who suggests that her problem is "all in her head," and seek out someone new who "understands" that she has a medical problem.

DSM-III-R
Diagnostic Criteria for
Somatization Disorder

A. A history of many physical complaints or a belief that one is sickly, beginning before the age of 30 and persisting for several years.

B. At least 13 symptoms from the list below. To count a symptom as significant, the following criteria must be met:

1) no organic pathology or pathophysiologic mechanism (e.g., a physical disorder or the effects of injury, medication, drugs, or alcohol) to account for the symptom or, when there is related organic pathology, the complaint or resulting social or occupational impairment is grossly in excess of what would be expected from the physical findings.

2) has not occurred only during a panic attack

3) has caused the person to take medicine (other than over-the-counter pain medication), see a doctor, or alter life-style

Symptom list:

Gastrointestinal symptoms:

1) vomiting (other than during pregnancy)

2) abdominal pain (other than when menstruating)

3) nausea (other than motion sickness)

4) bloating (gassy)

5) diarrhea

6) intolerance of (gets sick from) several different foods

Pain symptoms:

7) pain in extremities

8) back pain

9) joint pain

10) pain during urination

11) other pain (excluding headaches)

Cardiopulmonary symptoms:

12) shortness of breath when not exerting oneself

13) palpitations

14) chest pain

15) dizziness

The main objective in managing a patient with somatization disorder is to protect the patient from herself; in other words, to recognize and decrease the potential for iatrogenic or treatment-induced harm. Medications, invasive procedures, surgery, and other treatments should be undertaken conservatively. The establishment of a long-term relationship that is not conditional upon testing, diagnosing, and curing physical symptoms will gradually help shift the focus from exclusive attention to somatic complaints. Visits to the nurse or doctor should not be dependent on the status of the patient's symptoms. Rather, regular visits should be scheduled, perhaps with the doctor and nurse working as a team and alternating visits. As their relationship with the patient develops, attention can be redirected toward some of the problems and stresses of daily living, focusing on giving and mobilizing support and problem solving. Such an approach is much more likely to be successful than interpreting physical symptoms in psychological terms.

For instance, Marie was initially scheduled for a return visit to the clinic after one week. Her physician informed her that although her symptoms were to be followed very closely, she should not expect improvement right away. Visits were then scheduled two weeks apart and later decreased to once a month.

Conversion or pseudoneurologic symptoms:

16) **amnesia**
17) **difficulty swallowing**
18) loss of voice
19) deafness
20) double vision
21) blurred vision
22) blindness
23) fainting or loss of consciousness
24) seizure or convulsion
25) trouble walking
26) paralysis or muscle weakness
27) urinary retention or difficulty urinating

Sexual symptoms for the major part of the person's life after opportunities for sexual activity:

28) **burning sensation in sexual organs or rectum (other than during intercourse)**
29) sexual indifference
30) pain during intercourse
31) impotence

Female reproductive symptoms judged by the person to occur more frequently or severely than in most women:

32) **painful menstruation**
33) irregular menstrual periods
34) excessive menstrual bleeding
35) vomiting throughout pregnancy

Note: The seven items in boldface may be used to screen for the disorder. The presence of two or more of these items suggests a high likelihood of the disorder.

The doctor and nurse conveyed the attitude that they took Marie's symptoms seriously, but at the same time they tried to redirect her attention to problems at home and her relationship with her husband. Marie was ultimately able to accept the idea that there was a lot of stress in her life that could be affecting her health and was gradually encouraged to talk about it. Establishing a therapeutic alliance with this patient kept her from continuing her doctor shopping, as well as helped her to direct her attention to interpersonal problems.

Shifting attention away from somatic complaints and failing to accede to the patient's demands for fur-ther testing or medication may not always have positive results. The patient may get angry or exaggerate the seriousness of symptoms in an effort to manipulate the clinician. The patient may threaten to leave treatment and seek another doctor, or may even threaten suicide. The clinician should maintain an empathic but firm stance and not give in to such attempts at manipulation. However, if the patient expresses suicidal ideation which is more than a passing thought, a psychiatric consultation should be obtained. (See Chapter 18 on crisis for assessment and management of the acutely suicidal patient.)

CONVERSION DISORDER

Conversion disorder is characterized by the loss of all or part of some basic bodily function. The loss suggests a physical disturbance but is instead an expression of psychological conflict or need. Symptom onset is usually very sudden, follows some stressful experience, and is not voluntarily controlled by the patient. Usually the patient reports a sensory disturbance (such as anesthesias and parasthesias), a perceptual disturbance (such as blurred vision, blindness, or deafness), or a motor disability (such as paralysis, seizures, or loss of voice).

The psychodynamic interpretation of conversion disorder is most widely accepted today and has not changed much from Freud's early formulations. According to Freud (1938), the physical symptom is a defense that absorbs and neutralizes the anxiety generated by an unacceptable, unconscious impulse or wish. The psychic energy from the anxiety is transformed into a somatic loss. The anxiety is then detached from the impulse and the conflict it generates, thus rendering it neutral. The particular somatic loss symbolizes the underlying conflict associated with the unacceptable impulse or wish and defuses it. For example, if a woman develops (converts her unconscious anxiety into) a paralysis, she won't be *able* to leave her husband for another man. Current thought also recognizes the importance of psychological and personal gain (as discussed in somatization disorder) in conversion disorder. Behavioral theories assert that the symptoms are learned ways of communicating feelings of helplessness and manipulating the environment.

Conversion disorder is rare in today's population, although conversion symptoms may appear as *part* of a larger clinical picture such as in somatization disorder. Historically, "hysterical conversion" (as it was called prior to DSM-III) was a much more prevalent condition and has been important in the development of thought and theories on mind-body issues in psychology. However, because it is rarely seen currently, the discussion of conversion disorder will be brief.

Susan: A Patient with Conversion Disorder

Susan came into the emergency room with the report that she couldn't move her right arm and that she had lost all feeling in it. "From just below the shoulder," she said, "it's as if it just isn't there." The physician ordered a neurological workup, and Susan's psychotherapist, whom she had been seeing for several months, was called. The combination of a negative neurological workup (the anatomical distribution of the loss of function did not fit the innervation pattern of the arm, and the EMG was normal) and the information provided by the psychologist suggested that this might be a conversion symptom.

Susan had been divorced for three years and had two children, a son, age 12, who preferred to live with his father and thus was in his custody, and a daughter, age 6, who was with her. About one year ago, her ex-husband, who had remarried, began legal action to secure custody of their daughter. He maintained that he was more "stable" than Susan, who had a history of depression. Prior to going to court, Susan decided to give up custody of her daughter to her ex-husband. She felt weak, defeated, and as if she "just couldn't fight him anymore." Although she was deeply attached to her daughter (she had once stated to the psychologist that losing her daughter would be like losing her right arm), she felt she hadn't been a good mother. She felt guilty that, as a single parent, she hadn't been able to provide for her children as she would have liked. The onset of the symptom oc-

DSM-III-R Diagnostic Criteria for Conversion Disorder

A. A loss of, or alteration in, physical functioning suggesting a physical disorder.

B. Psychological factors are judged to be etiologically related to the symptom because of a temporal relationship between a psychosocial stressor that is apparently related to a psychological conflict or need and initiation or exacerbation of the symptom.

C. The person is not conscious of intentionally producing the symptom.

D. The symptom is not a culturally sanctioned response pattern and cannot, after appropriate investigation, be explained by a known physical disorder.

E. The symptom is not limited to pain or to a disturbance in sexual functioning.

Specify: single episode or **recurrent.**

curred the evening after her ex-husband took their daughter to live with him.

Susan was released from the hospital and continued her psychotherapy sessions. After a few sessions, in which her feelings of guilt and loss were brought out into the open, her symptom disappeared. A followup visit to the neurologist indicated there was no evidence of neurological disease.

The case of Susan illustrates some of the main features of conversion disorder. The symptom usually remits rapidly and with minimal suggestion. Psychotherapy can be helpful. If the symptom does not remit quickly, it may mean that neurological disease is present, and another medical workup is in order, or it may mean that the secondary gain obtained by the symptom is too important or too rewarding for the individual to "give it up."

Another feature of conversion disorder that historically has been emphasized is "la belle indifference." This refers to a patient's puzzling and incongruent lack of concern about even a major physical disability. Recent studies have shown this traditionally classic sign of conversion disorder to be of little use in making the diagnosis because this lack of emotional reaction or bland indifference is found only in a minority of patients (Pincus & Tucker, 1978).

SOMATOFORM PAIN DISORDER

A clear focus on pain distinguishes somatoform pain disorder (previously called psychogenic pain disorder) from other somatoform disorders. A complaint of pain, usually of a chronic nature, which is not substantiated adequately by laboratory findings, and which appears to be related to psychological factors, is the predominant clinical feature of somatoform pain disorder. Each patient may describe the pain in a variety of ways and it may occur in a variety of

sites, for example, lower back, abdomen, joints, and head. As with conversion disorder, patients may say that they can't walk, but this is because walking is too painful, not because their legs don't work.

As with somatization and conversion disorders, evidence of primary and secondary gain is a critical factor in the assessment and treatment of somatoform pain. The attention and sympathy given to the patient by family members, relief from responsibilities, and/or financial compensation for disability may sustain the pain and pain behavior. Individuals with psychogenic pain disorder may also be referred to as chronic pain patients.

Robert: A Patient with Somatoform Pain Disorder

Robert, a 42-year-old factory worker, had had severe, disabling lower back pain for nine months by the time he visited a medical clinic. The pain had begun when he lifted a large crate at work and was sent home by the employee physician for a few days of bedrest. When Robert returned to work, he was unable to perform his duties and began to take numerous sick days in order to visit a variety of doctors. Physical exams and laboratory findings suggested muscle strain at the time of the incident, but his symptoms seemed excessive considering the extent of his injury.

At the time of this clinic visit, Robert was no longer working and he and his wife were living on disability insurance. He was taking a number of medications for his pain, including Demerol and Valium, and was spending the majority of his day either reclining in bed or watching television on the sofa. His wife had taken over all of the household responsibilities and waited on him hand and foot.

Robert's case illustrates a number of important issues associated with chronic pain patients. First,

---

DSM-III-R Diagnostic Criteria for Somatoform Pain Disorder

A. Preoccupation with pain for at least six months.

B. Either (1) or (2):

1) appropriate evaluation uncovers no organic pathology or pathophysiologic mechanism (e.g., a physical disorder or the effects of injury) to account for the pain.

2) when there is related organic pathology, the complaint of pain or resulting social or occupational impairment is grossly in excess of what would be expected from the physical findings.

there is evidence of secondary gain in his receipt of financial compensation for his injury and in the attention given to him by his wife. Second, there is a drastic reduction in physical and social activity, which is commonly seen among these patients. Third, the patient is taking a number of analgesics and may even be addicted.

Behavioral treatments, like those first described by Fordyce (1976), are aimed at changing the patterns described above. The patient is started on a medication schedule that is not pain contingent, and gradually medications are withdrawn. The nurse or physician introduces other methods for dealing with pain and stress, such as relaxation training (see Chapter 25 on the intensive care patient for specifics). The patient learns that he or she can become more active and spends less and less time in bed or reclining. The importance of secondary gain is also addressed. Some treatment programs will not accept a patient who has litigation for financial compensation for an illness or injury pending, since it is unlikely that the patient will be motivated to comply with the program until the legal matter is settled. Family involvement is emphasized in order to discourage attention paid to pain behavior and to encourage attention and support for nonpain behavior.

In Robert's case, therapy sessions with him and his wife revealed that, prior to the injury, the marriage had been deteriorating; Robert's wife had had several affairs. His painful condition served the function of keeping his wife devotedly attached to him, and her caregiving role helped to alleviate her guilt about the affairs. In therapy these issues were brought out in the open and began to be dealt with in a more straightforward fashion.

Treatment of patients with somatoform pain disorder can be difficult and complex, for example, if the patient seems to need narcotics for pain relief but seems vulnerable to substance abuse. For this reason many hospitals have developed pain clinics comprised of a variety of medical specialists, nurses, psychologists, physical therapists, and others. A multidisciplinary approach seems better able to serve the complicated diagnostic and treatment needs of the chronic pain patient than would any individual practitioner.

HYPOCHONDRIASIS

The patient suffering from hypochondriasis has an unrealistic perception of bodily sensations as being abnormal and indicative of serious disease. He or she is preoccupied with physical health despite a physician's reassurance and the lack of physical findings.

This unrealistic fear of serious disease is the hallmark of hypochondriasis. The relationship that forms between the health care provider and the hypochondriac is characterized by the patient's dependency on the physician and feelings of hostility toward him or his nurse when needs are not met. Because they simultaneously demand and reject, hypochondriachal patients can generate intense feelings of anger and frustration in the physicians and nurses who work with them.

The difference between hypochondriasis and somatization disorder can be difficult to detect. Both involve numerous somatic complaints and the patient's belief that he has a serious illness. However, somatization disorder usually begins before the age of 30 and is seen almost exclusively in women, whereas hypochondriasis occurs more frequently during middle and old age and is equally common in men and women (Adler, 1981). Cognitive style may also distinguish somatization disorder from hypochondriasis. Anxious, obsessive attention to detail characterizes the hypochondriac, whereas the individual with somatization disorder is often a poor and inaccurate historian (Ford, 1983). Patients with somatization disorder tend to be preoccupied with symptoms rather than the fear of a specific disease; patients with hypochondriasis are preoccupied with the fear of serious illness.

Helen: A Patient with Hypochondriasis

Helen, a 52-year-old woman, was well-known to her family doctor and nurse as well as the local pharmacist. She made frequent doctor's appointments with a variety of complaints and symptoms over the years. A new symptom, or an exacerbation of an old symptom, might flare up for a period of months, during which her visits and calls to the doctor would increase. She would frequently excuse herself from work or social obligations because of ill health. She read popular medical journals and articles that she would share with her health care providers as well as those of her friends who tolerated listening to her many complaints.

On her latest visit to the doctor, Helen complained of constant pain in the left side of her abdomen, which she described as a dull ache. She had stopped eating red meat a few months before because of an article she read on stomach cancer. She was also concerned because a relative of a friend had just been diagnosed with stomach cancer.

Upon being questioned about her work situation and family life, Helen reported that there had been some changes. A supervisor at work with whom she

DSM-III-R Diagnostic Criteria for Hypochondriasis

A. Preoccupation with the fear of having, or the belief that one has, a serious disease, based on the person's interpretation of physical signs or sensations as evidence of physical illness.

B. Appropriate physical evaluation does not support the diagnosis of any physical disorder that can account for the physical signs or sensations or the person's unwarranted interpretation of them, **and** the symptoms in A are not just symptoms of panic attacks.

C. The fear of having, or belief that one has, a disease persists despite medical reassurance.

D. Duration of the disturbance is at least six months.

E. The belief in A is not of delusional intensity, as in Delusional Disorder, Somatic Type (i.e, the person can acknowledge the possibility that his or her fear of having, or belief that he or she has, a serious disease is unfounded).

---

had shared a close personal relationship had recently retired. The new, younger supervisor was more distant and demanding. At home, Helen's husband had been working long hours on an office project and had not been spending much time with her.

The case of Helen is an example of a hypochondriacal patient who has been managed well by her physician and nurse. Although Helen makes frequent visits to the clinic, she has remained with the same doctor and nurse over the years, apparently feeling that her needs will be met and her complaints will not be rejected by them. As with patients with somatization disorder, it is important to accept this patient's physical complaints without undertaking numerous and extensive diagnostic procedures and treatments.

In this case, it may be that the onset of symptoms and anxiety about cancer was stimulated by the loss of two important people in her life, her husband and her supervisor, on whom Helen had felt quite dependent. Helen's stomach pain may have been her "ticket" of entry into a system in which she could gain reassurance and security and thus meet some of her dependency needs.

It is helpful for the nurse to assume that neither she nor the physician will "cure" the patient with hypochondriasis. However, she, like the physician, can develop a long-term professional relationship in which the patient's physical complaints are respected and attended to. Within that relationship, the patient

can be encouraged gradually to discuss interpersonal issues and feelings. When the clinician experiences feelings of anger and frustration in the process (countertransference), she should wonder if the patient is experiencing these feelings as well and begin to explore this possibility. Sometimes the patient's most effective communication is nonverbal, and this is one example. (See Chapter 5 on psychosocial assessment for more on countertransference.)

The treatment and management of the hypochondriac is a difficult and lengthy undertaking. The health care professional needs to recognize the long-term nature of this patient's problems and their treatment, as well as her continuing role in maintaining the patient's sense of well-being. Initially, or during a flareup of symptoms, it is important to see the patient frequently. As the crisis resolves and the patient develops a sense that his or her needs will be met, the frequency of visits can be reduced without having the patient feel rejected or not taken seriously.

NURSING DIAGNOSES FOR SOMATOFORM DISORDERS

As with psychosomatic disorders, nursing diagnoses for somatoform disorders identify both the presenting "medical" complaint and the psychological factors that contribute to the problem. Nursing diagnoses for Helen (hypochondriasis) would include a) comfort (alteration in pain), b) activity intolerance, c) fear, d) ineffective individual coping, and e) dysfunctional grieving.

Box 13–3 ● Love, Medicine & Miracles

Bernie Siegel's best selling book, *Love, Medicine and Miracles,* is "about surviving and about characteristics survivors have in common. It is about healing and about how exceptional patients can take control in order to heal themselves. It is about courage—about patients who have the courage to work with their doctors to participate in and influence the course of their illnesses. It is about love and about how the journey to recovery begins by examining the role illness plays in your life and by examining your attitudes toward yourself," (book jacket, front flap).

The following excerpt illustrates psychological factors affecting physical condition in a positive way, more evidence of powerful mind-body connections.

Several years ago I received a letter from a remarkable woman named Lois Becker. After hearing of my work, she wrote to share her experience, thanking me for verbalizing what she intuitively knew.

After a terrible year in which her father died of cancer, her husband underwent surgery, her brother was divorced, and her mother and aunt were badly injured in an auto accident, Lois Becker decided to make something good happen by becoming pregnant with her second child. During an examination, her midwife discovered a lump in her right breast and sent her for an immediate biopsy. Her letter continues:

"A three-day wait for the results, which I already know in my gut. Three days lying flat on the couch, staring as the television changes programs hour after hour. The phone rings—they'll cut off my breast on Monday. I am thirteen weeks pregnant. I am 33 years old.

They do it. They really meant it. My right side has a 12-inch incision; no lymph glands, no breast. There are 12 more tumors in my glands.

I have three choices: immediate abortion, a caesarean section or induced labor at about 30 weeks, or a full-term delivery. My cancer is hormone-positive, and my body is lousy with hormones. I can't have any of the usual cancer therapy if I keep the baby. Even with an abortion and therapy, my chances are a shattering one in six for five more years of life.

I choose to go for 30 weeks. I don't choose it to save the baby. I choose it to get out of the hospital, so they won't do anything more to me now. They pull two long, sucking tubes out of my side, and I go home. It is January in Minnesota, as frozen as you can get, unless, of course, you are pregnant and have cancer.

When you are a human time-bomb, it is a lot longer than five months from January to May. Each day my baby grows, more of the hormones, so enormously dangerous to me, flood my body. There is little reason to hope that I will complete the pregnancy with no further cancer spread. I am so numb, so angry, so very, very sad that my face squeezes into an expressionless mask. I lose the ability to read (previously one of my greatest joys), because my concentration is completely destroyed. I don't expect to see my girl become eight years old on June 30, 1978. I buy all her gifts and wrap them in February. I plan my burial.

But I really was two people, each fighting hard for the upper hand. One heard what the doctors said and reacted as I have just described. But the other shouted obscenities at the hospital whenever her car passed by. This second person decided to fight, even though the first person was after her every day, sometimes every hour, to give up and give in.

Physically, my mastectomy didn't hurt very much. My chest, upper arm, and back were numb, but I healed fast, without complications. But my arm hurt from the beginning, sometimes so badly that I couldn't straighten it for days. Unfortunately it was my right arm, the one I used to strum my guitar. But it really didn't matter, because I wasn't happy enough to sing anymore.

As soon as I left the hospital, I tried to listen to my insides. I wanted my body and mind to tell me how to help them survive. I got some answers, and I tried to follow them even when I was too depressed to move or care. My body said, "Drink orange juice," a curious craving I'd never experienced before. I drank and drank, and it felt right. I put serious thought into what I put into my body. I told my food to make me strong. I told each vitamin, as it slid down my throat, to go to the right places and do the right things, because they were the only cancer pills I had.

My body said, "Move, Lois, and do it fast!" Thirty minutes after I came home from the hospital I went for a walk. It was hard. I was afraid of falling on my side. I was humped like an old lady. But my legs were strong. I bought a pedometer and walked off miles and miles. When spring came, I walked, ran, walked, and ran, until there was too much baby.

I told my body through exercise that I loved it and wanted it to be healthy. I started yoga again the week I came home. At first I could only move my arm about five inches from my side in any direction, but I stretched and stretched it. I got my three-pound weights out and made my arm muscles and tendons work even though they protested painfully. I got my arm back quickly and have full mobility and strength today. Reach to Recovery says, "Walk your fingers slowly up the door." I say, "Hang on the door, and then do chin-ups if you can."

My mind and body said, "Make love," and they were right. Making love (and other forms of exercise) gave me the only times I was free, the only times I was *me* again, the only times I didn't have cancer.

My mind said, "I need peace. I need some rest every day from the overpowering pressure. Rest me!" I had never meditated, but I went to the library and discovered the forms that worked for me. I practiced. Meditation dropped my tense body out of my waking turmoil into a sweet cradle, deep and dark and refreshingly peaceful. I literally lived for those moments.

Meditation also provided me with a chance to practice medicine without a license. I told my body to be well. I told my immunological system to protect me. I looked at my brain, my bones, my liver, and my lungs every night. I felt them and told them to be free of cancer. I watched my blood flowing strongly. I told the wound to heal quickly and the area around it to be clean. I told my other breast to behave, because it's the only one my husband and I have left. I still tell my body and mind every night, "I reject cancer. I reject cancer."

The doctors poke around, look at my x-rays, let me out into the world again. I make it into spring, into May.

We try an induction the last week in May. It goes on for 10 hours, hurts a lot, and accomplishes nothing. They, the ones not in the bed, want to try again tomorrow. Baby and I want to go home. We go, and I tell myself that three or four more weeks won't kill me! I am happy because, going full term, I can deliver with the midwives. Perhaps the birth, at least, will be beautiful even if the pregnancy was hell.

My college roommate had a baby on June 13, and I guess that I will, too. With amniotic fluid beginning to leak, I go to the hospital to a lovely room with plants and a big double bed. My midwife is good in all ways. The contractions are close and getting stronger, and I begin to lose the fear all women have. I am handling this well. I'm going to enjoy it.

She breaks the bag, and the bed and I are drenched. She says I'm six centimeters, but I watch her face change. I'm pushing the cord out before the baby. I know immediately that he could die—fast. She holds the baby's head off the cord, pushes him up as I push him down, and I now know what the word agony means. As we race to surgery, I hear them say that the baby's pulse rate is 60.

Maybe a C-section was a good idea. They spend another hour looking at my insides. They find nothing but insides, and when my husband tells me, I feel a moment of great relief.

The baby is an 8-pound, ½-ounce, 21-inch baby boy named Nathan Scott. He is very cute, with brown hair, long dark eyelashes—and a large ventricular septal defect, known among the lucky uninitiated as a heart murmur or hole-in-the-heart. It is congenital. It is serious. It will probably need surgery. It might kill him. And, worst of all for me, it means constant trips to a hospital I hate, trips that leave me exhausted and depressed for days. It means letting my baby be cut up, just like me, for his own good.

Nathan is in congestive heart failure for the first six months of his life. He takes digitalis twice a day. He sweats when he eats. His little bony chest rises and falls much too fast, and his liver and heart are enlarged. He goes into the hospital for awhile. I stay with him, and it causes me nearly to break. His original 50-percent chance of closure drops to 25 percent.

But then, sometime in his seventh month, he begins to improve. (I like to think it was during one of those moments when I was whispering in his little ear, "Nathan, you are *going* to get well!") *(continued)*

The doctors are surprised. The EKGs improve. He gains weight. His breathing slows and the liquid swelling leaves his liver.

In May 1979 Nate has his first normal EKG, a better event than a first birthday. The muscle has closed around the hole. Nathan pulls himself up on his feet and stands tall, and I begin to believe in his existence.

When my tummy flattened out, I had a big surprise. I really *didn't* have a breast on the right side. Now was the time when most new mothers love to put on their old clothes, or buy new ones, or dream of two-piece bathing suits. My tent clothes had protected me for six months. Now I had to confront my true feelings about my body, another struggle to add to all the rest.

To describe how I felt as depression is mild. But I kept pushing myself to continue the positive elements in my life. For seven months I didn't lose my baby fat, but when Nathan began to improve, I experienced a new wave of determination.

I lost 20 pounds. I continued to meditate and to swallow all my vitamins. Three months after the birth I rejoined my exercise group. Now I didn't have to walk; I could run. And I run so well I'm planning to enter some races. My exercise program consists of yoga, running, and biking. I do them every day. I have to. I believe they are helping me survive.

My figure is back, with clothes on anyway. I'm even beginning to think I don't look too grotesque with them off. My C-section scar didn't do much to help my self-image, but my husband is blind when he looks at my scars, and I am learning to see through his eyes.

I began to try to learn how to put *myself* first. No one helped me with this. No one suggested I even had a chance. The doctors totally depressed me with their statistics. Well meaning acquaintances practically destroyed me with their pity. But in spite of other people, what *I* did worked, and each day of continued good health makes me more confident of "mind over matter."

I think of cancer every day, but I also think of how strong my body is, how good it feels most of the time. I still talk to my insides. I have a feeling of integration of body, mind and, probably, spirit, which I have never before experienced. Cancer introduced me to myself, and I like who I met."

After six years in a remission of her own doing, Lois died, but the quality of her life during that time was something her doctors never predicted.

Source: Siegel, B. S. (1986). *Love, medicine and miracles*. New York, Harper & Row, pp. 119–122.

Case Study: Nonpsychiatric Setting

Joan was a 58-year-old woman who was married and had three grown children. She had been a housewife and mother most of her married life, but had worked in the family business for the past ten years, since her children had left home.

In May, a few days before Mother's Day, Joan had an "attack" in which she experienced chest pain, shortness of breath, and irregular heartbeats; she felt faint and passed out. Her husband brought her to the emergency room and she was admitted to the cardiac unit for further evaluation of her symptoms. Medical evaluation revealed no evidence of a heart attack and no abnormalities in her EKG. Joan's symptoms of chest pain and shortness of breath persisted but decreased in intensity during the next few days, after which she was released from the hospital. Her physician gave her a diagnosis of angina of unknown etiology, possibly related to hyperventilation. Joan was scheduled to be seen in a general medical clinic for outpatient followup of cardiac symptoms.

On her first outpatient visit, Joan reported having had several episodes of chest pain and shortness of breath since her release from the hospital. She also reported that thoughts of her mother's death at age 58 and feelings of anxiety preceded these attacks. She was afraid these attacks meant that she might have serious heart disease. Joan related, tearfully, that her mother had died of a heart attack on Mother's Day. Joan's relationship with her mother had been estranged; they lived quite a distance apart and communicated infrequently. Joan's mother died alone and unattended, and now Joan felt guilty that she had not made more of an effort to care for her.

Since there was no evidence that she had had a heart attack, Joan had begun to worry that she was having a "nervous breakdown." Twenty years before, she was hospitalized and put on "tranquilizers" following a "nervous breakdown." She had been doing well until recently, when she began seeing a psychotherapist concerning her feelings about her mother's death. When, after only a few weeks, the psychotherapist became seriously ill, Joan felt abandoned and deserted. She felt that this precipitated the current breakdown.

Joan grew up in a small rural community with her father, a country lawyer, her mother, a housewife, and her brother, two years younger than she. She described her father as a warm, quiet individual who always took an interest in her activities and well-being. She described her mother as strong willed, powerful, and always critical of her. Although Joan tried to please her mother, her brother always seemed to be the favorite, even though Joan felt that he didn't deserve to be preferred. While Joan worked hard to get good grades and did well in school, her brother was a discipline problem, and her mother often had to help him or bail him out of trouble. Although her parents argued infrequently, their relationship appeared distant and cool.

After her mother's death, Joan and her brother fought over their mother's estate. Her brother lived in the same town as her mother had and was supposed to be responsible for her care. Joan was angry at him for being negligent in this task, and for not fully informing her of her mother's condition. She was also angry at her mother for putting her brother in charge of her finances; ultimately he possessed the entire estate. Joan had considered initiating a lawsuit against her brother in response.

Joan described her own marriage as good and felt her husband had been concerned about her recent ill health. However, she felt her husband and children were becoming impatient with her because of her continuing preoccupation with her mother, her brother, and her mother's estate.

Joan's medical diagnosis according to DSM-III-R was as follows:

DSM-III Diagnosis

AXIS I Psychological Factors Affecting Physical Condition;
AXIS II None;
AXIS III Angina, hyperventilation, palpitations;
AXIS IV Psychosocial Stressors: death of mother, disputes with brother; Severity: 5—Extreme;
AXIS V Highest Level of functioning: 90

Nursing Diagnoses

*Ineffective breathing pattern (hyperventilation)
*Comfort, alteration in: pain (chest pain)
*Anxiety and fear
*Dysfunctional grieving (feelings of abandonment by mother, father, previous therapist)
*Alteration in family process (death of mother, disputes with brother, impatience of husband and children)
Anxiety (unresolved guilt and anger about mother's death)
Fear (of current episodes indicating heart disease)

*Nursing diagnoses developed in care plan that follows.

Nursing Care Plan for Joan

Nursing Diagnosis	Desired Outcomes	Interventions	Rationale
1. Ineffective breathing pattern	Joan will return to normal breathing and experience associated comfort.	Teach Joan systematic muscle relaxation (see Chapter 25 on intensive care), directing her to use onset of hyperventilation as stimulus to begin exercise.	Hyperventilation can be the first indication of heightened anxiety for some individuals. Using it as a stimulus to begin systematic muscle relaxation is a type of counterconditioning (see Chapter 8 on anxiety that allows the patient to counter anxiety with a physical state incompatible with it.
2. Alteration in comfort	Joan will experience increased levels of comfort and self-confidence.	Encourage Joan to practice systematic muscle relaxation when she is not anxious to increase her competence in dealing with anxiety.	When the patient learns this method of controlling anxiety, her fear of dying of a heart attack (secondary to the frightening experience of prolonged hyperventilation) will decrease.
3. Anxiety and fear	Joan will experience decreased anxiety and fear.	Supported exposure: Stay with Joan during attacks of hyperventilation, offering support while encouraging her to focus on her anxieties until her hyperventilation subsides.	Supporting Joan through an anxiety attack will help her learn that intense anxiety, though very uncomfortable and often frightening, does not cause heart attacks. Research has shown that facing the source of one's anxiety, rather than avoiding it, is most effective in reducing it. (See Chapter 8 on anxiety and anxiety disorders.)
4. Dysfunctional grieving	Joan will work through feelings about both positive and negative aspects of relationships with parents, brother.	Encourage Joan to express feelings about important people in her life. Label or ask about sadness, anger, and guilt as appropriate.	When grieving is arrested by associated anxiety and lack of support, it needs to be returned to through identifying and expressing feelings, positive and negative, about the lost love object or significant other. Sadness is usually easily identified and expressed, but anger at the person who has died and any guilt associated

Nursing Diagnosis	Desired Outcomes	Interventions	Rationale
			with his or her death, though normal, is more difficult to identify and talk about due to the associated emotional pain and fear of reprisal. (Also see Chapter 9 on mood disorders for more on the psychoanalytic view of loss and grieving that becomes pathological.)
5. Alteration in family process	Resumption of adaptive functioning in family.	Problem solve with Joan regarding her options for dealing with her brother, given her concerns about their mother's estate.	In addition to the need to help Joan with her feelings to facilitate the grieving process, cognitive intervention in the form of identifying her current realistic concerns and the options for dealing with them, along with their expected consequences, is also appropriate.
		Refer Joan and her family to a family therapist who may be helpful to them in resolving their differences which are likely to be secondary to feelings of anger and guilt regarding important losses.	In most dysfunctional families, one person's getting help through therapy is usually not enough to alter or interrupt maladaptive family dynamics. If Joan wants more than to learn how to cope with how her family *is,* if she wants to change how the family operates, family therapy is the best treatment option. (See Chapter 21 on families for more on family dynamics and family therapy.)

SUMMARY

Nowhere in the study of psychopathology does the mind-body connection come into focus more clearly than in the DSM-III-R classification of psychological factors affecting physical condition. This diagnostic category includes those bodily diseases that may be influenced by psychological and environmental factors. These illnesses are also called psychosomatic or psychophysiological disorders. Since these disorders include a bodily dysfunction with either demonstrable organic pathology or a known pathophysiological process, patients with these disorders are most often seen in general medical settings rather than psychiatric ones. Asthma, migraine headache, duodenal ulcer, irritable bowel, urticaria, hypertension, rheumatoid arthritis, and ulcerative colitis are diseases that are usually considered to be psychosomatic. Assessment, treatment, and management of patients with these disorders must include attention to both the organic pathology, or presenting medical complaints, and contributing psychological factors.

Psychodynamic, biological, and behavioral models focus on three factors that appear to be important in the development of disease: genetic disposition, personality, and life events.

Assessment and treatment of psychosomatic disorders is difficult due to three factors: 1) the patient's difficulty in making connections between physical symptoms and emotions or life problems; 2) the patient's feelings of rejection by the clinician, who conveys the message, "It's all in your head"; and 3) the patient's alexithymia, or difficulty recognizing and verbalizing feelings.

Although physical symptoms are attended to and alleviated if possible, for example, with medication, psychological factors should also be examined since they are likely to be important in the long-term management of the disease. Treatment aimed at the psychological aspects of the disease may reduce the need for medication as well as prevent relapse. Empathy, validation, and attention to the patient's symptoms, along with problem solving, practical suggestions, and support, are the main elements of treatment. Psychotherapy may benefit those patients who are motivated to explore their problems further.

Patients with somatoform disorders are similar to those with psychosomatic disorders. Their major complaints are about physical symptoms, and they are most often seen in medical rather than psychiatric settings. However, there is a lack of confirming medical evidence of organic pathology. The four diagnostic categories of somatoform disorders are somatization disorder, conversion disorder, somatoform pain disorder, and hypochondriasis.

Primary and secondary gain are important aspects of somatoform disorders. Primary (psychological) gain often serves a conflict-resolving purpose, such as alleviating guilt. Secondary (personal) gain often includes such things as relief from responsibility, manipulation of interpersonal relationships, or financial gain. However, the patient's behavior is not under voluntary control, as it is in malingering or factitious disorder.

Somatization disorder, or Briquet's syndrome, is characterized by multiple, recurrent, and chronic somatic complaints. Patients with conversion disorder have lost all or part of some basic physical functioning, often inexactly mimicking a "real" disease. Patients with somatoform psychogenic pain disorder have chronic and severe pain that is inconsistent with physical findings and that appears to be related to psychological factors. Patients with hypochondriasis are preoccupied with their physical health and an unrealistic fear of serious disease.

Treatment of patients with somatoform disorders is quite difficult because they consider their symptoms to be "medical" and resist the idea that psychological and emotional factors may be critically involved. They are often dependent on and demanding of the health care professionals who treat them. Treatment emphasizes long-term management of symptoms rather than a complete and rapid cure. In an inpatient setting, the nurse can lay the groundwork for such treatment goals by discussing the patient's expectations, offering support, and encouraging the patient to talk about his or her life stresses. Most of the long-term management of these patients occurs in the outpatient setting. Thus the development of a working relationship is an essential aspect of treatment.

This chapter attempts to provide an alternative to dichotomous thinking about these disorders by emphasizing the interactive nature of psychological factors and organic pathology. Though psychological factors influence disease, and the patient's perception of disease, it does not follow that the disease is not real. It is always real to the patient. The nurse's job involves not only helping patients obtain relief from their symptoms, but also helping them discover the role psychological factors play in their development and/or maintenance. Similarly, the nurse (as well as the physician) needs to remember that the patient with a history of somatoform or other functional disorder *can* develop organic illness.

KEY TERMS

psychosomatic or psychophysiological disorders

somatoform disorders

diathesis-stress

specific-organ vulnerability

general adaptation syndrome

alexithymia

somatoform disorders

somatization disorder

conversion disorder

somatoform pain disorder

hypochondriasis

primary gain

secondary gain

malingering

factitious disorder with physical symptoms

Munchhausen syndrome

Briquet's syndrome

STUDY QUESTIONS

1. Define and describe the critera for psychosomatic (or psychophysiological) disorders.

2. Name and describe the three etiological models of psychosomatic (or psychophysiological) disorders.

3. What three factors make assessment and treatment of psychosomatic disorder difficult?

4. Define and describe the criteria for somatoform disorders.

5. Name and describe the four types of somatoform disorders.

REFERENCES

Adler, G. (1981). The physician and the hypochondriacal patient. *New England Journal of Medicine, 304,* 1394–96.

Alexander, F. (1950). *Psychosomatic medicine.* New York: Norton.

Alexander, F., French, T. M., & Pollock, G. H. (1968). *Psychosomatic specificity: Experimental study and results,* Vol. 1. Chicago: University of Chicago Press.

American Psychiatric Association (1987). *Diagnostic and statistical manual of mental disorders,* Third edition, Revised. Washington, D.C.: American Psychiatric Association Press.

Couch, J. R., & Hassanein, R. S. (1979, November). Amitriptyline in migraine prophylaxis. *Archives of Neurology, 36,* 695–699.

Ford, C. V. (1983). *The somatizing disorders: Illness as a way of life.* New York: Elsevier.

Fordyce, W. E. (1976). *Behavioral methods for chronic pain and illness.* St. Louis: C.V. Mosby.

Freud, S. (1938). *A general introduction to psychoanalysis.* New York: Garden City Publishing.

Goodwin, D. W., and Guze, S. B. (1979) *Psychiatric diagnosis.* New York: Oxford University Press.

Grace, W. J., & Graham, D. T. (1952). Relationship of specific attitudes and emotions to certain bodily disease. *Psychosomatic Medicine, 14,* 243–51.

Graham, D. T. (1972). Psychosomatic medicine. In N. Greenfield & R. Sternbach (Eds.), *Handbook of psychophysiology.* New York: Holt, Rinehart & Winston.

Holmes, T. H., & Rahe, R. H. (1967). The social readjustment ratings scale. *Journal of Psychosomatic Research, 11,* 213–18.

Holmes, T. H., & Masuda, M. (1972). Psychosomatic syndrome. *Psychology Today,* April.

Kimble, R., Williams, J. G., & Agras, S. (1975). A comparison of two methods of diagnosing hysteria. *American Journal of Psychiatry, 132,* 1197–1199.

Lesse, S. (1967). Hypochondriasis and other psychosomatic disorders masking depression. *American Journal of Psychotherapy, 21,* 607–620.

McConnell, R. B. (1966). *Genetics of gastro-intestinal disorders.* London: Oxford University Press.

Parkes, M. C., Benjamin, B., & Fitzgerald, R. G. (1969). Broken heart: A statistical study of increased mortality among widowers. *British Medical Journal, 1,* 740–43.

Pincus, J. H., & Tucker, G. J. (1978). *Behavioral neurology,* 3rd Ed. New York: Oxford University Press.

Rich, V. L., & Rich, A. R. (1987). Personality hardiness and burnout in female staff nurses. *Image: Journal of Nursing Scholarship,* 19:2:63, Summer.

Rosenman, R., Brand, R., Jenkins, C., Friedman, M., Straus, R., & Wurm, M. (1975). Coronary heart disease in the Western Collaborative Group Study: Final follow-up experience of 8½ years. *Journal of the American Medical Association, 233,* 872–77.

Selye, H. (1956). *The stress of life.* New York: McGraw Hill.

Selye, H. (1976). *The stress of life* (rev. ed.). New York: McGraw Hill.

Sifneos, P. E. (1973). The prevalence of alexithymic characteristics in psychosomatic patients. *Psychotherapy and Psychosomatics, 22,* 255–62.

Sifneos, P. E. (1975). Problems of psychotherapy of patients with alexithymic characteristics and physical disease. *Psychotherapy and Psychosomatics, 26,* 65–70.

Tedesco-Carreras, P. (1988). Maintaining mental wellness. *NSNA: Imprint.* February/March.

Ziegler, D. K., Hurwitz, A., Hassanein, R. S., Kodanaz, H. A., Preskor, S. H., & Mason, J. (1987, May). Migraine prophylaxis, a comparison of propranolol and amitriptyline. *Archives of Neurology, 44,* 486–489.

14

EATING DISORDERS

LYN MARSHALL

LEARNING OBJECTIVES

After studying this chapter, the student will be able to:

- Recognize the symptoms of anorexia nervosa and bulimia nervosa.
- Describe the three theories regarding etiology of the eating disorders.
- Identify the principles underlying inpatient and outpatient treatment of patients with eating disorders.
- Identify and describe the specific cognitive-behavioral techniques for treating patients with eating disorders.
- Be aware of the special issues that may arise with the treatment of patients with eating disorders.
- Make nursing diagnoses and develop nursing care plans for patients with eating disorders.

INTRODUCTION

During the past twenty years, the rising incidence of eating disorders has become a grave concern for both health professionals and the general public. A study conducted in Monroe County, New York, by Jones et al. (1980), using the psychiatric case registry, showed that the incidence of reported cases of anorexia nervosa had doubled from 1960–1969 to 1970–1976. Recent studies of the incidence of bulimia nervosa offer variable estimates of occurrence. Reports include a range of four percent (Pyle et al. 1983) to thirteen percent (Gray & Ford, 1985) of college women who meet the DSM-III-R criteria for this syndrome. Although statistics differ depending on criteria for inclusion, it is clear that a growing number of women, and sometimes men, engage with varying frequency both in severe dieting measures (such as vomiting and laxative abuse) and in binge eating. (See Box 14–1.)

Eating disorders at one time seemed to the general public like bizarre excesses of dieting behavior (attributable to cultural pressure for thinness). The death of singer Karen Carpenter, however, became a shocking example of the serious and sometimes fatal consequences that may result from having an eating disorder. Health professionals are even more disturbed by the fact that both anorexia nervosa and bulimia have proven difficult to treat. Patients with eating disorders may require years of treatment in both inpatient and outpatient settings. Followup studies on patients with anorexia nervosa indicate that eating symptoms and preoccupation with weight, along with other problems such as mood disorders and impaired relationships, may persist after treatment (Garner & Garfinkel, 1982; Swift, 1982). Although followup research on bulimia is in its early stages, investigators report a wide range of results in outcome studies (Johnson & Conners, 1987). Clinicians generally agree that an ominous factor in predicting the outcome of treatment is that patients with bulimia often do not seek help until many years after the onset of symptoms.

HISTORY OF EATING DISORDERS

Although eating disorders have gotten attention in Western society only during the last decade, anorexia nervosa first appeared in medical literature in 1689. Even the earliest account, by Richard Morton, of a cachectic 17-year-old girl associated a psychological component with her refusal to eat. However, it was not until nearly 200 years later that Sir William Gull in England and Charles Lesegue in France independently but nearly simultaneously described the clinical picture of anorexia nervosa and named it as a specific disease entity. Then in 1909 a German pathologist named Simmonds discovered, during autopsy, a lesion in an emaciated subject's pituitary gland. Subsequently "Simmonds' disease" was the label used for patients with severe weight loss. It is thought that many deaths attributed to Simmonds' disease and pituitary failure were actually misdiagnosed cases of anorexia nervosa. By 1930, anorexia nervosa had been "rediscovered" and again identified as an illness occurring secondarily to a psychological disturbance. Specifically, psychoanalytic theorists began to view the disorder as originating in fantasies of oral impregnation (Lucas, 1981).

Few papers about anorexia nervosa appeared in the literature from 1945 to 1960. During the early 1960s Hilde Bruch began her now-classic contributions to the theory of etiology of anorexia nervosa. (Bruch's ideas are presented in more detail below, in the section on assessment.) Throughout the 1960s and well into the 1970s, eating disorders were viewed as a homogeneous group. However, as clinicians began to see increasing numbers of patients, they noted differences in personality factors.

In 1976 Beaumont compared "starving" anorexics with "vomiting or purging" anorexics. He noted more obsessional personality characteristics in the former group and thought the latter group displayed more histrionic traits (Beaumont, George, & Smart, 1976). The key factor in defining a "subgroup" of eating disorders was ultimately recognized in the symptom of bulimia or binge eating. Although Boskind-Lodahl (1976) had already published her theory of psychodynamic differences between anorexia and bulimia and had coined the term "bulimarexia," Gerald Russell (1979) published the first comprehensive clinical study of the unique features of patients with bulimia.

Extensive research has since evolved in an effort to refine the diagnostic features of bulimia. Controversy continues over whether or not bulimia should be considered a distinct clinical entity. Bruch (1984) held that bulimia is a symptomatic feature of other psychological conditions, including anorexia nervosa, rather than a disorder itself. Experts who maintain the validity of a separate diagnostic category for bulimia often criticize the DSM-III-R criteria for their limitations and broad definitions of symptomatology.

Box 14—1 ● In the 'Lite' Decade, Less Has Become More

It used to take so much time—days, sometimes weeks—to read a classic. "Moby Dick," alone, runs 710 pages. Today, thanks to a small publishing house called Workman, it takes a minute. Through abridging, reabridging and editing out "rambling soliloquies," Workman boasts that it has "cut down the literary canon to a lean pistol," producing an audio-cassette tape that offers listeners "Ten Classics in Ten Minutes."

The result is light literature, the latest demonstration that in the 1980's light beer is not the only thing that is less filling. What started out as a way to justify drinking three beers instead of two—the creation of a light beer with a third fewer calories—has become part of a broader phenomenon in which less is valued above more. This is the Light Decade, or as some would have it, Lite.

"Light is a way of thinking that we've come to in the 80's," says Dr. Robert T. London, a psychiatrist at New York University Medical Center. "It's an umbrella phenomenon where lightness transforms itself into the cars we drive, the lightness in a room, our diet, as well as lightness in the relationships we have."

Sociologists say that "lite," which started as a marketing term used to denote dietetic products, has become a metaphor for what Americans are seeking in disparate parts of their lives. In their relationships, for example, they have turned away from soul-searching and stress of emotional commitment; at the movies, they would rather watch an invincible hero, like Rambo or the Karate Kid, who never lets the audience down.

Attempting to bring itself up to date with today's expanded notion of light, the Federal Bureau of Alcohol, Tobacco and Firearms announced yesterday that it would try to determine just what constitutes "light" and "lite" in whiskey, wine and beer.

"The notion of the word 'lite' tends to follow what seems to be a trend in American culture," said Ray B. Brown, chairman of the department of popular culture at Bowling Green State University in Ohio. "That is for everybody to be utterly selfish about themselves, for people to want easy cures, easy riches, easy jobs and easy wealth."

The Light Decade is a time when men and women can "fall in love without paying the price," as a Honda Civic advertisement promises. They can undergo psychoanalysis in one sitting, because today's psychotherapy skips the formative years, namely childhood. For health care, busy executives can turn to a so-called Doc in a Box, a storefront medical clinic with extended hours, higher prices and no appointment, no referral—no medical history.

There is a light culture (books on tape), light shopping (buying clothes by video), light politics (candidates who run on image, not issues), light responsibility (the lowest voter participation rates of any democracy) and light music (Lite FM, where the heavy bass line has been removed so that the sound does not jar or stir listeners). And, of course, there is light food, with which people can cut calories without changing their diets by using products like Jell-O Light, Cornitos Light Corn Chips, Heinz Lite Ketchup and Glacé Lite, which, its manufacturer, Sweet Victory, says "gives you all the rich, delicious pleasures of 300-calorie premium ice cream" at 100 calories a scoop.

Food, notably dietetic food, is where the Light Decade started. It is also the clearest example of how the philosophy has caught on. "Lite," or "light," foods are now "one of the fastest growing segments of the American food industry," according to a recent Federal Food and Drug Administration report.

By the count of one market research company, Marketing Intelligence, 352 "lite" or "light" products have been added to the shelves of the nation's supermarkets and liquor stores since 1982.

Seven years ago the Miller Brewing Company tried to claim "Lite" as its own, part of its trademark for its low-calorie beer, and went to court to keep other brewers from using it. The courts ruled that "lite" was just an alternative spelling of "light."

There are light products for each meal of the day. For breakfast: Arrowhead Mills Griddle Lite pancakes topped with Log Cabin Lite syrup, a gob of Parkay Light Spread (a lower-calorie imitation margarine), and a side order of Jones Light Breakfast Meats.

For lunch: a Real Lite Cola, Trophy Lite Peanuts, a Lite Steak from BAR-S Lite Meats between two slices of Taystee Lite Bread and spiced with Miracle Whip Light mayonnaise, Lawry's Seasoned Lite Salt and some Heinz Lite Ketchup.

For dinner: a stir-fry of Hormel Cold'n Lite Breaded Vegetables, Lite Chef Tofu Mixers and Kikkoman Lite Soy Sauce, a salad with Wish-Bone Lite salad dressing, a glass of Christian Brothers Chateau La Salle Light Wine and David's Lite Cookies or a Whitman's Lite Coconut Bar. Top this off with a little relief—Lite antacid tablets from Rolaids, a salt-free form.

Before the 16th century, the word "lite" meant "little, not much, few" in English and was pronounced differently from "light," according to Traugott Lawler, a medievalist at Yale University. But the word fell out of use.

Today's "lite" is used to indicate fewer calories or less salt, and essentially refers to weight in the same way that light is a reference to weight, Mr. Lawler said.

"Its spelling has been simplified in the 20th century by advertisers who use it to suggest ease and simplicity," he said. "It's a light spelling."

The effect of light foods on weight loss has been, well, light.

"We know that the number of people who are obese has increased in the past 10 years," said Thomas A. Wadden, a psychologist at the Obesity Research Group of the University of Pennsylvania. "And the percentage of children who are obese is increasing."

Although one problem is that people do not exercise enough, the reliance on light foods may have contributed to the problem, for light foods are often not what they seem: They are not necessarily lower in calories, although they "generally" have low or reduced calories, according to the F.D.A. A box of Finn Crisp Lite crackers, for example, proudly claims "only 20 calories per slice." But the regular Finn Crisps have only 19 calories per slice.

Labeling foods "lite" can also give the impression that they are light in calories when they are actually low in salt, low in alcohol or, in the case of some whiskeys, light in color—the result of storing the liquor in uncharred new oak containers.

Bernard Phillips, a sociologist at Boston University, calls the Light Decade a "smorgasbord" approach to life, where people convince themselves that they can have the best of all worlds, immediately, by having a lightened version of everything.

Consider marriage, at a time when more than half of all marriages end in divorce. "It's come to the point where people who get married today don't have the deadly serious attitude of till death do us part," says Dr. London, a psychiatrist. "We want it to work, but if it breaks up, it'll break up."

Or the new brand of psychotherapy. "Many times, traditional exploration of unconscious longings toward mothers and fathers and aunts and uncles is as inappropriate as taking a horse and buggy on the Long Island Expressway," Dr. London said. Basically, society wants much more current needs solved without the arduous introspection of psychoanalysis."

Clinton R. Sanders, a sociologist at the University of Connecticut who studies popular culture, says the mobility of American society, both geographically and economically, has helped to bring about a Light Decade.

Dr. Sanders says that geographic mobility has increased the number of relationships based on daily routines and necessities, rather than on a shared background or common interests.

"The kinds of relationships we have most are secondary," he said. "They are light relationships, instrumental relationships. I don't go down to the grocery store to have a conversation with the checkout girl."

That same lack of attachment is evident in the appliances people buy today. Because modern technology has made them inexpensive, and because Americans generally have a high standard of living, appliances have become cheaper to replace than repair. They are what Dr. Sanders calls "light appliances, built to fall apart."

Source: William R. Greer, *The New York Times*, Wednesday August 13, 1986, p. 1.

DESCRIPTION OF EATING DISORDERS

Although since the late 1970s many clinicians and researchers have viewed bulimia nervosa as a separate entity from anorexia nervosa, many still feel that the two have more similarities than differences. It is important to keep in mind that an estimated fifty percent of patients with **anorexia nervosa,** or restrictive eating, also have the symptom of **bulimia,** which refers simply to **binge eating.** Another fifty percent of all patients with eating disorders move back and forth between symptoms of restrictive eating and binge eating (Garner, 1986). In addition, Johnson (1986) reports that fifty percent of all patients diagnosed with anorexia nervosa will develop symptoms of bulimia within two years of receiving the anorexia diagnosis.

Common to both groups of patients is a morbid fear of becoming fat. They also have a distorted body image (mental picture of the body)—patients in both groups are rarely able to estimate accurately their true body size, believing they are "fat" regardless of their weight or size. Patients in both groups organize measures of self-esteem around thinness; thus they share a sense of low self-esteem. Finally, the inaccuracies in body image and the fears of becoming fat contribute to an intense preoccupation with weight and dieting.

One clinical difference between the two disorders is starvation itself. Many patients with bulimia have attempted to diet in a restrictive fashion but have not succeeded. Thus a high percentage of patients with bulimic symptoms are at or above normal weight. In addition, many symptoms that are considered characteristic of anorexia nervosa are in fact side effects of the starvation process itself. Patients with either disorder who have reached subnormal weights exhibit behaviors related to starvation.

In 1950 a study was conducted on thirty-six men to assess the effects of starvation (Keys et al., 1950). The men, who were selected on the basis of physical and emotional health, were given a deprivation diet for six months. During the time that they were being starved, the men became preoccupied with food: they collected recipes, cookbooks, and cooking utensils; they changed their eating habits, mixing food together in unusual concoctions and cutting their food into very small pieces; and they dramatically increased their consumption of tea, coffee, and chewing gum. A small group of the men was unable to maintain the strict dieting and began to binge. This binge eating became worse in the rehabilitation phase of the study because these men would begin eating and be unable to stop. Many of the men in the study suffered changes in emotions and personality. They became depressed, anxious, irritable, angry, labile in affect, and socially withdrawn due to their preoccupation with food (Keys, 1950). This study is highly significant because it reveals that many behaviors seen clinically in patients with anorexia nervosa and in some bulimic patients are actually by-products of starvation and not manifestations of psychopathology. The implications of the study are important not only from a behavioral standpoint but from an emotional one as well. That is, some of the mood and cognitive changes seen in emaciated patients should be attributed to starvation.

ASSESSMENT OF ANOREXIA NERVOSA

Anorexia nervosa is characterized by deliberate starvation with the intention of becoming thin. The individual drastically reduces food intake and persists with rigid dietary patterns in spite of extreme emaciation. Dieting may be accompanied by self-induced vomiting, laxative abuse, and excessive activity and exercise. (See DSM-III-R Box.)

BRUCH'S THREE FEATURES OF THE ANOREXIC PATIENT. Hilde Bruch (1973) identified three features of the patient with anorexia that are central to the diagnosis. First is the body-image disturbance that often reaches delusional proportions. That is, although cachectic or wasted in appearance, the patient will firmly deny being too thin and will in fact refer to herself as being "fat." This severe distortion in body image motivates the individual to further weight loss. The person becomes obsessed with an attempt to achieve increasingly lower numbers on the scale. Weight-loss goals become more and more unrealistic. An anorexic person who is 5'2" and has reached ninety pounds will typically decide that only eighty-five pounds is satisfactory. If this goal is reached, the anorexic will then lower the goal to eighty pounds.

The following is an example of a typical day of eating for a patient with anorexia:

Breakfast:	two cups of black coffee
Snack:	one diet soda and one breath mint or piece of hard candy
Lunch:	small salad with low-calorie Italian dressing, one diet soda
Snack:	one breath mint and one diet soda

**DSM-III-R
Diagnostic Criteria for
Anorexia Nervosa**

A. Refusal to maintain body weight over a minimal normal weight for age and height, e.g., weight loss leading to maintenance of body weight 15% below that expected; or failure to make expected weight gain during period of growth, leading to body weight 15% below that expected.

B. Intense fear of gaining weight or becoming fat, even though underweight.

C. Disturbance in the way in which one's body weight, size, or shape is experienced, e.g., the person claims to "feel fat" even when emaciated, believes that one area of the body is "too fat" even when obviously underweight.

D. In females, absence of at least three consecutive menstrual cycles when otherwise expected to occur (primary or secondary amenorrhea). (A woman is considered to have amenorrhea if her periods occur only following hormone, e.g., estrogen, administration.)

Dinner:	one-half broiled chicken breast without skin, two spears broccoli, one cup black coffee, followed by vomiting
Snack:	one diet soda

The patient with anorexia thrives on the self-control and discipline associated with dieting. Thinness is equated with virtue. Restrained eating and constant activity become the means of achieving control over the person's inner world. A sense of mastery accompanies successfully meeting the increasingly lowered weight-loss goals. The rewards of acquiring a thin body override the harmful effects of starvation. Cues such as hunger, fatigue, and pain are either ignored or perceived as positive indicators of nearing weight-loss goals.

Failure to respond to bodily cues is one aspect of Bruch's (1973) second feature: disturbance in the perception of internal states. Patients with anorexia often lack the capacity to recognize and identify internal perceptions, both physical and emotional. Their experience is one of an inner void or emptiness. Many patients will speak of being and having "nothing" if they are not thin, denying or disavowing human emotions. Patients will describe having no reaction to events that would typically stimulate anger. When asked how they feel about an event, patients will frequently respond with "I don't know."

The final feature described by Bruch (1973) is a "paralyzing sense of ineffectiveness," a lack of a sense of competence in any area outside weight control. Many anorexics have spent their lives attending to the needs of others. They have been compliant, "good little girls" who have dedicated themselves to meeting the expectations of others and striving for perfection. As a result, they have little sense of their own needs and wants and how to go about meeting them. Although they maintain a superficially pleasant facade, they feel incompetent socially. In relationships they may assume the role of "listener" but rarely identify the need for support themselves. Eventually they may withdraw from others completely and devote themselves entirely to the pursuit of thinness. It is ironic that dieting meant to enhance a person in the eyes of others eventually leads to total social isolation. (See Box 14–2.)

ASSESSMENT OF BULIMIA NERVOSA

Bulimia nervosa is characterized by episodic bingeing on enormous quantities of food, followed by purging with vomiting, laxatives, and occasionally diuretics. In many cases the individual with bulimia will follow the binge-eating behavior with a period of restricted intake and sometimes excessive exercise. A self-perpetuating pattern develops, with alternating dieting and bulimic episodes. Attempts to diet lead to feelings of hunger and a sense of deprivation that heightens emotional responses. When faced with an emotionally triggering event, the individual succumbs to the urge to binge. Following the binge, she has feelings of panic associated with loss of control along with feelings of guilt, humiliation, and self-loathing. These feelings precipitate the purging behavior and lead to further attempts to gain "control" by dieting. The cycle continues and the individual feels helpless to stop, locked into this habitual sequence of behaviors. (See DSM-III-R Box.)

Box 14–2 • Male Anorexia

Anorexia nervosa, the self-star-vation disorder, is 10 times more common in women than in men. Men may be less vulnerable because of their biology (genes and hor-mones), their emotional develop-ment, their social situation, or all three. Researchers in Oxford, En-gland have attempted to identify characteristics that distinguish men vulnerable to anorexia from other men, and from women vulnerable to anorexia. They compared 13 male with 39 female anorectic patients seen between 1967 and 1983. The men were more likely to be physically overactive as well as anorectic; oth-erwise the symptoms were the same. Many of the men were also short (four of them were in the shortest 10 percent of the population) and, be-fore they stopped eating, fat (four of them weighed 25 percent more than the average for their height and age). Anorectic women were less likely to have been fat and were somewhat taller than average.

The women's and the men's families had about the same rates of mental illness and other problems. Five of the men had a parent, brother, or sister with a history of mental illness—mainly mood disor-ders—and five also had serious fam-ily problems. The authors suggest that a family vulnerability to mood disorders may take the form of an-orexia in people who are worried about the shape of their bodies. Be-cause men are both less subject to mood disorders and less concerned about body shape, they develop an-orexia nervosa much less often.

J. L. Margo. Anorexia nervosa in males: a comparison with female patients. *British Journal of Psychiatry,* 151:80–83 (July 1987).

Source: *The Harvard Medical School Mental Health Letter.* Vol 4 (11) May 1988, p. 7.

As with anorexics, bulimic patients strive to achieve thin bodies. Bulimics are often unsuccessful because of the nature of their symptoms. The patient may see herself as a "failed anorexic." She is ashamed of her bulimic symptoms and maintains them in se-crecy from others. In this way the patient differs from the anorexic, who develops a kind of pride in her symptoms. Individuals with bulimia may take great pains to prevent anyone from discovering their se-cret. Patients will have shopping marathons, traveling from store to store picking up binge foods so as not to be suspected in any one place; they will often re-fuse social events with friends in order to stay at home and binge in private. At the same time, the binge eating itself may be "useful" to the patient in that it serves as a means of soothing inner tension associated with painful mood states. Binge eating may even create a sense of euphoria similar to that of drug or alcohol abuse. Consequently, individuals with bulimia find their symptoms difficult to relin-quish in spite of their painful aspects.

It is not uncommon for other forms of substance abuse to accompany bulimia. Alcohol, drugs, and caf-feine can serve purposes similar to binge eating. In addition, a subgroup of patients are prone to shop-lifting to obtain food.

In most instances the individual with bulimia has accompanying symptoms of depression. Irritability, depressed mood, mood swings, and anxiety are com-mon. A significant number of patients have suicidal ideation and will actually attempt suicide. In fact, it is possible that the greatest potentially fatal risk for bulimics is suicide (Fallon, 1986).

Like the anorexic, the individual with bulimia feels ineffective and externally controlled. However, the bulimic may have had actual experiences of vic-timization, such as physical or sexual abuse. Some pa-tients come from family environments in which they experienced psychological or emotional abuse and were seen as "problem" children. Thus the feeling of powerlessness in these patients often has a history that involves victimization and loss of control over their world.

As with anorexia patients, individuals with buli-mia exhibit a wide range of psychopathology (partic-ularly mood disorders, personality disorders, and substance abuse) that coexists with eating-disorder symptoms. While some generalizations are possible,

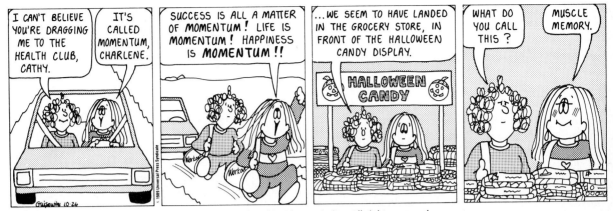

it is important to keep in mind that the degree of impairment in self-esteem and the capacity to relate to others varies considerably.

MEDICAL COMPLICATIONS OF BOTH DISORDERS

Prolonged starvation, vomiting, and laxative abuse all have serious medical consequences that are usually secondary to malnutrition, dehydration, and disturbances in electrolyte balance. First, in cases of weight loss of approximately twenty-five percent of average normal body weight, the patient may become amenorrheic. This loss of menses can be a particularly hazardous complication, especially if prolonged, because it causes infertility and estrogen loss. Over time, lack of estrogen may contribute to calcium deficiency and skeletal changes resulting in osteoporosis much like that found in older women. Weight restoration to at least ninety percent of average normal weight is usu-

ally necessary to ensure return of normal menses. Extreme emaciation also leads to additional, though less severe, changes, such as growth-hormone deficiency in the functioning of the hypothalamic-pituitary axes (Harris, 1983).

A second potentially dangerous effect of starvation over a prolonged period is decrease in myocardial muscle mass. Diminished cardiac functioning combined with dehydration leads to decreased heart rate, blood pressure, and cardiac output. Dysrhythmias secondary to electrolyte abnormalities caused by vomiting or laxative abuse may occur. Heart failure can ultimately result. Heart failure is also a potential problem if a patient is refed too rapidly and fluid overload occurs (Harris, 1983).

Less serious, though debilitating, side effects of starvation include lack of energy, weakness, intolerance to cold (occasional loss of shivering response), pain upon sitting or lying down due to lack of body fat, decreased ability to concentrate, and sleep distur-

DSM-III-R Diagnostic Criteria for Bulimia Nervosa

A. Recurrent episodes of binge eating (rapid consumption of a large amount of food in a discrete period of time).

B. A feeling of lack of control over eating behavior during the eating binges.

C. The person regularly engages in either self-induced vomiting, use of laxatives or diuretics, strict dieting or fasting, or vigorous exercise in order to prevent weight gain.

D. A minimum average of two binge eating episodes a week for at least three months.

E. Persistent overconcern with body shape and weight.

bances. The latter two are also associated with depression, which frequently coexists with anorexia nervosa and bulimia (Harris, 1983).

Purging either by vomiting or laxative abuse is a technique seen both in patients with anorexia nervosa and bulimia. Metabolic complications such as loss of potassium, chloride, and hydrogen are associated with purging. Hypokalemia is common, resulting in such symptoms as muscle weakness, constipation, headaches, palpitations, abdominal pain, tiredness, and polydipsia. Some patients will engage in a very dangerous method of inducing vomiting by drinking syrup of ipecac. This substance can remain in the system and lead to cardiac conduction defects, dysrhythmias, and myocarditis. Use of ipecac may be fatal and patients who complain of palpitations, skipped heartbeats, presyncope and syncope, chest pains, or shortness of breath are in serious danger (Harris, 1983).

Over time, vomiting and laxative abuse may also lead to alterations in renal functioning. Hypokalemia and dehydration impede the kidney's ability to function normally and eventually cause diminished capacity to concentrate urine. Laxative abuse also leads to problems in bowel functioning and after a while the bowels may become sluggish. Constipation and edema are frequently seen in patients early in treatment when they begin eating more normally and discontinue purging (Harris, 1983).

Finally, a non–life-threatening but common result of persistent vomiting is tooth erosion and damage to gums. Hydrochloric acid from the stomach repeatedly rushing over the teeth literally eats away teeth and gums. Patients frequently require extensive dental work.

PRIMARY AND SECONDARY PREVENTION OF EATING DISORDERS

Given the extent and severity of the medical and psychological complications of anorexia nervosa and bulimia, as well as the tenacity of the symptoms, it is necessary for health professionals to engage in a concerted effort to prevent young women and men from becoming anorexic and bulimic. The task of prevention is not easy because the individual susceptible to an eating disorder may be elusive. After all, countless adolescent and young adult women engage in some form of dieting behavior. In addition, those persons who are already symptomatic may appear to be healthy as they guard their symptoms in secrecy.

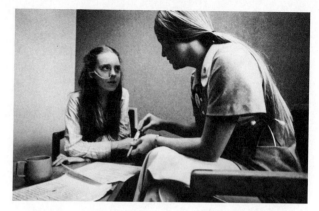

Continuing denial that there is a "problem" despite the anorexic woman's emaciation and food refusal (thus the need for tube feeding) in the experience of many clinicians is a *bad* prognostic sign.

Nurses, more than any other group of health professionals, may encounter susceptible individuals for several reasons. First, nursing is a profession that continues to be dominated by females and nearly ninety percent of patients with eating disorders are female. Thus, simply in peer interactions, nurses will be exposed to a higher percentage of vulnerable individuals. Also patients may feel more at ease revealing their preoccupation with thinness and dieting behavior to nurses. The general public tends to be somewhat more apt to engage in self-disclosure with nurses than with physicians or other health professionals. It is crucial to take advantage of this variable by educating women about the potential risks of eating disorders, identifying individuals at risk, and knowing how to help at-risk people to seek treatment. Schools, colleges, college health services, pediatric settings, dental clinics, and general medical settings are all potential sites for alerting the public and discovering individuals who may already be symptomatic.

It is important for nurses to pay attention to the degree to which any patient, particularly a young woman, is preoccupied with dieting and weight. Although many dieters focus on dissatisfaction with body size, this focus becomes exaggerated in the patient with an eating disorder. Body-size preoccupation has been shown to be the most effective predictor of successful or unsuccessful treatment (Johnson, 1986). That is, the degree to which an individual determines her self-esteem on the basis of body size, and the degree to which her body image is distorted (inaccurate), can be used as a barometer of the degree of her psychopathology.

In addition the individual may not be able to see positive aspects of herself aside from her diet. Patients with eating disorders share certain characteristic belief systems. For example, they may view specific foods such as dessert as "bad" and be terrified of taking even one bite of such a food. The person with anorexia may equate eating dessert with loss of control and dramatic weight gain, while the person with bulimia may see one bite as the trigger for a binge. Keep in mind that the most vulnerable time for onset of symptoms is following life changes that involve separation from significant others (such as starting high school or college or moving to a new city). This is based on object-relations theory which is described later in the chapter.

With these factors in mind, the nurse should be comfortable asking an individual directly about her dieting methods. A simple, straightforward question such as, "Have you ever tried vomiting or laxatives to lose weight?" is usually all that is needed to elicit an honest response from the bulimic patient. Many people suspect these measures to be harmful to themselves but feel embarrassed about having tried them. If the nurse highlights the physical dangers without projecting a judgmental attitude, the patient will be freer to discuss her feelings and behaviors.

The patient with anorexia, who typically denies the self-destructiveness of her behavior until late in the course of her illness, may be more difficult than the bulimic to engage in an open dialogue about her symptomatic behavior when it first appears. The nurse is mindful, however, that although the person may deny the severity of her condition, she may experience some relief in coming up against confrontation and urging from the nurse to seek treatment. Although some individuals have been able to halt symptoms without intervention, usually the person feels helpless to stop without assistance.

Often, a patient's family members seek assistance from their physician or nurse. There may be growing concern for a child or young woman in the family who continues to lose weight in spite of efforts to coax her to eat. In other cases the family may not realize the extent or severity of the problem. They may be unaware of how much weight their adolescent with anorexia has lost. Or, with a bulimic, they may not have paid attention to disappearing groceries and the amount of time their daughter spends in the bathroom. The nurse can help family members to recognize these indicators and to accept their need for specialized help for the individual in trouble, and for themselves.

THEORIES OF ETIOLOGY
PSYCHOANALYTIC/PSYCHODYNAMIC THEORY

Psychoanalytic theory describes the development of personality from infancy to adulthood. A number of theories have evolved since Freud conceptualized the internal psychic structure of id, ego, and superego. Each theory emphasizes different aspects of personality, such as the ego, and may focus on different stages of development such as infancy, toddlerhood, or adolescence. Theorists use terminology and language which is unique to their own thinking but which refers to similar phenomena. The result may be confusing when one attempts to integrate the various concepts in a unified approach to normal versus pathological personality development. There is common ground, however, in the belief that mother-child interactions influence the development of the self, and affect the way in which an individual views the world and relates to others.

Theories of cause and treatment of eating disorders parallel the evolution of analytic theories in general. Blending these theories is complicated, however, by the fact that the earliest writings pertained specifically to anorexia nervosa, and not to bulimia nervosa. In the following section we attempt to present the most significant and influential psychoanalytic thinkers and their theories about eating disorders.

EGO PSYCHOLOGY. Hilde Bruch (1973), renowned theorist in the field of eating disorders, rejected traditional analytic theory and focused instead on ego development, particularly in the area of self-image, body image, recognition of internal states (interoceptive awareness), and self-esteem. Her writings are based on the theory of **ego psychology** (a holistic, phenomenological, and social view of man [Masak, 1979]) and her extensive clinical work with patients with eating disorders. It should be noted that Bruch believed that bulimia was a variant of anorexia nervosa, and thus she did not distinguish between the two in her theory of etiology (Bruch, 1984).

Bruch (1973) recognized that the eating symptomatology of the patient with anorexia nervosa was closely related to problems in interpersonal relationships. That is, anorexic patients feel incompetent and ineffective in the social arena and often withdraw from relationships entirely. Bruch thought that the difficulties in relating to others stemmed from deficits in the individual's development, particularly in the area of self-image and body image. These two concepts are closely related and evolve from the child's interaction with the environment beginning in infancy in the mother-infant relationship.

In the ideal situation the mother responds in a timely manner to cues from the infant that convey physical and emotional needs. Consistent responses from the mother validate the infant's internal perceptions as well as satisfy needs for comfort and nurturance. This process forms the foundation of the developing sense of self and self-efficacy. Bruch theorized that patients with eating disorders have had mothers who inaccurately or inconsistently responded to their infants' signals. Thus as infants these patients did not get confirmation of internal perceptions. As a result, they failed to develop an ability to recognize internal states, and learned instead to respond to the needs and desires of their mothers.

Early in an anorexic's life, a pattern of relating to others emerges that is characterized by sensitivity and compliance. As children, anorexics typically maintain a pleasing facade with minimal awareness or expression of their own needs. Instead they focus on the needs and wants of others. They require little attention and are usually viewed by parents as problem free. Unfortunately, the patient's conformity to the expectations of others is not recognized by parents as a reflection of self-doubt (Bruch, 1973). Upon reaching adolescence, these young women are confronted with experiences they feel ill-equipped to handle. The advent of normal physiological changes and increasing sexuality coupled with the maturational tasks of adolescence, such as increasing independence from parents, are overwhelming to the preanorexic child. With a minimal sense of competence in the risky interpersonal sphere of adolescence, the young person turns instead to dieting as a means of effecting personal competency and improving relationships (Bruch, 1973).

OBJECT-RELATIONS THEORY. Like Bruch, **object-relations** theorists believe that problems in early childhood contribute to personality development that predisposes an individual to develop an eating disorder. The term "object" refers to "persons or things in the external environment which are psychologically significant to one's psychic life" (Brenner, 1974, p. 98). Using this language, object relations then refers to the style in which an individual perceives and relates to others based on the primary experience of her relationship with her mother or primary caretaker. Object-relations theorists hold that an individual will repeat this style of relating throughout life.

Many theorists feel that the preanorexic child never completely negotiated the process of **separation-individuation,** a concept that has sprung from the research of Margaret Mahler and colleagues (1975). They have detailed and organized observations of normal and pathological maternal-child interactions from infancy to approximately three years of age. The normal separation-individuation process described by Mahler is divided into stages during which the child gradually evolves from complete dependence on the mother for satisfaction of needs to having a rudimentary capacity to self-regulate in the absence of mother or other caretaker. **Self-regulation** refers to a person's ability to identify needs, manage impulses, tolerate frustration, organize a need-gratifying response, and delay gratification (Johnson & Connors, 1987). The mother who facilitates this process provides consistent, empathic responses for the child, giving her the experience of reliable caretaking that neither overwhelms, overcontrols, or neglects her (Johnson & Connors, 1987).

The process of separation-individuation parallels other developmental lines such as motor locomotion and cognitive and language development. For example, during the symbiotic phase (between the ages of one and four months) the child is still completely dependent on the caretaker for need gratification. The child of this age lacks the motor capacity to move away from the caretaker. In a sense, the child behaves as though she and mother are a single unit. During the first year of life, the child develops the cognitive ability to differentiate mother from other individuals, and the physical capacity to move away from mother and explore the environment. Intellectual and physical developments thus facilitate the child's beginning psychological separation. Gradually, the child begins to experiment by moving away from mother at times but "checking back" for reassurance that she is available. The child uses the mother as a kind of refueling station from which to explore and to return to for emotional refueling and security (Johnson & Connors, 1987).

During the toddler years, the child displays contradictory behavior that is thought to exemplify ambivalence about the process of psychologically separating from the mother. For example, the child will alternate between clinging to and darting away from her (Johnson & Connors, 1987). Language development at this time promotes the separation process, for example, through the child's use of the word "no," which becomes a concrete representation of the child's first assertion of psychological separateness. These years present the mother with the often challenging task of tolerating the child's efforts to become a separate individual. Limit-setting must be coupled with a willingness to let the child explore and take risks within a protected environment. Ultimately, the child develops an internal psychic image of the mother that serves to comfort or regulate in her absence.

Masterson (1978), another proponent of object-relations theory, has suggested that borderline personality syndrome (See Chapter 12 on personality disorders.) and eating disorders are associated. He feels that the mother of the anorexic was unable emotionally to tolerate her toddler's efforts to individuate. Instead, she was emotionally available to her youngster only for clinging, regressive behavior, and withdrew emotionally when the toddler displayed assertiveness or ambivalence. The toddler's immature ego then began to associate her mother's withdrawal of emotional supplies with aggressive energy, and defended against the fear of abandonment by maintaining the characteristic clinging, compliant behavior (Masterson, 1978).

This theory is complex but in essence describes a child who grows up fearing aggressive emotions, such as anger, which might drive away the mother and other important figures. Thus the child's attempts to relate to others are characterized by the desire to please. Any situation that threatens the pathological, clinging relationship triggers separation anxiety (related to fear of abandonment) and activates the ego's defense mechanisms. The onset of adolescence poses just such a threat to the future anorexic. The development of anorexic symptoms represents a defensive maneuver on the part of the ego. The symptoms, which ultimately present a picture of powerful fragility, become a maladaptive solution to the fears associated with the increasing demands for autonomy facing the adolescent that threaten her relationship with her mother and forecast tremendous emotional loss (Masterson, 1978). (See Box 14-3.) (Also see Chapters 4, 12, and 22 on theories, personality disorders, and children for more on object-relations theory.)

INTEGRATED DEVELOPMENTAL THEORY. Recently, Johnson (1986) has attempted to consolidate analytic theories and integrate them with family-systems theory (see page 504) to construct a model of intrapsychic organization that differentiates anorexia and bulimia. Simultaneously, Johnson has further subdivided the two groups along the lines of character or personality pathology. Both groups are seen as existing on a continuum of underlying psychic disturbance that includes at one extreme the psychotic patient and at the other the neurotic patient. He views the majority of patients as falling in the middle of the continuum in the categories of borderline and narcissistic personality disorders.

Johnson theorizes that the two groups differ in style as a result of their early experience of maternal involvement. Specifically, the anorexic has had the experience of maternal overinvolvement while the bulimic has grown up with maternal underinvolvement. The symptoms of anorexia and bulimia are viewed in a somewhat metaphorical way; that is, the patient with anorexia is engaged in both a conscious and unconscious effort to "keep things out" of the body and self while the efforts of the bulimic are directed at "taking things in" (Johnson, 1986).

To elaborate further, the patient with anorexia uses self-starvation in an attempt to define the self through rigid control of the body. Food refusal and the accompanying oppositional stance are a way to demonstrate autonomy and psychologically defend against the intrusive, overprotective caretaker. As Johnson points out, the effect is paradoxical. While the anorexia makes a statement of self-assertion, it ensures that the individual will remain "enmeshed" with her family. She will not have to face the expectations associated with psychobiological maturity. Instead, the illness will allow the patient to receive continuing care and protection from family and others (Johnson, 1986).

The bulimic, on the other hand, has had an experience of maternal disengagement; that is, her caretaker was typically emotionally unavailable for soothing her emotional needs. While usually not blatantly neglectful, this mother was overwhelmed by her child's needs. As a result, the child grows up with a rather shaky bond with the caretaker and develops a kind of emotional "emptiness." In an effort to fill that sense of emptiness, the individual eats. Johnson associates this use of food with the use by the child of transitional objects (such as teddy bears and stuffed animals) during the process of emotional separation from the mother. The child invests in these objects the capacity to soothe and comfort during the mother's absence. In the case of the bulimic, food is used to soothe and comfort when the individual experiences emotional needs and internal tension.

The symptomatic categories are further subdivided by Johnson into the borderline or narcissistic personality disorders on the basis of the child's experience of malevolent or nonmalevolent intent from her caretaker. If the behavior of the caretaker, whether overprotective or neglectful, has been tinged with aggression or deliberate hostility, the child is

Box 14—3 • Sugar and Spice and Everything Nice?

"I agree with much of the woman's liberation movement, but those angry women just turn me off!" Sound familiar? You've probably said as much yourself on occasion. According to Dr. Harriet Lerner, (1988, p. 60) a staff psychologist and psychotherapist at the Menniger Foundation in Topeka, Kansas, despite the feminist movement, our culture's definition of the healthy, "feminine" woman as one who is devoid of anger and aggressiveness, especially toward men, persists. Behind this attitude, she feels, are irrational fears (experienced by men *and* women) of woman's "omnipotent destructiveness" (p. 61), as well as the complex developmental task of separation-individuation for the female child. Lerner attributes the fearsome "power" that we imagine women to embody to the matriarchal world we grow up in. "It is the mother, along with a host of other women (governesses, baby-sitters, elementary school teachers), who provides rewards and punishments and narcissistic injuries[1] that are part of the day-to-day task of socializing a child" (p. 62). The relatively greater difficulty the daughter has in separating and individuating from her mother (as compared to the son), Lerner says, is a result of the girl's need to differentiate herself from the parent with whom she also is to identify. This is made even more difficult when the mother reacts to her daughter's assertion of differences as a "threatened 'loss', or as disloyalty or a violation of the bond between them" (p. 67). When this happens, healthy expressions of autonomy (such as anger) may be replaced by masochistic solutions (for example, an eating disorder), which enable the female child to become the hurt or dependent child, and so maintain a close mother-daughter bond. Avoiding our culture's tendency to blame the mother in situations such as this, Lerner points out that the overpossessive mother, or the one that envies (and, so, undermines) her daughter's youthful beauty and blossoming sexuality, who restricts her daughter's moves toward autonomy "may herself be the product of a distorting and constricting feminine socialization process which has left her with little else but her own children to possess" (p. 70).

The separation-individuation process which begins in early childhood continues throughout life in a variety of interpersonal relationships. Lerner holds that in the case of the woman whose individuation has been thwarted, she is likely to find for herself possessive and undifferentiated lovers or husbands who undermine her continuing struggle for autonomy, perceiving it as disloyalty and a threat to the security of their relationship.

[1] Narcissistic injury: disturbance in the sense of well-being that results from reaffirmation of one's core identity (Settlage, 1977).
Source: Lerner, H. G. (1988) "Internal prohibitions against female anger," *Women in Therapy,* New Jersey: Jason Aronson Inc., p. 59–75.

likely to develop a borderline personality, involving severe disturbance in the development of intrapsychic structure. This is characterized by significant impairment in ego functioning, such as the ability to self-regulate. There is also impairment in the ability to form and maintain relationships since others tend to be experienced as having sadistic or punitive intent. For example, when a nurse states a rule or sets a limit with such a patient, in a nonthreatening matter-of-fact style, the patient feels as though she is being punished and views the nurse as mean and hostile.

The narcissistic personality refers to an individual with a lesser degree of disturbance in internal psychic structure than the individual with borderline personality. These patients usually have developed an adaptive facade which gives them the appearance of a higher functioning personality. Overtly, these patients have good social skills and may be able to develop superficial relationships. Their attachments to others are not tinged with the hostility of the borderline individual because their experience of caretaking was probably without malevolence. That is, caretakers might have been controlling or neglectful but in a benign way. Thus the patients do not view the world as being dangerous or other people as punitive and retaliatory, as do borderline patients. They tend to view their caretakers as more ineffective and needing protection themselves as opposed to being hostile. Narcissistic patients often refer to themselves as "phony" or "fakes." The facade they maintain is not a representation of their experience of themselves, and thus they frequently struggle with a sense of identity. And despite not seeing the environment as dangerous, they have difficulty feeling as if they are involved in it or a part of the world. Table 14–1 illustrates the four categories that Johnson has delineated. (See Chapter 12 on personality disorders for more on borderline and narcissistic personality disorder and their management.) (Also see Box 14–4.)

FEMINIST PERSPECTIVE ON DEVELOPMENTAL THEORY. Orbach (1985) has criticized theories that essentially "blame" mothers for the development of problem behaviors in their children. Instead of targeting mothers for a failure in meeting the needs of their daughters, Orbach has attempted to understand the motives of mothers in light of the position of women in society. Specifically, Orbach sees the mother-daughter relationship as "ambivalent," in that the mothers are psychologically preparing their daughters for the social and psychological constraints they themselves face as women. She contends that women in general are taught to meet certain "basic demands" of society such as deference to others, caretaking, and identity through connection with another (Orbach, 1985; also see Chapter 19 on women). In order to meet these demands, the woman's own needs must be suppressed or go unrecognized. Women are also taught to display certain dependent behaviors and to refrain from expressing their own dependency needs. Orbach feels that defending against dependency needs, for example, through denial that they exist, is common to all women, and is frequently accompanied by concern for and taking care of *others*. Patients who have eating disorders carry this characteristic style of relating to the extreme of total denial of any need for help from others (Orbach, 1985).

Gilligan (1984) also holds that women are socialized to assume the role of tending to the needs of others; however, she emphasizes the positive aspects of the process. In her research, Gilligan found that adolescent girls equated the concept of dependence with reliability, caring, availability, and helpfulness. She theorizes that as a part of normal development, women develop sensitivity to others in an effort to connect with them and maintain affiliations. However, a conflict develops in adolescence if the age-appropriate emphasis on independence and autonomy is perceived as a threat to affiliation and connectedness. The conflict occurs in determining responsibility to self versus responsibility to others.

Gilligan sees the current eruption of eating disorders as tied to the new cultural value of indepen-

---

TABLE 14–1 Personality disorders associated with eating disorders

	Borderline: Malevolent Intent of Caretaker	Narcissistic: Benign or Nonmalevolent Intent
ANOREXIA Overinvolvement of caretaker	Self—Overwhelmed, in danger Other—Critical, harsh, punitive	Self—Extension of other, without identity, ineffective Other—Fragile
BULIMIA Underinvolvement of caretaker	Self—Worthless, unlovable Other—Withholding, punitive	Self—Fraud, inadequate Other—Incapable of adequately protecting, soothing

Source: Johnson, C. (1986, October). Treating the eating disorders patient with a character disorder. In *Being effective in assessment, treatment, and prevention.* The Fifth National Conference on Eating Disorders. Columbus, Ohio.

Box 14–4 ● Edie Sedgwick

Edie Sedgwick, playmate of Andy Warhol and Mick Jagger, was "one of the true personalities of the 60s." She was a *Vogue* model during the "Twiggy period" when "everybody slept with everybody like kittens...the pill changed the world" (p. 243). She died of an accidental barbiturate overdose at the age of 28 in 1971.

EDIE SEDGWICK (1943–1971)

I don't know how she did it.
Fire She was shaking all over.
It took her hours to put her
make-up on. But she did it.
Even the false eyelashes. She
ordered a gin with triple limes.

Then a limousine. Everyone knew
she was the real heroine of
Blonde on Blonde.
oh it isnt fair
oh it isnt fair
how her ermine hair
turned men around
she was white on white
so blonde on blonde
and her long long legs
how I used to beg
to dance with her
but I never had

a chance with her
oh it isnt fair
how her ermine hair

dence for women. She feels young women are torn between the pressure to be independent and the fear that autonomy will bring loss of affiliation with others. Consequently, eating disorders may not represent a failure of the individuation process but a response to conflict with cultural values (Gilligan, 1984).

FAMILY-SYSTEMS THEORY

MINUCHIN—FAMILIES OF ANOREXICS. Family-systems theory views the patient with an eating disorder within the context of her family as a whole. The family is viewed as having a structure consisting of a hierarchy that includes the parents, who are the executive subsystem, and the children, who are the sibling subsystem. Ideally, there is a clearly defined boundary between the two subsystems that maintains the leadership role of the parents. The boundary is supported by a mutually satisfying parental relationship that allows the parents to work as a team to foster the growth and development of the children. Conflict that occurs between the parents is addressed and resolved from within the parental subsystem (Minuchin, 1974).

Minuchin (1974) has identified several interactional patterns which he feels are characteristic of families of children with anorexia. One involves **enmeshment,** which is a lack of clear boundaries between the generations and between individual family members. Members are overly sensitive to one another. Emotions and needs of one individual are felt by the other members of the system (who feel endangered by associated conflict). There is also a tendency to avoid conflict, be overprotective of one another, and maintain a facade of harmony. While there are conflicts in any family, in the anorexic's family, according to Minuchin (1974), they are deflected onto the child, who becomes symptomatic. The family then focuses on the child with anorexia, which frees them from addressing their own problems. This system is self-perpetuating, and the family typically becomes locked into a rigid, unchanging pattern.

FALLON—FAMILIES OF BULIMICS. Patricia Fallon is a family therapist who has done extensive clinical work with families of patients with bulimia. She has identified three typical family types and their associated areas of conflict: the perfect family, the overprotective family, and the chaotic family. As with families of anorexics, Fallon feels families of bulimics have problems maintaining boundaries between individuals and between generational subgroups. In addition, she sees these families as having inequitable distributions of power and cites this as a focal point of conflict (Fallon, 1986).

The Perfect Family. In the **perfect family,** the conflicts center on expectations of female family members. While women are expected to demonstrate success in their careers and to achieve responsible, powerful positions, they are at the same time expected to behave in a more traditional, feminine way. That is, they are supposed to be sensitive to others and to refrain from expressing unladylike emotions such as anger. The female children in these families

used to swing so nice
used to cut the air
how all the men
used to dance with her
I never got a chance with her
though I really asked her
down deep
where you do
really dream
in the mind
reading love
I'd get
inside
her move
and we'd
turn around
and she'd

turn around
and turn the head
of everyone in town
her shaking shaking
glittering bones
second blonde child
after brian jones
oh it isnt fair
how I dreamed of her
and she slept
and she slept
forever
and I'll never dance
with her no never
she broke down
like a baby
she suffocated

like a baby
like a baby girl
like a lady
with ermine hair
oh it isnt fair
and I'd like to see
her rise again
her white white bones
with baby brian jones
baby brian jones
like blushing
baby dolls

—Patti Smith

Source: Stein, Jean. George Plimpton (Ed.) (1982) *Edie: An American Biography.* A Dell Book, pp. 344–345.

are often those who feel the pressure to be "superwoman." The expectations in the family are strong, and behavior inconsistent with these expectations is seen as a betrayal of family norms. Thus rebellion that is normally part of adolescent development is not an option for the female children. Bulimia offers a means of indirect expression of anger within the family, an alternative form of rebellion (Fallon, 1986).

The Overprotective Family. Overprotective families in many ways resemble the families of anorexics that Minuchin described. Females in these families are seen as needing protection from the world, often because the mother was abused, neglected, or abandoned as a child. In an attempt to protect her child from a similar experience, the mother may overcompensate and be unable to let go and launch her female children into the world.

In these families, bulimia serves as a means of keeping the child in a younger, less competent position and allows the parents to continue to protect her (Fallon, 1986).

The Chaotic Family. Chaotic families are the most disrupted families, in which there are extreme violations of boundaries in the form of physical or sexual abuse of the mother or daughter(s) by the males in the family. If the female child has undergone this kind of abuse, she feels unprotected and out of control of her life. Bulimia becomes for her a means of soothing and nurturing the self and defending against the pain associated with victimization. The

bulimic symptoms also serve as an expression of anger and disgust (Fallon, 1986).

HUMPHREY—FAMILIES OF BULIMICS. In addition to her extensive clinical work with families of anorexics and bulimics, psychologist Laura Humphrey (1987) has conducted studies of interactional patterns observed among their family members. Her findings thus far have shown that relationship patterns in families of bulimics differ considerably from those of an anorexic's family. The bulimic's family is usually more overtly conflictual, expressing anger and hostility openly toward one another. Bickering and use of humor and joking are common expressions of hostility. Less support and affection among the bulimic's family members was also found, as well as a greater sense of isolation in the identified patient.

BIOLOGICAL-PSYCHOLOGICAL-SOCIOLOGICAL PERSPECTIVE

Experts who have studied eating disorders generally agree that no single psychological theory can explain a disorder's development. Rather, psychological theory must be combined with an understanding of the biological effects of starvation and depression and be viewed in the sociocultural context. Certainly the rising incidence of eating disorders has been influenced by the cultural value of thinness and fitness. The degree to which advertising, television, and women's magazines affect the way women view themselves should not be underestimated. The slogan "You can

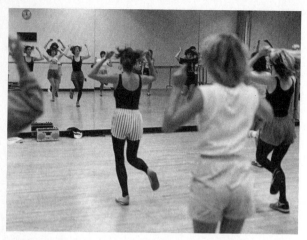

Everyone is participating in aerobics despite warnings about injury to bones, especially knees and hips in the vulnerable individual (the woman with a chronic eating disorder whose bones are often calcium-depleted [osteoporotic]). After aerobics, the anorexic will probably run or bike several miles—part of her daily routine—all on a diet of popcorn, lettuce, and black coffee.

never be too rich or too thin" seems to epitomize the degree of pressure women feel to have a thin body. Teenagers and women with low self-esteem are, no doubt, especially vulnerable to these influences. As health care professionals, we have a responsibility to help people to become more sensitive to the effect of this pressure, so the cultural value of thinness will begin to decrease and fewer individuals will be tempted to resort to extreme measures to achieve it.

TREATMENT OF EATING DISORDERS

The treatment of eating disorders is often a long-term process, extending over several years. Given the complex relationship between physical and psychological symptoms, it is necessary to treat both simultaneously. Simply restoring weight through behavioral management of the symptoms is insufficient for long-term recovery of the patient. In turn, a patient whose physical status is severely compromised by inadequate or chaotic eating patterns is difficult to engage in the psychotherapeutic process.

OUTPATIENT TREATMENT

If the physical and psychological condition of the patient are not so severe that the individual is at risk medically or unable to perform ordinary tasks of daily living, an initial trial of outpatient treatment is instituted. Modalities of treatment include individual therapy, family therapy, group therapy, or some combination of the three. Decisions about treatment interventions vary, depending on the philosophical orientation of the institution or the therapist. In most cases, if the patient is an adolescent or a young adult living at home, family treatment is warranted. In some cases it may be optimal to involve the family even if the patient has lived away from home for several years. The family therapist will aim interventions at determining the "function" the eating disorder symptoms serve in the family, redefining boundaries among family members, identifying conflict (for example, between parents), and helping the family to support the patient's separation and individuation. Group therapy may be a helpful adjunct to individual or family work by promoting supportive relationships with peers that further foster separation from the family. Groups are also useful for educational purposes as well as for symptom management. Peers can be extremely helpful in supporting one another in the attempt to "give up" eating disorder symptoms.

Most patients require individual therapy, and techniques of intervention vary considerably. There is controversy among mental health professionals about which type of treatment is preferable: psychodynamic, cognitive-behavioral, and/or psychopharmacological. The relative merits of each orientation and their compatibility continue to be debated by experts in the field. Those who believe in psychodynamic treatment feel that a patient is not truly "cured," even though she may be symptom-free, until the basic intrapsychic conflicts have been addressed. They believe that the relationship with the therapist will provide a new experience for the patient, one that does not repeat early traumatic or conflict-ridden relationship experiences. Through this relationship the patient will gain insight into how her self-destructive patterns may have developed while developing new, more adaptive patterns of living and relating to others. Issues that have interfered with both such as unresolved grief, experiences of victimization, or unrealistic parent expectations (for example, to be the perfect child) are uncovered in the process. This type of psychotherapy may involve years of treatment.

Cognitive-behavioral therapists focus interventions on changing "cognitive mediators"—thoughts that occur between an event and subsequent emotions and behavior. Therapists take an active and directive role with the patient and utilize questioning as a primary therapeutic tool. The patient is challenged to examine the validity of certain belief systems that have led to troubled feelings and self-destructive behaviors. Research on outcome of treatment of bulimia has shown that cognitive interventions help patients reduce the frequency of binges (Fairburn, 1984; Fairburn, 1986). This reduction of binges is associated with increased self-esteem. Thus cognitive-behavioral therapists feel that their approach is an effective one, and one that takes less time and money than psychodynamic treatment.

The third component in the debate involves the use of psychopharmacological treatment. Between forty and sixty percent of anorexic patients benefit from tricyclic antidepressants. Nonresponders may improve with the serotonin antagonist, cyproheptadine (Periactin) (Maxmen, 1986). Controlled studies are hard to find but in six out of seven studies antidepressant medications have been shown to be effective in controlling bulimic episodes in some patients (Hudson, 1986). Nevertheless, medication is used with caution as malnourished patients can be especially sensitive to drugs and experience untoward effects such as potentially fatal cardiac arrhythmias.

Bulimia has been shown to be highly responsive to tricyclic antidepressants and monomine oxidase inhibitors. About thirty percent of patients on TCAs and fifty percent of those on MAOIs have recovered completely according to researchers Pope (1983) and Walsh (1984) and their colleagues. Those not cured have reduced their binge episodes by over fifty percent. Because of this, MAOIs may be considered the preferred drug in the treatment of bulimics *except* those patients who will not or cannot follow a tyramine-free diet (Maxmen, 1986).

In most clinical settings some combination of these three approaches is used. For example, patients with an eating disorder and a concomitant depression are typically treated with an antidepressant as well as psychotherapy. Many psychodynamically oriented therapists use cognitive-behavioral techniques as well as psychodynamic ones. In some treatment settings, nurses use cognitive-behavioral techniques in their work with eating disorders patients. These are described in more detail on pages 509–510. The nurse works in conjunction with the patient's therapist, physician, and dietitian, who, as members of the treatment team, must have a strong working alliance and a good communication system. The team should be in agreement regarding treatment in any one case, for example, the criteria for hospitalization (such as weight below 100 pounds for two weeks, along with the desire to lose more weight), so that a consistent message is given to the patient.

INPATIENT TREATMENT

Hospitalization may be necessary in the early phase of eating-disorder treatment as well as in subsequent crisis periods. Conditions warranting inpatient treatment include extreme emaciation, medical complications (such as abnormal electrolytes), psychological distress, severe depression, an actual or threatened suicide attempt, and lack of response to outpatient treatment (Anderson, Morse, & Santmeyer, 1985). In the treatment of severe emaciation, dehydration, and electrolyte imbalances, the patient may first be hospitalized on a medical unit. Procedures such as nasogastric tube feedings, hyperalimentation, and intravenous fluids may be initiated. The relationship between the nurse and patient is important during this crisis period to establish the groundwork for a subsequent therapeutic alliance with the primary nurse in the eating-disorders treatment setting. In addition, nurses in the medical setting need to be familiar with symptoms and treatment of eating disorders in order to be able to anticipate and prevent problems. Patients have been known to disconnect tubing and discard feedings or solutions, to vomit, and to exercise if not monitored closely. For these reasons, it is rarely feasible to institute long-term management of the patient with an eating disorder on a medical unit.

Most often, the patient is hopitalized for intensive treatment in a psychiatric setting. However, the patient with an eating disorder will be a treatment challenge there as well. In recent years a number of specialized treatment units have been established. Nurses in the general psychiatric and medical areas can benefit from understanding the principles of intervention employed by nurses in these specialized treatment centers.

PRINCIPLES OF BEHAVIOR MODIFICATION AND THE NURSE

Most programs use principles of behavior modification to address the pathological behavior associated with eating disorders. A protocol for meals is established that usually begins with a low-calorie diet (1200 calories) proportioned into meals and snacks given to the patient at regular intervals. Food is treated as "medicine" and the patient is expected to eat the prescribed amount (Anderson, Morse, & Santmeyer, 1985). Liquid protein supplements are given to substitute for uneaten portions of food. If the patient refuses to eat, some programs initiate tube feedings immediately (Anderson, Morse, & Santmeyer, 1985). Others view this resistance as a treatment issue to be dealt with by the treatment team. It is generally considered preferable to advance the patient's caloric intake slowly (200–300 calories weekly). This promotes trust between staff and the patient, who worries that the treatment team will force a rapid weight gain. Although food preferences are taken into account, the dietitian selects menus for the patient in the early stages of treatment—this is consistent with the concept of food as medicine and helps minimize obsessive focusing on food.

Patients are monitored in a group by the nurse during meals and for at least one hour afterward to prevent postmeal purging. In order to avoid power struggles with patients, treatment programs typically involve mealtime rules to ensure consistency in staff responses. For example, condiments may be limited in number to prevent patients from using excessive amounts or from creating unusual combinations of condiments with food items, ultimately leading to food refusal. (Something with excessive salt, ketchup, mustard, and so on, could be declared unpalatable by the patient, and a power struggle over food and program rules would begin.) Other program expectations might include eating chicken skin, potato skin, and so on, while eating garnishes may be optional. These rules may appear to be obsessive; however, they effectively eliminate power struggles at mealtimes if they are stated clearly to the patient at the outset of inpatient treatment. It should be pointed out at that time that their purpose is to help the patient change her focus from food to feelings, a key principle of effective treatment.

Many programs establish a goal weight for the patient as well as demand that specific requirements for rate of weight gain be met before the patient is allowed certain privileges. To promote weight gain, the patient's physical activity is generally restricted in the early phase of treatment; later it may be used as a privilege or reinforcement for steady weight gain. Some programs incorporate a limited amount of regularly supervised exercise into the daily routine. Other privileges granted as the patient progresses in treatment might include decreased time under direct supervision by the staff and permission to leave the unit for meals or other unsupervised activities.

The role of the nurse in the inpatient setting primarily involves administering the protocol for nutritional rehabilitation in a supportive context. Nutritional rehabilitation is best facilitated with a clearly defined protocol for meals, as described above. It is important that the nurse convey a sense of confidence and authority in stating mealtime expectations. This will help to decrease the patient's anxiety at mealtime. Well-established program guidelines minimize the nurse's anxiety and enable her to exercise judgment and to set limits at mealtime on the eating-disorders unit.

Even with a nurse present at meals, it is not unusual for the patient to attempt to hide food or to obsess about what is on her tray. This behavior results from the anxiety, guilt, and panic the patient often experiences during and after eating. The patient is *not* malicious in her intent to thwart the program or the efforts of the nurse. Rather, it is the belief that all food is "bad" and will lead to excessive weight gain that results in the patient's clinging to the eating-disorder symptomatology.

The nurse should set limits for mealtime behavior in a nonpunitive, nonjudgmental manner. Sometimes simply reiterating expectations is all that is necessary. Providing external limits helps to contain the patient's anxiety. At the same time, it is important for the nurse to convey a caring and sensitive attitude toward the patient. A statement that indicates understanding of the patient's fears is likely to be experienced as reassuring and supportive. Skilled, confident nurses often use humor to coach patients through difficult moments. If, however, a power struggle ensues and the patient continues to protest, the nurse must decide whether or not to back down and avoid further provocation of the patient. A patient's chronic refusal to comply with expectations is an issue for the treatment team to grapple with. It may be necessary for them to ask the patient again to decide to work with the team and its program for weight gain, or to leave the hospital.

In group treatment settings such as the inpatient unit, peer group pressure to conform to mealtime routines can be a powerful treatment facilitator: patients who may be struggling with their own impulses want to avoid the disruption caused by watching another patient refuse food or engage in ritualistic behavior.

Weigh-ins are another particularly distressing part of the treatment program for most eating-disorders patients. Patients who have not achieved their goal weights may attempt to hide this by drinking excessive amounts of water prior to weigh-ins or by hiding heavy objects in their clothing or on their bodies. It is helpful to have the patient void before being weighed and wear a hospital gown with no underclothing. If the nurse suspects the weight is inaccurate, she questions the patient directly. The nurse conveys serious concern without seeming angry, shocked, or punitive when she discovers these attempts to get around the treatment program. A firm statement of the expectations for weight gain can be coupled with a willingness to listen to the patient's fears about it. Many patients have "magic" numbers, especially three-digit numbers (any weight 100 pounds or more), that are particularly frightening to them. Although a single pound of difference in weight may seem trivial to the nurse, the patient may be panicked at the thought of the increase. The nurse considers these fears with serious regard, giving empathic encouragement and support in order to motivate the patient to continue her efforts to gain weight.

COGNITIVE-BEHAVIORAL TECHNIQUES AND THE NURSE

The nurse should be familiar with cognitive-behavioral techniques that might be helpful to the patient (Fairburn, 1984; Johnson & Connors, 1987; Garner et al., 1984). These include psychoeducation, meal planning, introduction of avoided foods, self-monitoring, and stimulus control.

PSYCHOEDUCATION. Many interventions are designed to educate the patient by challenging the characteristic thinking patterns that motivate her self-destructive behavior. The nurse may offer to the patient information related to the physical complications of eating disorders. In addition, the nurse corrects inaccurate beliefs, such as the efficacy of laxative use for weight control. Patients are typically unaware that the majority of calories are absorbed into the small intestine before the laxatives take effect in the large intestine.

MEAL PLANNING. Dietary teaching includes stressing the importance of eating several times a day at regular intervals. Many bulimic patients defer eating until the end of the day, which heightens their hunger and increases the likelihood of binge eating. Dieting should be discouraged during the period in which the patient is attempting to stop binge eating (Garner et al., 1984). Often the patient is surprised to find that eating a balanced 1800–2400 calorie diet over the course of the day will not cause a weight gain. Patients with anorexia will frequently have great anxiety associated with planning a normal balanced meal and should practice this before leaving the hospital.

INTRODUCTION OF AVOIDED FOODS. Frequently patients avoid certain foods, such as pasta or sweets, because they consider these to be "bad" foods. The anorexic may avoid these foods completely; the bulimic may binge on them and then purge. The nurse encourages the patient to include small portions of these "high-risk" foods in her diet, and supports her as she gradually begins to eat. For example, the nurse can sit with the patient for the first trial of a "dangerous" food item. This process helps to desensitize the patient to eating these foods, and dispels the myth that certain foods will cause excessive weight gain or always lead to a binge.

SELF-MONITORING WITH BULIMICS. To reduce the frequency of binge-purge episodes, it is often helpful to begin with **self-monitoring.** This activity allows the patient and nurse to observe patterns that occur within the symptomatology. For instance, some patients may typically binge late in the evening or on certain days of the week. If possible, the patient should record any associated mood states or events that seem to trigger bingeing. Some patients may be more inclined to binge when they are angry or have experienced a rejection; other patients may binge because of boredom. Initial documentation of typical weekly patterns provides a baseline and a means of identifying alternatives in behavior that may help to interrupt the symptom cycle.

STIMULUS CONTROL. If predictable triggers typically precede a binge, the patient may be able to use **stimulus-control** techniques to delay the onset of the binge. This involves distraction accomplished by pairing the urge to binge with an activity different from bingeing, for example, exercise or social interaction (Wetherby & Baumeister, 1981). Many patients will find that this delay helps reduce the desire or necessity for a binge. The alternative behavior should be pleasant and rewarding in order to increase the likelihood that the patient will follow through with the process. The suggested alternative should be an adaptive means for coping with the identified mood state. For example, an individual who usually binges when agitated and upset might respond well to the alternative of taking a walk or run, or engaging in an activity that expends energy. If a patient binges when she is lonely and bored, calling a friend or listening to pleasant music may be suggested as an alternative. To be effective, the compensating behavior has to be individualized to reflect the patient's own situation or dynamics. It might be helpful for the patient to carry with her a card or notebook that lists alternatives to bingeing. The patient may also contract with the nurse to try two or three alternative activities before giving in to the impulse to binge. When successful, stimulus-control techniques result in managing the urge to binge more adaptively.

Typically, if these techniques fail and the patient binges, she feels guilt and failure. Often the patient believes that one relapse means total defeat. It is important to encourage the patient to continue trying even if binge eating occurs. The patient needs ongoing support to motivate her to continue in treatment despite such "failures." It is also important, however, to talk with the patient about times when she *chooses* to binge. That is, in spite of a willingness to give up the symptoms, there may be times when the patient actively decides to binge, for example, when she finds herself home alone for several hours. At these times, the individual must examine the secondary gains of binge eating (such as relief of tension) and accept responsibility for choosing to continue to use her eating disorder to achieve them (Wooley & Wooley, 1984).

FAMILY INTERACTIONS

Although dysfunctional family interactions have been cited as having a role in the development of eating disorders, it is important that the nurse not judge the families of these patients. The nurse remains sensitive to the fact that the parents of an anorexic patient may have been struggling for many months to get their daughter to eat. The distress of watching one's daughter willfully starve herself to death would cause chaos in any household. The parents are likely to feel guilty, ineffective, and depressed about the situation and will need support from the nurse. At the same time, the nurse needs to be aware that the parents of anorexic and bulimic patients may complain that the treatment is cruel and punitive and threaten to take the patient out of treatment. It is helpful to forewarn the parents about this phenomenon and encourage them to discuss such feelings with the nurse or the family therapist.

SPECIAL ISSUES IN TREATMENT

COUNTERTRANSFERENCE. Initiating and maintaining treatment with a severely emaciated patient frequently evokes emotional reactions in the nurse. If the nurse identifies these reactions, and understands what they may say about the patient, she may begin to comprehend those underlying dynamics with which the patient is struggling. Awareness of her reactions and willingness to self-examine during supervision helps the nurse resolve negative countertransferences and maintain sensitive and therapeutic communication with the patient. If she does not understand her reactions, they may impede the therapeutic process. (For more on countertransference, see Chapter 12 on personality disorders.)

FEELINGS OF IMPOTENCE. Nurses, like other health professionals, enter their careers with the intent of caring for others and helping to minimize and alleviate symptoms of illness, pain, and so on. The nurse receives personal gratification and validation of professional competence for her efforts when they are successful and when the patient expresses appreciation. The patient with an eating disorder not only challenges the nurse's skills, but also often acts as though it is the nurse's responsibility to improve the patient's physical status and promote weight gain. Few patients with eating disorders want to cooperate with the treatment process, let alone express appreciation for it. In addition a patient's continuing battles with the nurse over nutritional interventions can evoke feelings of impotence. Similarly, it is not unusual for the nurse to feel angry with a patient whose persistent symptoms feel like a personal rejection. Continued futile attempts to provide support may elicit the feeling that no matter what the nurse does, it is not enough. Peer support and conferring with the patient's therapist can help the nurse evaluate the situation and motivate her to keep trying.

OVERINVOLVEMENT AND UNDERINVOLVEMENT WITH THE PATIENT. A patient's resistance to treatment may be difficult to comprehend, given the outward appearance of many of these patients who were once bright, attractive, pleasant, and talented young women with many opportunities for success. It is not easy to accept the intractable nature of their symptoms while continuing to try to help them. It is difficult not to give up, especially if the nurse's hard work is held in contempt by the patient. The same patient who says "Leave me alone," however, may feel abandoned if she senses that the nurse is pulling out emotionally from their relationship, a situation that could trigger more self-destructive behavior.

On the other hand, many nurses share with the eating-disorders patient an understanding of society's pressure on women to be thin. This common understanding may give the nurse an advantage in developing a therapeutic alliance with the patient; however, the potential for overinvolvement and overidentification with her is also great. Maintaining a "safe" emotional distance, yet remaining empathically available, is not an easy task. In summary, the patient's response to the nurse varies from total rejection to the belief that she is the only competent professional on the treatment team, both of which threaten the patient's therapeutic relationship with the nurse as well as the one with her psychotherapist.

SPLITTING. Due to the patient's tendency to use the defense of **splitting** (see Chapter 12 on personality disorders), she may identify one or more nurses as "good" and the rest as "bad." Usually the nurse who calls the patient on symptomatic behavior and sets limits with the patient falls into the latter category. Efforts should be made by the treatment team to prevent splitting, for example, by ensuring that one nurse does not appear to be more lenient or strict than another. Some nurses will become annoyed or angry with the patient who complains repeatedly about food and program rules. Other nurses will have difficulty setting appropriate limits due to a fear of confrontation with the patient. Communication among the nurses is essential so that decisions made by the patient's primary nurse will be followed and supported by others. Similar "splits" may also develop between the nursing staff and the patient's primary therapist. Again frequent communication among treatment team members, including a willingness to discuss countertransference, is needed to counteract the patient's unconscious attempts to split them.

LACK OF CONFLICT RESOLUTION AMONG MEMBERS OF THE TREATMENT TEAM. Some of the countertransference reactions may mimic the patient's family dynamics. For instance, the nursing staff may become rigid in its thinking related to interventions with the patient. The nurses may insist on doing everything by the book to minimize their anxiety or prevent conflict. The hazards of this type of thinking, of course, include limiting spontaneity and creativity in the treatment process and in the patient. A nurse who remains flexible to new or changing treatment approaches (not to be confused with

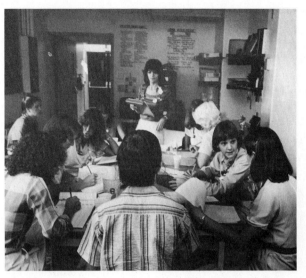

The staff on an eating disorders unit needs to identify and deal with patients' splitting (primitive defensive activity which involves seeing the world in terms of black and white; for example, there is the "good nurse" and the "bad nurse") before *they* get "sucked in" and become split as a staff. Countertransference issues can also be identified at this time, and needed support offered to one another.

inconsistency) may be singled out as a scapegoat for difficulties in the treatment process or the patient's lack of improvement. In fact, entire shifts may blame other shifts for not following the care plan exactly.

A forum such as report or weekly staff meetings should be designated to attempt to identify and resolve these inevitable problems. The staff can use these meetings to ventilate feelings, resolve differences, and support one another. Honesty and assertiveness are necessary qualities for the nurse who seeks to unify the group. Sharing humorous anecdotes about interactions with patients can provide a healthy means of tension release and bring the group closer together.

Despite all the problems and frustrations, working with the patient with an eating disorder can be a rewarding experience. Understanding and learning to use countertransference in treatment, engaging in successful teamwork, and helping young women who pay a high price for their extreme thinness, along with the increase in self-understanding that often develops in working with these interesting patients, are some of the intangible benefits that accrue to the nurse who specializes in eating disorders.

Case Study: Nonpsychiatric Setting

Nancy was a 16-year-old patient on a pediatric unit who had been hospitalized for a weight loss of thirty-five pounds in the last six months. She said that she "felt like a cow." She was 5'4" tall and had gone from 120 pounds to 85 pounds. She wanted to be even thinner. Her diet prior to hospitalization was limited to one bowl of dry bran flakes per day, diet soda (six–eight cans per day), unbuttered popcorn, and lettuce without dressing. Nancy chewed about three packs of sugarless gum per day and had been refusing to eat meals with the family. She was running five miles a day, regardless of weather, and did fifty situps morning and evening in addition to thirty minutes on an exercycle before bedtime.

Nancy's family (her parents, an older brother, and a younger sister) didn't realize that there was a problem until Nancy's weight dropped below 100 pounds. "Her clothes just seemed to hang on her and she seemed to be exercising constantly," said her mother. Nancy's family also began to be concerned about Nancy's obsession about being fat.

Nancy had always been an A student and was on the varsity track team. Recently, she seemed to be "driven" in both activities. She didn't go to a recent party, though she was invited, because she didn't want to be seen when she felt so fat, and because she felt that she didn't fit in with her peers. She also felt that they really didn't want to be with her either.

When Nancy's parents, over her protests, took her to the pediatrician, he found Nancy to be mildly hypokalemic, bradycardic, and amenorrheic. He said that she was dangerously underweight and suggested hospitalization for a medical assessment in order to rule out major physical illness. Since Nancy seemed to be obsessed with her diet and exercise regimen, denied depression, had a distorted body image, and seemed to be performing as well as ever in school, he suspected an eating disorder. Both Nancy and her mother were against hospitalization, Nancy because she wouldn't be able to do all her exercises, and her mother because Nancy would miss an important track meet and get behind in classes. Nancy's father was noncommittal but concerned. When Nancy's pediatrician promised her that she would only need to be hospitalized for a few days, and could go out for a walk once per day, she agreed to it.

Once in the hospital, Nancy refused to eat most of the food on her meal trays, saying she wasn't hungry, felt bloated, and was afraid of getting fat. She lost two pounds the first day in the hospital.

She talked with her primary nurse, Mary Gardner, about trivialities, denying feelings about everything. She said that she "felt fine," and didn't need to be in a hospital. She said that it would be easier for her to gain weight at home. She denied any conflict with the family, or within herself.

Nancy's medical assessment was negative and her doctor told her and her parents that he wanted to consult a child psychiatrist. Nancy's mother was outraged; Nancy shrugged her shoulders and said she didn't mind but didn't see what good it would do. She also promised that she would try to eat more. She said that this would be easier if she could go for a walk twice per day. The pediatrician agreed to this and requested a psychiatric consultation.

Nancy ate all of the food on her next meal tray, but was found vomiting shortly afterward in her bathroom. By the next morning she had lost another pound. Nancy's parents talked with her about the situation and the plan for them to see a child psychiatrist that day. They decided to remove her from the hospital since they had been reassured about her physical health and were concerned about her missing school; they agreed with Nancy that she would be more comfortable working on this eating problem at home, as long as she didn't have to eat with the family. "It's so gross to watch how much everyone eats."

While her father went to get the car and her mother to call the pediatrician, Nancy began to pack her suitcase. Her nurse, Mary, offered to help. While they packed, Nancy confided that she often felt very alone, at school and at home, and didn't care about anything but her dieting and exercising, which she said helped her feel better about herself. She said that she worried that her performance at school was slipping, and that if this continued, her mother would be very angry. The nurse told Nancy that the psychiatrist her doctor had consulted, Dr. Barbara Kelly, was easy to talk to, and understood about feelings like that and might be able to be of some help. Nancy said that it would be very hard for her to talk to anyone about these things. It would be embarrassing, and besides, she wasn't good at explaining things. In addition, even if she wanted to see Dr. Kelly, her mother was against "talking to strangers about problems." Nancy asked Mary, however, if she could talk to her again some time. Mary said that this would be difficult, since she only worked in the hospital, not in the pediatric clinic.

When Nancy's mother reached the pediatrician and told him about their decision to take Nancy out of the hospital, he said that if they did so, it would be against medical advice, and result in the termination of his involvement with them. He said that it would be impossible to help them if they refused to follow his recommendations.

Undaunted, Nancy's parents took her home that day. There Nancy continued to exercise and refuse food, losing another five pounds over the next week. She now weighed 80 pounds but continued to "feel fat" and see more weight loss as desirable. Her parents became alarmed and called the pediatrician, saying that they wished to cooperate with his treatment recommendations. He told them to take Nancy to the hospital immediately. He said he would admit her to pediatrics as before, but would request an immediate psychiatric consultation.

When they told Nancy all this, her parents were surprised to find her not only willing to be admitted to the hospital, but not at all upset about it. She only said that she hoped that her nurse, Mary, would be working that day.

Nursing Care Plan for Nancy: Nonpsychiatric Setting

Nursing Diagnosis	Desired Outcomes	Interventions	Rationale
1. Alteration in nutritional status	Nancy will establish acceptable patterns of nutrition as evidenced by (a) adequate intake, (b) normal eating patterns, and (c) normal body weight.	Help Nancy select menus with protein, fat, and carbohydrate requirements in mind. Divide the required intake into three meals and three snacks.	It is rare that a patient with an eating disorder will be able to change her pathological eating behaviors on her own, despite her knowledge of nutrition, even if she agrees that she is too thin and has an eating disorder.

Nursing Diagnosis	Desired Outcomes	Interventions	Rationale
2. Alteration in thought processes: (a) distorted body image, (b) distorted idea of eating and its relationship to weight gain, body size, and so on.	Nancy will see herself realistically as evidenced by her feeling positive about herself at a normal weight.	Communicate to Nancy that because of her eating disorder, she is not able to judge her appearance, adequate intake, etc. She needs to give up control of these things and allow others to determine what she needs right now to be healthy.	The patient with an eating disorder can be thought of as having a "psychosis" about food and eating and their effect on her. As with the psychotic patient, trying to convince Nancy that her beliefs are false is futile and may only agitate her. Empathizing with her anxiety while reassuring her that she is safe and that the treatment team will not allow her to get fat is more likely to be helpful. Encouraging Nancy to talk about her anxiety and other feelings, rather than about food and weight, and explaining that this is the way out of her unhappiness is important.
3. Disturbance in self-concept: (a) body image, (b) personal identity, (c) role performance, (d) self-esteem	Nancy will gain a positive self-concept as evidenced by (a) valuing her personal needs as she identifies them and (b) communicating her personal needs to significant others she trusts.	Talk with Nancy about what she wants and needs and legitimize those needs. Reinforce anything that qualifies as self-caretaking. Draw attention to Nancy's strengths. Communicate that even though many young women struggle with eating disorders, Nancy's situation is unique, one that she and her psychotherapist will work to understand and master.	The patient with an eating disorder denies needing anything but being thin. Helping the patient focus on feelings, beginning with those associated with being in the hospital, is the first step in the process of trying to understand this patient's psychological pain, the source of her denial. This as well as attention to her unique "self" and its nurturance counters anorexic thinking and behavior.
4. Social isolation	Nancy will establish and maintain satisfying social relationships as evidenced by her resumption of socialization with her peer group.	Involve Nancy in ward activities as well as occupational therapy. Talk with Nancy about her feelings toward her peers and about her social anxiety.	Social isolation encourages anorexic thinking and obsessing about food and weight. Positive social experiences counter negative thinking about the self and anxiety about rejection.
5. Ineffective individual coping	Nancy will develop effective individual coping as evidenced by verbalizing her feelings, rather than acting them out.	Help Nancy begin to make the connection between self-destructive behavior and feelings. Label her self-starvation and exercising to lose	Confrontation of the patient's self-destructiveness decreases its power and helps the patient trust that the nurse is strong

Nursing Diagnosis	Desired Outcomes	Interventions	Rationale
		weight as self-destructive.	enough to handle her, and is not intimidated by her "suicidality."
		Offer to help Nancy control these behaviors by being with her and offering support at mealtime and at times during the day when she usually exercises (supported exposure—see Chapter 8 on anxiety disorders).	Acknowledging Nancy's other feelings helps her to believe that the nurse (as well as the rest of the treatment team) is interested in more than just "feeding" her, a common assumption of the hospitalized eating-disorders patient.
		Ask Nancy about her feelings of anxiety, guilt, anger, and so on, and about the associated loss of control.	
6. Ineffective family coping	Nancy's family will develop effective family coping as evidenced by (a) verbalization of their needs, (b) their ability to support Nancy in her struggle, and (c) cooperation with treatment recommendations.	Talk with Nancy's family about what an eating disorder is, labeling her symptoms as evidence of deep-seated anxiety about herself and her relationships with other people.	The family of the patient with an eating disorder typically feels that what the patient needs is "to just eat." Their anxiety and guilt may interfere with their ability to understand how the patient may feel about herself and her family, and her related self-destructiveness. They also may not understand how being "tough" with their daughter despite her psychological pain can help her.
		Emphasize their need to work with the treatment team (the pediatrician, child psychiatrist, and primary nurse) and the need to prevent "splitting" (see Chapter 12 on personality disorders), which would occur if the parents again rescue Nancy from the hospital, something she is likely to demand.	The patient's family will need support as she begins to understand and express her underlying feelings, especially anger (at times, rage) at them.
		Help the family identify and express their feelings about having a daughter with an eating disorder, labeling as normal the guilt, anxiety, and anger that they feel.	
		Encourage them to participate in family therapy, offering to attend with their permission and that of Dr. Kelly and Nancy.	

Case Study: Psychiatric Setting

Nancy was readmitted to pediatrics, where she was put on a 1500-calorie diet that was to be gradually increased to 3000. She was told she had to refrain from any exercising until she reached 100 pounds. Mary Gardner continued as Nancy's primary nurse and enlisted another nurse, Ann, as co-primary nurse. Nancy was introduced to Ann and was told that she would function as Nancy's primary nurse when Mary was gone. As her primary nurse, Mary would meet with Nancy daily to help her identify and cope with feelings about being in the hospital, gaining weight, and so forth.

The psychiatrist, Barbara Kelly, met with Nancy and made the diagnosis of anorexia nervosa. She recommended both individual and family therapy. She felt that Nancy should remain on pediatrics rather than be transferred to the psychiatric unit because of her relationship with her primary nurse, which was very positive. She planned to meet Nancy for forty-five minutes twice a week. Family therapy would be held weekly in the hospital, and Nancy's primary nurse was invited to attend.

Nancy began to eat, but her weight did not change. After several days, she told Mary that she had been hiding some of the food she was given and vomited what she did eat. She said she felt frightened about eating, fearing that it would make her fat. Mary talked with Nancy about this and empathized with her but reiterated that she was dangerously low in weight and had to eat despite how painful that was. She suggested that Nancy think of eating as "surgery that was frightening and left her hurting temporarily, but which was needed for her survival."

Nancy began to eat. Her bathroom was locked and she was monitored for one hour after meals and a half hour after snacks. She began to gain weight. She met with her nurse daily and looked forward to their time together. She was not sure how she felt about Dr. Kelly, however, and was dreading the first family session. She was very happy that Mary would be there.

Nancy's progress was slow but steady over the next three weeks. By the end of the third week, she weighed 85½ pounds. At that time, Mary told her that she would be going on vacation for two weeks, starting the following week, but that Ann would continue to see her. (Ann and Nancy had been meeting when Mary was off duty.) Nancy seemed to take the news surprisingly well, but the day before Mary left, Nancy told her that she hated herself and she was thinking about suicide. Mary told Dr. Kelly about this, and, feeling guilty, left for her vacation.

Nancy again refused to eat. When she was threatened with tube feeding, she began to eat but vomited on the floor of her room, even when the nurse was present. It was suspected that she was also exercising whenever she was not supervised. By the end of the first week of Mary's vacation, Nancy had lost six pounds and Dr. Kelly determined, on the basis of Nancy's now depressed mood and the nurses' report that she was sleeping all the time and was very difficult to rouse in the morning, that she was clinically depressed (see Chapter 9 on mood disorders). When Nancy impulsively cut her wrists superficially with a glass she took from a meal tray and broke at change of shift, when the nurses were in report, Dr. Kelly transferred her to the psychiatric unit despite Nancy's protest. There Nancy was put on suicide precautions (see Chapter 18 on psychological crisis) and bed rest. Either a nurse or one of Nancy's parents was to be with her around the clock. If she vomited after eating, she would immediately be given a high-calorie liquid feeding, equaling the estimated amount of lost calories. If Nancy refused or vomited that, she would be refed the liquid supplement through a nasogastric tube.

Nancy was told that when she reached 85½ pounds, she would be allowed out of bed at intervals to participate in ward activities such as group therapy, supervised exercise, and occupational therapy. When she reached 90 pounds, she would be allowed a twenty-minute walk per day with her nurse. Nancy was introduced to her new primary nurse, Janet, a member of the staff who had special expertise in working with patients with eating disorders. During their first session together, Janet asked Nancy how she felt about being on the psychiatric unit. Nancy began to sob and say how badly she felt about Mary leaving her to go on vacation.

Nursing Care Plan For Nancy: Psychiatric Setting

Nursing Diagnosis	Desired Outcomes	Interventions	Rationale
1. Alteration in nutritional status related to anxiety regarding eating and weight gain	Nancy will achieve adequate nutritional intake as evidenced by gradual weight gain.	Monitor Nancy during meals and snacks, and for one hour after meals and one half hour after snacks. Offer empathy and support at that time (supported exposure). Refeed with Sustacal (a high-calorie liquid supplement) if food is refused or vomited. If Sustacal is refused, refeed the Sustacal through a nasogastric tube. Bathroom is locked and water turned off.	Even the motivated eating-disorders patient who agrees that she needs to gain weight must be closely monitored during and after meals as this is the most stressful part of this patient's day, and the time she is most likely to impulsively sabotage her treatment. This is also the time when she most needs the nurse's understanding and support. 　If necessary, tube feeding should be done in order to reassure the patient that the treatment program is stronger than she is.
2. Ineffective individual coping	Nancy will develop effective individual coping as evidenced by replacing acting-out of feelings via self-destructive behavior (vomiting, wrist cutting, and so on) with expressing them verbally to the nurse and/or her therapist.	Take suicide precautions, including a no-suicide contract to be signed each shift (see Chapter 18 on psychological crises). Arrange for a meeting between Nancy, her pediatric nurse (Mary), and her new primary nurse to discuss Nancy's transfer to psychiatry. Discuss her need for continuing supportive psychotherapy by primary nurse through daily contacts focused on identifying and verbalizing feelings of abandonment, anxiety, anger, and suicidality.	Nancy's recent suicide attempt puts her at risk for another. Continuing daily contacts with her primary nurse will be essential to the treatment program's success, as setting and enforcing limits on behavior are certain to stir up feelings that the patient will need help with understanding and expressing. 　Treatment team members need to be in close contact regarding the approach to Nancy to prevent or deal with splitting, the patient's attempt to "divide and conquer."

Nursing Diagnosis	Desired Outcomes	Interventions	Rationale
		Primary nurse to meet with Nancy and Dr. Kelly once a week in order to (1) prevent splitting (Nancy experiencing one as for her and the other as against her) and (2) talk with Dr. Kelly about a consistent approach to Nancy, and countertransference related to feelings about trying to "fill Mary's shoes."	Transfer to another unit and change of primary nurse is a set-up for a successful split by the patient.
3. Powerlessness and noncompliance (unwillingness to follow prescribed plan of treatment due to conflict with goal of treatment)	Nancy will develop a sense of personal effectiveness as evidenced by her ability to identify self-preservation needs and get them met.	Draw up a contract with Nancy regarding her program to gain weight and have her sign it. Breaking the contract will result in loss of time with primary nurse that day, as it will be interpreted as meaning that Nancy does not want her nurse's help, but prefers to manage her feelings her own way. (Repeated breaking of contract will lead to consideration by Dr. Kelly and staff of transferring Nancy to a long-term care psychiatric facility where she can be taken care of until she is ready to become actively involved in a treatment program).	Nancy's responsibility for her behavior and the success or failure of her treatment must be clear. The program and the team make it *possible* for Nancy to succeed in overcoming her eating disorder. Only she can make it happen.
4. Diversional activity deficit	Nancy will reduce the deficit of diversional activities as evidenced by a return to normal activities of daily living appropriate for Nancy's age group.	Arrange for regular contact between Nancy and the school, for example, through meetings with her teachers, homework, taping lecturers, and so on. Ask occupational therapist to suggest and provide for recreational activities while Nancy is on bed rest.	Diversional activities interfere with obsessing about food and weight and remind Nancy of a life outside the hospital and its incompatibility with a severe eating disorder.
		Suggest to Nancy that she begin a "feelings journal."	Focusing on *feelings* rather than on food and weight should be done at every opportunity.

Nursing Diagnosis	Desired Outcomes	Interventions	Rationale
5. Sleep pattern disturbance	Nancy will return to a normal sleep pattern as evidenced by 8 hours of sleep per night with no daytime naps.	Encourage Nancy to stay busy during the daytime, increasing physical activity as appropriate as she gains weight. Label her increased sleeping as "withdrawal" from her problems, something that will only make them worse. Remind her that, despite her feelings of abandonment, she is not alone in her struggle. Report continued withdrawal through sleep to Dr. Kelly who is considering starting Nancy on anti-depressant medication.	Sleeping excessively is often a defense against painful feelings, in this case, as a result of eating and weight gain. The sleep disturbance in the depressed adolescent typically involves increased sleeping rather than insomnia. (See Chapter 9 on mood disorders for more on symptoms and treatment of depression.)

SUMMARY

During the past twenty years, the rising incidence of eating disorders has become a grave concern for health professionals and for the general public. Although since the late 1970s researchers and clinicians have viewed bulimia (binge eating) as distinct from anorexia (restrictive eating), many still feel that the two disorders have distinct similarities. Many patients do, in fact, present with symptoms of both.

Patients in both groups have a terrible fear of becoming fat. Anorexia nervosa is characterized by the patient's deliberate starvation, with the intention of becoming thin. Psychiatrist Hilde Bruch identified three main features of the anorexic patient: 1) disturbance in body image; 2) disturbance in the perception of internal states; and 3) a paralyzing sense of ineffectiveness. Bulimia nervosa is characterized by the patient's binge eating, followed by purging, usually accomplished by vomiting or taking laxatives. Bulimic patients want to be thin but are often unsuccessful because of the nature of their symptoms. The bulimic patient is often depressed. Prolonged starvation, vomiting, and laxative abuse all have serious medical consequences that are usually secondary to malnutrition, dehydration, and disturbances in electrolyte balance.

Within the broad category of psychoanalytic theory, which concentrates on the development of the individual personality, there are three major theories regarding etiology of eating disorders: ego psychology, which emphasizes ego development, especially self-image, body image, recognition of internal states, and self-esteem; object-relations theory, which holds that problems in early childhood relationships contribute to personality development that predisposes an individual to the development of an eating disorder; and integrated developmental theory, which attempts to consolidate the analytic theories and integrate them with family-systems theory to construct a model that differentiates between anorexia and bulimia. The feminist perspective criticizes theories that blame patients' mothers for their psychological or emotional deficiencies.

Family-systems theory views the patient who has an eating disorder within the context of the family as a whole. Fallon identified three types of families and their areas of conflict: the perfect family, the overprotective family, and the chaotic family.

The treatment of an eating disorder is a long-term process. Patients may be treated on an outpatient or an inpatient basis. Most treatment programs use at least some of the principles of behavior modification to address the symptoms of eating disorders. Specific cognitive-behavioral techniques, such as psychoeducation, meal planning, introduction of avoided foods, self-monitoring, and stimulus control are also used.

The nurse may encounter some special issues when treating the patient with an eating disorder: intense countertransference, feelings of impotence, overinvolvement or underinvolvement with the patient, splitting, and lack of conflict resolution among members of the treatment team (similar to that often found in the patient's family).

KEY TERMS

anorexia nervosa

bulimia nervosa

binge eating

psychoanalytic theory

ego psychology

object-relations theory

separation-individuation

self-regulation

family-systems theory

enmeshment

perfect family

overprotective family

chaotic family

self-monitoring

stimulus control

countertransference

splitting

STUDY QUESTIONS

1. Define and describe the symptoms of both anorexia nervosa and bulimia nervosa.

2. Name and describe three theories which discuss the etiology of eating disorders within the broad category of psychoanalytic theory.

3. Describe family-systems theory, including three major subtheories.

4. Name and describe at least three of the specific cognitive-behavioral techniques for treatment of patients with eating disorders.

5. Name and describe at least three of the special issues a nurse may face when working with patients with eating disorders.

REFERENCES

Agras, S., & Werne, J. (1981). Disorders of eating. In S. Turner, K. Calhoun, & H. Adams (Eds.), *Handbook of clinical behavior therapy*. New York: John Wiley & Sons, pp. 214–239.

American Psychiatric Association. (1987). *Diagnostic and statistical manual of mental disorders*, 3rd ed., Revised. Washington, D.C.: APA.

Anderson, A., Morse, C., & Santmeyer, K. (1984). Inpatient treatment for anorexia nervosa. In Garner, D., & Garfinkel, P. (Eds.), *Handbook of psychotherapy for anorexia nervosa and bulimia*. New York: The Guilford Press.

Beaumont, P. J. V., George, G. C. W., & Smart, D. E. (1976). "Dieters" and "vomiters and purgers" in anorexia nervosa. *Psychological Medicine, 6,* 617–622.

Boskind-Lodahl, M. (1976). Cinderella's stepsisters: A feminist perspective on anorexia nervosa and bulimia. *Signs: Journal of Women in Culture and Society, 2*(21), 342–356.

Brenner, C. (1974). *An elementary textbook of psychoanalysis*. New York: Anchor Books.

Bruch, H. (1973). *Eating disorders: Obesity, anorexia nervosa, and the person within*. New York: Basic Books.

Bruch, H. (1984). Four decades of eating disorders. In Garner, D., & Garfinkel, P. (Eds.), *Handbook of psychotherapy for anorexia nervosa and bulimia*. New York: The Guilford Press.

Fairburn, C. (1984). Cognitive-behavioral treatment for bulimia. In Garner, D., & Garfinkel, P. (Eds.), *Handbook of psychotherapy for anorexia nervosa and bulimia*. New York: The Guilford Press.

Fairburn, C. (1986, October). Controversial issues in the diagnosis of anorexia nervosa and bulimia nervosa. In *Being effective in assessment, treatment, and prevention*. Columbus, Ohio: The Fifth National Conference on Eating Disorders.

Fallon, P. (1986, October). Treating bulimic families: A feminist family systems perspective. In *Being effective in assessment, treatment, and prevention*. Columbus, Ohio: The Fifth National Conference on Eating Disorders.

Garner, D. (1986, October). Introduction to eating disorders: Clinical considerations and medical issues. In *Being effective in assessment, treatment, and prevention*. Columbus, Ohio: The Fifth National Conference on Eating Disorders.

Garner, D., & Garfinkel, P. (1982). *Anorexia nervosa: A multi-dimensional perspective*. New York: Brunner/Mazel.

Garner, D., Rockert, W., Olsted, M., Johnson, C., & Coscina, D. (1984). Psychoeducational principles in the treatment of bulimia and anorexia nervosa. In Garner, D., & Garfinkel, P. (Eds.), *Handbook of psychotherapy for anorexia nervosa and bulimia*. New York: The Guilford Press.

Gilligan, C. (1984, November). Feminist perspective on eating disorder. In *center for study of anorexia and bulimia conference:* New York.

Gray, J., & Ford, K. (1985). The incidence of bulimia in a college sample. *The International Journal of Eating Disorders, 4*(2), 201–210.

Harris, R. (1983). Bulimarexia and related serious eating disorders with medical complications. *Annals of Internal Medicine, 99,* 800–807.

Herzog, D. (1988). Eating disorders. In A. M. Nicoli, Jr. (Ed.), *The new Harvard guide to psychiatry*. Cambridge: Belknap Press of Harvard University Press.

Hudson, J. (1986, October). Psychopharmacology in the treatment of eating disorders. In *Being effective in assessment, treatment, and prevention*. Columbus, Ohio: The Fifth National Conference on Eating Disorders.

Humphrey, L. (1987). Familywide distress in bulimia. In D. Cannon & T. Baker (Eds.), *Addictive disorders: Psychological assessment and treatment*. New York: Praeger.

Johnson, C. (1986, October). Treating the eating disorders patient with a character disorder. In *Being effective in assessment, treatment, and prevention*. Columbus, Ohio: The Fifth National Conference on Eating Disorders.

Johnson, C., & Connors, M. (1987). *The etiology and treatment of bulimia nervosa: A biopsychosocial approach*. New York: Basic Books.

Jones, D. J., Fox, M. M., Babigan, H. M., & Hutton, H. E. (1980). Epidemiology of anorexia nervosa in Monroe County, New York: 1960–1976. *Psychosomatic Medicine, 42*, 551–558.

Keys, A., Brozek, J., Henschel, A., Mickelsen, O., & Taylor, H. L. (1950). *The biology of human starvation*. Minneapolis: University of Minneapolis Press.

Lucas, A. (1981). Toward the understanding of anorexia nervosa as a disease entity. *Mayo Clinic Proc., 56*, 254–264

Mahler, M., Pine, F., & Bergman, A. (1975). *The psychological birth of the human infant*. New York: Basic Books.

Masterson, J. (1978). The borderline adolescent: An object relations view. In S. C. Feinstein & P. L. Giovacchini (Eds.), *Adolescent psychiatry* (v. VI). Chicago: University of Chicago Press.

Maxmen, J. S. (1986). *Essential psychopathology*. New York: W.W. Norton & Co.

Minuchin, S. (1974). *Families and family therapy*. Cambridge, Mass.: Harvard University Press.

Mosak, H. (1979). Adlerian psychotherapy. In *Current psychotherapies*. Stasca: F. E. Peacock.

Orbach, S. (1985). Accepting the symptom: A feminist psychoanalytic treatment of anorexia nervosa. In Garner, D., & Garfinkel, P. (Eds.), *Handbook of psychotherapy for anorexia nervosa and bulimia*. New York: The Guilford Press.

Pope, H. G., Hudson, J. I., Jonas, J. M., and Yurgelum, T. D. (1983). Bulimia treated with imipramine: A placebo-controlled double-blind study. *American Journal of Psychiatry, 140*, 554–558.

Pyle, R. L., Mitchell, J. E., Eckert, E. E., Halvorson, P. A., Newman, P. A., & Goff, G. M. (1983). The incidence of bulimia in freshman college students. *International Journal of Eating Disorders, 2*(3), 75–86.

Root, M., Fallon, P., & Friedrich, W. (1986). *Bulimia: A systems approach to treatment*. New York: W.W. Norton & Co.

Russell, G. (1979). Bulimia nervosa: An ominous variant of anorexia nervosa. *Psychological Medicine, 9*, 429–448.

Settlage, C. F. (1977). The psychoanalytic understanding of narcissistic and borderline personality disorders: Advances in developmental theory. *Journal of the American Psychoanalytic Association, 25*(4), 805–833.

Swift, W. (1982). The long-term outcome of early onset anorexia nervosa: A critical review. *Journal of the American Academy of Child Psychiatry, 21*(1), 38–46.

Walsh, B. T., Stewart, J. W., Roose, S. P., Gladis, M., & Glassman, A. H. (1984). Treatment of bulimia with phenelzine: A double-blind, placebo-controlled study. *Archives of General Psychiatry. 41*, 1105–1109.

Wetherby, B., and Baumeister, A. (1981). Mental retardation. In Turner, S., Calhoun, K., and Adams, H. (Eds.). *Handbook of clinical behavior therapy*. New York: John Wiley & Sons, pp. 635–664.

Wooley, S. & Wooley, W. (1984). Intensive outpatient and residential treatment for bulimia. In Garner, D., & Garfinkel, P. (Eds.), *Handbook of psychotherapy for anorexia nervosa and bulimia*. New York: The Guilford Press.

15

LEARNING OBJECTIVES

After studying this chapter, the student will be able to:

- Describe the difference between substance abuse and substance dependence.
- Assess patients for potential substance abuse and dependence.
- Discuss the different theories of substance abuse.
- Identify and compare the different modes of treatment of the substance abuser.
- Develop nursing diagnoses and nursing care plans for the substance abuser.

SUBSTANCE ABUSE

MEL HAGGART

INTRODUCTION

Substance abuse is a major, pervasive public health problem. It is endemic in most communities, reaches all levels of society, and affects people in all professions. It is a subject that, in recent years, has been the focus of nationwide campaigns and much debate by legislators, health-care professionals, and the general public. Yet there are few areas in mental health in which experts disagree so fundamentally.

Substance abuse is a melting pot in which genetics, culture, and psychodynamics intermingle. Substance abuse encompasses a complex array of conditions that vary widely in nature and clinical course. These conditions have been only marginally investigated and remain poorly understood, despite being among the most common problems presenting for treatment.

Substance abuse has been neglected in clinical practice as well. For example, a study by Westermeyer et al. (1978), which was conducted in an academic setting, demonstrated the failure of physicians and nurses to obtain even minimal information regarding the drug and alcohol use of their patients. Incredibly, this neglect occurred even for cases in which referral information suggested substance abuse as an underlying cause of a patient's problems.

Despite confusion regarding its causes, public bias against its victims, and the professional indifference exposed by Westermeyer, substance abuse remains one of the nation's foremost health problems. It is a substantial factor in the physical and emotional disorders of many patients and a ubiquitous presence in a number of our society's problems. Currently, the expanding consumption of psychoactive substances and the disastrous consequences of their use have led to greater public awareness of the problem, growth of treatment programs specializing in these conditions, and efforts at control and prevention from the local to the national level.

This climate has created concern and demand for services and underlined the responsibilities of health professionals to substance-abuse patients. Indeed, the task of recognition and treatment of substance abuse has become a major task of the health-care team. In most cases, nurses play a pivotal role due to their frequent contact with patients and their families, and the resulting opportunity to establish the clinical rapport needed to uncover this problem.

This chapter presents the information needed to assess, manage, and treat the substance-abuse disorders, and the role of the nurse in these three areas of clinical practice is explored. Discussion emphasizes a holistic approach to patients and a recognition of the complexities of their problems. Although the chapter presents information regarding all types of substance abuse, it focuses on alcoholism as the most familiar and best researched of the disorders.

PATTERNS OF USE

It seems difficult for most people to appreciate how common substance abuse is. Alcoholism has been called the most untreated treatable disease. Studies show substance abuse to be associated with at least 15 percent of the total health-care cost in this country and perhaps as much as 25 percent of general hospital admissions. In addition, substance abuse is linked with many problems other than physical illness. For example, more than one-third of suicides involve alcohol. Alcohol abuse has been identified in more than half of the families in which marital violence occurs, and it appears as a major causative factor in driving and industrial accidents, fires and arson, robbery, incest and rape, assaults, and homicides.

It is estimated that from 7–10 percent of the population in the United States is "alcoholic," and that 0.5 percent is addicted to narcotics. One-third of the families in our country are affected by substance abuse, and some estimates suggest that up to 50 percent of individuals seeking counseling services have a problem influenced by alcohol or other drugs.

The above statistics point to a problem with profound and widespread consequences. The substance abuser damages not only himself but his family, friends, and society at large as well.

Nonetheless, an expanding insight into substance use has permitted a view of the abuser not only as victimizer but victim as well, a person caught in the web of genetic predisposition, a drug tolerant culture, and a disturbed social milieu.

A knowledge of how these disorders interface with the community, and the ways in which they spread and change, can provide much insight into their nature and facilitate the planning of effective treatment programs. With the swell of attention focused on substance abuse, the epidemiology of these conditions has flourished and developed into a specialty in its own right. Two important issues have emerged: the importance of social and cultural factors in substance abuse, and the shifting nature of its prevalence in response to conditions outside the individual and his family. The history of cocaine abuse, currently a common disorder, is a case in point.

523

Gay and Sheppard (1973) and McLaughlin (1973), among others, have described the passage of cocaine into Western society. Before the arrival of Europeans in South America, the native Indian populations are believed to have used cocaine in ritualistic ways and to have restricted it to members of the upper classes. Following the conquest by the Spanish, the drug was interdicted for religious reasons. But once it was found that native workers could perform more work under adverse conditions if encouraged to chew the coca leaves from which raw cocaine is extracted, its use became progressively more extensive. Meanwhile, in Europe, cocaine was widely touted as a wonder drug by Sigmund Freud and others, an enthusiasm that only increased once its anesthetic properties were discovered. In the United States cocaine was at first sold openly and was an ingredient in many widely used patent medicines, such as the original Coca Cola. With experience, it was found that the benefits of the drug were primarily confined to its use as a local anesthetic, while its addictive and destructive effects became more obvious. Ultimately, at the turn of the century, the Pure Food and Drug Act, and a few years later, the Harrison Act, tightened controls on the use and possession of cocaine; it appears that from the 1920s to the 1950s, the use of cocaine was minimal and more or less confined to fringe subcultures. Since the 1960s, however, use of cocaine has been on the rise and has become socially acceptable in many areas of the country, particularly in the upper socioeconomic classes. In recent years, the price of the drug has

Box 15–1 ● It's Hard to Crack Down on Crack

Scientists doing research on drug addiction say that crack, the smokable form of cocaine, is the most troubling drug they have studied.

Once people become addicted, these experts say, it is nearly impossible for them to stop using crack and never go back to it again.

At the same time, researchers offer a modest message of hope—that various treatments may help restore crack addicts to functioning lives.

The researchers' new understanding of the biochemistry of crack addiction has led them to develop medical treatments that help quiet the craving for crack in the first few weeks of withdrawal, when addicts are particularly likely to relapse.

Researchers also are developing long-term programs to help crack users stay away from the drug and to help them escape its grip when they slip back to abusing it again.

But they think that the struggle to stay away from crack will be lifelong for former addicts and that the vast majority will relapse at least once.

"Crack is by far the most addictive drug we've ever had to deal with," said Dr. Charles O'Brien of the University of Pennsylvania School of Medicine in Philadelphia.

"It is highly, rapidly addictive. We see people who feel they lost control almost from the first time they used it. Most people who got started with crack were addicted in six months to a year. With heroin, the average time until people lose control is 10 years."

O'Brien estimates that "only a very small percentage, 25 percent or less" of crack addicts remain drug-free for even six months in most treatment programs.

Yet, he said, 60 percent of heroin addicts can stay away from the drug in methadone maintenance programs for at least six months. Eighty to 85 percent of alcoholics who come for treatment early in the course of their addiction can stay away from alcohol for at least six months and 50 percent of more chronic alcoholics can forgo alcohol for at least six months, O'Brien said.

To make matters worse, there is a shortage of treatment programs even for those crack addicts who are highly motivated and eager for help. Researchers say that they are still feeling their way in developing programs and that lack of money and resources is a severe problem.

Crack, like cocaine that is snorted, produces euphoria by stimulating a pleasure center in the base of the brain, in an area connected to nerves that are responsible for emotions. This area of the brain is stim-

fallen, due to an enormous increase in the supply of cocaine coming into the United States from South America. The decreasing cost has promoted its spread, and as a consequence of extensive abuse of the drug in various forms such as crack, centers specializing in the treatment of cocaine abuse have started to appear. (See Box 15–1.)

The history of cocaine is thus one of a complex series of events in the epidemiology of a substance-abuse condition based in part on availability and price of the substance, its acceptability in the social milieu of the user, legislative action, and originally, misunderstandings regarding the nature and potential of its harmful effects. Patterns of abuse of a substance may change in response to many factors, and effective management and diagnosis of these conditions requires professionals to keep up to date with current trends.

For example, heroin and other opiate use, traditionally believed to be confined to the inner city, has begun to cross class and cultural boundaries. There is evidence of growing heroin use by executives, and Flax (1985) has reported heroin use as one of the more underrecognized substance-abuse conditions. Part of the problem in recognizing narcotics abuse is both its low social acceptability, with abusers ashamed to come forward for help, and the stereotyped thinking of clinicians who neglect to ask middle- and upper-class patients for a drug history. (See Box 15–2.)

---

ulated every time a person feels joy or pleasure.

Cocaine stimulates this pleasure center to a far greater degree than it would ever normally be stimulated. The result is euphoria: a feeling of increased energy, of being mentally more alert, of feeling really good.

The dark side of crack, however, is that the euphoria fades quickly as cocaine levels drop, leaving the users feeling depressed, anxious, pleasureless.

Researchers say that because crack produces such an intense euphoria, people start associating the crack high with anything that happened to be in their surroundings when they smoked, specific people or locations, for instance.

Months, or even years later, they will experience urgent, and often irresistible cravings if they see these cues again. Such reactions to cues occur with other addictive drugs as well, experts say, but cues set off more intense longings in crack addicts.

With their growing knowledge of the biochemistry of cocaine addiction, researchers are having new success in helping addicts get through the first few weeks without crack.

Gawin and Kleber have been using an anti-depressant, desiprimine, on the theory that the addict's brain is altered by crack use so that, at least in the initial periods of abstinence, the addict cannot feel normal emotions.

At a recent scientific meeting, they described a study in which cocaine addicts were given desiprimine, lithium, which is another anti-depressant, or an inert substance for three weeks. Sixty percent of those taking desiprimine remained drug-free, 23 percent of the lithium patients could stay away from cocaine and 17 percent of those who got an inactive substance abstained from cocaine for at least three weeks.

But, Kleber said, these short-term treatments are no cure. "The major problem is not just getting off drugs but staying off," he said.

Source: Kolata, G. (1988). Crack worst drug, researchers say. *The Wisconsin State Journal,* July 26, p. 8A.

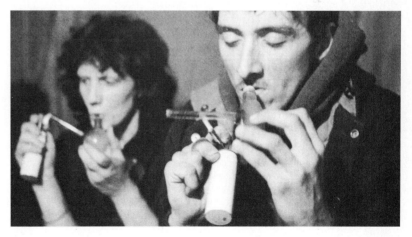

Crack is the drug of choice in most poor communities today because the initial purchases are so relatively cheap. As recently as one year ago, crack addiction was thought to be impossible to treat. But the experts' attitude has shifted. They now feel that treatment is possible, the key being "giving the addict a place in family and social structures where they may have never been before" or giving them "habilation rather than rehabilitation." (From Kolata, *The New York Times,* Aug. 24, 1989, p. 1)

Box 15–2 ● Marijuana

Although still illegal, marijuana is used regularly by millions and occasionally by millions more. Its use reached a high point in the late 1970s and early 1980s and has been declining ever since. Attitudes expressed in surveys show why habitual marijuana use is in decline. In 1978, 65 percent of high school students disapproved of it. In 1985, 85 percent disapproved. In 1978, 35 percent said it was very risky; in 1985, 70 percent said it was.

One risk is an acute anxiety reaction. The more common of disturbing reactions to marijuana, it is sometimes accompanied by paranoid thoughts or fear of dying or going insane. Mounting anxiety may lead to panic. The inexperienced user taking a high dose in an unpleasant or unfamiliar setting is especially vulnerable to this reaction, which is best

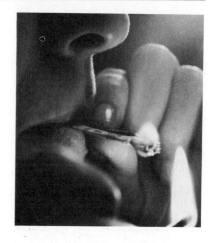

handled with calming support and reassurance while the effects of the drug fade.

Source: *The Harvard Medical School Mental Health Letter, 4,* No. 5, November 1987.

In general, there is an increasing number of women and teenagers, and even younger children, involved in substance abuse, especially in the form of alcohol abuse and dependence. The most common form of substance abuse at present is polydrug abuse. This is a pattern of drug use consisting either of the concurrent use of multiple drugs or the sequential use of a drug to counter the effects of another drug, for example, amphetamines to get going in the morning and sedatives to slow down at night.

A neotemperance movement countering the expansion of drug use in the United States has also appeared. Since the 1960s, this trend has advanced in a number of different directions. Prominent figures, such as former first lady Betty Ford, have made public their struggles with their own addictions and served as inspirations to others; legislative action has toughened drunk-driving laws; a national campaign has advertised the impact of abuse on our society and fostered public education; and national media, schools, churches, and other public organizations such as Mothers against Drunk Driving (MADD) have begun educating the public about these conditions and their early recognition. Associated with these efforts has been the first decline in alcohol consumption in the United States since World War II.

Nonalcoholic bars are enjoying success, and mineral water may be gradually replacing the martini as the favorite drink at the business lunch (Reed, 1985).

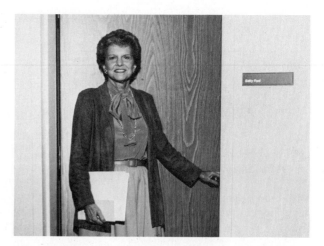

When former first lady Betty Ford admitted to having a problem with alcohol and pain-killers prescribed for a "pinched nerve" in her neck, she made quite an impression on the public who named her woman of the year for her courage in coming forward. She later founded the Betty Ford Center and today many people with substance abuse problems are treated there.

CLASSIFICATION AND DSM-III-R

Our ability to classify disorders to a large extent reflects our understanding of the disorders and their interrelationships. The more advanced our knowledge, the more meaningful our classifications, and the more helpful they will be to clinicians applying them in practice. As our experience and insight increase, our classifications of mental-health disorders will change, and as new conditions are discovered, new classifications will appear. The changes in the use of cocaine in our culture should underscore the important point that substance abuse has changed in nature and frequency over time. Along with these changes in substance abuse has come an evolution in social attitudes toward it.

During the 1800s, alcoholism was often regarded as a form of moral degeneration. Articles and pamphlets disparaging the "vice" of alcoholism were common. Although it is no longer acceptable in clinical settings to hold such a view openly, it unfortunately still remains as a prejudice in the minds of many clinicians.

A second view of many health professionals has been that substance abuse is a secondary problem, that is, a symptom of some other, more primary underlying disorder. For example, in DSM-I, alcoholism and drug addictions were listed under the personality disorders, reflecting the opinion that development of a personality disorder preceded the emergence of substance abuse.

Since the 1960s, the **disease concept of alcoholism** has become the dominant conceptualization of alcoholism by most professional organizations and prominent clinicians. In a sense, the disease model views the alcoholic as a victim, that is a person who, through no fault of his own, has acquired a "medical condition." Viewing alcoholism as a disease implies that it can be studied, diagnosed, and treated, in the same way that one approaches coronary artery disease, lung cancer, or any other physical ailment. It, however, does not imply that patients are not responsible for themselves. Hypertensives are expected to reduce salt intake, patients with emphysema are expected to stop smoking, and alcholics are expected to stop drinking. Vaillant (1983) has reviewed the disease concept of alcoholism, a point of view that still remains controversial, from both its theoretical and emotional standpoints. Essentially, the main objections against the disease model as a way of thinking about alcoholism have been that it has the appearance of a "volitional" disorder, is very strongly influenced by cultural and societal factors, and is difficult to define in a discrete way. The diagnosis of alcoholism is of course to some extent a subjective judgment, one that cannot help but be influenced by the examiner's own personal biases. Indeed, it seems almost impossible to decide where heavy drinking stops and alcoholism begins on the continuum of alcohol use.

Although the medical model (disease concept) may not completely account for all the features of alcoholism, it has much to add to the way we view substance abuse. Whatever the cause, once present, substance abuse takes on a life of its own, often requiring professional intervention, and in many patients, following a progressive or chronic relapsing course. The use of the medical model has substantially promoted the idea that alcoholics should be treated and that funding should be provided for this treatment, that research into its causes is a legitimate endeavor, and that those suffering from this disorder are victims, not villains.

The DSM-III-R classification system of substance abuse has been designed to develop a classification that is free from theoretical and personal bias; it adheres to the disease model and assigns the substance abuse conditions to the separate category of substance use disorders under the Axis I disorders.

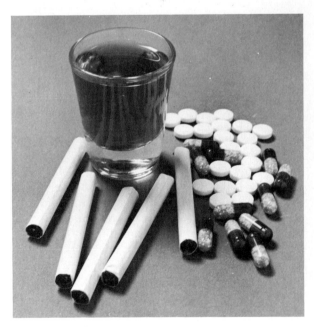

The adult version of a security blanket. We'd be better off with the real thing, as Gene Wilder did in *The Producers*, by carrying a small patch of the original in his back pocket.

DSM-III-R Diagnostic criteria for Psychoactive Substance Dependence

A. At least three of the following:

(1) substance often taken in larger amounts or over a longer period than the person intended

(2) persistent desire or one or more unsuccessful efforts to cut down or control substance use

(3) a great deal of time spent in activities necessary to get the substance (e.g., theft), taking the substance (e.g., chain smoking), or recovering from its effects

(4) frequent intoxication or withdrawal symptoms when expected to fulfill major role obligations at work, school, or home (e.g., does not go to work because hung over, goes to school or work "high," intoxicated while taking care of his or her children), or when substance use is physically hazardous (e.g., drives when intoxicated)

(5) important social, occupational, or recreational activities given up or reduced because of substance use

(6) continued substance use despite knowledge of having a persistent or recurrent social, psychological, or physical problem that is caused or exacerbated by the use of the substance (e.g., keeps using heroin despite family arguments about it, cocaine-induced depression, or having an ulcer made worse by drinking)

(7) marked tolerance: need for markedly increased amounts of the substance (i.e., at least a 50% increase) in order to achieve intoxication or desired effect, or markedly diminished effect with continued use of the same amount

Note: the following items may not apply to cannabis, hallucinogens, or phencyclidine (PCP):

(8) characteristic withdrawal symptoms (see specific withdrawal syndromes under psychoactive substance-induced organic mental disorders)

(9) substance often taken to relieve or avoid withdrawal symptoms

B. Some symptoms of the disturbance have persisted for at least one month, or have occurred repeatedly over a longer period of time.

In a culture in which alcohol is often an integral part of daily life and drug use is often termed "recreational" or "experimental," simple use of a substance can hardly qualify as sufficient to diagnose a disorder. This leaves the medical community with the difficult problem of determining how much is too much, or answering the question: When does use become **abuse?** DSM-III-R resolves this by distinguishing between dependence and abuse.

In DSM-III-R, the definition of **dependence** has been broadened to include behaviors, cognitions, and other symptoms that indicate a lack of control of substance use and continued use of the substance despite negative consequences. Dependence includes, but is no longer limited to (as in DSM-III), the physiologic symptoms of tolerance and withdrawal. **Tolerance** is

the need for increasing amounts of a substance to produce the desired effect. The absolute amount is less important than the fact that the patient needs more of the substance now than before to get high or to relieve tension or pain. **Withdrawal** is a syndrome precipitated by abrupt discontinuance of a substance that an individual has regularly used. Withdrawal is more than a hangover or a craving for the drug; it is a collection of signs and symptoms that are generally substance specific. Some patients who experience the symptoms of tolerance and withdrawal may not be dependent, hence the changes in DSM-III-R.

In DSM-III-R, abuse is a maladaptive pattern of substance use which does not meet the criteria for dependence. It is most often applied to people who

**DSM-III-R
Diagnostic criteria for
Psychoactive
Substance Abuse**

A. A maladaptive pattern of psychoactive substance use indicated by at least one of the following:

(1) continued use despite knowledge of having a persistent or recurrent social, occupational, psychological, or physical problem that is caused or exacerbated by use of the psychoactive substance

(2) recurrent use in situations in which use is physically hazardous (e.g., driving while intoxicated)

B. Some symptoms of the disturbance have persisted for at least one month, or have occurred repeatedly over a longer period of time.

C. Never met the criteria for psychoactive substance dependence for this substance.

have only recently started substance use and to substances which are less likely to be associated with withdrawal symptoms, such as cannabis and cocaine.

DSM-III-R recognizes nine classes of substances associated with both abuse and dependence: alcohol; amphetamine or similar acting sympathomimetics; cannabis; cocaine; hallucinogens; inhalants; opioids; phencyclidine (PCP) or similarly acting arylcyclohexylamines; and sedatives, hypnotics, or anxiolytics. Nicotine is associated with dependence only, as abuse is rare.

The actual diagnosis names the substance first and then states whether abuse or dependence is present. This can be followed by an optional number code that specifies the clinical course of the patient. A polydrug user would receive a different diagnosis for each psychoactive substance he uses and all combinations are possible. A diagnosis of polysubstance dependence would be applicable if the person has used at least three categories of substances (not including nicotine and caffeine), with no one substance dominating, for at least six months, and meets the criteria for dependence. There is a separate category for unspecified dependence or abuse that would be used if the specific substance used is not listed in DSM-III-R, such as anticholinergics. A patient being treated for narcotics withdrawal, who has a history of driving while intoxicated, and who smokes heavily, might receive the diagnoses of opioid dependence, alcohol abuse, and nicotine dependence.

Associated with substance abuse are a number of physical sequelae which are listed in DSM-III-R under a different category. These would be, for example, withdrawal syndromes, various acute psychotic conditions, conditions resembling depression, and organic brain syndromes. These are classified under

the organic mental disorders and will not be discussed further here, although the intoxication and withdrawal syndromes will be described. (See, instead, Chapter 11 on Organic Mental Disorders.)

BIOCHEMICAL SUBSTRATES OF COMMONLY ABUSED SUBSTANCES

The assessment and effective treatment of substance abuse requires an integrated approach based on an appreciation of medical, psychological, and social factors. Although substance abuse has been recognized as a significant problem since the time of the ancient Egyptians, it is only in recent decades that knowledge about it has progressed significantly, and much remains to be learned. Exact mechanisms of action of the various substances abused remain unknown. It is uncertain how these drugs cause a "high" and why some individuals can repeatedly use them socially without sequelae and others find themselves inexorably led into misuse and abuse. Nevertheless, clinical experience enables us to delineate both intoxication and withdrawal syndromes, and research continues to add to the fund of knowledge.

Each psychoactive substance has its own peculiarities, and the large number of substances precludes a complete discussion of them in this chapter. See Tables 15–1 and 15–2 for a summarized discussion. Texts on pharmacology, or more specialized works such as Mannaioni's (1984) provide more specific information. In this section, only an illustration of the type of material that is emerging from recent investigations will be presented. The mechanisms of action and the processes resulting in tolerance will be discussed only for the opioids, alcohol, and the amphetamines.

OPIOIDS

Perhaps the most exciting findings in the study of opioids have involved the detection of **opiate receptors** and the ensuing discovery of natural opioids in the body.

It has long been held that narcotics and their analogs work by binding to highly specific sites called receptors, on the surfaces of cells in the central nervous system. Indeed, many other substances are known to exert their physiologic actions by binding with protein molecules embedded in cell membranes. The effect of this binding is often to change the permeability of the membrane to ions, thereby changing its electrical characteristics, or to activate the cyclic AMP system and influence chemical reactions within the cell. Simon et al. (1973) exhibited stereospecific opiate binding sites in brain homogenate preparations. Similar work has established the presence of these receptors in all vertebrates studied to date. Extensive mapping studies have established high-density areas of these receptors in the limbic system, a part of the brain believed to be associated with emotions, and in pathways in the nervous system involved in mediating and modulating pain.

The discovery of opiate receptors in the nervous system led to the search for naturally occurring opioids in the body, and during the late 1970s such substances were found. These endogenous opioids, the enkephalins and the endorphins, are peptides and show essentially the same actions as externally administered narcotics. The enkephalins are found in the central nervous system in essentially the same locations as opiate receptors, although the correlation is not exact. The endorphins have a different distribution and are found primarily in the pituitary. These two groups of substances have opioid-like actions on smooth muscle, compete with exogenous opioids, cause analgesic effects, and produce tolerance. Much work has been done that suggests that these substances participate in an endogenous analgesic system, and it is widely hoped that, eventually, studies of these systems will lead to a better understanding of the mechanisms of tolerance and withdrawal as well as the experience of pain. (See Chapter 25 on Psychiatric Mental Health Nursing with the Patient in Intensive Care.)

Initial attempts to explain acquired tolerance to the effects of narcotics were in the context of the behavioral model. Although many specific theories have been offered, the core concept is that of **operant conditioning.** The term *operant* refers to behaviors spontaneously performed by the organism. For example, a monkey placed in a box with a lever will tend to explore his environment. From time to time, he may press the lever at random. If, each time he presses the lever, food appears in the box, he will tend to press the lever more and his initial random behavior is said to have been reinforced. In essence, the monkey trains himself to press the lever because of the pleasurable response produced. Monkeys have been confined in such environments where pressing the lever resulted in the administration of intravenous morphine. Within about two weeks, the monkeys increase their self-injections from three to four a day to thirty to forty a day (Shuster, 1970), thus mimicking to a certain extent the behavior of addicts. This group of theories proposes, therefore, that addiction is a learned behavior.

Although learned behavior certainly is a factor in the progression of substance use to substance abuse, there are convincing arguments that more fundamental factors are in play. The development of tolerance to narcotics has been shown to occur in many animal species, even those less susceptible to operant-conditioning techniques. Tolerance has been demonstrated in isolated organ preparations, and indeed even in the individual cells, and it is likely that tolerance to narcotics is a biochemical phenomenon.

With the putative role of the enkephalins in inhibiting pain and in modulating emotions via their role in the limbic system, it is likely that they play a role in the effects of the opioids, including that of acquired tolerance. A model proposed by Snyder (1975) gives an example of how these interactions might take place.

Snyder has proposed that, in the natural state, neurons with opiate receptors are constantly inhibited by a basal level of released enkephalin, although many opiate receptors remain unoccupied. When exogenous opiates are introduced into the body, the available sites become occupied and the neuron becomes more inhibited. To counteract this excess inhibition, reciprocal mechanisms come into play that suppress the natural enkephalin release, thus freeing up more opiate receptors. If the pleasurable effect the person feels is related to the extent that the neuron is inhibited, it will now take more exogenous opiate to produce the same amount of inhibition, and tolerance has occurred.

As appealing as the above theory may be, matters are certainly much more complex. Evidence suggests that catecholamines play a major role in withdrawal

TABLE 15–1 Commonly abused substances

Substance	Properties	Signs of Intoxication
(1) Alcohol	Depressant; the most commonly abused substance.	Poor coordination, impaired sensory function (decreased visual acuity, hearing, etc.), euphoria, release of inhibitions, loud speech, nystagmus, longer reaction time.
(2) Amphetamines	Stimulants; are common ingredients in diet pills; are used in treating hyperactivity; may be taken IV or PO.	Euphoria with dilated pupils, tachycardia, anxiety, hyperreflexia, tremor, and restlessness.
(3) Barbiturates	Depressants; very commonly prescribed drugs; are often used to alter the effects of other drugs such as amphetamines.	In general sedation and effects similar to those seen with alcohol. Some users experience euphoria.
(4) Caffeine	Mild stimulant and diuretic.	Tremors, insomnia, diuresis and tachycardia if taken in large doses.
(5) Cannabis	Normally smoked as marijuana; can be taken orally.	Resembles mild alcohol intoxication with injected conjunctiva and tachycardia. May cause panic reactions.
(6) Cocaine	A stimulant and local anesthetic; can be smoked, taken IV, or PO. At times is taken rectally or vaginally.	Brief sense of euphoria lasting minutes, followed by dysphoria; also tachycardia, hypertension, and hallucinations. Death from overdose can occur.
(7) Inhalants	A broad class of compounds including: gasoline, amyl nitrite, glues, thinners, liquid paper, PAM, various fluorocarbons (in sprays, etc.), nitrous oxide.	Brief sense of disorientation or "high"; effects similar to alcohol intoxication; mucosal irritation; various neurological changes.
(8) LSD	A hallucinogen; the effects of hallucinogens are basically similar. LSD is an acronym for lysergic acid diethylamide. Other hallucinogens are found in mushrooms; THC, an active ingredient in marijuana, is also a hallucinogen.	Intoxication of 6–8 hours; effects vary but include visual illusions and hallucinations, impaired attention, etc.; in some cases "bad trips" may lead to massive anxiety reactions and psychotic episodes. Physical findings of dilated pupils, tachycardia, and elevated temperature.
(9) Narcotics	Includes heroin, and many proprietary products, such as Demerol®, Dilaudid®, codeine, etc. Are taken IV or PO. Are basically sedative-like drugs but also cause euphoric-like states.	Often, nothing in addicts with tolerance, except that there is always miosis. In high doses, causes coma, respiratory depression, and death. If nystagmus is present, there is a high likelihood of concurrent alcohol or sedative-hypnotic use.
(10) Nonbarbiturate sedative hypnotic	Includes the commonly prescribed benzodiazepines.	Similar to alcohol and barbiturates.
(11) PCP	PCP is the acronym for phencyclidine; originally introduced as an anaesthetic. It is a hallucinogen but has special properties.	Usually a brief psychotic reaction with euphoria, disorientation, agitation or withdrawal, hypertension, ataxia, a rigid, fixed stare, nystagmus, and general muscle hypertonicity. Overdoses can lead to coma and death. May cause extremely violent, disorganized psychotic states of a paranoid type.

TABLE 15–2 Complications associated with commonly abused substances

Substance	Withdrawal	Complications	Special Features
(1) Alcohol	*	Numerous physical problems involving almost every organ system: cardiomyopathy, liver disease, pancreatitis, brain damage such as cerebellar syndrome, and Wernicke's syndrome.	*
(2) Amphetamines	*	Chronic users show social withdrawal, personal deterioration, and moodiness.	Can cause a paranoid psychosis indistinguishable from schizophrenia.
(3) Barbiturates	*	Chronic use can lead to personal neglect, confusion, disorientation, loss of emotional control, variable mood, decreased cognitive ability, ataxia, tremors, dysarthria, and nystagmus.	*
(4) Caffeine	*	A syndrome known as caffeinism is seen in chronic, heavy users which consists of: rambling thought, agitation, arrhythmias, and anxiety-disorder.	May aggravate ulcers or cardiac disease; caffeinism can mimic anxiety disorders and panic disorders.
(5) Cannabis	*	Chronic use may lead to a lack of motivation and involvement with others; physical effects of long-term use are only now being explored; these may include neurological damage.	THC, tetrahydrocannabinol, has been isolated as an active ingredient in marijuana, and can be used to increase the strength of cigarettes. Cannabis can cause psychotic reactions which are dose dependent.
(6) Cocaine	Agitation, severe depression, and, possibly, craving.	Chronic use can cause severe disturbances in life style. It can cause severe states of agitation and paranoid psychosis.	The sequence of "high" followed by a dysphoric period is very reinforcing for continued use.

from narcotics. The drug clonidine, a central alpha-adrenergic stimulant, has been shown by Gold et al. (1978) to block the symptoms of opiate withdrawal. There is also evidence that proteins in the serum of narcotic addicts can bind to circulating opiates, suggesting a role for the immune system in the acquisition of tolerance. Not only catecholamines, but most other neurotransmitters, such as serotonin, histamine, and others, are affected in terms of their production, release, and storage by chronic opiate use; and a single neurotransmitter is unlikely to account for the multiple effects of the opiates. Thus, in the case of narcotics, mechanisms of actions and acquisition of tolerance probably involve both the endogenous opiates and opiate receptors; however, the specifics are not well understood.

ALCOHOL

The mechanisms of alcohol's action are even less well explained by the available evidence than those of narcotics. Alcohol is known to interact with cell membranes, stabilizing them in low concentrations and destabilizing them in high concentrations. These effects involve changes in membrane permeability to various ions as well as inhibition of membrane ATPase. It is generally agreed that alcohol causes noradrenalin release both centrally and peripherally, and also affects other neurotransmitters in complex ways. Tolerance to alcohol, on the other hand, is believed to occur via changes in the efficiency of peripheral metabolism, probably through an increased activity of the liver microsomal system, and additionally, through some type of cellular adaptation in the brain.

TABLE 15–2 continued

Substance	Withdrawal	Complications	Special Features
(7) Inhalants	NA	Chronic use causes a wide variety of effects: neurologic damage, hematologic changes, poor school adjustment, etc.	The use of inhalants is probably extremely common.
(8) LSD	NA	Use can lead to personality disorders or permanent psychosis. Flashbacks can occur.	Acute intoxication with LSD may mimic schizophrenia.
(9) Narcotics	*	Overdose of narcotics is a common cause of death for addicts. Medical problems include: emboli, septicemia, and a high incidence of hepatitis.	*
(10) Nonbarbiturate sedative hypnotic	*	Similar to the barbiturates.	These are among the most widely prescribed drugs and abuse is very common.
(11) PCP	*	Chronic use can lead to recurrent psychotic states, changes in neurological functioning which include dysarthria, poor recent memory, and episodes of disorientation.	PCP can precipitate schizophrenia in vulnerable individuals.

*Withdrawal for these drugs is discussed in the body of the text.

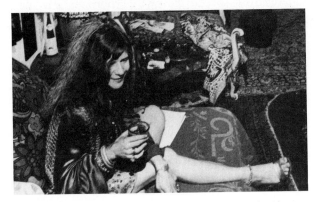

Janis Joplin, a famous singer of the 1960s, drank a fifth of whiskey as part of her act. She died at the age of 27 of what was probably an accidental overdose of alcohol (a *stimulant* as well as a CNS depressant) and barbituates (which she no doubt needed to counteract the alcohol's stimulant effects in order to sleep).

AMPHETAMINES

Amphetamines are a class of sympathomimetic drugs whose effects involve catecholamine release. This action is believed to be responsible for amphetamine psychosis, a paranoid schizophrenic-like reaction that is dose dependent. Tolerance to the effects of amphetamines builds rapidly, although the mechanism is not understood.

INTOXICATION AND WITHDRAWAL

In principle, intoxication and withdrawal syndromes are substance specific. In practice, however, intoxication syndromes overlap a great deal and are often difficult to evaluate on the basis of physical signs and symptoms alone. **Polysubstance abuse** is very common. Thus, in the acute situation, a mixed picture can be expected. In addition, given the number of substances being abused, an individual presenting to, say, an emergency room, may have taken anything from mushrooms to proprietary drugs, to any of a number of street drugs which can be impure, have multiple additives, and be misrepresented. The confusion may be reduced by local poison control centers, as they are usually very well informed as to drugs currently available in the community. Another mainstay is serum and urine testing for drugs and their byproducts, both of which are often obtainable on a stat basis.

A prototype for drug screening that law enforcement officials often use which has legal, as well as medical, implications is the **blood alcohol assay.** This is a standard and reliable test that is usually reported either as a mg/percent, that is, mg per 100 ml of blood, or simply as percent. A percent value such as 0.1 percent is converted to mg/percent by multiplying by 1,000. Thus, a 0.1 percent level is the same as 100 mg/percent. For legal purposes, a level of 0.1 percent is generally considered as evidence of intoxication, while levels of 0.35 percent and greater are considered life-threatening.

Because of the possibility of tolerance, it is not always possible to correlate behavior with the blood alcohol level, but most people will feel intoxicated at a level of 0.1 percent. A breath test is very well correlated with the blood alcohol level; urine testing is not reliable.

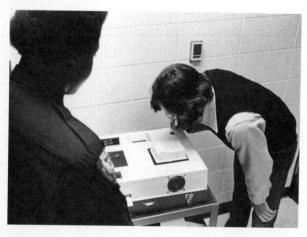

For legal purposes, a breath test along with a blood alcohol test showing a level of 0.1 percent is generally considered as evidence of intoxication and warrants a drunk-driving ticket. This typically involves a large fine, limited driving privileges, and alcohol and drug assessment and education.

In many cases, simple intoxication does not require treatment. In others, supportive management will be the main effort. In cases of overdose, measures to support airway and cardiac function and blood pressure may be needed. The triad of miotic pupils, coma, and respiratory depression, particularly if needle tracks or other signs of narcotic use are present, should engender suspicion of a heroin or other narcotic overdose and a trial of naloxone, a narcotics antagonist, which can reverse their effects.

Withdrawal syndromes are often more specific than symptoms of intoxication, although there is still overlap. Assessment is also complicated by polydrug abuse and the confusing clinical pictures that can occur.

A very specific syndrome is observed in the case of the opiates, although the mechanism is not well understood. Following cessation of narcotics, signs and symptoms of withdrawal begin to appear in about seven to eight hours and take the form of rhinorrhea, lacrimation, and mild perspiration. With time the symptoms intensify, and midriasis and piloerrection develop. Within twenty-four to thirty-six hours the patient begins to complain of back pain, hot and cold flashes, muscle twitching, and insomnia. Later developments include vomiting and diarrhea. Associated signs include elevated blood pressure and an increase in body temperature. Severity of these symptoms is somewhat related to the daily dose of narcotic, although anyone addicted to narcotics will experience them. Basically these symptoms peak at about three days and are mostly resolved by the end of a week. A dose of narcotic will abort the symptoms at any point in the process.

The above syndrome represents the primary withdrawal from narcotics. Following this, however, is a relatively specific secondary syndrome. This consists of a triad of anxiety, depression, and fluctuating moods, as well as recurrent craving for the drug. This syndrome causes the addict much subjective distress and often intensifies at times of emotional stress. It varies in intensity, but continues for months following cessation of drug use and is associated with relapse back to using. Newborns of mothers who have been on narcotics during pregnancy will exhibit a withdrawal syndrome that can be confused with other pathologies, particularly if the mother's narcotics use has been unrecognized by health-care professionals.

Withdrawal syndromes involved in alcohol and other drug abuse vary much more from patient to patient than the narcotic withdrawal syndrome. Most people who are dependent on alcohol will exhibit some form of minor withdrawal syndrome consisting of tremors, malaise, and sleep disturbance. These symptoms last about forty-eight hours and are relatively minor in medical severity. Roughly 5–10 percent of alcoholics admitted for detoxification, however, will progress to the more severe withdrawal syndrome of delirium tremens, the chief symptoms of which are severe tremors, an increased body temperature that progresses to the point of malignant hyperthermia, seizures, tachycardia, and agitation. Psychiatric symptoms include intense anxiety and restlessness, visual hallucinations, confusion, and disorientation. The prognosis for individuals with this condition involves a mortality rate of about 1–15 percent. These conditions are typically managed in an inpatient setting with supportive treatment, hydration, seizure medication, and vitamin replacement. Drugs that exhibit cross tolerance to alcohol, such as chlordiazepoxide, are usually administered to prevent the development of the more severe of these withdrawal symptoms.

Barbiturates and benzodiazepines are associated with a withdrawal syndrome that includes seizures and toxic psychosis, which appear within several hours to several days of abstinence. Although the benzodiazepine withdrawal is as a rule less severe, and occurs at a later time than the barbiturate withdrawal, the two syndromes have several other features in common. They include nausea, agitation, insomnia, muscle twitching, and tachycardia. The seizures are grand mal in nature; psychotic symptoms involve primarily vivid visual hallucinations which tend to be more severe at night.

Amphetamine withdrawal results in a syndrome of fatigue, depression, and disturbed sleep with increased dreaming. The depression can be severe and suicides have been reported.

Withdrawal from cannabis occurs in heavy users who stop abruptly and consists of irritability, sleep disturbance, poor appetite, and nausea. Similar symptoms occur with nicotine withdrawal.

ASSESSMENT OF SUBSTANCE ABUSE

The chief clinical skills required for the diagnosis of substance abuse are a basic knowledge of the individual conditions, a high index of suspicion, and a great deal of tact and patience.

The core information needed for assessment is contained in the DSM-III-R criteria, and an individual presenting for evaluation because of a concern about his alcohol and drug use, with sensitive and tactful questioning, will essentially diagnose himself. It should be emphasized that patients who are already concerned about their alcohol or drug use are highly suspect for being substance abusers and, on no account, should have their concerns dismissed without careful evaluation. To do any less is to play a direct role in maintaining a serious problem. Unfortunately, many persons do not present in this manner and there may be many hurdles to overcome in assessing the substance abuser.

Patients are frequently seen under adverse conditions. Many states have laws that require intoxicated drivers to have alcohol and drug assessments. Many school systems now require that students with suspect behavior be evaluated. Other individuals may be coerced into evaluation by concerned family members. It is understandable that such patients will be defensive, even hostile, and may lie or distort information in order to protect themselves from repercussions and continue to maintain their using lifestyles. Again, any expression of family or community concern about an individual's alcohol or drug use should lead the clinician to exercise the utmost caution before dismissing substance abuse as a diagnostic possibility.

Substance abuse can present in many less obvious ways. Recall that up to 25 percent of general hospital admissions are prompted by a problem related to substance abuse. While some patients have conditions obviously connected with substance abuse, such as cirrhosis or pancreatitis in the case of alcohol abuse, or septicemia or endocarditis in the case of heroin use, others have physical symptoms less obviously related to the problem, such as diarrhea, gastritis, or neuropathies, three common findings in alcoholics. As Westermeyer (1978) found, many of these kinds of patients are not recognized as substance abusers.

In addition to presenting with medical or legal problems, substance abusers can present with other individual or family psychopathologies. A family may be referred for counseling for incest that occurred while the perpetrator was intoxicated; a teenager may be referred for a learning evaluation following a period of poor school performance that is related to drug use; a patient referred for treatment of depression may turn out to have a major problem with alcohol and/or drugs instead. It is a relatively common experience in alcohol and drug treatment centers to find that patients with substance-abuse problems have been misdiagnosed, treated for other conditions, or told that their substance use is secondary to other conditions that must be treated first.

Major problems arise in interviewing and assessing patients when the nurse's own sense of values, personal history, and personal biases are activated in the course of an interview. The physician or nurse with a substance-abuse problem herself may avoid the unpleasant experience of seeing her own problems mirrored in her patients and may overlook, subconsciously, the signs and symptoms of substance use, or minimize them. One clinician may have feelings about her alcoholic father activated by alcoholics, and begin to act in hostile and derisive ways, destroying an already fragile rapport. Another, imbued with a *laissez faire* attitude toward drugs, may minimize her patients' problems because of her personal views.

Thus many practical and psychological problems may arise to interfere with identification of the substance abuser. The task is made even more difficult by the absence of specific diagnostic tests (such as the glucose tolerance test for diabetes) although efforts are being made in this direction.

There is an important distinction between alcohol, and perhaps also marijuana, though it is illegal, and other substances commonly abused. Alcohol is socially sanctioned and is used by many people without being abused. *Any* form of heroin use, however, on a regular basis, would be considered diagnostic of heroin abuse. Many people use alcohol on a daily basis without symptoms suggestive of any problems at all. Thus alcohol is one of the few substances for which normal and abnormal use must be distinguished. A relatively sophisticated approach is needed to separate the alcohol abuser from the alcohol user. Thus, the majority of this section will be devoted to assessment of the alcohol abuser.

There have been several approaches designed to establish reliable diagnostic criteria and/or tests for alcoholism. One of the most obvious is actually one of the least reliable: the amount and frequency of drinking. Many people simply do not know how much alcohol they drink. Few individuals actually measure their drinks, and one person's "single" may be another's "triple." Drinks served in bars and restaurants vary widely in alcohol content. In social settings, drinkers can lose track of their intake while having a good time, arguing with a spouse, or becoming so intoxicated as to forget an evening completely. Beyond this, there is wide variation in the individual response to alcohol, and some people may drink surprisingly large amounts of alcohol on a daily basis without appearing to have any problem. So, the amount consumed is only moderately helpful in establishing a diagnosis. More helpful, in a clinical setting, is the use of drug and alcohol screens. Urine screens can detect marijuana that was smoked a week before, for example.

Alice: A Patient with a Drinking Problem

Alice was an attractive, intelligent wife of a local attorney. She had been seeing her physician for a number of complaints throughout the years. At present she was complaining of recurrent abdominal cramping and diarrhea. As a part of his evaluation the physician asked Alice how much she drank. Her answer was two or three glasses of wine a day, usually with her husband before dinner. The internist followed up with standard lab tests and X rays that revealed no abnormality. At that point he prescribed symptomatic treatment, and Alice experienced some relief. The problem persisted, however, and on subsequent visits the nurse continued to ask about Alice's alcohol use, noting on one occasion that she had alcohol on her breath; but Alice continued to minimize her drinking.

In the case of Alice, one valuable assessment tool would be a blood alcohol level, a relatively inexpensive and reliable test. A particularly significant finding would be a high blood alcohol level with little to no clinical evidence of intoxication. This would be *prima facie* evidence of tolerance, almost certainly establishing a diagnosis of substance abuse.

Other laboratory tests are currently under evaluation as screening procedures to be used in the assessment of alcohol abuse. These techniques focus on abnormalities in liver enzymes which occur with heavy drinking, even in the absence of clinically significant physical problems.

Screening measures more elaborate and formalized than the DSM-III-R criteria are available. One of these is the Michigan Alcohol Screen Test (MAST) (see Table 15-3). This is a reliable test that provides a rapid and easy method of screening patients, and can be used as part of the evaluation process or as a mnemonic device for remembering the more common signs and consequences of troubled drinking. A person scoring five or more points on the MAST is assessed as having a problem with alcohol. The MAST or similar screening test might have been helpful in the evaluation of Alice, the patient described earlier.

Most of the items listed in the MAST are self-explanatory. The condition referred to as **blackouts,**

TABLE 15–3 Michigan Alcoholism Screening Test (MAST)

Points

	0. Do you enjoy a drink now and then?
(2)	*1. Do you feel you are a normal drinker? (By normal, we mean do you drink less than or as much as most other people?)
(2)	2. Have you ever awakened the morning after some drinking the night before and found that you could not remember a part of the evening?
(1)	3. Does your wife, husband, a parent, or other near relative ever worry or complain about your drinking?
(2)	*4. Can you stop drinking without a struggle after one or two drinks?
(1)	5. Do you ever feel guilty about your drinking?
(2)	*6. Do friends or relatives think you are a normal drinker?
(2)	*7. Are you able to stop drinking when you want to?
(5)	8. Have you ever attended a meeting of Alcoholics Anonymous (AA)?
(1)	9. Have you gotten into physical fights when drinking?
(2)	10. Has your drinking ever created problems between you and your wife, husband, a parent, or other near relative?
(2)	11. Has your wife, husband, (or other family members) ever gone to anyone for help about your drinking?
(2)	12. Have you ever lost friends because of your drinking?
(2)	13. Have you ever gotten into trouble at work or school because of drinking?
(2)	14. Have you ever lost a job because of drinking?
(2)	15. Have you ever neglected your obligations, your family, or your work for 2 or more days in a row because you were drinking?
(1)	16. Do you drink before noon fairly often?
(2)	17. Have you ever been told you have liver trouble? Cirrhosis?
(2)	+18. After heavy drinking have you ever had delirium tremens (D.T.s) or severe shaking, or heard voices or seen things that weren't really there?
(5)	19. Have you ever gone to anyone for help about your drinking?
(5)	20. Have you ever been a patient in a psychiatric hospital or on a psychiatric ward of a general hospital where drinking was a part of the problem that resulted in hospitalization?
(2)	21. Have you ever been seen at a psychiatric or mental health clinic or gone to any doctor, social worker, or counselor, for help with any emotional problem where drinking was part of the problem?
(2)	±22. Have you ever been arrested for drunk driving, driving while intoxicated or driving under the influence of alcoholic beverages? (If yes, how many times _____)
(2)	±23. Have you ever been arrested or taken into custody, even for a few hours, because of other drunk behavior? (If yes, how many times? _____)

*Alcoholic response is negative.

+Five points for delirium tremens.

±Two points for each arrest.

Source: Selzer, 1971, 1975
Scoring system: In general, five or more place the subject in an alcoholic category. Four points are suggestive of alcoholism, three or fewer points indicate that the subject is not an alcoholic.

however, is unique to alcoholism and has been the subject of some misunderstanding.

A blackout is the inability to recall a period of time during a drinking episode. While the blackout is occurring there is no impairment of consciousness or alteration in function, and neither the patient nor his companions are aware that a blackout is happening. In other words, a blackout is a form of amnesia. The amnesic period can last for several days, although several hours is more common. During the amnesic state the person may function more or less adequately and may not even appear intoxicated; however, the memory is not retrievable even with sodium amytal. Blackouts may result from gulping drinks and drinking without eating, and occur with highest frequency in heavy drinkers who have considerable tolerance and craving for alcohol. Although blackouts are associated with heavy drinking, many heavy drinkers never experience them, while other drinkers, including some who would not be classified as substance abusers, do have them. They are thus neither necessary nor sufficient for a diagnosis of substance abuse.

In general, application of the DSM-III-R criteria, supplemented by instruments such as the MAST, blood or urine drug screens, and a high index of suspicion will go far in identifying many substance abusers. Why did Alice's internist fail to diagnose her problem? At the time Alice saw her internist for diarrhea, she was drinking up to a fifth of vodka a day, along with the wine she reported having with her husband before dinner. No one, including her family, knew the extent of her problem. How could a problem this great have been missed? The relatively high incidence of alcoholism among physicians and nurses could be a significant reason for findings such as Westermeyer's. Remembering that one-third of all families are affected by substance abuse in some way, one realizes that a significant number of physicians and nurses attempting to diagnose alcoholism and drug abuse are as affected by it as the patients themselves. Many people harbor the stereotypes of the "bum" or the inner city hard-core drug abuser in mind when they think of substance abuse, and never quite manage to associate these conditions with the more affluent patient. Thus denial and bias are probably the two greatest stumbling blocks to diagnosing substance abuse.

SPECIAL DIAGNOSTIC PROBLEMS

TEENAGERS. Teenage substance abuse is a special problem. Drug and alcohol abuse among youth is

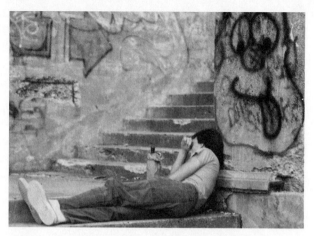

While marijuana use has declined among today's teen-agers (high school and college students), alcohol use has increased and begins as early as fifth or sixth grade. Parental denial that *their* child could be affected, despite decreasing school performance, moodiness, and increasing emotional distance from the family, is rampant. So also is the attitude (including that of many health-care professionals) that the alcohol-dependent teen-ager is a "bad child" rather than a sad one in need of help.

rapidly increasing and becoming more severe. In addition, it has been suggested that early onset alcoholism is more rapidly progressive. Thus the identification and treatment of teenage alcohol abuse is especially important. While some teenagers seek treatment on their own, perhaps as a result of one of the many programs designed to educate students and teachers about substance abuse, many teens, particularly those who are alienated from adults, enter treatment reluctantly, if at all, and then drop out. It can be extraordinarily difficult to establish rapport with such a patient. An attitude of acceptance, and willingness to allow him time to build up trust, can help. Although young people show the same signs and symptoms of alcohol and drug abuse as adults, patterns of abuse may differ. A common pattern includes changes in behavior and friends. A combination of the following symptoms is likely to indicate a substance abuse problem in a teenager: falling grades, new friendships along with the rejection of established ones, truancy, secretiveness, isolation from the family, running away, stealing money from a family member, unstable mood, and drug overdoses. A family history of substance abuse should always be explored in order to determine its relevance to the identified patient.

WOMEN. Substance abuse among women is increasing. There is some indication that the clinical course is a more rapidly progressive one than it is for men, and that treatment has a lower success rate. Clinical experience indicates that women alcoholics elicit less support from the family than men do as they go through the treatment process. Men are much more likely to divorce their alcoholic wives, even after treatment, than wives are to divorce alcoholic husbands. Women also seem to be more stigmatized by a diagnosis of alcoholism than are men, and so may be more reluctant to seek help. Women who remain alcohol users during pregnancy run the added risk of having an infant born with fetal alcohol syndrome. (See also Chapter 19, Psychiatric Mental Health Nursing with Women.)

THE ELDERLY. Alcoholism among the elderly often goes undetected, in part because of their isolated lifestyles and the fragmented medical care to which they are often subjected. Elderly patients are typically on multiple medications, many of which interact with alcohol. Additionally, they often have medical problems that are worsened by alcohol, making recognition of alcohol abuse in this population especially important. A propensity for falls, episodes of amnesia or confusion, unstable mood, irritability, or personal neglect may be due to dementia or other medical problems, but can also be due to substance abuse. The clinician should not overlook this possibility. (See Box 15–3.)

CLINICAL COURSE OF SUBSTANCE ABUSE

The clinical course of substance abuse is quite variable and many outcomes are possible. Some alcoholics will die from fires or car wrecks associated with drinking, while others die from cirrhosis or cardiomyopathy. Still others will be incarcerated because of crimes, *while some will spontaneously stop drinking.* Studies of Vietnam veterans have shown, for example, that many who abused drugs in Vietnam have not continued to do so on their return to the United States. Similarly, it is not unknown for previously heavy drinkers to return to social drinking without treatment.

These facts raise the issue of whether it is appropriate to speak of a clinical course at all. Yet studies of alcoholism are beginning to suggest that the variation in clinical course may be due to different forms of the problem. Goodwin (1985) cites studies that support a subtype of familial alcoholism characterized by a strong family history, a rapid clinical course with early deterioration, and absence of other psychopath-

ology. Other studies suggest that women may have a more rapid and severe acceleration of problem drinking than men. (See also Chapter 19, Psychiatric Mental Health Nursing with Women.)

While little can be said about the prognosis for individual patients, in general, the following is true. It takes most people years of social drinking to reach alcoholism. During these years of social drinking, there is a progression of the symptoms and signs enumerated in the MAST. The course of the illness is either progressively downhill, or is chronically recurrent. Many people continue in this way for a long time, until they either receive treatment, are forced to stop drinking because of associated problems that become unmanageable, or die of related complications. Regardless of how or why an individual stops drinking, there remains the ever-present threat of relapse. Thus any attempt to return to social drinking runs the risk of resulting in the same problems as before, or worse.

THEORIES OF SUBSTANCE ABUSE

Theories of substance abuse are manifold. Prevailing opinion, like substance abuse itself, has tended to change and evolve and usually has reflected popular theoretical leanings. Because much of the work on theoretical issues has been devoted to alcohol abuse, theories of alcohol abuse will occupy the bulk of this section.

Prior to the 1900s, a theory of acquired inheritance was widely accepted, and alcoholism was regarded as familial, being passed on to children via germ cells that had been altered by the drinking of the parents. Even in the professional literature, alcoholics were demeaned and looked upon with approbation. Thanks to Freud and other theorists, the thinking took on a psychodynamic perspective. When behaviorists appeared, so did behavioral theories of alcoholism. At the present time a multi-factorial theory is popular.

PSYCHOANALYTIC THEORIES

Psychoanalytic theories of substance abuse involve a three-tiered concept (Wurmser 1981). The substance abuse itself is on the most superficial level. It is thought to be an attempt on the part of the abuser to moderate unpleasant affects, such as anxiety or depression. The drug use becomes a defense against feelings, preventing their legitimate expression and

Box 15—3 ● Substance Abuse in the Elderly

How serious is the problem of substance abuse in old age? We asked Roland M. Atkinson, M.D., Chief of Psychiatry, Portland VA Medical Center and Professor, Oregon Health Sciences University. Dr. Atkinson has helped establish a model outpatient program for alcoholic World War II veterans.

Substance abuse in the elderly often differs from the patterns seen in young adults, and this has obscured the extent of the problem. It usually does not involve gross intoxication, abstinence symptoms, or antisocial behavior. Instead, it mimics symptoms of geriatric illness—paranoia, confusion, self-neglect, falls, incontinence, muscle weakness, malnutrition, diarrhea. It may cause memory and concentration problems, depression, anxiety, and insomnia. Heart disease and other medical problems may be aggravated. A clinician not trained to suspect alcohol or drug abuse is likely to make a diagnosis of depression, senile dementia, or a physical illness.

Many cases of alcohol and drug abuse are hard to identify for other reasons. Older people are biologically more sensitive to drugs, and therefore many reduce or stop their use. Those who continue may develop more problems than younger people at the same doses. The distinction between heavy drinkers, problem drinkers, and alcoholics begins to lose meaning with age. Older alcoholics are more likely to be middle class and to appear healthy on psychological tests. They may also be hard to identify because they have withdrawn from the social networks which bring younger abusers to professional at-

---

resolution, thereby creating a vicious cycle of unhappiness. According to psychoanalytic theory these feelings result from unconscious conflicts associated with disturbances in psychosexual or psychosocial development. While the details of these conflicts vary with the theorist, the basic concept of the "infantile neurosis," as set forth by Freud and modified by object-relations theorists, forms the essence of the purported disturbance. A failure of the mother-child relationship to pass through the "rapprochement phase" of development, as described by Mahler (1975), leads to an alteration in the development of a sense of self, and the maintenance of infantile defenses. This leads to a predisposition to intense affective states, particularly in the context of intimate relationships, persistent oral and narcissistic needs, insecurity, and dependency. Fixation at this level of development will also lead to persistent internal conflicts and their external expression, and defects in the ego and superego. These developmental defects result in difficulty delaying gratification, and a propensity to seek immediate relief from tension and certain affective states with drugs.

BEHAVIORAL THEORIES

Behaviorists have explored a number of issues related to substance abuse. Some of their concepts will be presented in the section on treatment, and others will be described here. All have in common the underlying belief that much of human behavior is learned. Meyer and Mirin (1981), for example, have studied **craving** and defined it as the feeling an addict has when he is in proximity to a drug, particularly in the context of previous use. They state that craving may be most intense in settings in which the person has actually received the drug, or during states of emotion he has used the drug to modify. Thus, according to these researchers, craving revolves around environmental cues associated with the pleasurable emotions and relief from tension the drug has evoked in the past.

Most behavioral theories are complex and involve factors such as past learning experiences both in and out of the family, styles of drinking, sundry environmental cues, and thinking patterns that interact to produce the behavior. Cognitive theorists, such as Beck (1976), have focused on maladaptive thinking patterns associated with drinking, such as a mind set that problems are unresolvable, or expectations that social drinking will help make friends. Caddy and Lovibond (1976) have evolved an elaborate treatment model based on self-regulation training using cognitive techniques as a basis.

Social learning theories of addiction have developed as a result of work with inner-city addicts, and

tention. Society also tends to overlook or excuse substance abuse in the elderly.

Given these problems of definition, detection, and attitude, it is not surprising that the extent of substance abuse among the elderly has not been well documented. Among people in their 60s, drug and alcohol abuse is probably as common as depression, and more widespread than senile dementia. It becomes progressively uncommon thereafter. Alcohol cases outnumber other drug cases among the elderly by 4:1 to 10:1. Five to 10 percent of elderly men admitted to acute medical wards are alcoholics, and 3 to 17 percent of elderly psychiatric clinic patients are active alcoholics.

Late-life alcoholism is often explained by stress, but there is little evidence for this. In fact, many late onset alcoholics have intact marriages and considerable financial resources. Discretionary money and time, and lack of social responsibility may foster alcoholism.

Persuading elderly patients to enter alcohol treatment programs requires gentleness and tact, but treatment works for them at least as well as it does for younger patients. After detoxification, most older long-term patients do well in supportive outpatient groups designed specifically for them. Family counseling and home visits are often helpful. Some abstinent alcoholics may benefit from antidepressant medication in low doses.

Fortunately, surveys show that most elderly patients receive no prescribed psychoactive drugs, the great majority who receive drugs use them properly, and underuse is more common than overuse. Besides alcohol, the drugs most often abused are prescription opioid analgesics, antianxiety drugs (mainly benzodiazepines) and sedatives. Illicit drug abuse is uncommon in old age. Little is known about over-the-counter (OTC) drug abuse, but cases like the following are common: An anxious 68-year-old woman reported taking 16 OTC caffeine tablets daily for bowel regularity. Cutting the dose to three a day reduced her anxiety without affecting her bowel habits.

As the population becomes older, the number of elderly alcohol and drug abusers will undoubtedly rise. Changing cultural patterns also suggest future increases in alcoholism among older women.

Source: *The Harvard Medical School Mental Health Letter*. Vol. 2, No. 1, July 1985, p. 8.

have formed a basis for the therapeutic community model of treatment. They emphasize the role of a life script that addicts learn in their communities of origin, that is reinforced by peers and negative attitudes of authorities, and that results in the development of deviant, often criminal, behaviors. The script becomes internalized and forms a part of the individual's life style. In short, the process of addiction is seen as an acculturation to a deviant environment.

BIOLOGICAL THEORIES

One of the most established facts about alcoholism is that it is familial. This is supported by almost every study that has addressed the issue since the late 1800s. A study by Winokur et al. (1970) showed a life-time expectancy rate for brothers of alcoholics to be 46 percent and for sisters to be 5 percent. These figures can be contrasted with the average male expectancy rate for alcoholism which is about 4 percent, and that of females which is about 0.5 percent, both of which clearly represent a significant familial influence. Although Winokur's figures are somewhat higher than the reports of others, almost all reports confirm that relatives of alcoholics have a substantially increased chance of developing alcoholism than the general population.

Since "familial" implies more than genetics, theories about the origins of substance abuse have been embroiled in the nature/nurture battlefield. Strategies used to resolve this issue have been the same as those used in studying schizophrenia and mood disorders, namely, twin and adoption studies. Goodwin (1985) has done an excellent job of summarizing these. The overall results tend to support the concept that genetics plays a role in the development of alcoholism, although the results are hardly decisive. Particularly convincing have been adoption studies which have shown that offspring of alcoholics have a higher incidence of alcoholism compared with the general population whether raised at home or in nonalcoholic homes.

That factors other than genetics are involved in the problem of substance abuse should already be clear from the history of cocaine use previously outlined. Evidence of cultural factors (nurture rather than nature) is readily supplied by epidemiology. A recurrent finding is that the prevalence of alcoholism varies widely from country to country. This finding can be compared with, for example, schizophrenia, which has a relatively uniform rate worldwide. Even within the United States, studies have consistently shown that Jews and Italian-Americans have relatively low rates of alcoholism while Irish-Americans have rates that are relatively high. Attempts to explain these differences have focused on differences in the way children from these two groups are first exposed to alcohol as well as attitudes toward drinking. Italian families are said to expose their children to drinking at an early age, within the family, at meals. This usage is moderate and associated with the sedate surroundings of the dinner table. In the case of the Irish, drinking among children is forbidden, and drinking practices are associated with taverns and expressions of manliness. Whether these explanations are valid or not, the influence of culture in addition to genetics (and, possibly, psychological development) on drinking patterns seems to be significant.

OTHER THEORIES

There are many more theories of drug addiction. Each has its own appeal, but no single theory explains even most of the available evidence. Theories that rely on predisposing pathology to explain alcoholism, such as object-relations theory, fail to explain findings suggesting that much of the psychopathology associated with alcoholism stems from alcohol itself. A study by Loper et al. (1973), involving a prospective analysis of the Minnesota Multiphasic Personalty Inventories (MMPI) of thirty-eight college students who later developed alcoholism, found that although psychophathology was elevated to pathological levels on MMPIs once alcoholism had developed, prealcoholic MMPI scores were normal. Other studies have failed to find indications of dependent personality in alcoholics, as has been suggested by some psychoanalytic theorists. Moreover, clinical experience seems to show that, despite obvious psychopathology on entry to alcohol-treatment programs, within six months of sobriety, as many as 25 percent of alcoholics no longer demonstrate such pathology.

A current issue is the possible relationship between alcohol abuse and mood disorders. Many alcoholics complain of variable moods and poor sleep, and often appear depressed at the time of evaluation. Many report that they drink when they get depressed in order to feel better, and so "treat" their mood fluctuations. However, alcohol itself is a depressant and interferes with sleep patterns. Thus many alcoholics develop problems with low mood as a result of drinking. In addition, alcohol has been shown to be a poor antianxiety and antidepressant agent. The exact relationship between alcoholism and mood disorders, if any, remains unclear. Winokur (1968) found increased rates of depression among female relatives of alcoholics; however, Goodwin and Erickson (1979) found that these relationships held up only if the females were actually raised in the alcoholic family. Increased rates of depression were not found when they were adopted or otherwise reared apart from the family. Other studies have indicated independence in genetic transmission of bipolar disorders and alcoholism. It has also been shown that the depression found in relatives of alcoholics has more in common with so-called "neurotic depression" and is associated with a lower incidence of abnormal DST suppression. (See Chapter 9, Mood Disorders.)

It should be clear that a unitary model of alcoholism has little to recommend it, and that, simply stated, we do not know why people drink too much or abuse drugs. It seems that genetic, cultural, social, and, probably, psychodynamic factors are involved. Many other factors may be involved as well; however, the significance of each possible factor has not been determined, and no clear etiologic conceptualization of alcoholism can be made. Nonetheless, the theories that exist represent a synthesis of a wealth of clinical experience, and provide a fund of knowledge to draw on in assessing and treating the substance abuser. The most prudent course is probably to keep all of them in mind, using one or more as resources as seems appropriate in the clinical situation.

TREATMENT OF SUBSTANCE ABUSE

The treatment of substance abuse is controversial and many approaches have been tried, with varying degrees of success.

In general, once a substance abuse condition has been recognized, which treatment the patient receives will depend on the need for medical intervention, availability of community resources, financial resources to cover the cost of treatment, and the willingness of significant others, such as the family, to become involved in the treatment process. Although conceptualizations of treatment vary widely, all agree that a thorough evaluation of the patient, which includes obtaining a history of the substance abuse, medical and psychiatric history, family, work, and legal history, and marital history is important.

Regardless of the treatment approach that is chosen by the clinician, the recovery process can be long and difficult. It is important to attempt to predict the problems the patient will face so that the skills and resources capable of remedying them can be identified and mobilized.

Patients present themselves for treatment in varying stages of difficulty. Some have pending legal problems, such as drunk driving charges. Others have severe financial problems as a result of mismanagement of their personal funds and/or expensive drug habits. Some have been fired from their jobs or are in serious trouble at work: these individuals often also have troubled marriages and families; their children frequently have problems; and there may be other substance abusers in the family as well.

Patients have different strengths and weaknesses that help or hinder their recovery. Some have had fairly intact premorbid lives, possess good work skills, and have a support network in friends and family. Others have had problems adjusting to the world as long as they can remember, and need much auxiliary help to get control of their substance-abuse problem.

INPATIENT TREATMENT

Initially, it must be determined by the clinician whether or not hospitalization is indicated for the patient. There is much controversy about how to make this decision. In the past, the initial step was usually hospital admission and inpatient detoxification. At present, there is a shift in focus away from the inpatient to the outpatient setting, that is, to outpatient **detoxification** or the process of withdrawal from the substance abused. Many alcoholics, such as those in good health with supportive family members, can be detoxified or withdrawn from alcohol on an outpatient basis. After discontinuing alcohol, the patient is started on a substitute, such as chlordiazepoxide, which prevents the more severe forms of withdrawal, and its dosage is gradually decreased over a period of several days. The patient's condition is monitored through daily visits to the doctor's office or home visits by a community nurse. Meanwhile, a standard alcoholism-treatment program, as described below, is instituted. These shifts are based in part on the expense of inpatient programs as well as a lack of evidence that they have more success than outpatient programs.

An inpatient treatment program should, at a minimum, provide a controlled environment in which withdrawal can proceed safely. For most alcoholics and substance abusers, this represents only a minimal first step in their rehabilitation, as relapses are common. In fact, for many, detoxification can just as well be accomplished on an outpatient basis. One of the primary functions of the initial assessment is the identification of those patients who require an in-

patient setting for medical or psychological reasons. Patients who have overdosed, who are significantly depressed or suicidal or have a history of suicide attempts, those with medical problems, those exhibiting symptoms of withdrawal, and those with high blood alcohol levels should be considered for hospital admission. Hospitalization may also be best for those patients who lack support systems in family and friends, who have a history of unreliability, and a history of delerium tremens with previous withdrawals from alcohol.

A substance-abuse treatment program that provides only inpatient detoxification rapidly becomes a revolving door. As a result, many hospitals have now formalized programs that emphasize a comprehensive approach to alcohol and drug abuse. These programs typically last about a month, and begin with whatever medical treatment is necessary for withdrawal syndromes. Most will attempt to involve the family in a comprehensive assessment, and provide education about alcohol abuse for the family as well as the patient.

Group treatment is often an integral part of the treatment program. In group therapy, each member of the group is encouraged to describe his drug and alcohol experience so that group members may better understand their problems, address each other's denial, and provide each other with support. Meanwhile, strategies for maintaining sobriety following discharge are developed through group process and the patients are introduced to available community programs by the group leader. Many inpatient programs encourage involvement with Alcoholics Anonymous (AA) and Al-Anon (an AA-sponsored support group for family members of alcoholics) while the patient is still in the hospital setting. The family and the individual begin therapy with the understanding that it will continue following discharge.

Some programs provide two weeks or so of initial assessment prior to treatment. This approach is especially helpful in difficult cases, for example, when adolescents are referred for assessment by the court. This gives the staff time to get to know the patient and build trust before making a diagnosis and recommending a treatment plan.

Similar, but more comprehensive, are the residential treatment programs usually referred to as **therapeutic communities.** This treatment approach was started in England during the 1940s, and was initially used with psychiatric patients. The essential concept is that of a protected and controlled environment in which patients share housekeeping and administrative duties with the staff. The result is a setting that resembles community living more than a hospital ward. The idea spread, and in 1958, Synanon, a community for the treatment of alcohol and drug abuse, was founded by Charles Dederich in Ocean Park, California.

Synanon has been a prototype for drug-abuse rehabilitation, and, since its founding, similar programs have arisen elsewhere. Some of these programs specialize in treatment of narcotics addiction; others accept substance abusers of all types. While the theoretical underpinnings of these programs are extremely varied, they do share certain characteristics. The staff usually is made up primarily of nondegreed professionals, often former addicts themselves, although the larger facilities have degreed staff as well. The patients live on the grounds and do much of the work of maintaining the facility, such as cooking and upkeep of buildings. The programs usually provide educational classes, group therapy, residential job training as well as more conventional job training, social skills building, remedial education toward high school degrees, and individual counseling. These programs emphasize abstinence from drugs, elimination of criminal behavior, development of employable skills, a new sense of self-reliance, and resocialization. They often employ the psychosocial-learning model, which views the abuser as the product of a disturbed social milieu.

OUTPATIENT TREATMENT

One of the most vital junctures in the treatment process is the transition from one treatment modality to another, for example, from inpatient to outpatient treatment. With time, the patient's sense of urgency that precipitated the initial contact abates, and his memories of problems fade. Return to the community brings temptation in the form of old drinking partners and, often, a lifestyle that includes socializing with an emphasis on alcohol and/or other drugs. The patient may have trouble learning to meet people in new ways and developing new living patterns. During the week between the initial outpatient appointment and the next one the patient may begin to again engage in denial and decide to drop out of treatment.

While some patients have support systems in family and friends, others need an extensive professional support network to maintain progress achieved in treatment and to prevent relapses. Fortunately, there are many community programs for substance abusers. The prototype, and certainly the most widely available, is Alcoholics Anonymous and the related programs of Al-Anon, Narcotics Anonymous, and Alateen.

Alcoholics Anonymous (AA) is a volunteer organization that was started by a stockbroker and a surgeon, both alcoholics who sought help at a time when formalized help was unavailable. Their initially small group has grown into a worldwide organization with over 48,000 chapters, each chapter having from four to six hundred members.

The volunteers who run AA are themselves recovering alcoholics. The organization is based on a philosophy of alcoholism contained in the "Big Book" (Alcoholics Anonymous, 1953), and summarized in a set of Twelve Steps and Traditions. Alcoholics Anonymous subscribes to the belief that alcoholism is a disease, and the program insists on the need for abstinence. The process of the program takes place partly in "meetings" that are held on a regular basis, and partly through contact with other AA members.

Most chapters hold several meetings a week, though the larger ones hold several meetings a day. AA members attend them on a voluntary basis. Members select a chairperson and a topic for discussion at each meeting. It may be related to alcoholism or it may be a topic such as anger, resentment, marriage problems, or the AA program itself. If new members are present, established members explain the format to them. The leader starts the discussion and then goes around the group, allowing each person the opportunity to comment on the topic or some other related problem or topic. Individuals may decline to comment and pass if they choose to do so.

Newcomers are often taken in tow by more experienced members, given information, and encouraged to return. Eventually, a member is expected to ask another member to "sponsor" him. A sponsor can be any same-sexed member of AA with more than a year of sobriety, who is willing to make himself available for support and what is essentially an informal counseling relationship, based on the philosophy and structure of the AA program.

In this context of group process and support, and the one-to-one relationship with a sponsor, members participate in the AA program. The essentials of the program involve a step-wise progression from personal recognition of one's alcoholism, to acknowledgement within the group setting, to commitment to sobriety. The program emphasizes the maintenance of sobriety "one day at a time," letting the months and years take care of themselves. The second phase of the program is a "searching analysis" of past and present behaviors, and the completion of the fifth step of the program which involves meeting with a minister, counselor, or sponsor, and relating past misdeeds in a process resembling confession. With time, insight, and healing, the recovering alcoholic is ready for the twelfth step of the program, which involves helping others achieve sobriety.

Although members proceed through a progression of steps within the AA program, they never really graduate. Instead, they regard alcoholism as a chronic condition that always carries the threat of relapse. For this reason, the steps of the program are linked together to form a model for daily living captured in the caveat: ". . . to practice these principles in all our affairs," (Step 12, *Alcoholics Anonymous*, 1953).

AA has been criticized for being nonprofessional, unscientific, and dependency fostering. Criticism has also focused on the fact that AA keeps no records and does little to promote research. Indeed, there can be a tremendous difference between one meeting and another, as well as a wide range of people attending them. The differences are important enough that it makes sense to recommend to patients that they try different meetings until they find one that they fit into comfortably. In any large city there will be many specialized meetings, some for professional people, some for women or men only. With a little effort, most patients can find one best suited to them.

Other complaints against AA are far outweighed by the enormous good it has done. Dependence of the members on the organization varies greatly, from considerable to almost none, and resembles the sort of dependence a congregation might have on its church. Perhaps the main problem with AA as a treatment method, however, is the ever-present group format. Patients with concomitant anxiety disorders, social phobias, or limited social skills can have insurmountable difficulties integrating themselves into the program. A second problem can be the emphasis on spirituality. While the spiritual side of most substance abusers often needs bolstering, some people are turned off by the word. AA is a nonreligious, nonsectarian organization, and there are atheists among its members who interpret spirituality in a nonreligious way. The program makes no demands on its members of a religious nature.

Some space has been devoted to AA because of its importance in the recovery process. Criticisms notwithstanding, there is no question that AA and its related organizations have proven to be one of the most successful community health programs ever devised. Its model has been adopted successfully by groups devoted to weight loss, gambling, overspend-ing, and eating disorders. For individuals who are self-motivated and can function at least minimally in a group format, AA represents one of the best chances alcoholics have for treatment success. AA is the only program available in almost every community on a seven-day-a-week basis. It is also the only program that is free of charge.

Al-Anon and Alateen are programs for the family members of alcoholics. They are organized along the same lines and principles as AA, and have proved to be of great value to family members seeking support, relief, and models for changing their situations.

Recently, another approach to dealing with the devastation of alcoholism has appeared. This method focuses on adults who have grown up in alcoholic families and suffer the consequences of chaotic and emotionally distorted childhoods. Woititz (1983) has researched these "adult children of alcoholics," and in her popular book of the same title presents her findings and recommendations for treatment. (See Box 15–4.)

These needy individuals are commonly encountered by health-care professionals in clinical settings. Recall that about one-third of adults are affected by alcohol abuse in some way, and share a number of common characteristics. Among these are a low self-concept, difficulty with intimacy, a constant need for approval, strong feelings of being different, and a basic difficulty in enjoying life. Groups using Woititz's findings and based on AA principles have appeared in many communities and are providing much needed support for the family victims of alcohol abuse.

Evaluation of the effectiveness of AA has been very difficult. Member abstinence rates of 34–75 percent have been reported; however, these figures are considered unreliable, since they do not take into consideration the fairly high dropout rate.

INDIVIDUAL COUNSELING

Neither clinical experience nor research findings (Gross, 1978) has much to recommend individual psychotherapy as a primary treatment of substance abuse. There are many reasons for this.

Substance abusers are prone to using denial and "acting out" as solutions to difficulties. Denial, as distinguished from lying, is an unconscious operation. In its pure form, the patient is not aware of engaging in it. It involves separating unpleasant aspects of reality from conscious awareness to such an extent that attempts by the therapist to challenge the denial often result in the patient's feeling attacked.

Box 15—4 ● Adult Children of Alcoholics

According to Janet Geringer Woititz, author of the nonfiction bestseller *Adult Children of Alcoholics* (1983), and inspiration of a new and growing national movement, Adult Children of Alcoholics (ACOA), children of alcoholics are robbed of their childhood. Yet, they display unflagging loyalty to their parents, paying the price with their self-esteem. They constantly seek approval and affirmation, have difficulty with intimate relationships, are super-responsible or super-irresponsible, and harbor a lot of anger.

The ACOA movement is six-years-old and growing rapidly. The concept of "co-dependency" is at the center of the movement. It involves the tendency of a family member to take responsibility for the alcoholic's drinking, and to believe that *he* or *she* can control, even cure, the problem.

Like the alcoholic, the co-dependent who does not admit his powerlessness over the substance is in a constant state of longing. Yet, Woititz says that many children of alcoholics "don't fall apart until they're in their 20s or 30s." Falling apart usually begins with a vague sense of failure or depression. Others begin having problems in childhood as a result of living in a state of constant anxiety. The evidence may be an ulcer, sleep disturbance, or other psychosomatic problem. Sometimes it is less subtle, for example, in the beer cans and drinking themes that appear in the drawings of children of alcoholics, or a sudden interest in class when the teacher talks about drinking.

Source: *Newsweek,* January 18, 1988, pp. 62–68.

Acting out refers to maladaptive behaviors a patient uses to deal with feelings in order to keep them out of conscious awareness. For substance abusers, the substance abuse itself constitutes primary acting out behavior. For example, a patient in treatment for substance abuse comes home to find his son suspended from school and his wife extremely upset. Immediately he has a few drinks "to settle his nerves" and then, his judgement clouded by the alcohol, he gets into an irrational fight with both his wife and son, ultimately leaving, exasperated, headed for the nearest bar to drown his sorrows. Later that evening, while driving home intoxicated, he is arrested for drunk driving. By the next therapy session, the main focus is likely to be the drunk driving charge. The therapist may never hear about the problems at home that precipitated the drunk driving itself.

John: A Patient with a Drinking Problem

John was brought to an initial counseling session by his wife, who had threatened to leave him because of his drinking. He had had two arrests for drunken driving, and admitted to drinking several beers before the session. While his wife recited a litany of marital and financial problems related to drinking, he said very little. At length he announced that he loved his wife and did not want a divorce. When asked if he had a drinking problem he said no, adding that he was unwilling to stop drinking. John had also acted out his feelings by drinking before this initial session in order to avoid the emotional pain likely to be associated with it; and he wasn't even in therapy yet.

Special techniques have evolved to deal with denial by the substance abuser, particularly in the beginning stages of assessment and treatment. Two of these are **confrontation** and **intervention.** Confrontation is not a sledgehammer approach. How a clinician confronts a patient is largely a matter of personal style; however, successful confrontation reframes the content of the therapeutic interaction, changing the patient's cognitive distortions into representations of reality while allowing the patient to maintain his personal integrity. Timing and tact are important. In the case of John, the therapist waited until a part of the session when his wife, exasperated, asked, "What has to happen before he will stop drinking?" The therapist replied, "Some alcoholics have to lose everything before they are willing to consider it." John's response to this exchange was to look at the floor with a sheepish, somewhat startled, look on his face.

While this therapist's comments may seem relatively low key, they proved to be useful, and contained the essence of confrontation, that is, a reframing of denial. In other situations, to be effective, confrontation must be more direct, even harsh, to be heard by the patient, the risk being that the patient will terminate therapy if he feels attacked. Whether such a risk is worth taking is a matter of clinical judgment. Some clinicians would say it is less a risk than a screening mechanism useful in sifting out patients who are serious about treatment.

An "Intervention" forms an important part of some treatment programs. Intervention consists of assembling the patient's family, along with friends, coworkers, employers, and significant others, asking each participant to tell both the patient and the rest of the group of his or her experiences with the patient's drinking, and what it has meant to him or her. Intervention emphasizes relating feelings, *not* laying blame; that is, exploring how each individual *feels* about the patient's behavior. The technique is very effective as long as care is taken that the patient is not overwhelmed. In the case of John, this type of intervention was in progress though it involved only John's wife. As she told her story, the therapist fostered a safe atmosphere by redirecting her away from expressions of blaming, and encouraging her to focus on her feelings, for example, the hurt, anger, and frustration she was experiencing.

Although individual psychotherapy for substance-abuse disorders is no panacea, it can be of some value. For example, John and his wife returned for a second assessment session. The therapist continued to focus on the need for a more formal alcohol and drug assessment, to which John ultimately agreed. Following an inpatient treatment program, John and his wife returned for further counseling. In counseling, the therapist initially focused on attendance at AA and Alanon meetings and the couple's relationship. As time progressed, the therapist relinquished her supportive role, relying on the AA programs for that function, and the sessions took on a more psychodynamic focus.

Therapy, if not handled with care, can be counterproductive. Alice, who was mentioned earlier, had been in both individual and family therapy at the time she was drinking heavily. Her therapist had had special training in dealing with substance abuse, and the therapy continued for more than two years. Despite the fact that Alice often had several drinks before the therapy sessions, only her husband's drinking was openly discussed. Ultimately, Alice sought help on her own, when the pain of her addiction could no longer be narcoticized by the enabling behavior of her family and her therapist. In this case, countertransference was the problem. The therapist had been subconsciously involved with Alice. He was having marital problems of his own and was able to deny his own wife's drinking problem as long as he avoided recognizing and confronting Alice's substance abuse. Although hardly to blame for Alice's problem, her therapist unconsciously became a part of the disturbed family system and perpetuated it.

While some substance abusers have problems that are easily managed in therapy, others have more profound personality disturbances such as those described in the section on psychoanalytic theories of alcoholism. The case of Alice, whose therapist saw her for more than two years without recognizing her alcoholism, illustrates the countertransference problems that can arise in assessment as well as therapy. Faced with a patient who deals with his problems by denying them and blaming others, and whose emotions are obscured by alcohol and/or drug use, the therapist may find herself operating with little real information in a therapy based on distorted feelings and half truths.

FAMILY THERAPY

Family therapy is often an integral part of the treatment of substance abuse. Most inpatient treatment programs involve the family, and many include other members of the patient's social network as well. While there is no typical family of the substance abuser, it is possible to discuss commonly encountered characteristics.

Many of these families have traveled a rough road. At best, they have experienced frequent discord, isolation, prominent use of denial and evasion by family members, and inhibited emotional growth. At worst, they have lived with violence, sexual abuse, extramarital affairs, several divorces, and chronically chaotic home life. Family members, not dealing directly with problems, tend to internalize conflicts. Guilt and resentment abound. Family members are rarely held responsible for their behavior, and are often unclear about their roles. The boundaries among them often become weakened and confused. Distorted relationships are the rule, and fear of emotional retaliation and even violence prevents self-assertion.

The wide variation in characteristics of alcoholic families has made it difficult to describe them in ways that consistently differentiate them from normal families. Kauffman and Pattison (1981), and Kauffman

(1984), have attempted to develop typologies that distinguish these disturbed families by means of four family reactivity types:

1. *The functional family system.* On the surface, this family appears stable and happy. Drinking is done outside the home or late at night. It is difficult for the clinician to learn the causative and maintenance factors involved, and the family's psychological defenses seem impenetrable. This family is typically supportive of treatment of their alcoholic member, and responds well to behavioral approaches. Therapy is best focused on education, setting limits regarding behavior, and the use of disulfiram, a drug which, taken regularly, prevents impulsive drinking. Great emotional insights should not be expected, as the defenses of these families are powerfully entrenched.

2. *The neurotic enmeshed family system.* Family functioning is severely affected by the alcoholic member. Stress in any family member affects everyone. There is pronounced blurring of roles. Communication often occurs through third parties. Conflicts are projected onto others and family members feel guilty and responsible for each other. Psychotherapeutic approaches to treatment turn out to be long and difficult. Often the therapist will become the family moderator, helping family members focus on the here and now, pointing out what is necessary for them to restructure their lives.

3. *The disintegrated family system.* In this family, the alcoholic is often completely disengaged, usually as a result of separation or divorce. In many cases, however, this is only a pseudoseparation; strong emotional bonds remain. Treatment of these families focuses on exploration of ruptured relationships and the establishment of new roles. Initially, the alcoholic receives treatment separate from the family. Once the patient has achieved sobriety, it is possible to have true family therapy sessions that explore the dynamics of existing interactions as well as the potential of family members' relationships with one another.

4. *The absent family system.* In this family, the alcoholic has been isolated for a long time. This patient probably has never had good coping skills, and there may be no family to work with. Treatment consists of helping the individual develop a social network and maintain sobriety. Longer-term goals for some of these patients, for example, the "street person", might consist of vocational training and help with developing independent living skills.

BEHAVIORAL APPROACHES TO TREATMENT

The advantage of the behavioral approach to the treatment of alcoholism lies in its flexibility and wide variety of available techniques. Behaviorists begin with detailed baseline assessments. This includes a detailed personal and family history, and a thorough investigation of patterns of drinking, precipitants of drinking, such as events at home that usually lead to a drinking episode, and environmental factors that promote drinking. This information is used in the development of a treatment plan which has as its goal the modification of the alcoholic's behavior.

Methods used have included: 1) chemical aversion, which involves giving an emetic along with alcohol to produce an aversive stimulus; 2) contingency contracting, an agreement providing rewards for the patient's sobriety, such as positive feedback from family and friends; 3) training in discrimination of blood alcohol levels; 4) videotape feedback; and 5) social skills and assertiveness training.

Some researchers from the behavioral school of treatment have challenged the traditional goal of treatment of alcoholism, sobriety. Sobell and Sobell (1973a, 1973b, 1976) have developed a broad spectrum treatment package designed to show that alcoholics can learn to modify their addictive behavior and become social drinkers. This concept has generated a great deal of controversy and media interest. The Sobells' treatment package involves a number of approaches directed at altering the patient's drinking behavior, the goal being "controlled" drinking rather than abstinence. While initial outcome studies were encouraging, at this point most agree that the accumulated outcome data do not justify such an approach, some because they believe the research is flawed. For this reason the standard treatment goal remains abstinence.

THE NETWORK APPROACH

Social network theory focuses on human beings as social animals. Favazza and Thompson (1984) define a **psychosocial network** as the sum total of all persons with whom an individual has a relationship; this includes family, friends, neighbors, coworkers, employers, and so forth. Networks provide an individual with social and emotional resources in times of crisis, a social framework within which to assess one's own functioning, and ongoing nurturing that provides a sense of well-being. Studies indicate that, in general, the more disturbed a person is emotionally, the fewer individuals in his social network, and the less useful that network is to him.

Studies of the social networks of alcoholics are in their infancy. However, the strategy of "intervention," behavioral techniques, and the concept of rehabilitation of the alcoholic with an absent family system all contain the essentials of a network approach to the treatment of alcoholism. Galanter's (1984) approach, which includes disulfiram and other standard techniques, such as involvement with Alcoholics Anonymous, also emphasizes regular meetings of the treatment team with network members, and an active attempt to restructure the patient's social network as a necessary part of treatment, encouraging him to ally himself with selected individuals the team views as helpful.

PHARMACOTHERAPY OF SUBSTANCE ABUSE

The two most commonly used drug treatments for substance abuse are **disulfiram,** used in the treatment of alcoholism, and **methadone,** used in the treatment of narcotic addiction.

Alcohol is normally metabolized in the liver, where it is first oxidized to acetaldehyde. Acetaldehyde is a toxic substance, but never accumulates in the body to any extent, as it is rapidly broken down into other, less toxic substances. Disulfiram blocks the breakdown of acetaldehyde, allowing it to accumulate. When a person is taking disulfiram, ingestion of even a small amount of alcohol results in a very unpleasant reaction as a result of the subsequent buildup of acetaldehyde.

The disulfiram-ethanol reaction is proportional to the amount of alcohol ingested. It includes headaches, flushing, nausea, vomiting, chest pain, palpitations, tachycardia, and confusion. The reaction lasts from several minutes to several hours and typically does not require more than supportive measures as treatment. In some cases, however, this reaction has led to arrhythmias, cardiovascular collapse, seizures, and death.

In principle, while taking disulfiram, an alcoholic is less likely to drink, knowing that he will have an adverse reaction. Impulsive drinking, in particular, is inhibited. Of course, disulfiram alone cannot prevent drinking. An abuser who decides to resume drinking will simply stop the drug and, within a week or two, start using alcohol without fear of a reaction. While

followup studies have not demonstrated a significant or predictable effect on treatment outcome, clinicians frequently prescribe the drug and many patients rely on it to help maintain sobriety.

Methadone, which is used in the long-term management of narcotics addicts, has been looked upon as a major clinical advance. Methadone is a narcotic that can be taken orally. Although it does not result in the same "high" as narcotics do, it prevents narcotic withdrawal symptoms and abolishes the craving for narcotics. It is a relatively safe drug and has few side effects. Methadone maintenance programs are in existence throughout the country. An addict accepted into such a program receives a dose of methadone in liquid form on a daily basis from the treatment center. In principle, this abolishes secondary withdrawal symptoms as well as the craving for the narcotic, and prevents relapse with street drugs. Patients are also offered other services such as counseling. One problem with this approach is a dropout rate of about 25 percent. Concurrent use of alcohol by patients treated with methadone has also been a problem. Withdrawal from methadone itself has been tried with little success. Thus it is likely that these patients need methadone maintenance for life. Those who stay with the program, however, and do not relapse with other drugs, show significant improvement in their social adaptation.

Interest in using lithium as a treatment for alcoholism has led to investigations designed to evaluate its effects, however it has not been shown to be an effective treatment. At present, lithium and antidepressants are indicated only for those alcoholics who have a concurrent diagnosis of mood disorder.

RESPONSIBILITIES OF THE NURSE IN THE ASSESSMENT AND TREATMENT OF SUBSTANCE ABUSE

The role of the nurse in the assessment and treatment of patients with substance-abuse problems will vary from setting to setting, depending on how responsibilities are shared. In recent years the concept of the treatment team has become more common, and the nurse involved in the treatment of patients with substance-abuse problems can expect to take a dynamic and responsible role in patient assessment and management. This role will include many aspects of evaluation, treatment, and aftercare.

Box 15–5 ● Suggested Readings

There is a lot of literature on substance abuse. Some sources are technical and review the scientific literature, attempting to give an accurate account for the technically minded person of the current state of the art. Other works consist essentially of personal experience and the individual viewpoints of the authors. A third subset of readings on substance abuse is aimed at a lay audience. Below are listed several suggestions for further reading which include each of the above types of material. It should be noted that in the case of clinical practice, personal experience is a valuable, indispensible learning process. Our ability to share these experiences with the authors of the references cited is an opportunity that should not be foregone.

1. Mendelson, Jack H., & Mello, Nancy K., Eds., *The Diagnosis and Treatment of Alcoholism*. New York: McGraw Hill Book Company, 1985. This is a comprehensive summary of the literature on alcoholism. It includes material on diagnosis, theories of etiology, and the various methods of treatment. It is an indispensable tool for the clinician who wishes an up-to-date reference. The material presented is both technical and practical.
2. Vallaint, George E., *The Natural History of Alcoholism*. Cambridge, Mass.: Harvard University Press, 1983. Vallaint is a psychiatrist with much experience in this field. His book describes a collaborative study that has been going on since the 1930s, which endeavored to explore

ASSESSMENT

The nurse is often responsible for the extended assessment of the patient, his family, and his social network. Many substance abusers are reluctant to accept a diagnosis of substance abuse. As a result they and their families may obscure and hold back information that would lead to such a diagnosis. The primary task of the treatment team initially is to maintain a positive relationship with the patient during the data-collection phase in order to avoid a rupture of the therapeutic alliance and resulting withdrawal of the patient and/or his family from the evaluation. The nurse has the primary role of establishing and maintaining a positive relationship with the patient and the important people in his life. She obtains a social history, ascertains the extent of the patient's social network, determines the composition and functioning of the immediate family, arranges family meetings, and actively participates in family discussions regarding the patient's activities and lifestyle. As rapport begins to build and family members become more comfortable in discussing sensitive issues, the nurse will be able to acquire a sense of the intimate lifestyle of the patient and his family. The more the nurse knows about the patient, the more able she will be to individualize treatment and nursing care.

ESTABLISHING NURSING DIAGNOSES

The establishment of a clinical diagnosis of substance abuse allows the treatment team to focus its efforts. A competent nursing diagnosis determines the specific needs of the patient to whom the team should direct those efforts. As we have seen, substance abusers present with a variety of problems that may affect many areas of their physical and psychological well-being. Nursing diagnoses will intersect all areas of their lives. In some cases there will be a number of physical problems, which, in their own right, will require assessment and diagnosis. These will not be considered in this chapter as their management is dealt with in other texts. Instead, the emphasis will be on the emotional and spiritual dysfunction of substance abusers which is often assessed and attended to by the patient's primary nurse.

The North American Nursing Diagnosis Association (NANDA) has established a corpus of approved nursing diagnoses that facilitate the assessment of the needs of the substance abuser. The following list of nursing diagnoses typically encountered in alcoholics and their families are listed in the order of NANDA's Taxonomy I.

ALTERATION IN NUTRITION. Under this heading are three possibilities in the NANDA diagnoses:

both the course and origins of alcoholism. The book, however, contains much more. Vallaint summarizes much of the research and gives an outstanding discussion of the theoretical and practical issues at stake. There is a superb discussion of the concept of alcoholism as a disease.

3. Lowenson, Joyce H., & Ruiz, Pedro, Eds., *Substance Abuse, Clinical Problems and Perspectives.* Baltimore, Md.: Williams and Wilkins, 1981. This is a comprehensive textbook on substance abuse and deals with virtually every aspect.

4. Mannaioni, P. F., *Clinical Pharmacology of Drug Dependency.* Forward by William W. Clendenin. Padua, Italy: Piccin Nuova Libraria, S.P.A., 1984. This is essentially a pharmacology text,

but includes much information regarding the etiology and treatment of substance abuse.

5. Wholey, Dennis, *The Courage to Change, Hope and Help for Alcoholics and Their Families.* Boston: Houghton Mifflin Company, 1984. This is superb general reading on alcoholism intended for a general audience. It contains the personal stories of many persons including celebrities and describes their process of addiction and treatment. A most valuable way to gain insight into the nature of alcoholism.

6. Mumey, Jack, *The Joy of Being Sober,* Chicago: Contemporary Books, Inc., 1984. A nice source book for alcoholics. Describes the

process of treatment and recovery and has much about AA.

7. Woititz, Janet Geringer, *Adult Children of Alcoholics,* Hollywood, Fla.: Health Communications, Inc., 1983. The definitive book for adult children of alcoholics organizations, this small volume is easy and practical reading based on Dr. Woititz's clinical experience.

8. Maxwell, Milton A., *The AA Experience, a Close-Up View for Professionals,* New York: McGraw Hill Book Company, 1984. This is the next best thing to actually attending an AA meeting, which of course is also recommended.

Less than body requirements

More than body requirements

Potential for more than body requirements

Substance abusers may exhibit any one of these diagnoses. Alcoholics and other drug abusers often present as malnourished. Bulimia is another problem frequently concurrent with alcohol abuse, especially in the young female alcoholic.

SOCIAL ISOLATION. This is a result of relationship disturbances and the primacy of alcohol in the patient's life.

ALTERED PARENTING. Actual and potential parenting problems abound in families where one or both parents are substance abusers. Effective management and prevention require assessment of parenting skills, and intervention and education as necessary.

SEXUAL DYSFUNCTION. Altered patterns of sexuality and sexual dysfunction can accompany substance abuse, either on a physiological or emotional basis and, of course, contribute further to relationship problems.

ALTERED FAMILY PROCESSES. As mentioned earlier, the family in which one or more members is

experiencing substance abuse will be under a great deal of stress and all members of the family will be affected.

SPIRITUAL DISTRESS. Guilt or shame as well as low self-esteem are often indicators of spiritual distress.

COPING. There are five diagnoses under the pattern of choosing that are related to coping and relevant to nursing management of substance abuse.

Ineffective individual coping

Defensive coping

Ineffective family coping: disabling

Ineffective family coping: compromised

Family coping: potential for growth

These diagnoses will apply to most abusers presenting for treatment and the material presented in this text should provide a basis for making these determinations. It is important to keep in mind that substance abuse tends to be familial, and many families will have more than one substance abuser.

NONCOMPLIANCE. An individual in a treatment program, either inpatient or outpatient, is expected to perform certain tasks, such as maintaining sobriety, avoiding bars, and so forth, and ascertaining compliance should be an ongoing part of the treatment and assessment process. It is important that family members support compliance and help with its assessment.

SLEEP PATTERN DISTURBANCE. This is common, especially during withdrawal from alcohol, but also often occurs with ongoing use.

DISTURBANCE IN SELF-CONCEPT. Disturbances in self-esteem, role performance, and personal identity commonly arise in the context of the disturbed, abusive relationships in families of substance abusers.

KNOWLEDGE DEFICIT. Many individuals in substance-abuse treatment have a surprising lack of knowledge about the effects of these substances on their physical and emotional well-being. Moreover, both they and their families lack an appreciation of the impact of the abuse on their lives. It is important to seek out and correct misunderstandings and misinformation so that effective treatment can proceed.

ANXIETY. Many patients who abuse drugs complain of anxiety. During periods of drug withdrawal, anxiety is a common symptom and can contribute greatly to the restlessness and discomfort of the patient. In addition, it is not uncommon for substance abusers to experience unease in social settings. Since many treatment programs utilize the group approach, it is important to identify this problem before it begins to interfere with treatment.

POTENTIAL FOR VIOLENCE. The alcohol-violence connection is significant. See Chapter 20, Psychiatric Mental Health Nursing with Men, and Chapter 24, Psychiatric Mental Health Nursing and the Violent Patient.

IMPLEMENTING NURSING CARE

The nurse is also responsible for helping patients and their families cope with difficult and complicated medical situations. In the case of substance abuse, there is often denial, resistance, and confusion when the diagnosis is presented. The rapport built during the evaluation phase of treatment will go a long way to overcome these hurdles.

The nurse is responsible for educating patients and their families about substance abuse, its effects, and its treatment. A tactful approach in presenting the relevant information will abate much of the confusion families and patients often feel initially. The nurse is responsible for distributing relevant reading material, explaining the resources that are available locally, facilitating the use of these resources, and helping to counter initial resistance the family might have in seeking help. A stratagem of tact, patience, and persistence will help to counter the denial and negativism that is often seen. It is important to remember that education in the face of denial is an ongoing process. The nurse may have to make many repetitions and must offer support.

The nurse will have many responsibilities around the medical care of the new patient. It is particularly important that the nurse be aware of an individual patient's potential for withdrawal. It is often the case that a patient will minimize or deny his drug use, and withdrawal may appear unexpectedly. Careful monitoring of the patient's vital signs and mental status is particularly important during the first few days of assessment and treatment. In addition, the nurse should do a nutritional assessment of the patient, monitor food and fluid intake, and prepare a treatment plan that will correct any nutritional deficiencies. Of course, there are many other medical disorders that can accompany substance abuse, for example, organic brain syndrome and pancreatitis, and the nurse will have to adapt the treatment plan to include the interventions needed for these problems.

At times, substance abusers will require medication, and it will usually be up to the nurse to provide information regarding the purpose, side effects, and necessity of any medications. Substance abusers are often treated with vitamin supplements, disulfiram, and in specialized centers, methadone, so the nurse needs to be familiar with these substances and their side effects.

During the treatment of substance abuse, patients commonly attend groups, individual counseling sessions, and family sessions. The nurse is often responsible for participating in these and takes an active therapeutic role. Again, the frequent contact between the patient and nurse is a valuable aid in facilitating these sessions. At times the nurse will be the group leader in educational groups and groups requiring self-disclosure.

The nurse plays an important role in aftercare. Many substance abusers will need long-term followup for their conditions, and much community support. The nurse can help organize community treatment and arrange for outpatient counseling and/ or her participation in outpatient counseling, and monitoring of nutrition, compliance, and family functioning. The nurse may need to provide specialized services for disorganized families such as home visits, parent training, teaching home economic skills, and well-child care. The nurse will also participate in ongoing medication management, monitoring vital signs and compliance with the treatment plan, and maintaining a relationship with the patient that promotes it.

The nurse will often be the member of the treatment team who has the most contact with the patient, and so may be the one to whom the patient turns in times of crisis. Thus it is not unusual for the nurse to be responsible for crisis management in working with the substance-abuse patient and his family.

ADDICTIONS NURSING

The Division on Psychiatric and Mental Health Nursing Practice of the American Nurses' Association set up a task force in 1983 to consider the practice of addictions nursing as a specialty area of nursing. The task force, consisting of members of the ANA Council on Psychiatric and Mental Health Nursing, the National Nurses' Society on Addictions, and the Drug and Alcohol Nursing Association, worked to define the parameters of this specialty area. The result is a document called *The Care of Clients*

with Addictions: Dimensions of Nursing Practice (ANA, 1987, p.1). The task force defines addictions nursing as the

> . . . Diagnosis and treatment of human response to patterns of abuse and addiction. The client's responses may be to actual or potential health problems related to abuse and addiction. Addictions nursing is a specialized area of nursing practice that employs theories of the biological, behavioral, and social sciences as well as theories and principles of nursing practice. The continuum of patterns of abuse and addiction elicits human responses. These responses are the essence of nursing diagnoses.

A central outlook in this specialty is the inclusion of the family, including significant others, as essential to the assessment, planning, and treatment of clients with addictions. Standards of addictions nursing are described in detail in the ANA publication, *Standards of Addictions: Nursing Practice with Selected Diagnoses and Criteria* (ANA, 1987).

It should be remembered that the material in the case history is not Fran's complete story. Again, this is the sort of information that one might expect from an initial interview. Actually, many patients are so defensive that little useful information can be obtained at first; the initial session is more of a basis on which to build trust than a fact-finding mission.

Case Study: Nonpsychiatric Setting

The following is an example of the information that might be obtained in a single interview with a patient who presents with family problems but who needs an alcohol and drug assessment. Notice that it is very easy to regard this patient's drinking problem as secondary; many patients who are substance abusers have such extensive problems with their personal lives that the alcohol use pales in comparison. In addition, very little information is forthcoming as to the amount of alcohol consumed, and there is a somewhat hazy quality about the nature of the drinking. These features are rather typical of many interviews, as patients often slant their presentations to suit their distorted perceptions of their lives. Diagnosing substance abuse is often more a matter of recognizing and interpreting somewhat subtle clues than engaging in a direct, straightforward interchange of information with the patient.

Fran was a single parent who arrived at The Family Practice Clinic for help with her son who was a behavior problem. Her life was a struggle from one crisis to another, and she had so many problems she hardly knew where to begin.

She had divorced her husband four years before and had been raising her two children alone. Her ex-husband, John, was erratic with child support and money was a major problem. Because she had little work experience, she could earn little better than minimum wage at a job that was unfulfilling and boring. Her son, Eric, was a major problem. For more than two years, he had been skipping school and making poor grades. He was also rude and noncompliant at home as well as at school. At the time of Fran's interview, he was in detention, having stolen a car. For the last few months, John had refused to take Eric on weekends, saying that Eric was too hard to manage. Her daughter, Amy, an excellent student, had become fearful, withdrawn, and clingy; Fran was relieved when Amy would visit her dad on weekends. Arguments with her ex-husband continued and Fran felt much anger and resentment toward him. The family had been in counseling with the school social worker on a number of occasions with very little progress; John often missed counseling sessions, and when he did attend, the sessions ended in screaming matches.

During the interview Fran agreed that her alcohol use had increased over the last year or so but didn't feel that it interfered with her life. She was quick to point out that her divorce was prompted by her husband's alcohol abuse, and proudly stated that she drove home from parties after he had had too much to drink. Fran was eager to talk about her nihilistic marriage, and the arguments, the confused lifestyle, her husband's affairs, and his verbal abuse of her and the children; but she was somewhat resistant to talking about her own behavior.

However, with some prompting, Fran revealed a pattern of increasing frequency of use and amount of alcohol over the last two years. Her coworkers often had drinks after work and many times on the job she looked at the clock, waiting for the end of the day, and her "break" from the tensions of work and raising children. After the children were in bed, she would have two or three drinks to "unwind" and help her sleep. Recently there had been times, particularly when Eric had been a problem to get off to school, when she would have a drink before work. This bothered her, but she felt it was a normal response to the kind of stress that she was living with. Eric complained about her drinking sometimes, but then Eric complained about everything.

Fran's relationships were limited to men, and on dates she usually went to bars or parties where drinking was accepted. She had had too much to drink at times and not remembered parts of the evening but said this was under control. She was sociable and attractive and fit easily into this milieu. Fran had no women friends, and in fact was uncomfortable around other women; she related much better to men. The parties and dating helped blot out the inner feelings of loneliness and pain that she was increasingly more aware of. It had become almost impossible for her to sit alone in her apartment when the children were gone. Their rooms were messy and the apartment was small and depressing. It was a place where she felt trapped and demoralized. Fran was thirty-five and felt that her life was going nowhere.

Fran began to talk about her childhood and wondered for the first time if her father were alcoholic. There was always drinking before, during, and after dinner. A few times, her father got drunk and her parents had terrible arguments. But these occasions were the exception rather than the rule. Actually, she remembered very little of the years before high school and knew very little about her extended family. Her mother and father were silent about their families and she never spent time with her grandparents alone. She did remember that her uncle was said to have a drinking problem.

In many ways, Fran's life lacked substance and meaning and her social skills only served to keep her relationships numerous but superficial. The past ten years had been times of continuous upheaval and turmoil as a result of her husband's drinking and Eric's problems. She experienced recurrent periods of low mood, intermittent anxiety, and frequently was unable to sleep without drinking. As a result, she found herself taking drinks when she didn't really want to. She felt totally isolated and rootless, as if she had nothing to stand on. The problems with her son had driven her to the wall, and she was ready to try anything. However, she was sure that if someone could help her son, and convince her ex-husband to act more responsibly, her drinking would take care of itself.

DSM-III-R Diagnosis

Axis I Alcohol abuse (305.00); parent-child problem (V61.20)
Axis II None known
Axis III None known
Axis IV Psychosocial stressors: single parent, financial difficulties; severity: 3
Axis V Current GAF: 60

Nursing Diagnoses

Ineffective family coping: disabling
Altered health maintenance
Knowledge deficit
Disturbance in self-concept: personal identity

Nursing Care Plan for Fran

Nursing Diagnosis	Desired Outcomes	Interventions	Rationale
1. Ineffective family coping: disabling.	Family communication will improve, with resumption of parental authority and a working relationship between Fran and her ex-husband will be established.	With Fran's permission, make contact with the school social worker and establish an alliance that will promote an exchange of information and an agreement as to treatment goals and methods.	The school social worker has had experience with Eric in school and with his family in counseling sessions. Her perspective may be useful to the nurse in treatment planning. Also, working with a multi-problem family often demands a team approach. The opportunity to talk with colleagues about countertransference issues can make an overwhelming situation manageable.
		Arrange family sessions to gather more data, and begin the building of rapport.	Encouraging the family to continue counseling with the social worker, despite the difficulties so far, is essential to the treatment of the dysfunctional system responsible for Fran's drinking and Eric's behavior problems.

Nursing Diagnosis	Desired Outcomes	Interventions	Rationale
			Eric's father needs to be told that his participation in counseling is so important to helping Eric that, if he doesn't plan to attend, it might as well not go on at all, in which case it is extremely likely that Eric's problems will get worse.
		Arrange an alcohol and drug assessment of Eric, who is exhibiting some of the common behaviors of adolescents who are substance abusers.	Substance abuse in adolescents is common. Their normal "grandiosity" prevents them from realizing that it can hurt them. They rarely present voluntarily for assessment and treatment, but are nevertheless responsive to treatment when it is offered, particularly if their families support and participate in it.
2. Altered health maintenance.	Fran will maintain normal weight and nutrition, and will understand the dangers of alcohol-related diseases.	Make initial assessment of body weight, nutritional status, cognitive functioning, and potential for withdrawal syndromes.	Physical sequellae of substance abuse need to be diagnosed and treated; potential for withdrawal in the case of addiction needs to be assessed and prepared for. Hospitalization may be necessary.
		Provide information about alcohol-related illnesses and nutrition.	Graphic description of the illnesses associated with alcoholism, for example, liver failure, may motivate the substance abuser to engage and stay in treatment.
		Monitor general health periodically.	Deterioration of health may indicate that substance abuse continues or has begun again, despite the patient's denial.
3. Knowledge deficit.	Fran will understand the basic facts about alcoholism and the impact of alcohol abuse on the lives of the patient and family.	Initial education about alcoholism through face-to-face contact, and supportive educational media, such as reading material and videotapes.	Presenting information through a variety of resources is likely to hold the patient's interest and break through denial that there is a problem.

Nursing Diagnosis	Desired Outcomes	Interventions	Rationale
		Introduction to AA and related community programs where further education may be obtained.	AA and Alanon are available, accessible, effective means of combating substance abuse and aiding its casualties (like Eric).
4. Disturbance in self-concept: personal identity.	Fran will exhibit an improved ability to take responsibility for herself and will allow others to take responsibilities for their own actions.	Encourage Fran to attend programs such as Alcoholics Anonymous which place emphasis on the needs and responsibilities of the individual.	The substance abuser often has a low sense of self-esteem due to relationship problems. The self-concept can also be disturbed in the other direction: the patient may feel grandiose and immune to the effects of substance abuse, especially addiction.
		Promote supportive individual counseling.	Individual as well as family counseling is often indicated for the substance abuser regardless of age. Support is essential during the important but difficult task of radically changing his or her lifestyle (which often revolves around the substance abuse) if this is to be successful. Also, once the abuse is under control, insight-oriented (psychoanalytic) or cognitive-behavioral psychotherapy may be helpful in understanding the underlying thoughts and feelings which are partly responsible for and/or maintain the drinking or drug problem.

SUMMARY

Substance abuse has a dramatic and devastating impact on a person's life. It also costs the nation billions of dollars a year in a myriad of ways and causes an immeasurable amount of human suffering and social turmoil. Over the last twenty years, there has been a steady increase in its incidence. Currently, it may be the country's most important public health problem; it is certainly one of the most common problems clinicians confront in their work.

Recognition of substance abuse is hampered by many factors, not the least of which are the conscious and unconscious attempts on the part of its victims to deny their involvement. This use of denial and other primitive defense mechanisms to cope with life stress has led many substance abusers into patterns of behavior that pile problem on problem, leading to chaotic and desperate personal lives.

The substance abuser often presents with a host of involved family, financial, legal, and medical problems that make a multifactorial approach a necessity for an adequate evaluation. The nurse must be prepared to assess a variety of physical health problems as well as mental status including suicide potential, and/or other psychiatric problems that may be present. She needs to meet the family members and evaluate family functioning, and explore the possibilities of family violence, incest, and child neglect; and ultimately take on a coordinator role, and help the family face the difficult times ahead. The family usually also needs help with financial planning, and assistance with employers and other relevant professionals, such as attorneys, probation officers, or child welfare workers.

Assessment, however, is only the beginning. There are many approaches to treatment, though there is little research to support one over another, and it is easy to be lost among the confusing claims and counterclaims to the different treatment models. At some point in time, however, the patient in any treatment program will become part of an outpatient program, and usually one involving a combination of approaches. It is likely that the patient and his family will be involved in both individual and family therapy of a supportive nature, and be expected to participate in group treatment modeled on the Alcoholics Anonymous approach. In fact, the consensus is that regular attendance at AA and Al-Anon offers the best chance for the average substance abuser to remain substance free. (See also Box 15–5 on pages 550–551.)

Treating the substance abuser is often frustrating and discouraging. In particular, these patients often bring out the clinician's own hidden fears and conflicts, and she may at times find herself in conflict with herself as well as the patient. It is important to keep in mind that nurses are human too. In fact, there is better than one chance in three that she may have been affected by substance abuse. As a result, each person has, during her lifetime, acquired a fund of prejudice and misconception about substance use and abuse that she may have to dispense with before she can comfortably and effectively treat these patients.

KEY TERMS

alcoholism	dependence
abuse	tolerance
withdrawal	acting out
opiate receptors	confrontation
operant conditioning	intervention
blood alcohol assay	family therapy
blackouts	social network theory
craving	psychosocial network
detoxification	disulfiram
therapeutic communities	methadone
Alcoholics Anonymous (AA)	

STUDY QUESTIONS

1. Define and describe substance abuse and substance dependence, including the three criteria for abuse.

2. Define and describe intoxication and withdrawal.

3. Name at least one special problem hindering diagnosis in each of the following population: teenagers; women; the elderly.

4. Describe the basic approach and techniques of treatment used by Alcoholics Anonymous.

5. Describe the basic role of the nurse in treating the substance abuser and his or her family.

REFERENCES

Alcoholics Anonymous. (1976). *Alcoholics anonymous,* 3rd ed. New York: Alcoholics Anonymous World Services.

Alcoholics Anonymous. (1953). *Twelve steps and twelve traditions.* New York: Alcoholics Anonymous World Services.

American Nurses' Association (1987). *The care of clients with addictions: Dimensions of nursing practice.* Kansas City, MO: American Nurses' Association.

American Nurses' Association (1987). *Standards of addictions nursing practice with selected diagnoses and criteria.* Kansas City, MO: American Nurses' Association.

Beck, A. T. (1976). *Cognitive therapy and the emotional disorders.* New York: International Universities Press.

Beck A. T. (1979). *Cognitive therapy of depression.* New York: Guilford Press.

Caddy, G. R., & Lovibond, S. H. (1976). Self-regulation and discriminated aversive-conditioning in the modification of alcoholics' drinking behavior. *Behavioral Therapy,* 7:223–23.

Favazza, A., & Thompson, J. (1984). A psychosocial network approach to alcoholism. From M. Gallanter, & E. Pattison (Eds.), *Advances in the psychosocial treatment of alcoholism.* American Psychiatric Press, Inc.

Flax, S. (1985). "The Executive Addict." *Fortune,* June 24, 1985.

Gallanter, M. (1984). The use of social networks in office management of the substance abuser. From M. Gallanter, & E. Pattison (Eds.), *Advances in the psychosocial treatment of alcoholism.* American Psychiatric Press, Inc.

Gay, G. R., Sheppard, C., Inaba, D., & Newmeyer, J. (1973). Cocaine in perspective: "Gift from the sun god" to "The rich man's drug." *Drug forum,* 2(4):409–430.

Gold, M. S., Redmond, D. E., & Kleher, H. D. (1978). Clonidine blocks acute withdrawal symptoms. *The Lancet,* September 16, 1978, pp. 599–601.

Goodwin, D. W. (1985). Genetic Determinants of Alcoholism. From J. H. Mendelson, & N. K. Mello, (Eds.). *The diagnosis and treatment of alcoholism,* 2nd ed. New York: McGraw-Hill.

Goodwin, D. W., & Erickson, C. K. (1979). (Eds.). *Alcoholism and affective disorders.* New York: Spectrum Books.

Kauffman, E. (1984). The current state of family intervention in alcoholism treatment. From M. Gallanter, & E. Pattison, (Eds.), *Advances in the psychosocial treatment of alcoholism.* American Psychiatric Press, Inc.

Kauffman, E., & Pattison, E. M. (1981). Differential methods of family therapy in the treatment of alcoholism. *J. Stud. Alcohol,* 42:951–971.

Loper, R. G., Kammeier, M. L., & Hoffmann, H. (1973). "M. M. P. I. characteristics of college freshmen males who later become alcoholics." *Journal of Abnormal Psychology,* 82: 159–162.

Mahler, M. S., Pine, F., & Bergman, A. (1975). *The psychological birth of the human infant: symbiosis and individuation.* New York: Basic Books.

Mannaioni, P. F. (1984). *Clinical pharmacology of drug dependency.* Forward by William W. Clendenin. Padua, Italy: Piccin Nuova Libraria S.P.A.

McLaughlin, G. T. (1973). Cocaine: The history and regulation of a dangerous drug. *Cornell Law Review,* 5813:537–572.

Meyer, R. E., & Mirin, S. M. (1981). A psychology of craving: Implications of behavioral research. From J.

H. Lowinson, & P. Ruiz (Eds.), *Substance abuse: clinical problems and perspectives.* Baltimore, MD: Williams and Wilkins, 1981.

Reed, M. *Time Magazine,* May 20, 1985, Vol. 25, No. 20.

Schuster, C. R. (1970). Psychological approaches to opiate dependence and self-administration by laboratory animals. *Fed. Proc.* 29, 2–5.

Simon, E. J., Hiller, J. M., & Edelman, J. (1947, 1973). Stereo specific binding of the potent narcotic analgesic 3H-etorphine to rat brain homogenate. *Proc. Natl. Acad. Sci.* USA 70.

Snyder, S. H. (1975). Opiate receptor in normal and drug altered brain function. *Nature,* 257, 185–189.

Sobell, M. B., & Sobell, L. C., (1973a). Individualized behavior therapy for alcoholics. *Behav. Ther.,* 4:49–72.

———, (1973b), Alcoholics treated by individualized behavior therapy: One year treatment outcome. *Behav. Res. Ther.,* 11: 559–618.

———, (1976), Second-year treatment outcome of alcoholics treated by individualized behavior therapy. *Results, Behav. Res. Ther.,* 14: 195–215.

Vallaint, G. E. (1983). *The natural history of alcoholism.* Cambridge, Mass.: Harvard University Press.

Westermeyer, J., Doheny, S., & Stone, B. (1978). An assessment of hospital care for the alcoholic patient. *Alcohol. Clin. Exp. Res.,* 2:53.

Winokur, G., & Clayton, P. J. (1968). Family history studies, IV. Comparison of male and female alcoholics. Q.J. Stud. Alc., 29:885.

Winokur, G., Reich, T., Renimer, J., & Pitts, F. (1970). Alcoholism III. Diagnosis and familial psychiatric illness in 259 alcoholic probands. *Arch. Gen. Psychiat.,* 23:104.

Woititz, J. G. (1983). *Adult children of alcoholics.* Hollywood, Fla.: Health Communication, Inc.

Wurmser, L. (1981). Psychodynamics of substance abuse. From J. H. Lowinson, & P. Ruiz (Eds.). *Substance abuse: clinical problems and perspectives.* Baltimore, MD: Williams and Wilkins, 1981.

16

SEXUAL HEALTH AND DISORDERS OF SEXUAL FUNCTIONING

DALMAS A. TAYLOR
FAYE GARY

LEARNING OBJECTIVES

After studying this chapter, the student will be able to:

- Define the two types of psychosexual disorders: paraphilias and sexual dysfunctions.
- Describe the four phases of male and female sexual response.
- Identify the roles of the nurse in promoting sexual health for patients in any health care setting
- Discuss the psychodynamic, behavioral, and biological theories of sexual dysfunction.
- Discuss the different methods of treatment of sexual dysfunctions.
- Define gender identity disorder.

INTRODUCTION

Sexuality is woven into the fabric of human life throughout the life cycle, playing a major role in everything from reproduction to childhood development, maturation, and adult lifestyle. Sexual feelings and behaviors comprise an important part of each person no matter what their age or situation and cannot be ignored by health care providers who see their clients and patients as whole beings. For the nurse, who often views the patient on a continuum of health and illness, sexuality is an essential element to be considered at every point along the continuum.

Because sexual health and illness may be relevant to patients at any given point in the health care system, this chapter will begin by discussing the myriad roles of the nurse—from counseling about sex education to helping patients cope with concerns about sexuality that are secondary to other illness. The sexual response cycle is briefly described, as are sexual disorders (sexual dysfunction and the paraphilias) and gender identity disorders as classified by the DSM-III-R (1987). Although generalist nurses will not practice sex therapy with patients identified to have sexual dysfunction, there are many opportunities for nurses to pursue advanced degrees that will allow them to practice as sex therapists or sex educators, as well as sex researchers (Poorman, 1988). Discussion of the sexual disorders, their assessment and management, should give the nurse increased understanding of the complexity of issues surrounding sexual feelings, behavior, and functioning. The two case studies at the end of the chapter cover issues of sexuality in non-psychiatric and psychiatric settings.

ROLES AND RESPONSIBILITIES OF THE NURSE

Nurses in all health care settings can play active roles in promoting sexual health and well-being, helping to prevent problems related to sexual functioning (including teaching about safe sex), assessing for potential problems, and helping their patients identify concerns related to sexual feelings or problems. This is a difficult role, however, since nurses can't be expected to be experts on sexuality (neither their education nor their clinical experience currently provides for this) nor are nurses automatically comfortable dealing with sexual issues with patients just because they are nurses (Kolodny, et al., 1979). Poorman (1988) suggests that nurses should not be expected to act as sexual encyclopedias but that they should have a sound theoretical base and knowledge of available resources for obtaining information on sexual issues when needed. The nurse works at becoming comfortable in talking about sexual issues with patients. Unless the nurse can overcome any feelings of discomfort she may herself have about sexual issues, it may be difficult for her to help the patient deal openly and honestly with his or her own concerns.

EDUCATIONAL NEEDS

Before they can be effective and knowledgeable with patients and their families, the nurse and other health care professionals must have some basic information about sexuality. During the nurse's education, she should be "given permission" to learn about human sexuality, including patterns of masturbation, the homosexual experience, exploration of myths about sexuality, and sexual enrichment. This content should assist the nurse in providing quality patient care, regardless of the patient's sexual orientation, diagnosis, culture, age, socioeconomic status, and other related variables (Vandervoot & McIlvenna, 1975; Hogan, 1980; Birk, 1988).

Nurses and other health professionals need to be trained in the identification and treatment of paraphilias and the sexual dysfunctions. If nurses were sensitive to potential and actual sexual disorders, health programs for the general public and high risk groups could be better planned and implemented. For example, recently divorced men frequently experience inhibited sexual excitement. Nurses, counselors, and physicians could counsel these men about the possibility of this and other problems (for example, arousal disorders, orgasm disorders, and so forth) and allay fears that the condition is permanent and enduring. Moreover, nurses should become more involved with educating the public about the paraphilias and the impact they have on society.

The operational definition of dysfunction needs to be further elaborated. The roles of age, gender, and ethnicity are factors that must be further explored in the service of determining normality of sexual functions, as well as the continuing refinement of treatment approaches.

The biological etiology of sexual dysfunctions is a growing field and involves a multidisciplinary approach to the assessment and comprehensive treatment of these disorders. Nurses should consider conducting research on sexual dysfunction with a variety of populations, including patients who present with specific illnesses such as heart disease, diabetes, cancer, paraphilias, or mental disorders as well as individuals who have no known medical and/or psychiatric problems.

SEXUAL SELF-AWARENESS

Before any assessment, teaching, or intervention related to sexuality can begin, the nurse must first become comfortable with discussing sexual issues with her patients. The effectiveness of education may well depend upon the nurse's own attitudes about sex and degree of comfort about sexual issues. Krozy (1978) has described an important goal for the nurse as becoming a "sexually comfortable person," defined by such characteristics as having a positive body image and self-esteem, being able to speak openly and honestly about any aspect of sexuality, respecting religious and sociocultural differences in sexual mores, and respecting confidentiality. Driscoll (1989) suggests that one way to overcome self-consciousness about sexual issues is to get supervised experience in discussing and exploring patients' sexual needs. In this safe, collegial environment, the nurse may not only gain experience and skill in communicating with others about sexual issues, but grow in terms of her own sexuality.

ASSESSMENT

Any general health history done on the patient should include questions about sexual health, though many nurses often avoid or skip over such questions (Poorman, 1988). As stated earlier, the nurse's own comfort with these issues will dramatically increase her ability to make the patient more comfortable with the topic. Good interviewing skills are another critical component in this process (Poorman, 1988). The same skills used in assessing other systems are appropriate for the sexual history—using language appropriate for that particular patient, asking open-ended questions and providing enough time for the person to respond completely. Some interviewing Dos and Don'ts are summarized in Table 16–1. Assuring confidentiality is especially important when asking questions about sexuality. It is not necessary to dwell on the topic of sexuality, especially if there is no reason to suspect that the patient has any problem in this area. Poorman (1988) suggests that one or two questions, such as "are there any changes in your sexual patterns since your illness?" or "are there any sexual issues or questions you would like to have answered or discussed while you are in the hospital?" should be sufficient for the patient who has not already brought up a specific sexual problem. Examples of sexual assessment questions for females and males are shown in Tables 16–2 and 16–3.

CARE OF HOSPITALIZED PATIENTS

The nurse working in a medical or surgical ward will often encounter patients with concerns over sexual functioning. Illness and/or hospitalization can have a profound effect on a person's sexuality. Positive self-esteem is essential for satisfactory sexual relations: it aids the person in feeling comfortable and secure in seeking and giving pleasure. Illness can occur and assault the individual's self-esteem (Hogan, 1980).

When a person is hospitalized, the nurse is the person the patient sees most frequently. The nurse should be aware of: 1) the patient's physical limita-

TABLE 16–1 Interviewing to obtain sexual information—some dos and don'ts

Do	Don't
1. Obtain information about all need areas.	1. Focus only on sexuality.
2. Provide privacy.	2. Obtain information when others are present or take copious notes.
3. Strive for an unhurried atmosphere.	3. Check your watch, tap your foot.
4. Maintain an attitude that is frank, open, warm, objective, empathetic.	4. Project discomfort, become defensive.
5. Use nondirective techniques when possible.	5. Ask many direct questions.
6. Have a prepared introduction to state purpose of interview.	6. Be vague about the purpose of the interview.
7. Use appropriate vocabulary.	7. Use street terms.
8. "Check out" words to ensure patient understands.	8. Assume the patient understands what you're saying.
9. Adjust the order of questions according to client's needs.	9. Follow a rigid format.
10. Give the client time to think and answer questions.	10. Answer questions for the client.
11. Recognize signs of anxiety.	11. Focus on getting information without recognizing patient feeling.
12. Give permission not to do something.	12. Have preset expectations of the patient's sexual activity.
13. Listen in an interested but matter-of-fact way.	13. Overreact or underreact.
14. Identify your attitudes, values, beliefs, and feelings.	14. Project your concerns or problems on to the patient.
15. Identify significant others.	15. Assume that no one else is involved in the patient's/client's sexual concerns.
16. Identify philosophical religious beliefs of patient/client.	16. Inflict your moral judgments on the patient.
17. Acknowledge when you don't have an answer to a question.	17. Pretend you know when you don't.

Source: Hogan, R. (1980). *Human sexuality: A nursing perspective.* New York: Appleton-Century-Crofts, p. 246.

tions, 2) the attitudes and beliefs he has about the limitations, and 3) the prescribed course of treatment and how it might (or might not) affect the patient's general psychological functioning as well as his sexual functioning.

The fears and fantasies that patients can have about the impact of an illness on sexual functioning are endless. For example, Mr. Reading, a 27-year-old oceanographer, was diagnosed as having diabetes. When the nurse saw Mr. Reading in the clinic approximately two weeks later, he confided in her that, "I can't get an erection anymore . . . I think I should stop taking my insulin because it is making me impotent." Similarly, Mrs. Morren, a farm worker, told

the public-health nurse that she could not take her penicillin tablets that were prescribed for an ear infection because she had been taught that penicillin "takes away the firmness of the inside of the woman's parts that give the man pleasure." She did not want her husband to become displeased with her, and therefore, could not risk taking the medications.

Thus, there are a myriad of circumstances and contexts within which a nurse can teach patients about their bodies, assist in values clarification, and provide factual information about their physical and mental disability, and its impact on sexual functioning.

TABLE 16–2 Sexual assessment: female

- Do you remember when you got your first period?
- Do you have any problem with your periods? Do you experience heavy bleeding, pain, irregularity?
- When did you have your last period?
- Have you ever been pregnant? If yes, how often? Any live children, abortions, miscarriages, stillbirths?
- When was your last Pap smear or GYN examination? Do you have regular GYN checkups?
- Do you perform breast self-exams? Any lumps, discomfort in the breasts? Any discharges?
- Currently, are you sexually active?
- Do you practice contraceptive methods/birth control? If yes, what type? Are you satisfied with this method? If no, is there a reason why you don't?
- Have you had any problems with vaginal infection, discharge, burning, or itching? If yes, encourage discussion regarding problem.
- Have you ever had any sexually transmitted diseases, e.g., syphilis, gonorrhea, chlamydia, trichomonas?
- Are you satisfied with your sexual abilities? If yes, proceed with next question. If no, is there anything you would like to share with me?
- Have you had more than one partner/lover in the last ten years?
- Are you aware of the AIDS epidemic?
- Can you share with me your understanding of how the AIDS virus is transmitted?
- Have you heard of safer sex techniques and/or risk reduction behaviors? If yes, please share with me your understanding of these. If no, it will be important to educate prior to discharge.
- Has this illness affected your sexual functioning?
- Do you have any questions/concerns regarding sexual behaviors and sexuality?
- Do you have any additional questions/concerns?

Source: Meisenhelder, J., & LaCharite, C. (1989). *Comfort in Caring: Nursing the Person with HIV Infection.* Glenview, IL: Scott, Foresman, p. 170.

Nurses can provide privacy and assist the patient to minimize guilt, desensitize himself against shame associated with normal behaviors, and overcome body-image disturbances.

WHEN NURSES ARE SEXUALLY ATTRACTED TO THEIR PATIENTS. Nurses sometimes do become sexually attracted to patients. When they act on that attraction in some way therapeutic nursing care is compromised. In this situation:

- Physical care can be embarrassing for the nurse and for the patient.
- The nurse should request that other professional nurses provide care for the involved patient.

- Nurses need to be aware of and acknowledge their own feelings of sexuality and sometimes seductive behaviors.
- Nurses who continually become sexually attracted to patients might need further counseling and support.

The following are areas of concern for the nurse and should be understood within the context of her practice (Hogan, 1980):

Touch:

- Touch is basic to nursing.
- Touch is a laying-on-of-hands.
- Touch conveys concern, love, and affection; it is associated with tasks; touch of genitals (male and

TABLE 16–3 Sexual assessment: male

- Have you ever had any urinary tract infections?
- Have you had any problems with urination (difficulty starting to urinate, pain, dribbling)?
- Have you noticed any lumps or changes in your testicles? Do you perform testicular examinations on yourself or does your partner?
- Have you ever been diagnosed with any sexually transmitted diseases? If yes, when and what treatment?
- Currently, are you sexually active?
- Have you had more than one partner/lover in the last ten years?
- Currently, do you use contraceptive methods during intercourse, i.e., condoms?
- Are you aware of the AIDS epidemic?
- Can you share with me your understanding of how the AIDS virus is transmitted?
- Have you heard of safer sex techniques and/or risk reduction behaviors? If yes, please share with me your understanding of these. If no, it will be important to educate you prior to discharge.
- Are you satisfied with your sexual functioning? If yes, proceed with next question. If no, is there anything you would like to share with me?
- Has this illness affected your sexual functioning? If yes, is there anything you would like to share?
- Do you have any additional questions/concerns?

Source: Meisenhelder, J., & LaCharite, C. (1989). *Comfort in Caring: Nursing the Person with HIV Infection.* Glenview, IL: Scott, Foresman, pp. 170, 171.

female) can be frightening for the nurse (and for the patient).

- Touch is culturally bound, with highly personal meanings for each individual.
- It is always a possibility that the patient or the nurse might falsely interpret a certain "touch" as flirtatious or sexual in meaning.
- Touch can be risk-taking.

Patient's Possible Responses to Touch:

- Covert expressions, as well as acting-out sexual behaviors (such as exposing oneself).
- Asking nurses for dates or personal information, such as phone number, address, and so on.
- Seductive comments, sexist jokes.
- Exposure of genitals during bath, use of urinals, sitting in chair, and so on.
- Touching the nurse in an inappropriate fashion (touching the hips, brushing against the nurse).
- Displaying dependency for the purpose of engaging the nurse for physical closeness.

PATIENT PRIVACY. The nurse should provide privacy for the patient and the patient's sexual partner to express their intimate feelings in the hospital setting. Closeness, touch, caresses, and other comforting behaviors should not be censored. Again, the privacy of the patient is important and should be respected. However, limits should be set by the nurse when the expression of sexual feelings is inappropriate because of place, time, circumstances, and so on.

Masturbation. The nurse who considers masturbation immoral or dangerous may overtly censor this behavior. Masturbation in the hospital (and other settings) serves a variety of purposes, including the relief of sexual tensions, the reduction of anxiety, providing pleasure, and recreating images of positive relationships, health, and positive self-esteem. Nurses should provide privacy for the patient (closed door) and knock before entering.

Homosexuality. The homosexual patient may create undue concern for the nurse. The nurse and other health professionals should remember that the homosexual patient ought to be treated with the highest regard, respect, and care as with any other patient. However, nurses and other health professionals may have difficulty with the homosexual patient not only because of his or her sexual orientation, but because of a fear about contracting AIDS. The patient may feel estranged from his or her mate/lover and feel a loss of independence and self-direction. He or she may be cautious about expressing intimacy, lest they provoke hostility or inappropriate humor from nurses and other health care providers.

In mental health settings, when the homosexual presents with depression or a crisis, there may be a propensity for the staff to want to treat the homosexuality rather than the depression. In other instances, the crisis is the homosexuality, rather than the psychiatric disorder.

CONFIDENTIALITY

Confidentiality remains an important aspect in the treatment of sexual disorders. The nurse must assure the patient that all information will be handled in a secure and professional fashion. The nurse will need to be judicious and highly selective about with whom she chooses to share this information. Because of the unusual, even bizarre, nature of some of the sexual disorders, particularly the paraphilias, there may be a tendency to discuss these cases with inappropriate persons, such as colleagues not involved in the case. This tendency must be stringently guarded against. The nurse should also be aware that men and women with sexual dysfunctions may feel embarrassed, angry, guilty, and frustrated, and deserve the most sensitive care.

The nurse must record patient information on the charts. She can provide information without specifying details or the names of others who might be adversely affected by this information. In some instances, special codes, rather than patient names, are used for filing purposes. In addition, some hospital clinics and others make special security provisions for the storage of these records. The nurse and other health professionals need to find the best solution for each situation (Group for the Advancement of Psychiatry, 1974). To complicate matters, the nurse is required by law in all states to report to child protective services any reasonable suspicion of sexual abuse of a minor. (See Chapter 28 for more on confidentiality and conflict of interest.)

CLIENT EDUCATION

Nurses have many opportunities to teach patients and their families about sexuality. In well-baby clinics, prenatal clinics, surgery clinics, and in public-health settings, nurses need to seize the opportunity to teach. The nurse can discuss the need for love and tenderness with a young couple, as well as with aging grandparents. She can work to dispel some of the myths that exist about sex with individual patients or with community groups (see Box 16–1). The nurse should also be alert for situations in which parents respond negatively to their children's sexual expression (such as occasional masturbation) and provide appropriate counseling (See Table 16–4). The nurse may observe for tensions and conflicts between cou-

---

Box 16–1 ● Myths about Sex

Masturbation causes physical and mental illness.

Masturbation is not practiced by children who grow up in a healthy environment.

Masturbation causes frigidity or the inability to have orgasm with a partner.

Teenage pregnancies (over 1/2 million) and abortions (250,000) occur because teenagers today are well-informed about sex.

Penis size is related to sexual adequacy.

Penetration by a very large penis will cause excruciating pain.

Men have greater sexual needs than women.

Older people are not, and should not be, sexually active.

Frequent intercourse will cause a woman to age rapidly.

Women do not conceive unless they have orgasm.

Sources: Adapted from Masters, W. H., & Johnson, V. (1970). *Human sexual inadequacy.* Boston: Little, Brown.
Nicholi, A. M. (1988). The Adolescent. In A. M. Nicholi, Jr. (Ed.), *The Harvard guide to modern psychiatry.* Cambridge: Harvard University Press.
Walker, I. (1981). *Clinical psychiatry in primary care.* Menlo Park: Addison Wesley, pp. 248–249.

TABLE 16—4 Teaching children about sexuality

The following suggestions are helpful for parents who have questions about the "hows" of teaching their children about sexuality:

1. Answer questions in a straightforward way.
2. Give the information the child requests.
3. Give the information at the time the child requests it—don't put off answering.
4. Avoid giving more information than the child requests at the time—the child will not be interested.
5. Don't worry about correct timing as to when to give information, for if the child is not psychologically or intellectually ready for the information, he/she won't be interested. Hearing it won't do any harm.
6. *Don't wait to give all information in one dose.*
7. Bring up the topic of sexuality casually and briefly when a child does not ask questions. (For example, when a pregnant woman is seen.)
8. Tell the truth—false stories about the stork or physician bringing babies more often confuse or frighten the child.

Source: Hogan, M. (1980). *Human sexuality: A nursing perspective.* New York: Appleton-Century-Crofts, p. 264.

ples and assist them in resolving their fears, feelings, and thoughts about a particular situation (Hogan, 1980).

The nurse is also often the health care provider with the greatest opportunity to teach patients about sexually transmitted diseases and should be familiar with the signs, symptoms, transmission and treatment of these conditions (see Table 16–5).

The Sex Information and Education Council of the United States (SIECUS) is an excellent resource for information about human sexuality. It encourages its members to know the basic facts about human re-

TABLE 16—5 Sexually transmitted diseases

Condition	Cause	Predisposing Factors	Symptoms	Treatment
Acquired immune deficiency syndrome (AIDS)	Exposure to HIV—containing body fluid, such as blood or semen	Frequent homosexual encounters among males in the United States Blood transfusions Hemophilia A Parenteral street drug abuse; use of volatile nitrites	T-cell immune deficiency	No cure or vaccine; zidovudine (AZT, Retrovir) to delay progression
Balanoposthitis/ balanitis (if circumcised)	Often a complication of gonorrhea, syphilis, trichomoniasis, or candidiasis	Diabetes mellitus	Inflammation of the glans penis and prepuce	Treat underlying cause

continued

TABLE 16—5 continued

Condition	Cause	Predisposing Factors	Symptoms	Treatment
	Can be caused by tight prepuce May be a drug reaction			
Candidiasis	*Candida albicans* (a yeast organism)	Use of oral contraceptives or broad-spectrum antibiotics; pregnancy; diabetes mellitus; pernicious anemia; corticosteroids; immunosuppressives	Vaginitis and vulvar pruritis; leukorrhea; males are usually asymptomatic carriers but may experience balanoposthitis	Female: Nystatin (14 days), clotrimazole (7 days), or miconazole (7 days) as vaginal gel, cream, or tablets Male: Nystatin cream on prepuce
Chancroid	*Hemophilus ducreyi* (a gram-negative bacillus)	None	Genital ulcers and swollen lymph nodes in groin	Sulfonamides (10–14 days)
Gonorrhea	*Neisseria gonorrhoeae*	None	Men: creamy yellow discharge; burning sensation on urination; lips of meatus red and swollen; epididymitis Women: often unnoticed; dysuria and vaginitis; salpingitis	Procaine penicillin G (one dose, 4.8 million units, IM); ampicillin and probenecid (3.5 g orally); or tetracycline (500 mg orally), qid for 5 days
Granuloma inguinale	*Donovania granulomatis* (gram-negative bacillus)	Mostly in tropical or subtropical areas	Red nodule progressing to granulomatous mass on penis, scrotum, groin, or thighs of males; vulva, vagina, or perineum of females; anus and buttocks in male homosexuals	Streptomycin or tetracyclines
Herpes simplex	Herpes simplex virus, mainly type 2	None	Painful, itchy lesions; flu-like symptoms; dysuria	Acyclovir for initial infections. No cure for recurrent infections. Lesions should be kept clean and normal saline applied twice daily
Lymphogranuloma venereum	Chlamydia	Mostly in tropical or subtropical areas	Genital lesions followed by lymphangitis	Tetracycline

Source: Swonger, A., & Matejski, M. (1988). *Nursing pharmacology.* Glenview, IL: Scott, Foresman/Little, Brown, p. 591.

production and sexual behavior and promotes the view that certain responsibilities are attached to one's sexual activity (Calderone, 1966).

TEACHING ABOUT SAFE SEX. One of the greatest opportunities for teaching about sexuality right now is the area of teaching about safe sex. Nurses should attempt to disseminate information about safe sex whenever the opportunity arises, for example, when doing a sexually active 16-year-old's camp physical, not just when she encounters a patient who may be at high risk for contracting a sexually transmitted disease (Driscoll, 1989). Providing accurate information to the public at large can only help to stem the increased rate of infection and enhance the protection of everyone. Public-health departments, school departments (in some areas), and the federal government are sponsoring a variety of AIDS education and training programs in communities all over the country, with nurses highly involved in both the organization and actual teaching. The content of the programs on safe sex is not complicated. There are some basic rules. Just as the Center for Disease Control's latest recommendation to health care workers is to consider the blood and body fluids from all patients to be potentially infectious (thus recommending universal precautions) (Centers for Disease Control, 1988:June 24), so it is recommended that all sex partners be considered as potentially infectious. One overall guideline for practicing safe sex is not to allow one person's semen, blood, vaginal secretions, or lactating mother's milk into another person's body (Shaw & Paleo, 1986). Using condoms and practic-

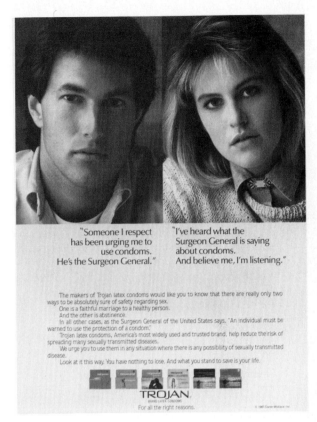

"Someone I respect has been urging me to use condoms. He's the Surgeon General."

"I've heard what the Surgeon General is saying about condoms. And believe me, I'm listening."

The makers of Trojan latex condoms would like you to know that there are really only two ways to be absolutely sure of safety regarding sex.
One is a faithful marriage to a healthy person.
And the other is abstinence.
In all other cases, as the Surgeon General of the United States says, "An individual must be warned to use the protection of a condom."
Trojan latex condoms, America's most widely used and trusted brand, help reduce the risk of spreading many sexually transmitted diseases.
We urge you to use them in any situation where there is any possibility of sexually transmitted disease.
Look at it this way. You have nothing to lose. And what you stand to save is your life.

TROJAN
BRAND LATEX CONDOMS
For all the right reasons.

With the advent of AIDS, condom manufacturers have become more explicit, and prolific, in their advertising methods.

ing sexual behaviors that limit the crossing of bodily fluids from person to person are recommended (see Table 16–6). Information sources on AIDS and AIDS organizations are listed in Box 16–2.

TABLE 16–6 Safe sex guidelines

Risk-free behaviors:

- Massage (without genital stimulation): As you discuss this behavior, you may also want to discuss with the client how massage can be a method of relaxation as well as shared intimacy. It may be helpful to discuss how both client and partner can use oils and lotions as well as create the environment to promote sensuality and eroticism.
- Mutual masturbation/pleasuring techniques: These behaviors are relatively safe as long as the skin is healthy and free of lesions/open areas. Many people have not learned to masturbate, or may view these behaviors as "dirty" or "sinful," depending on their cultural/religious upbringing. If this is the case, they may need to be referred to a counselor or sex therapist.
- Social kissing and hugging.
- Frottage (body-to-body rubbing): This behavior utilizes the erotic sensations of touch and can be combined with massage.

continued

TABLE 16—6 continued

Risk-free behaviors:

- The use of sex toys (dildos) that are not shared with partners.
- Casual contact: hand holding, arm holding, shaking hands, etc.
- Voyeurism and fantasy.

Low-risk behaviors:

- Intimate kissing (also known as deep kissing and/or French kissing): Penetration of tongue into partner's mouth. It is important that the mouth not have any open sores or lesions or any evidence of bleeding gums.
- Fellatio (oral sex) without ingestion of seminal fluid or semen. Risk is further reduced with use of condom.
- Cunnilingus (oral stimulation of the female genitals): Protective covering of the female genitalia will further reduce risk (dental dams, Saran wrap).
- Vaginal intercourse with the use of a properly applied condom
- Rectal intercourse with the use of a properly applied condom
- Use of shared sex toys that are cleaned in between uses and covered with a condom for penetration

High-risk behaviors:

- Ingestion of semen or vaginal/cervical secretions
- Vaginal and/or anal intercourse without the use of a condom
- Sharing sex toys without taking precautions
- Analingus (oral-anal contact, also known as "rimming")
- Piercing or drawing blood during sexual activity
- Fisting: Penetration of the anus with one's fist

Source: Adapted from Meisenhelder, J., & LaCharite, C. (1989). *Comfort in caring: Nursing the person with HIV infection.* Glenview, IL: Scott, Foresman, p. 173. Adapted from Bay Area Physicians for Human Rights, 1985; Bjorklund, 1987.

PREVENTION OF SEXUAL DISORDERS

The nurse's opportunities for communicating with patients in a variety of settings should be employed in the context of prevention of sexual disorders as well as education and treatment. The nurse can be a model for open communication; she must be able to discuss basic information, issues, concerns, and controversy with accuracy and empathy without embarrassment, moral judgment, intrapsychic conflict, and so forth (Birk, 1988). The nurse must not only be knowledgeable, but she should also carefully examine her own value system and learn to address the varieties of sexual disorders in a knowledgeable, empathic, and timely fashion.

When nurses lead group discussions with parents, patients, teachers, and other nurses, the following "Dos and Don'ts" in Table 16–7 might be helpful to facilitate a meaningful discussion.

SEXUAL DISORDERS

Beyond problems related to the lack of education about sexuality and sexual functioning and temporary disruptions in sexual health related to physical illness or disability, two major groups of sexual disorders have been defined in the DSM-III-R. These are the sexual dysfunctions and the paraphilias. The sexual dysfunctions are disorders in which there is an inhibition in the sexual appetite or an inhibition of the psychophysiological changes necessary to complete the sexual response sequence (American Psychiatric Association, 1987). The paraphilias are disorders in which sexual arousal occurs in response to "objects or situations that are not a part of normative arousal-activity patterns and that in varying degrees may interfere with the capacity for reciprocal, affectionate, sexual activity" (American Psychiatric Association, 1987, p. 279).

Box 16–2 ● Sources of Information about AIDS

Telephone Hotlines (Toll Free)

PHS AIDS Hotline
800-342-AIDS
800-342-2437

National Sexually Transmitted Diseases Hotline/American Social Health Association
800-227-8922

National Gay Task Force
AIDS Information Hotline
800-221-7044
(212) 807-6016 (NY State)

Information Sources

U.S. Public Health Service Public Affairs Office
Hubert H. Humphrey Building, Room 725-H
200 Independence Avenue, S.W.
Washington, D.C. 20201
Phone: (202) 245-6867

Local Red Cross or American Red Cross AIDS Education Office
1730 D Street, N.W.
Washington, D.C. 20006
Phone: (202) 737-8300

American Association of Physicians for Human Rights
P.O. Box 14366
San Francisco, CA 94114
Phone: (415) 558-9353

AIDS Action Council
729 Eighth Street, S.E., Suite 200
Washington, D.C. 20003
Phone: (202) 547-3101

Gay Men's Health Crisis
P.O. Box 274
132 West 24th Street
New York, NY 10011
Phone: (212) 807-6655

Hispanic AIDS Forum
c/o APRED
853 Broadway, Suite 2007
New York, NY 10003
Phone: (212) 870-1902 or 870-1864

Los Angeles AIDS Project
7362 Santa Monica Boulevard
Los Angeles, California 90046
(213) 876-AIDS

Minority Task Force on AIDS
c/o New York City Council of Churches
475 Riverside Drive, Room 456
New York, NY 10115
Phone: (212) 749-1214

Mothers of AIDS Patients (MAP)
c/o Barbara Peabody
3403 E Street
San Diego, CA 92102
(619) 234-3432

National AIDS Network
729 Eighth Street, S.E., Suite 300
Washington D.C. 20003
(202) 546-2424

National Association of People with AIDS
P.O. Box 65472
Washington, D.C. 20035
(202) 483-7979

National Coalition of Gay Sexually Transmitted Diseases Services
c/o Mark Behar
P.O. Box 239
Milwaukee, WI 53201
Phone: (414) 277-7671

National Council of Churches/AIDS Task Force
475 Riverside Drive, Room 572
New York, NY 10115
Phone: (212) 870-2421

San Francisco AIDS Foundation
333 Valencia Street, 4th Floor
San Francisco, CA 94103
Phone: (415) 863-2437

American Nurses Association
2420 Pershing Road
Kansas City, MO 64108
Phone: 1-800-444-5720

Source: U.S. Department of Health and Human Services, *AIDS-21*, October 1986.

TABLE 16–7 Do's and don'ts that help facilitate meaningful group discussions

Do	Don't
1. Provide an environment conducive to discussion: comfortable temperature, chairs arranged in circle.	1. Separate males and females.
2. Limit participants to 10 to 20.	2. Allow "observers" in the group.
3. Provide name tags, food, and drink.	3. Assume everyone knows everything.
4. Greet the participants.	4. Insist that "proper" language be used.
5. Plan for participants to get to know each other.	5. Moralize.
6. Start where the group is.	6. Be upset by giggling and silliness (ignore it or set limits if necessary).
7. Move the discussion if it starts to drag.	7. Be upset by individuals who try to put the leader on the spot for their own entertainment.
8. Remind the group to respect one another's opinions, feelings, and right to be heard.	8. Allow airing of personal problems.
9. Encourage contribution by praising appropriate comments.	9. Omit discussion of attitudes.
10. Ask quiet members' opinions.	10. Embarrass members by asking for direct information.
11. Relieve anxieties based on misinformation.	11. Monopolize the discussion, but guide by summarizing and questioning.
12. Be imaginative and keep the group involved.	12. Allow verbal attack on anyone, or domination of group process by any one member.

Adapted from Kempton, Winifred: *Techniques for Leading Group Discussion on Human Sexuality.* Philadelphia: Planned Parenthood of Southeastern Pennsylvania, 1973.

Before these disorders are discussed, a brief discussion of the normal sexual response cycle is given, in an effort to provide some background toward the understanding of the disorders.

THE SEXUAL RESPONSE CYCLE

The Masters and Johnson landmark study of human physiological response to sexual stimulation identified four phases of the sexual response in males and females—excitement, plateau, orgasmic, and resolution (1966). (See Figures 16–1, 16–2, and 16–3.)

EXCITEMENT PHASE. The **excitement phase** develops from physical or psychological stimulation. Given adequate stimulation, the response occurs rather rapidly. (See Figure 16–1.) During this stage, females will experience breast enlargement and nipples will become erect; voluntary muscles may become tense and heart rate and blood pressure increase. For males in the excitement phase, heart and blood pressure may increase, the penis becomes erect, and the testes become partially elevated.

PLATEAU PHASE. The **plateau phase** follows the excitement phase, and occurs if sexual stimulation is

effective. The sexual tensions intensify, and the person reaches a level where orgasm might occur. The duration of this phase is related to the effectiveness of the stimuli and the individual's drive for culmination of experience. If the individual fails to experience

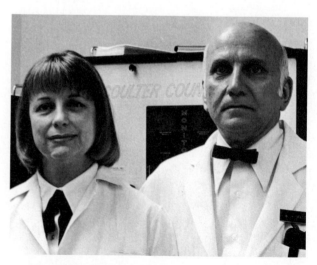

Masters and Johnson are considered by many to be the foremost authorities on sex therapy.

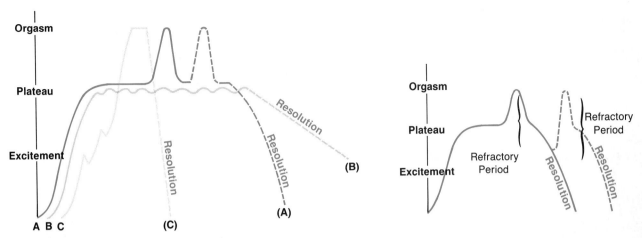

FIGURE 16–1 The Sexual Response Cycle
Left: Three variations of the female sexual response cycle.
Right: The most typical pattern of male sexual response cycle.

Source: Masters, W. H., & Johnson, V. E. (1966). *Human sexual response.* Boston: Little, Brown, p. 5.

orgasm, it is because the stimuli were withdrawn or were inadequate; the individual will then move from plateau to resolution phase.

ORGASMIC PHASE. The **orgasmic phase** lasts for a few seconds and the individual experiences vasoconstriction and myotonia, created by sexual stimulation. When maximum sexual stimulation occurs, the orgasm follows. The sensual awareness of the orgasm for the woman involves the clitoral body, vagina, and uterus. For the male, the sensual awareness involves the penis, prostate, and seminal vesicles. However, there is also a subjective sense of total body involvement for both males and females. During this phase the male will ejaculate; the female response is quite varied in intensity and duration.

RESOLUTION PHASE. The last phase of the human sexual response is the **resolution phase.** It is an involuntary period characterized by loss of tension and a return to the unstimulated state.

THE SEXUAL DYSFUNCTIONS

Sexual dysfunction is any condition which prohibits individuals from satisfying their personal sexual needs and which is not of organic etiology. Anyone can experience dysfunctional episodes, even though they are otherwise in good physical and psychological health. When, then, is a diagnosis of sexual dysfunction appropriate? Only when it can be established

that the disorder(s) is prohibitive to personal desires in one's sex life and the therapist is able to establish that the instances of dysfunction are beyond what may be considered "normal." A problem for one person may not be a problem for another.

Sexual dysfunctions are distinguished from the paraphilias, such as transvestism, fetishism, sadism, or pedophilia (American Psychiatric Association, 1987; Masters, Johnson, & Kolodny, 1988). The sexual dysfunctions can be conceptualized as either inhibitory (inhibited sexual desire) or hyperexcitatory (premature ejaculation) (Birk, 1988).

The DSM-III-R provides four categories of sexual dysfunctions: 1) Sexual desire disorders, 2) Sexual arousal disorders, 3) Orgasm disorders, and 4) Sexual pain disorders.

SEXUAL DESIRE DISORDERS

The Sexual desire disorders may have a biological basis. Androgens are critical for an adequate sexual desire in the male, and replacement therapy can trigger increased activity in sexual fantasies and rekindle the desire for male sexual activity. Among females, endogenous androgens have a significant role to play in sexual desire and sexual practice (Schiavi, 1985). Female and male sexual desire may also be hampered by naturally occurring biological processes, such as aging, fatigue, and pregnancy. Sexual desire disorders may also result from physical illness (diabetes, and so on), medication such as MAO inhibitors (powerful anti-depressant drugs), and psychiatric dis-

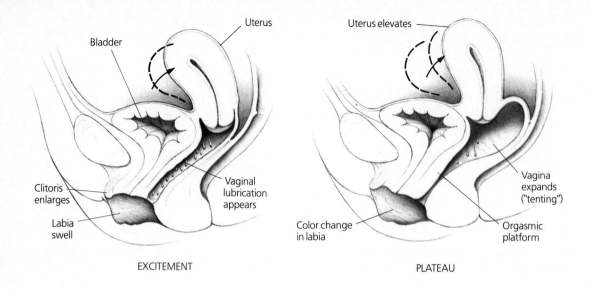

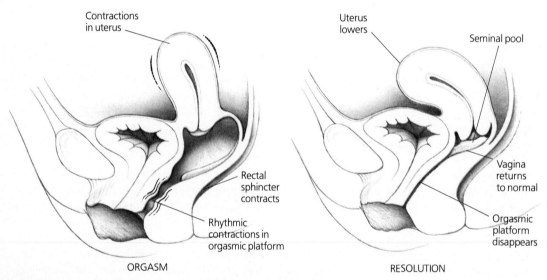

FIGURE 16–2 Internal Changes in the Female Sexual Response Cycle

Source: Masters, W. H., Johnson, V. E., & Kolodny, R. C. (1988). *Human sexuality,* 3rd ed. Glenview, IL: Scott, Foresman/Little, Brown, p. 84

orders (schizophrenia, depression, anxiety, etc.) (Schiavi, 1985). There are several questions that the nurse may ask to assist her in obtaining the patient's sexual history:

1. Is the primary complaint stated a loss of sexual desire? What is this complaint based on and compared to (statistics, previous sexual behavior, partner's complaints, partner's expectations, etc.)?

2. Is this desire general, or limited to specific circumstances and partners?

3. Does the loss of sexual desire encompass other forms of sexual activity such as masturbation, foreplay, and so on, or is it limited to specific sexual expressions such as copulation?

4. Is this low desire a recent occurrence, or is it chronic?

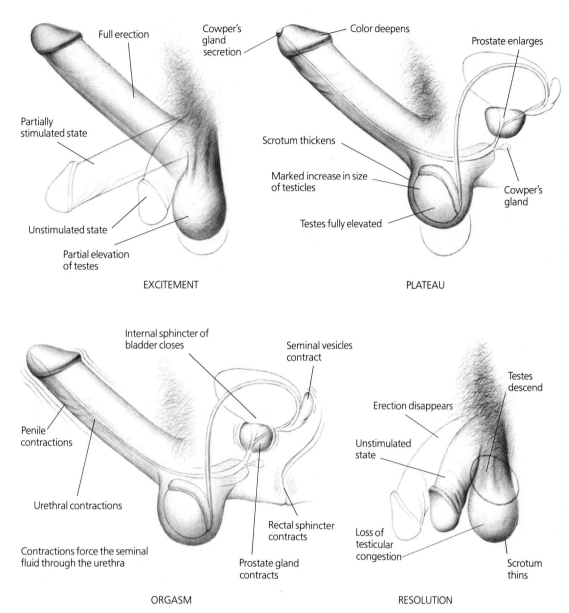

FIGURE 16—3 External and Internal Changes in the Male Sexual Response Cycle

Source: Masters, W. H., Johnson, V. E., & Kolodny, R. C. (1988). *Human sexuality,* 3rd ed. Glenview, IL: Scott, Foresman/Little, Brown, p. 85.

5. Are there specific medical, psychiatric, and/or environmental conditions that are possible antecedents to the condition? (Schiavi, 1985). For example, does the patient or his sexual partner bring a lot of work home? Is there a new baby in the house? Is Mom breastfeeding (decreases vaginal secretions)?

The Sexual desire disorders may also have bases other than biological. The couple (or an individual in a relationship) may not wish to engage in sexual ac-

tivity. There are asexual marriages. In these marriages, the partners sometimes cleverly arrange work schedules, travel, and so forth, to keep them separated from each other. Many times, these couples are otherwise compatible and attentive to each other. The absence of tension is related to the absence of sex. In such instances, the expression of sexual feelings in intercourse would be destructive to the relationship; sex is perceived, unconsciously, as dirty and a possible contamination of the loved one and/or the relationship. Thus, the relationship remains platonic to the mutual satisfaction of both partners (Strean, 1983).

Although problems of low sexual desire have been observed in both men and women, twice as many women report disinterest in sex or having an aversion to sex (Frank, Anderson, & Rubinstein, 1978). Two types of Sexual desire disorders have been identified.

HYPOACTIVE SEXUAL DESIRE DISORDER. Hypoactive sexual desire disorder, or arousal inhibition, is evidenced in women who are unresponsive to virtually all forms of sexual stimulation. Birk (1988) suggests that nurses and other clinicians who treat patients with this diagnosis assess for symptoms of depression, medical problems, and use of prescription and nonprescription medications, as well as alcohol abuse, and use of steroids, estrogen, progesterone. Arousal insufficiency in women results in a failure to lubricate.

SEXUAL AVERSION DISORDER. Sexual aversion disorder includes the avoidance of and withdrawal from all genital sexual activity with a partner and a completely negative attitude toward sexual activity. The disorder occurs in men and women. The individual may report hyperventilation, anxiety, and, ultimately, depression when expected to perform sexually. Causes associated with this disorder may be biological problems, incompatible sexual needs and proclivities in the sexual partners, loss of excitement in the relationship, marital problems (especially chronic, unexpressed anger), and previous sexual traumas (Gillan, 1987).

SEXUAL AROUSAL DISORDERS

Sexual arousal disorders may definitely be investigated from several perspectives. For example, men having a problem with desire should be queried about physical illness such as diabetes mellitus, liver and renal disease, low back pain, and so forth (Gillan, 1987; Birk, 1988). Sleep erections, "nocturnal penile tumescence," as proposed by Karacan (1978), can be measured in sleep laboratories to determine if the problem has organic causes (lack of erections) or is psychogenic. In the latter case, erections are likely to occur only when sleeping. It is also important to explore the sufficiency of blood supply to the pelvic organs and determine if there is adequate supply to support an erection (Katchadourian, 1987).

Women can also have blood flow problems that interfere with sexual arousal. Probes placed in the female's vagina that measure blood flow can help to diagnose this (Gillan, 1987).

Vasoconstriction occurs in males and females and can inhibit desire. Other types of conditions including chronic systemic disease, a history of sexual trauma, or endocrine disorders, can affect sexual arousal (Gillan, 1987; Birk, 1988). At times, women who fail to lubricate and engage in sexual activity will experience pain and damage to the vaginal tissues (Gillan, 1987). This can result in aversive conditioning to sex, especially penetration. Such conditioning is very difficult to overcome once it is established, even if the situation changes. However, estrogen replacement therapy and the use of commercial lubricants can assist in the alleviation of this problem.

Other concerns involve the quality and frequency of communication that occur between the couple; the nature of shared values about sexual behaviors; cultural norms that are considered acceptable/unacceptable to one or both partners; and the intricate relationship among hormonal, physiological, psychological, and sociocultural factors (Hogan, 1980; Barlow, 1986; Gillan, 1987; Masters, Johnson, & Kolodny, 1988). There are two types of Sexual arousal disorders: 1) Female sexual arousal disorder (previously referred to as frigidity) and 2) Male erectile Disorder (impotence) (American Psychiatric Association, 1987).

**DSM-III-R
Diagnostic Criteria for
302.71 Hypoactive
Sexual Desire Disorder**

A. Persistently or recurrently deficient or absent sexual fantasies and desire for sexual activity. The judgment of deficiency or absence is made by the clinician, taking into account factors that affect sexual functioning, such as age, sex, and the context of the person's life.

B. Occurrence not exclusively during the course of another Axis I disorder (other than a sexual dysfunction), such as major depression.

**DSM-III-R
Diagnostic Criteria for
302.72 Female Sexual
Arousal Disorder**

A. Persistent or recurrent extreme aversion to, and avoidance of, all or almost all, genital sexual contact with a sexual partner.

B. Occurrence not exclusively during the course of another Axis I disorder (other than a sexual dysfunction), such as obsessive compulsive disorder or major depression.

FEMALE SEXUAL AROUSAL DISORDER. Masters, Johnson and Kolodny (1988), in their discussion of female sexual dysfunction, point out that until recently women were considered less sexual than men. Now, however, "female sexual responsivity [has become] something of an expected accomplishment with women" (p. 504) and is assisted by the media, women's magazines, how-to-do-it books, peer groups, and radio and television talk shows. The end result of these changes is evidenced in the woman's perceptions of herself as an adequate and viable sexual partner. If there are perceived potential or real problems with her sexual performance, she, much like her male counterpart, can experience frustration, confusion, anxiety, and depression (Masters, Johnson, & Kolodny, 1988).

MALE ERECTILE DISORDER. Male erectile disorder is the inability to achieve or maintain an erection well enough, or long enough, for vaginal penetration and until the sexual activity is complete. This condition is often referred to as impotence. Primary erectile insufficiency is that condition in which a man has never been able to achieve an erection sufficient for penetration and ejaculation to his partner's sexual satisfaction. Secondary erectile insufficiency is that condition in which a male has experienced at least one instance of successful erection, penetration, and ejaculation, but is currently unable to produce or maintain an erection (American Psychiatric Association, 1987).

Prior to age 60 (when prostate difficulties and other medical conditions may occur), prolonged erectile insufficiency is rare. According to Kinsey and his colleagues (Kinsey, Pomeroy, & Martin, 1948), only about 25 percent of all males become impotent prior to age 70. Again, it is important to distinguish between organic and psychogenic causes of arousal dysfunction. Virtually all such cases were previously attributed to psychological causes. In many instances, the insufficiency appears to be a response to societal norms concerning proclivity in senior men. Recently, however, approximately a third of erectile dysfunctions have been attributed to organic causes (Shrom, et al., 1979). For the clinician, it is important to establish that even when adequate sexual stimulation is provided, arousal difficulties still persist.

ORGASM DISORDERS

Orgasm involves an intensely pleasurable response involving response from the entire human body at the end of the plateau phase of the sexual response cycle.

**DSM-III-R
Diagnostic Criteria for
302.79 Sexual
Aversion Disorder**

A. Either (1) or (2):

1) persistent or recurrent partial or complete failure to attain or maintain the lubrication-swelling response of sexual excitement until completion of the sexual activity

2) persistent or recurrent lack of a subjective sense of sexual excitement and pleasure in a female during sexual activity

B. Occurrence not exclusively during the course of another Axis I disorder (other than a sexual dysfunction), such as major depression.

**DSM-III-R
Diagnostic Criteria for
302.72 Male Erectile
Disorder**

A. Either (1) or (2):

1) persistent or recurrent partial or complete failure in a male to attain or maintain erection until completion of the sexual activity

2) persistent or recurrent lack of a subjective sense of sexual excitement and pleasure in a male during sexual activity

B. Occurrence not exclusively during the course of another Axis I disorder (other than a sexual dysfunction), such as major depression.

Physiological and psychosocial dimensions are always involved in orgasms (Masters, Johnson, & Kolodny, 1988), and both males and females do, at times, experience difficulties attaining orgasms.

Etiological factors contributing to orgasmic dysfunction in women include ignorance or misinformation, socialization to be passive, and fear of losing control (Barbach, 1980). On the other hand, positive parental attitudes toward sex, along with social and dating competence, have been linked to orgasmic responsiveness in females (Newcomb, 1983). Orgasm disorders include inhibited female orgasm disorder, inhibited male orgasm disorder, and premature ejaculation disorder.

INHIBITED FEMALE ORGASM DISORDER. Inhibited female orgasm is evidenced when a woman capable of experiencing sexual excitement is incapable of experiencing orgasm. In primary orgasmic dysfunction, the woman has never experienced orgasm under any form of sexual stimulation. Secondary orgasmic dysfunction refers to women who re-quire direct clitoral stimulation for orgasm in sexual intercourse. These conditions also correspond to primary and secondary erectile insufficiency in the male.

Evaluation of this condition is particularly complicated by the subjective quality of orgasm from woman to woman and its varying nature for each woman from experience to experience. Inability to achieve orgasm during intercourse in the absence of direct clitoral stimulation is quite common and is generally not considered a dysfunction in the absence of a patient complaint (Masters, Johnson, & Kolodny, 1988).

INHIBITED MALE ORGASM. Inhibited male orgasm is a condition in which males are incapable of ejaculation intervaginally or during intercourse. It is a relatively rare phenomenon and difficult to treat (Kaplan, 1974). Apfelbaum (1980) considers inhibited male orgasm to be coitus-specific since many clients are able to ejaculate in other contexts (for example, masturbation). There is a direct relationship,

---

**DSM-III-R
Diagnostic Criteria for
302.73 Inhibited
Female Orgasm**

A. Persistent or recurrent delay in, or absence of, orgasm in a female following a normal sexual excitement phase during sexual activity that the clinician judges to be adequate in focus, intensity, and duration. Some females are able to experience orgasm during noncoital clitoral stimulation, but are unable to experience it during coitus in the absence of manual clitoral stimulation. In most of these females, this represents a normal variation of the female sexual response and does not justify the diagnosis of inhibited female orgasm. However, in some of these females, this does represent a psychological inhibition that justifies the diagnosis. This difficult judgment is assisted by a thorough sexual evaluation, which may even require a trial of treatment.

B. Occurrence not exclusively during the course of another Axis I disorder (other than a sexual dysfunction), such as major depression.

**DSM-III-R
Diagnostic Criteria for
302.74 Inhibited Male
Orgasm**

A. Persistent or recurrent delay in, or absence of, orgasm in a male following a normal sexual excitement phase during sexual activity that the clinician, taking into account the person's age, judges to be adequate in focus, intensity, and duration. This failure to achieve orgasm is usually restricted to an inability to reach orgasm in the vagina, with orgasm possible with other types of stimulation, such as masturbation.

B. Occurrence not exclusively during the course of another Axis I disorder (other than a sexual dysfunction), such as major depression.

however between retarded ejaculation and the female disorder discussed above, inhibited female orgasm. The embarrassment and worry experienced by males suffering from inhibited male orgasm disorder compound the condition, as it can provoke within the male anxiety, depression, and confusion.

PREMATURE EJACULATION. Premature ejaculation is often associated with erectile insufficiency. In this instance, however, the male is incapable of refraining from ejaculation for a period of time sufficient to satisfy his partner. Obviously, an exact statement of the time interval involved in cases of premature ejaculation is specific to the complaining individuals.

However, based on the defined period of time it takes for the female to be ready for receipt of the sperm (for example, for the uterus to rise), and the male's reported feeling of inadequacy, some investigators have established a minimum time frame of four minutes of sustained erection without ejaculation (Jemail, 1977; LoPiccolo & LoPiccolo, 1978), or inability to reach orgasm during 50 percent of intercourse experiences (Masters & Johnson, 1970). According to this reasoning, a male incapable of tolerating four minutes of stimulation without ejaculating less than 50 percent of the time during sexual encounters is dysfunctional. Certainly, the specific desires of the partners, the age of the male and female, and prior sexual experiences must all be weighed in

assessing the efficacy of this estimation (American Pyschiatric Association, 1987).

SEXUAL PAIN DISORDERS

There are two types of sexual pain disorders: dyspareunia and vaginismus.

DYSPAREUNIA. Dyspareunia is painful coitus. There are certainly pathophysiological conditions which can cause dyspareunia in both males and females (for example, infection, tumors, continuous use of certain types of contraceptive devices). The woman might complain of discomfort at any time during sexual activity. The discomfort can be experienced as burning or piercing and can be experienced as being anywhere from localized in the vaginal area to deep in the abdomen and pelvic region (Masters, Johnson, & Kolodny, 1988).

Dyspareunia can also be associated with insufficient lubrication in the female that might have a physiologic basis, e.g., breastfeeding. Also, vaginal creams and foams used for contraception can irritate the male's penis and make intercourse extremely painful.

Fear and anxiety are associated with dyspareunia in that the woman may be afraid of the male's penis and generalizes these feelings to his fingers as well (Gillan, 1987). In these instances, sexual intimacy,

**DSM-III-R
Diagnostic Criteria for
302.75 Premature
Ejaculation**

Persistent or recurrent ejaculation with minimal sexual stimulation or before, upon, or shortly after penetration and before the person wishes it. The clinician must take into account factors that affect duration of the excitement phase, such as age, novelty of the sexual partner or situation, and frequency of sexual activity.

**DSM-III-R
Diagnostic Criteria for
302.76 Dyspareunia**

A. Recurrent or persistent genital pain in either a male or a female before, during, or after sexual intercourse.

B. The disturbance is not caused exclusively by lack of lubrication or by vaginismus.

---

foreplay, and overall psychological discomfort severely compromise the male's and female's ability to enjoy sexual activity.

Dyspareunia is often linked to aversion to intercourse and may be associated with sexual misinformation, correlating sex with shame, guilt, and/or strict religious upbringing. However, since sexual expression and desire can vary dramatically from one individual to another, it is more often than not presented as a relationship problem in which one partner is dissatisfied with the amount of interest and sexual response expressed by the other.

VAGINISMUS. Vaginismus is frequently related to performance anxiety. It is evidenced by persistent muscle constrictions of the outer third of the vagina, which prohibit penetration. Vaginismus can occur even under conditions where a woman experiences arousal. There can be considerable pain for both partners if intercourse is attempted under this condition. Milder forms of vaginismus can occur when the woman indulges in intercourse but experiences discomfort (Masters, Johnson, & Kolodny, 1988). Sexual trauma such as rape, violent sexual activities, and incest are often the cause of vaginismus.

EPIDEMIOLOGY

Sexual disorders occur most frequently during early adulthood, the early thirties. Clinicians recognize that this age group presents most frequently for help; it is after the establishment of significant sexual relationships that people begin to be concerned about their sexual functioning. The dysfunction may be abrupt

(single-episode), acquired (after a long period of normal functioning), or a life-long problem (American Psychiatric Association, 1987).

Prevalence data are scant. Sexual dysfunctions do not fit under traditional categories for which health statistics are collected and reported. These dysfunctions usually are not "disabling," are not the primary cause of death, are non-communicable, are not hereditary, seldom require hospitalization, and are not usually associated with job impairment (Nathan, 1986). However, the relationship with the sexual partner may be strained and fraught with tension (American Psychiatric Association, 1987).

ASSESSMENT

An initial task in considering a patient for therapy is the determination of the patient's suitability for treatment. This reminds the clinician to separate the specific sexual dysfunction from other complicating problems (for example, biological, interpersonal, situational). Failure to make this determination through proper diagnosis has been linked to treatment failure (Chapman, 1982).

Specifically, careful diagnosis is necessary in order to isolate specific non-sexual or sexually-related issues that may eventually intrude into the therapy, such as psychopathology (e.g., depression and/or anxiety) (Meyer, Schmidt, Lucas, & Smith, 1975), quality of relationship with mate (Frank, Anderson, & Kupfer, 1976; Sager, 1976), personal problems, such as failure to conceive, and medical problems (LoPiccolo & Lobitz, 1973; Masters, Johnson, & Kolodny, 1988). In the case of organic or physiolog-

---

**DSM-III-R
Diagnostic Criteria for
306.51 Vaginismus**

A. Recurrent or persistent involuntary spasm of the musculature of the outer third of the vagina that interferes with coitus.

B. The disturbance is not caused exclusively by a physical disorder, and is not due to another Axis I disorder.

ical problems that are not treatable medically, sex therapy is often possible with close coordination of a physician to advise on the extent and nature of the organic impairment. In some instances where there is an organic deficit, therapy may help the patient(s) to make an adaptive adjustment to the limitations imposed by the deficit, and begin to explore other options leading to the experience of sexual intimacy.

Once a specific diagnosis is made and the nature of the sexual disorder is understood, it is important to determine what role the disorder plays in the patient's relationship(s). A number of instruments are available for this assessment. The Minnesota Multiphasic Personality Inventory (MMPI) by Hathaway and McKinley (1967) can be useful in validating clinical impressions formed during a complete psychiatric interview and observation of the patient in a variety of situations.

Poor prognosis for sex therapy has been associated with, for example, psychiatric impairment (Meyer, Schmidt, Lucas, & Smith, 1975) and alcohol abuse (LoPiccolo & LoPiccolo, 1978). However, if the disturbance is not debilitating and does not interfere with the therapy, it is possible to proceed with the treatment process. Specific areas of sexual dysfunction that can be assessed are sexual history and background (Price, Reynolds, Cohen, Anderson, & Schochet, 1981; Schover, Friedman, Weiler, Heiman, & LoPiccolo, 1982a, 1982b); attitudes toward sex (Abramson & Mosher, 1975; Annon, 1975; Schneidman & McGuire, 1976; Warren & Gilner, 1978; Sewell & Abramowitz, 1979); and knowledge of sexual processes and behaviors (McHugh, 1967; Zuckerman, 1973; Derogatis, 1976; Zuckerman, Tushup, & Finner, 1976; Newcomb & Bentler, 1980; DiVasto, Pathak, & Fishburn, 1981).

Although these instruments have been quite useful in assessing patients' appropriateness for sex therapy, they should not be seen as an alternative to a good clinical interview. It is primarily through clinical interviews that therapists can create a supportive and non-threatening environment which, hopefully, will allow the patient to be honest and open with the therapist. Data regarding sexual history and other attitudinal and background information derived from questionnaires provide important clues to issues that can be examined more closely in a clinical interview. A proper and thorough assessment and diagnosis, consisting of a history and physical examination, are essential first steps in the treatment of any sexual dysfunction and remain the bedrock of the assessment process (Heller & Gleich, 1988). Stated more emphatically, it is not possible to provide appropriate treatment without a comprehensive assessment of the patient's sexual problems and his/her perceptions about them.

THEORIES OF SEXUAL DYSFUNCTION
BIOLOGICAL CONSIDERATIONS

The primary basis of all sexual function is biological, yet emotional, social, and cultural factors all contribute to sexual feelings and activity. However, organic causes of sexual dysfunction should always be investigated prior to attempting any therapy that presupposes psychogenic factors (Gillan, 1987; Birk, 1988).

SEXUAL DEVELOPMENT. Sexual dysfunctions can result when development proceeds abnormally. Developmental difficulties can arise at any point during the life span. The normal prenatal development of the human infant requires the coordination of many intricate mechanisms. A variety of anomalies can arise from errors during this period.

Another vulnerable period in sexual development occurs during puberty. At this time the reproductive organs begin to function, and secondary sexual characteristics are acquired. Deviations at this stage are often abnormalities in timing, either precocious puberty (early onset) or pubertal delay or failure. **Early onset** can be caused by a premature signal from the hypothalamic-pituitary alarm clock, or by a tumor or lesion. This is more common in girls and can occur as early as the first year of life. **Delayed puberty** refers to adolescents who develop much more slowly than their peers. Boys who have no testicular growth by age 14 and have not yet experienced a "growth spurt" by age 16 are considered delayed, as are girls with no breast development by age 14 (Kolodny, Masters, & Johnson, 1979). Boys are more likely to experience **pubertal failure** where the locus of the problem is a deficit in the sex glands themselves. When potentially dangerous tumors and lesions are ruled out, appropriate hormonal treatment may be indicated.

PHYSICAL ILLNESS. Injury, disease, illness, and organic causes are prominent among the biological factors affecting sexual functioning. The list is long and includes heart disease, diabetes, spinal cord injury, urological difficulties, some surgical interventions, and drugs for the treatment of a variety of medical/psychiatric illnesses (Birk, 1988). (See Table 16–8).

TABLE 16—18 Outline of organic factors in sexual dysfunction

Major Medical Causes of Sexual Dysfunction, Male and Female

Liver disease and renal disease	Decreased desire
Temporal lobe lesions (including temporal lobe epilepsy)	Decreased desire (or increased)
Diabetes	Arousal dysfunction
Endocrine disorders (e.g., hypothyroidism, hypopituitarism, Addison's disease, Cushing's disease)	Decreased desire and arousal dysfunction
Low back pain	Decreased desire and arousal dysfunction
Most chronic systemic diseases	Decreased desire and arousal dysfunction

Other Organic Factors, Male Dysfunction

Infectious mononucleosis	Decreased desire
Urethritis or prostatitis	Impotence, premature ejaculation
Local/physiological problems (e.g., phimosis, hypospadias, herpes simplex of penis)	Decreased desire, impotence
Mechanical/physiological problems (e.g., large inguinal hernia, or large hydrocele)	Impotence
Radical perineal prostatectomy	Impotence but desire normal
Abdominoperineal bowel resections	Impotence but desire normal
Abdominal aortic surgery	Ejaculatory disturbance
Lumbar sympathectomy	Ejaculatory disturbance
Some rhizotomies for pain relief	Impotence and ejaculatory disturbance
Castration	Loss of desire, impotence, and retarded ejaculation

Other Organic Factors, Female Dysfunction

Infectious mononucleosis	Decreased desire
Vulvitis and vaginitis; pelvic inflammatory disease, endometriosis; fibroids; ovarian cysts; uterine tumors; pelvic masses; Bartholin's cyst infection	Dyspareunia, with secondary decreased interest, arousal dysfunction, vaginismus
Painfully adherent clitoral hood; weak pubococcygeus muscles	Orgasmic dysfunction
Poor episiotomy; obstetrical trauma; poor hysterectomy	Dyspareunia and impaired sexual response but normal desire
Oophorectomy plus adrenalectomy	Decreased desire

AGING AND SEXUAL EXPRESSION. Sexual impairment or diminished enjoyment of sexual intercourse has also been associated with the aging process (for example, menopause in women, lengthened refractory period in men). In fact, research studies have consistently documented the decrements in sexual activity and enjoyment as a function of age in both men and women (Kinsey, Pomeroy, & Martin, 1948; Kinsey, 1953; Masters & Johnson, 1966; 1970; Masters, Johnson, & Kolodny, 1988).

However, growing old does not necessarily signal the end of normal sexual functioning and its concomitant pleasures. There are normal age-related changes, not identical for males and females, that are a function of changing physiological rhythms. The distinction between physical or biological changes in

Pharmacological Factors

Progesterone and estrogens (e.g., pregnancy, birth control pills)	Decreased desire
Alcohol and sedatives	Decreased sexual response, and decreased desire (high doses)
Narcotics (including methadone)	Orgasmic dysfunction
Antiandrogens (e.g., estrogens, ACTH, cortisone)	Decreased desire
Androgens (or high androgen/estrogen ratio)	Increased desire
Levodopa	Increased desire
Cocaine and amphetamines (acutely only)	Increased desire
Alcohol, sedatives and minor tranquilizers (low doses only, and weakly only)	Increased desire
Antipsychotics	
Phenothiazines	Retrograde ejaculation
Thioridazine	Retarded ejaculation; also impotence and arousal dysfunction
Fluphenazine (Prolixin)	Impotence
Haloperidol	Decreased desire, arousal and/or orgasmic dysfunction
Antidepressants (MAOI and tricyclics)	Arousal and/or orgasmic dysfunction
Lithium	Arousal and/or orgasmic dysfunction
Anticholinergic drugs (e.g., Banthin, Probanthine, Atropine, Cogentin, Artaine, etc.)	Arousal dysfunction
Antiadrenergic drugs (e.g., many antihypertensives especially guanethidine; ergot alkaloids)	Orgasmic dysfunction
Mellaril (Thioridazine)	Frequently causes retarded ejaculation

Index of Suspicion for Organic Factors, Ranked Highest to Lowest

Retrograde ejaculation	
Loss of desire	
Impotence	
Premature ejaculation	(If recent and acute, rule out infection)
Ejaculatory incompetence	Rule out psychotropic medications
Female arousal dysfunctions	Rule out psychotropic medications

Source: Birk, L. (1980). Shifting gears in treating psychogenic sexual dysfunction: Medical assessment, sex therapy, psychotherapy, and couple therapy. *Psychiatric Clinics of North America, 3* pp. 162–163.

sexual functioning due to age, as opposed to psychological reactions to these changes, is important to assess.

DRUGS AND SEXUAL DYSFUNCTION. Normal sexual functioning can also be altered by the intake of drugs or medications. Potentially, drugs can either enhance or hinder sexual functioning. Most evidence, however, suggests that more drugs hinder or interfere with normal sexual functioning than enhance it. Chemical substances can either directly affect the brain, which controls certain sexual functions, or they may cause changes in peripheral nerves and blood flow to the genital area (Kaplan, 1974).

Alcohol has been consistently linked to sexual dysfunction in both sexes (Braddell & Wilson, 1976;

Wilson & Lawson, 1978; Wagner & Jensen, 1981). Tobacco has also been shown to cause erectile problems in some men (Wagner & Green, 1981). Anticholinergic drugs (for example, atropine) have restraining effects on penile erection and vaginal lubrication (Kaplan, 1974). Finally, a host of drugs to control high blood pressure have been found to decrease normal sexual functioning and enjoyment (Kaplan, 1974; Koten, Wilbert, Verburg, & Soldinger, 1976; Masters, Johnson, & Kolodny, 1988). In many cases, the benefits of those medications outweigh the costs, and their adverse effects on sexual functioning may have to be tolerated. In such instances, efforts should be made to help the patients adjust to the undesirable side effects and explore other ways of experiencing intimacy.

Iatrogenic sexual dysfunction can be induced by drugs or medication for other conditions. Drugs which have an effect on parasympathetic or sympathetic nerve conduction and their synaptic mediators (for example, noradrenalin, acetylcholine) may interfere with ejaculatory response in the male through the lumbo-sacral sympathetic outflow. These drugs may also have equivalent orgasmic disturbances in the female. Overactivity of the autonomic nervous system may cause premature ejaculation coupled with partial impotence since the sympathetic and parasympathetic systems function in an antagonistic fashion (see Table 16–7).

PSYCHODYNAMIC THEORIES

Freud (1953) attributed sexual dysfunction to problems of poor psychosexual development. In agreement with Freud, Masters, Johnson, and Kolodny (1982) consider the vast majority of sexual dysfunctions to be psychogenic in origin. Freud placed particular emphasis on unresolved Oepidal (Electra) conflicts as being responsible for inadequate sexual functioning in adult life. Most proponents of this position employ therapeutic strategies that are psychodynamic in character.

Kaplan (1974) suggests that the following constructs are basic to sex therapy: the unconscious motivation, the childhood experiences that influence adulthood, and the Oedipal conflict.

Briefly, the unconscious can be a storehouse for irrational and conflictual forces that dictate the individual's sexual behaviors. The assessment and treatment of sexual disorders focuses on understanding conflicts, fears, and anxieties that were previously experienced and are enacted in adulthood. Repressed material is gradually brought to the conscious level and systematically explored.

Childhood experiences, defined by Freud (1953) (oral, anal, and phallic stages), have an effect upon the psychosexual development of the child. Special attention is given to the Oedipal phase when the child selects the parent of the opposite sex as the focus of his erotic feelings. Frustrations, conflict, and fears are associated with the parent of the same sex. The girl, for example, has intense feelings for the father; the boy, on the other hand, will have intense feelings for the mother. The resolution of the Oedipal (boy) and Electra (girl) conflict is the formation of the superego and sets the stage for future interpersonal and sexual relationships, including pathological sexual conditions such as pedophilia.

There is a tendency for some individuals to avoid sexuality through limited sexual contacts and other sexually provocative circumstances. This avoidance behavior is deleterious to sexuality and can elicit feelings of fear, anxiety, and guilt through the conditioning process (Kaplan, 1974). In fact, any individual who a) avoids sexual expression and b) fails to recognize and acknowledge his own sexual feelings and desires is not likely to have "normal" sexual responses (Wolpe, 1973; Kaplan, 1974). According to psychoanalytic theory, this individual is probably a victim of some type of sexual trauma at an early age.

Kaplan and Perelman (1979) state that an antierotic environment, created by the couple, inhibits sexual expression. They identify the following as causes of this type of environment: 1) fear and guilt about sexuality; 2) fear of failure (performance anxiety); 3) failure of communication; 4) anger that is sometimes hidden and directed at one another; and 5) concern judging sexual performance, rather than enjoying the sexual experience.

ANXIETY. Anxiety has been implicated as having a significant role in sexual dysfunctions among men and women (Barlow, 1986). Numerous therapists associated with various theoretical models have identified anxiety as playing a key role in sexual dysfunction (Wolpe, 1958; 1973; Masters & Johnson, 1970; Fenichel, 1945).

While experiencing anxiety, sexually functional and sexually dysfunctional men react differently to erotic stimuli (see Table 16–9).

THE ROLE OF CULTURE IN SEXUAL DYSFUNCTION. The role of culture has been implicated

TABLE 16–9 Reactions to erotic stimuli

Sexually Functional Men	Sexually Dysfunctional Men
Anxiety increases sexual arousal	Anxiety decreases sexual arousal
Neutral distraction decreases sexual arousal	Neutral distraction does not alter sexual arousal
When focused on sexual and performance-related cues, subjects achieve more arousal	When focused on sexual and performance-related cues, subjects evidence less arousal

Source: Adapted from Barlow, D. (1986). Causes of sexual dysfunction: The role of anxiety and cognitive interference. *Journal of Consulting and Clinical Psychology, 54*, 2, 140–148.

in sexual dysfunction through the inculcation of mores, religion, and other proscriptive conventions. Attitudes or behaviors that convey to young children that sex is dirty, unhealthy, or sinful can have long-range disturbing effects. Sexual expression in adult life is potentially pleasurable but can be traumatic due to conflicts created by early childhood rearing practices. Constant fears or anxieties about sex from childhood teachings can either impair adequate sexual functioning or make it completely impossible.

Moreover, the nurse needs to understand that different cultures prescribe and endorse different beliefs and practices about the sexual roles/behaviors of women, men, and children. The nurse should keep in mind that in order to provide effective care she will need to know about the patient's cultural perspective and its potential impact on the patient's sexual practices, dysfunction, and so forth (see Table 16–4).

BEHAVIORAL THEORIES

There are no delineated causal factors associated with the behavioral model. Instead, the focus is on the conditions under which the symptoms are acquired and maintained. Behavioral theory suggests that sexual dysfunctional symptoms are learned behaviors. Two mechanisms, conditioning and reinforcement produce these dysfunctions.

Conditioning involves learning that occurs outside the individual's awareness and, once in the repertoire of behaviors, is beyond conscious control.

This process develops through a series of negative contingencies. The man who has an erection and then experiences guilt, fear, or rejection from his mate can, over a period of time, learn to constrain and suppress his response.

Reinforcement can also produce sexual dysfunction, for example, if any secondary gain (his wife's sympathy and affection) is associated with sexual dysfunction. Even rejection, guilt, fear, or pain may be subtly rewarded. In a different vein, the man who has problems because of retarded ejaculation might, over time, experience some pleasure from his mate's frustration, complaints, and hostility and thereby satisfy his own unconscious anger with her or women in general (Kaplan, 1974; Annon, 1977; Wolpe, 1977; Masters, Johnson, & Kolodny, 1988).

TREATMENT OF SEXUAL DYSFUNCTION

There are three major approaches to the treatment of sexual dysfunction: biological, behavioral, and psychodynamic/behavioral. However, there is a great deal of overlap among these approaches since biological capabilities are always a factor, as are environmental stimuli or their lack, anxiety, the patient's need for increased self-awareness, education, and desensitization, and the effects of sexual dysfunction on the mate and their relationship.

The basic conceptual assumptions that the therapist holds will determine which theoretical model and associated therapeutic techniques will be employed. These assumptions determine how the therapist will approach a problem, where she will look for a solution, and how she will relate to a patient.

BIOLOGICAL TREATMENT

The biological approach to sexual dysfunction is highly specialized and can require the expertise of numerous specialists such as nurse therapists, gynecologists, urologists, endocrinologists, psychiatrists, and psychologists. In recent years, for example, there has been substantial progress in the treatment of erectile dysfunction as well as other types of sexual dysfunctions.

Nurses need to be knowledgeable about new scientific developments that are revolutionizing treatment strategies. The nurse and other health professionals will review all available patient assessment data before any treatment is initiated. Furthermore, there must be some determination, when at all possible, as to whether the patient's sexual dysfunction is physiologic, psychogenic, sociocultural, or a combination of the three. Only after there is a clear sense of etiology or contributory factors are the clinicians ready to proceed with a treatment regimen.

PHARMACOLOGIC INTERVENTIONS. Organic causes of male erectile disorders usually involve disturbances with the penile vascular reserve, innervation, and/or hormonal disruptions that contribute to biological impotence (Heller & Gleich, 1988).

For example, one type of treatment, the intracavernosal injection of vasoactive agents, such as papaverine and/or a combination of papaverine and phentolamine, phenoxybenzamine, and so forth, is thought to be rather effective in assisting the male to develop and maintain an erection sufficient for coitus (Watters, Keogh, Earle, Carati, Wisniewaski, Tulloch, & Lord, 1988).

After a thorough assessment is completed, the patient is given a trial of injections. Patients learn quickly how to self-inject the medication and are seen by health professionals rather infrequently, simply because of its effectiveness and limited side effects. There are some unpleasant side-effects worth mentioning: flushing, dizziness, nausea, vomiting, and general discomfort. There is also a possibility that injections will be viewed as so unpleasant that the patient will cease injecting himself (Watters, et al., 1988).

More recently, topical nitroglycerin has been used for the treatment of impotence; it functions as a vasodilator, is administered by placing the paste on the shaft of the penis, and is immediately absorbed into the area. In their study, Owen, Saunders, Harris, Fenemore, Reid, Surridge, Condra and Morales (1989) reported that of 26 males who were treated with nitroglycerin paste, 22 of them experienced an increase in penile circumference.

Prostaglandin E1, another vasoactive drug, when administered by injection can be used to treat erectile impotence and is especially recommended for men with psychogenic interference. After the administration of this drug, one researcher found that the patients could experience an erection in 2 to 3 minutes and the erection would last for 1 to 3 hours, with no reported episodes of priapism (Ishii, et al., 1989). The biological processes associated with the therapeutic actions of these drugs are not clearly understood. Over time, clinicians and researchers will be able to provide explanations about how vasodilators work in the treatment of erectile dysfunctions.

SURGICAL INTERVENTIONS. You will recall that the patient should have received a thorough physical assessment before any treatment is begun. This point is essential to remember because surgical and medical intervention may be the treatment of choice.

There are several popular types of surgical penile implant procedures for the treatment of impotence. One type of treatment is the penile prosthesis, which consists of cylinders that are implanted in each of the two corpora cavernosum. The patient and physician might elect to implant a semi-rigid prostheses, which remains firm at all times. Alternatively, one might elect the multicomponent inflatable penile prosthesis which consists of two inflatable cylinders, placed suprapubically, along with a pump located in the scrotum next to the testicle. Also, there is a choice of the self-contained penile prosthesis, which is inflatable with pumps and reserves located within the cylinders. This more recent innovation greatly diminishes the possibility of recurrent surgery because of technical and mechanical failure associated with the other two procedures (Heller & Gleich, 1988).

MECHANICAL TREATMENT. The penile-suction pump is another alternative in the treatment of impotence. This procedure involves placing a lubricated cylinder over the penis, withdrawing the air with a small hand pump (which creates the erection), and then placing a rubber band at the base of the penis to impede the flow of blood from the penis. The patient then removes the cylinder. Few complications associated with this method have been reported (Heller & Gleich, 1988).

BEHAVIORAL TREATMENT

There are almost as many treatments for sexual dysfunctions as there are psychiatric nurses, psychologists, psychiatrists, and sex therapists. In spite of the fact that each branch of psychotherapy has its own theories and approaches to treatment, some facts tend to support the concept that behavioral treatments are favored and most successful (Wolpe, 1958; LoPiccolo & Lobitz, 1973; Masters, Johnson, & Kolodny, 1988; Birk, 1988).

It is a fact, for example, that fewer people and care facilities can afford long-term treatment. Thus, most current therapies deal with specific symptomatology over an average of six to twenty sessions. Also, relatively permanent change in behavior is the only method for determining "cure." Therefore, the goals of most treatments are limited to what can be observed and clearly defined, as in behavior modification. That is to say, specific sexual dysfunctions are "targeted," and the therapist begins the assessment with a series of queries such as, "What specific problems bring you to treatment now? How long have you had those problems? Do *you* have any idea about what the problem is?" (Wolpe, 1958; Masters, Johnson, & Kolodny, 1988; Birk, 1988).

MASTURBATION DESENSITIZATION THERAPY. Masturbation, preferably referred to as self-stimulation, is used to sensitize the individual to his/her own sexual identity. Joseph and Leslie LoPiccolo and Charles Lobitz (1973) are credited with most of the work in this area. Groups are often used for feedback and support. However, total attention is paid to the subject—the relationship appears to be of secondary concern to the therapist.

Initially, diagrams and mirrors are used to acquaint the patient with his or her own anatomy. Next, tactile self-stimulation focuses attention on intensifying response levels. Step-by-step, patients guide themselves toward orgasm (a vibrator is sometimes suggested). The partner is allowed to act as observer as soon as the patient is comfortable with his/her body and responses. Gradually, patients are allowed to couple and learn each other's pleasuring techniques; occasionally, role-playing techniques are used to reduce inhibition. At this point, coitus usually occurs.

For women who have never experienced orgasm, LoPiccolo and Lobitz (1973) developed a nine-step masturbation desensitization program:

Step 1. Nude bath examination, genital examination; Kegel exercises for relaxation of the pubococcygeus muscle. (See Figure 16–4.)

Step 2. Tactile and visual genital exploration with no expectation of arousal.

Step 3. Tactile and visual genital exploration with the goal of locating areas that produce pleasurable feelings when stimulated.

Step 4. Manual masturbation of the areas identified as pleasurable.

Step 5. Increased duration and intensity of masturbation if no orgasm occurred in Step 4.

Step 6. Masturbation with a vibrator if no orgasm occurred as a result of activities in Step 5.

Step 7. After orgasm has occurred through masturbation, the male partner is allowed to observe the female masturbating.

Step 8. Male allowed to stimulate female partner in the manner she demonstrated in Step 7.

Step 9. Once orgasm has been achieved, the male continues stimulation during intercourse, manually or with a vibrator.

Masturbation desensitization is a form of behavioral therapy with its foundation in learning theory. The key assumption here is that orgasm is a learned response. Failure to achieve orgasm is, therefore, the result of inadequate learning. Behavioral therapists have reported from 86 to 100 percent success in the treatment of female orgasmic dysfunction (Lazarus, 1963; Brady, 1966; Lobitz & LoPiccolo, 1972; Madsen & Ullmann, 1967; Wolpe, 1969).

MASTERS AND JOHNSON TREATMENT STRATEGY. Masters and Johnson (1970; Masters, Johnson, & Kolodny, 1988) have developed a comprehensive treatment approach to the problems of sexual inadequacy including erectile, orgasmic, and ejaculatory problems. Their two-week therapy program using a dual sex therapy team has become the model on which a number of non-analytical treatment programs have been based. The Masters and Johnson approach is a rapid treatment program in which sexual problems are viewed as a metaphor for relationship problems and are treated within the partnership. Strained relationships are analyzed, and the sexual difficulties' relationship to the couples' hurt, anger, anxiety, etc. is explored. It is hoped that any damage done over the years can be mended and that the couple can learn to accept one another along with their imperfections. This lays the groundwork for improving the sexual part of the relationship.

According to Masters and Johnson, many of the problems couples experience with sexual inadequacy have a common base and the treatment program in many regards will be similar. A basic premise of the Masters and Johnson approach is that of the conjoint marital unit. That is, each partner is presumed to be implicated in the relationship in which there is a problem of sexual inadequacy. Therefore, it is imperative that both partners participate in the treatment program. Another premise of their treatment model is that sociocultural deprivation and ignorance of sexual physiology, not medical or psychiatric illness, are the cause of most sexual dysfunction.

FIGURE 16—4 Pubococcygeal Muscle Exercises

The purpose of this brief training program is to help you tone up your vaginal or PC muscles. The use of this muscle increases your pleasure during sexual intercourse. Both you and your partner will benefit from the new sensitivity from your vagina.

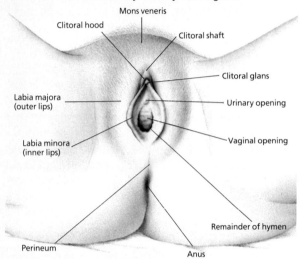

(1) *First week.* Locate the PC muscle by pretending to stop a flow of urine. If this is difficult then actually try this when you are urinating. Do this several times. Each time you urinate start and stop the flow of urine, and during urination only pass a teaspoon of urine at a time, stopping the stream by using the PC muscle.

(2) Lie down and put your finger in your vagina and contract the PC muscle. Feel the contraction around your finger.

(3) Practice 10 contractions on 6 different occasions each day. Each time you have a drink you could do this. No one else knows you are doing this, so you can do it anytime, e.g. when you answer the telephone at work or at home. Try to make each contraction last 3 seconds.

(4) *Second week.* Contract the PC muscle but release it quickly. This is called *twitching* or *fluttering.* Try to rapidly contract and release the PC muscle 6 times a day, increasing the number of contractions from 10 to 20.

(5) The next stage is to imagine you have a tampon at the opening of your vagina and that you use these muscles to suck it into your vagina. Continue the twitching 10 times a session and try to have 6 sessions a day. Continue with the ordinary paced contractions and increase these to 50 a session. When you are doing this try to enjoy some sexual fantasies and also try to picture your partner.

(6) The last exercise is to bear down, as if you were making a bowel movement, but with the emphasis more on the vagina than the anal area. Try holding this for about 3 seconds and practice it 10 times.

Source: Gillan, P. (1987). *Sex therapy manual.* Boston: Blackwell Scientific Publications, pp. 264–265.

A key aspect of the conjoint therapy is the use of a paired sex therapy team, with a member of each sex working with the couple. This arrangement allows the male and female patient each to have an objective interpreter of the same sex with no vested interest in the situation's outcome, and minimizes the complications of transference.

The couple is required to live in a hotel during the two-week treatment period. Mornings are spent in the clinic, with team discussions and a gradual introduction to the concepts of conjoint therapy. Each afternoon, the couple returns to their hotel room to practice the techniques which they have been taught.

The format for the morning sessions in the clinic is a round-table discussion in which the Masters and Johnson concept of "sensate focus" is introduced. Sensate focus is intended to establish the idea that touch is a vital part of personal relating through which feelings can be conveyed. The couple is instructed to engage in sensory exploration with each other during their afternoons in the hotel.

Specifically, they are instructed to return to bed at the hotel, where they are to disrobe completely and eliminate any distractions (television, radio). Once they are naked, they should fondle each other, initially avoiding the erotic areas, using moisturizing cream to enhance the quality of the sensation. As the week progresses, the couple is given permission to include the erogenous zones in their fondling experiences. A key aspect of this process is for the couple to maintain a completely non-demanding, non-anxiety producing atmosphere, give up their spectator role, and focus on giving pleasure to each other. Finally, intercourse is encouraged, but only after preliminary sex play.

Sensate focus techniques used for the treatment of impotence in men have success rates of 60 percent for primary impotence and 74 percent for secondary impotence. Masters and Johnson's "squeeze technique" during sensate focus sessions has yielded a success rate of 98 percent in men experiencing premature ejaculation.

The squeeze technique is a procedure in which the female partner squeezes the shaft of the penis just below the glans with her thumb and first and second fingers. After fifteen to thirty seconds, the partner resumes manipulation until erection is achieved and maintained. The male partner can usually achieve some degree of control over his ejaculations within a few days. The procedure is effective in causing the male to lose the immediate urge to ejaculate.

In treating the dysfunctional female, the same sensate focus procedure is employed with emphasis on the male partner giving non-demanding stimulation to the female. Using this procedure, Masters and Johnson report a success rate of 84 percent for women experiencing primary orgasmic dysfunction and a 78 percent success rate for secondary orgasmic dysfunction. These data were collected over a period of 11 years. A five-year follow-up study showed an overall success rate of 75 percent.

Utilizing learning theory, the therapist will assess each symptom targeted for modification. The goals are to remove the rewards associated with sexual dysfunction, extinguish undesirable sexual reactions, and, when appropriate, provide conditions for systematically extinguishing the impaired sexual response. Too, the behavior therapist might develop a program that focuses on substituting and reinforcing new, desirable behaviors (Kaplan, 1974).

Kolodny, Masters, Johnson and Biggs (1979) propose that the treatment approach to impotence shares certain common features with the approach to the treatment of any sexual dysfunction.

1. Blaming one's partner or oneself for sexual problems is not helpful.

2. Each partner is equally involved in the sexual activity, whether it is free and satisfying or constrained with problems.

3. Sexual problems are common and are grounded in physical, psychological, and sociocultural beliefs and practices.

4. Treatment can proceed even when the clinician is not able to determine the exact etiology of the dysfunction.

5. Sociocultural stereotypes about female/male sexual behaviors are extremely varied and frequently counterproductive.

6. Sex is a participatory activity, not a spectator activity.

7. Sex can be expressed in a variety of methods of physical contact and is not limited to coitus.

8. Sex is a form of highly personal and intimate communication. When sexual communication is not satisfying it usually indicates that other aspects of the couple's communication style are also faulty.

9. Focusing on past feelings, conflicts, and frustrations is not useful when the couple and therapist are trying to institute satisfactory sexual behavior change.

10. Each sexual partner in the relationship should be assisted in the development of the ability to be sensitive and responsive to the communication cues, needs, and desires of the partner.

11. Each partner should assume responsibility for his/her own sexual behavior (Kolodny, Masters, Johnson, & Biggs, 1979).

OTHER BEHAVIORAL TREATMENTS. It has been suggested that therapeutic techniques that occur in the couple's home are usually more effective than treatment in offices and other nonpersonal places (Kaplan, 1974). Premature ejaculation, for example, is frequently treated with in vivo desensitization. This treatment adheres to the principle that pairing a feared situation with a rewarding situation will yield a positive response (Kaplan, 1974). This technique has been employed by Wolpe (1969; 1973) and others and is described here.

Wolpe (1969) treated premature ejaculation, a problem one out of every three men claim to have (Nathan, 1986), and has written that impaired sexual response is related to anxiety regarding the sexual situation that must be alleviated.

1. First, the therapist should determine the point at which the anxiety begins. Is it when the man enters the bedroom, or at the point when he undresses?

2. In a stepwise progression:
   a) The man lies next to his wife (but takes no further action) until he feels free of anxiety.
   b) The man turns toward his wife.
   c) The man fondles her breasts while she continues to lie on her back.
   d) If the man is free of anxiety, he lies on top of his sexual partner in a face-to-face position, but there is no attempt at penetration.
   e) The penis is placed next to the vulva, but there is no attempt at penetration.
   f) A small degree of penetration can occur.
   g) Then, a greater degree of penetration can occur.
   h) There should be a minimum amount of movement.
   i) Increasing amounts of movement should follow.
   j) The wife or sexual partner manipulates the penis to the point of ejaculation and stops.
   k) A time lapse occurs . . . then she does the same thing again. (This procedure can be repeated several times during a session, and can provide delayed ejaculation from minutes to an hour or more.)

l) If either member of the couple begins to feel anxiety, they should stop what they are doing and return to the previous step.

The wife/husband can be taught to manipulate the penis (husband removing the wife's hand when he feels he is about to ejaculate). Stimulation through manipulation of the penis is begun again and discontinued just short of ejaculation. This technique will provide for the postponement of ejaculation almost indefinitely if the woman applies pressure gently, at the coronal sulcus, with one finger on the urethra and the other on the dorsum (see Figure 16–5).

Colonel Dyan: A Patient with Premature Ejaculation

Colonel Dyan has been in the Army for 21 years. He and his wife have had a harmonious relationship, raised two daughters, and lived all over the world. Because of his career arrangements, he had to spend long periods of time (as much as 2½ years in one instance) away from home. When Colonel Dyan returned home from his last assignment, about nine months ago, he experienced premature ejaculation during sexual activity with his wife. This was very upsetting to the Colonel and to Mrs. Dyan. Colonel Dyan

FIGURE 16–5 Two Forms of the Squeeze Technique

The Squeeze Technique Used in Treating Premature Ejaculation

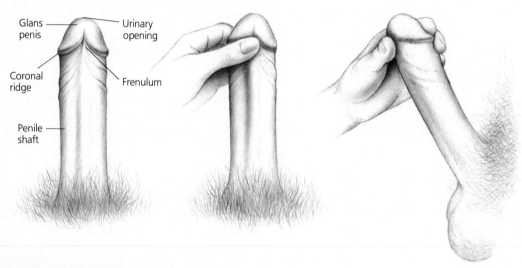

The Basilar Squeeze Technique Used in Treating Premature Ejaculation

Unlike the squeeze at the coronal ridge, the basilar squeeze can be applied by either the woman or the man. Firm pressure is applied for about four seconds and then released; the pressure should always be from front to back (as shown by the arrows), never from side to side.

Source: Masters, W. H., Johnson, V. E., & Kolodny, R. C. (1988). *Human sexuality*, 3rd ed. Glenview, IL: Scott Foresman/ Little, Brown, pp. 524–525.

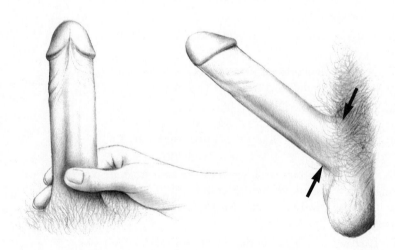

suggested that he was fatigued and "burned out." Perhaps a little rest, relaxation, and cessation of alcohol intake would help him regain his ability to make love to his wife.

After several weeks of continuous premature ejaculation, Colonel and Mrs. Dyan sought counseling at a nearby clinic. The following treatment was implemented after a psychosocial, physical, and psychiatric assessment and is based on the work of Semans (1956), Wolpe (1973), and Kaplan (1974).

The couple were instructed:

1. Both should lie in bed until Colonel Dyan felt completely relaxed and free of anxiety.

2. Colonel Dyan should caress his wife, fondle her breasts, kiss, and so on.

3. Then, Mrs. Dyan would fondle Colonel Dyan's penis.

Listed below is a recording of the time involved in penis stimulation with Mrs. Dyan applying pressure just short of ejaculation:

1st time; 10 minutes of stimulation until the point of ejaculation.

2nd time: 12 minutes

3rd time: 10 minutes

4th time: 7 minutes

After several days had passed, the time recording was:

1st time: 12 minutes

2nd time: 13 minutes

3rd time: 10 minutes

4th time: 15 minutes

By session ten, the Colonel had reached a near ejaculation state in 15 minutes and maintained it for 12 minutes.

PSYCHODYNAMIC/BEHAVIORAL TREATMENT

Psychoanalyst Helen Singer-Kaplan's therapeutic model combines some of the Masters and Johnson program (behavioral) with a psychodynamic approach. In 1974 with the publication of *The New Sex Therapy* and later *Disorders of Sexual Desire* (1979), she added a psychodynamic component to the treatment of sexual dysfunction. Kaplan (1974) described her approach as a "task-centered form of crisis intervention which presents an opportunity for rapid conflict resolution" (p. 199). Several sexual tasks are prescribed (for example, pleasuring), however, treatment also includes psychoanalytic psychotherapy in various formats (individual, couples, or family therapy) (Kaplan, 1974; 1978). A major feature in the Kaplan model is the contention that sexual dysfunction results from difficulties in the relationship that create frustrations and dissatisfaction, such as pressures from the environment (for example, in-laws, religious values, work stress, or children) or misunderstanding about what constitutes an appropriate sexual response.

One patient population with which Kaplan has reported success involves patients with inhibited sexual desire disorder (ISD). These patients have the physiological capacity to experience a sexual response but no desire to participate in activities leading to sexual arousal. In other words, the sexual "desire" has been lost. Consequently, the therapy focuses on the history of the relationship, often using psychodynamic techniques (for example, role playing). Goals in Kaplan's approach to therapy may well be a modification of the entire marital system or an enhancement of individual growth as a means of eliminating the dysfunctional behavior.

Kaplan (1974) reported that initial success in some instances is short-lived and is often accompanied by a "take-it-for-granted" attitude which in some couples leads to a reversal of positive changes. Ongoing therapy attempts to address these changes in attitude and behavior.

Relationships, not to mention intimacy, are difficult for many people. Initiating, establishing, and maintaining a viable relationship requires motivation, energy, concern and the ability to read accurately the cues given by a partner expressing feelings about the relationship. An individual who finds such relationships frightening or threatening or who harbors feelings that are inconsistent with general attitudes toward sex roles may experience performance anxiety. To regard such dysfunction as other than a treatable illness can result in an internalization of more guilt and compound the problem.

The sex roles of men and women in our society have remained fairly stable over a number of decades when compared to the changing boundaries of acceptable behavior. We have become more liberal than liberated. Many feel too much has happened too fast. "Casual sex" has left many feeling used and "empty." As a result of such feelings, and the increasing threat of AIDS, we as a society seem to be retuning to pre-1960's values, such as the desire to mate for life, committment, and family life.

The Masters and Johnson research confirms that the relationship and the individuals within that relationship are the focal points for successful resolution of sexual dysfunction. By addressing "the couple," the treatments focus less on a victim and more on a solution. Treatment tends to focus on learning one's own body and one's partner's body and then learning each other as parts of a unit.

You will recall that traditional psychotherapy for sexual problems has focused on the resolution of unconscious conflicts, which would lead to the relief of sexual dysfunction. The therapist's aim was to facilitate the patient's development of insight into his problems (Kaplan, 1974). However, Kaplan proposed an approach that operates on the assumption that the here-and-now conflicts, not the unconscious ones, should be, but are not required to be, addressed in order for resolution of sexual conflicts to be reached.

This technique focuses on modifying ". . . the results of the conflict between the patient's desire to have intercourse and the anxiety which arises at the moment of lovemaking" (Kaplan, 1974, p. 151). This technique is aimed at resolving the immediately-operating conscious conflicts that the individual is experiencing.

Other techniques focus on experiences that have the potential for aiding in unconscious conflict resolution. Touch, showing of affection, the exploration of erotic zones, and changing consequences evoked by sexual behaviors can yield behavioral change that is not dependent on insight into unconscious motivation.

More thorough and comprehensive treatment of sexual dysfunction will require couples therapy, according to psychoanalytic thinkers. It is evident that couples who experience marital conflict are likely to have sexual problems; it is also obvious that couples who have sexual problems might also be having other types of conflicts which affect the whole family. Even though family therapy and sex therapy emerged from different theoretical models and are practiced separately, professionals must begin to integrate the two modalities (Birk, 1988).

THE PARAPHILIAS

Paraphilias represent complex forms of sexual behavior that signify aberrations. According to the DMS-III-R (1987), paraphilias are characterized by unusual behaviors or bizarre imagery or acts that are necessary for sexual excitement. The imagery or acts are further categorized as involving either 1) preference for use of nonhuman objects for sexual arousal; 2)

repetitive sexual activity with humans that includes real, not merely simulated, suffering or humiliation; or 3) repetitive sexual behavior with nonconsenting partners. The eight specific categories of paraphilia include: exhibitionism, fetishism, frotteurism, pedophilia, sexual masochism, sexual sadism, transvestic fetishism, and voyeurism. A residual category of paraphilias not otherwise specified is also included.

EXHIBITIONISM

Exhibitionism is the act of obtaining sexual gratification from publicly exposing the genitals to others. The problem is primarily limited to males (who often achieve erection while exposing themselves). Some masturbate to orgasm at the time. The targets for most exhibitionists are innocent female passers-by.

Three motives have been attributed to the exhibitionist: 1) a primitive assertion of masculinity, 2) the naive assumption that their female victims will be sexually aroused, and 3) sexual solicitation. These men are typically insecure and uncomfortable with their sexuality, often suffering from impotence in heterosexual activity (Gebhard et al., 1965; American Psychiatric Association, 1987; Masters, Johnson, & Kolodny, 1988).

Exhibitionists are frequently apprehended by the police and have a tendency to "perform their act" in such a manner as to ensure that they get caught. For example, a man might exhibit himself in the same library, behind the same stacks, at the same time, once a week. Others will "flash" as they spring from behind a building or appear in a remote hallway (Snaith, 1983).

FETISHISM

The term "fetish" is used to describe an individual's recurrent and intense sexual arousal to an inanimate object (for example, panties, boots) or body parts that are neither primary nor secondary sexual organs. Fetishism is most often associated with female clothing, and the behavior primarily occurs in males (Brown, 1983). Occasionally, fetish objects are fondled, smelled, tasted, or rubbed against the skin (sometimes against the penis) in order to heighten sexual arousal. Fetish objects are also used as adjuncts to actual intercourse (American Psychiatric Association, 1987). The chosen object is not used as a substitute for the person; rather, it is chosen because it is available, silent, or safe (Stoller, 1977).

The nurse and other health professionals may find it extremely difficult to distinguish between fetishism and specific types of personal sexual prefer-

**DSM-III-R
Diagnostic Criteria for
302.40 Exhibitionism**

A. Over a period of at least six months, recurrent intense sexual urges and sexually arousing fantasies involving the exposure of one's genitals to an unsuspecting stranger.

B. The person has acted on these urges, or is markedly distressed by them.

ences. A rule of thumb might be to determine if the person is aroused by an individual with certain attire or if it is the attire that induces arousal independent of the individual (Masters, Johnson, & Kolodny, 1988).

In considering the origins of fetishes, Griffith and Hatfield (1985) discuss three factors: a) a powerful *conditioning experience* in which pleasure or sexual arousal is associated with the fetish object or items similar to it; b) *sexual symbolic value of the object* when the fetish is associated with a body part (or object) which symbolizes part or all of a human sexual partner; and c) *sexual maladjustment,* or doubts, regarding masculinity, adeptness, and potency. In addition, fears of rejection by one's sexual partner will lead to fetishes as a way of reducing threats associated with sexual experiences (p. 363). There is, however, no single explanation that accounts for this disorder, but the evidence, sometimes elusive or indirect, does point to an association between the fetish and some childhood experience of a traumatic nature (Meyer, 1980).

FROTTEURISM

Frotteurism is sexual behavior in which gratification is achieved by rubbing or pressing against women, usually in public places. The behavior ordinarily occurs in crowded situations where it is possible to feign inadvertence (Masters, Johnson, & Kolodny, 1988). Men who receive sexual gratification through this method are likely to frequent activities such as large public marches or crowded parks where their behaviors would not be suspect and they can easily escape arrest (American Psychiatric Association, 1987; Masters, Johnson, & Kolodny, 1988).

The specific act might include a man rubbing his genitals against a female's thigh or buttocks or fondling her breast and genitalia with his hands. Too, while fondling, he might develop mental images of having an intimate and caring relationship with the victim. Then, he escapes to avoid being apprehended (American Psychiatric Association, 1987; Masters, Johnson, & Kolodny, 1988).

PEDOPHILIA

A highly dramatized form of sexual pathology is evidenced in pedophilia. The term "pedophilia" is derived from the Greek word meaning "lover of children." The pedophile (almost always a male) is erotically aroused by, and seeks sexual gratification from children. DSM-III-R describes pedophilia as preferred or exclusive sexual activity (fantasized or actual) with prepubertal children. Additionally, there must be at least a five-year age difference between the victim and the perpetrator, unless the perpetrator is an adolescent.

**DSM-III-R
Diagnostic Criteria for
302.81 Fetishism**

A. Over a period of at least six months, recurrent intense sexual urges and sexually arousing fantasies involving the use of nonliving objects by themselves (e.g., female undergarments).

Note: The person may at other times use the nonliving object with a sexual partner.

B. The person has acted on these urges, or is markedly distressed by them.

C. The fetishes are not only articles of female clothing used in cross-dressing (transvestic fetishism) or devices designed for the purpose of tactile genital stimulation (e.g., vibrator).

DSM-III-R Diagnostic Criteria for 302.89 Frotteurism

A. Over a period of at least six months, recurrent intense sexual urges and sexually arousing fantasies involving touching and rubbing against a nonconsenting person. It is the touching, not the coercive nature of the act, that is sexually exciting.

B. The person has acted on these urges, or is markedly distressed by them.

Differences between same-sex and opposite-sex activity are important from a clinical perspective. Homosexual males are sexually attracted to the youth's masculine characteristics, whereas the heterosexual male is attracted to the youth's feminine characteristics. Since prepubertal children, male and female, are more likely to have feminine characteristics, exposure of these children to the heterosexual adult male constitutes a greater threat than exposure to homosexual males (American Psychiatric Association, 1987).

Heterosexual pedophiles are usually individuals whose occupational, peer, and adult sexual relationships are marginal. They typically resort to alcohol in dealing with stress, and sexual contacts with children frequently occur when they are intoxicated. Sexual deprivation from a partner is often a motivating influence as indicated in the following case:

DeWitt McClaren: A Quiet, Shy Husband

After a rather restrained premarital life, this shy and dependent young man married a woman who was more aggressive than he. She held a job, spent money freely, and went out frequently without her husband, leaving him at home to care for their child. He was periodically unemployed and felt perpetually jealous and inferior; the marriage continued to deteriorate. In a moment of depression, he tried suicide.

Not long thereafter while he was alone at home watching television, some neighborhood children came to the home. One child, a girl of ten, sat next to him and, according to him, "bugged" him. He became sexually aroused (sexual intercourse with his wife had become infrequent over the years due to her waning interest in him and his erectile difficulties) and ultimately took her into the bedroom and attempted to have sex with her.

Sexual and emotional deprivation, of course, are not sufficient to explain DeWitt McClaren's behav-

ior. Gebhard and his associates (1965) found a host of disturbances in men who initiate sexual contacts with children, including alcoholism, intellectual retardation, psychosis, organic brain syndrome, and severe personality disorders.

It is also important for the nurse to know that the pedophile expresses his sexual desires in numerous other ways. For instance, he might undress the child, expose his genitals, and possibly masturbate in the child's presence. Others might fondle a child, insert their fingers or objects into the child's anus, vagina, or mouth. The amount of force used during these acts varies greatly. Frequently, the pedophile will claim that acts perpetrated against the child are of valuable "educational significance" or provide the child with sexual pleasure or that the child "asked for it" through expressions of sexually provocative behaviors (American Psychiatric Association, 1987; Masters, Johnson, & Kolodny, 1988; Erickson, Walbek, & Seely, 1988).

Homosexual pedophiles exhibit marginal social experiences in dealing with adult peers but are specific about their preference for young boys whose bodies are smooth and hairless (that is, feminine) (Marshall, Barbaree, & Butt, 1988). The choice of prepubertal boys may be related to childhood masturbatory fantasies with young boys as a focus. The homosexual pedophile should not be confused with the homosexual, as the preference for prepubertal males is quite specific (Masters, Johnson, & Kolodny, 1988).

An especially damaging variant of pedophilia is father-daughter incest. In these instances, the father suffers from some of the psychopathology described above. However, his unique situation, in an unhappy (often sexless) marriage and disintegrating family circumstance, occasioned by a sexually maturing daughter, makes it possible for him to turn to his daughter for affection and sex. The father's position as head-of-household gives him power in these relationships, and the daughter might find him difficult to resist. Incest often goes on for years for a number of reasons, including the father's power, the daughter's ig-

**DSM-III-R
Diagnostic Criteria for
302.20 Pedophilia**

A. Over a period of at least six months, recurrent intense sexual urges and sexually arousing fantasies involving sexual activity with a prepubescent child or children (generally age 13 or younger).

B. The person has acted on these urges, or is markedly distressed by them.

C. The person is at least 16 years old and at least 5 years older than the child or children in A.

Note: Do not include a late adolescent involved in an ongoing sexual relationship with a 12- or 13-year-old.

Specify: same sex, opposite sex, or **same and opposite sex.**

Specify if **limited to incest.**

Specify: exclusive type (attracted only to children), or **nonexclusive type.**

norance regarding her rights and lack of support system, as well as shame, guilt, and fear of exposure (Masters, Johnson, & Kolodny, 1988; Erickson, Walbek, & Seely, 1988).

Pedophiles are typically conservative men who are highly moralistic but limited in exposure to adequate sexual outlets. Some are sexual thrill seekers, while others experience guilt concerning their wishes and actions (Gebhard, et al., 1965). Regardless, they exhibit little concern for their sexual partners, often using brute force and inflicting pain in their attempts to achieve coitus (American Psychiatric Association, 1987; Masters, Johnson, & Kolodny, 1988).

Finkelhor and Araji (1986) have pointed out that most theories about pedophilia are single factor theories and are not adequate to explain the complexities and diversities in this diagnostic classification. They do suggest, however, a four-factor model which can be summarized as a) emotional congruence (the pedophile manifests childlike emotional needs and lacks adult maturity); b) sexual arousal (the pedophile is thought to have had inappropriate sexual stimulation during his youth which, during adult years, results in being sexually aroused by children); c) blockage (characterized by the inability to get his adult sexual needs fulfilled by age-appropriate peers); and d) disinhibition (focuses on possible reasons why certain taboos or societal and legal restrictions regarding sexual behavior with children do not promote the inhibition and restrictions that they should).

Though not complete in its explanation about pedophilia, Finkelhor and Araji have come up with an excellent model for nurses and other health care professionals to use in their work with the pedophile and his victims and their families.

SEXUAL MASOCHISM

The essential feature of sexual masochism is the achievement of sexual satisfaction from receiving physical or psychological pain. Specifically, the individual experiences recurrent and intense sexual urges and fantasies that are acted upon and involve being humiliated, beaten, bound, and tortured. There are several forms of sexual masochism: a) physical bondage, in which the individual is physically restrained; b) blindfolding, in which the individual experiences sensory deprivation and/or bondage; c) flagellation, which includes beating, spanking, and so on; d) infibulation, which includes electrical shocks, cutting,

**DSM-III-R
Diagnostic Criteria for
302.83 Sexual
Masochism**

A. Over a period of at least six months, recurrent intense sexual urges and sexually arousing fantasies involving the act (real, not simulated) of being humiliated, beaten, bound, or otherwise made to suffer.

B. The person has acted on these urges, or is markedly distressed by them.

**DSM-III-R
Diagnostic Criteria for
302.84 Sexual Sadism**

A. Over a period of at least six months, recurrent intense sexual urges and sexually arousing fantasies involving acts (real, not simulated) in which the psychological or physical suffering (including humiliation) of the victim is sexually exciting to the person.

B. The person has acted on these urges, or is markedly distressed by them.

piercing; e) humiliation, whereby the individual is forced to bark like a dog, eat from the floor, or be urinated or defecated upon, f) infantilism, in which the individual experiences the desire to be treated as if he/she were a helpless infant; and, g) hypoxyphilia, which is a dangerous form of sexual masochism that requires oxygen deprivation (e.g., by hanging) in order for the individual to become sexually aroused (American Psychiatric Association, 1987).

SEXUAL SADISM

Sexual sadism is associated with recurrent, intense sexual urges and fantasies that involve inflicting physical or psychological suffering on the victim and experiencing sexual excitement and gratification from this behavior (American Psychiatric Association, 1987).

Sadism is the reciprocal of masochism. The sadist derives sexual gratification from inflicting physical or psychological pain on others. The key to understanding sadism rests in discovering the sadist's need to degrade and humiliate his sexual object while inflicting pain or otherwise making the victim suffer (Meyer, 1980).

TRANSVESTIC FETISHISM

Transvestism is the act of a heterosexual male obtaining sexual pleasure from cross-dressing (dressing in women's clothing) and is often accompanied by masturbation and mental images of other men being attracted to him as a "woman." This disorder should not be confused with gender identity disorder of adolescence or adulthood.

The extent to which the heterosexual male wears female apparel can range from one item, such as a garter or stockings, to dressing in all female apparel with a well madeup face and an immaculate feminine coiffure (American Psychiatric Association, 1987). It is believed that men who become transvestites have a history of having been punished by being made to dress in female clothing during their developmental years (Stoller, 1977; American Psychiatric Association, 1987).

VOYEURISM

The converse of exhibitionism is voyeurism. The voyeur derives sexual pleasure from looking at sexual objects or sexually arousing situations. No sexual activity with the observed persons is sought, only a viewing of unsuspecting people who are nude, in the act of dressing or undressing, or having sexual intercourse. In extreme instances in which voyeurism becomes a substitute for sexual gratification, it is called scoptophilia. Voyeurs, also called "Peeping Toms," receive sexual gratification without the complexities of interpersonal relationships. Although voyeurs have historically been perceived as harmless individuals because of their lack of social contact, evidence reveals that some have committed violent crimes such as rape and arson (Gebhard, et al., 1965; Masters, Johnson, & Kolodny, 1988).

**DSM-III-R
Diagnostic Criteria for
302.30 Transvestic
Fetishism**

A. Over a period of at least six months, in a heterosexual male, recurrent intense sexual urges and sexually arousing fantasies involving cross-dressing.

B. The person has acted on these urges, or is markedly distressed by them.

C. Does not meet the criteria for Gender Identity Disorder of Adolescence or Adulthood, Nontranssexual Type, or Transsexualism.

DSM-III-R Diagnostic Criteria for 302.82 Voyeurism

A. Over a period of at least six months, recurrent intense sexual urges and sexually arousing fantasies involving the act of observing an unsuspecting person who is naked, in the process of disrobing, or engaging in sexual activity.

B. The person has acted on these urges, or is markedly distressed by them.

Usually the individual masturbates and experiences orgasm during the voyeuristic event, or he engages in sexual fantasies at a later time and recalls the voyeuristic act and masturbates to orgasm. In the extreme form, "sexual activity" is limited to peeping (American Psychiatric Association, 1987).

PARAPHILIAS NOT OTHERWISE SPECIFIED

A number of paraphilias fall outside the officially designated types. They, nonetheless, have common elements with all of the paraphilias described earlier—objects or persons are used for sexual gratification in ways not ordinarily considered appropriate in this society. Atypical paraphilias include:

1. Telephone scatologia (lewdness)
2. Necrophilia (corpses) (See Box 16–3)
3. Partialism (exclusive focus on part of body)
4. Zoophilia (animals)
5. Coprophilia (feces)
6. Klismaphilia (enemas)
7. Urophilia (urine)

Box 16–3 ● Necrophilia

Necrophilia is from the Greek words "nekros" (meaning dead body) and "philia" (love of). It is a mental or emotional aberration nearly always found among men. Some authorities believe necrophilia occurs among men who seek sexual gratification with partners who are nonthreatening and totally subjugated (Mathis, 1972; Stoller, 1977). The two cases that follow are illustrative of these motives:

This morning our daughter phoned in hysterics. It seems her wedding night was a nightmare. Her husband asked her to take a very cold bath before coming to bed. He suggested that she soak in a tub for about half an hour. When she came to bed he asked her to close her eyes and be perfectly still. Then he said, "You may as well know that I am a necrophiliac. . . . I can only make love to dead women or women who look as if they are." . . . Our daughter fled in panic, packed her bags and checked into another room. She is at the mo-

ment in a state of shock and under a doctor's care. (Ann Landers Advises, January 4, 1976.)

KT was an embalmer by trade. . . . KT had been fired from his job only two times. Upon the first occasion he had incited the rage of the owner of the establishment when he had been discovered fondling the breasts of a young girl who had just been brought in. . . . His next and final apprehension came almost two years later when he was working in a small town in the southeast. He was discovered having intercourse with a female corpse which he was preparing to embalm (Mathis, 1972, p. 202).

Source: Mathis, J. L. (1972). *Clear thinking about sexual deviations*. Chicago: Nelson-Hall. Stoller, R. J. (1977). Sexual Deviations. In F. Beach (Ed.), *Human sexuality in love perspectives*. Baltimore: Johns Hopkins University Press, pp. 190–214. Landers, A. (1976). Ann Landers Advises (Jan. 4).

EPIDEMIOLOGY OF PARAPHILIAS

Little data exist on the prevalence of the paraphilias among individuals in our society. Most persons with paraphilias come to the mental health care system not because of their own distress, but at the behest of their partners or legal authorities (Masters et al., 1988). Consequently, these disorders are rarely seen in clinical practice settings, although the large market for paraphilic pornography and paraphernalia suggests that incidence in the greater community is high. With the exception of sexual masochism, those suffering from the paraphilias are overwhelmingly male. Even with sexual masochism, incidence is estimated to be twenty males for each female (American Psychiatric Association, 1987).

Individuals suffering from one of the paraphilias may actually exhibit more than one variety of the disorder at the same time. In addition, such persons are also often suffering from other mental disorders, such as psychoactive substance abuse disorder or personality disorder (APA, 1987). The degree of impairment of social and sexual functioning depends on several factors such as the severity of symptoms and the nature of the particular paraphilia. For example, mild fetishism would probably be less impairing than severe sexual sadism. In sexual masochism, serious injury, even death, can occur, and practices such as pedophilia, sexual sadism, exhibitionism, and voyeurism can lead to arrest and incarceration. (APA, 1987). While there are clear legal ramifications to the practice of these disorders (especially those which involve minors and non-consenting adults), more "sex-offenders" are candidates for therapy than for prison (Groth, 1979).

Tingle, Barnard, Robbins, Newman, and Hutchinson (1986) researched the childhood and adolescent characteristics of 42 pedophiles and 21 rapists who were in-patients at an evaluation and treatment center. Listed briefly are some of their findings:

1. The racial proportions of rapists and child molesters were similar; the molesters were older, better educated, and more likely to be in intact marriages at the time of their arrest.

2. Molesters reported more closeness to their mothers than did the rapists but neither group reported feeling close to their fathers.

3. Rapists reported more arguments with their mothers.

4. Violence was present in the homes of both groups, and both groups reported a history of physical abuse.

5. Both rapists and child molesters reported having run away from home during their formative years. Both groups (38% of rapists and 56% of child molesters) reported that during their youth, they had experienced sexual abuse by family and/or friends.

6. Rapists revealed more conflict in school, as demonstrated by expulsion, and so on, and more rapists than child molesters had participated in contact sports during high school.

7. Both groups reported that they had few friends during their youth and that they had interpersonal difficulties.

8. Both groups reported that they had family and friends who had difficulties with the law.

ASSESSMENT AND PRINCIPLES OF TREATMENT GOALS

Forensics of mental health is a new and growing field. In the past, sex offenders have been dealt with in the court systems of America. However, there is a growing trend for mental health professionals to treat child and adult sex offenders. Forensic institutions are being developed that encourage research, theory development, and testing of a variety of treatment approaches. It is evident that sex offenders need a variety of forms of treatment and rehabilitation, such as partial hospitalization, complete hospitalization, and outpatient and after-care programs (including the half-way house) (Groth, 1979).

Treatment for sex offenders remains a debatable issue. There are some clinicians who think that child offenders are not treatable, while others think that treatment is essential (Groth, 1979) and likely to be effective, especially in the case of incest (Giaretto, 1982).

Treatment for the sex offender consists of four basic components. First, the offender must acknowledge that he has committed a crime and take responsibility for his actions. Second, the offender must be held accountable for his actions. Third, the offender must become aware of the patterns and origins of his behavior. Finally, the offender must develop an alternative method of expressing his conflicts, impulses, and desires. Rehabilitation cannot begin until these four basic issues have been resolved (Groth, 1979).

TREATMENT STRATEGIES

Treatment for the paraphilias becomes very important when the individual's sexual urges and fantasies are expressed in behaviors that are potentially or actually harmful to themselves and others. Recall that, for example, sexual sadistic and masochistic behaviors can be extremely dangerous for partner and victim. Similarly, pedophilia, particularly incest, typically results in depression, dissociative disorders, even psychosis, in the victims. Young children are especially vulnerable (Ulman & Brothers, 1988). (See Fig. 16–6.) Thus, treatment always involves both the sex-offender and his victim, often a child. (Berlin, 1985; American Psychiatric Association, 1987; Fuller, 1989).

Finkelhor and Araji (1986) and Fuller (1989) suggest that between 100,000 and 500,000 children suffer from some type of sexual molestation each year, and most of these are in the category of incest.

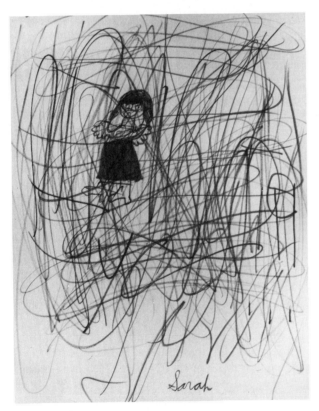

FIGURE 16–6 Childhood Incest

This drawing was done by a 7-year-old victim of incest. She portrays herself as small, dark, and mean—in a storm. Social services insisted she continue to visit her father who was big, poorly groomed, and lived alone in a dirty basement apartment. It was her word against his—and she was just a child.

Pedophilia is found almost exclusively in men, and the individual is often labeled as a sex offender if he has a history of associated entanglements with the law. (Berlin, 1985). The pedophile may not limit himself to one victim nor to one type of abuse. He commonly engages in exhibitionism, frotteurism, rape, sexual masochism, sexual sadism, and voyeurism (Fuller, 1989). Psychiatric evaluation of the pedophile is usually requested to determine if the offense is due to limited mental capacity, specific personality characteristics, or sexual orientation (Berlin, 1985; Fuller, 1989).

Treatment of pedophilia usually involves 1) psychotherapy, 2) behavior therapy, and 3) pharmacologic therapy.

PSYCHOTHERAPY. Berlin (1985) and Fuller (1989) suggest that the psychodynamic approach, including individual, family, and group therapy should be considered in treating child abusers, pedophiles, victims, and victims' families. Fuller does not think that one specific approach is superior but suggests that insight-oriented psychotherapy, supportive psychotherapy, sex education, assertiveness training, social skills training, and so forth, are helpful in the rehabilitation process.

BEHAVIOR THERAPY. The behavioral approach does not focus on psychodynamics associated with pedophilia. Rather, a common behavioral approach focuses on the extinguishment of erotic feelings directed toward children and, concomitantly, teaching the patient to become sexually aroused by age-appropriate partners (Berlin, 1985).

This modality involves self-observation and self-monitoring of targeted behaviors (Fuller, 1989). For example, the pedophile would be expected to heighten his awareness regarding current behaviors such as "cruising" for child victims, feelings/thoughts associated with sexual arousal, and so forth. The nurse therapist or other clinician can then work with the patient on 1) identification of the problem, 2) feedback about his abusive cycle and 3) developing contingencies associated with appropriate behavioral change (Fuller, 1989).

PHARMACOTHERAPY. Reversible chemical castration is another, though less common, treatment approach. The male patient is injected with the female hormone **medroxyprogesterone acetate (MPA; Depo-provera).** The typical dose is 400 mg.

per week given IM. It is gradually titrated to the most effective dosage for the patient. This drug is effective with rapists, child molesters, and pedophiles, because it lowers the male hormone, testosterone, and, thus, the male's sex drive (Spodak, Falck, & Rapperport, 1978). It is most frequently used with repeat offenders who have not responded to other treatments such as psychotherapy and behavioral therapy (Spodak, Falck, & Rapperport, 1978).

It is recommended that this drug be used along with concomitant therapies (that is, psychodynamic therapies, behavior therapies) (Fuller, 1989). Though always required, it is *imperative* that the patient thoroughly understands this treatment approach and gives his "informed consent" for treatment (Fuller, 1989). This point is of extreme importance to the nurse. She must be certain that the patient understands the treatment and the possible side-effects of the medication. The side-effects could include weight gain, increased sleep, and mood disturbance (including restlessness, fatigue, nervousness, and hot/cold flashes) (Spodak, Falck, & Rapperport, 1978). The nurse and other health professionals must also understand the ultimate goal of this treatment, to assist the patient in his control of socially unacceptable sexual impulses until he is able to control them without the aid of the drug (**MPA**).

SURGERY. In extreme cases, removal of the testes (surgical castration) for pedophilia, is recommended because it will substantially reduce testosterone production and lower the male's libido. This procedure leaves the penis intact (Berlin, 1985).

The nurse can surely understand the psychiatric implications of this procedure and will need to be fully aware of and knowledgeable about 1) issues regarding informed consent, 2) short-term and long-term effects of the procedure, 3) plans for additional therapies such as psychodynamic and behavioral therapy, 4) hospital ethics committee involvement in the decision-making process, 5) cultural implications, and 6) family involvement in the patient's treatment.

PREVENTION OF SEXUAL ABUSE

It is important for health professionals in all settings to focus their attention on prevention of the numerous forms of sexual abuse (Fuller, 1989). This should include 1) teaching children, women, and men how to protect themselves, 2) teaching the general public about the different types of sexual abuse and their

consequences, 3) teaching nurses and other health care professionals about the paraphilia disorders with information on early identification and appropriate referral, and 4) advocating for the establishment of state and national guidelines to regulate the screening, educating, and monitoring of individuals who work with children and other vulnerable populations (the retarded, incarcerated men and women, and so on).

PSYCHOSEXUAL DISORDERS NOT OTHERWISE SPECIFIED

DSM-III-R (1987) describes the following psychosexual disorders not elsewhere classified: feelings of inadequacy due to self-imposed standards of masculinity or feminity; distress due to abnormal and uncontrollable desires for sexual intercourse, in which people exist only as objects to be used (this classification should not be confused with promiscuity); and confusion about preferred sexual orientation.

These disorders are quite rare and require psychiatric treatment. Individuals with these disorders, like those with specifically designated psychosexual disturbances, also have relationship problems, personality disorders, and a lack of sexual satisfaction in sexual experiences.

GENDER IDENTITY DISORDERS

Although classified by DSM-III-R (1987) as disorders usually first evident in infancy, childhood, or adolescence because of their age of onset, **gender identity disorders** involve the psychological disequilibrium associated with an incongruence between biological sex assignment and subjectively experienced gender.

Sex is the biological designation of an individual as a function of certain physical characteristics (internal and external genitalia), along with chromosomal structure and hormones. Typically, most individuals can be classified as either male or female.

Gender, on the other hand, refers to an individual's sense of masculinity or femininity. Additionally, gender is partially defined in terms of how others react to or treat a given individual. Gender identity, the sense of being male or female, is determined by a variety of intrapersonal and extrapersonal factors, in-

DSM-III-R Diagnostic Criteria for 302.85 Gender Identity Disorder of Adolescence or Adulthood Nontranssexual Type (GIDAANT)

A. Persistent or recurrent discomfort and sense of inappropriateness about one's assigned sex.

B. Persistent or recurrent cross-dressing in the role of the other sex, either in fantasy or actuality, but not for the purpose of sexual excitement (as in transvestic fetishism).

C. No persistent preoccupation (for at least two years) with getting rid of one's primary and secondary sex characteristics and acquiring the sex characteristics of the other sex (as in transsexualism).

D. The person has reached puberty.

Specify history of sexual orientation: **asexual, homosexual, heterosexual,** or **unspecified.**

cluding anatomy and physiology of the genitalia and family and peer attitudes toward the individual (Stoller, 1968).

Money and Ehrhardt (1972) give an illustrative example of how critical the social environment can be in determining one's sense of being male or female. As identical seven-months-old male twins were being circumcised, the penis of one of them was irreparably destroyed through a surgical accident. With the parents' consent, the boy's genitals were surgically transformed into a vagina. His birth certificate was changed, and his parents began to rear him as a girl. In just a few years, this twin had developed a female identity, and, in contrast to his (her?) male brother, looked and acted in feminine ways. At puberty, female sex hormones will be administered to stimulate breast growth and other feminine characteristics. However, she will never menstruate or be able to give birth.

Although the above example may seem extreme, organic causes of ambiguous genitalia are not. For example, in congenital virilizing adrenal hyperplasia, the infant may look like a male child with undescended testes, or a female child with a large clitoris.

Social causes of gender identity problems include parents who reinforce cross-gender behaviors in their children. Reports from families with feminine boys often reveal instances of this, such as wearing mother's dresses and high-heeled shoes, and experimenting with makeup. Cross-dressing behaviors, when encouraged and reinforced by parents, can become emotionally, as well as sexually, gratifying, and are further reinforced by sexual pleasure if the boy masturbates while cross-dressed. It is highly likely that these activities contribute to conflicts between anatomical sex and acquired gender identity.

Throughout recorded history, individuals have attempted to manage gender identity crises in a number of ways. Classic is the tale of a Roman emperor who killed his pregnant wife by kicking her in the stomach while in a state of rage. Feeling lonely afterwards, he sought someone with a face that resembled his dead wife's. A young male ex-slave who met this description was surgically transformed into a woman, and the two were formally married. In a more recent case, Christine (formerly George) Jorgensen was surgically transformed from male to female in Copenhagen in 1952. Jorgensen, an ex-soldier, became the first transsexual whose operation was widely publicized (Masters et al., 1988).

TRANSSEXUALISM

Transsexualism is the DSM-III-R (1987) term for classifying individuals who undergo surgical procedures in order to achieve gender reassignment. The official criteria used in establishing transsexualism are: 1) a persistent sense of discomfort and inappropriateness with one's anatomical sex; 2) a wish, lasting longer than two years, to be rid of one's genitalia; and 3) absence of physical or genetic abnormalities, including other mental illness. However, the more general label, "gender dysphoria," has been recommended as more useful by some (Fisk, 1973; Cauldwell, 1949; Wise, 1983). Wise (1983) suggests that "transsexualism" be reserved for cases in which castration and cosmetic surgery have already

DSM-III-R Diagnostic Criteria for 302.50 Transsexualism

A. Persistent discomfort and sense of inappropriateness about one's assigned sex.

B. Persistent preoccupation for at least two years with getting rid of one's primary and secondary sex characteristics and acquiring the sex characteristics of the other sex.

C. The person has reached puberty.

Specify history of sexual orientation: **asexual, homosexual, heterosexual,** or **unspecified.**

---

been performed. The more general classification, therefore, allows for the successful elimination of individuals with ulterior motives (for example, winning back a lost homosexual lover) who might distort their histories in a desperate pursuit of gender reassignment.

The initial evaluation of candidates seeking gender reassignment surgery requires an assessment of the patient's life history in order to isolate the factors leading to the problem. The clinician must be in a position not only to understand the context in which the client's request is made, but also to validate, or rule out, suspected fabrications. Individuals with borderline personality are common among this population. Suicidal motives, fantasies of self-mutilation, and other mental aberrations require psychiatric management. These precautions allow the clinician to make referrals for hospitalization when appropriate and to avoid otherwise hasty recommendations for surgery (Wise, 1983).

Some individuals are indeed more suited for gender reassignment as a function of having an extended sense of being better suited as a member of the opposite sex. For males, there is often a lifelong history of feeling feminine and pursuing feminine activities. Females exhibit similar propensities for opposite sex activities and discomfort with the female role. In both instances, the crises seem especially acute during puberty. Development of secondary sex characteristics (breasts and pubic hair in the female; enlarged phallus and testes in the male) seem to emphasize the feelings of misfit and are reacted to with distress and depression.

Surgical procedures for gender reassignment have differential success rates for males and females (Markland & Hastings, 1978). The biological male requires augmentation mammoplasty, castration, and the surgical creation of a vagina. Female-to-male procedures include the creation of a male chest via breast removal, hysterectomy, and oophorectomy. Although without much success, an effort is typically made to create a functioning phallus for the newly transformed male. Hormone therapy is essential in both procedures. Research evidence to date indicates that sex change surgery for the male-to-female transsexual is the more successful (Markland & Hastings, 1978; Masters et al., 1988).

The long-term effectiveness of sex transformation surgery is difficult to evaluate. Some individuals who have undergone sex change surgery report feeling emotionally healthier; others do not. Meyer and Reter (1979) demonstrated that individuals who have had sex reassignment surgery are objectively no happier than a comparable patient group who did not have the surgery. More definitive evidence and conclusions await improvement in methodological problems, especially those involving appropriate control groups.

While various theories attempt to explain transsexualism in terms of biology or psychology, some sociologists consider rigid sex-role stereotypes to be responsible (Richardson, 1988). Society prescribes strict adherence to a narrow range of appropriate behaviors for each sex. Men are expected to be assertive, independent, competent, and stoic; women are expected to be passive, dependent, emotional, and nurturant. (See chapters 19 and 20 for more on this.) Social pressures to adhere to the appropriate stereotype are so strong, it is argued, that an individual whose personal characteristics do not fit may become so uncomfortable that gender reassignment surgery is sought.

Case Study: Nonpsychiatric Setting

Demographic Data

Name: Mrs. Barbara Bassant
Age: 43
Ethnicity: Irish
Religion: Methodist
Geographic locale: Denver, CO.
Occupation: Social Worker, MSW

Presenting Problem

Mrs. Bassant recently underwent surgery for the removal of an "abdominal mass." She had a total hysterectomy (removal of uterus body and the cervix). She returned to the Women's Clinic, as scheduled, for her four-week postsurgical checkup.

History of Presenting Problem

Mrs. Bassant is a married woman, mother of two daughters, age 20 and 23 (who currently live in Arizona). She had complained of irregular and painful menstruation for approximately six years. She had medicated herself for several years with over-the-counter pain medication and received some relief. At other times, she was prescribed aspirin with codeine and experienced complete relief of symptoms.

Mrs. Bassant had always made it a habit of having a yearly checkup with her gynecologist. During the routine pelvic examination, the gynecologist told Mrs. Bassant that a mass could be palpated. A sonogram was ordered for further exploration of the mass that was suspected. An additional examination was performed by another gynecologist for the purpose of confirming the diagnosis of "abdominal mass." Mrs. Bassant was told to prepare for surgery.

Initially, Mrs. Bassant rejected the possibility of surgery and stated that her work schedule and family responsibilities could not be interrupted. The gynecologist explained to Mrs. Bassant the difficulties associated with postponing the surgery. There was much discussion about the surgery—the physiology of the reproductive system was reviewed, along with an explanation of the surgical procedure and the rationale for it.

Mrs. Bassant stated that she had told her husband that she would have to undergo surgery, but did not discuss with him the details of the surgery. Instead, she mentioned to her husband in a matter-of-fact manner that the surgery would include the possibility of the removal of her uterus. There was no further discussion with him, as Mrs. Bassant felt that he would not be interested in "female problems."

Mrs. Bassant and her husband have been married for 25 years. Their relationship was described as strong by Mrs. Bassant. She had always been an independent working woman, and had made many of the family decisions.

There is no history of psychiatric illness in Mrs. Bassant's family.

Mental Status Examination

General appearance: Neatly dressed woman, who is four weeks postsurgical. She is returning to the clinic for her first post surgical checkup.

Orientation: Oriented to time, place, and person. Pleasant and alert.

Affect: Somewhat flat. Appears tired, but responds to questions.

Cognitive functioning: Normal, though formal testing not done. No sign of thought disorder.

Summary

Mrs. Bassant is a 43-year-old woman who recently had a total hysterectomy and is returning for her first postsurgical clinic visit.

After the checkup with the doctor, Mrs. Bassant was relieved to know that she was alright. However, she had many questions regarding her sexual desire and the possibility of not being a viable sexual partner because of the surgery. The gynecologist requested that the nurse in the clinic meet with Mrs. Bassant and discuss how healing occurs and to emphasize to Mrs. Bassant that she can resume her usual sexual habits.

During their session, Mrs. Bassant verbalized many fears and misconceptions about the surgery and how it would ultimately affect her sexual desire and ability to perform sexually and leave her with the feeling of being "not quite the woman she once was."

Having heard Mrs. Bassant's comments, the nurse in the clinic became very concerned about her. The nurse asked Mrs. Bassant to dress and to wait in the examination room for her. Having discussed her observations with the gynecologist, the nurse and gynecologist agreed that further assessment of Mrs. Bassant's perceptions and attitudes about the surgery, her own sexuality, and so forth, were essential.

The nurse decided to do a more detailed assessment, including a family history and a sexual history, as she was concerned about posthysterectomy syndrome of depression (The Boston Women's Health Book Collective, 1984). The highlights of the nurse's assessment are recorded here.

Family History

Mrs. Bassant was first married at age 17. This marriage lasted for about one year. There were no children born into the marriage. In less than one year after the divorce, Mrs. Bassant married her present husband. They have been married for 25 years.

Mrs. Bassant works as a social worker in a cardiac rehabilitation unit. Her husband is the registrar at a nearby community college.

Sexual History

Mrs. Bassant stated that her first marriage was to her high school sweetheart who was preoccupied with sex and that "she performed for his gratification." She was emphatic in stating that, "The marriage was a mistake for both of us. I had to get out . . . and did . . . and returned to my parents' home."

Mrs. Bassant stated that she was taught by her parents never to have sex before marriage and to always be truthful and loyal to your partner. She does not recall having received any additional information about sexuality, except how to bathe herself during menstruation.

During her current marriage, she and her husband have had sexual relations from 1–3 times each week. They tend to enjoy a private environment, free of noise and other distractions. The couple had thought that "Once the girls leave home we will really enjoy ourselves." Instead,

Mrs. Bassant became more and more disinterested in sex, focusing more on her pains and discomforts. Mr. Bassant was supportive but obviously disappointed.

Recently (within the last six months) the couple might have had intercourse 3–4 times, with Mrs. Bassant having to take pain medications after sexual intercourse on one or two occasions.

At present, she is anxious, perplexed, and depressed about the outcome of her surgery: How will sex feel to me? To my husband? Is it true that one becomes half a woman after a hysterectomy? Will my husband leave me for another woman? What about aging? My skin will really wrinkle! Her concluding comments were: "I hope my husband knows that I had absolutely no control over what happened to my body."

The nurse could clearly perceive that Mrs. Bassant was in need of additional counseling, teaching, and guidance.

Nursing Diagnosis

Anxiety
Impaired verbal communication
*Knowledge Deficit (lack of recall) related to sexuality
Powerlessness
Disturbance in body image
Disturbance in self-esteem
Sexual Dysfunction
Fear
*Alteration in family process
Family: coping, potential for growth
Ineffective individual coping
*Disturbance in self-concept

*Nursing diagnoses developed in the care plan that follows.

Nursing Care Plan for Mrs. Bassant

Nursing Diagnosis	Desired Outcomes	Interventions	Rationale
1. Knowledge deficit related to sexuality.	Mrs. Bassant will verbalize her understanding of: a) female reproductive organs; b) the surgical procedure; and, c) sexual functioning before and after surgery. Mrs. Bassant will express her beliefs and attitudes regarding past experiences that might be related to her reaction to the surgery.	Discuss with Mrs. Bassant sexual reproductive anatomy and physiology. Review the major functions of the uterus, ovaries, vagina, fallopian tubes, and so forth.	Information is basic to increasing Mrs. Bassant's understanding about the functions of her body.

Nursing Diagnosis	Desired Outcomes	Interventions	Rationale
		Diagram the major sexual organs in the body and highlight the uterus and cervix in the diagram. a) Review their functions. b) Explain what happens in sexual intercourse when these organs are removed.	Knowledge is necessary to combat feelings of powerlessness, anxiety, fear; to assist Mrs. Bassant in gaining a sense of control over her body; and to facilitate an attitudinal change about her ability to participate in a satisfying sexual relationship.
		Discuss the anatomy of the vagina and stress that it is still intact; highlight its characteristics such as: it stretches; possesses many nerve endings for increased sensitivity, etc.	This organ is a major component of the sexual act. Mrs. Bassant needs to understand that it is still there, as well as its characteristics and functioning.
	Mrs. Bassant will become active in the teaching-learning process as evidenced by verbalizing anxieties, asking questions, and making practical and informed decisions.	Encourage Mrs. Bassant to ask questions; provide a model so that Mrs. Bassant can see and study the anatomical structure of the sexual system.	These methods encourage discussion and facilitate learning and greater acceptance of the surgery.
		Suggest that Mr. Bassant join the teaching sessions and encourage Mrs. Bassant to invite him.	Encourages open dialogue between the couple; teaches Mr. Bassant about the sexual organs and sexuality; provides additional data base for the nurse: observations of the couple's relationship.
		When Mr. Bassant joins the sessions, ask him what concerns he has about his wife's surgery.	Talking about him first will capture his attention.
		Discuss with Mrs. Bassant the different options available for receiving hormone replacement therapy: patches on skin; suppositories; pill.	This teaching is rather straightforward and will assist in the control of some of her surgically induced menopausal symptoms.
		Explain the rationale for hormone replacement therapy and that it assists in the prevention of "hot flashes," reduced turgor of skin, etc.	

Nursing Diagnosis	Desired Outcomes	Interventions	Rationale
2. Disturbance in self-concept.	Mrs. Bassant will feel self-assured enough to engage in healthy sexual activity with her husband.	Encourage a discussion of concerns that both partners might have regarding their sexual relationship.	Assists the couple in improving their sexual expressions; enhances self-esteem for both individuals.
		Assist the couple in discussing ways of expressing love, concern, and support to each other (touching, kissing, hugging, etc.).	These behaviors communicate caring, are stimulating, and facilitate involvement and support for one another; militates against the chance that Mrs. Bassant will begin to feel isolated and fear that her husband is no longer interested in her as a sexual partner.
		Discuss with Mr. and Mrs. Bassant their understanding of the functions of the removed organs and the surgery. Explore with the couple their reactions to the surgery and assist them in developing healthy, useful responses.	These detailed discussions that focus on coping, communication, etc., can enhance the sexual functions of the couple.
	Mrs. Bassant will return to her job at the Cardiac Rehabilitation Center.	Discuss with Mrs. Bassant the possible return to employment. Assist in the identification of any concerns she has about her return to work.	Diminishes her feelings of being "sick, different, not in control of my body."
		Solicit Mr. Bassant's opinion.	Mrs. Bassant needs her husband's support and encouragement; he needs to feel she is getting better.
		Encourage Mr. and Mrs. Bassant to view and touch her incision; encourage them to talk about the scar.	Assists in eliciting thoughts and feelings from the couple about the surgery. Encourages the couple's acceptance of the surgery.
		Assure Mr. and Mrs. Bassant that they can have gratifying sexual relations.	No physical problem exists that precludes satisfying sexual activity.

Nursing Diagnosis	Desired Outcomes	Interventions	Rationale
		Encourage them to discuss their thoughts, beliefs, concerns, fears, etc., about sex and their marriage since the surgery.	Elicits feelings and data about their understanding and acceptance of the surgery, and the couple's ability to adapt to life stressors. This data can be used to determine future interventions.
3. Alteration in family process.	Family will return to the highest level of functioning as evidenced by support and concern for each other; return of a satisfying sexual relationship between the couple; verbalization of thoughts and feelings to each other; participation in presurgical roles such as wife, employee, sexual partner, etc.	Explore feelings of guilt, anger, blame, etc., that might exist between the couple.	Acknowledges feelings and provides opportunity for resolution.
		Discuss with couple the extent that they wish to involve their daughters as a part of their support system.	Suggests a source of support for couple; response indicates whether the couple feel they can "manage" or need additional help.
		Discuss with both wife and husband the roles and functions she will resume in the family.	Return to presurgical role functions helps to provide equilibrium in the family structure; enhances self-esteem and self-respect; enhances communication and intimate expressions.
	Mr. and Mrs. Bassant will elect to attend family therapy/sex therapy/counseling if needed.	Provide information about community resources; explain to the couple the types of treatment available should they feel the need for more intense long-term therapy.	Additional information provides options and assists couple in making informed decisions; alleviates anxiety and feelings of powerlessness.
		Give Mrs. Bassant the clinic number, nurse's name, and encourage her or Mr. Bassant to phone if they have additional concerns/questions.	A resource for support, information, referral, and so forth.

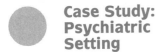

Case Study: Psychiatric Setting

Demographic Data

Name: Manuel Francisco
Age: 40 years
Address: Houston, TX
Occupation: Farmer
Ethnicity: Hispanic
Education: B.S., Agriculture
Religion: Catholicism

Presenting Problem

Mr. Francisco is a fourth-generation farmer who operates a small family farm. He, his wife, and their three children live in a home that Mr. Francisco built for his family. His farm has been a fairly lucrative business until recently at which time drought, disease, and a poor economic market have created near economic ruin.

He visited an outreach psychiatric clinic in his community for counseling. Mr. Francisco complained of "feeling nervous and jittery all of the time." The relationship with his wife had deteriorated to the extent that Mrs. Francisco had moved into their guest bedroom. Mr. Francisco stated that he has numerous problems: unpaid bills, crop failure, an estranged relationship with his wife who "bitches all the time," and adolescent children who have no respect for him.

Further exploration by the nurse revealed that Mr. and Mrs. Francisco have not had sexual relations in more than one year. Mr. Francisco stated, "I tried to have sex with Maria, but it won't work any more. I finish too early . . . and it won't stay hard long. I think I might lose my family! I feel like a beaten man! . . . Can you give me some medicine to help me be a man and satisfy my wife?"

History of Presenting Problem

Mr. Francisco stated he is proud of his children, and remembered the days when he and his wife had sex so frequently that they were continuously concerned about the possibility of her becoming pregnant. He further stated that he and Mrs. Francisco had always enjoyed sex until about three years ago. Though not able to identify a specific cause for "finishing too early," he did think it was associated with many other problems (near financial ruin, embarrassment because of infrequent sex, feeling humiliated and defeated, and so forth).

Psychiatric History

None.

Sexual History

Mr. Francisco stated that he had learned about sex from the guys in high school and college. "A man should have sex frequently; satisfy a woman; and desire more sex almost immediately!" was a part of his thinking; also, "A woman should be ready for her husband at all times, except maybe when she is very heavy and about ready to go down" (when a woman is pregnant and close to delivery).

Mr. Francisco stated that he feels he had a normal sexual development. He indicated that he had sex numerous times during his college days, but that he never discussed this with his wife. Since marriage, he has been faithful to his wife. This fidelity has been reinforced since there has been so much discussion about AIDS. In fact, Mr. Francisco had with him a pamphlet from the Surgeon General of the U.S. Department of Health and Human Services, Centers for Disease Control, that recently came in the mail. He showed it to the nurse and asked, "Why did I get this?" Lately, Mr. Francisco has begun to think that his limited sexual performance might be associated with HIV infection (AIDS); yet, at other times, he thinks that his wife might become interested in another man. He fears that she, too, could get AIDS, and ". . . goodness knows what else! She is a good looking woman, and I don't want her to get mixed up with another man!"

Health History

Mr. Francisco complains of back pain. He attributes this to heavy farm work. He has never sought medical care for this problem. He "medicated" himself with over-the-counter pain medication. Mr. Francisco also indicated that he sometimes drinks to relieve the jittery feeling and to "get some sleep."

Mental Status

General appearance: Neatly dressed; agitated and jittery; and experiencing difficulty discussing his concerns about himself.
Sensorium: Coherent; oriented to time, place, and person; responds to questions in a coherent fashion.
Mood: Sad and anxious.
Speech: Talked about his sexual concerns in a "whisper," while leaning toward the nurse. Other components of the interview were discussed audibly in a more natural tone.
Thought process: Coherent; easy to follow.
Thought content: Organized; focused; congruent with mood.

Medication

Nonprescription pain medications for back pain.

Potential for Violence

No evidence of suicidal or homicidal ideation or gestures.

Summary

Manuel Francisco is a 40-year-old Hispanic man who comes to the Outreach Mental Health Center with a complaint of feeling "nervous and jittery all of the time." Further exploration revealed that he is concerned about his inability to have sex with his wife. ". . . It won't work any more . . . I finish too early!" Recently, he has become concerned about AIDS and has been relating poor sexual performance with the remote possibility of AIDS. He is also preoccupied with problems related to financial matters and crop failure.

DSM-III-R Diagnosis

Axis I: 302.75, Premature ejaculation
             Generalized anxiety disorder (300.02)
Axis II: No diagnosis
Axis III: Back pain
Axis IV: Psychosocial stressors:
             Crop failure, financial problems, marital problems, three
             adolescent children who provoke concern
             Severity: 4-severe
Axis V: O (Inadequate information)

Nursing Diagnoses

Anxiety
*Alteration in family processes
Ineffective individual coping
Impaired verbal communication
Knowledge Deficit
Disturbance in self-concept
*Sexual Dysfunction
Sleep Pattern Disturbance

*Nursing diagnoses developed in care plan that follows.

Nursing Care Plan for Manuel Francisco

Nursing Diagnosis	Desired Outcomes	Interventions	Rationale
1. Sexual dysfunction.	Mr. Francisco will develop a trusting relationship with the nurse.	Listen intently to Mr. Francisco as he describes his situation to the nurse.	Active listening facilitates trust.
		Assure Mr. Francisco that all information will be held in confidence.	Allays fears and fantasies about who will receive this information, and how it will be used.
		Make appointment with Mr. Francisco for the purpose of discussing his problems. Be sure to arrive at designated place on time.	This behavior provides evidence that the nurse is interested in Mr. Francisco; alleviates tension, anxiety, and fear of rejection.
		Provide immediate positive feedback and supporting statements when appropriate.	Shows that nurse is listening, understands, and is committed to helping him (and his wife) work through their problems.

Nursing Diagnosis	Desired Outcomes	Interventions	Rationale
	Mr. Francisco will identify the stressors in his life, and begin to develop strategies and coping mechanisms that will assist in the resolution of these problems.	Encourage the expression of Mr. Francisco's feelings and provide support, clarification, and validation of feelings, as appropriate. Encourage Mr. Francisco to be as honest as possible in identifying all of the situations that are troubling him.	Data should be recorded in the patient's chart. However, details of sensitive subjects like sexual activity and proclivities should be left out unless the file can be made "restrictive."
	Mr. Francisco will become knowledgeable about the availability of a sex counselor, and be informed about the variety of services that can be provided.	Discuss the advantages of sessions with a sex therapist: explore Mr. Francisco's feeling about the intervention; discuss in detail the services that a sex counselor can offer; explain to Mr. Francisco the need to begin to discuss sex therapy with his wife. Request to discuss sexual problems with both Mr. and Mrs. Francisco.	Information is critical for generating options and making good decisions.
	The couple will gain factual knowledge about sexual functioning.	Sessions with Mr. and Mrs. Francisco will include: a) assessment of the couple's knowledge about basic anatomy and physiology related to sexual function, and normal male and female sexual response; b) discussions about anatomy/physiology related to sexual function and the normal male/female response, as well as the couples' *feelings* about all this. c) Exploration with the couple about their perceptions of specific problems that surround their sexual functioning; d) Encouragement of Mrs. Francisco to discuss her frustrations and disappointments about what seems to be her husband's limited sexual ability and the associated alienation between herself and her husband.	Mr. and Mrs. Francisco need factual information about human anatomy and physiology in order to assess their own functioning and make informed decisions. Information can decrease anxiety and help to control anger, suspicion, and so forth. Knowledge will provide enlightenment and insight, and will enhance cooperation with the therapist and between each other. Each partner will communicate his/her perception about the sexual dysfunction. Perceptions and feelings about premature ejaculation provide additional data and assist in enhancing communication between the couple; provides significant data for nurse to use in planning care.

Nursing Diagnosis	Desired Outcomes	Interventions	Rationale
	Couple will apply knowledge to their own situation.	Encourage the couple to share concerns about their sexless marriage.	Understanding of basic facts of life will assist the couple in setting realistic goals for themselves and enhances information base from which they make decisions and judgments.
		Help both individuals identify their needs for intimacy.	Mutual sharing of needs can enhance communication and cooperation for resolution of frustrations and conflicts; decreases feelings of estrangement, isolation, and loneliness.
	Mrs. Francisco will evaluate this alternative (sex therapy) and elect to become involved.	Explore with Mrs. Francisco her attitudes and thoughts about becoming involved in sex therapy. Discuss with the couple basic facts about premature ejaculation and methods of treating the problem. Discussion will include information about sensate touch, the squeeze method, etc.	Discussion about feelings and thoughts will assist Mrs. Francisco in self-exploration and provide the opportunity to explore a commitment to sex therapy with her husband.
	The couple will openly discuss with each other their frustrations, conflicts, fears, etc.	Encourage the couple to discuss other major stressors in their lives such as crop failure and consequent financial problems; concerns about guidance and limit setting for their three adolescent children; and severe back pain that Mr. Francisco experiences.	Information and help from the sex therapist can assist in alleviating anxiety, dispelling feelings of blame, inadequacy, shame, etc.
	The couple will explore and practice new methods of expressing intimacy and sensuality with each other.	Discuss with the couple their current methods of engaging in intimacy and sensual expression. Offer information about	An open and honest discussion about thoughts, feelings, attitudes, and behaviors is essential for improved

Nursing Diagnosis	Desired Outcomes	Interventions	Rationale
		the gratification that can come from touch (holding hands, kissing, rubbing husband's back, stroking, etc.).	coping, effective communication, and enhanced sexual activity that is mutually gratifying for each partner. These sensual activities can be very gratifying and can serve as antecedents to a mutually satisfying sexual relationship.
	The patient will verbalize an understanding of AIDS to include: signs and symptoms, methods of transmission, risk behaviors, safe sex, etc. The patient and his wife will verbalize their understanding about premature ejaculation and the methods used to alleviate it.	Acknowledge Mr. Francisco's concern about AIDS. Thoroughly discuss the contents of the publication, "Understanding AIDS," with Mr. Francisco and his wife. Explain that the publication on AIDS was provided to all people across the United States, and that there should be no connection at this time in his mind between premature ejaculation and AIDS.	This information is vital for the nurse and couple. Confusion about the two problems (AIDS and premature ejaculation) can forestall any activity toward intimacy, sharing, caring, loving, and so forth.
	The couple will verbalize concern for each other and for the relationship.	Assist the couple in labeling their feelings; discussing thoughts about why they had not communicated with each other and the impact that this behavior has had on their relationship.	Helps to restore trust, sexual activity; enhance self-esteem and self-concept; allay anxieties and fears. Knowledge about each other will assist the couple in communicating with each other, and will decrease isolation and alienation.
2. Alteration in family process.	Family will use this crisis as a potential for growth and to enhance the relationship.	Assist the couple in identifying their family struggles. The nurse might comment, "Mrs. Francisco, I commend you for joining your husband in these sessions!"; or, "I think the relationship means a great deal to both of you."	Helps to increase self-esteem, eliminate blame, guilt, and shame. Provides the couple with data about support within the family, and encourages the couple (and other family members) to give each other support.

Nursing Diagnosis	Desired Outcomes	Interventions	Rationale
		Facilitate the expression of blame, anger, guilt, humiliation, feelings of failure, etc.	The couple needs to acknowledge these feelings, and discuss situations and circumstances under which they occur.
	The couple will use knowledge in making decisions and in seeking sex and couples therapy.	Discuss the role of family therapy/couples therapy in assisting the couple to resolve these problems.	Assists the couple in realistically assessing their problems and available resources.
		Provide couple with information regarding financial counseling and agricultural assistance programs that are available for farmers.	
	Patients will identify community resources to assist them with financial stressors.	Refer the couple to a self-help group in the community.	Assists the couple in obtaining knowledge that will aid in planning realistic strategies.
	The couple will learn and practice stress-management techniques.	Teach the couple useful methods of managing stress to include: physical exercise, relaxation techniques, increased communication with each other, recreational activities (time away from the family), private time/space for each person, etc.	Provides sense of well-being.
	The couple will verbalize their thoughts and feelings about each of the children, and begin to develop strategies to deal with these concerns.	Discuss current patterns of limit setting, communication, roles of each family member, division of labor, expression of support, love, interdependency, and so forth.	The couple will develop alternative strategies for effectively communicating with the children.
	The couple will verbalize an understanding of overall functioning of their family.	a) Encourage the couple to discuss roles of each family member; methods by which responsibilities might be shared; budgeting; the future of the family; b) Assist the couple with the identification of their family's strengths and acknowledge how each might have participated in the development of those strengths.	Assists the couple in making decisions; knowledge of family enhances self-confidence and self-esteem. Helps couple to understand family structure and functions.

SUMMARY

Sexual functioning is a complex interaction of biological, psychological, interpersonal, and cultural factors. Sexual health and illness is a concern of the nurse no matter what the health care setting. Nurses have many opportunities to help educate their patients about sexuality, including clinics, group discussions, and inpatient settings. In addition, the Sex Information and Education Council of the United States (SIECUS) provides an excellent resource for information about human sexuality.

There are two types of sexual disorders as classified by the DSM-III-R: (1) the sexual dysfunctions which are disorders in which there is an inhibition in the appetite or psychological changes in the complete sexual response cycle and (2) the paraphilias, which are disorders in which sexual arousal occurs in response to nonhuman objects or in situations that are not normally arousing. Specific paraphilias include exhibitionism, fetishism, frotteurism, pedophilia, sexual sadism, sexual masochism, transvestic fetishism, and voyeurism. Sexual dysfunctions include sexual desire disorders, sexual arousal disorders, orgasm disorders, and sexual pain disorders.

The basis of all sexual function seems to be primarily biological. Biological causes of disorders might include injury and disease, aging, drugs and alcohol, and abnormal development (or abnormal timing of development). Psychodynamic theories of psychosexual disorders on the other hand, suggest that the following constructs are basic to the disorder and its treatment: unconscious motivation, childhood experiences, and lack of resolution of the Oedipus conflict. In addition, there can be emotional causes of the disorder as well as cultural catalysts. Behavioral theory posits that certain early negative or traumatic experiences involving sexual experiences can generate sufficient anxiety to produce a psychosexual disorder.

Behavioral therapies are the most favored of all therapies for the psychosexual disorders. One of the most prominent of these is Masters and Johnson's conjoint therapy, in which both partners must participate. Other therapies include: in vivo desensitization, masturbation desensitization, and pleasuring.

Gender identity disorders involve the psychological disequilibrium associated with an incongruence between biological sex assignment and assumed or felt gender. Sexual reassignment may take place after thorough psychological assessment.

KEY TERMS

paraphilia

sexual dysfunction

excitement phase

plateau phase

orgasmic phase

resolution phase

male erectile disorder

premature ejaculation

inhibited male orgasm

female sexual arousal disorder

inhibited female orgasm

vaginismus

dyspareunia

hypoactive desire disorder

sexual aversion disorder

gender identity disorder

exhibitionism

fetishism

frotteurism

pedophilia

sexual masochism

sexual sadism

tranvestism

voyeurism

transsexualism

conjoint therapy

sensate focus

in vivo desensitization

masturbation desensitization

pleasuring

STUDY QUESTIONS

1. What are the major differences between the two classifications of sexual disorders—the paraphilias and sexual dysfunctions?

2. What are the four phases of the male and female sexual response cycle, as delineated by Masters and Johnson?

3. List and briefly describe the four categories of sexual dysfunctions, as described by the DSM III-R.

4. Distinguish between sexual desire disorders and sexual arousal disorders.

5. How can nurses in nonpsychiatric settings help patients with sexual concerns and questions?

REFERENCES

American Psychiatric Association. (1987). *Diagnostic and statistical manual of mental disorders* (3rd ed. rev.) (DSM III-R). Washington, DC: American Psychiatric Association.

Abramson, P. R., & Mosher, D. L. (1975). Development of a measure of negative attitudes toward masturbation. *Journal of Consulting and Clinical Psychology, 43,* 485–490.

Annon, J. S. (1975). *The sexual fear inventory—female and male forms.* Honolulu: Enabling Systems.

Annon, J. S. (1977). The Plissit model: A proposed conceptual scheme for the behavioral treatment of sexual problems. In Fischer, J. & Gochros, H. L. (Eds.). *Handbook of behavior therapy with sexual problems, 1,* New York: Pergamon Press.

Apfelbaum, B. (1980). The diagnosis and treatment of retarded ejaculation. In S. R. Leiblum & L. A. Pervin, (Eds.). *Principles and practice of sex therapy.* New York: Guilford Press.

Barbach, L. (1980). Group treatment of anorgasmic women. In S. R. Leiblum & L. A. Pervin, (Eds.). *Principles and practice of sex therapy.* New York: Guilford Press.

Barlow, D. H. (1986). Causes of sexual dysfunction: The role of anxiety and cognitive interference. *Journal of Consulting and Clinical Psychology, 54:2,* pp. 140–148.

Berlin, F. S. (1985). Pedophilia: Medical castration and group counseling sessions help to modify this type of sexual behavior. *Medical Aspects of Human Sexuality, 19:8,* pp. 79–89.

Birk, L. (1980). Shifting gears in treating psychogenic sexual dysfunction: Medical assessment, sex therapy, psychotherapy, and couple therapy. *Psychiatric Clinics of North America, 3,* Table 1, pp. 162–163.

Birk, L. (1988). Sex therapy. In *The New Harvard Guide to Psychiatry.* Cambridge: Belknap Press, pp. 563–579.

Bjorklund, E. (1987). Prevention and reducing the risk of AIDS. In. J. D. Durham & F. L. Conen (Eds.). *The person with AIDS: Nursing perspectives.* (pp. 178–191) New York: Springer.

The Boston Women's Health Book Collective (1984). The new our bodies, ourselves: A book by and for women. New York: Simon and Schuster.

Braddell, D. W., & Wilson, G. J. (1976). Effects of alcohol and expectancy set on male sexual arousal. *Journal of Abnormal Psychology, 85,* 225–234.

Brady, J. P. (1966). Brevital-relaxation treatment of frigidity. *Behavioral Research and Therapy, 4(2),* 71–77.

Brown, J. R. W. C. (1983). Symposium of sexual deviation. Paraphilias: Sadomasochism, fetishism, transvestism, and transsexuality. *British Journal of Psychiatry, 143,* pp. 227–230.

Calderone, M. S. (1966). Sex education for young people and for their parents and teachers. In R. Brecher & E. Brecher (Eds.) *An analysis of human sexual response.* New York: New American Library.

Cauldwell, D. (1949). Psychopathia transsexualis. *Sexology, 16,* 274–280.

Centers for Disease Control (1988, June 24). Update: Universal precautions for prevention of transmission of human immunodeficiency virus, hepatitis B virus, and other bloodborne pathogens in health care settings. *Morbidity & Mortality Weekly Report, 37 (24),* 337–88.

Chapman, R. (1982). Criteria for diagnosing when to do sex therapy in the primary relationship. *Psychotherapy: Theory, Research and Practice, 19,* 359–367.

Cleveland, P., Walters, L., Skeen, P., & Robinson, B. (1988). If your child has AIDS . . .: Responses of parents with homosexual children. *Family Relations* (April) 37:2, pp. 150–153.

Dallas Times Herald, June 18, 1987, pp. F1–F3.

Derogatis, L. R. (1976). Psychological assessment of the sexual disabilities. In J. K. Meyer (Ed.). *Clinical Management of Sexual Disorders.* Baltimore: Williams and Wilkins.

DiVasto, P. V., Pathak, D., & Fishburn, W. R. (1981). The interrelationship of sex and guilt. Sex, behavior, and age. *Archives of Sexual Behavior, 10,* 119–122.

Driscoll, J. W. (1989). Teaching safer sex. In J. B. Meisenhelder & C. L. LaCharite (Eds.). Comfort in caring: Nursing the person with HIV infection (167–178). Glenview, IL: Scott, Foresman.

Dubovsky, S. L., & Weissburg, M. P. (1978). *Clinical psychiatry in primary care.* Baltimore: Williams and Wilkins.

Erickson, W. D., Walbek, N. H., & Seely, R. K. (1988). Behavior patterns of child molesters. Archives of Sexual Behavior, *17:1,* pp. 77–86.

Fenichel, O. (1945). *The psychoanalytic theory of neurosis.* NY: Norton & Company, Inc.

Finkelhor, D., & Araji, S. (1986). Explanations of pedophilia: A four-factor model. *The Journal of Sex Research, 22,* 145–161.

Fisk, N. (1973). Gender dysphoria syndrome—the how, why, and what of a condition. Interdisciplinary symposium on transsexuals Stamford University School of Medicine. Palo Alto, CA., Feb. 2–4.

Frank, E., Anderson, C., & Kupfer, D. J. (1976). Profiles of couples seeking sex therapy and marital therapy. *American Journal of Psychiatry, 133,* 559–562.

Frank, E., Anderson, C., & Rubinstein, D. (1978). Frequency of sexual dysfunction in "normal" couples. *New England Journal of Medicine, 229,* 111–115.

Freud, S. (1953). Three essays on the theory of sexuality. In the *Complete Psychological Works of Sigmund Freud, 7,* London: Hogarth Press.

Fuller, A. K. (1989). Child molestation and pedophilia, an overview for the physician. *Journal American Medical Association, 261:4,* pp. 602–606.

Furlow, W. L., & Goldwasser, B. (1987). Salvage of the eroded inflatable penile prosthesis: A new concept. *The Journal of Urology, 138,* pp. 312–314.

Gebhard, P., et al. (1965). *Sex Offenders: An analysis of types.* New York: Harper & Row.

Giaretto, H. (1982). *Integrated treatment of child sexual abuse: a treatment and training manual.* CA: Science and Behavior Books.

Gillan, P. (1987). *Sex Therapy Manual.* Boston: Blackwell Scientific Publications.

Griffith, W., & Hatfield, E. (1985). *Human Sexual Behavior.* Glenview, IL: Scott, Foresman/Little, Brown.

Groth, A. N. (1978). Guidelines for the assessment and management of the offender. In A. Burgess, A. N. Groth, L. Holstrom, & S. Sgroi (Eds.). *Sexual Assault of Children and Adolescents.* Lexington: Lexington Books.

Groth, A. N. (1979). *Men who rape: The psychology of the offender.* New York: Plenum Press.

Group for the Advancement of Psychiatry (1974). *Assessment of sexual function: A guide to interviewing.* New York: Jason Aronson.

Hathaway, S. R., & McKinley, J. D. (1967). *The Minnesota Multiphasic Personality Inventory.* New York: Psychological Corporation.

Hazelwood, K., Dietz, P., & Burgess, A. (1983). *Autoerotic fatalities.* Lexington: Lexington Books.

Heller, J. E., & Gleich, P. (1988). Erectile impotence: Evaluation and management. *The Journal of Family Practice, 26:3,* pp. 321–324.

Hogan, R. M. (1980). *Human Sexuality; A Nursing Perspective.* New York: Appleton-Century-Crofts.

Ishii, N., Watanabe, H., Irisawa, C., Kikuchi, Y., Kubota, Y., Kawamura, S., Suzuki, K., Chiba, R., Tokiwa, M., & Shirai, M. (1989). Intracavernous injection of prostaglandin E1 for the treatment of erectile impotence. *The Journal of Urology, 141,* pp. 323–325.

Jemail, J. A. (1977). Response bias in the assessment of marital and sexual adjustment. Doctoral Dissertation, State University of New York at Stony Brook.

Kaplan, H. S. (1974). *The new sex therapy.* New York: Brunner/Mazel.

Kaplan, H. S. (1979). *Disorders of sexual desire.* New York: brunner/Mazel.

Kaplan, H. S. (Ed.) (1985). *Comprehensive evaluation of disorders of sexual desire.* Washington, D.C.: American Psychiatric Press.

Kaplan, H. S. (1988). Anxiety and sexual dysfunction. *Journal of Clinical Psychiatry, 49,* 21–25.

Kaplan, H. S., & Perelman, M. A. (1979). The physician and treatment of sexual dysfunctions. In G. Usdin & J. Lewis (Eds.). *Psychiatry in General Medical Practice.* New York: McGraw Hill.

Karacan, I. (1978). Advances in the psychophysiological evaluation of male erectile incompetence. In J. LoPiccolo & L. LoPiccolo (Eds.). *Handbook of Sex Therapy.* New York: Plenum Press.

Katchadourian, H. A. (1987). *Biological aspects of human sexuality,* 3rd Ed. New York: Holt, Rinehart & Winston.

Kempton, W. (1973). *Techniques for leading group discussion on human sexuality.* Philadelphia: Planned Parenthood of Southeastern Pennsylvania.

Kinsey, A. C. (1953). Sexual behavior in the human female, by the Staff of the Institute for Sex Research, Indiana University. Philadelphia: Saunders.

Kinsey, A. C., Pomeroy, W. B., & Martin, G. E. (1948). *Sexual behavior in the human male.* Philadelphia, W. B. Saunders.

Kluz, R. (1986). Children with AIDS. *American Journal of Nursing, 86,* pp. 1126–1132.

Kolodny, R. C., Masters, W. H., & Johnson, V. E. (1979). *Textbook of Sexual Medicine.* Boston: Little, Brown.

Kolodny, R. C., Masters, W. H., Johnson, V. E., & Biggs, M. A. (1979). *Textbook of Human Sexuality for Nurses.* Boston: Little, Brown.

Koten, J., Wilbert, D. C., Verburg, D., & Soldinger, S. M. (1976). Thioridazine and sexual dysfunction. *American Journal of Psychiatry, 133,* 82–85.

Krozy, R. (1978). Becoming comfortable with sexual assessment. *American Journal of Nursing, 78,* 1036–1038.

Laker, B. (1987). *AIDS:* The youngest victims. *Dallas Times Herald,* June 18, 1987, pp. F1–F3.

Landers, A. (1976). Ann Landers Advises (Jan. 4).

Lazarus, A. A. (1963). Group therapy of phobic disorders by systematic desensitization. *Journal of Abnormal Social Psychology, 3,* 504–510.

Lobitz, C. W., & LoPiccolo, J. (1972). The role of masturbation in the treatment of orgasmic dsyfunction. *Archives of Sexual Behavior, 2,* 163–177.

LoPiccolo, J., & LoPiccolo, L. (1978). Perspectives in sexuality: behavior, research, and therapy. New York: Plenum Press.

LoPiccolo, J., & Lobitz, W. C. (1973). Behavior therapy of sexual dysfunction. In L. A. Hammerlynk, L. C. Handy, & E. J. Mash (Eds.). *Behavior change: Methodology, concepts, and practice.* Champaign, IL.: Research Press.

Macklin, E. (1988). AIDS: Implications for families. *Family Relations, 37,* p. 141–149.

Madsen, C. H., Jr., & Ullman, L. P. (1967). Innovations in the desenitization of frigidity. *Behavior Research & Therapy, 5*(1), 67–68.

Markland, C. & Hastings, D. (1978). Vaginal reconstruction using bowel segments in male to female transsexual patients. *Archives of Sexual Behavior, 7,* 305–307.

Marshall, W. L., Barbaree, H. E., and Butt, J. (1988). Sexual offenders against male children: sexual preferences. *Behavior Research & Therapy, 26*:5, pp. 383–391.

Masters, W. H., & Johnson, V. E. (1966). *Human sexual response.* Boston: Little, Brown.

Masters, W. H., & Johnson, V. E. (1970). *Human sexual inadequacy.* Boston: Little, Brown.

Masters, W. H., Johnson, V. E., & Kolodny, R. C. (1982). *Human sexuality.* Boston: Little, Brown.

Masters, W. H., Johnson, V. E., & Kolodny, R. C. (1988). *Human sexuality* (3d ed.). Glenview, IL: Scott, Foresman/Little, Brown.

Mathis, J. L. (1972). *Clear thinking about sexual deviations.* Chicago: Nelson-Hall.

McHugh, G. (1967). *Sex knowledge inventory.* Durham, N.C.: Family Life Publications.

Meisenhelder, J., & LaCharite, C. (1989). *Comfort in Caring: Nursing the Person with HIV Infection.* Glenview, IL: Scott, Foresman/Little, Brown, pp. 167–178.

Meyer, J. K. (1980). Paraphilias. In A. M. Freedman, H. I. Kaplan, & B. J. Sadock (Eds.). *Comprehensive Textbook of Psychiatry, 3,* Baltimore: Williams & Wilkins.

Meyer, J. K. & Reter, D. J. (1979). Sex reassignment: Follow-up. *Archieves of General Psychiatry, 36* (9), 1010–1015.

Meyer, J. K., Schmidt, C. W., Lucas, M. J., & Smith, E. (1975). Short-term treatment of sexual problems: Interim report. *American Journal of Psychiatry, 132,* 172–176.

Miller, P. (1984). Thou shalt not be aware. Afterword. (312–318) New York: Farrar, Straus, Giroux.

Money, J. & Erhardt, A. E. (1972). *Man and woman, boy and girl.* Baltimore: John Hopkins University Press.

Morin, S. & Batchelor, W. (1984). Responding to the psychological crisis of AIDS. *Public Health Reports, 99,* 4–9.

Nathan, S. (1986). The epidemiology of the DSM-III psychosexual dysfunctions. *Journal of Sex & Marital Therapy, 12*(4) Winter.

Newcomb, M. D. (1983). Orgasmic responsiveness in women: Attitude and behavioral determinants. Paper presented at the American Psychological Association meetings, Anaheim, California, August.

Newcomb, M. D., & Bentler, P. M. (1980). Assessment of personality and demographic aspects of cohabitation and marital success. *Journal of Consulting and Clinical Psychology, 44,* 11–24.

Nicholi, A. M. (1988). The adolescent. In A. M. Nicholi, Jr. (Ed.) *The Harvard guide to modern psychiatry.* Cambridge: Harvard University.

Owen, J. A., Saunders, F., Harris, C., Fenemore, J., Reid, K., Surridge, D., Condra, M., & Morales, A. (1989). Topical nitroglycerin: A potential treatment for impotence. *The Journal of Urology, 141,* pp. 546–548.

Poorman, S. G. (1988). *Human Sexuality and the Nursing Process.* Norwalk: Appleton & Lange.

Price, S., Reynolds, B. S., Cohen, B. D., Anderson, A. J., & Schochet, B. V. (1981). Group treatment of erectile dysfunction for men without partners: A control evaluation. *Archives of Sexual Behavior, 10,* 253–268.

Richardson, L. (1988). *The dynamics of sex and gender: A sociological perspective.* New York: Harper & Row.

Rudolph, A. (1987). Congenital adrenal hyperplasia. In *Pediatrics* (18th ed.) Norwalk, CT: Appleton & Lange.

Sager, C. J. (1976). The role of sex therapy in marital therapy. *American Journal of Psychiatry, 133,* 555–559.

Schiavi, R. (1985). Evaluation of impaired sexual desire: Biological aspects. In H. Kaplan (Ed.) *Comprehensive Evaluation of Disorders of Sexual Desire.* Washington, D.C.: American Psychiatric Association, pp. 18–35.

Schneidman, B., & McGuire, L. (1976). Group treatment for nonorgasmic women: Two age levels. *Archives of Sexual Behavior, 5,* 239–247.

Schover, L. R., Friedman, J. M., Weiler, S. J., Heiman, J. R., & LoPiccolo, J. (1982a). *A multi-axial descriptive system for the sexual dysfunctions: Categories and manual.* Stony Brook, NY: Sex Therapy Center.

Schover, L. R., Friedman, J. M., Weiler, S. J., Heiman, J. R., & LoPiccolo, J. (1982b). Multi-axial problem-oriented system for sexual dysfunctions. *Archives of General Psychiatry, 39,* 614–619.

Semans, J. H. (1956). Premature ejaculation: A new approach. *Southern Medical Journal,* Vol. *49,* pp. 353–357.

Sewell, H. H., & Abramowitz, S. I. (1979). Flexibility, persistence, and success in sex therapy. *Archives of Sexual Behavior, 8,* 497–506.

Shaw, N. & Paleo, L. (1986). Women and AIDS In. L. McKusick (Ed.), *What to do about AIDS.* (pp. 142–154). Berkeley, CA: University of California Press.

Shrom, S. H., Lief, H. I., & Wein, A. J. (1979). Clinical profile of experience of 130 consecutive cases of impotent men. *Urology, 13,* 511–515.

Snaith, Philip (1983). Symposium on Sexual Deviation, Exhibitionism: A clinical conundrum. *British Journal of Psychiatry, 143,* pp. 231–235.

Socarides, C. W. (1968). *Homosexuality.* New York: Brune & Stratton.

Spodak, M. K., Falck, Z. A., & Rapperport, J. R. (1978). The hormonal treatment of paraphiliacs with depo-provera. *Criminal justice and Behavior, 5:4,* pp. 304–314.

Stoller, R. J. (1968). *Sex and gender: The transsexual experiment.* London: Hogarth Press.

Stoller, R. J. (1977). Sexual Deviations. In F. Beach (Ed.). *Human Sexuality in Four Perspectives.* Baltimore: Johns Hopkins University Press, pp. 190–214.

Strean, H. (1983). *The Sexual Dimension: A Guide for the Helping Professional,* New York: Free Press.

Swonger, A. & Matejski, M. (1988). *Nursing pharmacology.* Glenview, IL: Scott, Foresman.

Tingle, D., Barnard, G., Robbins, L., Newman, G., & Hutchinson, D. (1986). Childhood and adolescent characteristics of pedophiles and rapists. *International Journal of Law and Psychiatry, 9,* pp. 103–116.

Ulman, R. & Brothers, D. (1988). *The shattered self: a psychoanalytic study of trauma.* Hillsdale, NJ: The Analytic Press.

Urwin, C. (1988). AIDS in children: A family concern. *Family Relations* (April) 37:2, p. 154–159.

U.S. Department of Health and Human Services, *AIDS-21,* October 1986.

Vandervoot, H., & McIlvenna, T. (1975). Sexually explicit media in medical school curricula. In R. Green (Ed.). *Human Sexuality: A Practitioners Text.* Baltimore: Williams & Williams, pp. 234–244.

Wagner, G., & Green, R. (1981). General medical disorders and erectile failure. In G. Wagner & R. Breen. *Impotence: Physiological, psychologic, surgical diagnosis, and treatment.* New York: Plenum Press.

Wagner, G., & Jensen, S. B. (1981). Alcohol and erectile failure. In G. Wagner & R. Breen. *Impotence: Physiological, psychological, surgical diagnosis, and treatment:* New York: Plenum Press.

Walker, I. (1981). Clinical psychiatry in primary care. (pp. 248–249). Menlo Park: Addison-Wesley.

Warren, N. J., & Gilner, F. H. (1978). Measurement of positive assertive behaviors: The behavioral test of tenderness express. *Behavior Therapy, 9,* 178–184.

Watters, G. R., Keogh, E. J., Earle, C. M., Carati, C. J., Wisniewski, Z. S., Tulloch, A. G. S., & Lord, D. J. (1988). Experience in the management of erectile dysfunction using the intracavernosal self-injection of vasoactive drugs. *The Journal of Urology, 140,* pp. 1417–1419.

Wiener, D. N. (1969). Sexual problems in clinical experience. A chapter in C. B. Broderick & J. Bernard (Eds.). *The Individual, Sex, and Society.* Baltimore: The Johns Hopkins Press.

Wilson, G. T., & Lawson, D. M. (1978). Expectancies, alcohol, and sexual arousal in women. *Journal of Abnormal Psychology, 87,* 358–367.

Wise, T. N. (1983). Evaluation and treatment of gender disorders. In J. K. Meyer, C. N. Schmidt, Jr., & T. N. Wise. (Eds.) *Clinical Management of Sexual Disorders, 2,* Baltimore: Williams and Wilkins.

Wolpe, J. (1958). *Psychotherapy by reciprocal inhibition.* Palo Alto: Stanford University Press.

Wolpe, J. (1969). *The practice of behavior therapy.* New York: Pergamon Press.

Wolpe, J. (1973). *The practice of behavior therapy* (2nd ed.) New York: Pergamon General Psychology Series; 1.

Wolpe, J. (1977). The treatment of inhibited sexual responses. In J. Fischer & H. L. Gochros (Eds.). *Handbook of behavior therapy with sexual problems, 1,* New York: Pergamon Press.

Zuckerman, M. (1973). Scales for sexual experience for males and females. *Journal of Consulting and Clinical Psychology, 41,* 27–29.

Zuckerman, R., Tushup, R., & Finner, S. (1976). Sexual attitudes and experience: Attitude and personality correlates on changes produced by a course in sexuality. *Journal of Consulting and Clinical Psychology, 44,* 7–19.

17

DISSOCIATIVE DISORDERS

BEVERLY A. BENFER
PATRICIA J. SCHRODER

LEARNING OBJECTIVES

After studying this chapter, the student will be able to:

- Describe dissociation as part of childhood development.
- Name and describe the different dissociative disorders.
- Discuss the special ethical and legal issues that may arise during the care of patients with dissociative disorders.
- Compare the roles of the nurse generalist and nurse therapist in the care of patients with dissociative disorders.
- Formulate nursing diagnoses for patients with dissociative disorders.

INTRODUCTION

The primary feature of **dissociative disorders** is a disturbance in the **integrative functions:** identity, memory, and consciousness (American Psychiatric Association, 1987). However, until the DSM-III was published in 1980 dissociative processes were considered to be within the framework of neurotic disorders and were most often seen as a variation of a **conversion reaction** (an involuntary loss, or alteration, of a function, which resembles a physical disorder but appears to arise from psychological mechanisms) (Maxmen, 1986). There are five types of dissociative disorders: 1) multiple personality (a disorder in which a person temporarily shifts from an original identity to another identity); 2) psychogenic fugue and 3) psychogenic amnesia (disorders characterized by the loss of memory about personal events of significance); 4) depersonalization (a disorder which is manifested by a compromise in or loss of a sense of one's own reality); and 5) disorders not otherwise classified. In this chapter we discuss each disorder, with emphasis on multiple personality because of its complexity and the increasing frequency of its diagnosis.

Dissociation is a defense mechanism that operates unconsciously to separate and detach emotional significance from an idea or situation. It begins as an individual's unconscious attempt to isolate him or herself from situations that cause anxious, uncomfortable, or fearful feelings. For instance, a student who is afraid of failing a course may go to sleep just when he needs to study. A business executive faced with inordinate demands in her job may engage in meditation as a way to get relief from feelings of pressure. A secretary who feels shy and isolated from her coworkers may daydream about another situation in which she is popular, sought out, and socially at ease. An accountant who is in personal financial difficulty may focus on a single task to shut out his concerns about money.

Dissociation serves as an ego defense to avoid feelings or situations that are unacceptable as part of an individual's self-identity. While the uncomfortable feeling or association is temporarily removed from

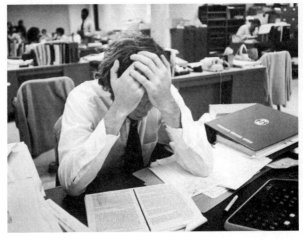

Dissociation serves as an ego defense to avoid feelings or situations that are intolerable to the individual. For example, a business executive may meditate to relieve stress.

consciousness by dissociation, the healthy individual has the ability to refocus on the problematic event or issue when necessary. For example, the business executive can return from meditation to think about her job demands and take appropriate action. The ability to refocus and bring into awareness the event or situation that has been dissociated is what differentiates the use of dissociation as a healthy coping mechanism from the use of dissociation in a maladaptive way. At the unhealthy end of the continuum, the degree of dissociation may be so extreme that the individual separates emotions and experiences into another personality. According to Peplau (1952), when a person's feelings and thoughts are not permitted expression or identification on a conscious level, they may seek expression outside of the person's awareness and control.

Since dissociation is a subtle disorder, difficult to diagnose, the nurse will seldom encounter it in a nonpsychiatric setting. The exception is the disorder of multiple personality. (Although the diagnosis of multiple personality is also rare, within the past few years more cases have been reported and patients are occasionally hospitalized.) The nurse is more apt to encounter the patient who has been hospitalized for another illness or injury, such as suicide threats, trauma, or depression, and is in a dissociative state.

While individuals can experience dissociative states due to a variety of physical causes, such as epilepsy, head injury, or a drug-induced state, only dissociative states with a psychological basis meet the criteria of a psychiatric disorder as outlined by the Diagnostic and Statistical Manual of Mental Disorders (DSM-III-R).

Altered states of consciousness (ASC) can be produced by a variety of factors including physical, environmental, psychological, and pharmacologic agents. These ASCs are recognized by the individual, and often others, as different from the norm for a particular person (Ludwig, 1966; Kaplan and Sadock, 1985).

Variables associated with altered sense of consciousness include:

1. Reduction of exteroceptive stimulation, such as reduction of sensory input, monotonous stimulation, and limited motor activity. These conditions occur in such situations as confinement in prison camps; highway hypnosis; flying at high altitudes; hypnogogic (the stage immediately preceding sleep) and hypnopompic (the stage immediately preceding awakening) states; and immobilization of body parts that occurs

when a person is in a body cast or other type of constraint.

2. Increase of exteroceptive stimulation, motor activity, or emotions such as excitement created by sensory overload and/or bombardment (emotional arousal and mental fatigue). These occur in such situations as brainwashing, trances associated with very intense groups (mobs or encounter groups), religious healing and conversions, certain rites-of-passage ceremonies, shamanistic trance states, tribal ceremonies, and glass or fire walking trances.

3. Increased alertness or mental involvement that results from situations of selective hyperalertness, leading to hypoalertness. This condition occurs during prolonged observation of radar screens; fervent prayer; concentrated enmeshment in a task such as writing or reading; intense involvement in listening to charismatic leaders; and watching a metronome or a revolving drum for long periods of time.

4. Decreased alertness or the relaxation of critical mental faculties. These behaviors occur when the individual has a "passive state of mind," with little evidence of active cognition and goal-directed thinking. Examples include mystical or transcendental states that occur during the relaxation of critical thought processes, or the adaptive regression in service of the ego; day dreaming; deep aesthetic experiences (profound appreciation of art work or music); free association (as experienced in psychoanalysis); and experiences associated with relaxation, such as floating on water or sun-bathing.

5. Presence of somatopsychological factors that occur primarily because of changes in body chemistry or neurophysiology. Such conditions may or may not be under the individual's control. Examples include hypoglycemia with postprandial lethargy; dehydration, thyroid and/or adrenal gland disorders; sleep deprivation; hyperventilation; toxic delirium; going "cold turkey" in treatment of a substance abuse addiction, narcotic, anesthetic, and stimulant drug use; and auras that occur preceding migraine headaches and epileptic seizures.

These features are varied and present with diverse duration and intensity. Yet, there are some common features associated with all of these behaviors that can aid in the conceptualization of these related occurrences. The common characteristics that are expressed to varying degrees include: a) alteration in thinking; b) disturbance in sense of time; c) feeling of loss of control; d) fluctuation in emotional expression; e) a rejuvenated feeling; and f) high suggestibility (Ludwig, 1966). The patient's memories, feelings, and fantasies are beyond his ability of conscious recall, but remain in his subconscious (Kaplan and Sadock, 1985).

Dissociation occurs on a continuum ranging from minor forms that happen on a frequent basis (day dreaming, intense concentration, meditation, and so forth) to the more pathological patterns as seen in multiple personality, amnesia, etc. (Ludwig, 1983; Bernstein and Putnam, 1986).

Dissociation is common, has widespread prevalence, and is seen in numerous forms, both adaptive and maladaptive (Ludwig, 1983; Bernstein and Putnam, 1986; Sanders, 1986). These observations led Ludwig (1983) to hypothesize that dissociation has a survival value for humans. From a clinical perspective, he has identified seven major psychobiological functions of dissociation.

DESCRIPTION OF DISSOCIATIVE DISORDERS

AUTOMATIZATION OF BEHAVIORS

Automatization of behaviors refers to the principle that the unconscious contains learned and instinctive behaviors that allow a person to function expeditiously on "automatic pilot." Behaviors associated with automatic-pilot functions include radar-screen trance, highway hypnosis, intensive piano playing, and so forth, while conscious thought is required to accomplish other tasks such as studying for an examination, making a speech, preparing a meal, and so forth.

ECONOMY AND EFFICIENCY

Similar to automatization, yet different, is the notion of economy and efficiency of effort. It allows the person to have a single-minded purpose; information, knowledge, and skills available in one level of consciousness are not available in another level. (Multiple personality is an extreme example.) Critical judgment might be suspended in the service of gaining immediate gratification. Because judgment is suspended, probabilities and consequences are not weighed. The deletion of judgment hastens the possibility of behaviors that bring gratification of needs, desires, frustrations, and so on.

RESOLUTION OF IRRECONCILABLE CONFLICTS

Dissociative states provide opportunities for the individual to express conflicts without having to deal with them. There is no integration or working through a problem. Instead, conflicts are expressed in sequence through altered states of consciousness. "Trance logic," for example, provides for the expression of conflicts; opposing forces such as thoughts of suicide versus the desire to live can exist harmoniously (as in multiple personality). The person may be able to participate in acts (taboos) with little regret or responsibility for his behaviors. These taboos can include incest, tantrums, spells, and satanic acts. Multiple personality, amnesia, fugue, and depersonalization disorders are all examples of this process.

ESCAPE FROM THE CONSTRAINTS OF REALITY

Reality is suspended for the patient who is in a dissociative state. For example, the patient believes that conquering diseases through ritualistic and religious dances is possible; that he can bring time to a halt; or that he can make contact with divine people through trances and intense meditation.

ISOLATION OF CATASTROPHIC EXPERIENCES

The psyche can experience extreme assault through humiliations, stressful life events, fatigue, and so forth. Since such experiences are difficult to reconcile, the psyche might seal off these problematic areas through repression and dissociation and allow the assaulted person to function freely without intense interference from problems. The dissociative state can be a repository for such unwanted feelings that then become accessible only through expression of altered consciousness.

Robert Louis Stevenson wrote a classic story, *The Strange Case of Dr. Jekyll and Mr. Hyde,* that told the story of a scientist, who through an induced chemical process, created extreme psychological changes in himself. There were two basic personalities: a dominant one, Dr. Jekyll, who was good (normal) and Mr. Hyde (the alter) who represented the bad (pathological) components of the total personality. Another example of multiple personality is *The Three Faces of Eve* (Thigpen & Cleckly, 1957).

ENHANCEMENT OF "HERD" SENSE

Individuals in a dissociative state can be easily led by charismatic leaders or authority figures rather than logic. A consequence of this is that large groups of individuals can be "led," in a cohesive fashion, to participate in a variety of religious, secular, and social activities. These activities provide an outlet for frustrations, conflicts, and desires in a socially acceptable manner.

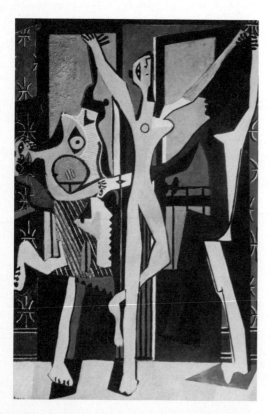

Dissociated emotions, such as frustration and aggressive urges, may be expressed in socially acceptable ways such as ritualistic dances and revival meetings. (*The Three Dancers* by Pablo Picasso.)

CATHARTIC DISCHARGE OF FEELINGS

A variety of stored-up emotions can be expressed through dissociative states. These usually follow culturally sanctioned folkways and behaviors, such as the ritualistic dances and revival meetings where aggressive urges, frustrations, and conflicts can be expressed in a culturally appropriate fashion.

Dissociation can serve an important function in a person's daily life. However, it is the profound, prolonged, and intensive use of this process that causes problems for the individual, his significant others, and society. Maladaptive expressions of an altered sense of consciousness are numerous and represent the individual's attempt to resolve emotional conflicts. The maladaptive expressions of needs, conflicts, desires, and experiences do occur and are seen in more disturbed patterns in dissociative disorders. This chapter will discuss those dissociative disorders that are maladaptive and create problems for the individual, his family, and society.

MULTIPLE PERSONALITY

The predominant feature of **multiple personality** is the presence of two or more distinct personalities or personality states within one person (American Psychiatric Association, 1987). The personality states consist of those secondary personalities that are not dominant and manifest at a given time. The fully developed personality(ies) can be termed the primary personality. There may be two or more fully developed personalities; there may also be one distinct personality and numerous other personality states. In fact, the frequency of personalities and personality states may range from two to more than one hundred (American Psychiatric Association, 1987). Given such a variety of personalities, it is understandable that the affected individual experiences unexplained complexities, frustrations, and conflicts.

The various personalities may be aware of the coexistence of the other personalities; however, the extent of the awareness may vary. The personalities might be friendly with each other, serve as companions, or function as adversaries. On the other hand, some personalities may not be aware of the other personalities. The personality that is dominant at any given time determines the person's behavior. Each personality is complex and integrated with its own behavioral patterns and interpersonal relationships (American Psychiatric Association, 1987). One hypothesis about multiple personality is that each sub-personality fulfills a precise function—to express anger, depression, and aggressive impulses, or to serve as a protector or a rescuer (Coons, 1984). The different personalities may also represent different traumatic events or developmental crises in the individual's life (Kluft, 1984c). For instance, one personality may appear antisocial, engaging in drug abuse, rebellious behavior, and resistance to authority, focusing on pleasure orientation. Another personality may show symptoms of an anxiety disorder, having a number of phobias, fears, and panic. The personality that is depressed, with thoughts of suicide, may be diagnosed with a mood disorder (Putnam et al., 1984).

Individuals with multiple personality usually have at least *some* insight about their condition, and know at some level that something is wrong with them. There is limited integration of personalities. The person will provide excuses for questionable behaviors.

Multiple personality represents one of the most complex disorders in the dissociative category. Clinical descriptions of multiple personality can be found in the literature as early as 1817 (Greaves, 1980). Freud also described this phenomenon, viewing it as an extreme form of depersonalization (Greaves, 1980). Scientific reports such as "Mrs. Beauchamp" (Prince, 1925) and books and movies have told the stories of persons with multiple personality, including *The Three Faces of Eve* (Thigpen & Cleckley, 1957), *The Minds of Billy Milligan* (Keys, 1981), and *Sybil* (Schreiber, 1973). Most mental health professionals, however, have not been directly involved in the treatment of patients with this disorder; thus even professionals sometimes share the public skepticism about its authenticity. (See Box 17–1.)

A common conceptualization of multiple personality is that it involves altered ego states or fragments of the personality (Coons, 1984; Kluft, 1984b; Stern, 1984). Each fragment contains a partial identification with people from the individual's past or serves a particular defensive function for the person (Clary, Burstin, & Carpenter, 1984).

Another theory of multiple personality is that because individuals can introject (withdraw emotion from an external person or event and make it part of themselves) not only attitudes and affects but also experiences, it is possible that the patient can introject the experience of sexual and/or physical abuse into a subpersonality who later contains that trauma as a partial self-view (Bliss, 1984; Coons & Milstein, 1986). Each personality may rely on a different ego defense, each of which is only partially successful. One personality may display a full-blown psychosis, although this is rare. (See Box 17–2.)

Many individuals with multiple personality find it difficult to give up the illness because the separateness has often resulted in some of the personalities operating autonomously. Secondary gains are powerful; to become integrated, the patient would have to deal with reality, which would require behavior changes. Also, there is considerable narcissistic investment in each separate identity (Kluft, 1984a).

Marian: A Patient with Multiple Personality

Marian Barkin was a 26-year-old executive secretary in a prestigious law firm. She was extremely skilled in office management and had been recently promoted to her current position in the firm. However, after her promotion she began making numerous mistakes, not following through with assignments, and complaining of feeling tired and "washed out." In therapy, it was revealed that Susie, another personality, was feeling neglected, abandoned, and spiteful.

DSM-III-R Diagnostic Criteria for Multiple Personality

A. The existence within the person of two or more distinct personalities or personality states (each with its own relatively enduring pattern of perceiving, relating to, and thinking about the environment and self).

B. At least two of these personalities or personality states recurrently take full control of the person's behavior.

Susie sabotaged Marian because of her own need for recreation and male companionship that was prohibited by Marian's long and tedious work hours.

EPIDEMIOLOGY

GENDER. Multiple personality occurs most frequently in females. The male to female ratio is about eight to one.

AGE. Multiple personality originates in childhood; clinical manifestations, however, begin during adolescence (Caddy, 1985).

MARITAL STATUS. Usually, the multiple personality patient will have been married at some time (Putnam et al., 1986)

LIFE EVENTS. The patient usually has a history of

Box 17–1 ● The Minds of Billy Milligan

The Minds of Billy Milligan is the fascinating, true story of a young man with 24 separate personalities. In his struggle to cope with a childhood filled with physical and sexual abuse, he split into "multiple selves."

Each personality is distinct, with a name and an identity. Three of them are female and several are children; some are dominant, others retiring. The original, or core personality was unaware of the existence of the other personalities for many years. However, some of the less dominant personalities were aware of each other as well as the dominant personalities.

From early childhood, Billy could remember "losing time," when he would close his eyes and open them to find that night changed to day, or the reverse. Often, this behavior would occur when an abusive episode was occurring. As a child, he would frequently find himself being punished for misdeeds he had no memory of performing. As he got older, some of the personalities began committing crimes, and then withdrawing to let Billy or one of the "others" take the consequences. It was this process that brought the bizarre case to light.

Billy Milligan was arrested in connection with a series of campus rapes at Ohio State University. During questioning as a suspect in the cases, other personalities began to reveal themselves, to the astonishment of his legal counsel and the evaluating psychiatrists. His illness became his defense, and for the first time in history, a diagnosis of dissociative disorder, multiple personality, was successfully used in a plea of not guilty by reason of insanity. This decision was reached on the grounds that Billy was unable to cooperate with his lawyers in his own defense.

Treatment for this disorder involves identifying the various personalities; making them aware of each other; and enlisting their cooperation in binding, or fusing them all into one intact personality. A long and tedious process, such therapy requires residence in a hospital facility, and the availability of a psychiatrist with expertise in treating multiple personality. Billy made progress when he received this treatment, and "The Teacher," or the "fused" Billy, began to make appearances. "The Teacher" had recall of the "others," and it was only through him that the whole sequence of events was recalled.

The story does not progress to a happy ending, however. The public, kept informed about the case by the enthusiastic media, was outraged that a rapist enjoyed the comparative comfort of a hospital rather than being confined in a maximum security prison. His treatment was interrupted as he was transferred from place to place, and the trauma he experienced resulted in serious setbacks. "The Teacher" appeared less often as Billy retreated into his unfused state and the hope of recovery gradually diminished.

Source: Keyes, Daniel (1981). *The Minds of Billy Milligan*. New York: Random House.

abuse, including sexual, physical, and emotional, as well as other traumas from childhood.

PERSONALITY CHARACTERISTICS. Frequently multiple personality patients have masochistic and depressive tendencies (Kluft, 1983). They are of above-average intelligence with IQs of 130 or higher (Schafer, 1986).

ASSESSMENT OF MULTIPLE PERSONALITY

MOOD. Depression, detachment, and sensations of derealization and depersonalization are mood states associated with multiple personality.

COGNITIVE CHANGES. Alterations in perception

Box 17—2 ● Considerations for Treatment

The Four Factor Theory of the Etiology of Multiple Personality Disorder

Kluft (1984) suggests that treatment of multiple personality disorders be guided by the Four Factor Theory of Etiology. This theory is undergirded with the "understanding that multiple personality is the final common pathway of a wide variety of combinations of influences," p. 13.

Factor 1 proposes that the individual who develops multiple personality disorder has the biological potential to dissociate (a characteristic seen in patients with high hypnotizability). If factor 1 is absent, the therapist should suspect that the individual may have some nondissociative condition, or may be malingering.

Factor 2 is the overwhelming stress or life experiences (physical, sexual, or psychological abuse, etc.) that occur during the developmental years, and cause the dissociation potential to become an active part of defensive functioning.

Factor 3 consists of experiences that help determine the formation of dissociative defenses. Those individuals who experience dissociation, and remain in that state, are influenced by Factor 4.

Factor 4 includes deficient stimulus barriers, inadequate nurturance, and limited soothing and growth producing experiences by significant others.

Focus of Therapy Based Upon the Four Factor Theory

Factor 1: Recognize that the dissociative process is occurring, interpret when appropriate, and restructure the dissociation. (Avoid trying to suppress or ignore the dissociation.)

Factor 2: Be gentle. Avoid imposing upon the patient any overwhelming experience that he may not be ready to deal with. Avoid becoming the "Traumatizer." Develop a therapeutic alliance with the patient, and, together, agree to unearth traumatic experiences; deal with relapses in a therapeutic manner.

Factor 3: Be cognizant of all shaping influences that helped to create the dissociative personalities. Do not generalize. Therapy must uncover all facets of the multiple personality.

Factor 4: Be empathic, listen to the patient, and allow the patient to internalize overwhelming experiences. The therapist should not take sides with any of the personalities, but must assure the psychological and physical safety of all personalities. The therapist must function as the individual's advocate when he is unable to help himself. Therapy should address the outcome of inadequate soothing and nurturance; the therapist should focus on restorative curative factors that she and significant others can provide for the patient.

Sources: Adapted from Kluft, R. (1984). Treatment of Multiple Personality Disorder: A study of 33 cases. *Psychiatric Clinics of North America*, Vol. 7, No. 1, pp. 9–29, and Kluft, R. (1984). Multiple Personality in Childhood. *Psychiatric Clinics of North America*, Vol. 7, No. 1, pp. 121–134.

can be severe: the patient hears the alternate personality's voice, visualizes the alternate, experiences auditory hallucinations, and experiences a disturbance in thought processes with thought withdrawals and insertions being present (similar to what the schizophrenic patient might experience).

MOTIVATION CHANGES. Motivational changes are determined by the dominant personality at any given time. The individual might be gregarious and outgoing one moment, and minutes later depressed, uninterested in the environment, confused, and so forth.

PHYSICAL CHANGES. A switch from one personality to another may be preceded by a sudden headache, arrhythmias, and/or stomach pain, particularly in those instances in which the transition from one personality to another occurs instantaneously. Recent research studies have focused on the physiology of patients with multiple personalities, with some startling results. Researchers have found differences in physiologic functioning among the subpersonalities of the same person, a finding which may have signif-icant implications for the study of mind and body connections in ordinary illness (see Box 17–3).

BEHAVIORAL MANIFESTATIONS. Abrupt personality changes occur as the individual assumes various personalities. These behaviors may range from helpless and childlike to exuberant, chaotic, and demanding. The person may have a history of depression, substance abuse, self-mutilation, suicidal ideation, gestures and attempts, and so forth (Maxmen, 1986).

SELF-RATING QUESTIONNAIRES. The Dissociative Experiences Scale is a relatively new instrument designed to 1) distinguish between patients who do have dissociative disorders and patients who do not, 2) provide for a method by which dissociative experiences might be reviewed as contributing to other psychiatric disorders, and 3) assess for a continuum of dissociation, ranging from minor dissociative experiences to major forms of dissociative disorders (Bernstein & Putnam, 1986).

Currently, only two instruments exist to quantify dissociative experiences. The Dissociative Experiences Scale (DES) is a relatively new instrument, created to

Box 17–3 • Probing the Enigma of Multiple Personality

When Timmy drinks orange juice he has no problem. But Timmy is just one of close to a dozen personalities who alternate control over a patient with multiple personality disorder. And if those other personalities drink orange juice, the result is a case of hives.

The hives will occur even if Timmy drinks orange juice and another personality appears while the juice is still being digested. What's more, if Timmy comes back while the allergic reaction is present, the itching of the hives will cease immediately, and the water-filled blisters will begin to subside.

Such remarkable differences in the same body are leading scientists to study the physiology of patients with multiple personalities to assess how much psychological states can affect the body's biology, for better or worse. The researchers are discov-ering that such patients offer a unique window on how the mind and body can interact.

Researchers feel that the study of these patients may also have significant implications for people with the medical disorders that are found to differ from one sub-personality to another. If the mechanisms through which these differences occur can be discovered, it may be possible to teach people some similar degree of control over these problems.

For more than a century clinicians have occasionally reported isolated cases of dramatic biological changes in people with multiple personalities as they switched from one to another. These include the abrupt appearance and disappearance of rashes, welts, scars, and other tissue wounds; switches in handwriting and handedness; epilepsy, allergies, and color blindness that strike only when

provide a reliable and valid method of measuring dissociative experiences. This instrument (DES) represents one of the first attempts to develop such a tool.

When administering the instrument, the clinician requests the subject to indicate his response to each item by marking a slash across the 100 mm line at the place that best represents his response. The mean of all items on the scale ranges from 0 to 100, and constitutes the Dissociative Experiences Scale (DES) score (see Box 17–4).

Normal adults tend to report five dissociative experiences, relatively infrequently. Conversely, adults with dissociative disorders reported a variety of dissociative symptoms, occurring rather frequently (Bernstein & Putnam, 1986; personal communication, June 28, 1988).

Sanders (1986) developed the Perceptual Alteration Scale (PAS) designed to identify modifications in ego functions that are associated with dissociative disorders and other types of psychopathology. The scale was initially developed to assist clinicians and researchers with the understanding of binge eating behaviors and the frequency and extent of dissociation in this population when compared to normals (non-binge eaters). Using a Likert scale, it presents response possibilities from one to four, and yields four scores. These scores consist of 1) a total score derived by summing the 60 scale items; 2) a control scale; 3) an affect scale; and 4) a cognition scale. It is hypothesized that disturbances in the latter three scales might be indicative of some dissociative activity (Sanders, personal communication, July 1, 1988).

FREQUENCY/INTENSITY DURATION. Multiple personality is usually a chronic condition, but over a period of time the frequency of switching from one personality to another decreases.

IMPACT ON INDIVIDUAL. Patients become emotionally enmeshed in nonuseful and pathological relationships. They experience enormous conflict between a wish to grow and mature and the demands of remaining the same.

IMPACT ON FAMILY SYSTEM. On numerous occasions, the individual is rejected by or estranged from family and friends. Continuous interpersonal relationships are, at best, difficult (Kluft, 1983).

---

a given personality is in control of the body.

Today, using refined research techniques, scientists are bringing greater rigor to the study of multiple personalities and focusing on a search for the mechanisms that produce the varying physiological differences in each personality.

Reactions to Medication

One of the problems for psychiatrists trying to treat patients with multiple personalities is that, depending on which personality is in control, a patient can have drastically different reactions to a given psychiatric medication. For instance, it is almost always the case that one or several of the personalities of a given patient will be that of a child. And the differences in responses to drugs among the sub-personalities often parallel those ordinarily found when the same drug at the same dose is given to a child, rather than an adult.

In a recent book, "The Treatment of Multiple Personality Disorder," published by the American Psychiatric Press, Dr. [Bennet] Braun, [a psychiatrist at Rush-Presbyterian-St. Luke's Medical Center in Chicago] describes several instances in which different personalities in the same body responded differently to a given dose of the same medication. A tranquilizer, for instance, made a childish personality of one patient sleepy and relaxed, but gave adult personalities confusion and racing thoughts. An anti-convulsant prescribed for epilepsy that was given another patient had no effect on the personalities except those under the age of 12.

In another patient, 5 milligrams of diazepam, a tranquilizer, sedated one personality, while 100 milligrams had little effect on another personality.

How Mind Regulates Biology

The medical phenomena being discovered in multiple personalities stretch the imagination, but researchers believe that they represent only the extreme end of a normal continuum. The effects found in these patients, they say, are graphic examples of the power of states of mind to regulate the body's biology. By studying them, researchers hope to find clues to links between mind and body that can help people with other psychiatric problems, as well as point the way to powers of healing that may one day be of use in treating normal medical patients.

Source: Adapted from Goleman, Daniel. Probing the Enigma of Multiple Personality, *The New York Times*, June 28, 1988.

Box 17—4 ●
Dissociative
Experience Scale

This questionnaire consists of twenty-eight questions about experiences that you may have in your daily life. We are interested in how often you have these experiences. It is important, however, that your answers show how often these experiences happen to you when you **are not** under the influence of alcohol or drugs. To answer the questions, please determine to what degree the experience described in the question applies to you and mark the line with a vertical slash at the appropriate place, as shown in the example below.

Example:

0% |————————/———————| 100%

1. Some people have the experience of driving a car and suddenly realizing that they don't remember what has happened during all or part of the trip. Mark the line to show what percentage of the time this happens to you.

0% |————————————————| 100%

2. Some people find that sometimes they are listening to someone talk and they suddenly realize that they did not hear part or all of what was just said. Mark the line to show what percentage of the time this happens to you.

0% |————————————————| 100%

3. Some people have the experience of finding themselves in a place and having no idea how they got there. Mark the line to show what percentage of the time this happens to you.

0% |————————————————| 100%

4. Some people have the experience of finding themselves dressed in clothes that they don't remember putting on. Mark the line to show what percentage of the time this happens to you.

0% |————————————————| 100%

5. Some people have the experience of finding new things among their belongings that they do not remember buying. Mark the line to show what percentage of the time this happens to you.

0% |————————————————| 100%

6. Some people sometimes find that they are approached by people that they do not know who call them by another name or insist that they have met them before. Mark the line to show what percentage of the time this happens to you.

0% |————————————————| 100%

7. Some people sometimes have the experience of feeling as though they are standing next to themselves or watching themselves do something and they actually see themselves as if they were looking at another person. Mark the line to show what percentage of the time this happens to you.

0% |————————————————| 100%

8. Some people are told that they sometimes do not recognize friends or family members. Mark the line to show what percentage of the time this happens to you.

0% |————————————————| 100%

9. Some people find that they have no memory for some important events in their lives (for example, a wedding or graduation). Mark the line to show what percentage of the important events in your life you have no memory for.

0% |————————————————| 100%

10. Some people have the experience of being accused of lying when they do not think that they have lied. Mark the line to show what percentage of the time this happens to you.

0% |————————————————| 100%

11. Some people have the experience of looking in a mirror and not recognizing themselves. Mark the line to show what percentage of the time this happens to you.

0% |————————————————| 100%

12. Some people sometimes have the experience of feeling that other people, objects, and the world around them are not real. Mark the line to show what percentage of the time this happens to you.

0% |————————————————| 100%

13. Some people sometimes have the experience of feeling that their

body does not seem to belong to them. Mark the line to show what percentage of the time this happens to you.

0% |————————————| 100%

14. Some people have the experience of sometimes remembering a past event so vividly that they feel as if they were reliving that event. Mark the line to show what percentage of the time this happens to you.

0% |————————————| 100%

15. Some people have the experience of not being sure whether things that they remember happening really did happen or whether they just dreamed them. Mark the line to show what percentage of the time this happens to you.

0% |————————————| 100%

16. Some people have the experience of being in a familiar place but finding it strange and unfamiliar. Mark the line to show what percentage of the time this happens to you.

0% |————————————| 100%

17. Some people find that when they are watching television or a movie they become so absorbed in the story that they are unaware of other events happening around them. Mark the line to show what percentage of the time this happens to you.

0% |————————————| 100%

18. Some people sometimes find that they become so involved in a fantasy or daydream that it feels as though it were really happening to them. Mark the line to show what percentage of the time this happens to you.

0% |————————————| 100%

19. Some people find that they sometimes are able to ignore pain. Mark the line to show what percentage of the time this happens to you.

0% |————————————| 100%

20. Some people find that they sometimes sit staring off into space, thinking of nothing, and are not aware of the passage of time. Mark the line to show what percentage of the time this happens to you.

0% |————————————| 100%

21. Some people sometimes find that when they are alone they talk out loud to themselves. Mark the line to show what percentage of the time this happens to you.

0% |————————————| 100%

22. Some people find that in one situation they may act so differently compared with another situation that they feel almost as if they were two different people. Mark the line to show what percentage of the time this happens to you.

0% |————————————| 100%

23. Some people sometimes find that in certain situations they are able to do things with amazing ease and spontaneity that would usually be difficult for them (for example, sports, work, social situations, and so on). Mark the line to show what percentage of the time this happens to you.

0% |————————————| 100%

24. Some people sometimes find that they cannot remember whether they have done something or have just thought about doing that thing (for example, not knowing whether they have just mailed a letter or have just thought about mailing it). Mark the line to show what percentage of the time this happens to you.

0% |————————————| 100%

25. Some people sometimes find evidence that they have done things that they do not remember doing. Mark the line to show what percentage of the time this happens to you.

0% |————————————| 100%

26. Some people sometimes find writings, drawings, or notes among their belongings that they must have done but cannot remember doing. Mark the line to show what percentage of the time this happens to you.

0% |————————————| 100%

27. Some people sometimes find that they hear voices inside their head that tell them to do things or comment on things that they are doing. Mark the line to show what percentage of the time this happens to you.

0% |————————————| 100%

28. Some people sometimes feel as if they are looking at the world through a fog so that people and objects appear far away or unclear. Mark the line to show what percentage of the time this happens to you.

0% |————————————| 100%

Dissociative Experience Scale

Subjects experiencing "normal" dissociative episodes have the lowest **DES** scores, and those with a diagnosis of multiple personality disorder were shown to have the highest **DES** scores. Instructions on the **DES** asks the subject to make a slash mark across a 100mm line to indicate where he or she falls on a continuum for each question. Items on the questionnaire refer to dissociative experiences, such as disturbances in identity, memory, awareness, and cognition and/or feelings of depersonalization. Scores for each item are determined by measuring the subject's slash mark to the nearest 5 mm from the left-hand anchor point of the 100mm line. The mean of all item scores ranges from 0 to 100 and is called the **DES score**. The **DES score** is an index of the duration of different types of dissociative experiences and the frequency of each experience. (For more in-depth discussion, see Bernstein, E. M., & Putnam, F. W. (1986). Development, reliability, and validity of a dissociation scale. *Journal of nervous and mental disease.* 174(12), 727–735.)

Source: Bernstein, E. M., & Putman, F. W. (1986). Development, reliability and validity of a dissociation scale. *Journal of Nervous and Mental Disease,* 174(12), 727–735.

NURSING DIAGNOSIS

A selected number of nursing diagnoses related to the symptoms of multiple personality disorders are listed below.

Alteration in thought processes

Ineffective individual coping

Potential for violence: self-directed or directed at others

Ineffective family coping: compromised

Self-esteem disturbance

Body image disturbance

Personal identity disturbance

Altered role performance

Anxiety

Additional nursing diagnoses include:

Impaired verbal communication

Pain

Chronic pain

Alteration in family processes

Fear

Knowledge deficit

Noncompliance related to anxiety

Altered parenting: actual/potential

Powerlessness

Sleep pattern disturbance

Because multiple personality disorders are often chronic but vary in intensity and duration of episodes, formulation of appropriate nursing diagnoses can be difficult. While the generalist nurse may not be able to address the issues of impaired communication and thought alteration without the help of a psychiatric specialist, she may be able to work with the patient to lessen anxiety or to improve conduct control, and with the family to improve family coping, and should certainly be aware of the patient's potential for violence.

PSYCHOGENIC FUGUE

A **psychogenic fugue** is a massive amnesia (Cameron, 1963). Fugues are generally precipitated by extreme stress (Beck, Rawlins, & Williams, 1984), with the individual taking actual flight in an attempt to escape whatever is overwhelming, threatening, or unacceptable. There is a sudden, temporary alteration in the integrative functions of consciousness (Beck,

Rawlins, & Williams, 1984), with the individual unable to recall personal information due to dissociation. A fugue occurs abruptly: for example, the individual may leave his occupation, family, and home and go to a new location. During this process, the individual develops amnesia about his old identity and assumes a new one. Precipitating events are frequently the same as those that precipitate psychogenic amnesia, with stress and major disruption of significant relationships being prominent (American Psychiatric Association, 1987).

Ron: A Patient with Psychogenic Fugue

Ron Chambers was a 22-year-old hospital technician. Although his coworkers described him as pleasant, kind, and gentle, no one knew him particularly well. Ron was plagued by financial difficulties, particularly the support of his wife and two children, ages three and six weeks. One day Ron failed to show up for work; his coworkers and wife were concerned. His car keys and billfold were still at home, and no clothes were missing. His wife feared that he had committed suicide or had been killed in an accident. Several weeks later, Ron was located using a different name, in California (several hundred miles from home) where he was working on the docks as a laborer for a shipping company. The police had discovered his identity when they checked his fingerprints after he had instigated a fight in a bar. With the aid of hypnosis, Ron was able to regain memory of his past life and returned home, where he continued psychiatric care on an outpatient basis for the marital and family issues that he had been unable to cope with at the onset of the fugue.

While in a fugue state, an individual's personality may be totally different from his prefugue personality. For example, the person who is usually shy may become outgoing; the individual who is usually passive may be argumentative and aggressive; the person who is usually reserved may become seductive; these changes express some of the desires that were kept under control in the prefugue personality. In prolonged fugue states, the individual can engage in quite complex activities, including work and new relationships. The person retains enough ego synthetic functioning to "invent" a believable past to replace the one lost with the fugue state (Cameron, 1963).

Fugue states differ from amnesia in that the person's behavior while in a fugue state is more complex; the individual engages in more activities calling for integration in spite of lack of recall. For instance, a person in a fugue state may be able to handle highly technical tasks, such as mathematics, or will not lose the knowledge of how to drive a car. At the same time, this individual is not as perplexed about his situation as the amnesic person is, which makes travel to new areas and altered behavior appear more purposeful. It is not uncommon to find a history of heavy drug or alcohol use prior to the development of the disorder; substance abuse can be another attempt to escape. In those instances, the fugue state may consist only of purposeless wandering with recall rapidly returning within a few hours (American Psychiatric Association, 1987).

EPIDEMIOLOGY

Psychogenic fugue is common among people who have suffered through war or natural disaster, severe stresses (such as marital difficulties or rejection), or psychological trauma. Alcohol abuse can also be associated with psychogenic fugue (American Psychiatric Association, 1987). The individual may experience the fugue for a few hours or days, engaging in limited travel. On occasion, however, it may continue for months and involve extensive international travel (American Psychiatric Association, 1987).

ASSESSMENT OF PSYCHOGENIC FUGUE

The individual's mood varies from aloofness to intense feelings of distress and he may become violent. (See Chapter 24 on the violent patient.) The individual experiences the lack of recall and the acquisition of another identity. He may flee, traveling long distances. However, the individual's travel and behavior have an outward appearance of purpose.

A problem with identity disturbances occurs at the time of the fugue. Usually there is not a developmental history of identity disturbances. Psychogenic fugue and malingering (an intent to deceive by simulating symptoms) are difficult to differentiate. At times, it is almost impossible to discern the difference (American Psychiatric Association, 1987).

The Dissociative Experiences Scale (Box 17–3) can be used to assess for specific behaviors and thoughts associated with this disorder.

The intensity and duration of this disorder consist of rapid onset and spontaneous recovery. An individual usually has only one episode of psychogenic fugue.

The impact of the illness on the individual varies. In some instances, the individual appears to function relatively well; at other times, however, the individual is confused, perplexed, has disruption in interpersonal relationships, and is dysfunctional to the extent that his employment is interrupted in some way. The illness also has an impact on the family; family members might be separated from the individual for long periods. The anxiety and apprehension associated with not knowing the whereabouts of the individual with psychogenic fugue can be extremely painful. Frequently, the family members become involved with the legal and health care delivery system for the purpose of aiding their loved one.

NURSING DIAGNOSIS

Nursing diagnoses related to the symptoms of psychogenic fugue include:

Self-esteem disturbance

Coping, ineffective individual

Personal identity, disturbance in

Alteration in thought processes

Potential for violence: self-directed or directed at others

Impaired verbal communication

Anxiety

Ineffective family coping

Alteration in family processes

Social isolation

Additional nursing diagnoses related to psychogenic fugue include:

Fear

Body image disturbance

Sleep pattern disturbance

Potential for injury

Personal identity disturbance

The nurse should be aware of the many behaviors associated with these nursing diagnoses and plan interventions specific to the individual's overall clinical state.

PSYCHOGENIC AMNESIA

Psychogenic amnesia is the sudden inability to recall important personal information, when there is no organic disorder present (American Psychiatric Association, 1987). This type of amnesia generally follows psychic stress (as opposed to amnesia resulting from head trauma or epilepsy). Familiar examples include extreme marital difficulties, a broken love affair, an accident that has resulted in the fatality of a loved one, or financial ruin. The individual is faced with a situation that threatens some aspect of his self-view, security, and relationships. During combat, it is not uncommon for soldiers to have amnesia when they are unable to deal with the possibility of killing or being killed. Such a situation is viewed as traumatic and unexpected (Coons, 1984). Normal coping mechanisms fail. Even in situations such as divorce or bankruptcy, in which the "disaster" may have been anticipated, denial may have kept thoughts about the situation from the individual's conscious awareness; thus the individual experiences the traumatic event as unexpected.

An individual may first use denial to deal with a crisis; for example, he may say, "It didn't really happen." When the denial fails as a defense, the mind represses the incident itself as well as information about personal history and relationships. Thus amnesia occurs.

There are four types of disturbance in the individual's ability to recall:

1. Localized amnesia, which is the failure to recall all events surrounding a specified time period. This is the most common type of amnesia.

2. Selective amnesia, which is the failure to recall some specific events, while remembering others, during a circumscribed time period.

3. Generalized amnesia, which is the failure to recall events associated with the individual's entire life. This is relatively rare.

4. Continuous amnesia, which is the failure to recall events during a specific time period through the present (American Psychiatric Association, 1987).

Bill: A Patient with Localized Amnesia

Bill Ferucci, a 33-year-old unemployed laborer, left a job interview angry because he was not offered the job. As he got in his car and headed home, he continued to think about the interview; he did not notice that he sped into a school area at fifty miles per hour. His car hit a child as she stepped into the school crossing. When the police arrived, Bill appeared to be in a daze, unable to identify himself or recognize his surroundings. Later, when asked questions at the police station, he kept repeating, "I don't understand." Upon the request of his lawyer, Bill was admitted to a forensic unit at the state hospital, where he did the specific things he was directed to do, such as eating, bathing, and dressing; but he did them in a detached manner. He sat on his bed staring at the wall, without showing emotion. The nursing staff observed him carefully as he wandered aimlessly about his room and sometimes in the hallway. He was disoriented as to time and place. Two nights later he suddenly, screamed, "No, no, no," appearing near panic, frightened, and agitated. A television news program was on in the next room, and the staff speculated that Bill may have heard the reporter give an update on the accident that had killed the child. The next morning Bill was able to recall what had happened, and he acknowledged it with guilt, remorse, and considerable apprehension. In fact, the nurses instituted extensive safety precautions to protect Bill as his behavior approached near-panic states. In fact, he became extremely violent and verbalized his belief that death was "on its way."

Amnesia may be limited to a single event and the period during which the event took place. Or it may be selective, allowing the person to recall some, but not all, of the details. After a shooting accident, an individual may be able to recall a conversation that took place before the accident and recall telephoning for an ambulance, but not recall the incident itself.

More complete, but less frequent, manifestations of amnesia are generalized amnesia, encompassing all of a person's life, or continuous amnesia, wherein everything from a certain point up to and including the present is obliterated from memory.

Francine: A Patient with Generalized Amnesia

Francine LeMayne, a 20-year-old girl from a rural family, was engaged to marry a boy whom she had known all through school. She was not outgoing or assertive and relied upon her fiance to make decisions for both of them. Her thoughts and plans focused on being married. Her fiance left for college in the fall and returned at Christmas, telling Francine that he was in love with someone else. Francine retired to her room for several days, unwilling to eat, sleep, or speak to anyone. When she did come out, she was unkempt, had not attended to hygiene, and was unable to recognize any of her family members—she simply stared blankly at them. She was admitted to a hospital where she continued to say, "I don't know," when asked about her past. Over a period of several weeks her memory returned in fragments, thus enabling her to recall events that had led to her amnesia.

All of us have some lack of recall of events in our lives, particularly of those that took place between ages three and six (Cameron, 1963). However, a person with amnesia does not have normal conscious recall.

During an amnesic episode, the individual looks and acts perplexed and is disoriented with regard to time, place, and person. Short amnesic episodes are an attempt to defend the self, and recall returns completely when there no longer seems to be a threat.

EPIDEMIOLOGY

Onset of psychogenic amnesia usually takes place during adolescence and young adulthood. It is most common among males in the military, during combat. Little information is available regarding the economic class of these patients. Patients from high socioeconomic groups tend to remain in therapy longer and have greater access to care than patients from the lower classes. Individuals in higher socioeconomic groups are also more likely to be diagnosed as having psychogenic fugue and depersonalization disorders. As a rule, people in lower socioeconomic groups are less frequently identified and treated. Such an individual will probably manifest florid symptoms before intervention by health care professionals occurs. Individuals from both groups may experience spontaneous recovery and never receive professional care for this disorder.

Life events triggering psychogenic amnesia include traumatic events such as seeing one's family and property destroyed by natural disaster or war, and personal events associated with internal feelings of guilt, shame, and anger such as being mugged or raped.

ASSESSMENT OF PSYCHOGENIC AMNESIA

The mood of the individual with psychogenic amnesia ranges from feelings of unrealness and indifference to bewilderment. Cognitive changes are evident in the individual's memory disturbances. Prior to the onset of amnesia, behaviors may consist of stupor or a "twilight-like" state which is a disturbance of consciousness during which time the patient may perform behaviors that appear to be outside of conscious volition. As a rule, he has no recall of these behaviors. The nurse may observe that the patient is acting abnormally. She might also observe that the patient is frightened and/or anxious (Kolb & Brodie, 1982).

Episodes of psychogenic amnesia are usually of short duration and they seldom reoccur. During a period of amnesia, the individual may feel perplexed and upset about not being able to recall what he wants to recall. He may also experience disorientation about time, place, and identity. The individual's aimless wandering, failure to recall events, and disorientation can be extremely upsetting to family members.

NURSING DIAGNOSIS

In addition to the nursing diagnoses identified for psychogenic fugue, the following are presented for use with psychogenic amnesia:

Ineffective family coping: compromised

Ineffective family coping: disabling

Family coping: potential for growth

Alteration in comfort

Dysfunctional grieving

Potential for injury

Disturbance in role performance

Knowledge deficit, lack of recall

DEPERSONALIZATION

During **depersonalization,** an individual's sense of self is altered, and he perceives parts of his body as increased or decreased in size or altered in form. Depersonalization also often involves the experience of being outside of one's own body, watching as an observer. Depersonalization can serve as a defense mechanism, protecting an individual's sense of self through detachment from an emotion, idea, or feeling. This "splitting off" of part of the ego produces a sense of alienation from the self or the environment, creating feelings of depersonalization (Munster, 1979).

Sally: A Patient Who Experienced Depersonalization

Sally, an 18-year-old patient, struggled to be accepted by her peers and sought an explanation for her discomfort with others. She attributed her discomfort to her weight. Upon leaving home for college, Sally's anxiety around others increased. On the day Sally was to attend a coffee at a sorority that she wanted to join, Sally noticed that her reflection in the mirror appeared grossly distorted. In fact, her face looked to be protracted and tilted to the right.

Depersonalization can have a multisensory impact; a person's visual, auditory, and olfactory perceptions can be influenced. While this experience may seem similar to a hallucination, a real hallucination occurs without external stimuli (Barile, 1984) and depersonalization involves a sense of unreality about the environment (Lego, 1984).

Most individuals who experience depersonalization have a sense of panic and fear that they are becoming psychotic and experience feelings different from any they have had in the past. During the depersonalization episode, the individual often experiences time as either accelerated or slowed dramatically, perhaps even standing still. It has been estimated that up to seventy percent of young adults experience depersonalization at least briefly at some time (American Psychiatric Association, 1987).

The individual experiencing depersonalization feels a loss of control over his own body and thoughts. Frequently, he experiences related physical symptoms at the time of depersonalization, including feeling faint, becoming anxious, or having temporary difficulty with recall and routine motor functions such as walking and talking. The individual may even attempt suicide due to the panic as a result of the experience (Sullivan, 1953). When the individual reaches this state of panic, the dissociation has, in fact, resulted in temporary psychosis (Arieti, 1955).

One episode (a one-time experience) of depersonalization does not necessarily mean that an individual has a dissociative disorder. For depersonalization to meet the criteria for a diagnosis of a dissociative disorder, there must be significant impairment in social or occupational functioning (American Psychiatric Association, 1987), and it must not be secondary to any other disorder. (See DSM-III Box.)

When depersonalization is associated with a major psychotic disorder such as schizophrenia, a mood disorder, or a personality disorder, the depersonalization is not viewed as a separate disorder, but as a symptom of the primary disorder. Minor episodes of depersonalization may occur when an individual is faced with life-threatening events or extreme anxiety.

Lauren: A Young Patient with Cancer

Lauren Geeson, a 24-year-old college student, was told that metastatic cancer was found in her body during a routine physical examination. Ordinarily quite emotional, Lauren's reaction to the illness was completely calm, and she went on with life and waited for surgery as if it were utterly routine. After her surgery, Lauren described the period of time beforehand: "It was as if it were happening to someone else; it wasn't really me."

EPIDEMIOLOGY

Depersonalization usually occurs during adolescence and young adulthood. In fact, it seldom occurs after age forty. Impairment may range from minimal to severe. Life events that precipitate depersonalization include disaster, military combat, auto accidents, threat to body image, and so forth. The personality characteristics of an individual with depersonalization are trait anxiety and extreme or unusual fear of the unknown.

The prevalence of this disorder is increasing, as approximately seventy percent of the young adult population may experience a single brief episode of depersonalization (American Psychiatric Association, 1987).

ASSESSMENT OF DEPERSONALIZATION

The mood of the individual with this disorder is likely to include depression, anxiety, and a general sense of bewilderment. The cognitive changes include a slowness in and difficulty with recall, and the individual may seem confused. The course of the illness

**DSM-III-R
Diagnostic Criteria for
Depersonalization
Disorder**

A. Persistent or recurrent experiences of depersonalization as indicated by either (1) or (2):

1) an experience of feeling detached from, and as if one is an outside observer of, one's mental processes or body

2) an experience of feeling like an automaton or as if in a dream

B. During the depersonalization experience, reality testing remains intact.

C. The depersonalization is sufficiently severe and persistent to cause marked distress.

D. The depersonalization experience is the predominant disturbance and is not a symptom of another disorder, such as schizophrenia, panic disorder, or agoraphobia without history of panic disorder but with limited symptom attacks of depersonalization, or temporal lobe epilepsy.

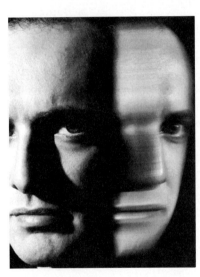

Diagnostic criteria for depersonalization disorder include persistent or recurrent experiences of depersonalization, where an individual experiences feelings of detachment from himself and his world. The person feels as if he is an outside observer, whereby his feelings and actions are isolated from his body.

is primarily chronic with periods of remission and exacerbation. The impact on the individual can be severe. Feelings of physical pain, losing control, anxiety, and depression are common. The individual may also experience distortion of common objects in the environment, which can be frightening.

The family observes impairment in interpersonal relationships and, on occasion, loss of employment; a general and slow deterioration of the family relationship with the individual occurs.

NURSING DIAGNOSIS

Additional nursing diagnoses for depersonalization include:

Impaired social interaction

Powerlessness

Sensory perceptual alterations: visual, auditory, kinesthetic

Sensory, perceptual alterations in

Sleep, visual, auditory pattern disturbance

Impaired physical mobility

Potential for injury

Ineffective individual coping

Family coping: potential for growth

Diversional activity deficit

Altered role performance

DISORDERS NOT CLASSIFIED ELSEWHERE

Most of the dissociative disorders have clearly defined symptomatology that is distinct for each specific disorder. Occasionally, there is evidence of dissociation that does not fit the criteria of a disorder. Ganser's syndrome,[1] trance states, derealization without depersonalization, and dissociative states associated with intense coercive acts such as brainwashing are all disorders in this category (American Psychiatric Association, 1987). Individuals who are held captive (such as prisoners of war), who have had intensive indoctrination (such as cult members), or who have unknown outcomes to their circumstances and minimal room for individual differences are likely to experience these types of disorders. Veterans returning from combat have reported episodes of flashback in which they awake from sleep with the sense that their nightmares are real. Post-traumatic stress disorders have also been identified with dissociative episodes (Coons, 1984).

Derealization frequently accompanies depersonalization and is characterized by a perception that the external environment has changed or become unreal. The patient will describe perceptions that indicate objects in the environment have changed in size and shape; the individual might also think that others have become unreal (Coons, 1986b; Nathan & Harris, 1980).

THEORIES OF DISSOCIATIVE DISORDERS

PSYCHOANALYTIC/PSYCHODYNAMIC THEORIES

Dissociation is one of an infant's earliest attempts at adaptation, that is, the infant learns to "ward off" his impulses and instinctual needs as he realizes that all of these needs will not be fulfilled immediately by others in the external environment. Dissociation, then, is closely allied with the development of the self-image system. The **self-image system** is that part of the personality born out of the influences of significant others on a person's feelings of well-being (Sullivan, 1954). All anti-anxiety defenses are security operations employed to protect that self-image system (Sullivan, 1954), and dissociation is one such defense. Psychoanalytic theory (Erickson, 1963; Jacobson, 1964; Mahler, 1968; Spitz, 1965) purports that the infant's development of a sense of self is di-

rectly influenced by interactions between the infant and primary care provider.

It is within the parent-child relationship that the child develops many of the values and beliefs that form his self-image system. The parental values and beliefs assumed by the child (Brenner, 1955) form the basis for the child's superego development, that is, the child learns behaviors accepted by family and society. For instance, if the parent conveys that it is wrong to curse or to hit another person, the child integrates that belief and sees those behaviors as bad, feeling guilty if he behaves contrary to what is viewed as good.

A discussion of the development of the superego requires an understanding of four basic terms: internalization, introjection, incorporation, and identification. These four terms are frequently used interchangeably in the psychiatric literature. Yet this usage is not correct, as these terms present different concepts (Bellak, Hurvick, & Gediman, 1973).

Internalization, the most general of the four concepts, describes the processes an individual utilizes when transforming real or imaginary interactions that occur in the external environment into inner guidelines, regulations, and self-governance mechanisms.

Introjection is a type of internalization, in which objects loved or hated are symbolically encompassed by the self. In fact, the individual places in his ego structure the pictures (mental images) as he envisions these objects (persons) really are. Hence, a person who introjects behaves toward these images as if they (the images) were the individual. This is an internal mental process.

Incorporation is a process in which an idea is not separated or differentiated from an act or deed. The individual indiscriminately takes a part or all of another person or thing and uses its components to gratify and/or upset his own impulses, sensations, feelings, and thoughts. This defense mechanism is considered to be relatively primitive in nature.

Identification refers to that process in which a person modifies his behavior in an effort to design himself after another person whom he admires, holds in high esteem, and wishes to use as a model for himself.

Most individuals with dissociative disorders have not been parented by people who manifested consistency in feelings, thoughts, values, mores, behaviors, and expectations. Thus the individual's introjection consists of conflicting feelings, thoughts, values, mores, behaviors, and expectations. These incongruities are hidden deep within the unconscious but are

---

[1]This is a relatively rare disorder; it is, however, frequently observed in prisoners. Its outstanding feature is the patient's incorrect and/or ridiculous reply. The patient might appear disoriented in time and place, but general behaviors indicate that he is alert and not confused (Kaplan & Sadock, 1985).

often expressed despite the psyche's struggle to seal them off. With a weak underpinning in which conflicts abound, the habitual defenses that the individual employs to avoid the most intense and difficult conflicts are more vulnerable. Under stress, the entire system of the ego's defense mechanisms is threatened, and the formation of dissociative symptoms is often the result.

Because dissociation is closely allied with the concept of the self, the development of the child's self-system is quite important. The period of infancy, with particular emphasis on the first eighteen months of life, is crucial to the formation of the self and influences whether or not the child will emerge with an integrated identity or a fragmented or only partially formed identity (Jacobson, 1964; Kernberg, 1975; Mahler, 1968; Spitz, 1965; and Sullivan, 1954). The parent-child relationship that leads to normal development is one that is mutually gratifying, with the child feeling adequately secure, able to trust, and relatively free of anxiety. With adequate parenting, the child is able to form a sense of self and others as good *and* bad, as well as a sense of things identified as *outside* of himself (Sullivan, 1954).

The child first identifies with attitudes and values of important others, such as parents, which are communicated through verbal and nonverbal interactions. Since the child is exposed to more than one experience with more than one person, there are multiple identifications, and the child experiences many overlapping self-images (Cameron, 1963). For example, a girl's relationship with her mother may foster an identification as "mommy's little helper," with the older brother it may be as a "tomboy," and with father it may be as "daddy's little girl." This process begins in infancy but continues through adulthood when the child's sense of self-unity and identity are more solid (Cameron, 1963).

Along with self-views, the child takes in images of significant others in relation to himself (Kohut, 1971). For example, a child may have one image of mother as a punitive figure and another image of her as a loving, nuturing figure. The conflict can create ambivalence within the child. Based in part on introjects, the images the child incorporates into his self-concept are what he perceives to be the expectations from others. Since the child relies heavily upon identification with significant others to gain a sense of self, he might experience blurring and uncertainty about which feelings, beliefs, and values belong to others and which belong to him. For example, if a parent is grieving over the loss of a friend, the child

(at about age three and upward) may take on the grief and experience it with intensity, even though he did not have a personal attachment to the parent's friend.

For the infant, dissociation is developmentally appropriate. It serves as a defense against anxiety and protects the developing self-system (Sullivan, 1954) by separating some parts of the self from other people (Cameron, 1963). The child's need to use dissociation decreases as he develops a more stable sense of self. Normal dissociation includes the process of **splitting,** in which the child views a person (such as a parent) as "all good" or "all bad" (Kernberg, 1976). However, if the splitting becomes extreme (if it continues into adulthood), the adult individual will have problems integrating identifications that he has taken on from others, which may put him at risk for the development of dissociative disorders (Blanck & Blanck, 1974). (Also see Chapter 12 on personality disorders.)

Since splitting and dissociation occur primarily in situations in which an individual perceives conflict or threat, he is often able to perform satisfactorily in conflict-free situations. To the casual observer there may be little evidence that problems exist. As a child, the individual may have been quiet, shy, clinging, fearful of others, and perhaps slow to learn. In addition, such children often engage in fantasy more than other children. Through fantasy, all children try on roles by pretending they are someone admired or that they have special relationships with their idols. From the variety of roles taken on through fantasy, children select some attributes to adapt to and incorporate into their own lives. Through pretending, children engage in attempts at problem solving. They can try out options and alternatives to a situation. They can reenact a situation so that it has a happier ending or better meets their emotional needs. For example, a little girl may in fantasy take on a parental role with her doll by reenacting a situation in which she was reprimanded. In pretending, dissociation of what is unacceptable about oneself and others occurs as the dissociated part is projected onto fantasy playmates or toys. This process occurs primarily in children between the ages of three and six, after which there is an abatement in this type of pretending. In a smaller percentage of children, the phenomenon may continue indefinitely.

The child with a fragile integration of self and poor ego boundaries may have trouble distinguishing between reality and imagination. When a child spends a lot of time alone and experiences isolation and loneliness, fantasy characters take on a greater sense of reality. Later, the child may use fantasy to substitute more and more for reality until eventually he has difficulty distinguishing between what is real and what is fantasy.

Some fantasy contains elements of denial. For instance, the ten-year-old girl who feels clumsy, awkward, and without social skills can deny those feelings while fantasizing that she is a popular dancer who is adored by her public. Her fantasy is pleasurable, and during the fantasy those aspects of herself that she doesn't like and that she denies are split off.

When the child substitutes fantasy for reality to the extent that the boundaries between the two become blurred, denial and vertical splitting continue as defenses, and denied aspects of the self are often projected onto real or imaginary persons and thus disowned as part of oneself. For example, a lonely eight-year-old girl who is sexually abused by her father and ignored by her mother may find escape in a fantasy in which she has loving parents and in which she transfers her feelings of guilt and anxiety to a younger sister whom she berates and gets into trouble.

The predisposition to later dissociative episodes is often rooted in the developmental period between ages one and a half and three and a half, in which the child attempts **separation-individuation** (Mahler, 1968). During the period of development, there may be traumatic events that result in either a real loss of a parenting figure or a loss in the parent's emotional availability to the child. Since the parenting relationship is central to the child's movement toward ego integration, without consistency the child may be forced either to substitute significant others in the environment or uses splitting and dissociation in order to cope.

Cindy: A Child Who Lost Her Mother

Cindy, a five-year-old child, was sent to live with her aunt and uncle when her mother was hospitalized for heart surgery. Cindy's mother died, and the arrangement with the aunt and uncle became permanent. Cindy withdrew from her friends, spending more and more time alone in her room. Cindy's aunt overheard her with her dolls, telling the dolls, "Mommy left because you were bad; but don't worry. I still love you and will take care of you."

The frightened, dependent part of Cindy's self was dissociated, split off from herself, and projected onto her dolls.

Once the child is past the separation-individuation stage of development, the use of dissociation usually diminishes and is replaced by other defense mechanisms, such as repression, sublimation, and displacement. Incidents that occur later in a person's life, however, may arouse old feelings that can precipitate a regression to the point where the person again uses the dissociative process.

Cindy: Grown Up

Cindy finished high school and entered her first year of college. Following an auto accident, she was hospitalized for injuries. This was the first time she had been to a hospital since her mother died. She was flooded with memories of her mother's death and feelings of abandonment, grief, and fear that she had experienced when she was five years old. She found relief from her severe anxiety by fantasizing herself as two different persons, talking to each other, one an older figure very much like herself offering words of comfort to a six-year-old version of herself, very much as she had comforted her dolls.

EGO STATES AND EGO FUNCTIONS. It is helpful to understand how **ego states** and **ego functions** relate to dissociative disorders. Watkins (1978, p. 525) defines ego states as "a body of behaviors and experiences psychologically bound together by some common principle and separated from other such states by a boundary, which is more or less permeable." Ego states can be likened to roles or moods wherein a person may have different feelings, experiences, and behaviors at different times, depending on the situation. For instance, a young woman may be flirtatious, daring, and intent upon having fun at a party, yet at work she may be serious, cautious, and task oriented. The boundaries between the different ego states are not rigidly set, and she is aware that she is the same person in one situation that she is in the other. The individual with a dissociative disorder also has different ego states, but they have the quality of being different identities. For instance, a patient with multiple personalities unconsciously assigns a different personality to each ego state. The business woman who conducts a successful fund drive for a local charity is separate from the woman who is timid in social situations with men and is separate from the frightened child within herself when her supervisor criticizes the way she carries out certain tasks on the job. The ego defenses of denial, repression, and splitting sharply differentiate one ego state from another to the point where there may be a complete lack of awareness of the split that has occurred.

Assessment of ego functioning provides a clinical framework for evaluation and description of the degree to which the functioning of the ego is adaptive to reality. Viewed on a continuum, the individual can be assessed for strength or weakness in each of twelve categories (Bellak, Hurvick, & Gediman, 1973). (See Chapter 5 on assessment.) Dissociative episodes can occur when there is a relative weakness in specific areas. For example, a fugue state may be exhibited when there is a disturbance in an individual's synthetic-integrative functioning (Webster, 1984a). Dissociative episodes are fleeting for the emotionally healthy individual and are related directly to a major life crisis, such as major surgery. Transient dissociative episodes can also occur at times when a person is extremely fatigued and suffering from emotional stress. However, unlike the individual with a dissociative disorder, these brief episodes disappear in a healthy person when the crisis is past (Kolb, 1973).

BEHAVIORAL THEORY

Psychoanalytic theories suggest that dissociative behaviors occur outside of the individual's awareness, that he has little control over these behaviors, and that these internal forces he experiences are powerful and all-encompassing. Conversely, behavioral theory suggests that behavioral response patterns depend on conditions or events in the environment. Furthermore, psychological functioning depends on interactions between environmental conditions and the individual (Bandura, 1969).

In his early work, Bandura suggested that observations of certain behaviors provide a model for the observer. (See the case of Audrey H., page 647.) Hence, an individual exposed to specific behaviors could acquire new response patterns to similar situations (Bandura & Walters, 1963; Nathan & Harris, 1980). Bandura further hypothesized that behavioral change occurs in two basic ways: 1) through changes in thought processes, the cornerstone from which behaviors are formulated, and 2) through learning by doing, the most effective method of effecting psychological change (Bandura, 1977).

Kohlenberg (1973) and Price and Hess (1979) reported the use of behavioral theory in the conceptualization and treatment of dissociative disorders in general and in multiple personality in particular. Kohlenberg wrote that individuals with dissociative disorders have learned their specific behaviors from others in their environment, have responded to a variety of personalities, and have learned how to manipulate their environment through the use of these behavioral patterns.

BIOLOGICAL THEORIES

Little evidence has been found of a link between biological determinants and dissociative disorders. However, one possible link may involve increased autonomic nervous system activity. It is also thought that brain function may be impaired in individuals with dissociative disorders. Brown (1981) has written that among right-handed individuals, the left hemisphere of the brain is dominant for verbal, logical processes and controls cognitive functions, while the right hemisphere of the brain is dominant for spatial processing and affective functioning. Galin (1974) has proposed that a disparate functioning between the left and right cerebral hemispheres of the brain in patients with dissociative disorders needs to be better integrated. Galin also suggests that among normal individuals, a functional disconnection between the left and right hemispheres might occur if the neural transmission across the corpus callosum is inhibited. Electroencephalographic findings of different dissociative states suggest a relationship between arousal and information input (West, 1967). In fact, multiple personalities in the same individual have produced different electroencephalographic results as well as different alpha-blocking and cortical-evoked responses (Ludwig, 1983).

THERAPIES FOR TREATING DISSOCIATIVE DISORDERS

Psychodynamic psychotherapy is the preferred modality for treatment of dissociative disorders. However, behavioral and biological approaches are also used (Maxmen, 1986; Kluft, 1982; Coons, 1986a, 1986b). (See Box 17–5.)

MULTIPLE PERSONALITY

PSYCHOANALYTIC/PSYCHODYNAMIC THERAPY. Because of the variety of symptoms that an individual with multiple personality can present, a diagnosis is usually based on the combination of detailed history, the results of interviewing the patient under hypnosis, and the administration of sodium amytal.

Box 17–5 ● The Perceptual Alteration Scale (PAS)

The following statements have been put together because we think they may provide information about a phenomenon which can be considered common and very normal in many cases, unusual in others, but which happens to most people at some time.

It is difficult to get honest reports on how often behaviors such as these occur in normal people, because these behaviors are very personal and not often spoken about. For this reason you are being asked to take this Scale seriously and respond to the sentences truthfully by circling the appropriate number. It is important that your answer describes experiences which have happened spontaneously in the natural course of living, and not as a result of hypnosis, drugs, or an experiment.

Please respond to every statement.

	NEVER	SOMETIMES	OFTEN	ALMOST ALWAYS
1. I feel as though things were not real.	1	2	3	4
2. I can't understand why I can get so cross and grouchy.	1	2	3	4
3. I feel out of touch with my body.	1	2	3	4
4. I automatically consume large amounts of food.	1	2	3	4
5. I find I cannot sit still.	1	2	3	4
6. I have fits of laughing and crying that I cannot control.	1	2	3	4
7. When I get tired or upset it seems like an outside force comes in to control my actions.	1	2	3	4
8. My body is too heavy.	1	2	3	4
9. I find myself in situations in which I do not wish to be.	1	2	3	4
10. I feel compelled to eat even when I am not hungry.	1	2	3	4
11. I feel hate toward members of my family whom I usually love.	1	2	3	4
12. My mind wants one thing but my body is determined to do another.	1	2	3	4
13. I am not aware of the passage of time.	1	2	3	4
14. I find myself doing several things at once.	1	2	3	4
15. I really enjoy eating alone.	1	2	3	4
16. It has been impossible for me to keep from stealing or shoplifting something.	1	2	3	4
17. In some situations my mind and my self just are not "together."	1	2	3	4
18. My moods can really change.	1	2	3	4
19. I have had periods in which I carried on activities without knowing what I had been doing.	1	2	3	4
20. I forget right away what people say to me.	1	2	3	4
21. If I am really set on doing something offbeat I can somehow make reality disappear.	1	2	3	4

	NEVER	SOMETIMES	OFTEN	ALMOST ALWAYS
22. I have had blank spells in which my activities were interrupted and I did not know what was going on around me.	1	2	3	4
23. I find myself concealing my activities from others.	1	2	3	4
24. I am glad that I can forget what I look like.	1	2	3	4
25. I do many things which I regret afterwards (I regret things more or more often than others seem to).	1	2	3	4
26. When eating, I read or watch television.	1	2	3	4
27. What my body is doing has nothing to do with "me."	1	2	3	4
28. I wake up and find that several days have passed.	1	2	3	4
29. Without any reason or even when things are going wrong I feel excitedly happy, "on top of the world."	1	2	3	4
30. I don't know how to stop myself from doing something.	1	2	3	4
31. I find myself in a strange place without knowing how I got there.	1	2	3	4
32. I find myself torn between doing one thing or another.	1	2	3	4
33. I find myself doing things without knowing why.	1	2	3	4
34. I feel compelled to think and act in a way that is out of character for me.	1	2	3	4
35. Bad words, often terrible words, come into my mind and I cannot get rid of them.	1	2	3	4
36. I find myself watching my every move.	1	2	3	4
37. Even when I have missed several meals I find that I am not hungry.	1	2	3	4
38. I find my mind blank.	1	2	3	4
39. I have one or more bad habits which are so strong that it is no use in fighting against them.	1	2	3	4
40. I find myself in social situations that I prefer to avoid.	1	2	3	4
41. When I go to sleep I find it easy to shut out external noise.	1	2	3	4
42. I have felt out of control.	1	2	3	4
43. I feel compelled to exercise much of the time.	1	2	3	4
44. Time passes so quickly when driving.	1	2	3	4
45. When driving, I have passed the street I meant to turn off on.	1	2	3	4

continued

	NEVER	SOMETIMES	OFTEN	ALMOST ALWAYS
46. When I eat I am aware of every bite.	1	2	3	4
47. After eating, I find it difficult to keep my food down.	1	2	3	4
48. I lose track of time.	1	2	3	4
49. I want to do two conflicting things at once and find myself arguing with myself.	1	2	3	4
50. I feel that my mind is divided.	1	2	3	4
51. I find I can tune out unpleasant sounds.	1	2	3	4
52. I have to pretend that I remember things.	1	2	3	4
53. I feel that there are two of me.	1	2	3	4
54. I do things without thinking.	1	2	3	4
55. I am not aware that I am eating.	1	2	3	4
56. In the middle of an activity, my mind goes blank.	1	2	3	4
57. I find that I have hidden something but don't know why.	1	2	3	4
58. I find myself more aware of pain than other people.	1	2	3	4
59. I do not notice the cold even when there are goosebumps.	1	2	3	4
60. I see myself differently than other people see me.	1	2	3	4

Perceptual Alteration Scale

The **Perceptual Alteration Scale (PAS)** was initially developed to discern dissociative behaviors among individuals who exhibited binge eating patterns (Sanders, 1986). The **PAS** utilizes a Likert-type scale on a continuum of 1 to 4: 1 represents those behaviors which rarely appear; 4 denotes those behaviors which occur frequently. The higher the **PAS** score, the greater the chances that the individual is exhibiting some sort of dissociative behavior. It is important to note that although this scale was initially developed to examine dissociative behaviors among individuals from a select population (eating disorders), Sanders (1986) has determined that this instrument can be advantageous in both clinical and research settings.

Source: Sanders, S. (1986). The perceptual alteration scale: A pilot study of a scale of dissociation. The University of North Carolina, Chapel Hill, North Carolina.

The sodium amytal or sodium pentothal interview is also known as **narcotherapy.** It consists of injecting intravenously 0.2 to 0.5 grams of the drug in a five to ten percent solution into the patient's vein. The drug induces relaxation and facilitates communication so that repressed memories, controlled affects, and conflicts can more easily be expressed by the patient (Campbell, 1981; Coons, 1986b). The patient undergoing narcotherapy should be observed closely for adverse reactions such as airway compromise or a psychotic reaction.

The patient may be hospitalized on a psychiatric unit for several reasons, the most common being suicidal behavior and/or poor impulse control on the

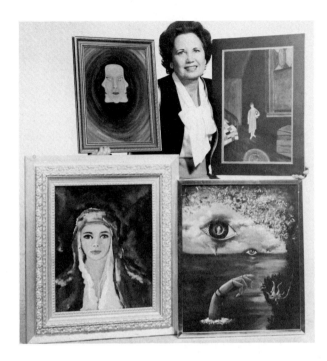
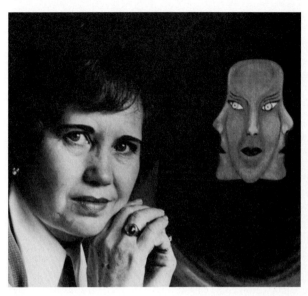

The "Three Faces of Eve," Chris Sizemore, displays some of her artwork which was completed during various phases in her treatment.

part of one or more of the personalities (Kluft, 1984b). (Suicidal ideation may result from illogical reasoning by one personality that "killing off" another would be a solution to dealing with "badness.") Increased anxiety or depression, fugue states, inappropriate behavior, or violence may also precipitate hospitalization (Kluft, 1984b). The patient may also be admitted on a nonemergency basis when a structured environment is needed for specific procedures such as hypnosis.

Hospitalization is usually brief, with the patient returning to outpatient therapy as soon as possible. In the rare instance when the patient is hospitalized for a longer period of time, it is essential that the treatment team have a well-formulated treatment plan and that the nursing care plan be congruent with that overall plan. (See the nursing care plan for Kay, p. 654.)

During the treatment, when conflicts and anxieties are being explored, it is not uncommon for the patient to have numerous physical complaints. Headaches, duodenal ulcers, tachycardia, back pain, and dysmenorrhea are common complaints. Because these complaints need to be managed medically and in keeping with the overall goals of treatment, a primary physician should be a part of the treatment team. This physician needs to have not only open communications with the psychiatrist, the nurse, and other members of the team, but also must have some un-

derstanding of the dynamics of multiple personality and the other types of dissociative disorders.

Numerous complications exist in the treatment process for multiple personality. Each personality has its own set of defense mechanisms in addition to the predominant one of dissociation. IQ test results vary according to the personality being tested. Psychological testing is of little help because a distinct personality does not emerge. The hostile personality can be lethal; the childlike personality can be seductive. Cues that suggest multiple personality disorder include changes in handwriting, time distortions or time lapses, amnesia about certain behavior or events, a report from others of noticeable changes, the use of "we" in speaking of oneself, a new possession that cannot be accounted for, headaches prior to a sudden behavioral change, and a report of hearing voices from within (Coons, 1980).

Depending on the specific personality being addressed in the individual, the patient may react to the therapist in different ways and the range of expressed behaviors and emotions can be wide. Hostile feelings can create murderous rage, and feelings of love can provoke behaviors of sympathy, caring, and protection. It is not uncommon, therefore, to observe that the patient has a chaotic and fluctuating relationship with the therapist.

The numerous personalities create havoc and crises through their attempts to control, sabotage, embarrass, abandon, and annihilate each other. Suicidal, homicidal, and other self-defeating behaviors enacted by an alternate personality can create crises through the expression of desires or through an altercation with one of the other personalities.

In treatment, the patient must come to terms with the alternate personalities (often called "alters") and hence with the internal conflicts that have given rise to them. The personalities have to be dealt with for the purpose of effecting compromise, cooperation, and synthesis. Although treatment, by its very nature, can create a crisis by disturbing an existing equilibrium and compromise among the personalities, the conflicts and dissociative experiences must be revealed to be treated.

The transference between patient and therapist is likely to change drastically as the therapist encounters each different personality. In fact, the transference may have to be "reestablished" each time the therapist works with the different personalities. Simultaneously, the therapist must be on the alert for countertransference. For example, the therapist may find herself relating (feeling, thinking, verbalizing, and responding) to each of the multiple personalities in a very different fashion, as the patient reveals them. In addition, her feelings can be numerous: anger, fascination, disbelief, exhaustion, confusion, and perplexity. Supervision for the psychiatric nurse or other therapist is essential.

Contracting with the patient is a useful therapeutic endeavor. The therapist should consider asking each alter to promise not to harm himself, others who exist within the patient's personality, and others external to the individual. The contract is linked to a specific time frame, for example, the therapist might ask the alters to agree not to harm the dominant personality, commit murder, become involved in child abuse, ingest large amounts of drugs, and so forth until the next session. A designated time period is helpful, especially if the patient is being treated in an outpatient facility. The designation of a time provides structure for the patient in an incremental and sequential fashion. These patients can be seen in therapy two and three times each week. They require close supervision because of their depressive tendencies and impulse-control problems. If a contract cannot be developed, then the patient should be placed in a secure environment such as a residential facility where controls can be provided.

In addition to being aware of problems with transference and countertransference, the therapist must be especially watchful of the following factors: patient response to suicidal ideation and behaviors; rejection by family and friends; the coexistence of two or more competing personalities; depression; fugue, amnesia, and switching of mood states and psychosis.

Coons (1986a) has described three phases in treatment therapy.

Phase One: Trust is the most important element in this phase of treatment. Factors that inhibit the establishment of trust include previous maltreatment of the individual during the formative years. In addition, there is usually a history of misdiagnosis and a tendency for therapists in the patient's past not to have believed the patient, to have thought he was fantasizing or lying about the abuse he'd suffered. The therapist must establish communication with all of the personalities, developing an understanding of their names, functions, behaviors, problems, and relationships to the other existing personalities. She establishes contracts with each of the personalities so that they do not act out against each other. In fact, a crisis might occur when alters threaten harmful acts such as child abuse, prostitution, murder, theft, and so forth. When these situations occur, the therapist must make it clear that such anticipated actions are unacceptable. The therapist must also communicate with the alters that they will be held responsible for their actions. The therapist must make it very clear that she will fulfill her obligation to the patient, and society, and practice in an ethical fashion (Kluft, 1983). The process might take several months.

Phase Two: This phase might extend over a period of several years. The primary focus of treatment is working with the original personality and the multiples. Those components of the original personality such as anger, rage, depression, aggression, and sexuality are treated. Treatment explores traumas that occurred during the developmental years.

Phase Three: This final phase focuses on the integration of all personalities. This is an arduous process. Moreover, the therapist must facilitate the patient's acceptance of and comfort with the "new self," with its different coping mechanisms and defenses.

HYPNOTHERAPY. Hypnosis is another method of treating multiple personality. As with narcotherapy, during hypnosis the patient's conscious mind is relaxed, and the therapist can more easily gain access to the "alters." Kluft (1983) has suggested that because individuals with multiple personality experience numerous crises in their lives, they will benefit from hypnotherapy. Several factors contribute to crises among multiple personality individuals, who tend to have depressive and masochistic features.

First, they have discontinuous memories—this deprives them of ongoing information about themselves and events in the environment. The individuals may also split off undesirable situations and not acknowledge a problem or crisis.

Second, they lack situational support from individuals in the environment. They often become isolated and estranged from family and friends or remain in pathological family relationships which hinder personal growth and development.

Third, they rely on a limited variety of coping or defense mechanisms. During a crisis, when these mechanisms are employed and fail the individuals withdraw, leaving themselves vulnerable to the personalities (alters) (Kluft, 1983).

BEHAVIORAL THERAPY. Although psychoanalytic/psychodynamic therapy is the preferred treatment for multiple personality, Caddy (1985) described behavioral therapy treatment of a patient with multiple personality. The approach is used frequently with depressed and severely anxious multiple personality patients.

The case of Audrey H. is presented (Caddy, 1985) as "the first successful cognitive behavioral treatment of multiple personality," (page 267). Briefly, Audrey H., a 29-year-old college student with two children, separated from her husband, sought therapy from her former teacher through his private practice. She complained of feeling as if she was going crazy, being "wacked out" on medications, suffering chest pain, depression, and anxiety. Audrey H. reported having been involved with more than 100 men in a six-year period.

Specific components in her therapeutic program included assessment, selection of treatment, and course of treatment. Each of the components will be briefly discussed here.

ASSESSMENT. The behavioral therapist became knowledgeable about the characteristics and behavioral patterns of Audrey's numerous personalities (alters).

Audrey was taking prescribed lorazepam (Ativan). She was administered the Minnesota Multiphasic Personality Inventory and the Thematic Apperception Test; these data along with continuous observation of her emotional state provided the assessment material that assisted in understanding her cognitions.

SELECTION OF TREATMENT. Audrey's dissociative process was conceptualized in a behavioral perspective that suggested that the multiple states of disruption representing distortions, confusion, and amorphous cognition coexisted within; thus, the patient experienced difficulties in interpersonal relationships. A program was implemented that highlighted "behavioral/interpersonal competence" and the integration of the various alters. Multiple Personality diagnosis requires that subpersonalities have a rich, unified, and relatively stable life of their own (Taylor & Martin, 1944).

COURSE OF TREATMENT. Audrey H. was prescribed a psychotropic medication at minimum dosage. Audrey and the behavioral therapist jointly developed four goals: 1) the therapy will be built on an honest and respectful relationship between Audrey H. and the behavioral therapist; 2) Audrey will decrease anxiety and tension by learning progressive relaxation and biofeedback methods; 3) Audrey will use imaginative and systematic desensitization to overcome her fears and phobias; 4) Audrey will learn effective assertive techniques to aid in her interpersonal relationships.

The therapist reported that Audrey showed slow but continuous progress toward goal attainment (Caddy, 1985).

Kohlenberg (1973) also used behavioral therapy with a patient diagnosed with multiple personality. In the treatment of a 51-year-old man with three personalities, Kohlenberg established a base line, contingencies, and extinction phase of therapy. He classified responses to a predetermined set of questions as belonging to the patient's high (aggressive, destructive activity), middle (relaxed and well-socialized), or low (depressed mood, slow speech and movements) personality. The investigator concluded that the three personalities either increased or decreased in frequency of expression (as seen in behaviors manifested by patient) depending on environmental contingencies such as tokens, touch, and nothing. Kohlenberg found that the occurrence of each personality was a function of the consequences attached to the appearance of the personality rather than a splitting of the ego. That is, if the appearance of the high personality was rewarded by touch or token, then it appeared more often.

BIOLOGICAL TREATMENT. Multiple personality patients with psychogenic amnesia who have not responded to other methods of treatment may be treated with barbiturates (sodium amytal or sodium pentothal) through intravenous infusion, along with a structured or supportive interview. The primary purpose of this procedure is to restore recall and provide the therapist with access to the unconscious (Ruedrich, Chu, & Wadle, 1985).

This procedure involves the administration of the barbiturate, which induces a feeling of well-being and relaxation, followed by the examiner exploring repressed thoughts, memories, conflicts, and affects in a gentle and gradual fashion. During this interview, it is anticipated that the patient will have some recall of memory. The nurse should carefully observe the patient until he is able to ambulate and is completely conscious.

The therapist is always cautious when prescribing medications of any type because of the possibility of overdose. Possibility of overdose increases if the person is diagnosed with multiple personality (Coons, 1986b) since one or more of the personalities may attempt suicide with little provocation.

PSYCHOGENIC FUGUE, PSYCHOGENIC AMNESIA, AND DEPERSONALIZATION

PSYCHOANALYTIC/PSYCHODYNAMIC THERAPY. Psychogenic fugue and amnesia have acute onset and brief duration; in many instances, individuals with these disorders recover spontaneously.

Most of the literature regarding the treatment of these disorders is based on anecdotal data and is, at best, scant. Treatment consists of close observation of behaviors and an in-depth review of the patient's history and mental status. Examination and treatment are conducted slowly, since the individual might recover spontaneously and without other interventions.

In instances in which recovery is not forthcoming, the therapist considers supportive therapy and provides the individual with opportunities for discussion about significant life events. The therapist's skill in gently prodding, persuading, and asking leading questions about those events that are difficult or impossible to recall can be used extensively with these patients (Maxmen, 1986; American Psychiatric Association, 1987).

Since amnesic persons are usually highly susceptible to hypnosis, hypnosis is a viable treatment for them. The therapist will probably be successful in engaging the hypnotized patient in an intensive discussion about traumatic events. Once the patient is awake, the objective is to keep him talking about those events.

When the intensity of the amnesia is severe, hospitalization might be required. The hospitalized patient who has amnesia needs assistance and direction in the activities of daily living, such as eating, grooming, and hygiene. The patient needs reality orientation to establish where he is and the date and year, with the information repeated as frequently as necessary. The nurse need not force the patient to accept information that is central to the amnesia, such as information about who he is or what has happened.

After regaining his memory, the patient may be agitated, anxious to the point of panic, and may need protection from suicidal gestures, depending on the nature of the precipitating event. For example, the patient may be quite distraught and overwhelmed with guilt feelings (Webster, 1984b). He may need an opportunity to discuss and sort out what happened and to discuss his feelings about what will now take place. In instances in which a tragedy is connected to the amnesia or fugue, the nurse will need to be sensitive to the normal grieving process that the patient may experience. However, psychiatric evaluation is often requested when there is a question of legal intent for an act committed during the period in which the person was amnesic. Medication generally does not have any therapeutic value for the amnesic.

A patient will rarely be hospitalized for symptoms of depersonalization without other accompanying symptoms. The patient who is hospitalized is likely to experience severe anxiety and disturbed reality orientation and be preoccupied with somatic complaints. More severe problems than just depersonalization are likely to exist, such as a severe personality disorder or schizophrenia.

When caring for a patient who experiences depersonalization in conjunction with a more severe disorder, the nurse is attentive to stimuli within the environment and is aware that the patient may have increased difficulty when there is excessive noise or activity. The nurse monitors the patient's sleep patterns, since fatigue may precipitate further depersonalization. Nursing interventions include assuring the patient of his safety, providing reality orientation, being attentive to environmental factors that may cause stress for the patient, and establishing a consistent relationship in which the patient can sort out the experience of depersonalization, validating reality as well as identifying precipitating stress factors. A careful patient history may reveal information about contributing factors such as the patient's use of illegal drugs prior to the depersonalization. Keeping in mind that the depersonalization is accompanied by impairment in social or occupational functioning, nursing care involves interventions to help the patient improve his interpersonal relationships as well as interventions to help identify and use his own personal strengths.

BEHAVIORAL THERAPY. The behavioral approach to treatment consists primarily of being careful not to reinforce the patient's maladaptive methods of coping. Instead, the healthy components of the patient's personality should be rewarded at all times. Token economy, modeling, and other reinforcement programs might be used with these disorders.

BIOLOGICAL TREATMENT. Amytal, administered intravenously, is also used to treat psychogenic fugue and amnesia. After the drug is administered, the therapist begins a gentle prodding in the areas in which the patient might be experiencing conflict and has dissociated feelings and emotions (Campbell, 1981; Coons, 1986b). In some instances, anxiolytics and major neuroleptics might be used to treat the severe anxiety that accompanies these disorders (Coons, 1986b).

RESPONSIBILITIES OF THE NURSE IN A PSYCHIATRIC SETTING

Although many nurses and other mental health professionals have not been directly involved in the treatment of a patient with a dissociative disorder, it is important for the nurse practicing in a psychiatric setting to understand the treatment process for patients with multiple personality.

PHASES OF TREATMENT

THE BEGINNING PHASE: ESTABLISHMENT OF TRUST. The nurse will need to expend the time and effort to establish trust and to develop a solid and consistent relationship with the patient. The nurse will need to gain the patient's alliance before progress toward the integration of the different personalities (alters) will occur. She must be prompt for appointments. Promises are sometimes difficult to deliver, and should be made with extreme caution. The patient will begin to participate in treatment only after he feels accepted and understood.

The nurse should provide support to the patient as the diagnosis is being shared with him. This information should be provided in a gentle and timely fashion, lest the patient abort treatment.

The nurse must establish contact with all personalities and become familiar with each alter's demographic data, including name, age, race, origin, function, conflicts, and the relationship to each of the other personalities.

The nurse must assess if any one of these personalities is thinking about harming another or itself. If there is a possibility of violence or any acting-out behavior, the nurse must establish contacts with the appropriate personality (personalities) and determine lethality, necessity for emergency measures, if changes in course of treatment are indicated, and so forth (Kluft, 1983; Kluft, 1984b; Coons, 1986A; Coons & Milstein, 1986). (Also see Chapter 18 on psychiatric crisis.)

MIDDLE PHASE. During the middle phase of treatment (which can extend for several years), the focus is on helping the patient deal with the "dissociated" components of the personality, which usually includes issues surrounding sexuality, aggression, anger, and depression.

FINAL PHASE. The fusion of the various personalities into one integrated person is the objective; successful termination of the relationship follows (Coons, 1986a; Spiegel, 1986; Coons, 1986b).

TRANSFERENCE AND COUNTERTRANSFERENCE ISSUES

The patient will experience a variety of transferences. Dependency, hostility, and seductiveness directed toward the therapist are common. These transferences might change from dependency to hostility, and so forth, without provocation from the therapist or other personnel in the milieu.

On the other hand, the nurse is likely to experience countertransference feelings. It is extremely difficult for the nurse to cope with being confronted with such an array of emotions. The nurse must be aware that feelings of overinvestment, underinvestment, fascination, anger, exhaustion, overwhelming anxiety, disbelief, and resignation will require that she monitor her feelings and thoughts very carefully. Additional clinical supervision and support from peers might be necessary during difficult phases in the treatment process. The nurse should be mindful to ask for support and supervision whenever these feelings surface (Kluft, 1982; Kluft, 1983).

THE DECISION TO HOSPITALIZE

Hospitalization usually occurs when the patient exhibits self-destructive behaviors; is psychotic or threatening a psychotic episode; or is dysfunctional to the extent that she experiences serious self-care deficits, such as the inability to feed and groom herself (Kluft, 1983; Kluft, 1984b).

MEDICATIONS

Antidepressive or antipsychotic medications may be prescribed for symptoms of depression or a psychosis. Minor tranquilizers are often used for treatment of anxiety. The nurse needs to keep in mind that there are no medications available for the specific treatment of multiple personality (Coons, 1986a; Schafer, 1986).

PREVENTION

Patients with multiple personality frequently have a history of childhood physical and sexual abuse. Similarly, multiple personality patients are likely to have a history of abusing their children (Coons, 1986a). The nurse should be alert to the possibility that the patient might be involved in child physical and sexual abuse. If the nurse is suspicious that abuse is occurring, she should discuss it with the treatment team and assist in determining what action must be taken. All states have explicit laws about reporting physical/sexual abuse of children.

MANAGEMENT OF CRISES

The nurse, responsible for patient care over the 24-hour period, will need to be prepared to deal with potential crisis. From a chart review of 106 multiple personality patients, Kluft (1983) identified and ordered in decreasing incidence the following types of crises (p. 76):

- Suicidal or self-injurious behaviors or urges
- Rejection and/or family uproar
- Co-presence phenomena[2]

- Depression phenomena
- Dysphoric switching of personalities, fugue, or amnesia
- Acute somatoform symptoms
- Impulses of destructive alters
- Loneliness
- Loneliness/depression after fusion
- Discovery of further, new, or relapsed separateness
- Acute phobias/panics
- Psychotic episodes
- Acute obsessive-compulsive phenomena

The patient might experience a discontinuous memory and be deprived of essential data to assist in effective problem solving. Confabulation might be used to supplement missing experiences and can precipitate crises. Also, the families of these patients are often estranged and not available to provide support in times of need.

In crisis situations, the alters present special problems: they tend to have limited skills; they withdraw abruptly, and leave another personality to deal with the crisis. The personality that deals with the dilemma may be distinctly different from the previous personality, and could have a different perception about the situation (Kluft, 1983).

Even the most skilled nurse can find crisis management perplexing, overwhelming, and exhausting.

POTENTIAL FOR SUICIDE AND ACTING-OUT BEHAVIORS

The nurse must be especially alert for suicidal behaviors. The patient with multiple personality disorder is prone to using one personality (alter) to kill or harm another personality (alter). Examples of actions the nurse might need to implement include: suicide precautions, no-suicide contracts; one patient/one nurse assignments; restricting activities to the psychiatric unit; assigning patient to space where observation is optimal and continuous; monitoring medications (patient might save them in preparation for overdosing); and removing glass or silverware from the environment.

COMMUNICATION WITH STAFF

Patients with dissociative disorders tend to create controversy within the staff. In order to elicit staff cooperation and participation in therapeutic activi-

---

[2]Co-presence phenomena are the existence of more than one psychological self within a single individual.

ties, the nurse will need to communicate to the staff the plan of care; discuss the dynamics associated with the patient's illness; inform the staff about changes in treatment strategies; and be attentive and sensitive to observations and opinions from other staff.

The hospitalized patient with amnesia and/or fugue might need assistance and direction concerning activities of daily living, such as eating, grooming, and hygiene. The patient needs reality orientation to place the date and year, and repetition of information should be provided as frequently as needed. The nurse should not attempt to force the patient to accept information about who he is or what has happened, which is central to the amnesia.

When memory has returned, the patient may need an opportunity to discuss and sort out what has happened, and to discuss his feelings about what will now take place. In instances where there is a tragedy connected to the amnesia, the nurse will need to assist the patient with the loss and grief (Coons, 1986a; Kluft, 1983; Coons, 1980; Coons, 1986b; Ludwig, 1983; Schafer, 1981; Bellak, et al., 1973).

LEGAL CONCERNS

The commonly used legal plea of "innocent by reason of insanity" in determining liability for a crime has particular pertinence to dissociative disorders (Lasky, 1982). Individuals have claimed amnesia or claimed to be in a fugue state during a crime. The nurse and other mental health professionals may feel that they are in a precarious position when doing a psychiatric evaluation for such an individual. It is important for the nurse to be able to detect when the person charged with a crime does not have a true dissociative disorder, yet at the same time to recognize when the patient is being truthful in stating a lack of recall for the period of time in question. Since there may be greater than average likelihood that this patient will at some point get into the legal system, it is even more important than usual for the nurse to pay attention to the accuracy of any information placed in the patient's record, since it could be subpoenaed by the court.

RESPONSIBILITIES OF THE NURSE IN A NONPSYCHIATRIC SETTING

The nurse is responsible for assessing dissociative disorders regardless of the clinical setting. For example, patients may display dissociative behaviors in numerous health care settings such as labor and delivery rooms or pediatric clinics. Thus the nurse should know how patients with dissociative disorders behave and how she could respond with further assessment and appropriate intervention. The nurse should seek opportunities to assess and plan treatment for those observed syndromes and symptoms that might be problematic to the individual and his family.

Similarly, the nurse is also aware of patients who experience crises and should assess individuals for the impact of the crisis on their lives. On occasion, individuals will experience a dissociative reaction that can range from psychogenic fugue (physical flight) to a feeling of depersonalization that lasts for a few seconds or minutes.

Assisting the individual in the development of appropriate defensive mechanisms is a most important task. Frequently the patient will not have a formal diagnosis of dissociative disorder. The nurse must be aware of the behavioral manifestations of these disorders, and give special attention to the patient's social and psychological history as it may reveal a set of common behavioral themes.

The nurse can help to allay a patient's anxieties and fears, can help the patient to ventilate fears and anxieties, and must, at all times, assess for suicidal and homicidal thoughts and plans. These behaviors require immediate therapeutic action, including 1) crisis counseling, 2) family involvement for support and management, 3) assistance with arranging hospitalization, and 4) reassuring the patient that he will not be abandoned.

In whatever setting the nurse functions, she can always assess for and document behaviors such as fear, anxiety, and difficulties in interpersonal relations and occupational activities. A psychiatric referral is often appropriate when the nurse's assessment reveals dissociative behaviors.

Case Study: Psychiatric Setting

Kay Lander, a 20-year-old college student in her junior year, had been in outpatient therapy for six months. She had experienced herself as different persons living within the same body since she was 13, but for many years had maintained this as a secret, even from her family. Kay's initial attempt at getting psychiatric help came when she was in her first year of college, which was the first time she had been away from home. She became depressed and sought help for suicidal ideation. Actually, it was one of the alter personalities who was suicidal, but this was not revealed in therapy. Antidepressant medication helped the symptoms but did not alter the personalities. Kay sought treatment this second time due to the emergence of a new personality—precipitated by forming a relationship with a young man at college, her fear of closeness, and sexual issues. The new personality was "Kathy," an outgoing personality who loved parties, used alcohol and drugs, and sought sexual activity. "Kathy" shared with the therapist that she was aware there were other personalities: "Connie," a 5-year-old who was afraid of men and of being hurt and who cried a lot; and "Chris," a 13-year-old who felt isolated at school, often dieted because people told her she was fat, and shied away from sexual issues. Another subpersonality, unknown to Kay, was "Betty," who was the patient's real age, held the suicidal ideation, and was punitive toward herself although concerned for the others. The patient herself, in the ego state she defined as the "real Kay," was a quiet, very proper, and hardworking student, although she received only average grades. She felt inadequate around others and was hypersensitive to anything she perceived as criticism. Kay was hospitalized after she ingested a large quantity of alcohol and an overdose of medication and was unable to state that she could control suicidal impulses. She was initially admitted to a medical unit where she was treated for the overdose, then transferred to a psychiatric unit.

Staff opinion of Kay was polarized even before her admission, based on the admission information and staff bias about multiple personality. Some of the staff wished to protect Kay while others resented the patient's "specialness" and believed that she was faking her illness. Staff members found it frustrating to interact with one personality, only to find that the patient had no recall of the discussion an hour later. Their sense of competence was threatened by Kay's lack of response to attempted interventions as she shifted from one personality to another. When "Connie," the proclaimed 5-year-old, appeared, staff members weren't sure whether to respond as they would to a child or whether to expect the patient to be an adult. They were uncomfortable with the patient's demands to be called "Connie." "Kathy" would be suggestive and seductive around male staff members, while "Connie" would cringe in fear of men. Nurses soon learned that when "Betty" was present, they needed to be especially alert to suicide potential, because she attempted to hoard her medication in order to take another overdose. Another patient on the unit announced that she, too, had multiple personality and mimicked having a "good" and "bad" personality.

In an effort to minimize secondary gains and reinforcement of the personalities, the treatment team limited discussion about the personalities to the primary therapist and to the physician as much as possible. The primary therapist met regularly with the team and clarified goals for the patient. In therapy, the goal was the ultimate fusion of the personalities with one another. The goal of hospitalization was to deal with the target symptom of suicidal behavior. Some issues had to be faced in both arenas: Kay was quick to develop transference feelings toward both the therapist and her treatment team with fear of parental-type disapproval while at the same time seeking nurturance from them. Kay's anxiety level was high and her suicide potential was an ever-present issue.

The treatment plan included many recommendations found in the writings of Kluft (1984b) including: assigning Kay to a private room; calling her what she wanted to be called; making sure not to infantilize her;

offering her frequent explanations, particularly when she was upset; including her in the planning of her treatment as much as possible; explaining rules of the unit and insisting on reasonable compliance; not including her in verbal groups but having her participate in activity groups; and minimizing splitting by clearly defining what would be handled in therapy and what would be handled on the unit, and with whom.

Since this was, for most of the staff, the first experience in treating multiple personality, meetings were held to help staff members understand the dissociative process, as well as to provide an avenue for them to deal with their own feelings about the case and to work together on a cooperative treatment program.

Many of the factors in Kay's history have been found to be common in patients with dissociative disorders. As a young child, Kay felt abandoned when her parents divorced, and clung to her mother, afraid that she, too, would leave. Since they lived in a rural area, Kay spent much time alone and had imaginary playmates in spite of her mother's disapproval. Kay reported to her therapist that she was raped by an uncle several times when she was seven, but her mother had refused to believe it, saying that Kay was imagining the incident. When Kay was twelve, her mother remarried, and the family moved to a new community. This marriage dissolved when Kay's stepfather physically abused both Kay and her mother. Kay described feeling guilty for the breakup of the marriage, feeling that if she had been "good enough," her mother would have been happy.

The team's assessment was that the separation from her father, the rape by her uncle, physical abuse, and loneliness were all factors contributing to Kay's vulnerability to ego splitting and dissociation. The personalities represented major unresolved conflicts and allowed Kay to escape from intolerable situations. The major treatment focus was psychotherapy, with the inpatient environment providing security, consistent relationships, opportunity to develop a sense of constancy in relation to herself, and opportunity to help her improve her self-image with emphasis upon her strengths. Kay's family was engaged in family therapy. A key factor in Kay's treatment was the staff members' acceptance of her need to dissociate some of her experiences and feelings. The team developed a nursing care plan for Kay that was consistent with the interdisciplinary treatment plan.

Nursing Diagnoses:

*Potential for injury: poisoning
*Ineffective individual coping
*Sexual dysfunction related to knowledge deficit
*Altered thought processes
 Knowledge deficit: information misinterpretation (sexual)
 Impaired verbal communication
 Anxiety
 Ineffective family coping: compromised
 Ineffective family coping: disabling
 Altered family processes
 Fear
 Dysfunctional grieving
 Altered health maintenance
 Rape-trauma syndrome

*Nursing diagnoses developed in care plan that follows

DSM-III-R Diagnosis

Axis I: Multiple personality disorder (300.14)
Axis II: (Borderline personality disorder (Betty) (provisional)
Axis III: Effects of alcohol and overdose of medication
Axis IV: Psychosocial stressors: formation of new romantic relationship;
severity: 2 (mild)
Axis V: Current GAF, 15; Highest GAF Past Year, 75

Nursing Care Plan for Kay

Nursing Diagnosis	Desired Outcomes	Interventions	Rationale
1. Potential for injury: poisoning.	Kay will avoid the ingestion of toxic substances in quantities sufficient to cause poisoning or intoxication.	Remove all potentially harmful items from Kay's environment. Place Kay in an area where she can be observed, but do not reinforce her for acting out hostile behaviors.	Kay has maladaptive coping behaviors and needs to be protected until capable of a higher level of functioning.
		Assist Kay in identifying her fears and concerns.	Kay needs the opportunity to ventilate feelings about anxiety and fear that led to her ingestion of drugs and alcohol.
		Always be alert to behaviors that might indicate suicidal behavior, gesture, or ideation. Observe, record, and report to other staff any change in mood, such as anger, elation, withdrawal, resignation, and so forth; although it may be helpful to form a no-suicide contract with Kay, her suicidal or violent personality may be one of the "alters" (e.g. Betty) and the contract may not be honored.	Patients with multiple personalities can abruptly change from one "state" to another. Impulses and uncontrollable behaviors need to be anticipated. Kay may or may not remember previous conversations with the nurse.

Nursing Diagnosis	Desired Outcomes	Interventions	Rationale
	Kay will develop a trusting relationship with the nurse.	Introduce yourself to Kay; explain your responsibilities to Kay; and, (a) Explore with Kay her perceptions of her recent problems. (b) Assess for the number of alters, and ask about their names, sex, age, race, personality characteristics, and relationships between and among them. (c) Determine if any alters have homicidal/ suicidal ideation/ attempts, and if other types of acting out behavior is a serious potential.	Alleviates anxieties and fears; helps Kay to understand the context of the relationship. Kay's behaviors, perceptions, needs, and so forth, need to be understood by the nurse. This information is essential for planning effective treatment.
		Communicate with Kay that you will work with her in the resolution of conflicts; do not make promises and do not agree to keep communications between nurse and Kay a secret. Make it clear that you (nurse) will communicate with staff.	Enhances security and facilitates self-esteem and communication; decreases anxiety and demonstrates acceptance of Kay, and empathy for her struggles.
	Kay will show increased impulse control as evidenced by decreased suicidal ideation and attempts at self-destruction.	Frequently assess Kay's potential for suicide and other impulsive ideation and acts.	Validation of nurse's care and concern; evidence that the environment will be made safe during times when Kay cannot control her impulses.
		Assure Kay that you are available to discuss her problems and concerns with her. Provide her with honest feedback.	Provides additional opportunity for Kay to develop trust and explore alternatives to previous behaviors.

Nursing Diagnosis	Desired Outcomes	Interventions	Rationale
		Assist Kay in identifying the thoughts and feelings associated with the personality that is destructive, impulsive, and frightening.	The "alters" switch quickly. There is potential for suicide through Betty's expression of her conflicts.
		Assure Kay that all staff are interested in her well-being; continuously assess for suicidal ideations and gestures.	Provides hope that Kay can function; addresses Kay's potential; focuses on Kay's strengths.
		Maintain Kay in the same room with the same roommate.	Provides a stable and familiar environment for Kay.
	Kay will return to the highest level of functioning as evidenced by an integration of the numerous personalities.	Assist Kay in the integration of the numerous personalities by providing: (1) Object constancy through assigning one nurse during eight-hour shift to assist in her care over the 24 hours. (2) Positive feedback when Kay accomplishes a task or engages in a meaningful interpersonal relationship. (3) Acknowledgment of the person that Kay states she is: Kay, Kathy, Connie, and so forth. (4) Frequent explanations about activities that occur in the environment. (5) Explain about ward rules and regulations, and encourage compliance.	Multiple personality patients have difficulty remembering events and are frequently confused. Assigning one nurse will help Kay decrease her anxiety and fears. Improves interpersonal functioning and provides Kay with a sense of hope. These alters are an authentic component of Kay's personality. Confusion occurs often when one personality forgets what the other remembers. Kay needs to understand the ward ground rules.
		Communicate with Kay about her behaviors and thoughts and feelings that staff observe.	Provides feedback essential to Kay's emotional development and sense of self.
2. Ineffective individual coping.	Kay will develop increased self-esteem and more wholesome methods of relaxation and problem solving.	Plan for periods of relaxation.	Helps prevent pent-up frustrations and emotions.

Nursing Diagnosis	Desired Outcomes	Interventions	Rationale
		Engage in methods of reducing stress such as jogging and swimming.	Provides a form of tension release.
		Assist Kay in dressing in proper attire. Emphasize that she does not have to be conservative, nor provocative.	Assists in the integration of needs and desires that are currently expressed through different personalities.
		Discuss with Kay situations that she thinks she has managed well; (a) explore with her why she thinks things went well; (b) assist her in identifying how she dealt with the conflicting demands at that time; (c) explore with Kay what she learned from the specific situations and how it can be applied to her life.	Focuses on effective conflict resolution; provides opportunity for Kay to understand her successes; provides continuous data for treatment.
	Kay will develop effective coping strategies as determined by a decrease in frequency that she employs personalities (alters) to express conflicts, frustrations, and so forth.	Determine Kay's present coping level; when appropriate, determine the coping level of Kathy, Connie, and Betty.	These personalities emerge and have their distinct profiles. For example, if Betty is the predominant personality, suicide attempt is a likely behavior. If Connie is the dominant personality, the nurse must be concerned about child-like and immature behaviors. Identifying behaviors will assist in anticipating the consequences related to each personality's maladaptive coping attempts.
		Assist Kay in verbalizing thoughts and feelings related to each personality. Observe and record their behaviors.	These data will assist the nurse in understanding Kay's behaviors and in planning for future interventions.
3. Altered thought processes.	Kay will have a decreased need to display alters as a coping strategy.	Provide opportunity for reality orientation that includes: Name, place, time, and reason for hospitalization.	Assists Kay in increased reality testing; decreases feelings of anxiety, fear.

Nursing Diagnosis	Desired Outcomes	Interventions	Rationale
		Assume that Kay's expressions of her thoughts and feelings are genuine, real, and significant to her. Do not laugh or make light of any components of her behavior.	The "alters" are real and necessary to her current ability to function.
		Be demonstrative of your care and concern for her; communicate that you want to understand her struggles, and will assist her in working through these difficulties.	Promotes feeling of trust and enhances self-esteem, both essential to the healing process.
	Kay will identify those situations that cause increased anxiety and compartmentalized feelings (personalities).	Assist Kay to verbalize her thoughts and feelings.	Forestalls the need for her to act out these thoughts and feelings.
		Encourage Kay to ask questions and seek explanations about the communications with nurse and other staff.	Alleviates the need to act out frustrations; clarifies distortions; assists in reality orientation.
4. Sexual dysfunction related to lack of knowledge.	Kay will verbalize an understanding of basic physiology of sexuality and discuss myths, fears, and anxieties regarding sexuality and intimacy with men. (The alter is Kathy.)	Determine Kay's baseline level of knowledge about female/male physiology and sexuality.	Provides a realistic beginning point for Kay, and gives nurse additional information that can be used in future planning for her care.
		Explore with Kay her source(s) of information about: (a) sexual functions, (b) intimacy, (c) pregnancy, (d) menstruation, (e) roles of men and women in intimate relationships, and so forth.	These data will assist nurse in planning present and followup (outpatient) treatment for Kay. Exploring the sources of her information with Kay will also help her become more knowledgeable about and comfortable with discussing this subject.
		Provide accurate information for Kay in the categories identified.	Healthy sexuality begins with correct information and clarification of any misunderstanding.

Nursing Diagnosis	Desired Outcomes	Interventions	Rationale
		Discuss with Kay a range of socially acceptable behaviors that are age and situation appropriate for her to be involved in.	Defines a framework within which Kay can judge and evaluate her own behaviors; increases self-esteem and autonomy.
		Discuss with Kay the impact of her cultural and familial beliefs and practices on her current behaviors.	Assists Kay in understanding her here-and-now behaviors; de-mystifies these behaviors that she has been struggling with.
		Correct and/or provide an alternative explanation of any distortions and erroneous thoughts and feelings that Kay might express.	Facts assist in building confidence, self-esteem, and the alleviation of fear and anxiety.
		Assist Kay in exploring the biopsychosocial components of sexuality, and how previous experiences during childhood might cloud her thoughts/attitudes about sexual experiences with males.	Sexuality is a basic part of the self-concept. Clarifies distortions; provides facts; and increases Kay's ability to make appropriate decisions for herself without having to dissociate.

Case Study: Nonpsychiatric Setting

Olive Thompkins: A Patient with Depersonalization Disorder

Demographic Data

Name: Olive Thompkins
Age: 40
Address: Rural Route 50, Homestead, Fl.
Ethnicity: Black and Hispanic
Referring Agency: Brought to hospital via ambulance
Occupation: High school principal and community leader

Patient's Perception of Problem

"I felt my body and mind lose touch with themselves. My legs no longer functioned; they became too small to hold me up. My head was just the opposite . . . it was big and round . . . like the moon. I was dizzy. I could not recognize where I was. My car stopped—I had no control over it. Speech that I had never heard before came from my mouth. I was watching myself have these experiences. I am frightened."

Olive's secretary stated, "I became concerned for Olive when she was late for work one morning. After several hours had passed, I went to look for her. Olive was found sitting in her car on the highway. I summoned an ambulance and Olive was taken to a nearby hospital."

History of Problem

Olive Thompkins is a single parent who lives in a small rural community. She claims to have "over-functioned" for many years. She took care of her mother who had Alzheimer's disease, supported her children (four daughters) through college and professional schools, served on numerous community boards, and volunteered for worthwhile activities in the community. Olive stated that for many years, work consumed all of her time.

Recently, she began complaining about a sensation in her chest and immediately placed herself on a self-designed exercise program, and limited her diet to complex carbohydrates, fish, chicken, and whole-grain cereals. Olive stated, "I actually had more energy and felt better."

In retrospect, Olive thinks that she was working even harder than usual because of her mother's rapidly failing health. She was losing sleep and felt stressed. Olive also stated that she had been a leader in the community for many years, and could not disappoint the parents and children whom she served.

Olive also commented that recently she had remained awake all night. She added, "I had to complete teacher evaluations, do my income tax return, and other things. Perhaps I just got too worn out."

Psychiatric History

Olive was hospitalized about five years ago because of a fear that she was too stressed. At that time, Valium 5 (diazepam) was prescribed for her. Olive did not feel the medication helped; she discontinued it.

Family History

Olive's father is deceased, and her mother has Alzheimer's disease. She describes them as hard working people with strong values. Olive's father was a field foreman on a sugar cane plantation. Her mother was a domestic worker who also "took in washing and ironing." Her parents managed to send Olive and her brother to a nearby university; they graduated. Olive's brother is a Certified Public Accountant (CPA). The two of them are considered to be very close.

Olive's husband died in the Vietnam War. Her daughters were quite small at the time of his death. After Olive's husband died, her mother and father moved into her home. They helped Olive care for her daughters.

Social History

Olive reports that she worked very hard during her formative years. She worked in the sugar cane fields with her father, and also helped her mother with the washing and ironing. She stated, "I learned how to work hard, and I have been doing just that for years."

Education

Olive completed high school and college, and received a master's degree in psychology. She graduated with honors from her baccalaureate and masters programs.

Substance Use

Olive denies using any type of psychoactive substance. (She acted embarrassed when the interviewer asked the question.)

Health Assessment

Relatively good health. Currently on a self-prescribed diet and exercise regime. She continues to complain of occasional tachycardia, weakness attacks, anxiety, and restlessness. Olive quietly commented, "Nurse, do you think I am going crazy?"

Present Status Examination:

General Appearance: Well dressed, looks perplexed and anxious; cooperative.
Emotions: Anxious and fearful. She continued to look across the room as if she were expecting someone to come in.
Voice/Speech: Quiet, deliberate, and barely audible speech. Coherent.
Motoric Behavior: Still, rigid, and slow.
Thought Process and Content: Deliberate, slow, and coherent.
Potential for Violence:
   Self, observe; no evidence. Other, observe; no evidence.
Summary:
   Olive Thompkins is a 40-year-old woman who experienced her "body and mind lose touch with themselves" as she drove to work. She is successfully employed as a principal of a small rural high school. Olive has a history of working extremely hard. She stated that she feels tired and is frightened.
   Olive was brought to the emergency room by ambulance, examined and hospitalized on a medical unit for further assessment and treatment.

Nursing Care Plan for Olive

Nursing Diagnosis	Desired Outcomes	Interventions	Rationale
1. Anxiety	Olive will recognize and acknowledge her anxiety, and develop appropriate coping strategies.	Be available to Olive when she is in the emergency room and on the medical unit: (a) observe her behaviors and record observations, (b) reassure her that she is not going crazy, and that she will be supported by the nursing staff, (c) remain with Olive, (d) validate her feelings of fear, (e) speak slowly and clearly.	Olive needs to know that she will not be abandoned, and that the nurse is empathic and understanding.

Nursing Diagnosis	Desired Outcomes	Interventions	Rationale
		Discuss with Olive methods she currently uses to manage her anxieties.	Information is essential for understanding Olive's behavioral patterns. Recognizes that Olive has been highly successful in the past; encourages her self-esteem.
		Help Olive identify those events that provoke feelings of anxiety.	Provides insights that are useful in conflict resolution.
		Assess the level of anxiety that Olive is expressing in the here-and-now: mild, moderate, extreme, or panic.	Information will assist in planning additional interventions.
		Support Olive's current adaptive coping behaviors: sadness, tearing, quietness, and so forth.	Olive needs support; she is dependent upon her habitual methods of solving problems.
	Olive will develop an interest in social activities that provide some pleasure.	Explore with Olive specific events that occur in the community, and assist her in selecting *one* activity per week that has the potential to provide relaxation.	Recreation and relaxation will assist in adaptive regression and provide an emotional outlet for Olive.
	Olive will review her diet and exercise regimen with the nurse.	Evaluate Olive's self-designed diet to assure that she is receiving adequate nutrition and request dietary consultation if needed.	Good nutrition is essential for physical and mental health. Diet should complement her activity level.
	Olive will discuss her exercise regimen with nurse.	Evaluate Olive's self-designed exercise program and request consultation if needed.	Exercises need to be safe. They should assist in relieving tension and anxiety.
	Olive will recognize if there is a relationship between anxiety and physical symptoms.	Tachycardia and dizziness will be discussed in terms of: (a) frequency, (b) duration, (c) time of day, (d) demands and stressors confronting Olive at time symptoms occur, and (e) types of behaviors that she implements to rid herself of psychological and physical symptoms.	Physical symptoms are common methods the body uses to express anxiety. Depersonalization may be accompanied by physical symptoms, e.g., Olive's cardiac symptoms.

Nursing Diagnosis	Desired Outcomes	Interventions	Rationale
		Provide health teaching related to physical symptoms, stress, and anxiety.	A cognitive understanding should assist in compliance with recommended methods of relaxation.
		Teach Olive relaxation techniques such as breathing and stretching techniques, muscle relaxation.	These are brief and effective methods of stress reduction.
	Olive will seek support for caring for mother with Alzheimer's disease.	Discuss with Olive that support is available through community agencies to assist with mother's care.	Provides support and alleviates physical and psychological strain for Olive. Gives "permission" to Olive to "let go" of some of her responsibilities.
		Assist Olive in beginning to assess support services for mother.	Validates that support is available and appropriate. May assist in alleviating guilt feelings associated with not being the all-involved caregiver.
		Explore with Olive the notion of discussing their mother's condition with her brother, and ways that he can be supportive to Olive. Role play with Olive how she can communicate this information to him.	Olive needs a respite from the constant demands of providing care for her mother.
		Encourage expression of feelings and the acknowledgment that she is anxious/stressed.	Helps validate Olive's feelings and recognizes her role strain.
	Olive will experience a greater degree of psychological and physiological comfort.	Explore with Olive her unmet needs when she begins to experience uncomfortable sensations such as tachycardia, fatigue, dizziness, or fear of going crazy.	Facilitates the expression of anger, helps Olive become comfortable with her feelings and her body.
		Assist Olive in linking feelings to these events, and encourage her to describe them.	Promotes a sense of self-awareness and control; provides a base for exploring future alternatives.

Nursing Diagnosis	Desired Outcomes	Interventions	Rationale
2. Ineffective individual coping	Olive will develop a plan for elimination of stress and role strain	Assess for suicidal risk: gestures and attempts. Determine the risk of self-harm. Include: (a) history of ideation, gestures, and attempts; (b) status of job, faculty relations; (c) changes in interpersonal relationships in the community, relationships with daughters and brother; (d) mother's health and needs, additional care demands; (e) appetite and sleep habits; and (f) sexual activity.	Assists staff in understanding Olive's coping strategies; provides additional data for future planning; helps nurses determine what their priorities should be in the here-and-now.
		Role play with Olive in problematic situations (Olive will provide the context).	Role playing is a form of behavioral rehearsal, a method of showing Olive that she can execute new behavior.
		Explore Olive's support system and, if indicated, assist in the development of an active one. Consider: (a) establishing a core of friends with whom Olive can talk and share feelings; (b) giving information about the Alzheimer's family support group that meets twice a week in the community; (c) involving brother as a support; (d) ongoing therapy after discharge in an outpatient clinic. Count and evaluate commitments in the community; consider withdrawing from some; suggest participation in a stress reduction workshop (a one-time/all-day workshop).	A support system will enhance the overall treatment process, providing a network of individuals who can listen, share experiences, and assist in problem solving. Allows Olive to try out new social roles.

Nursing Diagnosis	Desired Outcomes	Interventions	Rationale
	Olive will evaluate her strengths and explore behaviors that enhance her coping.	Encourage Olive to describe how she manages conflicts and pressures competing for her time: (a) What were those conflicts? (b) How did you manage them? (c) What was the outcome? (d) What were your thoughts/feelings about the outcome? (e) Did you experience feelings of heightened self-esteem, elation, and pride, or defeat, anger, hostility, and so forth?	Olive's strengths and previous successes can be used to enhance overall functioning.
		Identify and reinforce adequate and effective coping mechanisms that Olive has used. Also, assist Olive in identifying coping strategies that were not useful and explore alternatives.	Olive needs to understand her strengths and weaknesses.
	Olive will experience restful sleep at night.	Teach breathing and relaxation techniques (see Chapter 25 on the ICU patient for specifics) to be implemented near bedtime. Encourage Olive to play relaxing music when retiring.	At least 7½ hours of restful sleep is essential for Olive. Relaxation is difficult for her, but essential. Sleep and relaxation will aid in decreasing physical symptoms (tachycardia, dizziness, etc.).
		Explore the possibility of employing sitters or paraprofessionals to attend to Olive's mother at night.	Olive thinks she will not be attentive to her mother if she completely relaxes and goes into a "deep" sleep.
	Olive will understand basic health data and use it in making adjustments in her daily activities.	The nurse will: (1) Explain dietary and exercise programs; (2) Teach Olive about basic structures and function of heart and vascular system; discuss	Information assists with compliance, enhances autonomy, increases self-esteem, helps Olive understand the consequences of her behaviors, and their

Nursing Diagnosis	Desired Outcomes	Interventions	Rationale
		headaches, and dizziness; (3) Review relaxation techniques with Olive; (4) Provide names of professionals whom she can contact after discharge. (5) Assist in arranging follow-up appointments in the cardiac clinic and outpatient psychiatric clinic; (6) Explain the purpose of any prescribed drugs, other treatment, and so forth.	impact on her physical and psychological well-being.
3. Disturbance in self-concept	Olive will experience improved self-concept as evidenced by her ability to accomplish her short-term goals and satisfy her personal needs.	Encourage Olive to share her perceptions and expectations of herself and significant others such as community leaders, staff at school, her daughters, and her brother.	The self-concept involves a sense of self, perceived competence in role performance, internalized mental pictures of body, personal identity that determines who Olive thinks she is, and so forth.
		Explore with Olive her responses to failed expectations associated with significant others, and the coping strategies she employs to deal with these disappointments.	The exploration of coping strategies will assist Olive in further self-examination of useful vs. non-useful strategies.
	Olive will develop increased self-esteem and an appreciation of her own accomplishments.	Explore with Olive her subjective sense of her self-worth. Assist Olive in exploring the relationship between her work schedules and her sense of self-worth.	Self-esteem is related to Olive's self-evaluation of satisfying interpersonal relationships and achievements.
		Discuss with Olive her assessment of her past role performance as a mother, principal, adult-child caretaker, community leader, and so forth.	A positive assessment reflects high self-esteem, provides direction for further interventions, provides opportunity to identify conflicts and introduce alternative strategies, facilitates autonomy and independence.

SUMMARY

Dissociation is used as an ego defense by individuals who need to remove themselves from feelings or situations that result in anxiety, discomfort, or fear. As part of normal ego development, dissociation can be understood as an early attempt at adaptation. The excessive or continued use of dissociation, however, creates problems for the individual that may be expressed in the form of multiple personality, psychogenic fugue, psychogenic amnesia, depersonalization, or derealization. Dissociation may also occur as one of the symptoms of other major psychiatric disorders.

Multiple personality represents one of the most complex dissociative disorders. The individual with multiple personality usually has one primary personality and one or more subpersonalities. The dominant personality at any given time determines the individual's behavior.

Psychogenic fugue is also precipitated by extreme stress, but the person in a fugue state usually flees whatever is causing stress by leaving his or her family, job, and home. He or she is suddenly unable to recall any personal information and manufactures new information.

Psychogenic amnesia is the sudden inability to recall important personal information, without the presence of an organic disorder. This type of amnesia generally follows psychic stress.

Depersonalization is an altered sense of self, while derealization is an altered perception of the environment; these two states may occur together.

Trance states, derealization without depersonalization, brainwashing, and post-traumatic stress disorders are all atypical dissociative disorders; their symptomatology does not fit a specific dissociative disorder.

There are some special issues in the care of patients with dissociative disorders. Sometimes staff members are skeptical that a patient with one of these disorders is really ill. Further, a patient may be charged with a violent crime and may be pleading innocent "by reason of insanity," claiming dissociation during the time of the crime. Thus it is important for professionals to be able to determine whether or not an individual actually has a dissociative disorder.

Finally, the nurse therapist exposed to patients with dissociative disorders should have as her primary goals the fusion of alternate ego states and dealing with the patient's intolerable conflicting feelings.

KEY TERMS

dissociative disorders

integrative functions

conversion reaction

dissociation

automatization of behaviors

multiple personality

psychogenic fugue

psychogenic amnesia

localized amnesia

selective amnesia

generalized amnesia

continuous amnesia

depersonalization

derealization

self-image system

internalization

introjection

incorporation

identification

splitting

separation-individuation

ego states

ego functions

STUDY QUESTIONS

1. Define *dissociation*. What role does it play in the development of a child?

2. Name and describe the four major dissociative disorders (excluding the atypical disorders).

3. Why are dissociative states considered to be common among a large percentage of the population? Give examples of behaviors that would substantiate your response.

4. How can the nurse generalist help care for the patient with a dissociative disorder?

5. What special ethical and legal issues may arise during the care of patients with dissociative disorders?

REFERENCES

American Psychiatric Association. (1980). *A psychiatric glossary*. Boston: Little, Brown.

American Psychiatric Association. (1987). *Diagnostic and statistical manual of mental disorders* (3rd ed. revised). Washington, D.C.: American Psychiatric Association.

Arieti, S. (1955). *Interpretation of schizophrenia*. New York: Robert Brunner.

Bandura, A. (1969). *Principles of behavior modification*. New York: Holt, Rinehart and Winston.

Bandura, A. (1977). Self-efficiency. Toward a unifying theory of behavioral change. *Psychological Review, 84*, 191–215.

Bandura, A., & Walters, R. (1963). *Social learning and personality development*. New York: Holt.

Barile, L. (1984). The patient who is hallucinating. In S. Lego (Ed.), *The American handbook of psychiatric nursing*. New York: J. B. Lippincott, pp. 446–449.

Beck, C. M., Rawlins, R. P., & Williams, S. R. (1984). *Mental health—psychiatric nursing*. St. Louis: C. V. Mosby.

Bellak, L., Hurvick, M., & Gediman, H. K. (1973). *Ego functions in schizophrenics, neurotics, and normals*. New York: John Wiley & Sons.

Bernstein, E. M., & Putnam, F. W. (1986). Development, reliability and validity of a dissociation scale. *Journal of Nervous Mental Disorders, 174*(12), 727–735.

Bernstein-Carlson, E. M. (1988). Personal communication, July 6, 1988.

Blanck, G., & Blanck, R. (1974). *Ego psychology theory and practice*. New York: Columbia University Press.

Bliss, E. L. (1980). Multiple personalities. *Archives of General Psychiatry, 37,* 1388–1397.

Bliss, E. L. (1984). A symptom profile of patients with multiple personalities including MMPI results. *The Journal of Nervous and Mental Disease, 172,* 197–202.

Boor, M. (1982). The multiple personality epidemic. *The Journal of Nervous and Mental Disease, 170,* 202–304.

Bowman, E., Blix, S., & Coons, P. (1985). Multiple personalities in adolescence, relationship to incestual experiences. *Journal of American Academy of Child Psychiatry, 24*(1), 109–114.

Bradlow, P. A. (1973). Depersonalization, ego splitting, non-human fantasy and shame. *International Journal of Psychoanalysis, 54,* 487–492.

Brenner, C. (1955). *An elementary textbook of psychoanalysis*. New York: Doubleday.

Brown, S. L. (1981). Dissociation of pleasure in psychopathology. *Journal of Nervous and Mental Disease, 169*(1), 3–17.

Caddy, G. (1985). Cognitive behavior therapy in the treatment of multiple personality. *Behavior Modification, 9*(3), 267–292.

Cameron, N. (1963). *Personality development and psychopathology*. Boston: Houghton Mifflin.

Campbell, R. (1981). *Psychiatric dictionary*. New York: Oxford University Press.

Caul, D. (1984). Group and videotape techniques for multiple personality disorder. *Psychiatric Annals, 14*(1), 43–51.

Clary, W. F., Burstin, K. J., & Carpenter, J. S. (1984). Multiple personality and borderline personality disorder. *Psychiatric Clinics of North America, 7*(1), 89–99.

Coons, P. M. (1980). Multiple personality: Diagnostic considerations. *Journal of Clinical Psychiatry, 41*(1), 330–336.

Coons, P. M. (1984). The differential diagnosis of multiple personality. *Psychiatric Clinics of North America, 7,* 51–67.

Coons, P. M. (1986a). Child abuse and multiple personality disorder: Review of the literature and suggestions for treatment. *Child Abuse and Neglect, 10,* 455–462.

Coons, P. M. (1986b). Dissociative disorders: Diagnosis and treatment. *Indiana Medicine, 79*(5), 410–415.

Coons, P. M. (1986c). Psychosexual disturbances in multiple personality: Characteristics, etiology, and treatment. *Journal of Clinical Psychiatry, 47,* 106–110.

Coons, P. M. (1986d). Treatment progress in 20 patients with multiple personality disorder. *Journal of Nervous and Mental Disease, 174*(12), 715–721.

Coons, P., & Milstein, V. (1986). Psychosexual disturbances in multiple personality: Characteristics, etiology, and treatment. *Journal of Clinical Psychiatry, 47,* 3, pp. 106–110.

Crisp, P. (1983). Object relations and multiple personality: An exploration of the literature. *The Psychoanalytic Review, 70*(2), 221–234.

Erickson, E. H. (1963). *Childhood and society*. New York: W. W. Norton.

Galin, D. (1974). Implications for psychiatry of left and right cerebral specialization. *Archives of General Psychiatry, 31,* 572–583.

Goodwin, J. (1987). Developmental impacts of incest, pp. 103–106 in *Basic Handbook of Psychiatry* (Editor-in-chief, Joseph Nostipitz), Vol. V, New York: Basic Books.

Greaves, G. (1980). Multiple personality: 165 years after Mary Reynolds. *Journal of Nervous and Mental Disease, 168,* 577–596.

Gregory, I., & Smeltzer, D. (1983). Anxiety, somatoform, and dissociative disorders (nematic disorders). In *Psychiatry*. Boston: Little, Brown.

Horewitz, R. P., & Braun, B. G. (1984). Are multiple personalities borderline? *Psychiatric Clinics of North America, 7*(1), 69–87.

Jacobson, E. (1964). *The self and the object world*. New York: International Universities Press.

Kaplan, H. & Sadock, B. (1985). *Modern synopsis of comprehensive textbook of psychiatry/IV*. Baltimore: Williams & Wilkins.

Kernberg, O. (1975). *Borderline conditions and pathological narcissism*. New York: Jason Aronson, Inc.

Kernberg, O. (1976). *Object-relations theory and clinical psychoanalysis*. New York: Jason Aronson, Inc.

Keys, D. (1981). *The minds of Billy Milligan*. New York: Random House.

Kim, M., McFarland, G., & McLane, A. (1984). *Classification of nursing diagnosis*. St. Louis: C. V. Mosby.

Kluft, R. P. (1982). Varieties of hypnotherapeutic interventions in the treatment of multiple personality. *American Journal of Clinical Hypnosis, 24,* 230–240.

Kluft, R. P. (1983). Hypnotherapeutic crisis intervention in multiple personality. *American Journal of Clinical Hypnosis, 26*(2), 73–83.

Kluft, R. P. (1984a). An introduction to multiple personality disorder. *Psychiatric Annals, 14,* 19–23.

Kluft, R. P. (1984b). Aspects of the treatment of multiple personality disorder. *Psychiatric Annals, 14,* 51–55.

Kluft, R. P. (1984c). Multiple personality in childhood. *Psychiatric Clinics of North America, 7*(1), 121–134.

Kluft, R. P. (1984d). Treatment of multiple personality disorder. *Psychiatric Clinics of North America, 7*(1), 9–29.

Kohlenberg, R. J. (1973). Behavioristic approaches to multiple personality: A case study. *Behavior Therapy, 4,* 137–140.

Kohut, H. (1971). *The analysis of self*. New York: International Universities Press.

Kolb, L. C. (1973). *Noyes' modern clinical psychiatry*. Philadelphia: W. B. Saunders.

Kolb, L. C., & Brodie, H. K. (1982). *Modern clinical psychiatry* (10th ed.). Philadelphia: W. B. Saunders.

Lasky, R. (1982). *Evaluation of criminal responsibility in multiple personality and the related dissociative disorders.* Springfield: Charles Thomas.

Lego, S. (1984). *The American handbook of psychiatric nursing.* New York: J. B. Lippincott.

Ludwig, A. M. (1966). Altered states of consciousness. *Archives of General Psychiatry, 15,* 225–234.

Ludwig, A. M. (1983). The psychobiological functions of dissociation. *American Journal of Clinical Hypnosis, 26*(2), 93–99.

Mahler, M. S. (1968). *On human symbiosis and the vicissitudes of individuation.* New York: International Universities Press.

Maxmen, J. (1986). *Essential psychopathology.* New York: W. W. Norton.

Moore, B. E., & Fine, B. D. (1968). *A glossary of psychoanalytic terms and concepts.* New York: The American Psychoanalytic Association.

Munster, A. J. (1979). Altered and dissociative states of consciousness. In M. M. Josephson & R. T. Porter (Eds.), *Clinician's handbook of childhood psychotherapy.* New York: Jason Aronson, pp. 241–251.

Nathan, P., & Harris, S. (1980). *Psychopathology and society.* New York: McGraw-Hill.

Peplau, H. E. (1952). *Interpersonal relations in nursing.* New York: G. P. Putnam.

Price, J., & Hess, N. C. (1979). Behavior therapy as precipitant and treatment in a case of dual personality. *Australia-New Zealand Journal of Psychiatry, 13*(1), 63–66.

Prince, M. (1925). *The dissociation of a personality.* New York: Longmans, Green.

Putnam, F., Guroff, J., Silberman, E., & Barban, L. (1986). The clinical phenomenology of multiple personality disorder: Review of 100 recent cases. *Journal of Clinical Psychiatry, 47,* 285–293.

Putnam, F., Lowenstein, R., Silberman, E., & Post, R. (1984). Multiple personality disorder in a hospital setting. *Journal of Clinical Psychiatry, 45*(4), 172–175.

Ruedrich, Chu, & Wadle (1985). The Amytal interview in the treatment of psychogenic amnesia. *Hospital and Community Psychiatry, 36*(16), 1045–1046.

Saltman, V., & Solomon, R. (1982). Incest and the multiple personality. *Psychological Reports, 50,* 1127–1141.

Sanders, S. (1986). A brief history of dissociation. *American Journal of Clinical Hypnosis,* Vol. 29, No. 2, 83–85.

Sanders, S. (1986). *The perceptual alteration scale: A pilot study of a scale of dissociation.* The University of North Carolina, Chapel Hill, North Carolina.

Sanders, S. (1988). Personal communication, Friday, July 1, 1988.

Schafer, D. W. (1981). The recognition and hypnotherapy of patients with unrecognized alter states. *American Journal of Clinical Hypnosis, 23* (3), pp. 176–183.

Schafer, D. (1986). Recognizing multiple personality patients. *American Journal of Psychotherapy, XL*(4), 500–510.

Schreiber, R. (1973). *Sybil.* New York: Henry Regnery Press.

Schultz, J. M., & Dark, S. L. (1986). *Manual of psychiatric nursing care plans.* Boston: Little Brown.

Shader, R., & Greenblatt, D. (1986). Some practical approaches to the understanding and treatment of the symptoms of anxiety and stress. In P. Berger & K. Brodie (Eds.) *American handbook of psychiatry.* New York: Basic Books.

Spiegel, D. (1986). Dissociating damage. *American Journal of Clinical Hypnosis, 29* (2), pp. 123–129.

Spitz, R. A. (1965). *The first years of life.* New York: International Universities Press.

Stern, C. (1984). The etiology of multiple personalities. *Psychiatric Clinics of North America, 7*(1), 149–159.

Stevenson, R. L. (1979). *The strange case of Dr. Jekyll and Mr. Hyde.* New York: Dodd-Mead.

Sullivan, H. S. (1953). *Conceptions of modern psychiatry.* New York: W. W. Norton.

Sullivan, H. S. (1954). *The psychiatric interview.* New York: W. W. Norton.

Swanson, A. R. (1984). The client who is experiencing sleep disorder. In S. Lego (Ed.), *The American handbook of psychiatric nursing.* New York: J. B. Lippincott, pp. 455–466.

Taylor, W. S. and Martin, M. F. (1944). Multiple personality. *Journal of Abnormal and Social Psychology, 39,* pp. 281–300.

Thigpen, C. H., & Cleckley, H. M. (1957). *The three faces of Eve.* New York: McGraw-Hill.

Watkins, J. G. (1978). Ego states and the problems of responsibility II: The case of Patricia W. *Journal of Psychiatry and Law, 6,* 519–536.

Webster, M. (1984a). Differential diagnosis. In S. Lego (Ed.), *The American handbook of psychiatric nursing.* New York: J. B. Lippincott, pp. 17–18.

Webster, M. (1984b). Psychiatric nursing assessment. In S. Lego (Ed.), *The American handbook of psychiatric nursing.* New York: J. B. Lippincott, pp. 3–17.

West, L. (1967). Dissociative reaction. In A. M. Freedman & H. I. Kaplan (Eds.), *Comprehensive textbook of psychiatry.* Baltimore: Williams & Wilkins.

Wilbur, C. B. (1984). Multiple personality and child abuse. *Psychiatric Clinics of North America, 7*(1), 3–7.

Wilbur, C. B. (1984b). Treatment of multiple personality. *Psychiatric Annals, 14,* 27–31.

Wilson, H., & Kneisel, C. (1979). *Psychiatric nursing.* Menlo Park, CA: Addison-Wesley.

18

PSYCHOLOGICAL CRISES
KEM LOUIE

LEARNING OBJECTIVES

After studying this chapter, the student will be able to:

- Describe the concept of psychological crisis.
- Assess patients in psychological crisis related to physical trauma including AIDS, attempted suicide, violence and abuse within the family, and rape.
- Describe the theories that provide a framework for treating patients in psychological crises.
- Identify the responsibilities of the nurse toward patients in crisis.
- Develop and implement nursing care plans for patients in crisis.

CONCEPT OF CRISIS

DESCRIPTION OF CRISIS

Crisis situations are an integral part of a person's growth and experience in life. These situations have the potential for stimulating positive growth in individuals and their families. The concept of crisis is partly a theory and partly a methodology that nurses and other health professionals use to assist their patients. Crisis techniques are not limited to psychiatric inpatient units; they are utilized in telephone crisis units, general hospital units, and community settings. This chapter deals with selected crisis situations: physical trauma, suicide, spouse and child abuse, sexual abuse, and rape.

In order to understand the concept of crisis, it is important to differentiate the terms *stress, predicament,* and *emergency* which have been used interchangeably with the term crisis. The following discussion clarifies the meaning of each term and addresses the meaningful differences and relationships among them. According to Hoff (1978), **stress** can be defined simply as a tension, strain, or pressure; a **predicament** is a situation that is unpleasant, dangerous, or embarrassing; an **emergency** is an unforeseen event that requires immediate action. Hoff continues, "Predicaments and emergencies lead to stresses which carry the potential of becoming crises. Whether such predicaments and emergencies become crises depends on our ability to handle these stresses" (p. 6). Therefore, a traumatic event does not necessarily become a crisis situation. The determining factor of whether an event will be a crisis is the individual's ability to cope with or adjust to the stressful event. If the stress is overwhelming and an individual is unable to cope with the situation, a crisis will result. It is not just the event or situation that activates the crisis, but the interpretation of the situation that leads to the experience of stress and inability to cope.

The word *crisis* is derived from the Greek words for *decision* or *turning point.* In addition, the Chinese ideograph or character for crisis is interpreted both as a "danger," a threatening situation which may result in serious consequences, and as an "opportunity," in which the individual is receptive to influence (Golan, 1978). Caplan (1964) presented a commonly accepted definition of crisis. He defined a **psychological crisis** as the ". . . psychological disequilibrium in a person who confronts a hazardous circumstance that for him constitutes an important problem which he can for the time being neither escape nor solve with his customary problem-solving

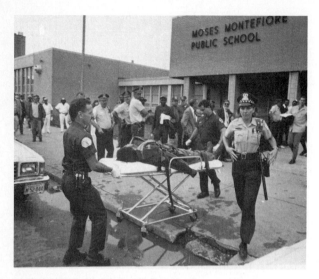

An example of psychological crisis: A schoolyard shooting in Chicago on September 22, 1988 resulted in the homicide of a policewoman.

resources" (p. 53). The crisis is precipitated by situations related to loss (perceived or real), as in an illness, or change in status or responsibilities. These situations can be classified as maturational or situational crises. A **maturational crisis** is any event that is related to the normal growth and development process, such as becoming a parent, conflicts during adolescence, and retirement. Sheehy (1976) describes potential maturational crises as transition periods in life. **Situational crises** are events that are precipitated by unanticipated stress. These events include such occurrences as death of a loved one, acute physical or mental illness, and any type of serious physical or psychological trauma.

THEORIES ABOUT RESPONSES TO CRISIS

Crisis theory was initially derived for the most part from the work of Eric Lindemann (1965). He studied grief responses in families of victims of the infamous Coconut Grove fire in Boston in 1943. In his study and observations, he found that grieving responses followed a sequence of defined stages. These stages were applicable to any situation in which individuals experienced loss—of self-esteem, function, independence, position, or a significant other. Lindemann suggested a process whereby individuals learn to cope with the stressful event. The duration and severity of bereavement were associated with the

survivors' ability to grieve for the deceased, readjust to the environment without the deceased, and form new relationships. **Crisis intervention** began to be known as brief, active, and collaborative therapy that utilized the individual's own coping abilities and resources within the community.

Gerald Caplan (1964) added to the concept of crisis in his early work with immigrant mothers and children after World War II and his work in community mental health. Caplan noted the importance of crisis periods for individuals and groups. He viewed individuals as being in a state of emotional equilibrium, and when usual or customary problem-solving techniques failed, this balance or equilibrium was altered. He postulated three levels of crisis intervention and maintenance of mental health: they include primary, secondary, and tertiary interventions. The primary level of intervention includes methods which reduce or eliminate stress in the lives of individuals, families, and/or communities, such as education and consultation. The secondary level of intervention is designed to reduce the number of existing crisis cases by early diagnosis of the problem and prompt and efficient treatment. The goal of this level is to provide services that would prevent lengthy periods of disability. Crisis intervention is viewed as part of the secondary level of prevention, its goal being to restore the individual to a stable, or precrisis, state of functioning. The third level of intervention, tertiary, includes methods that reduce or decrease long-term mental problems or disability.

In contrast, Pasquali et al. (1985) recognized that crisis intervention is an important part of each of the three levels of prevention. In the primary level of prevention, the stress that can precipitate a crisis is identified, and through education and referral, it is reduced. In secondary prevention, active crisis-intervention techniques are employed to assist individuals to cope with the stressful situation. The third level of prevention involves assisting the individual in learning new coping behaviors and resources.

Crisis is not a pathological state and can occur in anyone's life. Individuals faced with similar situations may not respond in the same manner, and some situations are so acutely stressful that a crisis may not be preventable (Golan, 1978).

ASSESSMENT OF CRISIS

Crisis periods are time limited, generally lasting from four to six weeks (Caplan, 1964). During this time, the person passes through predictable reactions. First, psychological and physical unrest occurs. For example, the individual experiences aimless activity or immobilization, disturbance in body functions, and/or mood and intellectual functioning. He may be preoccupied with events associated with the crisis. Gradually, he readjusts to the altered situation.

Caplan (1964) has described four phases of crisis:

Phase I: The individual perceives a threat (stressor) which causes anxiety. He utilizes normal coping strategies to deal with the threat. If these strategies are not effective, the individual moves into Phase II.

Phase II: The individual experiences a sense of increased anxiety and disorganization.

Phase III: The individual is most amenable to assistance from professionals during this phase. The crisis situation is redefined, avoided, or altered by the individual, and new coping strategies may be employed. If resolution of the crisis occurs, the individual returns to his precrisis level of functioning.

Phase IV: If resolution does not occur, the individual suffers increased disorganization that may reach a panic level of anxiety.

Aguilera and Messick (1982) have proposed a paradigm that can be useful in the process of crisis assessment as well as in predicting its outcome. (See Figure 18-1.) The successful or healthy resolution of a crisis is a function of three factors as seen in Figure 18-1: realistic perception of the stressful event, availability of support systems, and availability of individual coping strategies.

Burgess and Baldwin (1981) further developed a classification system based on the severity of the crisis situation, as well as strategies for each classification:

Class 1: Dispositional crisis: involves problematic situations that present a sense of immediacy, such as the need to provide the family of an alcoholic with education and information, or to refer a family without housing to social service agencies. Interventions to reduce stress may include clarifying the issues, providing necessary support, strengthening coping abilities, and referral to other professionals.

Class 2: Crisis involving life transitions: includes situations occurring in normal growth and development, such as job changes, divorce, or the diagnosis of a chronic illness. Interventions include anticipatory guidance, identifying the effects and helping the individual

interpret the meaning of the transition, and exploring and developing coping strategies with him, for example, joining a support group.

Class 3: Crisis resulting from sudden unexpected traumatic stress: involves external stressors. Individuals experience increased anxiety and immobilization. Examples include sudden death of a spouse, rape, or catastrophic illness. Interventions involve providing immediate support, encouraging the expression of thoughts and feelings concerning the situation, and helping the individual develop coping strategies.

Class 4: Maturational or developmental crisis: involves stress that is internal and based on psychosocial issues. These developmental issues occur across the life span and include dependency, power, intimacy, sexual identity, and psychodynamic conflicts. Child abuse, incest, marital difficulties, or interpersonal problems may be involved. Interventions focus on understanding the underlying developmental issues and needs while developing strategies to deal with the current situation.

Class 5: Crisis resulting from psychopathology: preexisting psychopathology (such as severe anxiety or mood disorders, personality disorders, and schizophrenia) precipitates a crisis or impairs crisis resolution. Affected individuals present multiple problems involving several areas of functioning. Intervention includes identifying the underlying psychopathology and determining effective coping strategies. It is important not to focus on the underlying psychological problems that cannot be resolved during the crisis therapy. Instead, the goal is to reduce the individual's stress to a level sufficient to prevent further regression or decompensation. Referral to a psychotherapist may be appropriate.

Class 6: Psychiatric emergencies: include attempted suicide, acute psychosis, out-of-control anger and aggression, and severe drug overdose or alcohol toxicity. Individuals in these emergencies experience total psychological disorganization resulting in grossly impaired functioning. In a psychiatric emergency, the individual is usually considered dangerous to himself or others. Interventions are directed toward immediate assess-

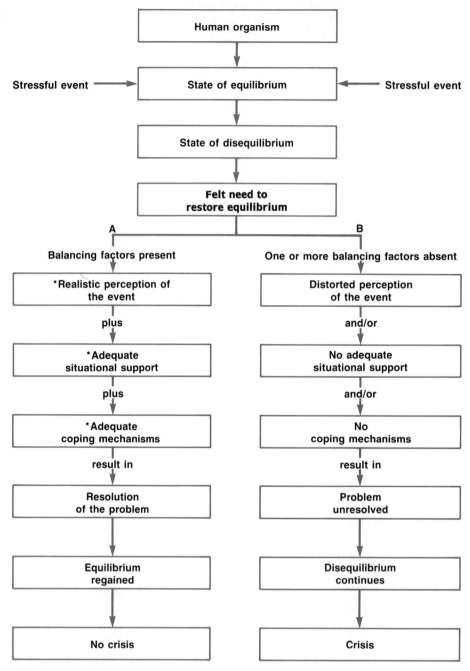

*Balancing factors

FIGURE 18–1 Crisis Assessment Paradigm
Source: From Aguilera, D. C., & Messick, J. H. (1982). Crisis intervention: Theory &
methodology, 4th edition. St. Louis: The C. V. Mosby Co., p. 65.

ment and acute treatment of the mental and
physical condition of the patient and the prevention of harm or injury.

This classification system facilitates crisis assessment
and provides a basis for intervention. As the crises
proceed from Class 1 to Class 6, increased clinical

skill and training is required to deal with the crisis
and resolve it therapeutically.

Data collected in the process of crisis assessment
include:

1. Specifics of the hazardous event or those reactions
and stresses that culminated in a crisis. These hazard-

ous events can be anticipated or unanticipated and internal or external to the individual. Involving the patient in this aspect of assessment helps him make some order out of what seems to be chaos.

2. Precipitating factors involved in the crisis. Precipitating factors and behavioral responses to them may have been long-standing problems. It is important to separate the current crisis from long-established pathological patterns (Everstine & Everstine, 1983). Obtaining an individual and family psychiatric history will help identify preexisting problems.

3. The patient's degree of anxiety and thoughts and feelings related to the crisis. The patient may be experiencing overwhelming guilt, anger, or embarrassment, all of which demand an immediate response from the clinician. An example of an anxiety rating scale is one from 1–5, with 1 being mild anxiety and 5 representing overwhelming anxiety that causes the individual to panic and become dangerously dysfunctional.

4. The patient's previous and present coping abilities. Observation of the patient's current behavior helps to determine the type and degree of emotional stress that the patient is experiencing, as well as the adaptive or maladaptive coping mechanisms he is using.

5. The patient's resources and available support system. Assessing the patient's relationships with family members and/or friends helps to determine the patient's support system and provides information about the need for followup. Spiritual support can be very helpful to some patients, but assessment of spiritual resources is often overlooked by professionals in times of crisis (Ryan, 1984).

NURSING MANAGEMENT OF CRISIS

PLANNING. Following the collection and analysis of the assessment data, the nurse formulates a plan to address the problems of the patient in crisis. Rapoport (1970) identified the following goals of crisis intervention:

1. Alleviation or relief of symptoms, for example, anxiety, disorganization, and immobilization;

2. Restoration to at least the precrisis level of functioning;

3. Understanding of the relationship of the precipitating events and the state of crisis and disequilibrium;

4. Identification of family and/or community resources;

5. Understanding of the relationship of past life experiences to the current stress; and

6. Development of new coping strategies that the patient can use in future situations.

The nurse develops the care plan in collaboration with the client in crisis and significant people. According to Caplan and Grunebaum (1967), a good plan is one that is:

1. Problem oriented. The plan focuses on the immediate, concrete problems related to the crisis. Referrals for psychotherapy are appropriate after resolution of the immediate crisis.

2. Appropriate to the patient's functional level and dependency needs. The patient's behavior and thoughts and feelings at the time of the crisis are considered by the nurse as she determines which immediate decisions can be made collaboratively with the patient and which need to be made without him.

3. Appropriate given the patient's culture and lifestyle. Interventions should not conflict with the patient's cultural, ethnic, and/or religious background or affiliation. (See Chapter 6 on sociocultural diversity.)

4. Inclusive of significant other(s). A plan that has the support of the patient's significant others is likely to be more effective.

5. Realistic, time limited, and concrete. The patient's available resources as well as needs must be taken into consideration. Also to be effective, the plan needs to be concrete in terms of time, place, and circumstances.

6. Dynamic and renegotiable. The plan is ongoing, should be flexible, and subject to revision after evaluation.

7. Includes follow up. Follow up ensures that the crisis support system will not be withdrawn too soon.

IMPLEMENTATION. Implementation of the nursing care plan for the patient in crisis involves the following activities (Hoff, 1978):

1. Listening actively and with concern.

2. Encouraging open expression of feelings.

3. Helping the patient gain an understanding of the crisis.

4. Helping the patient gradually accept reality.

5. Assisting the patient in exploring new ways of coping with problems.

6. Linking the patient to a social network and support system.

7. Utilizing problem-solving techniques such as generating and evaluating options.

8. Reinforcing newly learned coping strategies and evaluating them on followup after resolution of the crisis.

EVALUATION. In the evaluation phase, the nurse reviews the effectiveness of the intervention strategies and determines whether the goals of the plan were met, in whole or in part. According to Jacobson (1974), the patient's continued or increased use of such coping mechanisms as projection, introjection, and denial indicates unsuccessful crisis resolution. Successful or adaptive resolution of the crisis is evident if the patient ultimately experiences feelings of mastery and increased self-esteem.

CRISIS RELATED TO PHYSICAL TRAUMA

DESCRIPTION OF CRISIS RELATED TO PHYSICAL TRAUMA

Situational crisis involves hazards or threats to physical health, self-image, or life itself. Physical illness, disease, or an accident often precipitate crisis. In addition, the hospitalization and treatment that result from the physical illness or accident can also precipitate crisis situations for the individual and family.

EPIDEMIOLOGY OF CRISIS RELATED TO PHYSICAL TRAUMA

In 1984, the number of reported disabling injuries was 8,700,000, resulting from motor vehicle accidents, work and home accidents, and accidents in public places (National Safety Council, 1987). Accidental deaths in 1984 were estimated to be 92,000, which increased by 500, or 1 percent above the 1983 total. Accidents are the fourth leading cause of death in the United States and the major cause of death in children.

The National Center for Health Statistics (1988) reported the ten leading causes of death as follows (all but two involve physical illnesses and disease):

1. Disease of the heart

2. Malignant neoplasms

3. Cerebrovascular disease

4. Accidents

5. Chronic obstructive pulmonary disease

6. Pneumonia and influenza

7. Diabetes mellitus

8. Chronic liver disease and cirrhosis

9. Atherosclerosis

10. Suicide

ASSESSMENT OF CRISIS RELATED TO PHYSICAL TRAUMA

Welty, Rosillo, and Graham (1973) identified three groups of psychosocial stressors of individuals diagnosed with cancer:

1. Loss of health induced by the disease: feelings of shame, punishment, retribution, loss of control, and impending death;

2. Stresses related to the treatment: fear of injury, mutilation, pain, and disfigurement;

3. Stresses related to hospitalization: diminished contact with family, friends, and usual surroundings, and loss of employment and identity.

Krouse and Krouse (1982) found that mastectomy patients experienced emotional stress, with their most profound period of crisis during the initial weeks following hospital discharge. By the sixth and seventh week, the women experienced less emotional turmoil and preoccupation with physical changes. Thus, in concordance with Caplan (1964), the crisis period was limited to six weeks in duration. In some situations, the crisis period may be extended due to continued psychological and physical stressors.

According to Hoff (1978), the signs and symptoms of crisis resulting from threats to physical integrity and self-image include:

1. Shock and anger: "Why me?"

2. Helplessness and hopelessness in regard to future normal functioning: "What's left for me now?"

3. Shame of obvious scar, handicap, or reduced physical ability and dependence on others: "What will my husband or lover think?"

4. Anxiety about the welfare of spouse or children who depend on them: "How will they manage at home without me?"

5. Deep sense of loss of body integrity and loss of goals the person hoped to achieve before the illness or accident: "I don't think I'll ever feel right again."

6. Doubt of acceptance by others: "No one will want to be around me this way."

7. Fear of death, which may have been narrowly escaped in an accident or that now must be faced in the case of cancer: "It was almost the end" or "This is the end" (p. 160).

Aguilera and Messick (1982) report that a chronic illness such as heart disease can precipitate a series of crises for the individual and his family. The medical interventions for the rehabilitation of the individual with heart disease include severe changes in lifestyle and occupation, use of medications, and, possibly, surgery. Compared with other serious illnesses, cardiac disease has three unique features: 1) it is associated with sudden death; 2) there is an onslaught of anxiety and restriction of physical activity which increases feelings of vulnerability, depression, and helplessness; and 3) depression and emotional regression may develop. Other responses may include aggression, anger, and projection of feelings or denial. An individual will react to a life-threatening situation with a variety of coping mechanisms that may be appropriate at one stage of recovery but will be inappropriate at another. For example, denial is adaptive when it initially acts as a buffer against the shock of the trauma and provides time for the individual to gather together his internal resources and respond to the reality of the situation. Denial can be inappropriate or indicate maladjustment, for example, when it leads to self-destructive behavior such as rejection of or noncooperation with treatment or therapy.

The assessment should be aimed at identifying the individual's emotional strengths, motivations, and coping abilities. Information concerning the unique meaning of the illness or accident to the individual should be ascertained. In a study of cancer patients, Capone et al. (1979) found that cancer represented punishment, weakness, loss, damage, death, pain, or abandonment to patients.

Previous stressful experiences and how the individual coped with the situation can influence his perception of his ability to deal with the present illness or accident. An individual's ability to cope with the disease and treatment is also influenced by his personality, premorbid emotional status, values, activities, and relationships as well as previous and present life events (Krumm, 1982). The patient's cognitive abilities such as intellectual capacity, memory, and orientation need to be assessed. Spiritual and religious needs and practices can provide a basis for hopefulness.

NURSING MANAGEMENT OF CRISIS RELATED TO PHYSICAL TRAUMA

PLANNING. The nursing-care plan focuses on those areas that are most disturbing to the patient. Immediate physical and psychological goals are collaboratively determined by the patient and health care team members. The patient's psychological strengths and adaptive defenses will assist him in identifying and mobilizing his support system. Initial treatment goals include developing and maintaining adaptive coping mechanisms, fostering independence and responsibility for self-care practices, strengthening supportive relationships with family and friends, and a return to normal activities of daily living.

IMPLEMENTATION. Nursing intervention in crisis therapy during the acute stage of an illness or an accident can decrease the psychological and emotional stress encountered during treatment and recovery. Specific interventions (Capone et al., 1979) include:

- Identifying and reducing anxiety, for example, by clarifying the patient's physical condition, proposed treatment, and prognosis.
- Reinforcing healthy coping mechanisms as well as identifying nonadaptive coping mechanisms such as prolonged denial, extreme regression, and withdrawal.
- Instilling reality-based expectations, with a focus on special concerns of the patient.
- Knowing what information the patient has received and how he has processed it, and clarifying misperceptions, distortions, and confusion the patient may have concerning the medical problem and treatment regimen.
- Assisting the patient with formulating and asking questions about his illness, treatment, and recovery, as this can diminish the patient's anxieties and fantasies regarding the many unknowns.
- Encouraging the patient to take responsibility for solving his emotional problems, in order to reduce helplessness and increase the patient's sense of control.
- Facilitating contacts with self-help groups. These groups provide a forum for patients and/or their families to share their thoughts and concerns with other people who have similar problems. Spiegel, Bloom, and Yalom (1981) found that weekly support group meetings attended by women with metastatic breast cancer resulted in improved mood, coping, and self-esteem. Self-help groups may also provide ongoing social support in the future.

It is the role of the nurse to attempt to understand the individual patient's reactions to his illness or trauma and his efforts to cope with it. She also needs to understand how these reactions are influenced by the individual's sociocultural attitudes and beliefs (Boyle & Andrews, 1989). She provides a model of coping with crisis for the patient by focus-

Box 18–1 ● Caring for the AIDS Patient: Confidentiality Versus Disclosure

The nurse caring for the HIV-infected individual may face the dilemma presented by the need to protect her patient's confidentiality and at the same time to prevent injury from coming to a potentially vulnerable third party (such as a spouse or significant other). Because of the potential for discrimination and mistreatment of HIV-infected individuals, health professionals have been advised to take extraordinary measures in preserving the confidentiality of their patients' HIV status (National League for Nursing, 1988). However, when there is an identifiable third party or parties at risk (and

when state law dictates), it may be necessary for the nurse or physician to disclose this information to the at-risk individual.

The Association of State and Territorial Health Officials, together with the National Association of County Health Officials and the United States Conference of Local Health Officers (1988), have put together some guidelines to help health care providers handle these situations. They recommend invoking the privilege to disclose when all four of the following criteria have been met and documented:

ing on and understanding the illness or accident, identifying adaptive and maladaptive coping mechanisms, and encouraging the appropriate use of support systems.

CRISIS RELATED TO AIDS

In recent years, AIDS has become a far-reaching concern for nurses, other health professionals, families, and society. The effects of AIDS are not limited to the infected individual. Sexual partners, spouses, parents, grandparents, siblings, and children of victims are affected in various ways. Family members suffer some of the same stigma and isolation experienced by the person with AIDS. Lack of understanding of the methods of transmission can lead to the unfounded fear of contracting the disease from the victim or an uninfected family member of the victim. Even health professionals who treat AIDS patients may find themselves and their families experiencing discrimination (Macklin, 1988).

The sexual partner of the victim is at risk for infection, and needs counseling to cope with fear and to minimize risk through safe sex practices. While the partner's fear is realistic, other family members may also experience fear for their own health, even when they know such alarm is unfounded. Sometimes the fear becomes so great that the AIDS sufferer is abandoned by his or her family at a time when loving

support is crucial to well-being. Abandoning a loved one can lead to acute guilt for the family member which complicates the grieving process (Macklin, 1988).

Often, telling the family of the AIDS diagnosis entails the revelation of the victim's homosexuality. This can lead to a double load of shock and grief. Parents react in a variety of ways when confronted with AIDS in a gay adult son. While most are supportive, many express the intention of maintaining secrecy and a few are completely rejecting (Cleveland, et al., 1988).

The family is often called upon to assume financial responsibility for the medical treatment. Treatment costs are high and earning ability of the AIDS sufferer is reduced because of deteriorating health and/or the loss of employment and attendant benefits due to discrimination against persons with AIDS. AIDS victims and their families are subject to unique difficulties and stress in addition to the anger and grief that would be felt by the family with a member who was suffering from any other terminal illness. Help should be sought for victims and families in the form of counseling and support groups. (See Box 18–1.)

AIDS AND CHILDREN

When children have AIDS, the tragedy deepens. While adults have the opportunity to modify their behavior to minimize their risk of contracting AIDS,

1. The provider knows of an identifiable third party at risk.

2. The health care provider believes that there is a significant risk of harm to the third party.

3. The provider believes that the third party does not suspect that he or she is at risk.

4. The index patient has been urged to notify the at-risk partner, and has refused or is considered to be unreliable in his or her willingness to notify the partner.

It is every health care provider's responsibility, however, to keep abreast of new state or federal legislation regarding disclosure; the laws governing disclosure and confidentiality vary among the states and seem to be changing frequently. (See Chapter 27, Legal Considerations in Mental Health Nursing Practice, and Chapter 28, Ethical Considerations in Mental Health Nursing Practice for a broader discussion of these issues.)

References and for Additional Information

The Association of State and Territorial Health Officials, the National Association of County Health Officials, and the United States Conferene of Local Health Officers. (September, 1988). *A guide to public health practice: HIV partner notification strategies.*

National League for Nursing. (1988). *AIDS guidelines for schools of nursing.* New York: National League for Nursing.

Centers for Disease Control. (April 1988). *AIDS recommendations and guidelines.* Atlanta: U.S. Public Health Service, Department of Health and Human Services.

---

children have no such ability. The majority of children with AIDS (80%) have mothers who are also infected or who are at high risk for contracting the disease. Another 15% acquire AIDS through blood transfusions, and 4% from infected clotting factor in the treatment for hemophilia (Laker, 1987; U.S. Department of Health, 1986).

The long latency period often seen in adult victims of AIDS is not found in infants. These babies are often small, fail to thrive, and exhibit such symptoms as enlarged liver and spleen, respiratory disease, fevers, rashes and diarrhea. Characteristic facial features include a small head with a box-like forehead, flattened nose bridge, expanded lips, and wide-set eyes. Fewer than 20% survive longer than two years after being diagnosed with AIDS (Kluz, 1986).

In addition to the discrimination and isolation endured by other AIDS patients, children with AIDS must deal with interference with mastery of developmental tasks. Both physical and psychological development can be compromised by the disease and its social consequences (see Box 18–2).

Since, as we noted earlier, children with AIDS often have an infected mother, the family frequently must cope with the illness and death of multiple members. If a parent transmitted the disease to the child, grief and guilt must be dealt with by a person who may also be infected with AIDS.

A Family with AIDS

Sandra and James, ages 32 and 33, are a white, college educated, religious couple who have been married 10 years. They both have had professional careers. Sandra was in an automobile accident 6 years ago and had a transfusion. Subsequently, she had two children. Her infant son became ill and tested HIV positive. Since then, she and her 4-year-old daughter have been tested, and both carry the virus but are asymptomatic. Stunned at the diagnosis, Sandra and James question why this happened to them.

When they decided to have children, Sandra resigned from her job to remain at home to care for them. Even though her husband helps her, she wishes there were more alternatives for child care to give her an occasional break. When his employer learned of the AIDS diagnosis, James was given a permanent leave of absence. He took new employment, lost his group insurance coverage, and had to purchase personal insurance coverage at an annual premium cost of $6,000 per year. In addition, out-of-pocket medical expenses for one year were $3,000. Sandra and James have vacillated in feelings of confusion, frustration, guilt, and helplessness. Their one solace has been the medical professionals who have been helpful and caring to them.

Sandra and James decided to move to a larger nearby city to receive better medical care and have access to more resources. Initially, they felt very

Box 18–2 • Eliana goes to school for first time

Entering a classroom with her mother, Eliana squealed with glee. Another child, oblivious to the controversy surrounding the frail new girl, rushed forward and hugged her. Other children gathered around.

With that simple welcome, almost three years after Hillsborough school officials first refused to let the AIDS-afflicted girl into a classroom, Eliana Martinez's school days had begun.

"Finally, she's where she belongs and where she should have been a long time ago," said Rosa Martinez, later describing her 7-year-old daughter's first moments in class.

The barriers to Eliana Martinez's enrollment were removed Wednesday, when U.S. District Judge Elizabeth Kovachevich ordered the Hillsborough County School Board to allow Eliana to attend school.

The risk that the mentally handicapped child could transmit AIDS to other students is too remote to justify excluding her from school or separating her from other children, the judge ruled.

For Eliana, the decision meant venturing into such strange new experiences as learning songs with classmates, eating macaroni and cheese in a cafeteria and slipping her delicate body down a playground slide.

"It's just a whole new world for her," Eliana's mother said. "It's not just watching the world on television anymore."

In addition to the benefits for Eliana, the judge's decision sends a message of compassion and intelligence to all victims of AIDS, said Stephen Hanlon, the attorney who has represented Mrs. Martinez since she filed a federal lawsuit against the School Board in 1987.

"I think the case establishes, once and for all, that children with AIDS cannot be excluded from school rooms unless they pose a significant risk to other children." Hanlon said. "The risk they pose is nothing more than a remote and theoretical risk."

That risk didn't frighten most of the parents of children attending Manhattan Exceptional Center in Tampa. Only two of the 11 children in Eliana's class for the trainable mentally handicapped stayed home Thursday. Overall, 60 of the school's 201 students were absent, about

alone. They now have a wide circle of family and friends but have told very few persons about their situation. They are worried about the stigma that AIDS provokes. Sandra has been learning about AIDS and has helped develop a support group for parents, which she feels has been her lifeline. She also volunteers time with other parents and AIDS children.

Their son died this past year. His death is still hard for them to accept, and Sandra says helping others aids in the healing process.

Source: Urwin, C. (1988). AIDS in Children: A Family Concern. *Family Relations, Journal of Applied Family and Child Studies.* Vol. *37,* No 2, p. 155.

All family members are affected and may experience sadness, anger or fear. Fewer support groups exist for families with young AIDS victims, so family and friends are more often the main support than in the case of adult victims (Urwin, 1988).

The financial burden can be greater for families of young victims because the lack of out-of-hospital care facilities results in longer hospitalizations. Often, one parent must withdraw from employment in order to care for the child, severely reducing the family's income (Urwin, 1988).

NURSING MANAGEMENT OF AIDS PATIENTS

The person diagnosed with AIDS experiences the same psychosocial stressors as others with chronic or incurable illnesses—fear of death, denial, anger, social isolation, and depression. The emotional stress, however, is heightened by the stigma surrounding this disease and, in some cases, a lack of support and

twice the usual number, said Sandra Kilpatrick-Williams, the school's principal.

Some parents are keeping their children home until they can attend a meeting on Monday with school officials and doctors about Eliana's condition and AIDS, she said.

Judi Cook, whose 8-year-old son attends the school, said she wasn't concerned about Eliana's presence.

"I figure there are other things in the environment and in society that are just as threatening," Ms. Cook said.

Some faculty members at the school, however, were less comfortable with the school's newest student.

When Eliana's class arrived in the playground, the two classes already there immediately left, said Peggy Kelly, Eliana's teacher. Although school officials said the classes were leaving anyway, Ms. Kelly said she has sensed fear and hostility from a few aids and teachers.

"People are still deathly afraid," said Ms. Kelly, who's been teaching Eliana at home after school for the past two years.

One of the teacher's aides assigned to work in Eliana's class requested a transfer and refused to walk into the classroom on Thursday to gather her belongings, Ms. Kelly said. The aide who volunteered Thursday morning to replace her, Verdell Poole, said she was snubbed by other aides who couldn't believe she had volunteered for the position.

"With a lot of kids, we don't know; they could have AIDS," Mrs. Poole said, explaining her actions. "The fact that we know (with Eliana), we know to take the precautions."

So far, those precautions include placing Eliana's used diapers in a special box for medical wastes. The box stands in the corner of the room, beside a changing table with disposable covers and a small potty-seat. Eliana is not toilet-trained, but her teacher expects her to follow examples of the other students and learn that skill soon.

Initially shy with her classmates, Eliana began showing signs of progress Thursday. For two years, she has refused to go near a playground slide. But when she saw her new classmates sliding easily down, she tried it herself. Now that Eliana will be interacting with other children daily, Ms. Kelly expects to see other improvements in the child's social skills and severely limited speech.

It's that kind of learning Mrs. Martinez was seeking during three years of battling the School Board to enroll Eliana in school. It's also why she appealed Judge Kovachevich's initial ruling last summer that Eliana could attend school only if she remained in a special glass booth.

The victory seemed to agree with Eliana.

At three o'clock, her teacher picked her up and asked if she liked school. The child nodded. The teacher laughed, hugged Eliana and planted a kiss on her cheek.

Source: Dukess, K. St. Petersburg Times, Friday, April 28, 1989, P. 1–A.

empathy from family and significant others as well as the world at large. Nursing care for HIV-infected persons must focus on helping them cope with both the specific physical illnesses caused by the disease as well as the emotional stressors (Locke, 1989). Helping HIV-infected patients maintain psychological stamina in the face of acknowledged (and realistic) fears about the illness and death may provide them with the strength to live full and positive lives. Maintaining some hope, if not for a cure for AIDS, then for newly established short-terms goals, such as accomplishing a specific career objective or attending a family event can allow the person to "begin to think of themselves as living with AIDS instead of dying with AIDS (Locke, 1989, p. 215)." Specific interventions for dealing with the emotions associated with AIDS are summarized in Table 18-1. The nurse, because of her role as direct care provider, will need to be sensitive not only to the AIDS patient's conflicts, but to the conflicts and struggles that occur in their families as well. The nurse must take the necessary action to provide services that assist the patient and family.

When a homosexual adult contracts AIDS, the nurse might find it extremely difficult to seek support from his family of origin. Acknowledging that he has the disease might mean that he has to disclose his homosexuality. For those who have disclosed this information already, parental support appears to be available. Cleveland, Walters, Skeen, and Robinson (1988) systematically queried 736 parents (28% fathers and 72% mothers) of homosexual children to determine how these parents would feel if their children contracted AIDS. Their results revealed a variety of responses with the majority of the parents indicating a desire to support their children. Examples

---

TABLE 18–1 General interventions for people with HIV infection

---

1. *Communicate Acceptance and Concern:*
   - Touch: make physical contact when greeting, talking, or caring for client.
   - Eye contact: shows acceptance and increases trust.
   - Physical proximity: stand close to the client.
   - Body language: gestures that show openness, desire to connect, such as leaning forward, arms open.
   - Avoid judgmental-sounding language. Terms such as "high-risk behavior" or "homosexual" can sound condemning within some contexts. Speak openly about a gay lifestyle, sexual contacts, or drug use.

2. *Establish a Trusting Relationship:*
   - Take all concerns seriously, such as pain, guilt, fatigue.
   - Follow through on everything that you say you will do.
   - Do everything possible to relieve concerns, including physical interventions for comfort and psychological ones.

3. *Encourage Verbalization of Emotions:*
   - Avoid the temptation to dismiss fears as unrealistic. All negative emotions (fear, anger, grief) must be felt and expressed in order for them to be resolved and fade.
   - Help the client determine how to vent the emotions: making an audio or video tape, writing a journal, making a quilt panel, organizing a self-help group, volunteering for legislative work for persons with AIDS, talking to a friend, counselor, or nurse.

4. *Give the Client Control:*
   - Keep clients and families fully informed.
   - Encourage clients to make all decisions possible, ranging from the type of treatment to the time of day for bathing.
   - Encourage clients to do everything they can for themselves, and maintain as "normal" a life as possible, even within the hospital (i.e., hobbies, seeing friends, working, spiritual activities).

---

included, "When and if appropriate, I would get him to the best AIDS clinic immediately, and see that his partner was present, involved, and not blamed," (p. 151). Another comment: "Get help, medical and psychological, for him and for me," (p. 151). Yet, there were some parents who indicated some ambivalence as evidenced by such responses as, ". . . be grief stricken . . . be afraid . . . wouldn't accept my love and loyalty and care . . . pray for a cure . . . fight to carry on" (p. 151).

Parents of patients with AIDS have indicated that they would want counseling to help them cope with feelings of anxiety, depression, and fears. Too, conjoint family therapy might assist the family in the resolution of old familial conflicts.

Support groups are effective in the treatment process with the AIDS patient as well as his family. This modality is effective in "touching" the family's pain that frequently includes anger, fear, guilt, and so forth (Morin and Batchelor, 1984; Cleveland, Walters, Skeen, and Robinson, 1988).

Education about AIDS and HIV infection needs to be available to parents and other family members and friends. Self-help groups and other organizations that encourage self-help are available and can be of great assistance to their families.

The National Council on Family Relations (1987) uses the following principles to support their policies on AIDS (Macklin, 1988, pp. 141–149).

1. AIDS affects the individual and the family.

2. The family plays a major role in education, prevention, and assisting in attitudinal change about AIDS.

3. Families should be viewed as a component of the treatment of AIDS; families need to have information about AIDS.

- Introduce the concept of complementary therapies as a way of gaining control over one's treatment and well-being, such as relaxation techniques, guided imagery, and hypnosis. . . .

5. *Reinforce a Positive Self-Concept:*
   - Give positive feedback for all accomplishments, such as reaching the goal of getting out of bed.
   - Ask clients, and encourage them to focus on, what they like about themselves, or what they do/did well.

6. *Help Clients Continue Roles and Relationships:*
   - Encourage them to continue their work as much as possible, or to undertake any task that is important to them.
   - Help clients see new ways to continue relationships such as:
     1) even if they cannot physically care for their children, they can provide essential affection, counsel, and reinforcement.
     2) even if they cannot provide physical intimacy, they can give emotional intimacy to a spouse.
   - Provide privacy for clients when visiting with all others in order to invite the expression of affection with friends and family.

7. *Facilitate a Positive Body Image:*
   - Facilitate exercise programs.
   - Minimize the display of invasive intervention such as IV lines.
   - Encourage clients to dress in street clothes.
   - Encourage and facilitate the client's usual grooming habits, such as seeing a hairdresser or manicurist.
   - Facilitate the use of attitudinal healing methods (i.e., affirmation, meditation, positive thinking) to fortify self-concept and self-image.

Source: Meisenhelder, J. & La Charite, C. (1989). *Comfort in caring: Nursing the person with HIV infection.* Glenview, IL: Scott, Foresman/Little, Brown, pp. 214–215.

4. AIDS' impact on the family continues long after the infected member's death.

5. Low-income and inner-city families of color must be given special attention because of the AIDS epidemic in these groups.

6. Discrimination, stigma and isolation of HIV infected member and family must be eliminated.

7. Educational and prevention activities must be rational, practical, and supportive of safe and healthy sexuality.

8. Prevention and treatment should reflect the application of solid research and theory promulgation.

9. Social policy must consider the needs of the family, its varieties, strengths, etc.

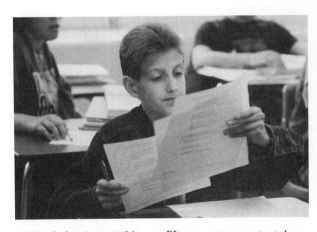

AIDS victim Ryan White, at fifteen, prepares to take a test in his high school math class. Ryan was unable to attend school with his classmates until he obtained a special health certificate. Many children with AIDS are also victims of discrimination and isolation, because of the public's fear and the various myths about the disease.

SUICIDE

DESCRIPTION OF SUICIDE

Attempted or completed suicide is a crisis. The suicidal crisis passes through the four stages described by Caplan (1964) and represents a disequilibrium within the individual.

Understanding the dynamics of suicide involves knowledge drawn from many disciplines. The population at risk for suicidal behavior is highly heterogeneous, and no single theory can fully identify its cause. Suicide is defined as "the human act of self-inflicted, self-intentioned cessation [of life] . . . which involves tortured and tunneled logic in a state of inner-felt, intolerable emotion" (Shneidman, 1976, p. 5). This definition encompasses the intention and conscious wish to be dead; it also focuses on the conscious and unconscious psychological state of the suicidal individual. Several theories that attempt to explain this phenomenon will be discussed later in this chapter.

EPIDEMIOLOGY OF SUICIDE

The number of suicides reported in the National Safety Council, Accident Facts (1987) was the following: 22,689 males and 6,507 females. However, a large number of suicides are never reported and are certified falsely as accidents or natural deaths.

Identified high-risk factors include age, gender, family status, race, religion, employment, health, personality styles, and predisposing conditions.

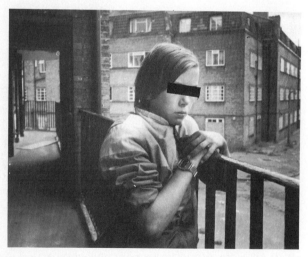

The incidence of suicide increases with age but is also high among adolescents.

AGE. The incidence of suicide increases with age and is highest in elderly white males, but is also a major cause of death in adolescence.

GENDER. Three times as many men commit suicide as women. However, more women *attempt* suicide than men.

FAMILY STATUS. Families who are separated, divorced, widowed, or those who have experienced a recent loss are susceptible to suicide. So also are families who are socially isolated and lack a support network or personal resources.

RACE. Racial groups that are at highest risk include whites, American Indians, and urban blacks.

RELIGION. Protestants have the highest rates of suicide.

EMPLOYMENT. Unemployed persons are at higher risk than those who are employed.

HEALTH. Individuals in poor health or experiencing physical illness, depression, or the effects of alcohol/drug abuse are vulnerable to suicide.

PERSONALITY STYLES. Those at high risk include individuals with impulsive personality, and/or risk-taking personality.

CHRONIC PREDISPOSING PSYCHIATRIC CONDITIONS. These include past history of suicidality and mood disorders, particularly manic-depressive illness.

ASSESSMENT OF SUICIDALITY

Assessment of the patient for risk of suicide is a critical part of the initial step of the nursing process. Realistic goals and a care plan may save the patient's life. The following information should be obtained in the assessment (Hatton, Valente, & Rink, 1977, pp. 43–57):

1. Demographic data—age, sex, race/culture, education, religion, and family members.

2. Clinical characteristics:
   - Precipitating factor—a recent event within the past three weeks that poses a threat to the patient, especially any loss through separation or death. During this phase, the nurse assesses what the loss means for the patient.

- Crisis—degree of anxiety, tension, anger, or depression that interferes with the patient's ability to cope with the crisis.
- Coping strategies—how the patient has handled previous stressful situations, and how this problem differs from a previous one.
- Significant others—the person(s) on whom the patient can rely during stressful situations. The nurse should help the patient identify significant others and encourage the patient to contact them.
- Social and personal resources—the patient's ability to provide for his basic needs such as food, shelter, clothing, and health care, and his access to other resources such as employment, hobbies, and a support system.
- Past suicide attempts—the number of serious previous attempts and their treatment.
- Past psychiatric history—previous emotional and mental conditions that might influence the outcome of the present crisis, specifically, how the condition was viewed by the patient and treated.
- Current psychiatric/medical history—any present physical or psychiatric problems for which the patient is being treated. It is important here to listen for clues to "cries for help" in the suicidal patient who is attempting to seek assistance. Always investigate psychosomatic complaints. (Also see Chapter 13, Psychophysiological Disorders.)
- Lifestyle—the stability of the patient's job, support system, and coping abilities may help to predict how the patient might succeed in adjusting to the present situation.
- Suicide plan—the method, availability of means, specificity, and lethality of the suicide plan. The patient's ability to carry out the plan and its specificity will predict the risk to the patient. Hatton, Valente, and Rink (1977) summarized the risk factors and arranged them in order of intensity based on behaviors/symptoms presented by suicidal patients (see Table 18-2).

THEORIES OF SUICIDE

Several models have emerged that are useful in the investigation of suicide: psychoanalytic, behavioral, biological, and sociological.

PSYCHOANALYTIC. In contrast to Durkheim, (1951), Freud's (1957) psychoanalytic explanation proposed that suicide was *intrapsychic,* or within the mind. Specifically, suicide represents an unconscious hostility toward an introjected love object who has been regarded ambivalently by the individual. Litman's (1967) analysis of Freud's thoughts on suicide enumerates other psychodynamic correlates related to suicide. These include rage, guilt, anxiety, dependency, and feelings of helplessness, hopelessness, and abandonment. Menninger (1938) contributed to the understanding of suicide by expanding on the psychodynamics of hostility as developed by Freud. He believed that the hostile drive in suicide is composed of three dimensions: the wish to commit suicide, the wish to be killed, and the wish to die. Menninger went further and identified situations in which the lifestyle of a person is self-destructive. This group of behaviors may alter one's activities, as well as cut short one's life (Farberow, 1980). Examples of such self-destructiveness include alcohol or drug addiction, multiple surgeries, risk-taking behavior, frequent "accidents," and mismanagement or sabotage of recommended treatment for disease. (See Chapter 13 on psychophysiological disorders).

Shneidman (1976) has identified three main psychological characteristics related to suicide:

1. The acute suicidal crisis is a dangerous period of self-destructiveness that is of relatively short duration (twenty-four hours or less).

2. Ambivalence may be paramount: an individual can make plans for suicide and at the same time entertain fantasies of rescue.

3. Most suicides are considered a two-person, or dyadic, event. Usually, the significant other is a parent, child, spouse, or lover who is involved in the interpersonal dynamics of the individual. In addition, in the case of completed suicide, the emotional needs of the "survivor victim" need to be addressed.

BEHAVIORAL/COGNITIVE. Another way to understand suicide is through the behavioral model and learning theory. The behavioral model does not consider behavior to be a symptom of unconscious conflict, as does psychoanalytic theory, but as a learned response to the situation or environment. The underlying premise is that all behavior is learned. Frederick and Resnik (1971) wrote that suicidal behaviors including suicidal threats, attempts, and competition are associated with previously learned associations or responses to crises. They further noted that the suicidal act functions as both reward and punishment for the suicidal individual. Therefore, nonreinforcement of suicidal behaviors should extinguish them.

TABLE 18—2 Assessing the degree of suicidal risk

Behavior or Symptom	Intensity of Risk		
	Low	Moderate	High
Anxiety	Mild	Moderate	High, or panic state
Depression	Mild	Moderate	Severe
Isolation/withdrawal	Vague feelings of depression, no withdrawal	Some feelings of helplessness, hopelessness, and withdrawal	Hopeless, helpless, withdrawn, and self-deprecating
Daily functioning	Fairly good in most activities	Moderately good in some activities	Not good in any activities
Resources	Several	Some	Few or none
Coping strategies/devices being utilized	Generally constructive	Some that are constructive	Predominantly destructive
Significant others	Several who are available	Few or only one available	Only one, or none available
Psychiatric help in past	None, or positive attitude toward	Yes, and moderately satisfied with	Negative view of help received
Lifestyle	Stable	Moderately stable or unstable	Unstable
Alcohol/drug use	Infrequently to excess	Frequently to excess	Continual abuse
Previous suicide attempts	None, or of low lethality	None to one or more of moderate lethality	None to multiple attempts of high lethality
Disorientation/disorganization	None	Some	Marked
Hostility	Little or none	Some	Marked
Suicidal plan	Vague, fleeting thoughts but no plan	Frequent thoughts, occasional ideas about a plan	Frequent or constant thought with a specific plan

Source: From Hatton, C. L., Valente, S. M., & Rink, A. (1977). *Suicide: Assessment and intervention*. New York: Appleton-Century-Crofts, p. 56. Reprinted with permission.

Concomitantly, nonsuicidal behaviors (such as constructive physical activity and seeking out assistance) must be learned and reinforced in order for new, more adaptive behaviors to be acquired.

Other behavioral theorists view attempted suicide as an attempt at interpersonal manipulations or control of the behavior of significant others. In this framework, the suicidal individual has learned maladaptive ways of seeking help or getting attention (Bostock & Williams, 1974).

Cognitive-behavior theorists emphasize the impact of attitudes, beliefs, and expectations on behavior. This view considers the power of individual expectations and interpretations on behavior and interpersonal relations. Beck, Kovacs, and Weissman

(1975) found that hopelessness is a significant influence in the development of suicidality. They postulated that hopelessness results from distorted cognitions which result in an extremely negative attitude toward self, others, and the environment. Cognitive-behavioral therapy involves changing these attitudes to more positive and hopeful ones (also see Chapter 9 on mood disorders).

BIOLOGICAL. Three areas of biochemical research involving individuals with suicidal depression have yielded interesting findings. They involve norepinephrine metabolism, adrenal cortical function, and electrolyte metabolism (Gibbons, 1960; Gibbons, 1964; Bunney & Fawcett, 1965; Fawcett & Bunney,

1967; Carpenter & Bunney, 1971; Sachar, 1982). These three neuroendocrine systems are all interrelated in the biological activity and functioning of the brain.

Gibbons (1960) and others pioneered research into the role of electrolyte metabolism in depressed patients. It has been found that depressed patients have significantly elevated sodium levels within the nerve cells. These findings are consistent with the pharmacological studies using lithium in the treatment of manic depression where lithium interferes with sodium exchange at the cellular level.

Research examining the role of the neurotransmitter norepinephrine in depressed patients has found that monoamine oxidase (MAO), an enzyme, breaks down biogenic amines like norepinephrine in the body. MAO inhibiting drugs prevent the enzyme from metabolizing biogenic amines; these amines therefore accumulate, increasing the concentration of neurotransmitters released upon nerve stimulation.

The dexamethasone suppression test (DST) has been useful in confirming a diagnosis of depression. An abnormal DST indicates a dysfunction in the limbic system and hypothalmus and is found exclusively in depressed patients, though it does not occur in *all* depressed patients.

Further biological support for depression is addressed by Prange, et al. (1972) and Loosen & Prange (1982). According to these researchers, the use of the thyrotropin-releasing hormone (TRH) in a majority of depressed patients resulted in lower levels of thyroid-stimulating hormone (TSH). For more information about depression and related biochemical research, see Chapter 9 on mood disorders.

SOCIOLOGICAL. From the sociological perspective, Durkheim (1951) classified and described three categories of suicide in terms of the individual's relationship to society. Suicide is believed to be a result of society's degree of control over the individual. Durkheim's theory was based on inferences he made while studying suicide rates in the Western world. They are described below:

1. Altruistic suicide involves the rigid obedience to customs or rules of a society. The practice of suicide has been expected under certain circumstances; for example, **Hara-Kiri** as practiced by the traditional Japanese and suttee as practiced by Hindu widows were once considered honorable behaviors (Shneidman, 1976).

2. Egoistic suicide involves the lack of an individual's involvement with or connection to his society. This individual is characterized by his loneliness and isolation from family and friends. Most suicides that occur in the United States belong to this category (Shneidman, 1976).

3. Anomic suicide occurs when the relationship between an individual and his society is severed or abruptly changed. For example, the death of a friend or loss of a job could lead to an anomic suicide (Durkheim, 1951).

TREATING ATTEMPTED SUICIDE

A cognitive/behavioral treatment approach is common during the crisis of attempted suicide and its aftermath. Interventions aimed at changing the patient's suicidal ideation include ". . . confronting the patient's helplessness as soon as possible and then helping him recognize the degree of illogical thinking, overgeneralization, and erroneous assumptions that go into the hopeless thinking" (Beck, Rush, & Kovacs, 1977, p. 82).

Depression is strongly associated with suicide, and Lewinsohn (1975) has summarized the major components of behavioral treatment of depression and suicide. Its goal is to restore an adequate schedule of positive reinforcement in the individual's life through altering the level, quality, and range of the patient's activities and social interactions. It involves:

1. Initially, examining the environment and reinforcing all positive self-concepts;

2. Increasing the patient's activity level by means of self-monitoring and social reinforcement;

3. Reducing negative self-verbalizations through social reinforcement of positive ones; thought stopping (a loud noise is introduced concurrently with the word "stop" at the beginning of a negative thought); and discrimination training (the patient is provided with consecutive two-minute intervals in which he may or may not express negative statements);

4. Relaxation training and encouraging affective expression (expression of feelings of amusement, humor, and sexual excitement); and

5. Assertiveness training and training in social skills that would enhance interpersonal and social behaviors.

Patient monitoring and videotape confrontation (Burgess & Lazare, 1976) offer two innovative techniques used in the treatment of suicidal patients. Patient monitoring involves obtaining a definitive commitment in the form of a contract from the patient that he will not act on suicidal feelings for a certain time period. This technique, also called a no-suicide contract, depends on the nurse's or therapist's evaluation of the patient's ability to make and keep the contract. The videotape confrontation technique involves presenting the patient with segments of a videotape recorded upon admission to the hospital in the emergency room that depicts his condition, professional intervention, and family's reactions. The videotape is presented to challenge an individual's denial of despair and suicidal intent. It is believed that this technique also serves as an aversive consequence of suicidal behavior that may help to extinguish such behavior.

The education, training, philosophy, and goals of nursing and medical professionals involved determine the specific cognitive behavioral techniques implemented. Nurses should be familiar with the theory and predicted outcome of the prescribed treatment in order to evaluate the appropriateness of the goals for an individual patient and the effectiveness of the nursing care plan.

NURSING MANAGEMENT OF THE SUICIDAL PATIENT

Caring for the suicidal patient is complicated and involves many personal and ethical as well as theoretical conflicts for nurses and other health-care professionals. The nurse must be aware of these issues (applicable to patients in any crisis situation) in order to provide objective and sensitive care. Hatton, Valente, and Rink (1977) have identified nine critical areas of conflict for the nurse:

1. *Developing trust and rapport.* Conflicts can arise concerning the patient's honesty and the truth of the information he presents. A patient's problem should be accepted as true and accurate in the absence of information to the contrary. The nurse may seek further verification during the family assessment, however.

2. *Feelings of professional inadequacy.* The crisis or suicidal situation may trigger feelings of anxiety in the nurse. The patient's psychological and emotional symptoms may be overwhelming. Experienced as well as beginning nurses may at times feel that they don't know enough or aren't competent to care for the suicidal patient.

3. *Anxiety regarding responsibility for decisions* in the course of assessing and planning the suicidal patient's care. The nurse may overcome her concern about mistakes and misjudgments with interdisciplinary consultation, personal experience, and support from other professionals.

4. *Suicidal feelings in the nurse.* Identification with the thoughts and feelings of a suicidal patient can result in the nurse's doubting her own coping abilities.

5. *Resentment of the patient* for causing the crisis. Countertransference of this type (anger) must be acknowledged and examined. Consultation can, again, be helpful.

6. *Subjective comparisons.* The patient's value system may conflict with the nurse's, resulting in additional negative countertransference.

7. *Listening difficulties.* Any of these issues or conflicts can present blocks in listening and communication.

8. *Confidentiality and protection.* The nurse needs to know the policies of the institution, the rights of the patient, and legal regulations relevant to the crisis situation.

9. *Sociocultural stereotyping.* Demographic statistics can sensitize the nurse to the need for assessment of the suicidal patient, but care should be taken to avoid stereotyping.

Hendin (1982) addresses other issues. He states that the nurse's own attitudes toward death, dying, and suicide are almost as important as the patient's in determining the clinical outcome. Dealing with suicidal patients arouses uncomfortable and anxious feelings that the nurse copes with in a variety of ways. These include avoiding the patient's depersonalizing, demonstrating excessive compassion or empathy, and being overly solicitous. Other reactions include:

1. Anxiety over the possibility of having to cope with the suicidal patient's death and related guilt.

2. Anxiety and confusion about whether a patient is seriously suicidal or just testing the nurse or therapist.

Nurses must provide a supportive and caring attitude but need to be attuned to the patient who sets up a savior-victim relationship. The nurse's countertransference should be explored if she has rescuing fantasies. **Countertransference** is especially likely to occur in professionals working with suicidal children and adolescents. In these instances, the nurse could view the patient as a significant person from her past, or perceive in the patient conflicts and frustrations that she herself has experienced.

Feinsilver (1983) points out that health professionals may have difficulty relating to suicide patients because their problems often seem to be self-induced.

In such a situation, the staff will exhibit feelings of anger and guilt as well as sorrow toward the patient.

Mr. Hommer: A Suicide Patient Not Taken Seriously

Mr. Hommer appeared in the emergency room after ingesting his wife's insulin in a suicide attempt. During the treatment process in the emergency room, the staff told the patient that oral ingestion of insulin was not harmful. The staff quietly made negative comments to each other about Mr. Hommer, such as "he can't even do this right." His suicide attempt was not taken seriously. Instead, the staff made light of his behavior. The patient was aware of the staff's attitude and behaviors.

Several nights later, Mr. Hommer returned to the emergency room via an emergency vehicle. This time he was in an insulin coma. Apparently, he had injected himself with his wife's insulin. The social history provided by his wife revealed that Mr. Hommer had, just two days ago, questioned her vigorously about the difference between oral and injectable insulin.

PLANNING. The primary goal in planning nursing care for the suicidal patient is to understand the acute problems or issues that are motivating the patient's behavior. Long-term goals should be specific, realistic, and directed toward ensuring the patient's continual safety and assisting him in developing more adaptive coping abilities.

IMPLEMENTATION. The nurse has an opportunity to begin to establish the therapeutic relationship as soon as the patient requests help. Every suicide attempt or threat, regardless of the seriousness of the intent, should be taken seriously. Active listening for verbal and nonverbal clues is essential. The nurse acknowledges the patient's thoughts and feelings of hopelessness, anger, and ambivalence and empathizes with his feelings. By showing concern, empathy, and support the nurse enables the patient to identify the source of his distress and begin to develop more adaptive solutions for it. The nurse provides genuine assurances that assistance is available and that the crisis will only last for a limited period of time.

Initial treatment strategies focus on the current degree of risk to the patient. The lethality of the suicidal intent must be determined immediately, and interventions, such as making a no-suicide contract, implemented promptly. **Lethality** of the situation is determined by assessing how specific and well-thought-out the patient's suicide plan is and whether or not the means to implement the plan are available to him. The degree of current risk increases if the patient has a history of suicide attempts, has demonstrated impulsivity, is socially isolated, and/or has thoughts about "joining" a deceased significant other.

After gaining an understanding of the crisis, the nurse reduces the dangerousness of the situation by removing or destroying the means that the patient has intended to use to carry out the suicide, for example, drugs, weapons, belts, knives, or other sharp objects. Table 18–3 outlines appropriate intervention techniques based on the risk of lethality.

Hospitalization within a controlled environment is necessary for patients who are assessed as having high suicide lethality, for example, severe depression with impulsive self-destructive behaviors or a history of the same, and/or psychosis. One-to-one supervision or frequent (every 15 minutes) observational checks usually provide sufficient monitoring of the patient to ensure his safety. Suicide precaution policies vary from institution to institution, although searches of the patient and his room for potentially harmful objects such as glass, matches, belts, ties, razors, and drugs are usually conducted periodically. Elopement precautions are also usually implemented both when the patient is on the psychiatric unit and when he is taken off it for special procedures. The staff may need to lock the unit door to prevent the patient from leaving the hospital. It is important for the staff to communicate to the patient about why these safety precautions are taken. Some patients will welcome these protective measures and others will resist or be suspicious of them.

If the patient's suicidal risk is assessed as being moderate or low, the staff may plan less intense precautions. Hospitalization may still be warranted to resolve the immediate crisis when an individual makes a suicide attempt or gesture. A "no-suicide" contract should be implemented whether or not the patient is hospitalized. This agreement between the primary nurse or therapist and the patient conveys the idea that the patient has the responsibility for controlling his behavior. As previously mentioned, the "no-suicide" contract specifies that the patient will not act on his suicidal feelings in any way. The contract specifies the length of time of the agreement (usually, one shift) and is renewable. The nurse and the patient both sign the agreement. If the patient wants to alter the wording of the contract, by stating, for example, "I will *try* not to kill myself," he is show-

TABLE 18–3 Intervention techniques based on lethality

	Lethality of Suicide Plan or Attempt		
Technique	**Low**	**Moderate**	**High**
Assess emergency	No plan to commit suicide within next 24 hours	No plan within next 24 hours	Plans suicide in next 24 hours; what, when, where: what has already been done?
Focus on hazard and crisis	Primary	Primary after emergency is ruled out	May be secondary until client is safe
Clarify the hazard/crisis	Assist client to arrive at clearer idea	Client needs more help from caregiver	Client needs most help from caregiver
Reduce imminent danger	Help client reduce future danger; obtain verbal contract to avoid suicide	Help client reduce danger; obtain verbal contract	Direct client to reduce danger; provide first aid if necessary; obtain verbal contract
Assess need for medication	Evaluate	Evaluate	Most often—but must be monitored!!
Assess need for someone to stay with client	Often a good idea to have someone available for support	Frequently necessary	Essential precaution to prevent hospitalization or suicide
Mobilize internal and external resources	Very important; usually can mobilize internal resources	Very important; can mobilize some internal resources	Essential; few internal resources; needs help to mobilize external resources
Contact significant others	Important	Very important	Essential
Harness coping devices	Minimal help needed	Needs more help	Needs commands and directions
Give structure	Minimal help needed	Needs more help	Needs specific directions
Continue daily activities	Needs encouragement	Needs encouragement and some direction	Needs directions and assessment of what is possible
Direct to planned/ organized action	Needs encouragement	Needs encouragement and some direction	Needs commands

Source: From Hatton, C. L., Valente, S. M., & Rink, A. (1977). *Suicide: Assessment intervention.* New York: Appleton-Century-Crofts. p. 78. Reprinted with permission.

ing ambivalence, and further discussion is warranted. If the patient refuses to sign the contract, increased supervision and observation are indicated. The agreement usually also includes other conditions, such as "I will talk to the nurse or call my therapist if I feel like hurting myself" and "I will cooperate with restrictions and remain in the sight of the nurse."

Identifying the patient's present coping strategies, exploring new ones, and testing alternatives offer the patient healthy methods of coping with crisis. This process teaches patients to respond to crisis situations and conflicts with problem solving and ra-

tional decision making rather than with emotion. Involving the family or significant others in the care plan is essential. Observing their reactions to and interactions with the patient may shed light on the emotional dynamics of the patient's suicidality (Shneidman, 1976).

Structuring or organizing the patient's activities and responsibilities during hospitalization helps the patient regain a sense of control and direction in his life. This may be accomplished through the use of a behavior contract. It is important for the nurse to bear in mind that the suicidal gesture or attempt may

1) be associated with secondary gain, for example, attention or avoidance of the conflict or 2) be a manipulative attempt to have needs met. Medication may be warranted for the agitated and depressed suicidal patient. If this is indicated, close surveillance of the patient's swallowing of medication is necessary as patients have been known to horde medication by collecting it in the cheek or under the tongue when it is administered until there is enough to use in a suicide attempt.

Hendin (1982) asserts that surveillance and taking precautions is not as effective in preventing suicide as trying to understand the meaning of the individual patient's use of the suicidal threat. He recommends assisting the patient with identifying and dealing with the problems associated with his suicidality. "Only in psychotherapy does the nature of the suicidal individual's involvement with death and self-destructiveness become fully apparent" (Hendin, 1982, p. 162).

Case Study: Nonpsychiatric Setting

May Sue Sing: Suicide Attempt

May Sue Sing
Age: 28
Residence: San Francisco, CA
Ethnicity: Chinese
Occupation: Postdoctoral Fellow at University of California

Present Problem:

May Sue Sing, a 28-year-old woman was admitted to an intensive care unit because of a drug overdose. She was recently transferred from the intensive care unit to a medical floor within the same hospital.

When the nurse questioned her about the overdose, and asked about suicidal intent, she denied it. She indicated, however, that she did have severe back pain. The nurses on the medical unit noticed that May appeared withdrawn and isolated. She ate very little and was up late at night. She complained of headaches, which she had had since coming to the U.S. May had only one visitor during the two weeks she was hospitalized.

May Sue Sing had been in the United States six months pursuing postdoctoral study in chemistry. She was from China and felt it was an honor to be given a fellowship to study in the United States; she was also a competitive and capable woman. May had some difficulty expressing herself in English, but comprehended and read English very well.

May's professor had recently indicated to her that he was somewhat disappointed in her overall performance as a postdoctoral fellow. May responded by studying longer hours. She had recently lost about fifteen pounds; she slept three to four hours each night; and she further withdrew from friends, thereby limiting her activities to only studying.

About two months ago, May had injured her back while roller skating and was prescribed analgesics for back pain. The psychiatrist who evaluated May felt that she had accidentally overmedicated herself.

Previous History:

May denied any previous psychiatric problems. She did indicate that she was lonely for her family and friends. May had always made excellent grades. Her family was proud of her. She felt that she "should continue to perform well, regardless of the amount of effort required."

Family History:

May's father is a 55-year-old government official who lives in Beijing, China. He is described by May as kind and loving, with high expectations for all of his children. May's mother is part owner of a small export business in Beijing. She, too, is described as loving, supportive, and hard working. The two of them are very proud of May. According to May, they are in excellent health.

Employment History:

May's work consists of studying. She has, since coming to the United States, concentrated on her studies. Only on one or two occasions has she directed her attention from her studies. One such occasion was the roller skating activity where she injured her back.

Health History:

Generally, good health. May voiced concern about the recent weight loss. May also stated, "My back hurts much of the time."

Present Mental Status:

Dressed in hospital gown; quiet, withdrawn, and slow to respond to interviewer's questions. Coherent, responds appropriately to interviewer's questions on 1) time, 2) place, 3) date, 4) person. Memory and recall are intact.

Affect: sad, withdrawn, frightened looking; eyes tend to search the room continuously.

Voice/speech: Voice is barely audible; at times, difficult for interviewer to understand May's speech.

Thought content: back pain: Concern about getting behind in studies

Thought process: organized and articulate thoughts in a clear and concise fashion.

Medication: analgesics, Tylenol #3 (acetaminophen and codeine) and muscle relaxants (Norflex) to be taken every 4 hours, prn, for back pain.

Suicide potential: The staff was not in agreement about whether May accidentally overdosed herself or if she had actually attempted suicide. She admitted to taking "over ten" tablets of the Tylenol #3 in "a couple of hours" on the evening she was admitted to the hospital. May explained that she "just wanted the back pain to go away," and the prescribed dose "wasn't working well enough." She "didn't think the extra tablets would hurt her." May had been brought to the hospital by a friend who found her weak and vomiting in her apartment that evening. She had been admitted to the ICU for initial treatment and observation and had been transferred to the medical unit when she stabilized and showed no signs of long-term liver damage and stated she was not suicidal.

One nurse, whose own background was Chinese, shared her knowledge of some relevant cultural characteristics with the other staff members. She stated that depression is a common manifestation among Chinese, but that Chinese are not likely to verbally state, "I am depressed," or "I feel sad"; they are more likely to complain of physical symptoms because this is a more culturally acceptable behavior. The nurse felt strongly that the overdose was a suicide attempt. The team accepted these observations and agreed to include "suicide attempt" in the differential diagnosis.

DSM-III-R Diagnosis

DSM-III-R axis diagnosis deferred because of inadequate information.

Nursing Diagnoses

Ineffective individual coping
Fear
Social Isolation
Anxiety

Nursing Care Plan for May Sue Sing

Nursing Diagnosis	Desired Outcomes	Interventions	Rationale
1. Ineffective individual coping.	May Sue Sing will verbalize her feelings about difficulties adjusting to life in the United States, begin to develop a support system, and experience less depression.	Establish a supportive relationship with May Sue Sing.	Increases communication; displays concern for May's welfare; increases the possibility that May will provide more information about herself.
		Assess present degree of suicide risk.	Provides vital information about May that will be used in planning her care while in hospital (she may need to be transferred to the psychiatric unit) and after discharge.
		Explore the meaning of failure and shame within May's culture.	Ventilation and verbalization are useful as therapeutic agents; the nursing staff will gain information to be used in planning May's treatment; the nursing staff gains a cultural perspective about May's behaviors that will assist them in providing culturally congruent nursing care.
		Maintain direct observation and implement suicide precautions.	Ensures safety.
		Explore how May handled stress in China; determine what is different/the same about the two situations.	Assists in mobilizing effective defense mechanisms and coping strategies.

Nursing Diagnosis	Desired Outcomes	Interventions	Rationale
		Develop a no-suicide contract with May if she is found to have been or to be suicidal.	Encourages May to verbalize her feelings about suicide.
		Assist May in understanding that suicidal behaviors include suicidal ideation and suicidal gestures.	Expressions of feelings are acceptable; suicidal behaviors are not.
	May will identify effective and ineffective coping methods.	Assist May in the outward expression of anger.	Outward expression of anger in a socially acceptable manner helps to develop effective coping, increases self-esteem, and so forth.
		Encourage May to participate in pleasurable activities. Assist May in selecting foods she enjoys. Provide dietary consultation for May. Provide specially prepared meals for May.	Assists May in adapting to a new culture; provides autonomy, demonstrates nurse's respect for and sensitivity to May's cultural differences.
		Make arrangements for May to join a support group after hospitalization.	Enhances socialization, provides support, interpersonal learning, a sense of belonging, and so forth.
2. Fear.	May's fear will decrease.	Orient May to the environment and give brief and concise explanations.	Increases orientation and promotes psychological comfort.
		Avoid details, give clear explanations of any procedures, activities, expectations.	Minimizes anxiety; promotes safety and predictability.
		Encourage May to share problems with staff.	Increases social contact, self-esteem.
		Encourage May to face the events that she is fearful about and assist her in facing them.	Increases sense of competence; autonomy; decreases feelings of helplessness and powerlessness.
		Encourage straight-forward responses such as "yes . . . my back hurts me now."	Encourages effective communication; facilitates expression of feelings; decreases depression.

Nursing Diagnosis	Desired Outcomes	Interventions	Rationale
3. Social isolation.	May will develop meaningful interpersonal relationships and begin to participate in recreational activities.	Assist May in describing her feelings of isolation and loneliness.	Helps to identify feelings.
4. Anxiety.	May will recognize 1) when she is anxious and 2) the types of behavioral responses she employs to manage her anxiety.	Assess the levels of anxiety that May experiences (mild, moderate, severe, panic) and intervene accordingly.	Information needed in planning treatment.
		Teach May to monitor problems, frustrations, and conflicts and their relationships to physical back pain.	Anxiety may be manifested through physical pain which is culturally acceptable for May.
		Encourage May to seek alternative methods of coping with frustrations and anxiety, to include verbalization, recreational outlets, realistic appraisals of what she can/cannot do, increase interpersonal support system.	Assists in developing new behavioral responses to anxieties.

SUCCESSFUL SUICIDE

SURVIVORS. When a person commits suicide, the survivors experience an initial period of denial, followed by guilt, blame, anger, and depression. McClean (1982) states that "families tend to respond to a loss by suicide as a rejection due to lack of trust or love, or even hatred" (p. 595). In a study by Dorpat (1972), children who lost a parent by suicide were particularly vulnerable to the development of psychological problems. The seventeen children studied exhibited guilt, depression, morbid preoccupation with suicide, self-destructiveness, absence of grief, and developmental arrest. However, Henslin (1972) found that significant others did not experience severe adjustment problems if they interpreted the cause of the suicide as nonattributable to them. Conversely, those who believed they contributed to or could have prevented the suicide showed significant problems in dealing with it.

The after-effects of the completed suicide need attention from health-care professionals. Psychological support is needed to allow the bereaved survivors, such as children, parents, and spouses, to express their feelings and understand the suicidal death. Studies have shown that they are more likely to have higher morbidity and mortality rates in the year following the death of their loved one. Therefore ". . . the major public mental health challenge in suicide lies in offering . . . help to the survivor-victim" (Shneidman, 1976, p. 21).

Nurses and other health-care professionals experience intense reactions when a patient they knew or cared for has committed suicide, for example, in the hospital or immediately after discharge. The staff goes through the grieving process which includes anger, guilt, helplessness, and hopelessness (McClean, 1982). A supportive group forum for the nurses and other staff to vent and share their feelings can help to work through the many and complex feelings associated with a completed suicide.

ASSESSMENT OF SUCCESSFUL SUICIDE. In an effort to understand a successful suicide, a psychological autopsy is often performed. The psychological autopsy retrospectively recreates events in the individual's life history which may help to answer several important questions in regard to the decedent's mode of death (how the death occurred), why the death occurred at this particular time, and why the individual may have committed suicide (Schneidman, 1976). Schneidman suggests that the mode of death is especially important since it determines whether the individual's death was intentional or accidental.

The information in the psychological autopsy is gathered through interviews with close survivors, relatives, and friends of the deceased. If the suicide is completed in the hospital unit, nurses and other professionals on the staff are also used as resources (see Table 18–4).

ADOLESCENT SUICIDE

DESCRIPTION OF ADOLESCENT SUICIDE

Suicide at any age is tragic but suicide committed by young people is probably the most difficult to deal with, especially for the victim's family, friends, and teachers. While adolescence is characterized by emotional and behavioral changes and a search for identity and independence, a suicide attempt is never a "normal" response to a developmental crisis. It is always an indicator of psychopathology in the adolescent or his or her family.

EPIDEMIOLOGY OF ADOLESCENT SUICIDE

The highest incidence of suicide in young people is reported to be in the fifteen to twenty-four age group. It was on the increase for the twenty years prior to 1977, but has decreased and leveled off since then. It has been hypothesized that the decrease in numbers of adolescents in the population over the last twelve years is responsible for the decline. If this is true, then we can expect the adolescent suicide rate to begin to increase again in the 1990's when the number of adolescents in the population is expected to take an upward turn, and they face increased com-

---

TABLE 18–4 Outline for psychological autopsy

1. Identifying information for victim (name, age, address, marital status, religious practices, occupation, and other details)

2. Details of the death (including the cause or method and other pertinent details)

3. Brief outline of victim's history (siblings, marriage, medical illnesses, medical treatment, psychotherapy, previous suicide attempts)

4. "Death history" of victim's family (suicides, cancer, other fatal illnesses, ages at death, and other details)

5. Description of the personality and life style of the victim

6. Victim's typical patterns of reaction to stress, emotional upsets, and periods of disequilibrium

7. Any recent—from last few days to last 12 months—upsets, pressures, tensions, or anticipations of trouble

8. Role of alcohol and drugs in (1) overall life style of victim and (2) his death

9. Nature of victim's interpersonal relationships (including physicians)

10. Fantasies, dreams, thoughts, premonitions, or fears of victim relating to death, accident, or suicide

11. Changes in the victim before death (of habits, hobbies, eating, sexual patterns, and other life routines)

12. Information relating to the "life side" of victim (upswings, successes, plans)

13. Assessment of intention, i.e., role of the victim in his own demise

14. Rating of lethality

15. Reactions of informants to victim's death

16. Comments, special features, etc.

Source: Shneidman, E. S. (1976). Suicide Among the Gifted. In E. S. Shneidman (Ed.), *Suicidology: Contemporary developments*. New York: Grune and Stratton. p. 353.

---

petition for admission to colleges and universities, for academic and athletic honors, for jobs, and so on (Hollinger, Offer, & Ostrov, 1987). (See Box 18–3.)

Pfeffer (1985) has identified risk factors associated with adolescent suicide from her work with adolescents. Two specific social factors involved increased family mobility and the increasing number of divorced and separated families. Adolescents in these situations are under a fair amount of stress as they have to adjust to and cope with the associated major life changes such as attending new schools, making new friends, or taking on new responsibilities.

Box 18–3 ● Suicide Among Youth (Ages 15–24)

● Suicide now ranks as the second leading cause of death among young persons aged 15–24. In the U.S. about 5,000 suicides occur annually among this age group. That means that each day, 13 young people kill themselves. Many more of them attempt suicide and fail.

● While deaths from all other causes in the U.S. have declined among youth since 1950, the suicide rate increased nearly threefold by 1980. In 1950, the rate was 4.5 per 100,000. By 1980, the rate had risen to 12.3, exceeding the rate for the population as a whole for the first time.

● By 1985, the number of suicides among young persons had dropped to 4,760 or 12.0 per 100,000, for unknown reasons. There have been slight increases again since that date.

● Suicide attempts among youth are estimated at 5 to 20 times greater than completed suicides; between 1 and 10 percent of those who attempt suicide succeed.

● Violent deaths among young people, which include suicides, homicides and accidents, are the leading cause of potential years of life lost in the U.S. Suicide alone is estimated to account for 200,000 potential years of life lost annually among 15–24-year olds.

● In 1980, suicide in the young was more common among males than females by a ratio of approximately 5 to 1. By far, most (89.5%) young male suicide victims are white. Rates for young white men have increased in each of the past three decades.

● While fewer in number, the suicide rate in young black males tripled from 4.9 per 100,000 in 1950 to 12.3 in 1980. The 1984 rate stood at 11.2.

● The highest suicide rate among Hispanics occurs in the 20–24 age group. Data from five southwestern states show that the rates for Hispanics are lower than for whites, but higher than for blacks.

● For young Native Americans, suicide is the second leading cause of death, following accidents. The average rate reported for 1981–1983 was 27.9 for 15 to 24-year-old Native Americans, compared to 12.2 for all Americans in this age group. Suicide rates vary considerably among individual tribes, and suicide victims are usually younger than the general population, peaking at ages 20 to 24.

● Many medical examiners and coroners believe that the reported number of suicides among youth, as well as in the general population, may be less than one-half the true number.

● The western states currently have the highest adolescent suicide rates; the northeastern states the lowest.

● The most common methods of suicide are by firearms, hanging, and drug overdose. The most frequent method of suicide for males 15–24 was firearms during the period 1970–1980. For young females, the leading method changed from drugs to firearms during that period.

Source: U.S. Department of Health, Education, and Welfare. Update. (1987). Data from Secretary's Task Force Report on Youth Suicide. Washington, D.C.: U.S. Government Printing Office.

Another risk factor is clinical depression, especially when associated with poorly managed anger and aggressive behavior (Poznanski & Zrull, 1970). Adolescents at risk exhibit intense preoccupation with death and may live with depressed parents, especially if a parent is a suicidal "model," that is, talks about or attempts suicide (Toolan, 1975).

ASSESSMENT OF ADOLESCENT SUICIDE

Adolescent suicide can be a gesture without intent to die, an attempt with the hope of intervention (cry for help), or a completed act. It is important to be able to identify the clues of potentially suicidal adolescents. DeMaio-Esteves and Shuzman (1983) have provided a list of such clues:

Withdrawal from family and friends

Giving away valued possessions

Notable history of substance abuse (marijuana, alcohol, other drugs)

Anorexia or overeating

Changes in personality and moods (aggressive, defiant, isolated, lonely, sullen)

Loss of interest in old activities and friends

Change in school performance

Psychosomatic complaints

Preoccupation with death and suicide in thought, drawings, poems, scribbles, and letters to friends.

THEORIES OF ADOLESCENT SUICIDE

There is no comprehensive theory to explain adolescent suicide. However, various theorists have examined adolescent suicide in the context of the family systems perspective, looking at communication patterns and reactions to loss and grief. For example, since the suicide rate is higher among college students than those people of the same age who are not in college, it has been suggested that separation from the family as well as academic pressure are contributors (Hendin, 1982). It is thought that these individuals may devote themselves to academic study as a means of obtaining love and approval from their parents and are devastated when they don't "make the grade."

Another correlate of adolescent suicide is found in a study by Dorpat, Jackson, and Ripley (1965). Their research shows that the death of a parent is more common among adolescent suicide victims who die than those who attempt, but do not succeed, in suicide. These researchers have also noted, however, that the majority of young people who have lost a parent are not suicidal.

Hendin (1982) also reports that the suicidal behaviors of high school students differ from that of college students. Factors associated with suicidal high school students include provocative and defiant behaviors toward parents, drug abuse, and lack of interest in school. It is postulated that these rebellious and self-destructive behaviors attract attention, with the result that the adolescent's depression is missed. This problem has resulted in the term "masked depression." However, the depression, often about "unstable and unhappy family relationships" (p. 48), is not so much masked as not noticed or attended to.

Speck (1968) studied families with a suicidal member and proposed that suicidal symptoms may

function to meet family needs and goals. For example, Schut (1964) found that parental communication that is demeaning, likely to contribute to a negative self-concept, or induces guilt feelings has been associated with self-destructive behavior in the adolescent. Noncaring or indifferent parents, and those who seem incapable of empathy, have also been associated with adolescents who commit suicide (McIntire & Angle, 1973).

Hellig (1983) studied five families with an adolescent who exhibited suicidal behavior. The study's findings revealed the following common characteristics of the families:

1. Separation and loss were perceived as threats to survival.

2. Parents had difficulty in allowing the child or adolescent most involved in the family to separate, even if the "separation" was normal or age appropriate; for example, if the adolescent became involved with a boyfriend or planned to go away to college, the family felt threatened.

3. The seriousness or frequency of suicidal behaviors were an indication of the level of dysfunction in the family system.

A developmental perspective on adolescent suicide is advanced by Gilead and Mulaik (1983). They view adolescence as a developmental phase characterized by many role changes and social, cultural, and biological pressures. As a result the adolescent is often preoccupied with a search for independence, identity, and maturity. The adolescent is unable or has difficulty in adjusting to the role changes and becomes suicidal for the following reasons:

1. absence of a role model,

2. lack of internal resources (for example, the emotional development necessary to carry out the role), and

3. nonsupportive significant others who do not recognize or allow these role changes.

That is, crisis can occur during adolescence when there is a lack of external support, alienation from family and friends, and feelings of hopelessness and helplessness in resolving problems. DeMaio (1983) states that the stress on adolescents in our technological society has increased and exacerbates the normal turmoil in adolescence associated with developing and learning maturity. The stress confronting today's youth is "marked by turbulent political, social, and economic change, and a high degree of geographical and social mobility" (DeMaio, 1983, p. 55). High

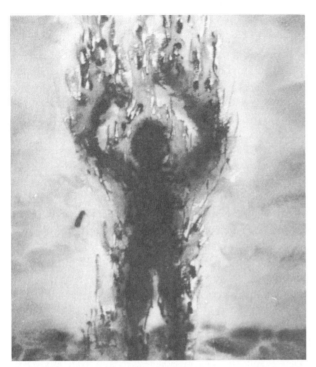 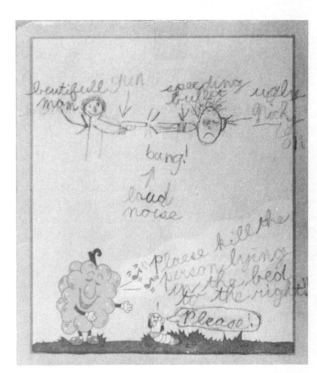

Two artistic examples of what children feel when suicide is contemplated. Left: the shadowy figure in flames is a painting done by a sixteen-year-old boy the night of his third suicide attempt. It was not successful and he responded well to treatment and ultimately did well. Right: This drawing/note is a suicide note left by a nine-year-old boy for his parents. They found it before he carried out his plan. He, too, is currently doing well. He had been suffering from major depression, as was his mother, at the time the note was written.

economic goals and a thrust toward involvement in adult experiences such as sex and use of alcohol as well as the threat of nuclear war may predispose the youth in our society to depression and suicide.

Keidel (1983) has proposed three intrapsychic factors associated with adolescent suicide:

1. Manipulation by the adolescent as a form of coping with frustrations and getting his own needs met (this is often learned from a parent or significant other who has modeled maladaptive behaviors).

2. Anger at or an attempt to get even with a significant other (implies that death is not seen as final).

3. An overwhelming sense of real or imagined loss.

NURSING MANAGEMENT OF THE SUICIDAL ADOLESCENT

Nursing intervention with suicidal adolescents is dependent upon the setting and specifics of the individ-

ual patient. The setting may be a telephone call via a crisis hotline, an emergency room, a hospital, a clinic, and so forth. Crisis intervention in the case of a serious suicide threat or attempt is implemented as it is in the case of the adult patient. Gilead and Mulaik (1983) suggest the following general interventions:

1. assess the immediacy and potential lethality of the suicidal threat,

2. express a concern and willingness to help,

3. encourage verbalization of thoughts, feelings, and events leading up to the crisis situation,

4. explore ways in which the adolescent can feel more in control of his life, and

5. refer the adolescent to counseling.

(If the patient is already in therapy, the therapist should be notified immediately. It is also important to get in touch with the adolescent's parents, not a breach of confidentiality in this case.)

Although confidentiality is usually a requirement for any effective counseling to take place, no such pledge should be made in the event of a possible suicide (Curran, 1987). When working with adolescents, one is faced with an additional responsibility. The therapist may need to contact those caretakers of the adolescent, such as the parents or, if the adolescent is currently in treatment, the primary therapist (Curran, 1987). The adolescent may initially react with anger and fear and may attempt to manipulate the therapist into maintaining secrecy concerning the suicidal intent. If the therapist feels strongly, however, that danger sincerely exists and that the adolescent is capable of harming himself, every opportunity should be made to allow the primary caretakers to shoulder some of the responsibility (Curran, 1987).

Obtaining the address of the patient's residence is important when conducting crisis intervention on a telephone hotline. Police or emergency personnel should be notified if the adolescent is considered to be at high risk for suicide. (See Fig. 18-2.)

If the patient has made a serious suicide attempt in the presence of the nurse, first aid measures are implemented. These include preventing hemorrhaging from gunshot or stab wounds, artificial respiration and cardiopulmonary resuscitation with hanging or drowning victims, prophylaxis for shock, and inducing vomiting in the case of drug overdose. If the victim is found hanging, the nurse immediately supports the victim's body weight, calls for help, and loosens or releases the noose from the victim's neck.

Once the adolescent is admitted to the hospital unit, staff will maintain surveillance or constant observation. These restrictions will be curtailed as the adolescent is able to take more appropriate control of his life. Medications may be ordered for anxiety and/or depression, and the psychiatrist, psychologist, social worker, or psychiatric nurse begins or continues psychotherapy, usually both individual and family therapy. Parents' reactions to their adolescents' self-destructive behavior include shock and disbelief, denial, anger, and resentment (DeMaio-Esteves & Shuzman, 1983), all feelings that the nurse can assist the parents in verbalizing.

CHILD SUICIDE
DESCRIPTION OF CHILD SUICIDE

It is difficult to comprehend that children are capable of suicide. The incidence of completed suicides among children six through twelve years of age is relatively low, but a reality. Children use methods sim-

ilar to those used by adults. In addition, it has been shown that children are capable of understanding the lethality of the suicide methods used and the meaning of suicidal acts (Orbach et al., 1983). They tend, however, to underestimate their own vulnerability to death. Even adolescents, in some cases, might not realize how final death really is. They may wish to kill themselves, but not to die. Moreover, children and youth who are suicidal tend to place life-like qualities onto death and dying (Seiden, 1972; Pfeffer, 1984; and Benenati, 1988). In the same vein, Orbach et al. (1983) found that "children's misconception about death (i.e., death as another form of life) [may be] a defensive maneuver to cope with the anxiety of planning suicide rather than a reflection of cognitive immaturity" (p. 661). (See also Chapter 22, Psychiatric Mental Health Nursing with Children, for more on the child's concept of death).

ETIOLOGY OF CHILD SUICIDE

As a result of clinical observations, Orbach, Gross, and Glaubman (1981) found that suicidal children live with a high degree of internal and external pressures in families familiar with the experience of crisis (especially violence or abuse), and are unable to develop satisfying relationships with adults. In their investigation, these researchers found that suicidal children exhibited particular attitudes toward life and death that are significantly different from nonsuicidal children. These children revealed:

1. A moderate degree of attraction to life; that is, life is at times enjoyable for them and they feel some acceptance by parents, teachers, and peers.

2. A high degree of repulsion by life, indicative of an unsatisfying family life and rejection by significant others.

3. A high degree of attraction to death, which may be based upon various cultural and religious beliefs about death. Some children's perception of death is distorted, their fantasies about death involving a better life or continuation of life.

4. A moderate or low degree of repulsion by death, which suggest that death does not arouse fear and anxiety in these children.

These attitudes may serve as a partial explanation of the motivating forces for suicide in children and suggests that suicide in children may involve a specific set of personality attributes and not merely a reaction to a specific problem.

Kazdin et al. (1983) examined suicide cases and compared suicidal children with psychiatrically disturbed nonsuicidal children to see if a sense of hope-

FIGURE 18–2 Psychological First-Aid

The following are preventive steps for the mature adult dealing with the suicidal youngster:

Step 1: **Listen**
The first thing a person in a mental crisis needs is someone who will listen and really hear what he is saying. Every effort should be made to understand the feelings behind the words.

Step 2: **Evaluate the seriousness of the youngster's thoughts and feelings.**
If the person has made clear self-destructive plans, however, the problem is apt to be more acute than when his thinking is less definite.

Step 3: **Evaluate the intensity or severity of the emotional disturbance.**
It is possible that the youngster may be extremely upset but not suicidal. If a person has been depressed and then becomes agitated and moves about restlessly, it is usually cause for alarm.

Step 4: **Take every complaint and feeling the patient expresses seriously.**
Do not dismiss or undervalue what the person is saying. In some instances, the person may express his difficulty in a low key, but beneath his seeming calm may be profoundly distressed feelings. . . .

Step 5: **Do not be afraid to ask directly if the individual has entertained thoughts of suicide.**
Suicide may be suggested but not openly mentioned in the crisis period. Experience shows that harm is rarely done by inquiring directly into such thoughts at an appropriate time. As a matter of fact, the individual frequently welcomes the query and is glad to have the opportunity to open up and bring it out.

Step 6: **Do not be misled by the youngster's comments that he is past his emotional crisis.**
Often the youth will feel initial relief after talking of suicide, but the same thinking will recur later. Follow-up is crucial to ensure a good treatment effort.

Step 7: **Be affirmative but supportive.**
Strong, stable guideposts are essential in the life of a distressed individual. Provide emotional strength by giving the impression that you know what you are doing, and that everything possible will be done to prevent the young person from taking his life.

Step 8: **Evaluate the resources available.**
The individual may have both inner psychological resources, including various mechanisms for rationalization and intellectualization which can be strengthened and supported and outer resources in the environment, such as ministers, relatives, and friends whom one can contact. If these are absent, the problem is much more serious. Continuing observation and support are vital.

Step 9: **Act specifically.**
Do something tangible; that is, give the youngster something definite to hang onto, such as arranging to see him later or subsequently contacting another person. Nothing is more frustrating to the person than to feel as though he has received nothing from the meeting.

Step 10: **Do not avoid asking for assistance and consultation.**
Call upon whomever is needed, depending upon the severity of the case. Do not try to handle everything alone. Convey an attitude of firmness and composure to the person so that he will feel something realistic and appropriate is being done to help him.

Additional preventive techniques for dealing with persons in a suicide crisis may require the following:

- Arrange for a receptive individual to stay with the youth during the acute crisis.
- Do not treat the youngster with horror or deny his thinking.
- Make the environment as safe and provocation-free as possible.
- Never challenge the individual in an attempt to shock him out of his ideas.
- Do not try to win arguments about suicide. They cannot be won.
- Offer and supply emotional support for life.
- Give reassurance that depressed feelings are temporary and will pass.
- Mention that if the choice is to die, the decision can never be reversed.
- Point out that, while life exists, there is always a chance for help and resolution of the problems, but that death is final.
- Focus upon survivors by reminding the youngster about the rights of others. He will leave a stigma on his siblings and other family members. He will predispose his friends and family to emotional problems or suicide.
- Call in family and friends to help establish a lifeline.
- Allow the youngster to ventilate his feelings.
- Do not leave the individual isolated or unobserved for any appreciable time if he is acutely distressed.

These procedures can help restore feelings of personal worth and dignity, which are equally as important to the young person as to the adult. In so doing, the adult helping agent can make the difference between life and death. A future potentially productive young citizen will survive.

Source: Frederick, C. J. (1976). *Keynote, IV* (3), pp: 3–5 and Boy's Clubs of America.

lessness discriminated between them. They found that the suicidal children showed significantly greater feelings of hopelessness (negative expectations toward themselves and toward the future) between five and thirteen years of age. Their findings also suggest that depression in childhood is similar to that experienced by adults. The authors concluded that "hopelessness, depression, and suicidal intent appear to be related in a similar manner for children and adults" (p. 510).

In her review of the literature, Pfeffer (1984) discussed factors that appear to contribute to the risk of suicidal behavior in children. They include:

1. Problematic family communication patterns and psychopathology (suicidal preoccupations and behaviors) in the family. This may include the "expendable child" hypothesis that suggests that "a parental wish, conscious or unconscious, spoken or unspoken, that the child interprets as their desire to be rid of him, for him to die" (Sabbath, 1969, p. 273) is associated with suicidal behavior among children.

2. Conflicts involving the mother and identification with her depression, or a culmination of the stress resulting from the associated lack of nurturing by the mother which often leads to a sense of worthlessness and self-hatred in the child (Pfeffer, Conte, & Plutchik, 1980).

3. Depression in children (Toolan, 1975; Pfeffer, Conte, & Plutchik, 1980).

4. The child's perception in some cases that death is temporary and a pleasant state of pain alleviation.

5. Motivations including conscious and unconscious fantasies about suicide and associated wishes, fears, and prohibitions, such as the wish to manipulate and punish the parents. The fantasy of joining a deceased parent or relative, or the hope of finding "the all-giving and loving mother" in death can promise to fulfill a suicidal child's search for love (Ackerly, 1967). According to Pfeffer (1984), there are similarities between the suicidal motivation of children and that of adults.

ASSESSMENT OF THE SUICIDAL CHILD

Assessment of potential suicide in children is similar to that done with adolescents. Some children will express directly their wish to die and are openly preoccupied with death. Other children will exhibit signs of depression, such as being irritable, sad, tearful, and unhappy. Changes in eating and sleeping patterns are also significant. Some children stop eating or begin to overeat. Depressed children cannot sleep, or sleep restlessly, waking up during the night or early morning. They may exhibit changes in motor activity. Physiological complaints such as headaches and stomachaches along with these behavioral changes are common among suicidal children. (See Chapter 22, Psychiatric Mental Health Nursing with Children, for more on depression in childhood).

NURSING MANAGEMENT OF THE POTENTIALLY SUICIDAL CHILD

The treatment plan and its implementation for potentially suicidal children is similar to that for adolescents. Generally, a child who is depressed and/or displays aggression as a primary emotion ought to be considered a high suicide risk (Pfeffer, 1985). The safety and protection of the child is paramount. Once the child is brought to a health care or mental health facility, it will be determined whether the child should be treated in an inpatient or outpatient facility. The developmental and cognitive levels of the child are taken into consideration when planning care. The family is always included; in some cases, individual family members may also need treatment.

VIOLENCE WITHIN THE FAMILY

DESCRIPTION OF VIOLENCE WITHIN THE FAMILY

Spouse and child abuse are probably the most common crises occurring within families today. Violence in the home has been in the national attention since the early 1960's when Kempe et al. (1962) first identified the battered child syndrome. According to the National Committee for Prevention of Child Abuse, 2.2 million cases of abuse were reported in 1988 (Leavitt, 1989). Spouse and child abuse are treated as separate entities for discussion here, but most researchers believe that there is a relationship between the two types of violence in the home.

When studying abusive or violent relationships, one may discover that a number of terms, such as battering, abuse, and violence are used interchangeably. Therefore, it is important to develop an operational definition that will adequately describe the phenomenon of abuse.

The term **violence** usually implies only the use of physical force, whereas the term **abuse** may include both violent and nonviolent interactions. A victim of abuse may or may not have evidence to indicate physical injury. Battering is specifically related to serially repeated forceful actions, with resultant physical injuries (Brown, 1987). Other forms of abuse include physical and emotional neglect, and sexual abuse.

Family violence is commonly understood using the sociological theoretical model. Within that model, family violence is related to modern industrial society in which the extended family once predominated and now the nuclear family predominates. Glick (1975) found that there tends to be less violence in large, extended families than in nuclear families. He feels that the support system that often served to prevent intrafamily conflicts no longer exists, and as a result, families today focus their difficulties upon each other or their children.

ASSESSMENT OF VIOLENCE WITHIN THE FAMILY

Women who have been physically and emotionally abused are seen in a variety of health-care settings, including emergency rooms, prenatal and maternal care units, community health agencies, clinics, and inpatient services. Hilberman (1980) noted that abused women came to the attention of health-care professionals because of mixed anxiety and depressive symptoms, usually related to marital difficulties or physical problems. The marital difficulties included alcoholism, as well as the husband's financial irresponsibility and infidelity. These women rarely mentioned the abusive situation. During the assessment of a woman whom the nurse suspects has been abused, the nurse asks directly, "Has anyone hit you or tried to hurt you in some way?" The nurse then can incorporate the information obtained into the health history. It may also be useful to ask about current conflicts in the family and how stress is usually handled by family members.

Complaints of abused women include psychophysiological symptoms such as fatigue, insomnia, headaches, anorexia, gastrointestinal problems, hypertension, and palpitations. Physical injuries noted include contusions, lacerations, burns, scars, hematomas, joint tenderness, limited range of motion, edema, dental injuries, or spontaneous abortions. Drake (1982) found in her sample of twelve abused women a correlation between being battered and being pregnant. If the nurse suspects the patient has been abused, it is important that she assess the situation in a private room with the patient alone. Specifically, the nurse assesses the pattern of the abuse, its duration, any use of weapons, and the current level of danger. Assessment of the stressors and violence in both spouses' families of origin, as well as the support system and the wife's level of dependency on the marriage relationship for her self-worth provides further "soft evidence" of a possibly abusive situation. (See Table 18–5 for other factors that increase the probability of violence in an intimate relationship.) Table 18–6 identifies phases of the assessment and responses that, when occurring together, indicate a high probability of an abusive situation.

THEORIES OF VIOLENCE WITHIN THE FAMILY

PSYCHOANALYTIC. Early psychoanalytic theorists held that women were masochistic. Waites (1977–78), in her critical review of theories of female masochism, argues that these explanations are inadequate because they do not consider the external constraints placed upon women. Masochism only

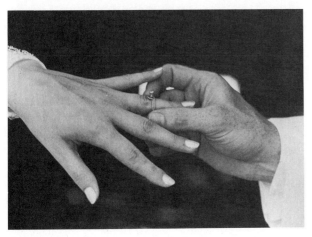 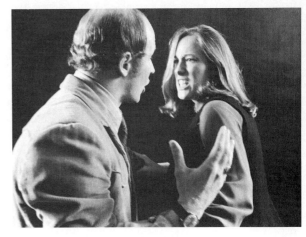

The wedding day . . . the beginning of a lifetime of happiness . . . or a lifetime of violence.

TABLE 18–5 Factors that increase the probability of violence in an intimate relationship

---

Dating violence: continuation of intimate relationships in which any degree of courtship violence has occurred.

Youth: marriage or cohabitation at a young age, especially after a brief courtship period.

Premarital pregnancy: dependency is already established; a combination of youth and premarital pregnancy is extremely dangerous.

Stepchildren: entering a new relationship with a dependent child or children by another man.

Isolation: breaking off close contact and relationships with friends and family; lack of support systems.

Unknown history: lack of knowledge about the man's former intimate relationships whether they be with lovers, wives, or parents.

Dependence: lack of ability to function independently because of health, education, or occupational deficits.

Source: Pagelow, M. (1984). *Family violence.* New York: Praeger Special Studies, p. 305.

considers the internal motivation of women. Just as important are external constraints such as the lack of social and financial resources necessary to escape the abusive situation.

BEHAVIORAL. Walker (1979) applied the concept of learned helplessness (Maier & Seligman, 1976) (see Chapter 9 on Mood Disorders for a review of the concept) to the psychological response of the abused woman. The behavioral results of learned helplessness include anxiety, depression, and dependence, a symptom picture similar to that of the battered woman. According to Walker (1979), once women believe they are unable to control or prevent their abuse, the perception of helplessness becomes a reality.

In her studies of abused women, Walker identified a pattern of violence. The first, or "tension-building," phase involves minor battering incidents in which the woman generally allows or submits to her husband's abuse. Her feelings of helplessness and fear increase over time. This phase can last from a few weeks to years. Phase two is the "acute battering incident" in which serious violence, lasting from two to twenty-four hours, is committed. The woman then tries to hide to avoid further injury. In the third phase, the "aftermath," the abuser becomes loving

and promises not to batter her again. This phase reinforces the woman's hope that the beating will end, but the cycle repeats itself when the abuser again begins to experience tension.

SOCIOLOGICAL. Much research on spouse abuse utilizes the sociological perspective. In the United States there is a high level of visible violence; for example, violence against individuals appears on television, in newspapers, in movies, and on the streets. This exposure to violence has contributed to our society's desensitization regarding violence and acceptance of it as a normal part of life. Culturally, most families typically engage in some form of violence in the home, for example, spanking children. Corporal punishment in our schools has been condoned by the Supreme Court (Newberger & Bourne, 1978). Straus (1974) points out that people can also be socialized to use violence for conflict resolution.

Our society still harbors sexist attitudes about the role, worth, and function of women, particularly spouses or mates. Germain (1984) refers to spouse abuse or battering of women as a "transcultural phenomenon that grows naturally out of ancient, honored, and sometimes legal traditions found in patriarchal societies" (p. 64). (Also see Chapter 19, Psychiatric Mental Health Nursing with Women.)

NURSING MANAGEMENT OF VIOLENCE WITHIN THE FAMILY

The primary goal in planning nursing care is to provide a safe environment. Support systems such as family or friends can help by providing shelter. If such support is not available, the nurse or other health-care team member locates safe temporary residence for them. The woman may not want to leave her husband/mate; many abused women are seen for treatment of their injuries several times before they seek shelter. Gelles (1976) has identified three major factors that influence an abused woman's decision regarding whether or not to stay in her marriage or the abusive relationship: 1) violence that is less severe and frequent, 2) a history of being assaulted by her parents when she was a child, and 3) limited financial and social resources.

IMPLEMENTATION. Drake (1982) suggests that the ideal time for the nurse to intervene (and the time when the woman is most likely to seek assistance) is between the end of phase 2, the acute battering incident, and the beginning of phase 3, the

TABLE 18–6 Indicators of potential or actual wife abuse from history

Area of assessment	At-risk responses
I. Primary Concern/ Reason for Visit	Unwarranted delay between time of injury and seeking treatment
	Inappropriate spouse reactions (lack of concern, overconcern, threatening demeanor, reluctance to leave wife, etc.)
	Vague information about cause of injury or problem; discrepancy between physical findings and verbal description of cause; obviously incongruous cause of injury given
	Minimizing serious injury
	Seeking emergency room treatment for vague stress-related symptoms and minor injuries
II. Family Health History	
A. Home of Origin	Traditional values about women's role taught
	Spouse abuse or child abuse (may not be significant for wife but should be noted)
B. Children	Children abused
	Physical punishment used routinely and severely with children
	Children are hostile toward or fearful of father
	Father perceives children as an additional burden
	Father demands unquestioning obedience from children
C. Spouse	Alcohol or drug abuse
	Holds machismo values
	Experience with violence outside of home, including violence against women in previous relationships
	Low self-esteem; lack of power in workplace or other arenas outside of home
	Uses force in sexual activities
	Unemployment
	Extreme jealousy of female friendships, work, and children as well as other men; jealousy frequently unfounded
	Stressors such as death in family, moving, change of jobs, trouble at work, etc.
	Abused as a child or witnessed father abusing mother
D. Household	Poverty
	Conflicts solved by aggression or violence
	Isolated from neighbors, relatives; few friends; lack of support systems
III. Past Health History	Fractures and trauma injuries
	Depression, anxiety symptoms, substance abuse
	Injuries while pregnant
	Spontaneous abortions
	Psychophysiological complaints

Source: From Campbell, J., & Humphreys, J. (Eds.) (1984). *Nursing care of victims of family violence.* Reston, Va: Reston Publ. Co., pp. 251–252.

aftermath. At this time, the victim is in an active stage of crisis and disequilibrium and is more willing to seek and receive assistance.

The crisis-intervention model is helpful in working with the acutely abused woman. Initially, the abused woman's symptoms are characteristic of loss and grieving (Campbell, 1984). These include shock, disbelief, and guilt. Interventions are based upon where the patient is in the grieving process. Educating the patient about spouse abuse can be helpful to her in gaining understanding of the dynamics of battering in her case. The nurse also helps the abused woman decrease her anxiety and enhance her self-concept with crisis counseling, empathy, and referral to a support group and/or individual or group psychotherapy (Weitz, 1982). The nurse also encourages the woman to maintain existing healthy relationships with supportive significant others; couples therapy or marriage counseling can be helpful if the husband or mate is willing to take responsibility for the violence and to work toward change. In the sessions, the couple is taught alternative methods of coping with anger and stress and more adaptive ways of communicating with each other.

Information and assistance from a variety of community resources is essential to the long-term management of spouse abuse. These include the following:

1. Medical facilities, which provide physical and mental health care

2. Social services for financial assistance, housing, food stamps, daycare, and child protection services

3. Criminal justice agencies for protection against further injury and violence

4. Legal aid for assistance with warrants, court procedures, separation and divorce agreements

5. Vocational rehabilitation for job training and employment counseling

6. Women's support or self-help groups for a sense of belonging.

Case Study: Nonpsychiatric Setting

Maria: A Victim of Spouse Abuse

Maria, age 31, was married for six years and had three children, ages 5, 3, and 1. Her husband John, age 35, worked in a business management firm. Maria had little time to socialize because of the young children; her husband worked long hours and drank occasionally. Maria and John had frequent fights that began with screaming. Within the last three years, John started to slap and punch Maria, at times shoving her against the wall. Most of the time, the fights began because Maria or the children did not carry out his wishes. Once, Maria's arm was broken. (She told hospital nurses that she tripped while running after the children.) After that incident, her husband did not batter her for four months. Maria had thought about leaving a few times, but did not know where she could go with three young children.

One day, John came home from work early because he was feeling ill. John, Jr., his oldest son, wanted to play with him but John explained he was tired, wanted to have an early dinner, and go to bed. As John, Jr., began to cry, John started to hit him. Maria pleaded with John to stop. John started to punch her. The neighbors, who witnessed the fight, called the police. In the emergency room, where Maria was treated for facial cuts and eye trauma, she was not talkative; she felt guilty about the incident and wanted to go home. She expressed feelings of hopelessness and loss of control in her marriage. John verbalized regret about what had happened and recognized his need for help.

Nursing Diagnoses

Potential for injury related to husband's abuse
Ineffective individual coping
Disturbance in self-concept: self-esteem
Powerlessness
Pain

Nursing Care Plan for Maria

Nursing Diagnosis	Desired Outcomes	Interventions	Rationale
1. Potential for injury as a result of husband's violence, and related to the husband's inability to cope with stress.	Maria will find a safe environment.	Provide Maria with the appropriate resources, such as a woman's shelter or social services.	Allowing Maria to make the initial contact with support agencies will enhance her self-care role, as well her self-esteem. Furthermore, it will minimize her victim role.
		Provide legal alternatives for restraint order to prevent further abuse.	Allows Maria to have several options available to protect her and her family.
	Maria will evaluate her own danger and situation.	Assess realistically for potential abuse.	Allows practitioner and Maria to understand possible danger and to plan for subsequent action related to potential abuse.
	Maria will state realistically the pattern of abuse in the past and make projections for the future.	Help Maria identify patterns of past abuse and seek assistance from legal aid.	Allows Maria to develop insight in regard to the abusive relationship with her husband and to develop a more autonomous self-care role.
2. Ineffective individual coping.	Maria will establish an appropriate support system to alleviate stress.	Consult with hospital social worker to help Maria find new support networks in the community.	Allows Maria to identify alternate support systems, thereby increasing her available resources.
	Maria will express feelings of anger and helplessness.	Tell Maria she will need counseling to deal with her feelings about what has happened.	Gives Maria alternatives for expressing such unacceptable emotions as anger and helplessness.
3. Disturbance in self-concept: self-esteem	Maria will develop a more positive self-concept and self-esteem.	Help Maria identify her strengths. Refer Maria to marriage and individual counseling.	Allows Maria to place her marital relationship in proper perspective. Problems are not all her fault.
		Tell Maria that her husband must take responsibility for his behavior.	Will minimize Maria's "victim" role.

Nursing Diagnosis	Desired Outcomes	Interventions	Rationale
		Encourage Maria to express her feelings of anger, hopelessness, and fear; be supportive and nonjudgmental.	Giving positive feedback and affirmation of Maria's feelings will make her feel worthwhile and important.
4. Powerlessness	Maria will competently demonstrate more adaptive behaviors.	Allow Maria to make decisions concerning her life situation. Give Maria positive feedback for autonomous behaviors exhibited.	Maria will function more independently. This will decrease feelings of powerlessness and need for dependency.
		Provide appropriate referrals for legal and financial aid.	Allows Maria to take responsibility for her life.
5. Pain	Maria will receive appropriate medical treatment, as well as social supports for her protection.	Provide for appropriate medical follow-up.	Physical trauma is often present in victims of abuse.

CHILD ABUSE

DESCRIPTION OF CHILD ABUSE

Historically, child abuse and neglect have permeated many cultures, but in the early 1960's it was increasingly recognized and identified in the United States as a clinical problem referred to as the **battered-child syndrome** (Kempe & Helfer, 1972a). The Child Abuse Prevention and Treatment Act of 1973 (Public Law 93-247) defines "child abuse and neglect" as "the physical or mental injury, sexual abuse, negligent treatment or maltreatment of a child under the age of eighteen by a person who is responsible for this child's welfare under circumstances which indicate that the child's health or welfare is harmed or threatened thereby" (U.S. Congress, 1974). At this time, all fifty states have enacted legislation each of which differs in its definitions and emphasis, but all of which mandate the reporting of suspected cases of child abuse by nurses and other professionals such as physicians, teachers, and psychotherapists. With this enactment, legal involvement is now recognized as an integral component of the professional and community treatment of child abuse.

EPIDEMIOLOGY OF CHILD ABUSE

Child abuse and neglect occur in families from all socioeconomic classes, cultures, religions, and geographical areas. However, the majority of reports of abuse occur in the lower socioeconomic class. This is the case, in part, because these families tend to utilize public health facilities much more frequently than their counterparts in higher socioeconomic classes. These families also face more environmental and situational stressors, such as lack of housing, overcrowding, and lack of financial and psychosocial resources (Gelles, 1987; Starr, 1988); in turn, these stressors may precipitate violence.

Kempe and Helfer (1972b) have utilized a social-psychological model to try to understand what factors contribute to child abuse and neglect. The conditions or characteristics that have been found to be associated with physical abuse include the following:

1. *The special parent*. The parent who has the potential to become abusive, most often because of his history of having been abused as a child; he has been described as emotionally immature, lacking self-esteem, inexperienced in parenting, and having unrealistic expectations of the child, for example, that the child be "someone to love me and never leave me."

2. *The special child*. This child is viewed differently from the other children in the family. The child may be physically different (handicapped, chronically ill, small at birth), or special meaning may be attached to him (for example, if he is the child of a former marriage/partner, or if he resembles a significant negatively regarded person).

3. *The stressful situation*. A perceived crisis situation, involving either acute or chronic stress, precipitates the act of aggression.

Blumber (1974) has identified the following characteristics of parents who abuse their children:

1. They frequently come from violent families.

2. They exhibit inadequate parenting skills and lack knowledge concerning normal child development.

3. They demonstrate emotional immaturity, with poor impulse control.

4. They are socially isolated, especially from community resources, and lack a social support system.

Justice and Justice (1976) found in their study that 95 percent of the adults who abuse and neglect their children are not severely mentally ill. Usually these individuals suffer from personality disorders and benefit more from supportive social services than insight-oriented psychotherapy. Table 18–7 outlines the factors that increase the probability of child abuse by mothers.

ASSESSMENT OF CHILD ABUSE

Schmitt (1978) has provided a diagnostic tool designed to be sensitive to situations in which child abuse is suspected. Evidence of two or three of the following indicators qualifies a case for further investigation by social services as well as involved health-care professionals.

1. An unexplained injury or reluctance to explain an injury.

2. A discrepancy between parents' and child's description of the incident which led to the injury.

3. A discrepancy between the type of injury or wound the child has and the report of how it occurred.

4. Suspicious injuries that are reported to be self-inflicted.

5. Injuries reported to be caused by a third party.

6. A delay in obtaining medical care for the child's injuries.

7. A history of suspicious injuries (pp. 39–57).

The first time the nurse encounters a family in which there is suspected abuse, she needs to be as nonconfronting and nonthreatening as possible. Her primary goal is to convey empathy and a desire to help. The nurse also needs to learn as much as possible about the family, its members, the home situation, family stressors, and the available support system. Once she completes this initial assessment, depending upon the status of the child, she conducts a physical, emotional, nutritional, and developmental

---

TABLE 18–7 Factors that increase the probability of child abuse by mothers

1. young mother
2. single mother
3. unwanted pregnancy
4. difficult birth
5. other young children at home
6. low birth weight infant
7. low education level of parent(s)
8. mother's health problems
9. child's health problems
10. lack of respite from child care
11. social isolation
12. irritable or unresponsive infant
13. poverty (substandard environment; poor medical care; malnutrition, and so forth)

Source: Pagelow, M. (1984). *Family violence*. New York: Praeger Special Studies, p. 197.

assessment of the child. (See Chapter 28, Ethical Considerations in Psychiatric Mental Health Nursing Practice for the ethical issues involved in this situation.)

Common injuries to abused children include head injuries, internal injuries, lacerations and contusions, multiple contusions, and any type of burn, especially a burn in the genital area or on the buttocks, rope burns, hematomas, and human bite marks. Emotional symptoms of the acutely abused child include excessive fearfulness or stoicism, depression, extreme withdrawal, aggressiveness, and inappropriate affect (for example, lack of appropriate protest to invasive procedures) (Drake, 1982).

THEORIES OF CHILD ABUSE

SOCIAL LEARNING/FAMILY SYSTEMS. The social-learning model and family-system model have been used to attempt to understand the behavioral dynamics of individuals who abuse a spouse, children, or parents. Straus, Gelles, & Steinmetz (1980) studied the extent and dynamics of violence in the home. They found that violence or aggression is learned through vicarious or direct experience. Their findings support the belief that transmission of violence continues through family generations (Gayford, 1975). In other words, parents who are physically and/or verbally abusive toward their children probably had parents who abused them. Straus, Gelles, and Steinmetz (1980) report other factors in society that contribute to the social learning of violence, for example, structural violence inherent in our society, so-

cial frustration, social disorganization, population density, a subculture of violence, and machismo. Garbarino (1977) has offered a human ecological model based upon culture, family, parents, child, and stress factors. Physical abuse and neglect of children are seen as part of a larger problem involving parent-child relations.

Drake (1982) reports that individuals who abuse their spouses are more likely to abuse their children; however, this is not always the case. Abused children in turn show greater violence toward their siblings and peers. As these children become adults, they will continue to develop the potential to abuse their spouses and/or children. The abuser and the victim share similar personality characteristics, namely, poor self-concept, feelings of helplessness and powerlessness, dependence and insecurity, and inability to contain anger.

Reactions of the victims of abuse to their abusers include:

1. Feeling responsible for bringing on the abuse.

2. Accepting the blame or blaming themselves for the abuse.

3. Feeling guilty for the abusive situation even though there is confusion or lack of clarity about their reasons for feeling guilty (Drake, 1982).

SEXUAL ABUSE OF CHILDREN

DESCRIPTION OF SEXUAL ABUSE. Faller (1988) has written that there are several types of sexual abuse that affect children and youth. **Non-contact sexual abuse** might include sexy talk (whereby a perpetrator makes statements to a child about his or her sexual attributes), or exposure (when the perpetrator displays his/her private parts [breasts, penis, etc.] or masturbates in front of the child). **Voyeurism** occurs when the perpetrator subtly or blatantly observes the victim in an incident that provides the perpetrator with a sense of sexual gratification. **Sexual contact** involves touching or "feeling" intimate body parts (breasts, anus, vagina, penis, etc.). **Oral-genital sex** occurs when the perpetrator licks, kisses, sucks, or bites a child's genitals or when the perpetrator induces the child to orally copulate with him. Faller's description of sexual abuse also includes **cunnilingus** (oral activity with vagina), **fellatio** (oral activity with penis), and **anilingus** (oral contact with anus). **Interfemoral intercourse** occurs when the perpetrator puts his penis between the child's thighs. The perpetrator may rub his penis against the child's

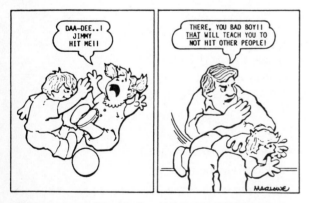

When a parent hits his/her child, the child learns to associate love with violence. This association continues into the child's adulthood, when he/she uses violence in times of stress and frustration, or to attain what he/she wants.

vulva, but there is no penetration. **Sexual penetration** occurs when there is some intrusion into the child's body orifice. There are numerous types of sexual penetration, and they include digital penetration (fingers are placed in the vagina or anus or both); penetration with objects (rulers, dildos, vibrators, bananas, cucumbers, etc.); genital intercourse (perpetrator's penis is inserted into the victim's vagina); and anal intercourse (the perpetrator inserts his penis into the victim's anus).

In a study of 190 victim-perpetrator dyads, Faller (1988) reported that 92 percent of the perpetrators were male while 84 percent of the victims were female and that families were of lower socioeconomic backgrounds. Specific characteristics of sexual abuse as described in this study follow.

The perpetrators (59.25%) typically abuse more than one person, and some victims (17.5%) were abused by more than one person. The age of onset of victims was approximately 5 years or younger, and they reported being abused from one to twenty times. The type of sexual abuse tended to be varied (non-contact, sexual contact [41.2%, being the most frequent]), child pornography and prostitution, and so forth.

Most sexual abuse situations that occurred in the family involved the step-father or mother's in-residence lover. The second most frequent situation consisted of the polyincestuous family; that is, a family in which incest is occurring among several family members (mother-son, father-daughter, and sometimes between siblings). Faller (1988) also observed that sexual abuse was reported to have existed in the family of origin in more than 50% of the families studied, and 52% of the perpetrators were characterized as having problems with drugs and alcohol. More than 80% of the subjects reported some type of intrafamilial violence, such as spouse abuse, child abuse and neglect, and so forth. Interestingly, few couples reported that they had hostile marriages but in 35% of the families, the perpetrator was perceived as the dominant person. Some families (35%) reported obsessional-type rituals that were associated with the abuse, while 34% reported no obsessive behaviors and 29.5% reported other rituals. Finally, the study indicated that all families experienced some isolation from support structures: 37% reported some support, 38.5% reported few supports, and 4.7% reported no support.

A study conducted by Finkelhor (1979; 1986) indicates that, of the 796 university students interviewed, approximately 1/2 of the population had experienced incest. In the same study, Finkelhor (1984) found that the majority of incest victims were female, whereas the majority of perpetrators were male.

ASSESSMENT OF SEXUAL ABUSE. Children who report sexual abuse or who act out sexually should be handled in a caring and sensitive manner by all professionals involved. Children will react in different ways to sexual abuse, but many will have physical symptoms. (See Table 18–8.) A physical examination should be completed for the purpose of documenting and diagnosing the possibility of sexual abuse. Frequently, acute psychiatric services are needed for the child and family; attitudes and behaviors of the child victim and family should be carefully observed and documented. The nurse might find that families of sexually abused children are not always cooperative in the treatment. The resistance must be overcome if treatment is to be effective. Working with these families and children can sometimes be emotionally draining and extremely frustrating for the nurse (Fontana, 1984). (See Box 18–4.)

NURSING MANAGEMENT OF THE ABUSED CHILD AND FAMILY

Sideleau (1982) has identified several reactions a nurse may have toward the victim of family violence and his family. Initially, the nurse may be outraged, shocked, and angry and may unconsciously act those feelings out in dealing with the parents of the injured child. She may, for example, reject the parents overtly by ignoring them or covertly by becoming indifferent to their needs. The nurse also may project her own emotional needs onto the child as well as entertain rescue fantasies. Since treatment resources available

---

TABLE 18—8 Children's reactions to sexual abuse

Clinging	40%
Fear of specific people	35%
Sleep disturbances	30%
Loss of appetite	25%
Anxiety	25%
School problems	85%
Physical symptoms	90%

Source: April, 1988. *Harvard Medical School Mental Health Letter.* Vol. 4, No. 10, p. 7.

**Box 18–4 ●
Assessment of
Allegations of Child
Sexual Abuse**

In assessing allegations of child sexual abuse, mental health professionals should be aware that in up to 30% of cases the allegations may be unfounded. Types of unfounded allegations include:

1. Charges arising in divorce cases with disputed custody or visitation rights. The anxious mother may misinterpret the father's conduct with the child; the vindictive mother may fabricate allegations.

2. Children, especially adolescents, may fantasize or fabricate allegations

of abuse for attention or to manipulate.

3. Allegations of abuse at day care centers may "snowball" and be for financial gain.

4. Public attention to child abuse may result in unfounded complaints filed out of an abundance of precaution.

5. Children's normal curiosity about their bodies may be misinterpreted.

Source: *The Harvard Medical School Mental Health Letter.* November, 1987. Vol. 4, No. 5, p. 4.

---

to abused children and their parents are lacking and inadequate, it is crucial that nurses respond with empathy and resourcefulness when presented with individual cases of child abuse. It does not help abused children for the nurse to reject the child's parents nor does it help to give up on the possibility of treatment when organized treatment resources are not immediately available. Many communities have done much to treat and prevent child abuse and battering of women by mobilizing existing professional resources (for example, the local hospital) and starting volunteer service programs, such as the Lay Health Visitor program first developed by Kempe and Helfer (1972a), with the assistance of mental health professionals acting as consultants. Federal, state, and private monies have helped to finance such programs, demonstrated to be effective in preventing first time and repeated physical abuse in many communities. Table 18–9 identifies some guidelines for effective crisis intervention during the initial interview of abused children and their families.

IMPLEMENTATION. The primary nursing goal is early identification of child abuse and neglect and prevention of its reoccurrence. Treatment initially focuses on the safety of the child; ultimately it involves caring for the dysfunctional family. Sideleau (1982) suggests that treatment in cases of child abuse focus on:

1. The resolution of old conflicts.

2. The maintenance of a stable home environment.

3. Developing parenting skills and feelings of adequacy as parents.

4. Developing adaptive ways of dealing with stress.

5. Increasing self-esteem and self-acceptance.

6. Reducing social isolation.

7. Ameliorating a faulty attachment process between child and parent.

8. Integrating the child into the family system.

9. Developing a healthier family system that more adequately meets the needs of its members.

Horowitz and Wintermute (1978) found interventions aimed at reducing acute stress were effective in early treatment of abusive families. These included emergency housing, supplemental food, and short-term child care.

RUNAWAY CHILDREN AND YOUTH

Only a small number of studies have been done to address the problem of runaway and homeless youth in America, although the problem has become serious enough to come into national attention (Committee on Health Care for Homeless People, 1988). While public concern is increasing, there is little research on why these children and adolescents leave their homes. In a study involving 199 youth in one shelter, 78% reported serious physical abuse from a parent approximately one year before the runaway occurred (Farber et al., 1984). In another study, Janus et al. (1987) reported that of 87 runaways living in their parents' homes when they ran away, 44% stated they had been sexually abused and 35% reported that their decision to run away was directly associated

TABLE 18–9 Effective crisis-intervention techniques for suspected child abuse

Maintain a neutral, matter-of-fact attitude about the alleged maltreatment.
> Be particularly careful to avoid words or body language which convey shock or
> disapproval in relation to the incident or the actions of the parents.

Be supportive whenever possible.
> Use responses such as "Young children can be very stubborn," or "I know it's difficult for
> you to talk about this," to convey support and understanding.

Provide validating statements and recognize positive intentions.
> For example, the statement "You really got your child to the hospital in a hurry" can
> provide reinforcement for positive action taken by the parent when it occurs.

Keep the focus upon the welfare of the children and the parental caretakers.
> For example, avoid talking about why the report was made and concentrate on what can
> be done about the situation.

Keep attention upon what the parental caretakers themselves reveal and what is directly observable.
> Avoid accusation and interpretations made on the basis of information from other sources.

Be reassuring.
> Parental caretakers need to be reassured that the worker is approaching the situation with
> an open mind and is soliciting evidence that will confirm adequate care and treatment of
> children if that is the case, not just evidence of maltreatment. The worker may give a
> description of the procedures usually followed in determining incidence of neglect or
> abuse if the family shows concern about them. When it is appropriate, assure the parents
> of their right to legal counsel. If it appears that the family will need continued service, it
> is important to point out the various options and kinds of resources and help the agency
> and community can provide, especially services to families and children in their own homes.

*Be acutely aware of nonverbal communication and look for signs of hostility, fear, and affection
among family members.*
> Careful observations and response styles can yield more information than verbal responses
> to questions.

If possible, talk to family members separately at first.
> Following this, they can be brought together again as a group.

Use open-ended questions.
> For example, instead of asking who hit the child, ask how the child's face was bruised.

Recognize and label feelings.
> Statements such as "That must have really been confusing and frustrating" will help the
> parents feel that the intervenor really understands how they feel in the situation.

*Restate the parents' answers to make sure they are understood and to give the parent a chance to
provide more information.*
> For example, say "Now let me make sure I understood. You got upset because Peter
> spilled paint over the floor right after you finished washing it."

*Avoid agreeing with or seeming to condone everything, but make it clear that facts and feelings are
understood.*
> Use statements like "That really made you mad" or "That was really upsetting," but avoid
> such comments as "Anyone would have done that," or "No wonder you got so mad."

Do not take verbal abuse personally.
> Parents are in a stressful situation, and their hostility is focused on the intervenor's role,
> not on the person in that role.

Convey a desire to alleviate the stress and help change the situation.
> Express confidence in the parent's ability to act responsibly, but make it clear that you are
> prepared to take charge of the situation to the extent necessary.

Source: Borgman, R., Edmunds, M., & MacDicken, R. A. (1979). *Crisis intervention: A manual for child protective workers.* National Center on Child Abuse and Neglect Children's Bureau: Administration for Children, Youth and Families Office of Human Development Services. U.S. Department of Health, Education and Welfare. DHEW Publication No. (OHDS) 79-30196.

with physical abuse they had experienced from their families. Significantly, approximately 60% of the adolescents in this study had made some contact with mental health professionals or social service workers prior to making their decision to run away.

Once these youth leave home, they are likely to experience a variety of dangers and problems. Runaway children have a high mortality rate. Many runaways suffer from malnutrition, venereal disease, and are frequently sexually exploited. Runaway youth will often resort to prostitution (Brenton, 1978). Many commit suicide (Brenton, 1978; Institute of Medicine, 1988).

Each year the runaway youth served at shelters and other types of agencies become more troubled with multiple complex problems (The National Network of Runaway and Youth Services, Inc., 1985). More research on spotting potential runaways and developing more effective strategies to help troubled youth before they leave home is clearly needed.

RAPE

DESCRIPTION OF RAPE

Rape is a severe and complex form of assault. It affects the victim's physical and emotional integrity, competence, and trust in others and the environment. A sexual assault also affects and exaggerates preexisting personal problems, particularly with spouses or mates who are often a major part of the victim's support system (Foley & Davies, 1983).

Published statistics identifying the occurrence of rape are misleading. For example, according to National Crime Survey Data (U.S. Department of Justice, 1986), 138,000 rapes (out of a total 35 million estimated number of crimes) were reported in 1985. However, only 87,340 of these were classified by the Federal Bureau of Investigation as forcible rapes (U.S. Department of Justice, 1988) with only 36,970 arrests (out of a total 11.9 million arrests for all crimes reported by law enforcement agencies). The actual number of rapes far exceeds even the highest of these statistics (reported rapes) because many victims do not report the crime.

EPIDEMIOLOGY OF RAPE

Identified risk factors for victims include age, race, marital status, sex, occupation, and socioeconomic status (Katz & Mazur, 1979; Foley & Davies, 1983).

AGE. Rape happens to persons of all ages. The youngest reported rape victim was 5 months old and the oldest 93 years old. High risk groups are teenagers (13 to 17 years) and young adults (18 to 24 years).

RACE. Most reported rapes occur within the victim's race. No one race is more vulnerable to the problem of rape than the others.

MARITAL STATUS. Statistics indicate that the majority of rape victims are unmarried when they are raped, and they live with one or both parents or with a roommate.

SEX. Most rape victims are female but male rape has been reported.

OCCUPATION. The majority of victims are students. Also, women who work late hours or travel alone are at risk.

SOCIOECONOMIC STATUS. In general, persons from the lower socioeconomic classes are more vulnerable to rape.

MOTIVATION OF THE RAPIST

Understanding the motivation of the rapist can be helpful in caring for the assailant as well as the victim. This discussion focuses on the female victim because the majority of research on rape has examined this population.

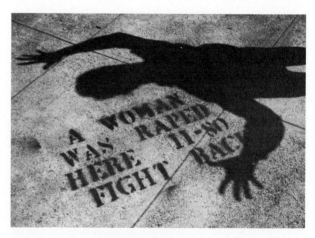

Rape is a violent crime which not only affects the victims but also their families, other potential victims, and society as a whole.

The male rapist is usually not sexually motivated, nor is he sexually gratified when he has assaulted a victim. Rape serves primarily nonsexual needs. Groth and Birnbaum (1980) believe that a person who rapes has serious psychological difficulties and expresses his anger, frustration, resentment, and rage through the sexual assault. These authors have identified three basic patterns of rape:

1. *Power rape* compensates for the assailant's feelings of inadequacy and incompetence concerning his masculine identity. He seeks to assert his mastery over the victim sexually but without intent to harm. This is the most common form of rape.

2. *Anger rape* is characterized by physical brutality. The rapist is able to release and feel relief from pent-up anger. His motives are retaliation and revenge against a transgression by a significant female in his life (such as mother, or wife).

3. *Sadistic rape* involves the eroticization of aggression. The assailant finds that sexual abuse of a victim is sexually gratifying and exciting. The rape may include bizarre ritualistic behaviors, torture and bondage, or symbolic victims (victims who share common characteristics in appearance or professional identity with a rapist's significant other). In extreme cases the rapist may murder the victim and mutilate the body to express his anger, power, domination, and retaliation.

Anyone can be a victim of rape. As mentioned previously, the sexual assault can aggravate or create serious emotional problems, particularly those related to developmental issues such as the search for identity in adolescence, or the ability to achieve adequate coping skills in adulthood (Foley & Davies, 1983).

ASSESSMENT OF RAPE

According to legal criteria, three essential elements must be present to define an act of rape (Foley and Davies, 1983):

1. The use of force, threat, intimidation, or duress.

2. Vaginal penetration, however slight.

3. Lack of consent of the victim.

During the assessment phase in a case of rape, the nurse collects data on the physical and emotional effects of the trauma. A complete physical and gynecological examination should be conducted and emergency treatment provided for the patient. The patient at this time will be informed of her legal rights. The nurse caring for a victim of rape needs to inform the woman of the evidence needed for legal prosecution, such as torn clothing, seminal fluid, and the assailant's hair or tissue. The nurse acts as the victim's advocate during the legal process of obtaining evidence. Rights of the rape victim are summarized in Table 18–10.

According to clinical observations made by Burgess and Holmstrom (1974), victims of rape consistently demonstrate significant immediate physical and emotional symptoms, which may persist over time. This is called the **rape-trauma syndrome** and specific symptoms occur during 1) the immediate or acute phase and 2) the reorganization phase (pp. 38–47).

IMMEDIATE OR ACUTE PHASE

1. The victim displays two types of emotion: controlled (masked, calm, or composed affect) and expressed (feelings of anger, fear, and anxiety).

2. Physical symptoms include general soreness of the body and/or specific concern for parts of the body that were the focus of the assault.

3. The victim experiences disturbances in sleeping and eating patterns.

4. The victim has emotional reactions that are similar to those associated with acute stress disorders, in which the victim has been threatened with death. The primary feelings generally are fear of physical injury, mutilation, or death. Other feelings include disbelief, shock, guilt, shame, embarrassment, self-blame, anger, and revenge. PTSD (Post Traumatic Stress Disorder) which involves persistent flashbacks of the rape, nightmares, and high levels of anxiety, may develop (see Chapter 8, Anxiety Disorders).

The acute phase may last from a few days to a few weeks, and these symptoms will overlap with those of the reorganization phase.

REORGANIZATION PHASE

1. The individual is able only to resume a minimal level of functioning and generally relies on family for support, even if she has not told the family about the incident. Some victims change their permanent residences in the hope that they can stop worrying about being raped again.

2. The victim often experiences two types of dreams and nightmares. She either dreams that she is in a similar rape situation and is unable to free herself, or she herself commits violence or murder in the dream.

3. The patient often develops fear and phobias specific to the circumstances of the rape situation (for

TABLE 18–10 Rights of the rape victim

Rights of the Rape Victim

1. To transportation to a hospital when incapacitated.

2. To emergency room care with privacy and confidentiality.

3. To be carefully listened to and treated as a human being, with respect, courtesy, and dignity.

4. To have an advocate of choice accompany her through the treatment process.

5. To be given as much credibility as a victim of any other crime.

6. To have her name kept from the news media.

7. To be considered a victim of rape regardless of the assailant's relationship to the victim, such as the victim's spouse.

8. To *not* be exposed to prejudice against race, age, class, life-style, or occupation.

9. To *not* be asked questions about prior sexual experience.

10. To be treated in a manner that does not usurp her control, but enables her to determine her own needs and how to meet them.

11. To be asked only those questions that are relevant to a court case or to medical treatment.

12. To receive prompt medical and mental health services, whether or not the rape is reported to the police, and at no cost.

13. To be protected from future assault.

14. To accurate collection and preservation of evidence for court in an objective record that incudes the signs and symptoms of physical and emotional trauma.

15. To receive clear explanations of procedures and medication in language she can understand.

16. To know what treatment is recommended, for what reasons, and who will administer the treatment.

17. To know any possible risks, side effects, or alternatives to proposed treatment, including all drugs prescribed.

18. To ask for another physician, nurse practitioner, or nurse.

19. To consent to or refuse any treatment even when her life is in serious danger.

20. To refuse to be part of any research or experiment.

21. To reasonable complaint and to leave a care facility against the physician's advice.

22. To receive an explanation of and understand any papers she agrees to sign.

23. To be informed of continuing health care needs after discharge from the emergency room, hospital, physician's office, or care facility.

24. To receive a clear explanation of the bill and review of charges, and to be informed of available compensation.

25. To have legal representation and be advised of her legal rights, including the possibility of filing a civil suit.

Source: Foley, T. and Davies, M. (1983) *Rape: Nursing care of victims*. St. Louis: C. V. Mosby Co., p. 298–299. Used with permission.

example, global fear of everyone, fear of sex, and fear of being alone or being in crowds).

4. The rape victim may exhibit pseudoadjustment involving denial, suppression, or rationalization (Sutherland & Scherl, 1970). The nurse must be aware that further treatment may be necessary.

Many rape victims experience problems with sexual adequacy and sexual identity after their trauma. These problems can include aversion to all sexual activity, reduction in vaginal lubrication, loss of sensation in the genital area, vaginismus (sexual dysfunction), and loss of ability to have orgasm. Not every victim experiences these problems, but often when her partner makes an overt sexual gesture, a victim relives or has flashbacks to the rape. The types of responses are highly individualistic, and the length of each phase is unpredictable.

The rape assault also affects the victim's relationships with her family and friends. Silverman and McCombie (1980) state, "Abrupt changes in the balance of interpersonal relations and family functions may occur in direct parallel to the intrapsychic disharmony experienced by the rape victim" (p. 173).

Amir (1971) reports that family members and friends close to the victim generally share the same misunderstandings and prejudices about the crime of rape as the general public. They usually react more to the sexual aspects rather than the violent aspects of the rape. The feelings of resentment, anger, and blame toward the victim generate the **revictimization** of the woman. Opinions such as "Nice girls don't get raped" or "Women who are raped asked for it" are examples of attitudes that blame the victim, a maladaptive response of some family members and associates of the victim trying to cope with their own feelings about the trauma of rape. These are examples of the attitudes and opinions that need to be explored with family members and male mates; misconceptions and myths can make it difficult for the victim to gain support from family and mates. See Table 18–11, "Myths and Facts about Rapists."

MARITAL RAPE

Little is known about marital rape; in recent years, however, research on family and spouse violence has produced more information on marital rape. This type of sexual abuse is not legally recognized in some states, which means that a man cannot be held legally accountable for raping his marital partner. Too, there are many definitions for marital rape. Generally speaking, marital rape is said to occur when there is forced sexual activity between husband and wife. Whatever the definition, the wife, guided by her definition, will determine if she has been raped (Hanneke and Shields, 1985).

Research on marital rape has focused primarily on incidence and prevalence. One study suggests that as many as 600,000 to 900,000 women are raped and battered by their husbands each year. There are also a group of women who are raped and not beaten; the total number of marital rape victims then becomes much higher. It is difficult to determine the number of women who are victims of marital rape. Fear of retribution by the assailant, avoidance of the stigma of victimization, fear of being blamed for

their own victimization, and most important, the victims' refusal to admit that the incident was rape all contribute to the victims' unwillingness to report marital rape (Hanneke and Shields, 1985, p. 487).

Women do react to rape and battering that occur in the marriage. Their responses include lowering of the woman's feelings and opinions of herself; change of her feelings and acts toward her husband (or lover); and her feelings and behaviors toward others (Hanneke and Shields, 1985). Shields and Hanneke (1983) found that marital rape was related to the victim's responses of inadequate self-esteem; pessimistic attitudes toward men in general; withholding sex from their partners, and not desiring sex with their partners; and using alcohol to treat their depression.

Marital rape is now seen as a growing problem in today's society and is worthy of future research. Yet, professionals face numerous problems in providing services to this group of women. Kilpatrick (1983) has identified three major problems that professionals are likely to confront when working with marital rape victims. It can be extremely difficult for nurses and other counselors to view rape in the context of a marriage. Furthermore, these women are difficult to work with because of the impact of the violence on them. Some of the women will present as confused, disoriented, and detached, and display inconsistent attitudes and behaviors about their situation. Depression is frequently present among the women. Marital violence should alert the nurse and other professionals to the possibility of family violence, as it is very unlikely that marital rape is the only problem (Hanneke and Shields, 1985).

NURSING MANAGEMENT OF THE RAPE VICTIM

In order to obtain an accurate and sensitive assessment of the rape victim, the nurse must be knowledgeable about the legal, psychological, social, and physical aspects of sexual assault. The myths and misconceptions of rape and society's sexist attitudes toward it also need to be explored. Anger at the victim or assailant as well as feelings of anxiety over the threat of rape and other forms of violence or a sense of helplessness could impede providing therapeutic care. It is not uncommon for the nurse and patient both to feel uncomfortable, initially, because of the transference and countertransference issues involved in this type of trauma (McCombie & Arons, 1980). Some countertransference issues nurses may confront include helplessness, rage, guilt, shame, fear, and vulnerability. Sexual issues for the nurse may be evoked

TABLE 18–11 Myths and facts about rapists

Myths	Results	Facts
Rapists are sex fiends releasing pent-up impulses.	Belief in this myth excuses the offender for behavior misperceived as a crime of passion. Normal behaviors (e.g., sleeping nude) are labeled as provocation or precipitation even when the victim is attacked by surprise in her own home. Rapists are not brought to trial nor charged with offenses.	All rapists report readily available sexual partners. In no case has sexual provocation on the victim's part been found. Rapists report sexual dysfunction (e.g., impotency, retarded ejaculation) during the assault but not with consenting sexual partners.
Rapists would not rape if prostitution were legalized or if castration were the punishment for such acts.	This myth perpetuates notions of rape as a sexual crime rather than a violent one.	Motives for rape are power, anger, and sadism; therefore castration and legalized prostitution do not treat the underlying conflict that perpetuates the behavior.
Rapists will flee if the woman resists.	One who believes this myth subscribes to a blame-the-victim model and perpetuates notions of the crime as an act of passion.	Force (e.g., verbal threats or physical force) is used to subdue the victim in all rapes. Lack of resistance does not imply consent or provocation; it reflects women's socialization to be passive and submissive, to feel fear and terror when faced with aggression, to defer to men rather than fight back. Women aim to survive by whatever means seems appropriate, given the assailant encountered. Resistance by the victim is essential for some offenders to become sexually aroused and may cause more harm rather than the expected release to safety.
Rapists are "dirty old men" or just young boys "sowing wild oats."	This myth minimizes the violation of a woman's rights, the situational crisis imposed on the victim, and the long-term resolution process.	Rapists are most often between the ages of 15 to 24 years; almost none are found over the age of 45.
Raping is a one-time act reflecting a momentary lapse of judgment; it is not a serious offense.	Belief in this myth fails to acknowledge the offender's inadequacy in interpersonal relationships, gender identity, impulse management, and chronic immaturity.	Raping is a repetitive offense; convicted offenders report 13 rapes for every convicted offense. Even in the majority of reported rapes, no suspect is apprehended and convictions are rare.
Rapists are mentally ill or mentally retarded and not responsible for their acts.	Society does not consider rape abnormal unless it is extremely brutal and the victim has physical proof of that brutality. One who believes this myth excuses the offender for his behavior.	Rapists exhibit defects in their personality structure, including denial of their behavior and projection of responsibility for their acts. These defects in psychologic functioning do not exonerate them from their behavior; to do so would corrupt

Myths	Results	Facts
		their treatment and rehabilitative therapy.
		Alcohol and drug abuse are common secondary diagnoses that reflect the offender's difficulty with impulse management, his dependency, and his demands for immediate gratification.
		There are more descriptive similarities than differences between rapists and nonrapists: married or previously married, moderate to heavy drinking, skilled and semiskilled trades, and not provoked by the victim.
All rapists have similar characteristics.	Belief in this myth results in applying a treatment approach that may be contraindicated and fails to meet the offender's individualized needs.	Equalizing all rapists objectifies their personhood and fails to recognize the uniqueness of different human beings.
		Definitions of the rapist's characteristics depend on the source—popular literature, the rapist, researchers . . .
		Men rape for different reasons: power, anger, sadism. Personality structure is unique to the offender.
Rapists are not treatable.	One who believes this myth supports outdated laws that lead to incarcerating the offender and function solely as preventive detention, not treatment. With the underlying conflict for rape untreated, the incarcerated offender continues to rape while in prison and when released.	Current research suggests that rapists can benefit from some form of specialized treatment based on a comprehensive assessment and a wide selection of approaches that meet individualized needs.
		The effectiveness of any given treatment approach, including measurement of recidivism, has yet to be established.
		Most rapists are "treated" in maximum security prisons, an environment not conducive to meaningful psychologic change.

Source: Foley, T., & Davies, M. (1983). *Rape: Nursing care of victims.* St. Louis: C. V. Mosby Co., pp. 28–30. Reprinted with permission.

when asking or listening to the explicit details of the rape. The nurse's awareness of her feelings and reactions enables her to contain them in counseling sessions with the victim.

Burgess and Holmstrom (1974) provide four models that guide the nurse in planning and implementing nursing care for the rape victim:

1. The medical model, which includes care and follow-up of the physical sequellae of the trauma.
2. The social-network model, which is characterized by assisting significant others in supporting the rape victim during and after the crisis period.
3. The behavioral model, which involves treating those behaviors that are the outcome of rape, specif-

TABLE 18–12 Goals of crisis intervention for families of rape victims

- Helping the family to openly express their immediate feelings in response to a rape—as a shared life crisis
- Helping the family to be supportive of and reassuring to the victim
- Helping the family work through immediate practical matters and initiate problem-solving techniques
- Helping the family develop cognitive understanding of what the rape experience actually means to the victim and to the family
- Explaining the possibility of future psychologic and somatic symptoms that characterize a rape trauma syndrome and what the family can do to minimize these symptoms
- Activating qualities characteristic of healthy family functioning during the impact and resolution phases of the shared crisis
- Educating the family about rape as a *violent crime,* not a sexually motivated act, and eliminating focus on the victim's guilt or responsibility
- Eliminating the family's sense of guilt for not protecting the victim by assuring them that they could not have anticipated or prevented the rape
- Discouraging violent, destructive, or irrational retribution toward the rapist (under the guise of being on the victim's behalf) by encouraging a sharing of feelings of helplessness, sadness, hurt, and anger
- Encouraging discussion of the sexual relationship between partners; suggesting that the man let the victim know (a) that his feelings have not changed (when this is true) and that he still sexually desires her, (b) that he will wait for her to approach him, and (c) that sex therapy is available if they have difficulties that persist and want assistance in reestablishing normal sexual relations
- Explaining the possibility of venereal disease and pregnancy that may result from a rape, the preventive care necessary for the victim and spouse or boyfriend, and the follow-up care indicated

ically phobic reactions, stresses, and anxiety. The rape victim is also helped to resume activities of daily living through the use of desensitization techniques.

4. The psychological model, which incorporates crisis intervention and counseling principles. This model focuses on the experience of the assault. The goals of this model are to assist the rape victim in expressing her thoughts and feelings about the experience, understanding the experience, and coping with the effects of it.

Silverman and McCombie (1980) have identified four interventions that apply to work with family members of the rape victim in order to increase their support of her during the acute and reorganization phases of the rape trauma syndrome:

1. Encouraging the expression of thoughts and feelings regarding the rape, as in treatment of PTSD.

2. Assisting with the understanding of the violent nature of rape and what this means to the victim.

3. Teaching about the nature of the crisis including future psychological and somatic sequellae of rape.

4. Emphasizing the concept of **containment** of the victim's feelings within therapy. Containment results in a safe and noncritical environment for the rape victim to express her feelings. Containing behaviors include reassurance, empathy, willingness to address painful information, and at times being directive with the victim. Silverman and McCombie (1980) also suggest educating family members, spouses, and mates of the victim about the nature of the crisis of rape to enable them to be truly supportive of the victim. Providing counseling to individual family members may be necessary if their responses to the rape experience interfere with their ability to cope adaptively. (See Table 18–12, Goals of crisis intervention for families of rape victims.)

- Explaining that early crisis intervention often prevents long-term problems in resolving the crisis and that to seek counseling at this time does not imply mental illness (the nurse specifies that crisis intervention usually lasts for 3 to 6 hours during the first few weeks post-rape)

- Giving families, lovers, and friends a copy of "A Note to Those Closest to Rape Victims"

- Referring the family for direct counseling when members' shared responses to the crisis interfere with their ability to cope adaptively

- Providing factual data, resource lists for counseling, and follow-up care *in writing* (because highly stressed persons do not hear or recall information verbally communicated)

- Letting families know that some decisions, such as whether to prosecute the rapist or move to a safer residence, can be postponed while more immediate needs, such as medical care, are taken care of. (This action helps the family (1) set priorities and organize decisions about what has to be done now, and (2) gain emotional distance from the urgency and confusion felt during a crisis state to permit sound decision making later.)

- Identifying how the family has handled crises in the past and encouraging members to use adaptive coping mechanisms for this crisis

- Encouraging contact with persons identified as supportive to the family and offering to contact such persons

- Assigning a primary nurse to spend time talking with the family in the emergency department waiting room while the victim receives medical care

- Allowing time for thoughts and feelings in a decision-making process

- Using empathic listening to convey understanding of the family's feelings and concerns

- Asking if the nurse can check back with the family the next day to see how they are getting along and answer any questions they may have

Source: Foley, T., & Davies, M. (1983). *Rape: Nursing care of victims.* St. Louis: C. V. Mosby Company, p. 137. Reprinted with permission.

Case Study: Nonpsychiatric Setting

Alicia: A Victim of Rape Trauma

Name: Alicia Torres
Age: 16
Ethnicity: Hispanic
Marital Status: Single
Referring Agency: Self/Parents
Occupation: High School Student
Religion: Catholic
Geography: Homesville, Alabama

Present Problem

Alicia, a 16-year-old majorette in the high school band, was a popular student. She had a steady boyfriend who was an excellent football player. He was injured in the game on a Friday night. The boyfriend usually walked Alicia home after each football game, but did not on this particular night because of his injury.

As Alicia walked to the bus stop, she was approached by a young man who began making lewd remarks about her body and his desire to undress her. The young man, who had alcohol on his breath, grabbed

Alicia, dragged her into a nearby park, took her behind a building in the park, undressed her, made obscene comments as he disrobed himself, and began to rape her. Alicia struggled to get away . . . she wept, screamed, and fought back.

Seemingly, the harder she fought, the angrier her assailant became. He continued the rape and squeezed her breasts while continuing to yell obscene comments at her.

Alicia managed to get away after the rape. She ran home and, in a hysterical fashion, described what had happened to her. Her parents immediately took her to the emergency room of a community hospital.

Alicia had had no previous psychiatric hospitalizations.

Family History:

Alicia's mother was a certified public accountant, and her father was a high school guidance counselor. They stated that they had an excellent relationship with Alicia.

Alicia had an older brother who was away at college. They were reported to have a close relationship. In fact, Alicia's brother, a former band member, encouraged Alicia to become a majorette in the high school band. He was very proud of her (and so were her parents) when she succeeded in being selected for the majorette position.

Alicia had a history of normal growth and development. Her grades were consistently about average. She always maintained positive relationships with peers at school and in the neighborhood.

Her greatest support system consisted of her parents, brother, and a neighborhood family. She did have several female friends who were majorettes. Her boyfriend (a football player) of one year, was considered to be warm, respectful, and supportive, also.

Alicia denied any use of alcohol or street drugs. Her parents stated that they were not aware of Alicia ever using any type of drug.

Alicia had no known medical problems. She was very conscientious about her diet and physical exercise, and jogged about three times each week.

Present Mental Status:

General Appearance: Alicia's clothing was torn and covered with dirt and spots of blood. Her hair and face were covered with dirt and grass. She also had dirt on her legs and feet. Her left foot had a deep gash.

Sensorium: Alicia was sobbing and crying uncontrollably; she was able to state, "I am in the emergency room at Community Hospital."

Mood: Alicia was extremely anxious and agitated.

Speech: Alicia's speech was rapid with intermittent silence that lasted for 30–40 seconds.

Motor Behavior: Alicia remained agitated; her hands were trembling. Alicia clenched her chest and held on to her clothing; she was hypersensitive to touch.

Thought Processes: Alicia was somewhat disorganized; she said over and over as she cried quietly, "Please, don't touch me . . . please don't touch me—Help me . . . nurse . . . please help me . . ."

Thought Content: In trying to explain the incident, Alicia became confused but, with support, was able to describe the circumstances of her rape. She seemed unable to talk about much else.

Other Data: The patient was not taking prescription medications. She had no history of psychiatric illness.

Nursing Diagnoses

*Rape Trauma Syndrome
Impaired verbal communication
Fear
Dysfunctional grieving
Powerlessness
Ineffective individual coping
Pain
Anxiety

*Nursing diagnosis covered in care plan that follows.

Nursing Care Plan for Alicia

Nursing Diagnosis	Desired Outcomes	Interventions	Rationale
1. Rape trauma syndrome.	Alicia will return to and function at prerape level within a 6–8 week period.	Encourage Alicia to discuss her reactions to rape, including: anger, fear, anxiety, depression, guilt, rage, helplessness, and so forth.	Alicia needs to know that her reactions are normal; that staff support her and accept these feelings.
		Observe for outbursts of crying spells, extensive periods of silence, and behaviors that indicate she feels unclean, including frequent bathing, washing mouth, changing clothes, and so forth. Support Alicia by expressing concern for her when she manifests any of these behaviors. Record Alicia's behaviors in her medical records.	These responses are normal reactions to a rape and indicate Alicia's need for reassurance and support. If they persist, treatment of obsessive-compulsive disorder may be implemented. (See Chapter 8 on anxiety.)
		Provide Alicia with opportunity to ask questions and to respond to the nurses' questions about her rape.	Alicia may be experiencing a variety of emotions such as anxiety, guilt, anger— she will need time to assimilate and articulate her thoughts and feelings.
		Reassure Alicia that she is in a safe environment.	The nurse has responsibility of creating a safe environment for Alicia.

Nursing Diagnosis	Desired Outcomes	Interventions	Rationale
		Alicia should have someone with her at all times at first. All procedures should be explained to her beforehand.	Alicia also needs to be reassured that nursing staff will assist her in understanding procedures that she will undergo in the emergency room. Knowing what the evaluation (physical and psychological) will consist of will increase the predictability of Alicia's environment and, so, decrease her anxiety.
		Empathize with the difficulties and frustrations Alicia feels at this time.	Empathy will decrease Alicia's sense of isolation and vulnerability.
		Encourage Alicia to discuss her personal perceptions of the meaning of rape in her life.	Provides Alicia additional opportunity to ventilate her feelings; provides nurse and health-care team with additional information for assessment and interaction purposes.
		Explore Alicia's personal beliefs and value system as related to the rape.	Provides clarification/information about how the rape experience impacts upon her total functioning, perspective, and philosophy of life.
		Discuss with Alicia the expectation that she will return to her prerape level of functioning.	Lets Alicia know that you have confidence in her returning to her normal level of functioning: maintain academic performance and participation as a majorette.
		If Alicia does not wish visitors/friends, respect and support her decision.	It is important to respect the rape victim's right to privacy. She may need time to deal with feelings of shame, guilt, rage, and so forth.
		Assist Alicia in mobilizing effective coping mechanisms she has used previously in stressful situations.	Identification of effective coping mechanisms will increase Alicia's feelings of autonomy, self-esteem, and control.
		Assist and encourage Alicia to participate in	Alicia will be reassured by autonomous

Nursing Diagnosis	Desired Outcomes	Interventions	Rationale
		normal activities of daily living.	functioning in as many areas as possible.
		Provide Alicia with information: followup appointments, names and telephone numbers of crisis counseling centers and other mental-health services, pastoral counseling (if appropriate), legal representation, support groups.	Assists Alicia in mobilizing appropriate support services that will assist her in returning to the highest possible level of functioning.
		All observation of physical and psychological responses to rape trauma must be recorded in Alicia's health records. All required forms should be completed and signed.	These nurses' recordings could be subpoenaed for legal purposes.
		Discuss with Alicia the need for followup physical assessments and the possibility for treatment of sexually transmitted diseases.	Alicia needs information about the possibility of somatic responses such as muscular tension, vaginal discharge, burning sensation upon urination, and so forth.
			Prophylactic treatment of sexually transmitted disease (if needed) will aid in prevention and ensure prompt treatment for Alicia.
		Provide support and health teaching for Alicia's family: encourage them to ventilate their anger, disgust, and contempt surrounding the rape incident. Teach them how to respond to feelings and thoughts Alicia might express about men (mistrust), the rape experience, and other long-term responses such as nightmares and other symptoms of anxiety. (Also see Chapter 8 on Anxiety Disorders, especially, post traumatic stress disorder.)	Since her family is Alicia's major support system, they can provide guidance and support for Alicia during the acute phase and the long-term resolution phase. They need to know what to expect from Alicia and how to deal with her.

TREATMENT OF THE SEX OFFENDER

Recent research has focused on treatment of those who commit violent crimes against women, and treatment programs for those offenders are increasing (Annis, 1980–1982; Watts & Courtois, 1981; Scott, 1983–1984; and Shorts, 1985–1986). Treatment in maximum security prisons (Shorts, 1985–1986) and residential settings (Annis, 1980–1982) consists of psychological therapies (group, individual, sex education, etc.); vocational therapies (food service, small engine repair, office management education); occupational therapies (art, music, ceramics, carpentry); recreational therapies (individual and team sports, dances, ward parties); and other activities (school, library, civic organization participation [Jaycees]) (Annis, 1980–1982). Groth, Burgess and Holstrom (1977) have suggested that treatment for sex offenses (rape, incest, exhibitionism) should be based on the assumption that the perpetrator experiences serious intrapsychic and interpersonal conflict.

A team of researchers ranked rape episodes that were described by 133 offenders and 92 victims and found that all rapes against the victims were motivated by the need for power (when sexuality was used as the major vehicle for expressing power and anger). The team concluded that none of the rapes perpetrated by the men in their sample described sex as the central problem (Groth, Burgess, and Holmstrom, 1977).

Annis (1980–1982) observed that sex offenders in a Florida State Hospital usually manifested poor impulse control, experienced difficulty handling frustration and expressing emotions, and had inadequate assertive behaviors. He also observed that the offenders experienced continuous anxiety and depression, low self-esteem, and were highly sensitive to perceptions of rejection.

In the case that follows, the nurse is one of several mental health professionals who provide therapy for sex offenders in a variety of settings which include prisons, hospitals, and other residential and outpatient facilities. It is important that she understand basic approaches to treatment of men who rape women.

Case Study: Psychiatric Setting

James Cobin: Rapist

Name: James Cobin
Age: 18
Ethnic Background: Caucasian
Religion: Protestant
Referring Agency: Courts
Occupation: High School Student
Home: Homeville, Alabama

James Cobin stated that he raped a fellow schoolmate as she walked home from a football game. He further stated that he needed help.

James Cobin was found guilty of the rape of Alicia Torres, age 16, in the criminal court of Marion County. The presiding judge presented him the option of participating in an intensive treatment program for sex offenders or going to a state prison for four years (without parole) and consideration for parole after an intensive evaluation. James Cobin elected the intensive residential treatment program. The psychiatric nurse's first contact with James followed.

History

James did not have a history of psychiatric problems. He recalled, however, wishing that he had someone to talk to him and his mother after his father left home. He stated that "it has been a long time since I felt close to anyone."

Family History: James' father was a dentist who divorced James' mother and left the area four years ago. Within the last two years, James' father remarried and became the father of a new son. James' mother was forced to seek employment as a secretary in order to make ends meet after the divorce. She was very bitter about the divorce, and over the past few years, had begun to drink excessively evenings and on the weekends.

James was his mother's only child. He had one half brother from his father's second marriage. James had never seen his brother. Little history about James' extended family was available. He was fond of an aunt who lived in Georgia. His fondness developed for this aunt during the time his mother and father were fighting. The fights became severe and his aunt suggested that James spend a year with her and attend school in Georgia. He reported this period to be the best time of his life.

James started dating at age sixteen. He was popular at school, physically well built, an average student, and very polite and courteous to peers and teachers. He had a part-time job at a nearby theater where he worked approximately twenty hours per week. James stated that he was saving his money to buy a car. He hoped to "feel better about things when I get my own 'wheels.'"

James was 14 years old when his mother and father divorced. He remembered that the divorce was a traumatic experience for his mother and him. He and his mother felt betrayed by his father, and very alone.

Mrs. Corbin was an attractive woman who had a habit of disrobing and "skinny dipping" in their backyard pool, or sun bathing on the deck of the pool; she had little regard for James' feelings about this. When James suggested that she wear a bathing suit, she would respond, "You have no appreciation for a woman's body." On several occasions, while nude, she slipped into James' bed, lay beside him, and gently took his hands and placed them over her breasts and genitals. James become sexually excited and experienced a heightened sensation of pleasure along with anxiety. He enjoyed the experience, but felt intense shame and guilt.

James began to experience feelings of sexual excitement when he went to bed each night. He also began having dreams about nude women. In fact, he learned to mentally undress any woman and envision her body as he had in reality seen his mother's body. Later, he began to add to these images the feel of a woman's breast and genitals and all of the sexual excitement that accompanied his experience with his mother. Over the last year he began to have intense sexually sadistic fantasies.

James had always had difficulty developing and maintaining a relationship with any one girl. He felt frustrated and restless as a result. At the same time, he was afraid to become involved intimately with anyone.

Nursing Diagnoses:

*Ineffective individual coping
*Ineffective family coping
 Disturbance in self-concept
*Sexual dysfunction
*Potential for violence
 Grieving
 Fear
 Anxiety
*Social isolation

Nursing Care Plan for James

Nursing Diagnosis	Desired Outcomes	Interventions	Rationale
1. Ineffective individual coping.	James will learn to control his assaultive impulses.	Assist James in understanding the consequences of his behavior.	James needs to take responsibility for his behavior and its consequences.
		Talk with James about the areas of difficulty in his life; home (mother), friends, father, peers at school, and so forth. Assure James that you will support him as he begins to work through these conflicts.	One-on-one discussions can provide James structure for the exploration of his conflicts and the development of insight into his behavior in order to increase his motivation to control it. Reassurance can forestall feelings of hopelessness and fear of abandonment.
		Encourage James to attend group therapy that meets twice each day on the unit. (One group consists of offenders; the other also includes rape victims.)	James can experience a sense of belonging and caring from the group, some responsibility for the group process, the healing power of the group process through interpersonal understanding and group cohesions.
2. Ineffective family coping.	James will begin to understand the relationship between familial conflicts and his pathological behavior.	Assist James in exploring his feelings of anger and resentment toward his mother and father.	James needs to verbalize his negative and positive thoughts and feelings about his mother and father.
		Observe James for periods when he becomes angry and feels like committing a violent act; discuss these feelings with James and reassure him that while he *cannot* control his feelings, he *can* control his behavior.	James will need support, reassurance, and help with self-control as he works through his conflicts.
		Encourage James to write down thoughts and feelings when he gets angry and share them with the nurse.	Helping James to become aware of his anger is the first step toward developing effective coping strategies to manage it.
3. Sexual dysfunction/knowledge deficit.	James will learn about the physiology and psychology of sexuality.	Explore with James the sources of his information about sex and women.	Myths and cognitive distortions about sex and women need to be clarified and challenged.

Nursing Diagnosis	Desired Outcomes	Interventions	Rationale
		Provide James with information about male and female reproductive anatomy and physiology.	Knowledge about anatomy and physiology of male and female reproductive systems will assist James in understanding his sexual feelings and gaining control over them.
		Assess the sexual experiences that James had as a child.	Parental influence is likely to have had a profound impact upon James' attitude toward sex and women.
		Reassure James that there will be no recrimination as a result of honestly discussing his perceptions and feelings about sexuality, women, and so forth.	Feelings of humiliation and embarrassment about sexual issues are common among young adult sex offenders.
4. Social isolation.	James will identify reasons why he feels isolated and develop effective methods for alleviating feelings of isolation.	Discuss with James specific behaviors that lead to isolation.	Identification of specific incidences should assist James in developing strategies for improving the frequency and duration of meaningful interpersonal contacts.
		Encourage James to discuss his feelings of loneliness and isolation.	Expression of feelings can lead to insights into behavior and behavior change, such as increasing social contacts.
		Focus on James's responses to thoughts of intimacy with women: anger, rage, hostility, fear, and so forth.	These responses have helped to create social isolation; exploration and resolution of these feelings are necessary for better functioning in relationships with women.
		Offer James the opportunity to release energy in a socially acceptable manner through recreation—for example, team sports such as basketball.	Exercise can provide the opportunity to sublimate feelings of anger.
5. Potential for violence (inability to control behavior).	James will control his violent behavior.	Assist James in identifying situations and incidents that provoke his tendency to be angry and violent; then assist	James needs to understand the relationship between his feelings, thoughts, and his behavior.

Nursing Diagnosis	Desired Outcomes	Interventions	Rationale
		him in developing effective methods to deal with these feelings and associated behaviors.	
		Identify factors in family relationships and community contacts that may perpetuate thoughts of violence in James's life.	James's behaviors are to some extent learned and possibly reinforced by others in his environment.
		Evaluate James's use of alcohol and assess for abuse of other chemical substances.	Alcohol lowers impulse control, can disrupt functioning of defense mechanisms, can distort reality, and so forth.
		Discuss with James what personal beliefs, ideas, and opinions he holds about violence against others.	It can be helpful to James to depersonalize to some extent his rage and feelings about women and violence.
		Offer James the opportunity to role play a problematic interpersonal situation (ask James to provide the scenario).	Role playing can assist James in developing new ways of relating interpersonally with others, especially women.
		Encourage James to participate in occupational therapy, recreational therapy, physical therapy, and so forth.	These resources provide alternative methods of expressing frustrations, conflicts, and so forth.

SUMMARY

While crisis is an integral part of everyone's life, situational crises are events that are precipitated by unanticipated stress; these events can cause psychological crisis. The nurse can help patients cope with psychological crises related to physical trauma, attempted suicide, violence within the family, and rape. Crisis intervention is brief, active, collaborative therapy that uses the patient's own coping abilities and resources within the community.

Crisis periods are time limited, usually lasting from four to six weeks. During the time of crisis, an individual passes through distinct phases. In addition, there are six types of crisis: 1) dispositional crisis; 2) crisis involving life transitions; 3) crisis resulting from sudden traumatic stress; 4) maturational crisis; 5) crisis reflecting psychopathology; and 6) psychiatric emergencies.

Physical illness, disease, or an accident may precipitate crisis. The nurse utilizes principles of crisis intervention to help the patient identify and reduce anxiety, develop healthy coping mechanisms, instill reality-based expectations, and take responsibility in solving emotional problems.

For the suicidal patient, assessment of suicide risk is a critical part of the initial step of the nursing process. An assessment should include demographic data as well as clinical characteristics, such as precipitating factors, coping strategies, past suicide attempts, and past psychiatric history. A thorough assessment could save a patient's life. A patient may have attempted altruistic, egoistic, or anomic suicide, according to sociological theories. Or the attempted suicide may have been a result of intrapsychic conflict, according to psychoanalytic theory. Interventions in the case of attempted suicide include making a no-suicide contract with the patient, mobilizing the patient's personal and professional support system, thorough psychological assessment, and therapies for anxiety and depression.

If a nurse treats a woman whom she suspects has been abused, she needs to assess the situation with the woman alone, without her husband. Complaints of abused women include psychophysiological symptoms and physical injuries. The nurse also assesses the stressors in the woman's life. The primary goal of the nursing care plan is to provide a safe environment for the woman and her family. The nurse may note child abuse by an unexplainable injury, a delay in obtaining medical care for the child, and a discrepancy between the parents' and child's description of the circumstances of the injury.

Rape is a severe and complex type of assault; contrary to popular belief, it is usually not sexually motivated. Rather, it falls into one of three categories: power rape, anger rape, or sadistic rape. A victim often suffers from rape-trauma syndrome, which is comprised of two distinct phases: the acute phase and the reorganization phase. The nurse may use any or all of four models to plan and implement care, but it is important for her to be knowledgeable about the psychological, legal, and physical aspects of sexual assault in order to assess and care for a patient effectively.

KEY TERMS

stress

predicament

emergency

psychological crisis

maturational crisis

situational crisis

altruistic suicide

egoistic suicide

anomic suicide

lethality

countertransference

battered-child syndrome

rape-trauma syndrome

revictimization

containment

STUDY QUESTIONS

1. Define *maturational crisis* and *situational crisis*.

2. Name and describe the four phases of crisis.

3. Name and describe some of the interventions that a nurse can make to help a patient cope with the acute stage of an illness or accident.

4. Describe some of the strategies a nurse could use to help an AIDS patient maintain some hope in his or her life.

5. Name and discuss the conflicts the nurse may face in caring for the patient who has attempted suicide.

6. Name and describe the four models a nurse can use to help her plan and implement care for the rape victim.

REFERENCES

Ackerly, W. C. (1967). Latency age children who threaten or attempt to kill themselves. *Journal of the Academy of Child Psychiatry, 6,* 242–261.

Aguilera, D. C. & Messick, J. M. (1982). *Crisis intervention: Theory and methodology,* 4th ed. St. Louis: The C. V. Mosby Co.

Amir, M. (1971). *Patterns of forcible rape.* Chicago: University of Chicago Press.

Annis, L. (1980–1982). A residential treatment program for male sex offenders. *International journal of offender therapy, 24–26,* 223–234.

Basch, M. F. (1988). *Understanding psychotherapy.* New York: Basic Books, pp. 65–99.

Bassuk, E. L. (1980). A crisis theory: Perspective on rape. In S. L. McCombie (Ed.), *The rape crisis intervention handbook.* New York: Plenum Press.

Beck, A. T., Kovacs, M., & Weissman, A. (1975). Hopelessness and suicidal behavior: An overview. *Journal of the American Medical Association, 234,* 1146–1149.

Beck, A. T., Rush, J., & Kovacs, M. (1977). *Individual treatment manual for cognitive behavioral psychotherapy of depression.* Philadelphia: Department of Psychiatry, University of Pennsylvania.

Benenati, M. (1988). *Antecedents of adolescents' suicidal behaviors: Differences between levels of suicidal behaviors exhibited by a psychiatric in-patient population and adolescent.* Unpublished Masters Thesis. University of Florida.

Blumber, M. (1974). Psychopathology of the abusing parent. *American journal of psychotherapy, 28,* 21–29.

Bostock, T., & Williams, C. L. (1974). Attempted suicide as an operant behavior. *Archives of general psychiatry, 31,* 482–486.

Bowen, M. (1976). Theory and practice of psychotherapy. In P. Guerin (Ed.), *Family therapy: Theory and practice.* New York: Garden Press.

Boyle, J. S. & Andrews, M. M. (1989). *Transcultural concepts in nursing care.* Glenview, Illinois: Scott, Foresman and Co.

Brenton, M. (1978). *The Runaways: Children, husbands, wives and parents*. Boston: Little, Brown.

Brown, A. (1987). *When battered women kill*. New York: The Free Press.

Bunney, W. E., Jr., & Fawcett, J. A. (1965). Possibility of a biochemical test for suicidal potential. *Archives of general psychiatry, 13*, 232–239.

Burgess, A. W., & Baldwin, B. A. (1981). *Crisis intervention: Theory and practice*. Englewood Cliffs: Prentice Hall, Inc.

Burgess, A. W., & Holmstrom, L. L. (1974). *Rape: Victims of crisis*. Bowie, MD: Robert J. Brady Co.

Burgess, A. W., & Lazare, A. (1976). *Community mental health: Target populations*. Englewood Cliffs: Prentice-Hall Co.

Campbell, J. (1984). Nursing care of abused women. In J. Campbell and J. Humphreys (Eds.), *Nursing care of victims of family violence*. Reston, VA: Reston Publishing Co.

Caplan, G. (1964). *Principles of preventive psychiatry*. New York: Basic Books, Inc.

Caplan, G., & Grunebaum, H. (1967). Perspectives on primary prevention: A review. *Archives of general psychiatry, 17*, 331–346.

Capone, M. A., Westie, K. S., Chitwood, J. S., Feigenbaum, D., & Good, R. S. (1979). Crisis intervention: A functional model for hospitalized cancer patients. *American journal of orthopsychiatry, 49*(4), 598–607.

Carpenter, W. T., & Bunney, W. E. (1971). Adrenal cortical activity in depressive illness. *American journal of psychiatry, 128*, 31–40.

Cleveland, P., Walters, L. H., Skeen, P., & Robinson, B. (1988). If your child has AIDS . . .: Responses of parents with homosexual children. *Family Relations* (April), *37* (2), 150–153.

Committee on Health Care for Homeless People, Institute of Medicine (1988). Health problems of homeless people. *Homelessness, Health, and Human Needs*. Washington, D.C.: National Academy Press.

Curran, D. K. (1987). *Adolescent suicidal behavior*. New York: Hemisphere Publishing Corporation.

DeMaio, D. (1983). Technological society: its impact upon youth. *Topics in clinical nursing, 4*, 37–58.

DeMaio-Esteves, M., & Shuzman, E. (1983). Adolescent suicide in a technology society. *Topics in clinical nursing, 4*, 59–65.

Dorpat, T. L. (1972). Psychological effects of parental suicide on surviving children. In A. D. Cain (Ed.), *Survivors of suicide*. Springfield: Bannerstone House.

Dorpat, T., Jackson, J., & Ripley, H. (1965). Broken home and attempted and completed suicides. *Archives of general psychiatry, 121*, 213–216.

Drake, V. K. (1982). Battered women: A health care problem in disguise. *Image, 14*(2), 40–47.

Durkheim, E. (1951). *Suicide*. Translated by J. A. Spaulding and G. Simpson. New York: The Free Press.

Engle, G. L. (1964). Grief and grieving. *American journal of nursing, 64*, 93.

Everstine, D. S., & Everstine, L. (1983). *People in crisis: Strategic therapeutic interventions*. New York: Brunner/Mazel Publishers.

Faller, K. C. (1988). *Child sexual abuse: An interdisciplinary manual for diagnosis, case management and treatment*. New York: Columbia University Press.

Farber, E. D., Kinast, C., McCoard, W. D., & Falkner, D. (1984). Violence in families of adolescent runaways. *Child abuse and neglect, 8*, 295-299.

Farberow, N. L. (Ed.) (1980). *The many faces of suicide: Indirect self-destructive behavior*. New York: McGraw-Hill.

Fawcett, J. A., & Bunney, W. E. (1967). Pituitary adrenal function and depression. *Archives of general psychiatry, 16*, 517–535.

Feinsilver, D. L. (1983). The suicidal patient: Clinical and legal issues. *Hospital practice, 18*, 48E-48L.

Finkelhor, D. (1984). *Child sexual abuse: New theory and research*. New York: The Free Press.

Finkelhor, D. (1979). *Sexually victimized children*. New York: The Free Press.

Finkelhor, D., with Araji, S. (1986). *Sourcebook on child sexual abuse*. Beverly Hills, CA: Sage Publishers.

Foley, T. S., & Davies, M. R. (1983). *Rape: Nursing care of victims*. St. Louis: Mosby.

Fontana, V. J. (1984). When systems fail: Protecting the victim of child sexual abuse. *Children today, 13*, 14–20.

Frederick, C. J., & Resnik, H. L. P. (1971). How suicidal behaviors are learned. *American journal of psychotherapy, 25*, 37–55.

Freud, S. (1957). *Mourning and melancholia*, Standard Edition, XIV. London: Hogarth Press.

Garbarino, J. (1977). The human ecology of child maltreatment: A conceptual model for research. *Journal of marriage and the family, 39*(4), 721–735.

Gayford, J. J. (1975). Battered wives. *Medicine, science and the law, 15*, 237–245.

Gelles, R. J. (1976). Abused wives: Why do they stay? *Journal of marriage and the family, 38*, 659–668.

Gelles, R. J. (1987). *Family violence*, 2nd edition. Newbury Park: Sage Publications.

Germain, C. P. (1984). Sheltering abused women: A nursing perspective. *Journal of psychosocial nursing, 22*(9), 24–31.

Gibbons, J. L. (1964). Cortisol secretion rate in depressive illness. *Archives of general psychiatry, 10*, 572–575.

Gibbons, J. L. (1960). Total body sodium and potassium in depressive illness. *Clinical science, 19*, 133–138.

Gilead, M. P., & Mulaik, J. S. (1983). Adolescent suicide: A response to developmental crisis. *Perspectives in psychiatric care, 21*(3), 94–101.

Glick, P. C. (1975). A demographic look at American families. *Journal of marriage and the family, 37*, 15–27.

Golan, N. (1978). *Treatment in crisis situations*. New York: The Free Press.

Groth, A. N., & Birnbaum, H. J. (1980). The rapist: Motivations for sexual violence. In S. L. McCombie (Ed.), *The rape crisis intervention handbook*. New York: Plenum Press.

Groth, A. N., Burgess, A. W., & Holstrom, X. (1977). Rape: Power, anger, and sexuality. *American journal of psychiatry, 134*(11), 1239–1243.

Hanneke, C. R., & Shields, N. A. (1985). Marital rape: Implications for the helping professions. *Social casework: The journal of contemporary social work, 66*(8), 451–458.

Hatton, C. L., Valente, S. M., & Rink, A. (1977). *Suicide: Assessment and intervention*. New York: Appleton-Century-Crofts.

Hellig, R. (1983). *Adolescent suicidal behaviors: A family system model*. Ann Arbor, Michigan: UMI Research Press.

Hendin, H. (1982). *Suicide in America*. New York: W. W. Norton.

Henslin, J. (1972). Strategies of adjustment. In A. Calin (Ed.), *Survivors of suicide*. Springfield: Bannerstone House.

Hilberman, E. (1980). Overview: The wife-beater's wife reconsidered. *American journal of psychiatry, 137*(11), 1336–1347.

Hoff, L. A. (1978). *People in crisis: Understanding and helping*. Menlo Park, CA: Addison-Wesley Publishing Company.

Hollinger, P. C., Offer, D., & Ostrov, E. (1987). Suicide and homicide in the United States: An epidemiologic study of violent death, population changes, and the potential for prediction. *American journal of psychiatry, 144*(2), 215–219.

Horowitz, B., & Wintermute, A. (1978). Use of emergency funds in protective services. *Child welfare, 57*(7), 432–437.

Institute of Medicine (1988). *Homelessness: Health and human needs*. Washington D.C.: National Academy Press.

Jacobson, G. F. (1974). Programs and techniques of crisis interventions. In S. Arieti (Ed.), *American handbook of psychiatry,* 2nd edition. New York: Basic Books.

Janus, M. D., McCormack, A., Burgess, A. W., & Hartman, C. (1987). *Adolescent runaways: Causes and consequences*. Lexington, Massachusetts: Lexington Books.

Justice, B., & Justice, R. (1976). *The abusing family*. New York: Human Sciences Press.

Katz, S., & Mazur, M. A. (1979). *Understanding the rape victim: A synthesis of research findings*. New York: John Wiley and Sons.

Kauffman, C. K., & Neill, M. K. (1975). The abusive parent. In S. A. Johnson (Ed.), *High risk parenting*. Philadelphia: J. B. Lippincott Co. pp. 227–242.

Kazdin, H. E., French, N. J., Unis, A. S., Esveldt-Dawson, D., & Sherick, R. B. (1983). Hopelessness, depression and suicidal intent among psychiatrically disturbed inpatient children. *Journal of consulting and clinical psychology, 51*(4), 504–510.

Keidel, G. C. (1983). Adolescent suicide. *Nursing clinics of North America, 13*(2), 323–332.

Kempe, C. H., & Helfer, R. E. (1972a). Innovative therapeutic approaches. In C. H. Kempe and R. E. Helfer (Eds.), *Helping the battered child and his family*. Philadelphia: J. B. Lippincott Co.

Kempe, C. H., & Helfer, R. E. (Eds.), (1972b). *Helping the battered child and his family*. Philadelphia: J. B. Lippincott Co.

Kempe, C. H., Silverman, F. N., Steele, B. F., Droegemuller, W., & Silver, H. K. (1962). The battered child syndrome. *Journal of the American Medical Association (JAMA). 181,* 17–24.

Kilpatrick, D. G. (1983). Rape victims: Detection, assessment & treatment. *Clinical psychologist, Summer,* 92–95.

Kluz, R. (1986). Children with AIDS. *American Journal of Nursing, 86,* 1126–1132.

Krouse, H. J., & Krouse, J. H. (1982). Cancer as crisis: The critical elements of adjustment. *Nursing research, 31,* 96–101.

Krumm, S. (1982). Psychosocial adaptation of the adult with cancer. *Nursing clinics of North America, 17,* 729–737.

Kubler-Ross, E. (1983). *On children and death*. New York: Macmillan Co.

Laker, B. (1987). AIDS: The youngest victims. *Dallas Times Herald,* June 18, 1987, pp. F1–F3.

Leavitt, P. (1989). USA Today. March 31, 1989.

Lewinsohn, P. M. (1975). The behavioral study and treatment of depression. In M. Hersen, R. M. Eisler, and P. M. Miller (Eds.), *Progress in behavior modification*. New York: Academic Press, Inc.

Lindemann, E. (1965). Symptomatology and management of acute grief. In H. J. Pared (Ed.), *Crisis intervention: Selected readings*. New York: Family Service Association of America.

Litman, R. E. (1967). Sigmund Freud and suicide. In E. S. Shneidman (Ed.), *Essays in self-destruction*. New York: Science, pp. 324–344.

Locke, A. M. (1989). The Psychosocial Impact of HIV Infection: Minimizing the Losses. In J. B. Meisenholder and C. L. LaCharite (Eds.) *Comfort in caring: nursing the person with HIV infection*. Glenview, Illinois: Scott, Foresman and Company, pp. 213–221.

Loosen, P. T., & Prange, A. J. (1982). Serum thyrotropin response to thyrotropin-releasing hormone in psychiatric patients. *American Journal of psychiatry, 139,* 405–416.

Macklin, E. (1988). AIDS: Implications for families. *Family Relations,* (April), 37 (2), 141–149.

Maier, S., & Seligman, M. (1976). Learned helplessness: Theory and Evidence. *Journal of experimental psychology, 105,* 3–46.

McClean, L. J. (1982). Guilt and fear of self-destruction. In J. Haber, A. M. Leach, S. M. Schudy, and B. F. Sideleau (Eds.), *Comprehensive psychiatric nursing,* 2nd ed. New York: McGraw-Hill.

McCombie, S. L., & Arons, J. H. (1980). Counseling rape victims. In S. L. McCombie (Ed.), *The rape crisis intervention handbook*. New York: Plenum Press.

McIntire, M. S., & Angle, C. R. (1973). Psychological biopsy in self poisoning of children and adolescents. *American journal of disease in children, 126,* 42–46.

Menninger, K. A. (1938). *Man against himself*. New York: Harcourt, Brace.

Morin, S., & Batchelor, W. (1984). Responding to the psychological crisis of AIDS. *Public Health Reports, 99,* 4–9.

National Center for Health Statistics. (1988). *Vital statistics of the United States, 1986.* Vol. II, Mortality, Party B. DHHS Pub. No. (PHS) 88–1114. Public Health Service. Washington, D.C.: U.S. Government Printing Office.

The National Network of Runaway and Youth Services, Inc. (1985). A profile of America's runaway and homeless youth and programs that help them. Oversight hearing on runaway and homeless youth. 94th Congress, 1st Session. July 25, 1983.

National Safety Council. (1987). *Accident facts, 1987* edition. Chicago: National Safety Council.

Newberger, E. H., & Bourne, R. (1978). The medicalization and legalization of child abuse. *American journal of orthopsychiatry, 38*(4), 594–607.

Orbach, I., Carlson, G., Feshbach, S., Glaubman, H., & Gross, Y. (1983). Attraction and repulsion by life and death in suicidal and in normal children. *Journal of consulting and clinical psychology, 51*(5), 551–670.

Orbach, I., Gross, Y., & Glaubman, H. (1981). Some common characteristics of latency age children: A tentative model based on case study analyses. *Suicide and life-threatening behavior, 4,* 180–190.

Pasquali, E. A., Arnold, H. M., DeBasio, N., & Alesi, E. G. (Eds.). (1985). *Mental health nursing: A holistic approach,* 2nd edition. St. Louis: C. V. Mosby Co.

Pfeffer, C. R. (1984). Clinical aspects of childhood suicidal behavior. *Pediatric annals, 13,* 56–61.

Pfeffer, C. R. (1985). Self-destructive behavior in children and adolescents. *Psychiatric clinics of North America, 8*(2). 215–226.

Pfeffer, C. R., Conte, H. R., & Plutchik, R. (1980). Suicidal behavior in latency age children: An outpatient population. *Journal of the American academy of child psychiatry, 19,* 703–710.

Poznanski, E., & Zrull, J. P. (1970). Childhood depression: Clinical characteristics of overtly depressed children. *Archives of general psychiatry, 23,* 8–15.

Prange, A. J., Lara, P. P., Wilson, I. C., Alltop, L. B., & Breese, G. R. (1972). Effects of thyrotropin-releasing hormone in depression. *Lancet, 2,* 999–1002.

Rapoport, L. (1970). Crisis intervention as a mode of brief treatment. In R. W. Roberts and R. H. Nees (Eds.), *Theories of social casework.* Chicago: University of Chicago Press.

Ryan, J. (1984). The neglected crisis. *American journal of nursing, 84*(10), 1257–1258.

Sabbath, J. C. (1969). The suicidal adolescent—the expendable child. *Journal of the American academy of child psychiatry,* 272–289.

Sachar, E. J. (1982). Endocrine abnormalities in depression. In E. S. Paykel (Ed.), *Handbook of affective disorders.* New York: Guilford. pp. 191–201.

Schmitt, B. D. (1978). *The physician's evaluation in the child protection team handbook.* New York: Garland STPM Press. pp. 39–57.

Schut, F. (1964). Suicidal adolescents and children. *Journal of the American medical association, 18,* 1103–1107.

Scott, E. (1983–1984). Treatment of the rapist: A case illustration. *International journal of offender therapy and comparative criminology, 27–28,* 11–21.

Seiden, R. H. (1972). Studies of adolescent suicidal behavior. In B. Q. Hafen and E. J. Faux (Eds.), *Self destructive behavior: A national crisis.* Minneapolis: Burgess. pp. 153–191.

Sheehy, G. (1976). *Predictable crises of adult life.* New York: E. P. Dutton and Co., Inc.

Shields, N. A., & Hanneke, C. R. (1983). Battered wives' reaction to marital rape. In D. Finkelhor, R. J. Gelles, G. T. Hotaling, and M. A. Straus (Eds.), *The dark side of families: Current family violence research.* Beverly Hills, CA: Sage Publications, pp. 132–148.

Shneidman, E. S. (1976). Suicide among the gifted. In E. S. Shneidman (Ed.), *Suicidology: Contemporary developments.* New York: Grune and Stratton.

Shorts, I. (1985–1986). Treatment of a sex offender in a maximum security forensic hospital: Detecting changes in personality and interpersonal construing. *International journal of offender therapy and comparative criminology, 29–30,* 237–249.

Sideleau, B. F. (1982). Abusive families. In J. Haber, A. Leach, S. M. Schudy, and B. F. Sideleau (Eds.), *Comprehensive psychiatric nursing,* 2nd edition. New York: McGraw-Hill Book Co.

Silverman, D. C., & McCombie, S. L. (1980). Counseling the mates and families of rape victims. In S. L. McCombie (Ed.), *The rape crisis intervention handbook.* New York: Plenum Press.

Speck, R. V. (1968). Family therapy of the suicidal patient. In H. Resnick (Ed.), *Suicidal behaviors: Diagnosis and management.* Boston: Little, Brown, and Co. pp. 341–347.

Spiegel, D., Bloom, J. R., & Yalom, I. (1981). Group support for patients with metastic cancer. *Archives of general psychiatry, 38,* 527–533.

Starr, R. H., Jr. (1988). Physical abuse of children. In V. B. van Hasselt, R. L. Morrison, A. S. Bellack, and M. Hersen (Eds.), *Handbook of family violence.* New York: Plenum Press, pp. 119–156.

Straus, M. A. (1974). Violence in the family. *Nursing digest, 2.*

Straus, M. A., Gelles, R. J., & Steinmetz, S. (1980). *Behind closed doors: Violence in American family.* New York: Doubleday, Anchor Press.

Sutherland, S., & Scherl, D. J. (1970). Patterns of response among victims of rape. *American journal of orthopsychiatry, 40,* 503–511.

Toolan, J. M. (1975). Suicide in children and adolescents. *American journal of psychotherapy, 29,* 339–344.

Urwin, C. (1988). AIDS in children: A family concern. *Family Relations, Journal of Applied Family and Child Studies, 37* (2), 155.

U.S. Congress. (1974). *Child abuse prevention and treatment act.* Public Law 93–247, 93rd Congress, Senate 1191.

U.S. Department of Health, Education, and Welfare. Update. (1987). Data from Secretary's Task Force Report on Youth Suicide. Washington, D.C.: U.S. Government Printing Office.

U.S. Department of Justice. (1986). *Criminal victimization, 1985.* Washington, D.C.: Bureau of Justice Statistics Bulletin, October, 1986.

U.S. Department of Justice. (1988). *Report to the nation on crime and justice,* 2nd edition. Washington, D.C.: Bureau of Justice Statistics.

Waites, E. A. (1977–78). Female masochism and the enforced restriction of choice. *Victimology: An international journal,* 2(3/4), 535–544.

Walker, L. (1979). *The battered women.* New York: Harper and Row.

Watts, D. L., & Courtois, C. A. (1981). Trends in the treatment of men who commit violence against women. *Personnel and guidance journal, 60,* 246–248.

Weitz, R. (1982). Feminist consciousness raising self concept and depression. *Sex roles, 8,* 231–237.

Welty, M., Rosillo, R., & Graham, W. (1973). The patient with maxillofacial cancer-II: Psychologic aspects. *Nursing clinics of North America, 8,* 153–158.

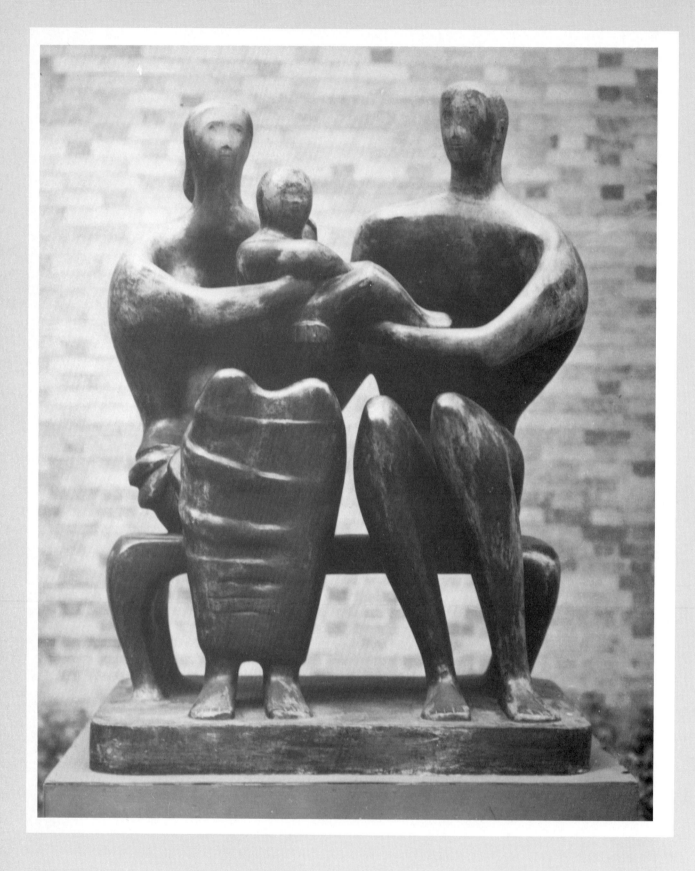

Part Three

PSYCHIATRIC MENTAL HEALTH NURSING THROUGHOUT THE LIFE SPAN

19

PSYCHIATRIC MENTAL HEALTH NURSING WITH WOMEN

HANNAH LEE

LEARNING OBJECTIVES

After studying this chapter, the student will be able to:

- Describe the concept of victim behaviors.
- Identify the different types of victim behaviors and how they express or reflect women's place in U.S. society.
- Describe the ways in which women may change their position in U.S. society.
- Recognize victim behaviors in patients, and develop nursing interventions to help patients change these behaviors.
- Discuss other important areas of possible research related to mental health needs of women as a group.

INTRODUCTION

The Women's Movement and other economic and social changes in our society over the last thirty years (especially the increase of women in the workplace) have made a great impact on lifestyle and roles for women today. However, many people believe that in spite of these changes, Western culture is still basically structured as a **patriarchal hierarchy.** This label denotes 1) concentration of power at the top of a vertical social structure (hierarchy) and 2) concentration of power in the hands of males (patriarchy). The hierarchical structure ensures that those in whom power is concentrated will be able to keep other groups relatively powerless. The patriarchal characteristic ensures that one of the relatively powerless groups will be women. "The problems inherent in developing a female sense of identity in a situation of male domination . . . are the problems of all women in a social context of female inequality" (Greenspan, 1983, p. 35).

While the specific mental health care needs of women are discussed throughout this book, this chapter will focus on one topic: mental health ramifications for women living within a patriarchal hierarchy. The chapter addresses how women, as cultural subordinates, behave in order to compensate for their relative powerlessness and to meet the needs that are not acknowledged by the culture or by themselves. (Needs are not met by women themselves insofar as they have internalized the attributes of inferiority assigned to them by the culture.) There exist many other important mental health issues specific to women that need to be addressed in our society, and readers are encouraged to pursue these issues as well. Some of these include issues related to family, parenting, and the effects of multiple roles on women's mental health. This last issue is addressed briefly at the end of the chapter.

VICTIM BEHAVIORS

Behaviors used by **cultural subordinates** or social outgroups in situations in which survival (physical or emotional) is or is perceived to be threatened may be called **survival mechanisms** (Allport, 1958; Pierce, 1978). They may also be called **victim behaviors** since they are utilized by persons who have been victims—of crime, economic and social oppression, discrimination, and violence (Steinem, 1983). "Victim behaviors" is probably the best label, since euphemizing may delay change.

Victim behavior seeks compensation for the power that the victim has been denied. Such behavior seeks to meet basic needs such as the need for self-worth, the need to be heard and acknowledged, the need for privacy, and the need to feel competent and effective. These are needs that cultural subordinates themselves often ignore. Women may forget that they have these needs, or they may resign themselves to perpetual unfulfillment. They may then unconsciously seek ways of satisfying them. For example, a woman who is unconscious of her need to be heard and/or assumes that the need will not be met, may end sentences with requests for confirmation ("right?", "see?"), raise her voice slightly, and lean forward demanding immediate response. Or she may talk far more than necessary to get her idea across, thus not only attempting to satisfy her unmet need to be heard but unconsciously venting some anger by not allowing others to express themselves. Men may reinforce the overtalking by keeping their facial expressions impassive, as men in this culture are trained to do, or by other lack of response. Other women may reinforce it by indulging the overtalker out of kindness or empathy (Pierce, 1978).

It might be argued that labeling some behaviors as "victim behaviors" blames the victim. Blaming the victim holds the recipient of abuse or disadvantage—rather than the perpetrator—responsible for the

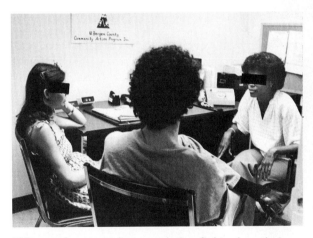

This couple stopped an escalating fight when their two-year-old awakened from his nap and started to cry: "Mommy, daddy—no fight!" They called their county's crisis intervention unit and were given an appointment later that afternoon. Here they are shown talking to a crisis counselor for the first time. Once this crisis is defused, she is likely to refer them to the community's "Alternatives to Domestic Violence" family-oriented treatment program.

abuse. However, labeling certain behaviors as "victim behaviors" is *not* the same as blaming the victim; it in no sense implies that change must be unilateral, nor that victims deserve whatever fruits of cultural subordination fall to them. Women are already told in myriad ways by the culture that something is wrong with them; labeling certain behaviors as "victim" behaviors can help women look at these behaviors in their cultural context, so that they can begin to discern their responsibility realistically and direct their efforts toward change in an effective way.

Victim behaviors are not totally negative; in fact, Allport (1958) noted that some victim behaviors, such as enhanced striving, have results that are extremely beneficial. The pressure to survive and succeed under adverse conditions often makes victims very resourceful people (Pierce, 1978). Moreover, victim behavior is basically realistic; for example, a woman may agree to the demands of her drunken and abusive husband in order to mollify him until she can get the children safely out of the house. Nevertheless, women do have to change; they need to identify introjected feelings of inferiority and inadequacy

that are by-products of their position of subordination, so that they can value themselves more highly and participate more equally in their own destinies. Women need to change, not because something is wrong with them, but because much that is right with them is not available to themselves or others in their search for solutions to problems that plague them and the modern world, for example, interpersonal, societal, and international violence. The personal and cultural cost of the waste of women's resources is too high. Victim behaviors reflect and reinforce feelings of powerlessness and helplessness, and they help to maintain the position of women as the primary consumers of psychiatric treatment for depression, as the most frequent heads of households operating at or under poverty level, and as the most frequent victims of crimes against person.

This is not to say that men do not have to change. But to wait for members of the dominant class, no matter how sensitive and sympathetic, to initiate change on their own, especially change that may threaten their power, is unrealistic. Men have the responsibility to examine the behaviors that com-

Box 19–1 ● The Nurse as Victim?

Nurses have one of the highest rates of participation in the labor force among workers in predominantly female occupations. Almost 80% of registered nurses are actively employed (full-time or part-time) as compared with 54% of all American women. Hospitals are employing more registered nurses than ever. In 1972, hospitals employed 50 nurses per 100 patients; by 1986, the figure had increased to 91 nurses per 100. Nurses today account for 58 percent of hospitals' total nursing service personnel, compared with only 33 percent in 1968. Yet we continue to read and hear about the "nursing shortage." The reason for it is not a declining supply of nurses (though this is a problem that will need to be faced in 1995 when the number of new nurse graduates will have fallen from 83,000 to 69,000 or less), but a changing demand for them. This is a result of hospitalized patients being sicker and needing more during shorter hospital stays, increased hospital budgets (and, so, more budgeted nursing positions), and low

wages. Regarding the wage factor, labor economists have described nursing as a "captured" labor market since there is no demand for nurses outside the health care field that is sufficient to create competitive pressures on the hospital industry. Since most nurses work in hospitals, they must accept the terms offered by the hospitals who do not *need* to compete with one another by offering nurses higher salaries.

The result, especially in the small community, is that hospitals have a real bargain in the nurse. Her salary is less today than a teacher's or any other female professional and technical worker's despite her ever-increasing workload, patient-care responsibilities, and need for advanced technical skills and continuing education. In addition she doesn't need much supervision, and she functions as secretary, lab tech, pharmacist, physical therapist, and social worker as well as nurse.

It is no wonder that there is a tremendous drop in nursing school enrollment, and that several excellent

plement women's victim behaviors—that is, the ways they use their positions of dominance. Many men can recognize the behaviors described below as means they have used to cope with being dominated at work or in other situations in which they regularly find themselves invalidated (Pierce, 1978). (See Box 19–1.)

CATEGORIES OF VICTIM BEHAVIOR

Victim behaviors have been categorized according to whether the behavior is basically directed outward toward others (extropunitive) or inward toward the self (intropunitive) (Allport, 1958). This categorization describes a direction of energy flow and helps in discerning some of the consequences of a given victim behavior. Most victim behaviors have both extropunitive and intropunitive characteristics. Most significant about these terms, however, is the *punitive* suffix, which recognizes the rage that underlies all victim behavior, no matter where it is directed or how it is disguised. "Anger is energy—the deep energy of the life-force that arises in response to threat"

(Starhawk, 1982, p. 66). Competitiveness and excessive need to control others are examples of extropunitive victim behavior. Internalizing and personalizing are examples of intropunitive victim behavior; hence Greenspan's (1983) suggestion that depression is a victim behavior. Several common victim behaviors are described below in further detail; this list is not intended to be exhaustive, but it should give the reader an idea of how to identify victim behavior and its consequences. Note the ways in which the behaviors overlap and interlock to reinforce the victim role.

EXCESSIVE NEED TO CONTROL SELF AND OTHERS

The need to control, or feel in control, is innate and legitimate (Pierce, 1978). In a hierarchical structure, control becomes dominance, or power over others (Starhawk, 1982). "Those who are controlled by others learn to control . . . in return" (Pierce, 1978). A woman who feels dominated may seek to dominate others to compensate for the powerlessness she feels. If, in addition, she feels that her need for power is

---

schools of nursing are closing. It is understandable that there has been a 50% decline since 1974 in the proportion of full-time women students planning to pursue nursing careers, in contrast to an almost threefold increase in the proportion interested in careers in business. These things may also explain the recent finding that SAT scores of high-school students interested in nursing careers are well below the national average for college-bound students, with the SAT gap between prospective nurses and non-nurses widening over time.

Other contributors to the nursing shortage include 1. the increasing numbers of women pursuing more lucrative careers in business, engineering, law, medicine, and science, few of which require night or weekend work or rotating shifts; 2. the nursing profession's continuing struggle with definitional issues; 3. AMA opposition to nursing's pursuit of independent practice; 4. substantial cuts in federal funding of nursing education; 5. little involvement of nurses in hospital management deci-

sions regarding standards of practice and support services; and 6. lack of salary advancement (in one American Hospital Association study, it was found that the average difference between a nurse's starting salary and the maximum she can earn in the same position is about $8,000.00, regardless of length of service).

All of this has led to the current worrisome situation: the number of women intending to be physicians in a 1986 survey done by the American Council on Education surpassed the number intending to be nurses by a ratio of 10 to 8. This is in contrast to the one to three ratio of doctors to nurses in 1968. Kenneth Green, associate director of UCLA's Higher Education Research Institute, has said that "by 1990 or 1991 American colleges will award some 14,500 BSN degrees (compared to almost 16,000 MD degrees)."

What isn't stated directly but is implied in scholarly analyses of the "nursing shortage" is that surely some of nursing's plight has to do with nursing's embodiment of the

traditional mothering role for many, if not all, professionals and patients, and the fact that 97% of nurses are women. The ideal mother takes care of everything, works tirelessly in the service of others, and wants little to nothing in return for herself. The questions we are left with include: Is this *really* good for anyone? Are women who strive for this ideal self-destructive? Or are they being destroyed by a society that wants too much? Is the nurse an example of woman as victim?

Sources: Aiken, L. H. & Mullinx, C.F. (1987). The nurse shortage, myth or reality? *New England Journal of Medicine, 317,* 10. 641–645.
Inglehart, J. K. (1987). Health policy report, problems facing the nursing profession. *New England Journal of Medicine, 317,* 10. 646–651.

illegitimate (or "unladylike") she may manipulate others in order to meet her need without having to acknowledge it. For example, a woman who is constantly interrupted by husband or children, and feels she has no right to personal privacy or time alone, may keep tight control over the scheduling of activities that keep other family members occupied outside the home (Pierce, 1978). If she is self-aware enough so that her motivation—to gain some private time—is not completely repressed, she will be likely to feel inner conflict between guilt about her deviousness and helplessness about her inability to change it. In order to change the situation enough so that she can identify her need and ask for private time directly, she must grant herself the right to have a legitimate personal want, and convince herself that she is not depriving her family by doing so.

If a woman is in a position that legitimizes her need for control to some degree, she may seek to meet this need more directly. For example, a female supervisor in a work situation, such as a head nurse on a busy surgical unit, has her need to control legitimized by her position. She is responsible, in charge, and therefore not only entitled but obliged to ask people to carry out her wishes. To be an effective supervisor, she must identify herself as having power and ask directly for what she wants from others. This authority, however, is a characteristic of the position, not a personal attribute; if her supervisory role is the only area of her life in which this woman can feel such authority, she may use the supervisory role to meet some of the need for personal power lacking in other areas. As a result, she may supervise too closely, make inappropriate demands, or exercise her authority too rigidly (Pierce, 1978).

Female frigidity, or low sexual response, may be interpreted as a control issue. The standards for sexuality in Western culture are set by males. Female sexuality is either repressed ("Nice girls don't") or defined in a way that suits male sexual requirements ("If I don't have an orgasm, *he* feels inadequate, so I fake it"). Frigidity is an inevitable result of sexual repression, and can also represent a woman's conscious or unconscious refusal to make herself vulnerable to male sexual demands. "In the long battle between the sexes and the consequent power struggle called making love, this is the woman's way of not allowing the man to win" (Greenspan, 1983, p. 198).

LOW SPONTANEITY

Excessive control needs of victims interfere with spontaneity and with intimacy. Self-consciously preoccupied with trying to adjust herself to accommodate others while maintaining a sense of self, the victim expends a great deal of attention on her ego boundaries, often exaggerating them so that she can sense herself as effectively resisting invasion or attack. This sense of unsafety combined with such intense self-preoccupation greatly inhibits spontaneous expression. Gaining a degree of control results in the loss of ability to respond naturally. Spontaneity is a power issue. Dominant power discourages spontaneous behavior (Pierce, 1978). When natural expression is inhibited, the energy associated with it is lost to consciousness; thus the absence of energy, or fatigue, may be a clue that one's position is the subordinate one in a given situation. Spontaneity is associated with energy, excitement, and power; its lack is associated with boredom, lack of naturalness, limited options, reduced creativity, depression, and loss of ability to respond naturally (Greenspan, 1983).

Furthermore, spontaneity is often associated with sexuality in U.S. culture. "Our socialization patterns contrive to keep natural energy from flowing, out of fear that sexual energy will be tapped. This fear keeps all kinds of other energy under control in such a way that a broad range of ways to act is lost in both work and social relationships" (Pierce, 1978, p. 11).

DISCOUNTING FEEDBACK

Because dominants control the flow of information in the culture, they can withhold information from women and disregard women as resources. The woman who neither gives nor receives information is invalidated; her enthusiasm is dampened, lowering spontaneity, and her self-esteem is undermined. Resentment builds, making her ego boundaries even more brittle, and decreasing her openness to whatever trickle of information may come her way, particularly if the information includes feedback about herself or her performance that she may interpret as criticism (Pierce, 1978). Discounting feedback is a particularly unfortunate victim behavior because all people need feedback to grow professionally and personally. Because of women's general invisibility in jobs that are primarily support functions for men, feedback is rare and often given in a form that is not useful, such as praise or criticism based on factors which are irrelevant to job performance, like appearance or maternal role functioning (for example, taking care of the office coffee pot). Irrelevant feedback does not help the woman understand what her impact has been. Ironically, a woman who discounts useful feedback will often accept criticism that is not useful because it supports her negative self-concept (Pierce, 1978).

ENHANCED STRIVING

The victim behavior that Allport has called **enhanced striving** has been a successful and culturally approved mode of compensation for many social subordinates, or outgroups, as Allport termed them. People generally like to hear success stories about an underdog who has overcome a handicap through hard work (Allport, 1958, p. 152). Trying harder in the face of obstacles is seen as virtue. Insofar as the effort arises from and ultimately enhances a solid base of self-care it is a positive and healthy response to life's difficulties. However, the grim determination of enhanced striving exacerbates the self-rage of the victim and puts off those around her. And it fails to satisfy; whatever she may accomplish on the outside is of little use to her within herself. Carried to the extreme, such striving can result in the fierce perfectionism of anorexia and other eating disorders (Herzog & Copeland, 1985). A less extreme form can be seen in a woman's preoccupation with appearance; no matter how beautiful she may be, she never feels that she is beautiful enough. (See Box 19–2.)

The sequelae of enhanced striving merit close attention. In extreme forms, enhanced striving goes beyond ordinary goal-oriented effort and may express the victim's self-blame for her victim position. The woman sees herself as embodying the negative characteristics that the culture has attributed to women (see the section on internalizing and personalizing, page 746) and strives to correct them in herself, even though one of the cultural attributions may be that her fault is innate and, therefore, irreversible. Not only is she "faulty" and, therefore, doomed to strive; but the fault is, also, innate, so her striving is forever in vain—a depressing, even schizophrenogenic (psychosis-inducing) situation. (See Box 19–3 on p. 746.)

HYPEREMOTIONALITY

Two factors contribute to the generally elevated emotional level of women as compared to men. One is the cultural permission given to women to express a greater range of emotions than men are allowed to express. However, as has been pointed out, because the ability to express a wide emotional range is seen as a feminine trait, it has been devalued in the culture and used to ridicule women as being unstable and immature (Greenspan, 1983). Women attempt to compensate for supposed emotionalism, when trying to be taken seriously, by keeping their facial expressions impassive and narrowing their range of vocal pitch to a " 'reasonable' monotone" (Steinem, 1983, p. 188). The result is often not being heard at all. On the other hand, when men withhold emotions, they usually strengthen their identification with the dominant class.

The other factor contributing to hyperemotionality is the pain of persistent invalidation that keeps the emotions of subordinates continually on the verge of arousal (Pierce, 1978). Elevated emotional levels are a survival mechanism, the energy that arises to react to oppressive dominant energy (Starhawk, 1982). The most usual emotions hovering near the surface are the negative ones, such as hurt, anger, and fear (Pierce, 1978). A woman who tries to keep her elevated emotions from erupting, so that her vulnerability to ridicule or punishment is not increased, risks falling prey to depression.

Hyperemotionality exacerbates women's frequent inability to make and carry out long-term plans, especially plans on their own behalf. Living with their emotions on edge, women expend a great deal of time and energy simply dealing with their own responses and those of others in the present, leaving little leisure for gaining perspective or planning initiatives for the future. An insecure economic base may add even more limitations to a woman's ability to plan: "Planning ahead is a measure of class. The rich and even the middle class plan for future gener-

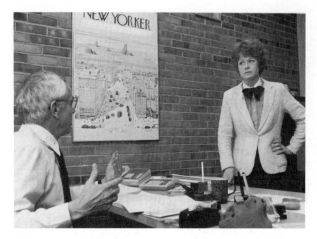

This seasoned career woman is about to try something new, saying "no" to her boss. She has just completed an assertiveness-training program and is thinking about entering psychotherapy in order to understand where her tendency to put the needs of others before her own comes from.

Box 19–2 ● The Resurgence of Anorexia, the Emotional Disease of Young Women Bent on Self-starvation

Can history help us come to grips with one of the most devastating emotional disorders of modern young women, the self-imposed starvation that is the hallmark of anorexia nervosa?

Yes, says Dr. Joan Jacobs Brumberg, author of "Fasting Girls: The Emergence of Anorexia Nervosa as a Modern Disease" (Harvard University Press). A historical perspective, she insists, can both help us to understand the origins of eating disorders and suggest guidelines for stemming the current epidemic, which Dr. Brumberg believes has not yet reached its peak.

Anorexia nervosa is not a new disease, said Dr. Brumberg, who is director of women's studies as well as associate professor of human development and family studies at Cornell University. The disease did not emerge with the fashion industry's focus on emaciated female bodies, although the modern imperative to be thin is feeding the epidemic of eating disorders. Although no precise statistics exist, an estimated 10 percent of American women have eating disorders, including anorexia, and on college campuses the number often exceeds 20 percent, she said.

Dr. Brumberg demonstrates that women have been fasting for various reasons at least since medieval times, when some young women starved themselves in a quest for religious perfection. It resurfaced in a more secular form in Victorian times. At that time, changes in family and social dynamics, especially the emergence of a bourgeois class that treated young girls and women as delicate creatures, put pressure on privileged women to deny their appetites for food, which they tended to equate with an appetite for sex.

Characteristics

Anorexia nervosa, meaning emotionally caused loss of appetite, was first identified by physicians in England, France and the United States in the 1870s, long before any modern preoccupation with dieting.

But not until after World War II did the incidence of anorexia begin to rise, under the combined influences of growing affluence, greater availability of food, increased expectations for achievement and rising social pressures on young women. And not until the 1970s did it take off, receiving the attention that led to both a greater likelihood of diagnosis and a significant increase in the number of girls who learned about anorexia and "chose" it to express their emotional and social turmoil.

Any theory about the underlying causes of anorexia must take into account characteristics of the disease that have prevailed since at least the mid-19th century. Dr. Brumberg said that anorexia is prevalent only in affluent societies when the economy is thriving. The incidence was very low in the Depression and World War II.

It is a syndrome almost exclusively limited to adolescent girls and young women from middle- and up-

ations, but the poor can plan ahead only a few weeks or days" (Steinem, 1983, p. 173). This raises stress and emotionality levels even further. Women's lives are reactive, lived "from one emergency to the next" (Steinem, 1983, p. 174).

As a woman becomes aware of her subordination and begins to make efforts to move away from it, the anger that underlies the culturally stereotyped subordinate roles she is rejecting can be expected to surface. Greenspan sees this repressed rage as the seed of health that can, with help, transform the "woman as victim" (Greenspan, 1983, p. 35). Without this anger to goad them, many women would lack the impetus to break the expected patterns of role behavior. "Righteous" anger can be a heavy burden for the woman who has the courage to allow herself to feel it, as well as for those around her, even those who support and encourage her (Pierce, 1978, p. 17). It

per-class families. Although some young men develop anorexia, 90 to 95 percent of current victims are women or girls. Victims of anorexia are nearly always conscientious, hard-working, dependable overachievers who were trouble-free until they got sick.

"Today there is a whole new set of stresses that are added to the ordinary sexual pressures on young women," Dr. Brumberg said in an interview. "We have raised women's expectations without giving them adequate social support. They are fearful about many things: integrating career and family, changes in sex and gender roles, sexually transmitted diseases, commitment, family instability as evidenced by the high rate of divorce."

It is not surprising, then, that so many young women develop a disease that strips them of their sexuality and physical maturity. Dr. Brumberg also sees anorexia as "a perfect psychopathology" for the "Superwoman" of the 1970s and 80s.

"For the modern woman, being thin is the ultimate form of perfection," she wrote. "The kind of personal control required to become the new Superwoman parallels the single-mindedness that characterizes the anorectic."

Overemphasis on Beauty

Dr. Brumberg views anorexia as a "secular addiction to a new kind of perfectionism, one that links personal salvation to the achievement of an external body configuration rather than an internal spiritual state."

But the biggest push has come from society's overemphasis on beauty and a degree of slimness that is abnormal for most women, combined with the constant availability of tempting foods.

Dr. Brumberg sees college campuses as the perfect breeding grounds for eating disorders.

"There are no required sit-down meals anymore," she said. "Students today eat everywhere, every hour of the day and almost anything you can imagine." Everywhere a student turns, there are vending machines, delis and fast-food establishments, some of which will even deliver in the middle of the night.

"For a youngster prone to an eating disorder, it can be an extraordinary struggle to stick to an eating pattern," Dr. Brumberg said, adding that "college students today are more promiscuous about food than they are about sex."

Since millions of young women are exposed to the same cultural conditions, why don't many more develop anorexia? Clearly, Dr. Brumberg said, cultural pressures alone do not cause the disorder. Rather, culture interacts with individual psychology, biology and family influences, resulting in an "addiction to starvation" among vulnerable women.

Fighting the Epidemic

How can the epidemic of eating disorders be stemmed? As a historian and feminist, Dr. Brumberg supports efforts to foster emotional and social development of women, some of which have already taken root. Among other things, she suggests the following:

- More emphasis should be put on intellectual activities and creativity.
- Women's magazines, which promote an endless stream of weightloss plans and beauty makeovers, should place less emphasis on the social presentation of self.
- Society should not be afraid to extol the more traditional virtues of women as feeling, caring, healing beings. In the process of rejecting sexist stereotypes, society has de-emphasized these attributes and fails to present them to young women as a source of satisfaction.

"I'm not suggesting that women should pay no attention to their physical well-being," she said. "We should all try to eat healthfully and keep ourselves physically fit. But we have to lose that intense preoccupation with the external body as the be-all and end-all of a woman's worth."

Source: Brody, J. (1988). The resurgence of anorexia, the emotional disease of young women bent on self-starvation. *The New York Times*, May 16, p. 24.

is essential to understand this anger as a necessary stage. At this point, affiliation with other women in support and friendship networks can be of crucial importance.

COMPETITIVENESS

When dominants withhold power, subordinates' attention is normally given more to dominants than to other subordinates. Blaming women for "cattiness" and other forms of competitiveness with each other obscures the fact that competitive behavior is inherent in the subordinate position and is an example of "identification with the aggressor" (Steele & Pollock, 1980), which, like depression, is a frequent consequence of abuse. Men may reinforce women's competitiveness by paying attention to some women in a group and ignoring others, making the ignored

Box 19–3 ● Women as Survivors of Incest

At least one in three females and one in seven males are sexually assaulted before the age of 18 in the United States. According to Sandra Butler, a counselor who works with survivors of incest and sexual abuse, when a girl is sexually abused, she learns several lessons about what it means to be female in a misogynist society. "She learns to live in the service of others. She learns that her emotional role in this world is to maintain harmony, even at the price of her own continued victimization" (Dehli, 1987, p. 6).

Butler also contends that women who, as children, were sexually abused by a family member or a trusted caretaker typically carry into adulthood a profound feeling of powerlessness, an inability to determine who is trustworthy, confusion about sexuality, and a feeling that they are unable to withstand the intrusion of others.

The abused child also learns that she is bad from the person who abuses her or from other family members who may blame her in order to reduce their own feelings of guilt. Because of this, the survivor of abuse feels worthless, may not take care of herself, and may gravitate toward people who are uncaring. Perhaps this explains in part why forty-

four percent of females who survived sexual assault as children will be the victims of rape or attempted rape at least once in their adult lives.

Sexual abuse is also associated with eating disorders. According to Mary Jo Barrett, director of the Midwest Family Resource Center in Chicago, 65% of the women who attend her clinic for an eating disorder have also been sexually abused (Dehli, 1987, p. 7).

Survivors of sexual abuse typically have a poor image (or a distorted one) of their bodies and often try to emotionally detach themselves from them. A woman who starves herself is literally ridding herself of a body she has learned to loathe. Other abuse survivors use the tremendous control they have over their bodies to compensate for pervasive feelings of powerlessness.

In contrast, the incest survivor who compulsively overeats "may be adding layers of protection between herself and the outside world; it was, after all, the boundary of her body that was initially violated," (p. 7) according to Ms. Barrett.

Source: Dehli, Joyce. (1987) Sex abuse counselor stresses self-healing; Eating disorders often tied to sex abuse. *Wisconsin State Journal*, section 3, p. 6–7.

women feel left out, particularly when the attention has sexual overtones. The bases upon which attention is allocated are the standards of looks, success, and power as set by the culture. Women, insofar as they, too, sort other women on dominant criteria—avoiding both those they judge to be superior and those they judge to be inferior—keep themselves separated from each other, competing for male attention and precluding the support and power of networking (Pierce, 1978). (See Box 19–4.)

INTERNALIZING AND PERSONALIZING

Internalizing is the taking on of an externally imposed value and treating it as one's own (Greenspan,

1983). **Personalizing** is a similar process, but more specific; it involves taking on the events in a given situation as if they were directed at oneself personally (Pierce, 1978). "Patriarchal society has contempt for women; so the depressed woman hates herself," is an example of internalizing. "As a child, I used to feel that if only I were *good* enough, the overwhelming sorrow that my parents suffered as victims of the Holocaust would disappear" (Greenspan, 1983, p. 201), is an example of personalizing. The two work in tandem: for example, because women internalize the societal injunction that it is their job to keep interpersonal interactions flowing smoothly in "the labor of relatedness" (Greenspan, 1983, p. 205), they often feel that they are personally responsible for

Box 19–4 ● Are Women Better Doctors?

Dr. Marjorie S. Sirridge, physician and assistant dean of the University of Missouri Medical School at Kansas City, worries that female medical students don't pursue leadership roles as readily as their male colleagues. On the other hand, she thinks women do much better when it comes to human interaction. "For the women, relationships with patients are very important, a very positive thing," she says. "Many men also have this quality, but men in positions of power in medical education and government by and large do not." (p. 46)

One place where this difference shows is the operating room. According to Dr. Marilyn R. Richardson, a 39-year-old obstetrician-gynecologist specializing in reproductive gynecology, the way that women run an operating room *is* different: "Men are often arbitrary, demanding, and disrespectful, and the level of efficiency suffers. Women don't usually command quite as fiercely. . . . You get camaraderie with other staff members." (p. 46)

Dr. Susan Love agrees. One of the first female surgical residents at a major Boston teaching hospital, now, at age 40, a surgeon in private practice with a specialty in breast disease, Dr. Love says she had to suppress many of her basic values in order to get through her surgical residency: "Surgeons don't really like having women, and don't make it comfortable for them. Things that women like—talking to patients—aren't important. It's how many operations you've done, how many hours you've been up. . . . If you get through your five or six years of training, you can regain your values, but it's a real 'if.' . . . "(p. 56)

Dr. Love offers an example of something she does differently, something no one taught her: before a patient is put to sleep, she makes it a practice to hold that person's hand. "I'm usually the only person in the room they know, and it's the scariest time," she says. "The boys scrub,

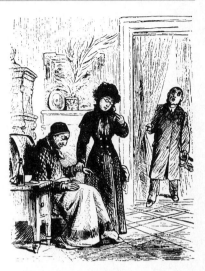

"Women as Competitors." A cartoon depicting the predominantly male medical profession's reaction to a woman physician.

then come in when the patient's asleep. I got razzed for it, but they're used to it now." (p. 48)

Perri Klass, a pediatric resident in Boston and author of *A Not Entirely Benign Procedure: Four Years as a Medical Student* (Klass, 1988), the author of this *New York Times Magazine* article, closes with an anecdote: "Recently, I told my 4-year-old son he was due for his annual check-up with his pediatrician. He looked distinctly nervous (rumors about shots had obviously been making their way around the day-care center), and asked me anxiously, 'Is she a nice doctor?' I thought about the doctors my son knows best—me and my close friends, most of them female. I picked my words carefully. It was clearly one of those critical moments requiring all a mother's wisdom and tact. 'Benjamin, I have to tell you something,' I said. 'Boys can be doctors too if they want to. If they go to school and learn how, boys can be very good doctors, really.'" (p. 97)

Source: Klass, Perri (1988). Are women better doctors? *New York Times Magazine,* April 10, pp. 32–97.

everything that goes on around them (Pierce, 1978). It is easy to see how this dynamic can result in enhanced striving and compulsive perfectionism. The woman can control herself; she cannot always control the environment. If she can internalize the environment, she may be able to feel some measure of control over her own life, no matter how illusory or mistaken these feelings of control may be. A particularly poignant example of this is found in relationships that have gone wrong wherein the woman perceives herself—as, often, does the man—as being too needy and dependent. If only she were more independent, she believes, more able to satisfy her own needs for warmth, emotional responsiveness, and intimacy, without having to rely on the man, the relationship would not have failed. She does not notice that her needs for warmth and emotional responsiveness are legitimate, and that what she may be experiencing is hyperemotionality in the face of male impassivity; she does not notice that the envied self-sufficiency of her partner may be based on the fact that he is, true to cultural form, denying his own dependency needs while at the same time getting them met, through her, without ever having to acknowledge them. She has turned her legitimate emotional requirement into a self-criticism through internalizing and has personalized the situation as her fault. This may give her a false sense of control—"all she has to do is get her head together" for the relationship to work (Greenspan, 1983, p. 294n).

DEPRESSION

It is normal for women to hate themselves in a culture that idolizes femininity but devalues women.

The feelings associated with depression—helplessness, worthlessness, and so forth—are in some sense adaptive to the cultural reality. "Oppression is depressing" (Greenspan, 1983, p. 193). Depression is a culturally acceptable way for women to be protected and taken care of; it works when a direct appeal for nurturance and protection may not.

Gaining self-esteem involves becoming angry about one's powerlessness, but the cultural ideal of femininity disallows anger. A woman who is able, perhaps as a result of psychotherapy, to allow herself to feel power and anger may suffer profoundly from a sense of social isolation and lack of protection. She may also experience disorientation in her gender identity, fearing that as she deviates from femininity by allowing herself anger or power, she may become a lesbian, or at least lose her attraction and attractiveness to men. This situation may be complicated by

her sense of growing closeness with other women and possible, if temporary, need to withdraw from relationships with men in order to break patterns of subservience in relationships with them. In order to overcome depression, however, she must acknowledge her underlying rage; but rage, like power, is seen as masculine. There are as yet few models for power that are not based on aggressive, other-diminishing, and often abusive models of power that the patriarchy fosters (Starhawk, 1982). Women may quite rightly resist these models and, lacking new ones, remain caught in the depression of femininity (Greenspan, 1983). See Chapter 9 on mood disorders for additional information on depression.

THE SEEDS OF CHANGE

Labeling victim behaviors changes the way we view them. Considering the context of the behavior elucidates both the behavior and the culture that gives rise to it, so that indications for effective change become clearer. Seeing victim behaviors as cultural phenomena rather than individual shortcomings calls for cultural alterations that ensure that women do not merely replace men at the top of a hierarchical structure supported by the subordination of other persons. Different societies require different kinds of egos (Greenspan, 1983). Our patriarchal hierarchy, requiring rigid ego boundaries and ruthless goal orientation, has reached an impasse in its ability to deal with the current political, social, and interpersonal crises in all areas of the world—crises created largely by the extreme elaboration of patriarchal ego values. The affiliative, empathic, and mediatory ego qualities consigned by the culture to females are badly needed now by everyone.

The concept of "woman-as-victim" will exist as long as women actually *are* victims. Helping a woman acknowledge her rage about her powerlessness is not enough (Greenspan, 1983). Beyond it lies the task of seeding the changes that will realign the culture toward a positive valuation of the very qualities assigned to women that have been so devalued by the patriarchy, undoing the myth of female inferiority.

AWARENESS

Women as individuals must identify and make explicit to themselves their own victim behaviors, the ways in which they themselves internalize and comply with oppression. They may find that some of their needs may be met more directly as they observe themselves and their daily contexts. (During the late 1960s and early 1970s this was called "consciousness raising," a term that now sounds naive compared to the level of mindfulness required to monitor one's own habitual thought and behavior patterns.) Where possible, women need to find more direct means of expressing anger and getting needs met.

BONDING WITH OTHER WOMEN

The importance of female bonding to successfully enduring and constructively channeling rage has been mentioned. In addition, the support and insight of other women is crucial to every phase of these changes. Learning to value oneself as a woman entails learning to value the friendship of women and respect its requirements as much as one respects the requirements of relationships with men. Woman-as-victim has learned to compete with other women for the attention of men; but woman-as-female-human-being can experience herself as validated by the attention of a person she respects, regardless of gender.

COURAGE

A woman who chooses to move away from a victim-based femininity and becomes aware of her compliance with the victim role will need courage to make changes—to be patient with herself, endure her anxiety, avoid giving up on herself in the midst of redefinition, and suspend judgment on a gender identity that may be in flux.

MODELS

Women need models for femaleness after femininity has been discarded. Acknowledging rage without knowing how to direct it or what to put in its place may be worse than not acknowledging it at all. Such models have been evolving over the last century and are more available to women than ever before. Artists, poets, novelists, film makers, theologians, and Jungian psychologists tend to be the current holders and purveyors of the images around which the shape of selves to come is molded. More and more, these image shapers are women, many of whom are finding ways through their rage to forge new models of personal power (for example, see Alice Walker, *The Color Purple*; Marion Zimmer Bradley, *The Mists of Avalon*). The Jungians and many theologians are bringing about a revival of interest in ancient goddess imagery (see Jean Shinoda Bolen, M.D., *Goddesses in Every Woman*; Merlin Stone, *When God Was a Woman*; Edward Whitmont, *The Return of the Goddess*), supported by the growth of popular interest in Eastern religions, many of which honor female as well as male aspects of deity.

But models for victim-based femininity are abundant (for example, see Marabel Morgan, *The Total Woman,* and Phyllis Schlafly). Women must take care about the models they choose for themselves, and be clear in themselves about why they choose the models they do. They must begin viewing themselves as models, aware that other women might be looking to them, ready to become what they behold. (See Box 19–5.)

MANAGING MULTIPLE ROLES

As women's roles become more diverse, the availability of real-life models may decrease. The roles and behaviors associated with traditional motherhood have changed a great deal in the last twenty or thirty years, and yet many women still feel the pressure of conforming to a traditional model that may no longer be relevant for them (See Box 19–6). McBride (1988) describes the work of expert panelists convened by the National Institute of Mental Health in 1986 for the purpose of setting an agenda for women's mental health. Some of the most interesting studies have focused on role conflicts and burdens for women who choose "career-accommodating" lifestyles. Some researchers have found that the healthiest women are those who have combined roles in career, marriage, and parenting (McBride, 1988). Others have studied the stresses of women who are caught in the middle, trying to excel in all realms (the syndrome of the "SuperMom") and also the stresses for women who must care for the needs of elderly relatives while trying to raise their own families. Much of the research carried out has focused on the competing demands on women brought on by the existence of multiple roles, with an associated risk of role strain and psychological disturbances such as depression, anger/hostility, and anxiety (McBride, 1988). (See also Case Study/Care Plan on Olive in Chapter 17, Dissociative Disorders.) McBride proposes a commitment of further research related to the mental health consequences of women's multiple roles and based on the the stated objectives of the National Institute of Mental Health's 12 research branches (1986) (see Table 19–1 on p. 753).

Box 19—5 ● Margaret Sanger, a Role Model for, and on Behalf of Women and Nursing

Margaret Sanger (1879–1966), mother, trained nurse, and leader of the American birth control movement, has done more than any other individual to give women control of their bodies. By 1912 she had established herself among radicals as a speaker and writer on sexual reform, a response to the urgent demand among women of all classes for information about venereal disease, birth control, and sex education.

A midwife and visiting nurse who practiced on the Lower East Side of New York, Sanger was horrified by the numerous deaths from self-induced abortions among her patients. As a result, she began to focus all her energy on the single cause of reproductive autonomy for women.

One of her first projects was an investigation of birth control methods with the goal of discovering a safe, effective, female-controlled contraceptive. She also campaigned for the legalization of birth control, for example, by opening the Brownsville Clinic in Brooklyn in 1916, the first birth control advice center in the United States, which provided 488 mothers with contraceptive advice during the ten days before it was closed by the police. In the same vein, Sanger organized the American Birth Control League, the national lobbying organization which later became the Planned Parenthood Federation of America in 1942.

In 1923 Sanger opened the Birth Control Clinical Research Bureau in New York City, the first doctor-staffed birth control clinic in the United States. A model for the nationwide network of over 300 birth control clinics established by Sanger and her supporters by 1938, it was staffed mainly by women doctors and supported by the efforts of women volunteers.

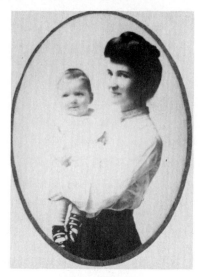

Pictured here is Margaret Sanger with one of her children.

Throughout her career, Sanger raised large sums of money for research on her dream, a female-controlled physiological contraceptive. In 1952 she played a key role in the development of the birth control pill by bringing the work of biologist Gregory Pincus to the attention of Katharine Dexter McCormick, who subsidized the research that led to its first marketing in 1960.

Source: Reed, J. (1980) "Sanger, Margaret. Birth control reformer," in B. Sicherman and C. Green (eds), *Notable American Women: The Modern Period.* Cambridge: Harvard University Press, pp. 623–627.

Box 19–6 ● Mothers With Babies—and Jobs

A Transforming Change, in One Generation

Among women who had a child in the year preceding the June 1987 survey, 51 percent were in the labor force . . . as compared with 31 percent in June 1976.

These calm words from a new Census Bureau report denote another dramatic social transformation. In the last three or four decades, America has experienced unimaginably rapid changes involving race, gender, sexual mores, and smoking. The rising number of mothers with jobs creates equally monumental change as it is altering the way Americans raise their children.

Not many years ago, working mothers were made to feel guilty, reproached with truisms: Even a bad mother is better than good day care. But look who's in the labor force now—a vast majority of mothers, a majority of those with young children, a majority even of those with babies. A transformation is at hand.

Except for one thing. It's a transformation society does not yet accept. More mothers work for fulfillment and many more do so for income, but whatever the reason, the phenomenon is barely acknowledged by employers, government, and other institutions.

Perhaps passing this newest milestone finally will jolt America into confronting the reality: What was once unusual is now the norm.

Most of Them Work Because They Must

For many women with families, a job outside the home is nothing new. Those from lower-income families have always been under pressure to bring home a second income.

What is new is the entry into the labor force of women who have young children and whose wages are not always necessary to keep the wolf from the door.

Few educated Americans of either sex would choose to reverse this social revolution even if they could. It began as highly educated women with no financial need challenged social norms to join the white-collar elite. Their success has made it easier for middle-class women to break out of "women's work" and aspire to fulfilling careers.

Equality is still far from real; women typically earn 20 to 30 percent less than men, even after adjusting for age, education, and hours worked. But even the prospect of equality creates a benign impact on the culture of the work force.

Even so, there are blunter reasons for millions of middle-class women having deserted housework for office and factory work. Their entry into the paid work force reflects the special obstacles young families must overcome to hold onto the middle-class living standard taken for granted by their parents. For these women and their families, the 1970s and 80s have been a time in which they have had to run just to stay in place.

What explains their difficulties? The social acceptability of divorce plays a part. Divorced middle-class women, as well as poor women, often must assume financial responsibility for children. According to census figures, just half of all divorced mothers receive child support; and for those, the average annual payment in 1985 was a pitiful $2,500.

But as Frank Levy, an economist at the University of Maryland and the author of "Dollars and Dreams,"

continued

Box 19—6 continued

points out, the pressure on women to work also reflects deep problems in the economy. Between 1947 and 1973, the average worker's inflation-adjusted earnings rose 61 percent, reflecting a rise in productivity. Since 1973, however, productivity has stagnated and average earnings have fallen 15 percent. Family incomes have remained virtually constant only because many more women have joined the paid work force.

Even these pre-tax figures mask some inequities imposed on women of child-bearing age. Social Security taxes have risen sharply, reflecting massive income transfers from young families to old. And younger families, who had not bought homes by the early 1970s are being ravaged by housing costs. In 1973, mortgage payments represented 21 percent of an average 30-year-old male's income. In 1984, the figure was 44 percent.

The explosive increase of wives and mothers in the labor force reflects a welcome change in social attitudes: Society is beginning to treat women as equals in the workplace. They can now aspire to work in any occupation because they want to. But that fact is harshly linked to another: Women who work, even in the most fulfilling professional jobs, do so because they have to.

When Will Society Escape the Myths?

This revolution is not news to individual women and families. They've been adjusting in a host of ways—patching together day care by calling on grandparents, hiring illegal aliens, organizing nurseries. Yet society, from the local workplace to Washington, looks on blankly, fixed on romantic images of Mommy in the kitchen watching over Baby in the playpen, learning how to count.

Most families need institutional help to keep daily life livable—employers willing to be flexible about hours, governments willing to monitor and support child care. Such accommodations to the rearing of its children ought to be hallmarks of a decent society. Yet society still dithers, even amid the signs of dramatic change.

A school for nannies begins. Restaurateurs who once winced at children now eagerly proffer crayons and crackers. Takeout food services are booming. Housekeeping standards relax; consider the rapid rise of no-iron fabrics, microwave ovens, and tolerance for clutter around the house. Individual women create ways to cope, like "sequencing": moving in and out of the work force to balance family and professional needs.

Studies show that women who "have it all" are among the happiest Americans, free from stifled homemaker's depression and martyred motherhood. But their lives are hard, too. Work takes a toll at home; home is on their minds at work. About two-thirds of salaried women either support themselves, are their families' sole supporters, or have husbands who earn less than $15,000. For them, the struggle is harder. And it's harder still for poor single mothers who can't have it either way, let alone both. Many lack parenting skills—and lack even the *prospect* of steady work.

The work force has been transformed, but hours, expectations, and responsibilities have not. Extensive leaves, paid or unpaid, for childbirth and early child care remain the exception, far more than in other industrialized nations. On-site day care, flexible benefit options, flexible hours, job-sharing: such adjustments, contemplated for decades, remain unrealized.

The political campaign has brought some proposals, notably from Bruce Babbitt: tax incentives for businesses to establish day care centers, a child care voucher program and the expansion of Head Start. But when people realize that such reforms cost money, the discussion quickly dissipates. Some companies find that caring about family issues brings more benefits than costs. They notice that the double burden on women lowers productivity. They find that they are losing recruits or expensively trained employees by not helping to accommodate child care needs.

For now, however, women are still being pressed to keep on meeting all, or most, of their old responsibilities to home, family and community. Each responsibility suffers accordingly. The changes in social life are real, as real as the 11-year progression from 31 percent to 51 percent of women with babies and jobs. Perhaps now, at last, employers, government, and society will accept it.

Source: *The New York Times,* Sunday, June 19, 1988, p. 26E.

TABLE 19–1 Women's concerns in need of study superimposed on objectives of NIMH research branches

NIMH Research Branch	Women's Concerns in Need of Study
Behavioral sciences	Development of competence and adaptive behavior, vulnerability, stress reactivity and coping.
	The relationship of stressful life transitions to mental health and mental illness, especially as influenced by specific environmental or systems factors.
	Development and maintenance of interpersonal networks and support systems as they affect individual and family functioning.
	Psychosocial stressors and coping mechanisms in families at risk because of caregiving burden.
	Family and individual factors that facilitate self-efficacy, resilience and self-regulation.
	Individual and family structures mediating the effects of family disruption.
	Learning processes and strategies related to successful and unsuccessful coping with transitional stress.
Health and behavior	The development of objective measures of stress (e.g., endocrinological, cardiovascular and psychophysiological) and measures of coping capacities.
	Identification and specification of stressors.
	Individual variability in stress vulnerability.
	Methods useful for combating stress and stressful situations.
	Stressful life events and their outcomes in terms of mental or physical disorders.
Health and behavior	The interrelationships between psychological–social-behavioral processes and immune function.
	Methods to assess altered immune function as a result of stressful behavior states.
Neurosciences	Environmental influences on brain function including the response of neural substrates to acute and chronic stress.
	Neural mechanisms underlying behavior including the neural basis of integrative brain activities such as response selection, attention, symbolic/linguistic representation and problem-solving behaviors.
Epidemiology and psychopathology	Identification and assessment of risk factors influencing the development of mental disorders, especially the presence or absence of a particular premorbid characteristic.
	Distribution and association of clinical phenomena (e.g., depression) in specified populations.
Mental disorders of aging	Effects of families and support systems on the care of older persons with significant mental disorders including family stress and care of Alzheimer's disease victims.
Prevention	Strategies for reducing the incidence of mental and emotional disorders/dysfunctions through promoting coping skills or mobilizing naturally occurring support systems.
	Validating and refining procedures for targeting "true-positive" individuals among known or presumed risk groups.

continued

TABLE 19–1 continued

Affective/anxiety disorders	Description, etiology, prediction and clinical course of depression and anxiety secondary to stressful life events. Psychosocial and pharmacologic treatment of depression and anxiety secondary to stressful life events.	in the building and maintenance of supportive social networks. Basic social processes related to response to stress and the effects of stressors on the development of mental disorders.
Child/adolescent disorders	The effects of child/adolescent disorders on the well-being of families providing care.	
Schizophrenia	Assessment of patterns of family response to care of schizophrenic relatives.	
Biometric/clinical applications	Assessment of the need for and access to services of family caregivers.	
Antisocial/violent behavior	The effects of violence/abuse on stress, coping, strain and mental disorders.	
Minority	Investigations of community characteristics, socioeconomic status, social roles, social coping skills and other personal and social characteristics as possible factors	

Source: McBride, A. (1988, Spring). Mental Health Effects of Women's Multiple Roles. Image: *Journal of Nursing Scholarship. Vol. 20, No. 1,* 45.

References

Aldwin, C. M., & Revenson, T. A. (1987). Does coping help? A reexamination of the relation between coping and mental health. *Journal of Personality and Social Psychology, 53,* 337–348.

Allen, K. R., & Pickett, R. S. (1987). Forgotten streams in the family life course: Utilization of qualitative interviews in the analysis of lifelong single women's family careers. *Journal of Marriage and the Family, 49,* 517–526.

Allen, V. L. (1984). A role theoretical perspective in transitional processes. In V. L. Allen & E. Van de Vliert (Eds.), *Role transitions: Explorations and explanations* (pp. 3–18). New York: Plenum Press.

Antoni, M. H. (1987). Neuroendocrine influences in psychoimmunology and neoplasia: A review. *Psychology and Health, 1,* 3–24.

Baruch, G. K., Biener, L., & Barnett, R. C. (1987). Women and gender in research on work and family stress. *American Psychologist, 42,* 130–136.

Baucom, D. H., & Weiss, B. (1986). Peers' granting of control to women with different sex role identities: Implications for depression. *Journal of Personality and Social Psychology, 51,* 1075–1080.

Case Study: Nonpsychiatric Setting

Amy was an RN in the emergency room of a large metropolitan hospital. She was taking care of a female patient, Marilyn, who had just returned from X ray, where she was found to have two broken ribs and some torn cartilage. In addition, Marilyn had facial and upper body bruises on the front and back, and a badly sprained right wrist. Her left eye was swollen shut. She did not have a concussion, though there was a bump on her head that was painful to the touch. Marilyn was very thin and dishevelled, but her soft wool slacks and sweater were tasteful and obviously expensive. When Amy asked how the injuries occurred, Marilyn told her in a voice that was almost inaudible, and, without making eye contact, that she tripped and fell down a long flight of stairs at home.

Amy was trying to understand whether Marilyn's injuries were explained by her story, and asked for details, but as Marilyn related more of her story, the details made less sense. Marilyn finally broke down in sobs, and began to tell a different story. She said that her husband had beaten her and left the home. She feared that he might not return, and she worried that she would not be able to survive without him. She had no marketable skills, having dropped out of college to get married. He had insisted throughout their marriage that her place was in the home and forbade her to work or continue her education. It was a point of honor for him that his family relied solely on his—now considerable—income for their support, and that he maintained complete control over all their activities outside the home. Amy was shocked to learned who Marilyn's husband was: a highly successful attorney who was well-known in the community.

Marilyn stated that her husband had never beaten her before, though he frequently slapped her and yelled at her. She said that when this happened she saw it as a positive occurrence in that at least she knew she had his attention and could reach him emotionally. Most of the time he appeared indifferent toward her. This time, however, she was frightened — not because she was more injured than ever before, but because he might not return home. Marilyn was sure that she and their two adopted children could not survive materially without him and hinted that she might kill herself if he did not return. She was also extremely fearful that people in the community would learn about this incident because of her visit to the hospital, and he would be angrier than ever. She begged Amy not to reveal the truth to social services, the physician, or police.

Although Marilyn stated that she had had no problems with sleeping or eating, she was quite underweight and appeared fatigued. She stated that her most recent abuse occurred when she returned from running that afternoon (she ran approximately 10 miles per day). Her husband had come home from the office early to pack for a business trip and expected to find some shirts that he had asked her to iron for him. When he did not find them in his drawer, he went after her. After criticizing her housekeeping skills and going on to berate her sexual ability and her family, he resorted to more physical means of expressing himself. Marilyn stated that she never struck back in situations like this because she feared it would only make him angrier. "Besides," she said, "he is right, I should have had the shirts done; I am a bad housekeeper, probably not very sexy, and my family can be hard to take."

As she listened to this story, Amy noted the symptoms of a dependent personality disorder, and observed the following symptoms of depression: low self-esteem, a sense of helplessness and hopelessness, dropped head, lack of eye contact, and chronic unhappiness. She also wondered whether the patient's thinness and compulsive exercising were symptoms of an eating disorder.

Throughout this narration, Amy responded empathically, labeling the patient's anxiety and low self-esteem, and encouraging her to talk about it. When Marilyn paused, apparently relieved of some of her emotional burden, Amy expressed concern about the situation and suggested that she at least share this information with the physician so that a psychiatric evaluation could be obtained. It seemed that at the very least, Marilyn needed someone to talk with about her many problems.

Marilyn refused, however, fearing that this would be admitting she was "crazy" and her husband would never stand for such a stigma. In addition, he did not believe in seeing psychiatrists.

Amy was having difficulty listening to all this; she was becoming angry herself, angry at Marilyn's husband for his treatment of his wife, and, strangely, angry at Marilyn for what seemed to be her unwillingness to act on her own behalf. Amy wondered how Marilyn even managed to get to the emergency room. Marilyn said that she would not have come, but the pain from her injuries made housework impossible, and she worried that she might not be able to run tomorrow. She only wanted something for pain so that she could continue both. Her husband would be furious with her if the housework wasn't finished by the time he returned from his trip. He might even leave again. It was also likely that he would be angry about this emergency room visit if he found out about it.

Amy excused herself in order to get Marilyn something for pain and to speak with the physician about how they should handle this very complicated situation. She doubted that they would be able to help Marilyn, given her denial and dependence on her abusive husband. But she felt they should try. The following is her nursing care plan.

Nursing Diagnoses

Anxiety
Ineffective family coping
Self-esteem disturbance

Nursing Care Plan for Marilyn

Nursing Diagnosis	Desired Outcomes	Interventions	Rationale
1. Anxiety regarding staying in the hospital and going home.	Marilyn will be able to consider alternatives to facing her husband alone in the hospital or at home.	Empathize with Marilyn, labeling her anxiety as a solvable problem. Offer to consult social services, pointing out that any *services* are optional. She doesn't *have* to do anything. There is no harm in finding out what is available in the community for couples and families with this kind of problem: anger that gets out of control and results in hurting someone you love. For example, there is a battered women's shelter staffed by counselors and women who are former victims themselves.	Since Marilyn seems to be headed home, Amy's only option is to try to make interpersonal contact with her through empathy, label her situation as a problem, and educate her about community services that could be of help to her and her husband.
2. Ineffective family coping	Marilyn's husband will seek treatment for the purpose of learning to verbalize feelings rather than act them out; control his aggressive impulses; and begin to use community resources available to families with problems with violence.	Respond to Marilyn's negative feelings about herself by asking how she came to have such a low opinion of herself, as it does not develop in a vacuum; point out that even if it were accurate, it did not justify the injuries inflicted on her.	It is essential to maintain that physical violence in the home is never justified and always indicates that at least two individuals (in this case, Marilyn and her husband) are in need of social support or psychological help. Emphasizing treatment

Nursing Diagnosis	Desired Outcomes	Interventions	Rationale
		Label Marilyn's husband as in need of help, not punishment; whether or not he is still angry, he is probably now frightened and ashamed of what he has done; label his *problem* with violence as treatable and the treatment as confidential and available. Offer to talk more with her and her husband about this.	rather than punishment as the solution to the problem of physical violence in the family may help to reassure abusers and their victims about the consequences of "asking for help."
3. Self-esteem disturbance	Marilyn will recognize that her low self-esteem is a result of her chronic abuse and possible depression, both of which are treatable.	Tell Marilyn that low self-esteem and chronic dysphoria may be symptoms of depression, another treatable correlate (as well as often a precipitant) of family violence. Explain what treatment usually involves (see Chapter 9) and offer to refer Marilyn to a mental health professional.	Depression, a common sequela of physical abuse in the victim, only leads to more abuse as the depressed victim feels that her abuse is justified and that she is helpless to do anything about it. Labeling these feelings as symptoms of a treatable illness and referring Marilyn for psychiatric treatment may interrupt the dynamics of abuse in this family.

SUMMARY

Because U.S. culture is a patriarchal hierarchy, men are relatively powerful and women are relatively powerless. As cultural subordinates, women are rewarded for behaviors that keep them powerless and negatively reinforced for being or seeming powerful; thus the structure maintains itself. Women often resort to means that are indirect, overdone, and ultimately self-limiting to accomplish their goals while avoiding retribution.

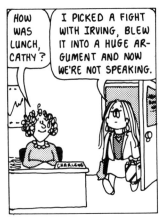
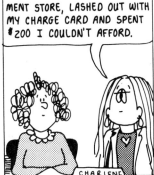
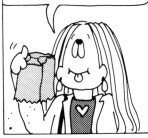
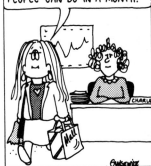

Viewing many of the dysfunctional behaviors prevalent in women in their cultural context can show these behaviors to be in large part cultural adaptations rather than symptoms of personal defect. Such a view can lighten the burden of self-blame for individual women and reduce the hopelessness that prevents change. It can give indications for changing the culture as well, so that the personal changes the individual woman makes can be maintained and in a way that ensures that women will not merely replace men at the top of a system based on the subordination of other persons. The effects of multiple role demands on the mental health of women is another important investigation topic for nurses and other health professionals.

KEY TERMS

patriarchal hierarchy

cultural subordinates

survival mechanisms

victim behaviors

extropunitive

intropunitive

enhanced striving

internalizing

personalizing

STUDY QUESTIONS

1. Define the term victim behaviors.

2. Name and explain the two categories into which victim behaviors fall.

3. How does enhanced striving affect a woman's view of herself?

4. How would a woman use internalizing and personalizing to explain her commitment to a relationship that is unsatisfying and perhaps even abusive?

5. How might role models and bonding with other women help women improve their position in U.S. society?

REFERENCES

Allport, G. (1958). *The nature of prejudice*. New York: Doubleday Anchor.

Greenspan, M. (1983). *A new approach to women and therapy*. New York: McGraw-Hill.

Herzog, D. B., & Copeland, P. M. (1985, August). Eating disorders. *New England Journal of Medicine, 313,* 5.

McBride, A. B. (1988). Mental health effects of women's multiple roles. *Image: Journal of Nursing Scholarship, 20* (1), 41–47.

National Institute of Mental Health. (1986). *Extramural research support*. Rockville, MD: The Institute.

Pierce, C. (1978). *Women and victim behavior*. Laconia, NH: New Dynamics.

Starhawk, (1982). *Dreaming the dark: Magic, sex, and politics*. Boston: Beacon Press.

Steele, B. F., & Pollock, C. B. (1980). Parents who abuse children. In S. I. Harrison and J. F. McDermott, Jr. (Eds.) *New directions in childhood psychopathology*. New York: International Universities Press.

Steinem, G. (1983) *Outrageous acts and everyday rebellions*. New York: Holt, Rinehart and Winston.

20

PSYCHIATRIC MENTAL HEALTH NURSING WITH MEN

DANIEL G. SAUNDERS

LEARNING OBJECTIVES

After studying this chapter, the student will be able to:

- Define the concept of hypermasculinity and how it affects men.
- Describe the effects of patriarchy on men.
- Identify the special problems that men have, including their resistance to counseling.
- Describe methods for counseling men.
- Develop nursing care plans especially designed to help men cope with problems brought on by hypermasculinity.

INTRODUCTION*

Masculine behavior, when taken to the extreme, has negative consequences for men's physical and emotional health. The adoption of extreme forms of masculine traits such as competitiveness and ambition is called **hypermasculinity.** Engaging in hypermasculinity is also why men often hurt those who are closest to them. Nurses are encouraged to see the male patient as a product of strong cultural messages that push men to be emotionally restricted, possessive, and achievement oriented. Men end up feeling alienated from their own needs, from other men, and from their families. Although men often avoid looking at the connection between their behavior and their health, sensitive interview techniques can help men see the underlying factors that may result in poor health and premature death.

On the average, men have higher rates than women of all major diseases leading to death, especially heart disease (USDHEW, 1979; Waldron & Johnson, 1976). In general men:

- Die almost eight years younger than women (USDHEW, 1980).
- Have higher rates of accidents than women (Waldron, 1976).
- Have significantly higher rates of drug and alcohol abuse than women (Goodwin & Guze, 1979).
- Have higher rates of suicide than women (although women have higher rates of *attempted* suicide) (Harrison, 1984).

A startling number of men also turn their violence outward:

- Men have higher rates of assault and murder outside the home than do women, most often victimizing other men (Harrison, 1984).
- Inside the home, men's physical and sexual abuse of women and children is at epidemic proportions (Finkelhor, 1986; Straus & Gelles, 1986).

Why are men so damaging to themselves and others? This chapter describes men's socialization into a "masculine mystique" that leads to problems with intimacy, alcoholism, poor health, and violence to themselves and others. Chapter 19, "Psychiatric

*The author would like to thank Ginger Alberts, David Allen, Patricia Cumbie, and David McKee for their helpful comments on an earlier draft of this chapter. Writing of this chapter was supported in part by NIMH Grant MH–17139–02.

Mental Health Nursing with Women," describes how patriarchy keeps women in a one-down position and affects their mental health. This chapter illustrates how men are also affected by patriarchy, especially those men who adopt rigid masculine traits and end up oppressing women, other men, and themselves.

Nurses can play an important role in improving the health of men. David Forrester (1986) emphasizes that "Opportunities exist in virtually every practice setting to encourage men to care for their health. Nurses encounter men as patients, fathers of patients, and partners of patients. They are all deserving of expert care which considers their unique needs as men in today's complex society" (p. 20).

THE EFFECTS OF PATRIARCHY ON MEN

To say that men are oppressing themselves and other men is not to diminish the oppression of women. Indeed, the cause of women's oppression can be traced beyond individual men to men's socialization. In the overall scheme of **patriarchy,** or a social organization marked by the supremacy of men, women are the most oppressed. However, understanding the effects of patriarchy on men can lead to positive changes for everyone. In the words of Stan Taubman, " . . . There is no need to assume that a man's disadvantages under the present social system in any way offset those of a woman. Men and women experience different kinds of disadvantages, have different levels of awareness of their respective disadvantages, and have different options available to them in resolving their respective problems" (p. 13, 1986).

THE INFLUENCE OF THE ABSENCE OF A FATHER

In support groups, men often reveal the pain of growing up barely knowing their fathers. To their surprise, this is almost a universal experience among men. Shere Hite's (1981) national survey of more than 7000 men revealed that most men had not been close to their fathers. Since the Industrial Revolution, men's work has been separated from the home, which has kept sons from working as partners with their fathers. Even when the modern father is at home, he may be preoccupied with thoughts of work and pressures to succeed.

When fathers are asked how they show caring for their families, they might say simply, "I bring home the bacon." The distance between father and son is not only physical, but emotional (Osherson, 1986). Sons feel the emotional connection with their mothers but may lack this connection with their fathers. They do not realize that their fathers have difficulty trying to put emotions into words or feeling that it is all right to do so. One dilemma for men is feeling a need to identify with their fathers but not really knowing who their fathers are.

Scientific support regarding the effects of the absence of a father is not totally clear (see Pleck, 1981, for a review). During the last two decades, there has been an increase in the level of paternal involvement in child rearing, but the effects of this involvement appear to be positive only when both parents want it (Lamb, Pleck, & Levine, 1986). Naturally, the quality of father-son interaction is crucial. For example, the idyllic scene of sons working on their fathers' farms may in reality mean working long hours for little pay and receiving harsh punishment from the fathers rather than emotional closeness.

There are a number of indirect effects that the absence of a father has on the health of a son, and many of these are described on page 762. A nurse may observe some direct effects. In one case, for example, a patient, Carol, confided in the nurse at a pediatric clinic that she felt that her marriage was falling apart. Her husband, Mike, showed almost no interest in their son, who was now two years old. Carol did not know whether Mike's behavior was due to his "immaturity," a lack of love for her, or a hatred of children.

The nurse found that she could identify with Carol's plight but she had difficulty understanding Mike's behavior. Carol was becoming increasingly depressed. After talking more with Carol and then with her husband, the nurse learned that Mike's father had treated him the same way. Mike had some yearning to be close to his son but was unsure how to play with him or show him affection. He also harbored fears that such behavior would make him look effeminate.

ALIENATION FROM WORK

Another source of pressure on men is their work. During the Industrial Revolution, work in open fields, cottages, or small shops was replaced by work in foul-smelling factories and, more recently, impersonal, technological and corporate settings. Men are usually not as connected to the total production of

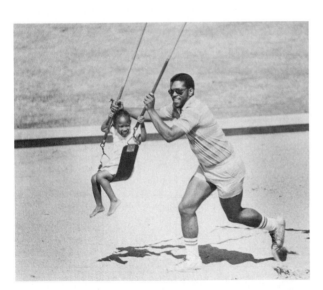

It is common today to see fathers "fathering" in the park, in restaurants, and even accompanying their children to school on the first day. While divorce and "visitation" and joint custody account for some of this, the increased appreciation of the child's need for a *father* and the distinct role he plays in the child's emotional growth and development is, no doubt, beginning to affect behavior.

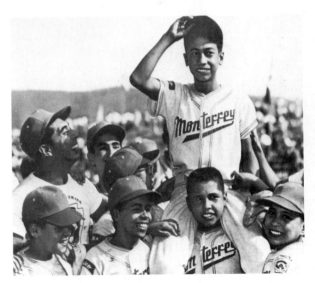

The scramble for success starts early. These boys and their coach are having *fun*, too, actually more important at their age than athletic development, learning how to be a *team* player, and experience in competitive sports. If the child is too young or the pressure from parents or coaches too great, the fun stops, and a "game" becomes associated with anxiety, frustration, and low self-esteem.

their work as they once were, and they do not have the satisfaction of putting their names on their articles of craftsmanship.

The other major source of stress for men is the pressure to scramble for traditional signs of success. "Be a *Success*" is an extremely potent message that men receive in our world. This pressure is compounded by the practice, and belief, also stemming from the Industrial Revolution, that men should be the sole breadwinners in their families. In the drive for success, masculinity becomes equated with the size of a man's paycheck, office, car, or other material possession (Gould, 1973).

The scramble for success is fueled by competition. Cooperation is seen as a feminine trait by many men. Parents sometimes reinforce competition by giving their young sons praise only when they win at sports or succeed at school. Even blue-collar workers seek status through seniority, work skills, or influence with management (Shastak, 1969). Therefore, most men live in a world where they can only be one-up or one-down—where everyone desires to be on top, but where there is room for only a few at the top. The price men often pay for their competitiveness is chronic depression, carefully hidden from sight, because they persist in jobs they despise and feel alienated from and distrustful of fellow workers.

Today, many men seriously question the costs of getting ahead—costs to their health, peace of mind, and family life (Gerzon, 1982). For example, more and more men now refuse promotions when it means transferring to another city. The more that men realize the high cost of an identity equated with success at work, the more they refuse to be "success symbols" and are stepping off of the workaholic treadmill.

ALIENATION FROM OTHERS

The lack of an expressive, same-sex role model during childhood and competition in the workplace seem to spill over to men's nonwork relationships (Weiss, 1985). In both childhood and adulthood, men are told, "be tough" and "stand on your own two feet." Rugged individualism is a theme that runs deep in U.S. culture. The frontiersman was the movie and TV hero for many men during their boyhoods. One result of rugged individualism is that men have fewer deep friendships than women (Stein, 1986); men may appear to have many male friends, but most of these relationships lack depth. Hidden beneath male camaraderie are competitiveness and the fear of seeming weak if feelings are revealed. Many men indicate that they talk to women when they want to share

feelings. However, both men and women tend to disdain men who reveal that they are depressed (Warren, 1983). For example, more than one male presidential candidate has lost votes or the candidacy itself as a result of looking depressed or admitting a history of treatment for depression.

Men also have a hard time developing platonic friendships with women, partly because they tend to sexualize their relationships with women, and they have a hard time making a commitment to an intimate relationship. Like women, they often fear hurt or loss, but men seem to have other fears as well: of "being exposed" for who they "really are," of showing imperfection, of being mothered and hating it, and also the opposite, of being mothered and loving it (Wolfman, 1985).

Men who make the commitment to marriage appear to be physically and psychologically healthier than other men, but this may not be the result of marriage. There is evidence that men who marry had happier childhoods and better family relationships (Duncan, 1986) than those who do not, and thus mentally healthy men may be more likely to marry in the first place.

There is a stereotype that when men are in intimate relationships they are more jealous than women. Yet the evidence shows they may be no more jealous than their partners. What seems to differ is that men, when suspecting a partner's unfaithfulness, react with more dominance or avoidance, thus increasing the feelings of alienation in the relationship (Buunk, 1986).

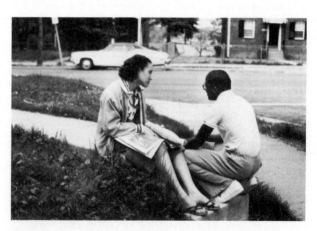

Though we talk a lot about the importance of expressing feelings, research has shown that there exists a double standard. Both men and women "tend to disdain" men who reveal that they are depressed. Perhaps we've lived with "macho" for so long, we think it's the norm, and desirable.

Today, there are signs that the primary reasons that men marry are changing. Once, men sought a strong woman who could farm and bear many children; today there is more emphasis on wanting a friend with whom to talk (Lewis, 1986). As fathers and husbands, more men today are fulfilling the nurturing roles that were discouraged twenty or more years ago. The dilemma for the "new male" is that he may be judged negatively if he shows his own need for affiliation and affection (Stein, 1986). (See Box 20–1.)

ALIENATION FROM SELF

Modern men are often confused and distressed about what it means to be a man (Komarovsky, 1976). For traditional men, striving for symbols of success and for what they think women want denies them the awareness of their own emotional needs and desires. More liberated men, on the other hand, may feel identity confusion between nurturing roles and traditional "macho" roles.

Men are also usually out of touch with their feelings, which is not surprising given their socialization. Erikson describes how social pressure leads to shame and self-alienation: "There is a limit to a child's or an adult's endurance in the face of demands to consider himself, his body, and his wishes as evil and dirty and to his belief in the infallibility of those who pass judgement" (1950, p. 253).

Many feelings become distorted; for example, the message "Don't be a crybaby" becomes the internalized message, "I can't feel sadness." Many boys learn to block out pain after repeated, harsh physical punishment from their parents. Adult men learn to do the same thing, for example, blocking out the pain of broken bones and torn ligaments on the football field. In the short run, pain suppression helps men through tough spots; in the long run, however, the results may be life-threatening.

Therapists working with men note the difficulty in uncovering men's feelings. When the "fight-flight" response is activated, men note their actions rather than their inner arousal. For example, a man may be aware that when frustrated he hit a wall with his fist, but not the way his anger rose. For most men, to become angry means to be aggressive. Marital therapists sometimes hand a list of "feeling" words to men to help them express various types and gradations of feelings. They are also taught about the possibility of having a mixture of feelings. In summary, being cut off from awareness of feelings means that men tend

to be alienated from themselves without really knowing it.

IS HYPERMASCULINITY HARMFUL TO MEN'S HEALTH?

Why is it that men die at a younger age than women? A look at the major causes of death for men provides some clues (Waldron, 1976). Table 20–1 lists the major causes of death for men in the United States. The following sections focus on those causes of death that are most likely related to hypermasculinity and characteristics of male socialization that make it difficult for men to be patients.

"TYPE A" PERSONALITY AND HEART DISEASE

Diseases of the cardiovascular system are at the top of the list of the diseases that kill men (Foreman, 1986). While genetics certainly plays an important role in heart disease, lifestyle and the ability to handle stress are also important causes. A personality profile, called the Type A personality, is associated with heart disease and is most commonly seen in men. It has many features of hypermasculinity

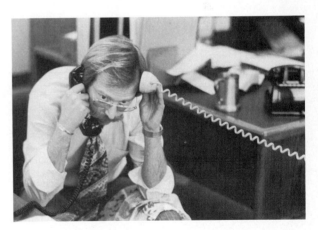

The nurse working with this man *after* his heart attack as he recuperates in the cardiac ICU, may get through to him by challenging him to be a "Type-A Health Nut" when he goes home: i.e., to work at being the *best* among his peers at eating right, giving up cigarettes, drinking alcohol in moderation, exercising, and *relaxing*. It will be the hardest thing he's ever had to do—but then, again, he *is* a Type A. If anyone can do it, he can. He can make his personality work *for* instead of against him.

Box 20–1 ● The Truth Is Not Simple

I don't know exactly how long we lived together. (Which is one way we were different. She remembered the moment we met and precisely when we took our first apartment.) I think it was about 10 years, give or take a couple.

We met at a summer resort where I had gone for a weekend alone and she had gone with friends. We were both recent refugees from bad marriages and, when I discovered her, I thought a miracle had happened. She was my ideal woman: independent, cheerful, optimistic, able and willing to take care of herself, and full of spontaneous warmth and affection. All this in stark contrast to my own habitual reserve.

Almost from the beginning, the pattern of our relationship established itself. We worked all week, and on the weekends jumped into a breathless round of good food, good fun and good sex. Then, on Sunday night, she'd drive away, and we'd go from the glamorous to the prosaic until the next weekend.

When we had seen all the shows, done all the museums, picnicked in all the parks, we took weekend excursions out of the city. She took me to Bar Harbor, Cape Cod. I showed her Tanglewood and Fire Island. To-gether, we discovered Nantucket, Block Island, Bermuda.

When something interesting happened in her life away from me, she would phone and talk, chatting animatedly about this event or that. These calls were hard for me. After the intensity of our weekends, I wanted time to myself, but when she called, wanting to share her good feelings, I didn't know how to say "Please stop."

We lived like this for more than a year, a fantasy existence of meetings and partings. It came to an end when she decided to move to the city and go to graduate school, and she moved in with me.

At first I was terrified. I had lived with only one other woman in my adult life, and it hadn't worked. Here we were in a small sublet apartment. She was gregarious, I was aloof. She was warm, I was cool. I didn't see how it could last.

That it did was because of our real and deep caring. There was some profound need that we fulfilled, each for the other, and this took precedence over the equally real differences that, for the time being, took second place.

For several years we lived as a married couple without benefit of

TABLE 20–1 Major categories of death for men: by rank

Cause of Death	Number of Men Who Died	Rate per 100,000
1. Heart Attack	397,097	345.2
2. Cancer	242,790	211.1
3. Accidents	64,053	55.7
4. Stroke	61,697	53.6
5. Chronic obstructive lung disease	44,013	38.3
6. Pneumonia/influenza	29,440	25.6
7. Suicide	22,689	19.7
8. Liver disease	17,558	15.3
9. Homicide	15,038	13.1
10. Diabetes	14,859	12.9

Source: National Center of Health Statistics (1986). Vital Statistics of the United States, 1984. Washington DC: U.S. Government Printing Office.

marriage. From time to time we argued, she accusing me of not wanting to make a commitment, I agreeing, saying that I could make no promise for the future, that I only knew how I felt at that moment.

The fights were symptoms, not causes, of the tension that had arisen between us. We were living in the real world now, and our differences were making themselves felt. We had a traditional middle-class life, but, more and more, I felt that I was trying to be someone I was not, and periodically I fell into a depression and would withdraw from her until it passed and I felt better. Then the cycle began again.

I wanted to understand why this was happening, whether this apparent inability to give her what she needed was unique to me. I knew, because she had told me, that when women get together they often complain about their men, and often the complaints come down to this: in one way or another the men are withholding.

The more I thought about it, the more I was convinced that, despite contemporary efforts to make us alike, there are real and enduring differences between women and men, and there always have been. I believe that women actually are more feeling. They do thrive on intimacy, have more and closer friendships with others of their sex, are more likely to reach out and touch with their emotions. What they do naturally, they naturally do well.

Men, by and large, relate very differently. When we gather socially, we talk about things, not feelings. We view life as a challenge, other men as threats. We are more private, less communicative, more interested in goals than relationships.

As if in some cruel joke, it seems that whatever one sex needs most, the other is least equipped to provide (with the single exception of sex itself), so men and women keep coming together and bouncing off each other like the wrong ends of a magnet.

In the blush of first romance, the differences seem unimportant, but if a relationship continues, inevitably one partner emerges as the dominant force. In our case, we each wanted our own way, but our ways were not the same. So she exerted steady, unrelenting pressure, while I let resentment build until it surfaced in periodic outbursts.

Now that I had it all figured out, surely we could repair the mess we were in. But too much had happened on the journey to where we now stood. The old feelings just weren't there anymore.

It seemed like such a waste to throw it all away. Some of the best moments of our lives had been spent together. But for all the laughter and tenderness and love, the basic insurmountable differences were stronger at last.

Perhaps, I thought, if we went back to the beginning we could work it out. We could live in separate apartments and have separate lives during the week, coming together on weekends. She would have the companionship of her women friends. I would have my quiet, my precious solitude. We could be together because we wanted to, not out of routine or habit or outdated custom. We would create a relationship to accommodate our differing needs and all would be well again.

But it was a fantasy years ago, when we had it, and it was a fantasy now, when I dreamed it. The truth was not so simple; the reality was not so nice. And so it ended.

Source: The *New York Times,* "About Men," by Robert Ragaini, Jan 11, 1987, p. 38.

(Grimm & Yarnold, 1985), including the endorsement of traditional male-role norms (Thompson, Grisanti, & Pleck, 1985). The prime example of the Type A personality is the highly competitive business executive who narrows his life to the single goal of success at work, or "compulsive achievement" (Garamoni & Schwartz, 1986). Brusqueness and hostility are additional features of this personality type (Strube, 1984). Type A behavior may also sometimes be adaptive. Recent research indicates that although Type As are more prone to develop heart disease, after having a heart attack they appear no more likely to die than other men. It is not known for certain, but they may use their hard-driving personality to lower their cholesterol and blood pressure and get their smoking under control (Roberts, 1988).

A number of studies confirm that the systolic blood pressure of Type A persons rises significantly just prior to a challenging or ambiguous task, as though they were getting "psyched-up" for battle (for example, Blumenthal, Lane, & Williams, 1985; Contrada, Wright, & Glass, 1984). These findings extend even to elementary school boys, showing that the pattern begins early in life (Mathews & Jennings, 1984).

Obviously, the nurse who cares for cardiac patients is in a good position to detect signs of Type A behavior. Regardless of whether the patient shows signs of Type A behavior, he is likely to progress through the emotions typical of cardiac patients: from anxiety, to denial, and then to depression (Cassem & Hackett, 1978). Hostility and dependency are also common reactions. Male patients have the

Box 20–2 ● Taking It

In 1944, at the age of eleven, I had polio. I spent the next two years of my life in an orthopedic hospital, appropriately called a reconstruction home. By 1946, when I returned to my native Bronx, polio had reconstructed me to the point that I walked very haltingly on steel braces and crutches.

But polio also taught me that, if I were to survive, I would have to become a man—and become a man quickly. "Be a man!" my immigrant father urged, by which he meant "become an American." For, in 1946, this country had very specific expectations about how a man faced adversity. Endurance, courage, determination, stoicism—these might right the balance with fate.

"I couldn't take it, and I took it," says the wheelchair-doomed poolroom entrepreneur William Einhorn in Saul Bellow's *The Adventures of Augie March.* "And I *can't* take it, yet I do take it." In 1953, when I first read these words, I knew that Einhorn spoke for me—as he spoke for scores of other men who had confronted the legacy of a maiming disease by risking whatever they possessed of substance in a country that believed that such risks were a man's wagers against his fate.

How one faced adversity was, like most of American life, in part a question of gender. Simply put, a woman endured, but a man fought back. You were better off struggling against the effects of polio as a man than as a woman, for polio was a disease that one confronted by being tough, aggressive, decisive, by assuming that all limitations could be overcome, beaten, conquered. In short, by being "a man." Even the vocabulary of rehabilitation was masculine. One "beat" polio by outmuscling the disease. At the age of eighteen, I felt that I was "a better man" than my friends because I had "overcome a handicap." And I had, in the process, showed that I could "take it." In the world of American men, to take it was a sign that you were among the elect. An assumption my "normal" friends shared. "You're lucky," my closest friend said to me during an intensely painful crisis in his own life. "You had polio." He meant it. We both believed it.

Obviously, I wasn't lucky. By nineteen, I was already beginning to understand—slowly, painfully, but inexorably—that disease is never "conquered" or "overcome." Still, I looked upon resistance to polio as the essence of my manhood. As an American, I was self-reliant. I could create my own possibilities from life. And so I walked mile after mile on braces and crutches. I did hundreds

most difficulty with feelings of anxiety and dependency, which they often express as hostility (see Box 20–2).

While the stress-management programs of many coronary-care units will help men change their stress-related habits, they may not go far enough in evaluating hypermasculinity as an underlying trait. David Allen and Marianne Whatley (1986) make this point well:

Adaptation/coping models fail to question the nature of what is beng adapted to. Certainly the emphasis on cardiovascular fitness and the emotional benefits of aerobic exercise are important, but often the assumption is that men should exercise to achieve social identities as males—often defined as status, material success, and power over others. Rather than assume men should adapt to those models of male identity, a men's health movement should open those issues for debate, asking whether to transform the executive, his workplace, or both (p. 9).

ACCIDENTS

For men under age 45, death and disability are more likely the result of accidents than heart disease or cancer (Committee on Trauma Research, 1985). Many of these accidents are due to the dangerous occupa-

of push-ups every day to build my arms, chest, and shoulders. I lifted weights to the point that I would collapse, exhausted but strengthened, on the floor. And through it all, my desire to create a "normal" life for myself was transformed into a desire to become the man my disease had decreed I should be.

I took my heroes where I found them—a strange, disparate company of men: Hemingway, whom I would write of years later as "my nurse"; Peter Reiser, whom I dreamed of replacing in Ebbets Field's pastures and whose penchant for crashing into outfield walls fused in my mind with my own war against the virus; Franklin Delano Roosevelt, who had scornfully faced polio with aristocratic disdain and patrician distance (a historian acquaintance recently disabused me of that myth, a myth perpetrated, let me add, by almost all of Roosevelt's biographers); Henry Fonda and Gary Cooper, in whose resolute Anglo-Saxon faces Hollywood blended the simplicity, strength and courage a man needed if he was going to survive as a man; any number of boxers in whom heart, discipline and training combined to stave off defeats the boy's limitations made inevitable. These were the "manly" images I conjured up as I walked those miles of Bronx streets, as I did those relentless push-ups, as I moved up and down one subway staircase after another by turning each concrete step into a personal insult. And they were still the images when, fifteen years later, married, the father of two sons of my own, a Fulbright professor in the Netherlands, I would grab hold of vertical poles in a train in The Hague and swing my brace-bound body across the dead space between platform and carriage, filled with self-congratulatory vanity as amazement spread over the features of the Dutch conductor.

It is easy to dismiss such images as adolescent. Undoubtedly they were. But they helped remind me, time and time again, of how men handled their pain. Of course, I realized even then that it was not the idea of manhood alone that had helped me fashion a life out of polio. I might write of Hemingway as "my nurse," but it was an immigrant Jewish mother—already transformed into a cliché by scores of male Jewish writers—who serviced my crippled body's needs and who fed me love, patience and care even as I fed her the rhetoric of my rage.

But it was the need to prove myself an American man—tough, resilient, independent, able to take it—that pulled me through the war with the virus. I have, of course, been reminded again and again of the price extracted for such ideas about manhood. And I am willing to admit that my sons may be better off in a country in which "manhood" will mean little more than, say, the name for an after-shave lotion. It is forty years since my war with the virus began. At fifty-one, even an American man knows that mortality is the only legacy and defeat the only guarantee. At fifty-one, my legs still encased in braces, and crutches still beneath my shoulders, my elbows are increasingly arthritic from all those streets walked and weights lifted and stairs climbed. At fifty-one, my shoulders burn with pain from all those push-ups done so relentlessly. And at fifty-one, pain merely bores—and hurts.

Still, I remain an American man. If I know where I'm going, I know, too, where I have been. Best of all, I know the price I have paid. A man endures his diseases until he recognizes in them his vanity. He can't take it, but he takes it. Once, I relished my ability to take it. Now I find myself wishing that taking it were easier. In such quiet surrenders do we American men call it quits with our diseases.

Source: Klein, E., & Ericson D. (Eds.) (1987). *About men: Reflections on the male experience*. NY: Pocket Books, pp. 250–252.

---

tions men hold such as mining and construction (Ossler, 1986), but many are due to daredevil recklessness. For example, when states repeal laws mandating the wearing of helmets for motorcycle riders, the number of men wearing helmets decreases to fifty percent despite the forty percent increased risk of death or disability they face (Watson, Zador, & Wilks, 1980). As another example, one wonders how far we have come from the duelling knights when we hear of teenaged boys trying to show their fearlessness by playing deadly driving games such as "chicken." We also know that some deaths labeled as accidental are actually from suicide or the abuse of alcohol.

SUICIDE

Although more women attempt suicide, more men succeed (Goldberg, 1980). Even when taking their own lives men are "macho" and tend to use lethal, violent means such as guns and hanging. Men's suicides are often dramatic, in extreme cases taking family members with them or staging a shoot-out with the police. It may be understandable why the man who loses a job or intimate relationship sinks into despair, but the man who appears to "have everything" may become so lonely at the top that his life becomes meaningless.

Signs of suicidal intent need to be taken seriously by family, friends, or health care professionals in a

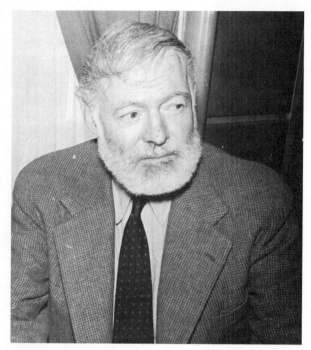

Many celebrities find it "lonely at the top." Alcohol is often turned to by the "macho" man, first, as a source of relief from the pain of loneliness, and, then, for some, as a means to the end: "slow suicide." Hemingway lived life in the fast lane until 1961, when, at age 62, he shot himself through the roof of his mouth with a hunting rifle.

position to observe them. If these signs, such as jokes about dying and organizing life affairs, are not responded to, the man may have his feelings confirmed that no one cares for him.

ALCOHOL AND OTHER DRUGS

Alcoholism has been called "slow suicide." Men turn to the bottle for relief from depression, for a social lubricant, and for one more chance to prove their manliness; however, after the initial lift, they only experience the depressant effects of alcohol. Men may attempt to use alcohol to become charming to women and feel sexual, but often end up being the opposite—obnoxious and impotent. With continued abuse, it may only be a matter of time before alcohol leads to a serious automobile accident or cirrhosis of the liver (see Chapter 15 on substance abuse.)

Promoted by advertising, the ties between manliness and the ability to drink a lot create great pressure on men. For example, the rite of passage in col-

lege fraternities known as hazing sometimes includes coercing initiates to drink large quantities of alcohol. The results are sometimes lethal. Men may also be attracted to drugs that have a higher risk and stronger "kick," such as cocaine. The highly publicized deaths of collegiate and professional athletes from cocaine overdoses may help men realize that cocaine is far from being a recreational drug. (See Chapter 15 on substance abuse.)

ASSAULTS AND HOMICIDE

Civilization's written history is a history of wars, riots, bloody crusades, duels, and torture, mostly among men. It is tempting to conclude that men are innately aggressive, yet there is plenty of evidence that aggression is learned. There are, for example, cultures in which peace is the norm, for example, the Tasaday tribe in the Philippines; but in our patriarchal society, the norm is quite different (Sanday, 1981). The United States is particularly violent, being one of the world's leaders in homicide rates. Some authors have analyzed connections between the need to show masculine toughness and the warring behavior of recent United States presidents (Fasteau, 1980). On an individual level the escalation of conflict leading to violence is related to the difficulty men have in backing down from confrontation (Toch, 1969).

SEXUALITY

Sexuality strongly affects the emotional health of men. The first information men receive about sex is from peers and is usually misinformation. The notion that men naturally know what sex is all about, combined with their reluctance to ask for advice, keep many sexual myths intact (Zilbergeld, 1976). Even though the sexual revolution has provided boys and men with more information about sex, the changes may be superficial. Instead of trying to have sex with many partners, men may now try to be "technically" proficient in pleasing one partner. When the man simply strives for competence he may suffer from impotence or premature ejaculation because the focus is on performance rather than intimate exchange (Gross, 1978).

The growing fear of sexually transmitted diseases, in particular AIDS, is making sex education available to a larger number of boys. This fear has also meant that men are restricting the number of their sexual partners. It is not yet known if the anxiety over sexually transmitted diseases will lead to more sexual disorders. (See Box 20–3.)

THE MIDLIFE CRISIS

Doubts about sexual performance are a major source of worry for most men, and these doubts are most likely to occur during the middle of their lives. It is in the turmoil of the midlife crisis that men also become preoccupied with their health. These health concerns are described by Nancy Mayer:

> This is the time of life . . . when a man begins to worry about his body. Suddenly he suffers from prostate troubles and pulled muscles. Suddenly he needs glasses or root canal work. His cholesterol count goes up, his energy level down. His body is less reliable on the tennis court, less resilient under stress. He can no longer work such long hours or travel at his usual hectic pace.
>
> He finds it maddening, this loss of control. He feels that his body has betrayed him.
>
> High blood pressure develops and so do ulcers. Psychosomatic illnesses erupt: A man is suddenly beset by chronic fatigue, acute indigestion, mysterious backaches, painful joints, and migraine headaches. He complains a lot or even becomes hypochondriacal, convinced that every cold is the forerunner of pneumonia, every pain the sign of cancer, and every rapid heartbeat the precursor of a coronary (1978, p. 22).

Despite the high rate of morbidity for men, they are less likely to seek medical help than are women, perhaps because men do not readily perceive or admit to somatic distress (Forrester, 1986). Sometimes a self-help book can be a useful adjunct to nursing intervention. The book *Men's Bodies, Men's Selves* (Julty, 1979) is especially useful because it was written specifically for men and covers all of the male problems discussed above, plus many more.

IS HYPERMASCULINITY HARMFUL TO WOMEN'S AND CHILDREN'S HEALTH?

While they are growing up, boys are encouraged to fight with other boys, but they are often told they should not pick on girls or anyone else smaller than they are. Somewhere on the road to adulthood, an opposing message often takes precedence—that women and children are the property of men, property to control and protect. For some men, the pattern of control is continuous while for others it appears to erupt when their own lives are out of control. Men's restricted emotionality can be a factor. The fear and hurt they feel are not manly emotions, and so are quickly channeled into anger and then aggression. When men realize the damage they cause to loved ones, they may react with guilt and shame; however, they will need to go beyond these emotions and become aware of the hurt and rage that is theirs as a result of living in our society.

VIOLENCE AGAINST WOMEN

Men who rape women or beat their partners were once thought to be deviant and "sick" or reacting to extreme provocation from their victims. We now know that neither of these notions is true. These men often look perfectly normal and don't necessarily have DSM-III-R diagnoses. Approximately one-third of all married women experience some form of physical abuse sometime during their marriages (Straus, Gelles, & Steinmetz, 1980). We also know that dating and divorced women are not immune from this violence (Makepeace, 1983) and that the violence includes sexual assault in the form of "date rape" and marital rape (Finkelhor & Yllo, 1985; Russell, 1982). Sexual assault by strangers continues to be a problem but we are more aware today that the home is often not the peaceful sanctuary we would like to think it is.

The differences between the wife abuser or rapist and other men may be slight. Studies of male college students show that their attitudes about rape and wife beating do not differ greatly from those of rapists and wife abusers (Malamuth, 1981; Saunders et al., 1987). Abusers are more likely to have experienced abuse in childhood (Straus, Gelles, & Steinmetz, 1980), be nonassertive (Rosenbaum & O'Leary, 1981), and be in autocratic types of relationships (Yllo, 1983). There is some evidence that they suffer from low self-esteem. Men who batter their partners are more likely than other men to abuse their children (Hotaling & Sugarman, 1986); thus, it is important for the nurse to ask about all types of family violence if any one type is detected.

Men who batter may show many different types of psychiatric disorders, but rarely seek help voluntarily. Alcoholism, dependent personality, and narcissistic personality disorders seem to be common; severe mental disorders appear to be rare. There is some speculation that there is more than one type of man who physically abuses his wife (Hofeller, 1980). One type of batterer is very dependent on his partner and is violent only at home and on the occasions during which he fears abandonment; he may show a great deal of affection most of the time. The other type has a dominant, antisocial personality and is violent both inside and outside of the home. His general attitudes

Box 20–3 ● AIDS and Mental Health

The first cases of AIDS were discovered in the United States in 1979. By 1981 it was apparent that most patients were homosexual men, and the complex of symptoms was identified as a new disease, the acquired immune deficiency syndrome. Medical care of the earliest patients was complicated by fears of contagion and prejudice against homosexuals. As the number of cases grew, the ethical, social, political and psychological ramifications became more extensive. Intravenous drug users emerged as a second socially stigmatized risk group. Studying the transmission of AIDS meant exploring sexual practices and drug use—sensitive areas in which confidentiality was a major issue. National hysteria grew when 'innocent victims' were found among hemophiliacs and other recipients of blood transfusions.

After the virus that causes AIDS was identified in 1984, the blood supply could be protected and people carrying the AIDS antibody could be notified and counseled. Infection control guidelines reduced the anxiety of medical personnel and fellow employees of AIDS patients. It remains important to educate the public about safe sex and hygienic drug use, and to reduce fear by means of clear and accurate medical information. Each case provides an opportunity to teach health care workers and the patient's family and friends about AIDS and mental health.

The AIDS Patient

The patient must confront an uncertain progression of painful and debilitating symptoms. Slow thinking and poor memory are early signs that the virus has affected the brain. Repeated hospitalizations are required to treat opportunistic infections, especially a rare form of pneumonia (*Pneumocystis carinii*). Patients who develop Kaposi's sarcoma have purple skin lesions on exposed parts of their bodies. Antibiotics, steroids and interferon used to treat the symptoms may produce emotional symptoms and physical side effects. The few promising new drugs have not yet proved themselves.

The social effects are also painful. Patients commonly suffer discrimination in health care, housing, public assistance and employment. Fear of contagion may make them pariahs. When concealed homosexuality becomes known to the patient's family, the impact can be overwhelming. Patients often feel guilty about having exposed others. A number of children have been born with the disease, usually to parents who are intravenous drug users. In caring for these patients, individual or family counseling must be part of the plan.

AIDS patients respond to their illness in much the same way as people with cancer or any other illness likely to be fatal. One difference is that a person with AIDS has usually

---

about women are more negative and he is likely to have multiple marriages and a criminal lifestyle (see Box 20–4).

Because most abusive men do not usually present themselves to medical facilities, it is usually the women who first reveal the abuse. Due to her feelings of shame about being a battered woman, she may only hint about the abuse and present vague somatic complaints and show signs of depression. The detection of abuse is best accomplished with the use of direct and detailed questions. If abuse is detected in the presence of both partners, it is best to separate them for further assessment so the victim can feel comfortable talking about the abuse. Separate assessments are also needed because men have been shown to minimize the abuse even more than the women.

There is at least one practical handbook for guiding emergency medical personnel with the problem of domestic violence (NJDCA, 1985). However, emergency rooms are not the only medical units in which battered women appear (Braham et al., 1986; Campbell & Humphrey, 1984). For example, a

been anticipating the diagnosis for months, and therefore may greet it with a kind of relief instead of denial. But anxiety and depression persist throughout the course of the illness. Common symptoms are agitation, tension, insomnia, loss of appetite and panic attacks. The patient may develop a clinical depression, with intense feelings of hopelessness, helplessness, isolation and guilt. Awareness of lost mental capacity also causes depression. Thoughts of suicide are common; in our experience, AIDS patients are more likely to attempt suicide than cancer patients. Many people with AIDS contemplate future refusal of life support measures after witnessing the death of a friend from the disease.

Patients may understandably be suspicious of others' motives and expect rejection. They are often angry at their doctors and the public. A psychiatrist is most often consulted for depression, anxiety, delirium, dementia, or assistance in home care. The most common diagnosis is adjustment disorder with depressed or anxious mood; the second most common is major depression. . . .

Clinical Management

All patients should have access to social workers to plan physical and financial assistance and referral to local AIDS self-help crisis organizations. Early psychiatric consultation is recommended for anxiety and depression and for evaluating mental status. Mental health professionals caring for people with AIDS should become aware of any possible fears and prejudices of their own that might interfere with their work. Having the latest available information about AIDS is important to avoid misinforming patients and others. The health professional treating an AIDS patient must feel comfortable in discussing sexual matters and know enough about bisexuality and homosexuality to understand the problems involved. Familiarity with the typical psychological problems of intravenous drug users is essential in caring for them. Health professionals should learn to recognize and evaluate early signs of dementia and other brain diseases and distinguish them from depression and anxiety. Benzodiazepines can be used to control anxiety and insomnia; antidepressants are useful for insomnia as well as depression. In most communities the local AIDS self-help group is the best source of social, practical and educational services for people with AIDS. Health care professionals should maintain relationships with these organizations and use them to make referrals to support groups and psychotherapy.

Health care workers must also be prepared to help AIDS patients with practical and psychological problems. Anxiety and panic should be anticipated and discussed. Patients should be informed about available treatments and research. They should be encouraged to explore their feelings about sexual practices and develop a sense of responsibility about spreading contagion. Anal and vaginal intercourse are the riskiest practices, but the disease can also be transmitted by oral intercourse. People with AIDS should be advised to abstain from sexual intercourse, or, failing that, to use a condom and withdraw before ejaculation. Intravenous drug users must be urged to enter drug treatment programs or at least to sterilize injection equipment and avoid sharing needles.

Patients should be encouraged to express anger and direct it constructively, perhaps through volunteer service and political activism. They must be assured that care will be continuous and that the symptoms will be controlled as much as possible. A home care program should be designed to provide 24-hour monitoring of physical symptoms and emotional distress. The patient should be allowed an opportunity to discuss concerns about death and terminal care. . . .

Source: Holland, J. C. & Tross, S. (1987). Aids and mental health. *The Harvard Medical School Mental Health Letter, 4*(1), p. 4-5.

---

woman confided to a nurse at an infertility clinic that she had been "shoved around" by her husband. That was the reason that she was sobbing—not the fact that she had been unable to conceive. Her husband, Bill, had been blaming her for her inability to become pregnant. The nurse asked the physician to help interview Bill to see if he would admit to abusing his wife and accept a referral to a specialized treatment program. The section on counseling will illustrate some statements that can be made to the abuser to help him to open up.

ABUSE AND NEGLECT OF CHILDREN

As described earlier, the absence of a father takes an emotional toll on boys. Girls also suffer from this absence. Fathers often withdraw further from daughters or act harshly toward them when their daughters reach puberty, fearing their own sexual feelings—again, men's difficulty in separating sex from affection plays a part.

Abuse of children can take two forms: physical abuse and incest. **Physical abuse,** defined here to include slaps and spankings, occurs in nearly every U.S.

Box 20–4 ●
Picasso: A Man's Man

War was in his pictures—not this war, not any particular war, but the darkness and the anger and the hatred that cause wars. In June the German army marched into Royan and Picasso painted one of his most brutal and vengeful images of womanhood: Dora as the *Nude Dressing Her Hair*. The brutality was no less present in his life. He often beat Dora, and there were many times when he left her lying unconscious on the floor. The transformation of the princess into a toad and of sensuality into horror was complete. And in the dog-face portraits he painted of Dora, he completed the transformation of woman into servile animal. As the art historian Mary Gedo put it, Dora, like his Afghan hound Kazbek, "came whenever he whistled." More than two thirds of his work during 1939 and 1940 consisted of deformed women, their faces and bodies flayed with fury. His hatred of a specific woman seemed to have become a deep and universal hatred of all women.

"He had a warrior's mentality," Picasso's cousin Manuel Blasco said. "Fight during the day and fornicate at night." In November of 1965, in conspiratorial secrecy, Picasso was taken to the American Hospital in Neuilly for gall-bladder and prostate surgery. From then on there would be only fighting. For a warrior who had worn his virility like a badge, the end of his sexual life was a terrible calamity. It looked as though the operation might signal the end of his fighting days, too. During the rest of 1965 and up to December of 1966 he drew and he etched, but he did no painting. It was the longest he had ever been away from the battlefield. "When a man knows how to do something," he told the bullfighter Luis Miguel Dominguín, "he ceases being a man if he stops doing it."

Source: Huffington, Arianna Stassinopoulos (1988). Creator and destroyer. *The Atlantic*, June, p. 37–78.

---

family. This so-called "minor" physical punishment needs to be addressed because it is associated with child abuse and wife abuse later in life (Straus, 1983). Although more mothers than fathers are physically abusive toward their children, fathers are more likely to have proviolence attitudes. In addition, this increased frequency of abuse of children by their mothers is largely due to the greater time mothers are with children (Pagelow, 1984) and the displacement of aggression they receive from their husbands (Walker, 1984). (See Chapter 18 on crisis.)

Father-daughter incest is more prevalent than other types of parent-child incest (Finkelhor & Russell, 1984). Compared to physical abuse, however, sexual abuse is cloaked by stronger taboos and thus is more difficult to detect. Some assumptions about incest have recently been challenged; for example, the notions that incest is caused by marital conflict and the mother's complicity, or that incest offenders are quite different from child molesters (pedophiles) (Conte, 1985).

In addition to the difficulties in detecting signs of incest, both professionals and nonprofessionals are likely to avoid suspected cases because of the strong emotions elicited by the topic of incest.

Kerry: A Victim of Incest

Kerry was a 6-year-old girl who was evaluated several times at the hospital for urinary tract infections. She was also not doing well in first grade and was being evaluated for a possible learning disability. During her morning bath Kerry told the nurse that she and her father played a "game" when they took a bath together. At first the nurse wanted to ignore her suspicions of sexual abuse but she knew that she had to ask Kerry some specific questions about the "game." Kerry began to cry, saying that she didn't want to get her father in trouble and that he had threatened to hurt her if she told anyone.

The nurse obtained enough details of sexual abuse to contact the hospital's child protection team.

A county child protection worker could also have been contacted. Because she had some rapport with Kerry's father, the nurse asked to meet with the child protection team when they confronted the father with the suspicion of sexual abuse. Before the meeting, the nurse found it useful to talk with her supervisor and fellow nurses about the revulsion she felt toward the father. In the meeting, she became angry when the father denied the abuse, and then saw some hope when he broke down and showed how revulsed he was by his own behavior. After many weeks of therapy at a sexual abuse treatment center, the father was able to reveal that he had compulsive sexual urges toward many children and often felt helpless in trying to control them.

RESISTANCE TO PSYCHOSOCIAL TREATMENT

It is enough of an ego bruise for many men to find they have a physical problem and are in need of medical help. The mere suggestion that a man may need psychiatric help can send him scurrying the other way. The value that men place on self-reliance, the fear they have of the unknown, and their focus on external reality make them reluctant users of mental health services. It is no wonder that women are the most frequent initiators of individual and couples therapy. Special clinical skills are often required to lower the defenses of men who refuse to look at psychological issues. This becomes especially true when men are acutely ill, feeling out of control, and facing female nurses who have some control over them (see Box 20–5).

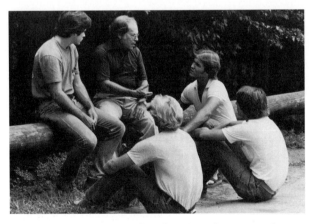

While individual counseling has its advantages (e.g., privacy), peer group counseling can be both appealing and effective in modeling the way to find help by helping someone else.

Swanson and Woolson (1973) trained nursing students to use psychotherapeutic techniques with unmotivated patients. Among the principles they used for enhancing motivation were:

- To have the patient actively involved in setting goals for therapy and prioritizing those goals
- To focus on the patient's satisfying memories and present feelings
- To set concrete goals in the patient's terms
- To fantasize about positive results of therapy
- To use a sequence of definite, practical steps for trying out changes
- To give regular feedback, with a large dose of it being positive

METHODS FOR COUNSELING MEN

Whether seeking help voluntarily or involuntarily, men come to the helping relationship with the pain of their alienation coupled with a need for intimacy. The need for intimacy is usually hidden because of a simultaneous desire to maintain autonomy. Nurses need to be aware of the powerful forces on men today to change and yet remain the same.

DeHoff and Forrest (1984, p. 20) suggest several points to keep in mind when identifying the health care needs of men:

- Giving them permission to have health concerns and to openly talk about them
- Assistance and support in considering male role influences on their physical and mental health
- Attention to lifestyle factors that may result in an illness (for example, occupation, leisure patterns, personal/sexual relationships)
- Recognition that a sense of confusion is normal and may even be adaptive during times of rapid social change (for example, changes in sex roles)
- A flexible health care system that adjusts to constraints imposed by men's occupations and makes it possible for men to obtain health care.

For men who are fathers, an important role for the nurse is to understand the uncertainty and anxiety with which they face this role. Fathers need to be supported in their attempts to become directly involved with their children and to feel more fulfilled in their role as father. For example, the increased attendance of fathers at childbirth classes and visits to obstetrics clinics provides an early opportunity to understand their fears and sense of isolation. Although reluctant to reveal their feelings, expectant fa-

Box 20–5 ● Men and Couples Therapy

Fifteen years ago, divorce was most often initiated by men; couples therapy was almost always initiated by women. Today, most divorces are initiated by women; and therapy is increasingly initiated by men.

According to marital therapists across the country, therapy issues have changed as well. Ten years ago the major theme was "self-fulfillment." Today the issues include "bonding," dual-career marriages, roles, and how to spend what little leisure time the couple has. Then and now common relationship problems have to do with communication, conflict resolution, and sexual dissatisfaction.

Another change is that couples are seeking therapy sooner these days. In fact, there is a growing interest in *pre*marital therapy, especially, for the previously married who don't want to make the same mistake twice. Here, again, increasingly, it is the men who are initiating the therapy.

The next thing you know, they'll be eating quiche.

Source: Lear, M. W. (1988) Men and therapy, *New York Times Magazine*, March 6, pp. 63-64.

thers are likely to have queasiness about the birth process, fear about increased financial responsibility, fear of the mother and/or child dying during childbirth, and fear of being replaced by the infant (Shapiro, 1987).

Whatever the presenting problem, male nurses are in a unique position to disclose their own struggles with gender-role strain (Morgan, 1981). A prerequisite, of course, is that they have developed an awareness of their own gender-role issues (Collison, 1981).

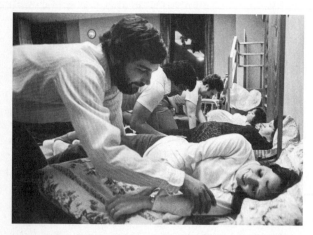

Lamaze teaches an expectant father to attend to his wife's every sound and movement. Perhaps this is a way of preparing her to do exactly the same for her baby, in the service of the development of a strong and healthy sense of *self* (Stern, 1988).

While men may tend to disclose more to female nurses (Feldstein, 1979), female nurses face their own set of challenges (Carlson, 1981). For example, they may need to learn to feel comfortable when men cry. They may find it necessary to deal with men's anger over their fear of dependency and simultaneous wish for female attachment. Finally, female nurses need to avoid the trap of giving simple assurances to men about their worth.

Female nurses may also have difficulty dealing with the chauvinism of male patients. Men may react to the female nurse as someone who "cannot possibly understand the unique male experience" (Forrester, 1986). The men may exhibit evasive or dishonest communication, or worse, the view that male physicians and male nurses are more competent.

The interview process needs to move slowly in identifying issues associated with physical and psychic pain. Male patients may need "permission" from a nurse to feel physical pain and then to express emotions about it. Some humor might be useful, for example, to say "Death will be your body's way of telling you to slow down." Most men find it easier to express anger than hurt or fear, and the anger may be expressed about seemingly irrelevant topics. When asking about feelings the nurse may have to repeat the question several times. It is usually best to avoid asking questions beginning with "why" because they are likely to elicit endless explanations but little emotional awareness.

Feelings may have to be elicited indirectly by asking about thoughts first; for example, "What thoughts do you have if you think of this (condition/

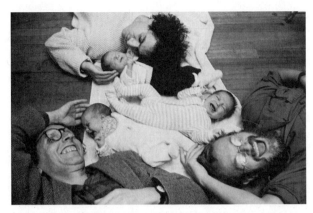

It is important for fathers to become involved in their children's development as early as possible and to have the support of others in the process.

illness) returning? . . . or not going away?" Grief reactions are likely to be triggered and should be dealt with whether or not full health is restored. Illness and recovery still mean that the man may have lost his sense of invulnerability and thus he has a need to grieve.

If a behavior harmful to another person, such as wife or child abuse, is detected, then a combination of empathy and confrontation is likely to motivate the man to seek further help. Either empathy or confrontation alone will not be enough. The following is an example of a nurse-patient dialogue combining the two (for more on assessment, see Saunders, 1982):

Man: She was probably out chasing men. I caught her once with another man.

Nurse: You thought she was with another man, and you felt upset and angry? (empathy) Even if she was, what you did to her was clearly against the law. (confront)

Man: She deserved it. If she wants to leave, good riddance.

Nurse: Does it upset you to think of her leaving you? (empathy)

Man: Yeah, I don't know what's happening.

Nurse: You seem to let your fears get to you, then you boil over and want to control her. (empathy and clarification)

Man: Yeah, sometimes my mind goes pretty far out.

Once the problems are identified, the consequences of continued maladaptive behavior can be explored and alternatives generated (Collison, 1981). Men will feel more comfortable if therapy is structured and concrete decisions result from it. Thus behavioral and cognitive therapies that take the mystery out of the therapy process seem more palatable to most men, at least initially. Pharmacological and unstructured, psychoanalytic approaches are likely to threaten their sense of self-control. Strategies for change may involve an appeal to the male patient's self-interest, his sense of altruism, or his need to make compromises within an intimate relationship (Lewis, 1981).

Men may need some direct permission to feel vulnerable with a statement such as, "It's OK to admit you can't always be on top of things." After some awareness of the harmful consequences of hypermasculinity develops, a summary of this progress is in order, for example, "You are starting to see that long-term pain outweighs the short-term gains in status and thrills." For a patient who has had a close call with death, it may help to encourage him to think about life goals, potential years remaining, and what he can expect realistically to accomplish in that time.

Case Study: Nonpsychiatric Setting

Ronald Blake was a 39-year-old radio talk show personality at the time he went into the hospital for a corneal transplant operation. He was known throughout the South as "The Tennessee Iron Man" for his all-night program, which he often conducted without any accompanying guests. He was at the peak of his career at the time of the surgery. It bothered him that he would be laid up for at least a week after.

"I really feel restless," he told his wife, while chain-smoking in his private room only one day before surgery. "I'm gonna go crazy just lying here. I'll try and talk them into letting me broadcast live from my bed."

Blake loved the idea. He would be a model for all of the sick people who wallow in self-pity, and that excited him. He was sure his audience would love him for his courage, and that his audience would grow. It would reinforce his "Iron Man" image and at the same time reassure his wife that she didn't have a middle-age invalid on her hands.

Six days after surgery, he was discharged from the hospital, and by then he had become "fast friends" with most of the staff. He had proven to everybody that the "Iron Man" label was no hype by turning his recovery into a party without any complaining, self-pity or special attention.

Three months later he collapsed right after his nightly program and was taken to the hospital with double pneumonia. Two years later he died, "unexpectedly" and suddenly of a heart attack.*

Nursing Diagnoses

Anxiety
Ineffective individual coping
Dysfunctional grieving
Altered health maintenance

*Adapted from Herb Goldberg, *The New Male.* Copyright © 1979 by William Morrow & Company. Reprinted by permission of publisher.

Nursing Care Plan for Ronald

Nursing Diagnosis	Desired Outcomes	Interventions	Rationale
1. Anxiety	Ronald will be able to recognize and effectively manage his anxiety. Ronald will be able to experience and accept his dependency needs and emotional support.	Encourage Ronald to verbalize anxieties about his condition and hospitalization, labeling them as normal. Correct any distorted views he may have about what he is going through. Encourage Ronald to let you know if he feels uncomfortable or anxious; check on him regularly, even if he doesn't call. (Also see Chapter 8 on anxiety disorders.)	Identifying and talking about anxiety and its sources are the first steps in any attempt to master it. (Also see Chapter 8 on anxiety and its treatment.) Attending to Ronald during a bout with anxiety is likely to be more effective than just discussing it with him afterwards. The nurse needs to check on him, not just wait for his call, since this is a patient who resists demonstrating any evidence of dependency.
2. Ineffective individual coping	Ronald will adaptively cope with feelings of inadequacy and temporary dysfunction.	Explore Ronald's feelings about his eye surgery three months ago and his possibly premature return to work. Help him look at the meaning of his behavior as well as its apparent	Helping Ronald see connections between feelings (for example, anxiety about dependency) and behavior, and their consequences (in this case, hospitalization) is

Nursing Diagnosis	Desired Outcomes	Interventions	Rationale
		consequences, including rehospitalization at this time, allowing him to come to his own conclusions.	essential to any attempt to change his maladaptive behavior. Allowing him to come to his own conclusions is likely to be more successful than "preaching" to him would be.
3. Dysfunctional grieving	Ronald will begin and be able to resolve the grieving process associated with the loss of normal vision, health, youth, and so on.	Encourage Ronald to verbalize his feelings about health-related losses, labeling anger, sadness, anxiety, and so on as appropriate; empathize with the difficulties he faces. Help him identify present and potential compensatory attributes, abilities, and so on.	The hospitalized cardiac patient's behavior is often best understood and dealt with in the context of the psychoanalytic model of loss and grief. Empathy is a means of making interpersonal contact with the patient, the essential prologue to a cognitive-behavioral approach to changing maladaptive behavior. (See Chapter 9 on mood disorders for more on dysfunctional grieving and its treatment.)
4. Alteration in health maintenance	Ronald will resume effective health maintenance.	Explore with Ronald his current lifestyle and the health risks it involves. What is the potential for altering diet, quitting smoking, beginning a supervised exercise program, and scheduling adequate rest and relaxation? Examine cost-benefit ratio of present and alternative acceptable lifestyles, allowing Ronald to reach his own conclusions.	A cognitive-behavioral approach is likely to appeal to Ronald more than a focus on feelings (which he may resist out of fear of looking like a "wimp").
		Challenge Ronald to become a success at being healthy, a *new* type of male role model.	Building on the adaptive components of Ronald's personality type (for example, achievement-orientation) rather than trying to change it is an achievable goal. (See Chapter 12 on personality disorders.) Also, there is evidence that the hard-driving Type A man can redirect his energy and motivation to succeed toward health rather than self-destruction.

SUMMARY

It is important for the nurse to understand better the pressures on men in the modern world and try to respond to their special needs. Social pressures on men often lead to their alienation from their work, families, friends, and even from themselves. Most of men's health and psychological problems may be traced to these forms of alienation. The socialization of men also explains why they are reluctant to seek help.

Among the health problems related to the male syndrome of hypermasculinity are heart disease, accidents, suicide, and alcoholism. When men externalize their problems, they all too often hurt the very people they care about—their wives and children. Nurses in all types of settings and roles are in a position to detect the ways in which men harm themselves and others. An understanding of the reasons that men may not appear to need or want help can reduce the nurse's frustrations when she detects or suspects problems in men.

Allen and Whatley (1986) describe the advantages of a socially focused role for nurses and its relationship to men's health: "A central strength of nursing is its attempts to maintain a holistic perspective, to view clients in their social context. Gender is a primary aspect of anyone's social existence" (p. 11). They add that,

> A men's health movement cannot ignore the fact that gender identity is a social process, not a biologic given. . . . This may be somewhat troublesome to nurses since many have unconsciously adopted a vision of nursing as scientific with the concomitant ideal of being value free. . . . [However] if nurses are to participate in a men's health movement that is anything beyond an examination of genitals, they will have to struggle with these social issues (p. 9).

The challenge in providing nursing care to men, therefore, comes from the need to confront men's self-destructive and other-destructive behavior, balanced with the knowledge that there is a pained child inside saturated with years of patriarchal conditioning. The process is likely to be slow at first, but when the bravado finally melts, tremendous change is likely to occur.

KEY TERMS

hypermasculinity   physical abuse

patriarchy

STUDY QUESTIONS

1. Define and describe hypermasculinity.

2. Name and discuss the four major ways in which patriarchy affects men.

3. How does hypermasculinity contribute to the midlife crisis in men?

4. How does hypermasculinity contribute to male violence against women and children?

5. Name several methods that the nurse can use in counseling male patients.

REFERENCES

Allen, D. G., & Whatley, M. (1986). Nursing and men's health: Some critical considerations. *Nursing Clinics of North America, 21,* (1), 3–13.

Blumenthal, J. A., Lane, J. D., & Williams, R. B. (1985). The inhibited power motive, Type A behavior, and patterns of cardiovascular response during the structural interview and Thematic Apperception Test. *Journal of Human Stress, 11*(2), 82–92.

Braham, R., Furniss, K., Holtz, H., & Stevens, M. E. (1986). *Hospital protocol on domestic violence.* Jersey Battered Women's Services, 36 Elm St. Morristown, N.J.

Buunk, B. (1986). Husband's jealousy. In R. A. Lewis & R. E. Salt (1986). *Men in families.* Beverly Hills, CA: Sage.

Campbell, J., & Humphreys, J. (1984). *Nursing care of victims of family violence.* Reston, VA: Reston Publishing.

Carlson, N. L. (1981). Male client—female therapist. *Personnel and Guidance Journal, 10,* 228–231.

Cassem, N. H., & Hackett, T. P. (1978). The setting of intensive care. In N. H. Cassem & T. P. Hackett (Eds.), *MGH handbook of general hospital psychiatry.* St. Louis: C. V. Mosby, pp. 319–341.

Collison, B. B. (1981). Counseling adult males. *Personnel and Guidance Journal, 10,* 219–222.

Committee on Trauma Research (1985). *Injury in America.* Washington, D. C: National Academy Press.

Conte, J. (1985). Clinical dimensions of adult sexual abuse of children. *Behavioral Sciences and the Law, 3*(4), 341-354.

Contrada, R. J., Wright, R. A., & Glass, D. C. (1984). Task difficulty, Type A behavior pattern, and cardiovascular response. *Psychophysiology, 21*(6), 638-646.

DeHoff, J. B., & Forrest, K. A. (1984). Men's health. In J. M. Swanson & K. A. Forrest (Eds.), *Men's reproductive health.* New York: Springer.

Duncan, S. F. (1986). Why some men do not marry. In R. A. Lewis & R. E. Salt (Eds.), *Men in families.* Beverly Hills, CA: Sage.

Erikson, E. (1950). *Childhood and society.* New York: Norton, p. 253.

Fasteau, M. (1980). Vietnam and the cult of toughness in foreign policy. In E. H. Pleck & J. H. Pleck (Eds.) *The American man.* Englewood Cliffs, NJ: Prentice-Hall.

Feldstein, J. C. (1979). Effects of counselor sex and sex role and client sex on client's perceptions and self-disclosure in a counseling analogue study. *Journal of Counseling Psychology, 26,* 437-443.

Finkelhor, D. (1986). *A sourcebook on child sexual abuse.* Beverly Hills, CA: Sage.

Finkelhor, D., & Russell, D. (1984). Women as perpetrators. In D. Finkelhor, *Child sexual abuse.* New York: Free Press.

Finkelhor, D., & Yllo, K. (1985). *License to rape.* New York: Free Press.

Foreman, M. D. (1986). Cardiovascular disease: A men's health hazard. *Nursing Clinics of North America, 21* (1), 65–73.

Forrester, D. A. (1986). Myths of masculinity: Impact on men's health. *Nursing Clinics of North America, 21* (1), 15–23.

Garamoni, G. L., & Schwartz, R. M. (1986). Type A behavior pattern and compulsive personality: Toward a psychodynamic-behavioral integration. *Clinical Psychology Review, 6,* 311–336.

Gerzon, M. (1982). *A choice of heroes: The changing face of American manhood.* Boston: Houghton Mifflin Company.

Goldberg, H. (1980). *The new male.* New York: New American Library.

Goodwin, D. W., & Guze, S. B. (1979). *Psychiatric diagnosis* (2nd ed.). New York: Oxford Press.

Gould, R. (1973). Measuring masculinity by the size of a paycheck. *Ms. 1*(12).

Grimm, L. G., & Yarnold, P. R. (1985). Sex typing and the coronary-prone behavior pattern. *Sex Roles, 12*(1-2), 171–178.

Gross, A. E. (1978). The male role and heterosexual behavior. *Journal of Social Issues, 34*(1), 87–107.

Harrison, J. B. (1984). Warning: The male sex role may be dangerous to your health. In J. M. Swanson & K. A. Forrest (Eds.), *Men's reproductive health.* New York: Springer.

Hite, S. (1981). *The Hite report of male sexuality.* New York: Knopf.

Hofeller, K. H. (1980). Social, psychological and situational factors in wife abuse. Unpublished doctoral dissertation, Claremont Graduate School.

Hotaling, G., & Sugarman, O. (1986). An analysis of risk marker in husband to wife violence: The current state of knowledge. *Violence and Victims, 1*(2), 101–124.

Julty, S. (1979). *Men bodies, men's selves.* New York: Dell Publishing.

Komarovsky, M. (1976). *Dilemmas of masculinity.* New York: Norton.

Lamb, M. E., Pleck, J. H., & Levine, J. A. (1986). Effects of increased parental involvement on children in two-parent families. In R. A. Lewis & R. E. Salt (Eds.), *Men in families.* Beverly Hills, CA: Sage.

Lewis, R. A. (1981). Men's liberation and the men's movement: Implications for counselors. *Personnel and Guidance Journal, 10,* 256–259.

Lewis, R. A. (1986). What men get out of marriage and parenthood. In R. A. Lewis & R. E. Salt (Eds.), *Men in families.* Beverly Hills, CA: Sage.

Makepeace, J. (1983). Life event stress and courtship violence. *Family Relations, 32,* 101-109.

Malamuth, N. (1981). Rape proclivity among males. *Journal of Social Issues, 37,* 138–157.

Mathews, K. A., & Jennings, J. R. (1984). Cardiovascular responses of boys exhibiting the Type A behavior pattern. *Psychosomatic medicine, 46*(6), 484–497.

Mayer, N. (1978). *The male mid-life crisis.* Garden City, NY: Doubleday.

Morgan, R. M. (1981). Counseling the uncoupling male. *Personnel and Guidance Journal, 10,* 237–241.

New Jersey Department of Community Affairs (1985). *Domestic violence: A guide for emergency medical treatment.* Division on Women, New Jersey Department of Community Affairs, 379 West State St., Trenton, NJ 08625.

Osherson, S. (1986). *Finding our fathers: The unfinished business of manhood.* New York: Free Press.

Ossler, C. C. (1986). Men's work environments and health risks. *Nursing Clinics of North America, 21*(1), 25–36.

Pagelow, M. D. (1984). *Family violence.* New York: Praeger.

Pleck, J. (1981). *The myth of masculinity.* Cambridge, MA: MIT Press.

Roberts, M. (1988). Can what harms also heal? *Psychology Today, 22*(2), 8–10.

Rosenbaum, A., & O'Leary, K. D. (1981). Marital violence: Characteristics of abusive couples. *Journal of Consulting and Clinical Psychology, 49*(1), 63–71.

Russell, D. (1982). *Rape in marriage.* New York: Macmillan.

Sanday, P. R. (1981) *Female power and male dominance: On the origins of sexual inequality.* Cambridge: Cambridge University Press.

Saunders, D. G. (1982). Counseling the violent husband. In P. Keller & L. G. Ritt (Eds.), *Innovations in clinical practice: A source book,* Vol I. Sarasota, FL: Professional Resource Exchange.

Saunders, D. G., Lynch, A., Grayson, M., & Linz, D. (1987). The inventory of beliefs about wife-beating: The development and initial validation of a measure of beliefs and attitudes. *Violence and victims, 2*(1), 39–56.

Shapiro, J. L. (1987). The expectant father. *Psychology Today, 21*(1), 36–43.

Shastak, A. (1969). *Blue-collar work.* New York: Random House.

Stein, P. J. (1986). Men and their friendships. In R. A. Lewis & R. E. Salt (Eds.), *Men in families.* Beverly Hills, CA: Sage.

Straus, M. A. (1983). Ordinary violence versus child abuse and beating: What do they have in common? In D. Finkelhor, R. J. Gelles, G. T. Hotaling, & M. A. Straus (Eds.), *The dark side of families.* Beverly Hills, CA: Sage, 17–28.

Straus, M. A., Gelles, R. J., & Steinmetz, S. K. (1980). *Behind closed doors.* New York: Anchor.

Straus, M. A., & Gelles, R. J. (1986). Societal change and change in family violence from 1975 to 1985 as revealed by two national surveys. *Journal of Marriage and the Family, 48,* 465–479.

Strube, M. J. (1984). Interpersonal aggression and the Type A coronary-prone behavior pattern: A theoretical distinction and practical implications. *Journal of Personality and Social Psychology, 47*(4), 839–847.

Swanson, M. G., & Woolson, A. M. (1973). Psychotherapy with the unmotivated patient. *Psychotherapy: Theory, research and practice, 10*(2), 175–183.

Taubman, S. (1986). Beyond the bravado: Sex roles and the exploitive male. *Social Work, 31*(1), 12–18.

Thompson, E. H., Grisanti, C., & Pleck, J. H. (1985). Attitudes toward the male role and their correlates. *Sex Roles, 13*(7-8), 413–414.

Toch, H. (1969). *Violent men.* Chicago: Aldine.

U.S. Department of Health, Education and Welfare (1979). *Monthly vital statistics report—Advance report—Final mortality statistics, 1977.* Hyattsville, MD: National Center for Health Statistics.

U.S. Department of Health & Social Services (1980). *Monthly vital statistics report.* Hyattsville, MD: Author, National Center for Health Statistics.

Waldron, I. (1976). Why do women live longer than men? Part I. *Journal of Human Stress, 2*(1), 2–13.

Waldron, I., & Johnson, S. (1976). Why do women live longer than men? Part II. *Journal of Human Stress, 2*(2), 19–30.

Walker, L. E. (1984). *The battered woman syndrome.* New York: Springer.

Warren, L. W. (1983). Male intolerance of depression: A review with implications for psychotherapy. *Clinical Psychology Review, 3,* 147–156.

Watson, G. S., Zador, P. L., & Wilks, A. (1980). The repeal of helmet use laws and increased motorcyclist mortality in the United States, 1975–1978. *American Journal of Public Health, 70*(6), 579–585.

Weiss, R. S. (1985). Men and the family. *Family Process, 24,* 49–58.

Wolfman, I. (1985). The closer you get, the faster I run. *MS, 14*(3), 34–36 plus 112.

Yllo, K. (1983). Sexual equality and violence against wives in American states. *Journal of Comparative Family Studies, 14*(1), 67–86.

Zilbergeld, B. (1976). *Male sexuality.* New York: Bantam.

PSYCHIATRIC MENTAL HEALTH NURSING WITH FAMILIES

DAVID KEITH

We shall not cease from exploration
And the end of all exploring
Will be to arrive where we started
And know the place for the first time.

—T. S. Eliot

INTRODUCTION

When we talk about psychopathology in families we enter a very different world, one in which there are no individual people because the smallest organisms are families. The individuals in our usual world are like the family's anatomical components; the interpersonal process compares with the family's physiology. In this world we will be a little like Alice in Wonderland. We cannot always tell the meaning of what we see. We cannot always be sure of who *we* are. Just when we think we have the key to unlock the family's mystery, a small shift occurs and we are confused again.

This chapter attempts to help the nurse see the individual patient as a fragment of a family and see how families with psychopathology interact. Clinical work with families demands a creative approach to human experience. When dealing with families, it is often difficult to name what one sees. If the oldest son in a family is depressed, should the clinician consider this a depressed family? If the father is obese, should the clinician call the family obese? Or, because the family includes both of these people, should the clinician describe the family as depressed and obese?

There is no adequate system for discussing family pathology. In early research on families, an effort was made to describe families in relation to the pathology of the identified patient. Thus families were identified as, for example, schizophrenic or anorexic. However, the discriminating features of these families do not hold up. While families with a schizophrenic member have certain patterns in common, the differences are not solid enough to develop a diagnostic system. Part of this trouble is that once it enters the clinic, the family is affected by and reacts to the therapist (de Schazer, 1983). For example, families with a schizophrenic member were once described as "cold and hostile." However, in a clinical setting, these families are frightened; their self-protection may give the appearance of coldness and hostility, eliciting coldness and hostility from caretakers. Continued experience has shown that, as a working relationship is formed, "cold and hostile" family members are often found to be naive about relationships and hungry to learn more (Whitaker, 1978).

Keeney (1983) indicates some of the complications of describing psychopathology in families.

> It is incorrect to assume that psychiatry has "named" all symptomatology. . . . When "pathology" is identified in any social setting, it is likely that other connected members are sites of pathology. A wife diagnosed as "depressive" often signifies to the therapist a husband who is excessively enthusiastic, rational, hopeful, or well-behaved. These complementary forms of . . . behavior suggest other labels for the diagnostician that might include "neurotic normality," "psychotic hope," and "involutional happiness." (Keeney, 1983, p. 125).

Another example of the family's complexity is the hyperactive child with a learning disability. His parents may have a "perfect marriage" and "never fight," yet they seem angry, diverting their attention to him and away from themselves. His hyperactivity keeps them focused on him. His learning problems are related to learning *not* to see what he sees. This is an example of an abnormally normal family, with pathologically innocent parents.

To illustrate this point further, a therapist worked with the family of a severely entrenched anorexic daughter. The father, a prominent corporate executive, would inquire repeatedly about whether his daughter had a "thought disorder." In a way, she did, especially when she talked about how she viewed her own body. On the other hand, the father had another "thought disorder," characterized by an unemotional, condescending, narrow-mindedness. His pattern of expressing himself was appropriate in the board room; however, it was inappropriate when he was discussing family relationships. His daughter's "craziness" was, in part, "caused" by, or a reaction to, his intense rationality. The whole family participated in this disordered way of thinking about people, vacillating between hysterical distortion and overlogical distortion.

To repeat, the whole family can participate in a thought disorder. The behavioral qualities belong to the **family system**. In a family with an acutely psychotic person, there are usually several persons who are overrational. It is no easier for them to act crazy than it is for the psychotic person to act sane. The implication is that even psychotic behavior is role determined. A therapist can help a family to reverse roles in order to gain insight. Consider, for example, a family in which the father, an overrational executive, dressed in a three-piece suit, left a psychiatric interview in bare feet and his daughter's baseball cap,

782

while his "psychotic" son pleaded with his father not to make a fool of himself. The father took over the son's role, temporarily driving the son sane.

In a family in which there is a suicidal person, all members are either suicidal or homicidal. It helps to understand that, while the symptoms are overt in one family member, they are covert in the others. Likewise, health is a quality that describes families more than individuals.

The most important point here is that *every* patient has a family and the family is the arena of *psychological development*. It is also crucial to understand that the family has qualities which drive people crazy and it also has qualities that promote healing. When the treatment does not bring about the expected effect, we should suspect the influence of the former. When the patient gets better before treatment is commenced it is probably because of the latter.

Thinking about families in relation to psychopathology involves a mental jump, from thinking in linear terms more common to our culture (A causes B, but B has no effect on A) to thinking in terms of systems (A causes B, which also causes A). The change in thinking is comparable to the jump from playing football to playing baseball. The rules, the equipment, and the skills are different. There are few skills that translate from one sport to the other. Similarly, if family-oriented clinicians set out to write a diagnostic manual, they would not end up with a DSM-III-R diagnosis.

Kramer (1985) suggests that all families are "masterpieces"; each family is coherent in reference to itself, but idiosyncratic in reference to other families. Each family is its own best explanation (Kramer, 1985). The concept creates a feeling for looking at a whole rather than simply fragments. Keeney (1983) says it neatly when he suggests that a "balance of diversity" is a way of talking about health. A pathological family is a distorted one.

When talking about psychopathology, it is important to consider classification systems developed for the purpose of describing it. Any system developed to describe and classify psychopathology includes the diagnostician's system of morals, personal values, and personal symbols and philosophy. We have the most access to our own system when we look at our own family backgrounds. Contemporary psychiatric diagnostic patterns (such as DSM-III-R) attempt to eliminate these features from diagnosis, viewing them as distortions of objectivity. They fail to take into account the family-systems components of what we call psychopathology. DSM-III-R is a use-ful guide, but it is limited. It limits imagination, curiosity, and understanding. Its objectivity can result in another kind of distortion (Faust & Miner, 1986).

In summary, the family's dynamics add to the complexity of patient-centered care because the patient's family is his or her context. Often, when medical treatment and nursing care do not go well, or the patient's response is not as expected, it may be because of some background interference generated by the family dynamics.

PATHOLOGY IN FAMILIES

Pathology is a medical science that studies disease and its origins. It is interesting to note that the most important root in the word *pathology* is *pathos*, a "quality that arouses pity or sadness." Thus we could say that pathology is the study of conditions that arouse pity or sadness. This is not to say that there are not such experiences as "self-pity" or intrinsic (biological) depression; but *pathos*, the arousal of pity or sadness, implies a relationship with another person. Further, if there is pity and sadness, there must be caring, a variation of loving. We don't feel pity or sadness toward a person if we do not care about him. It follows that pathology is the study of patterns for seeking love. Something important to bear in mind, however, is that any effort devoted to *seeking* love has patterns for *avoiding* love built into it. This is because loving always involves risk, specifically, the risk of losing the loved one.

Warkentin (1972) pushes thinking further in this direction with his idea, "Where there is caring, all pathology is sharing." When a therapist begins to work with a family, she may ask herself what the interpersonal implications of the symptoms are. Is the hyperactive boy trying to activate his emotionally dead family? Is the anorexic girl starved for love? Examining a family in this light involves keeping in mind at least three generations of the family's relationship to the community. This is because the extended family is like a recursive algorithm,[1] or one whose output is fed back into it as input.

It makes little difference whether a symptom is biological, psychological, or social. The problem is pathological to the extent that it inhibits family

---

[1] An algorithm is a fixed procedure for converting input into output, for taking one body of information and turning it into another (Wright, 1988).

growth. The family-systems view provides a way to move beyond the dichotomy of mind and body. "Every mental adjustment . . . has its somatic component" (Meyer, 1908, p. 585). In other words, family living is a psychosomatic experience.

At this point, clinicians have no unified theoretical view of families. Nor do they have a diagnostic system that takes into account the complexity of life in a family. Family therapists are united not by shared truths so much as unsettling questions. One approach to this chapter might have been to review efforts at developing diagnostic systems for families; but it seems more crucial to communicate that there is no single system: "It is easier to know ten lands than one man" (Rosten, 1976). The family is made up of numbers of people who are not easy to know. In addition, the family consists of the relationships among these persons, and the relationships among these relationships. If a therapist or nurse only knows the family through an interview with one family member, she may find a completely different reality when she meets the other family members.

Marjorie: A Depressed Patient with a Depressed Husband

Marjorie, a 56-year-old woman, was referred after evaluation of a lump in her right breast since a negative diagnostic assessment did not relieve her apprehension. During the psychiatric consultation interview, she told a long story about her husband, a railroad engineer, who "had a woman at every whistle-stop." The therapist asked that he come for an interview the next day, expecting Casey Jones, macho hero of the railroad, to arrive. Instead, Marjorie's husband was a bewildered, timid, skinny man. At 58, he seemed old for his age and planned soon to retire from the railroad. He described feeling discouraged about himself and his recent sexual impotence. His wife "caught" her depression from him. It infected her defective self-esteem and appeared as a fantasied cancer. The man the therapist had expected was created by Marjorie's projections (Keith & Whitaker, 1988).

The example of Marjorie and her husband shows how pathos enters into the family distress. The physiologies and psyches of the couple are involved. Even though we do not have a specific diagnosis for the family, we must concern ourselves with the whole rather than just the individual.

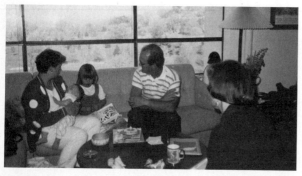

Family therapy can take many forms, but the focus is always the "family system." Here a young family and their therapist try to understand where the older child's anxiety is coming from. Family therapy can involve the extended family (e.g. all siblings and their families) as well. In the case of the divorced family, it can involve the two new couples and all the children. A complex treatment format, and a challenge for the most experienced therapist, family therapy is a powerful way to treat many disorders.

A FRAMEWORK FOR UNDERSTANDING THE FAMILY AND THE DEVELOPMENT OR MAINTENANCE OF PATHOLOGY

The nurse needs a framework for her thinking about the families she sees in the clinical setting. What she needs is a kind of "loom" that will enable her to weave her observations and responses to the family into a special tapestry. The discussion below shows how multiple components are woven into the fabric of symptomatic or pathological behavior in a family.

THE WHOLE IS GREATER THAN THE SUM OF ITS PARTS

The relationships among family members are part of the family itself. For example, in a family with one child, the family includes the relationship between the parents, the relationship between the mother and the child, the relationship of the child to the parent's relationship, and so forth. It is not possible to predict what will happen when the parts are mixed together (see Box 21–1).

This point can be demonstrated in the family practice clinic, with the clinician first taking a patient's history in a one-to-one format. She then adds

Box 21–1 ● Only Children: Well Enough Alone

You might think that in the late 1980s birth control, high divorce rates, and the strain of double careers would favor single-child families. In fact, the American family is shrinking, down from an average of 2.6 children per family in 1969 to 1.8 in 1985—the lowest it has ever been.

But it's the two-child families that are becoming more common. Families with one child are increasing only slightly. Right now just 14 percent of American women between the ages of 18 and 34 intend to raise an only child, according to the Census Bureau. The signals are clear: many of us still believe only children are worse off than children with siblings.

Many of us are wrong.

At the National Institute of Child Health and Human Development in Bethesda, Maryland, psychologist Gloria Kamenske cited the 11 only-child studies her organization has funded. These have ranged from in-depth reviews of individual cases to surveys of thousands, from babies to middle-aged adults. "In not a single one," Kamenske says, "have onlies been shown to have any disadvantage."

One study has defied not only the conventional wisdom but the preconceptions of the researcher himself. "I guess I was a bit surprised," admits John Claudy of the American Institutes for Research in Palo Alto, California. He compiled personality profiles of 4,000 high school students and then followed the students for 11 years. He expected the only children to develop at least a few more psychological problems than their peers.

Instead, the only children did no worse when measured against any standard of competence and actually fared slightly better in educa-tional achievement and cognitive test scores. They suffered no apparent social problems either, Claudy says, although they were a bit more likely to enjoy solitary activities such as reading and painting. They also tended to marry slightly more educated spouses. But, Claudy emphasizes, it was the groups' similarities, not their differences, that were most striking.

Famous Only Children

Clark Gable, Indira Gandhi, Charles Lindbergh, Lauren Bacall, Joseph Stalin, Franklin Roosevelt, and Upton Sinclair were all only children—but don't search for any personality pattern. While tests show that only children are a bit more motivated and confident than others, history reveals that they're no more likely to find fame and fortune. Some of the famous have remarked on their childhoods, however. Here are just a few:

I was not meaner or more ungenerous or more unkind than other children, but I was off balance in a world where I knew my grand importance to two other people who certainly loved me for myself, but who also liked to use me against each other.
LILLIAN HELLMAN

A great many only children were born in 1932. I make no apologies. I do not remember ever feeling the space for a competitor within the house.
JOHN UPDIKE

My truth, my character, and my name were in the hands of adults. I had learned to see myself through their eyes. I was a child, that monster which they fabricated with their regrets.
JEAN PAUL SARTRE

Source: Martin Lasden (1988). *Family Hippocrates*, March/April, pp. 30–32.

the patient's wife and two of his children and reviews the history again. If she were able to videotape both sessions, she could compare not only how the patient behaves and what he says in and out of his family context, but the changes in her own style as well.

The consciousness of the family is not the same as the consciousness of the individual, and it cannot really be described by individual family members. It takes the family group to describe the family, just as it takes the *group* to *be* the family.

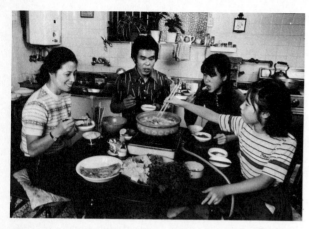

Regardless of nationality, social class, or identified patient, families are systems and behave accordingly. In family therapy, the *system* is the patient to be assessed and treated.

THE HEALTH OF THE WHOLE IS EXPRESSED IN THE FAMILY MORALE

Some families enjoy being together, and they include outsiders easily. They have the feeling of a team that enjoys playing together and has a winning record. In contrast, families with poor morale cannot even get everyone to the psychiatric interview; and when they do, they are overcautious in their self-description. There is usually dissension within the team and a tendency to blame the team's "losses" or dysfunction on one member.

In recent years, the New York Yankees baseball team has provided an example of how team spirit expresses the health of the whole. The autocratic team owner (father) has infinite financial power and has filled his roster with star players (teenage kids), but the *team* has not done well. The relationship between the players, the feeling of being a team, has developed poorly because of the owner's interference and rapid player turnover. The team has the *quality* of players needed to win, but the *relationship* between the players is defective. Keeping this perspective, health belongs to families rather than individuals and is rooted in group morale.

FAMILY SYSTEMS ARE POWERFULLY STABLE

Families change little, if at all; living patterns have a continuity that bridges generations. The process that maintains this stability is called **homeostasis**. Families can remain stable despite stressful extremes of rage, drunkenness, unemployment, moving, illness,

divorce, and death. The stability is in the family's self-defined sense of normality, which, in some cases, involves pathology.

SYMPTOMS ORGANIZE THE FAMILY

Symptoms can occur as an organizing response to a crisis or any process that **disrupts** the family. One way to think of it is that the **family phobia systems** (the family's hidden fears) are covered over by the symptoms. The specific symptom makes little difference in thinking about the family. The beginning symptom can be behavioral: a hyperactive boy, a school-phobic girl, a suicidal impulse in the father. The symptom may be psychosomatic: father's back spasms or daughter's abdominal pain. The symptom may be an accidental injury or even a major somatic illness. Or the first symptom may have to do with a battle between the community and the family.

In any case, it is important to remember that in the family framework, all illness is psychosomatic, and the presenting symptom is usually the least dangerous.

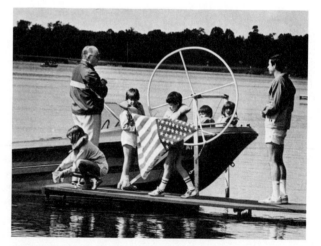

The influence of one generation on another is a powerful one. For example, in treating a young woman suffering from borderline personality disorder and bulimia, the therapist saw the family regularly. At one session, the father remembered that when he was a boy, his tyrannical father locked all the cupboards before leaving for work in the morning so the family could have no food until his return; he alone would distribute it. The patient's father went on to say that this made him so furious that when he ravenously ate his supper allotment, he often vomited, strangely feeling a sense of victory over his tyrant father (personal communication, Kavanagh, 1988).

THE MOST DISTURBED FAMILY MEMBER MAY NOT BE THE IDENTIFIED PATIENT

An example would be an anorexic young woman with a hypertensive, obese, 50-year-old father who chain-smokes. The father's mortality risk is much higher than the daughter's, but the family is more overtly troubled about the daughter. In fact, when the nurse mentions her concern about the father's health, the family dismisses her concern.

To further illustrate, a family was seen in a psychiatric clinic because the father was angry with his 16-year-old son's school performance. A 10-year-old daughter was eight months postsurgery for a brain tumor. During the first five interviews, the family was unable to discuss any topic related to the daughter's illness without ultimately returning to the ways that the son was a disappointment.

It is often the case that the most disturbed family relationship is the marital relationship. However, this relationship must be handled delicately at first, in the process of addressing the family's concern about the identified patient, while the treatment alliance is developing.

WHEN SYMPTOMS DIMINISH, ANXIETY INCREASES

When symptoms diminish, anxiety increases and symptoms may emerge in other family members.

Vicky: The Linchpin in a Family System

A 15-year-old girl was admitted to the hospital after sudden onset of bilateral paralysis of the lower extremities. The neurological exam suggested an hysterical conversion reaction. A psychiatrist interviewed the girl alone, found no clear precipitant, and suggested individual psychotherapy and a low-dose antidepressant. The girl's primary nurse knew something about family systems and suggested a consultation with a family therapist. During the consultation interview with ten family members from three generations, it developed that the daughter was involved in balancing most of the other family relationships. Metaphorically, it was no wonder that she was paralyzed. Her concern about her family had figuratively and literally tied her up. Within two days of the interview, her paralysis began to disappear. However, her mother went to bed with back spasms and her father's ulcer symptoms recurred. The secondary gain for her symptoms was not hers, but the family's.

SYMPTOMS CAN BE A WAY TO CONTROL THE EMOTIONAL TEMPERATURE OF FAMILY RELATIONSHIPS

This is most clearly seen in a rigid family or in the overinvolved, enmeshed family. Symptoms occur when the possibility of more loving appears, for example, when the husband or wife wants to increase the intimacy in their relationship, or when there is danger of separation. Children profoundly affect the temperature of family relationships, which can range from frigid to too hot to handle, and any growth steps children make can disturb the emotional balance of the family and lead to symptomatic behavior.

A single psychiatric interview with an oppositional teenager and his parents illustrates this point. The teenager chronically refused to go to school and now was refusing to cooperate with the court's sentence for driving while intoxicated (suspension of driving privileges and assessment and treatment of his substance abuse). Cross-generational anger was a long-standing family tradition and, in this case, had turned cold. The parents were fed up and wanted their son placed in long-term, residential treatment. At the beginning of the interview, the young man was sullen and disrespectful. The emotional temperature in the family was just above freezing. But after about thirty minutes, the son changed. His anger lifted, he began to talk, and then suddenly, he started crying. The emotional temperature in the family began rising. The boy's mother choked up and could not speak. Oddly, the father began scolding the boy. The father viewed his son's tears as a trick on the family, an attempt to manipulate them. His anger at his son restored the son's angry demeanor, allowing the mother to regain her composure. The emotional temperature in the family fell back to the initial level. Everyone was relieved that the mother's tears had ended. Did this mean that the family would rather see the son stay angry and go to residential treatment, than have the mother cry? Perhaps. Families can go through endless contortions in order to avoid being upset. (Also see Box 21-2.)

SYMPTOMS DEVELOP AROUND REPRESSED AFFECT OR MISLABELED FEELINGS

Health demands the free flow of affect in spontaneous living. Affect might be viewed as the REM sleep equivalent of daytime living. When it is suppressed for too long, it leads to symptoms of psychiatric illness or other tension patterns.

Box 21–2 ● Craziness Is Where Life Is

Carl Whitaker, one of the founding fathers of family therapy, believes that there is no such thing as an individual, only fragments of families. His therapeutic technique, which evolved over forty years of practice and is now known as symbolic-experiential family therapy, consists of two major elements: Using paradox, mystification, and spontaneous craziness, he seeks to raise the anxiety of the family group, to provoke a crisis by "raising the affective thermostat." Simultaneously, he provokes, badgers, and seduces family members into changing their customary ways of responding to crisis toward the direction of a greater maturity. Whitaker's approach emphasizes the biological rootedness of psychological maturation and the goal of helping individual family members toward a higher level of differentiation of self within the family (p. 19).

Whitaker on the family:

The greatest ordeal in life is marriage—it is the central focus for enlightenment and the natural therapeutic process in the culture (p. 366).

The secret of being a good parent is in the enjoyment of being hated (p. 367).

Marriage is a horrible state, and the only thing that's worse is being single (p. 370).

A dead mother is more demanding than a live one (p. 370).

Just as the three year old played at being mama with dolls, the four year old plays at being sexy with papa. If papa can play in turn, instead of being adult sexy, the child will know what love is and never confuse it with sex (p. 372).

I believe craziness is where life is (p. 375).

Source: *From Psyche to System: The Evolving Therapy of Carl Whitaker*, John R. Neill and David P. Kniskern (Eds.) (N.Y.: The Guilford Press, 1982).

The Marlboros: Mislabeled Feelings

The Marlboros sought psychiatric treatment for their 15-year-old son, Jerry, whom they regarded as a chronic underachiever and, recently, as destructive (he had shot out the yard lights with his BB gun). The initial history suggested that Jerry was a competent young man with an edge of frustrated anger at his parents. The parents' description of him did not fit the young man the clinicians saw in the clinic. As they developed the family history, they discovered that Jerry's mother had Hodgkin's disease two years previously. She was treated successfully, and, to date, had no recurrence of the illness. However, the mother allowed no one in the family to talk about any feelings or thoughts they had about her disease. Yet it could be seen from Jerry's restlessness that the topic of her illness tapped into very deep feelings. At the next interview, Jerry's 13-year-old sister, Maureen, burst into tears as she recalled how she felt when her mother was ill and her prognosis was guarded. Both Maureen's and Jerry's anger and sadness flowed over their parents' attempts to block the discussion. When the family returned to the clinic two weeks later for the third session, they reported that Jerry's school performance had improved significantly.

The Conroys: A Substructure of Rage

The Conroy family was referred to a psychiatric clinic because one of their three daughters was anorexic. The family was determined to maintain the fantasy that they were a "normal" family, without conflict. Any discussion of personal issues caused the mother to become defensive. In each of the first four interviews she and the therapist got into heated arguments. The arguments were distressing; the therapist even noted that his hair prickled on the back of his neck. "We might as well give up on these interviews if you are going to fight me all of the time like this," he said. "These aren't fights," she replied, "just disagreements." The therapist could then see what she meant when she said that the family never fought. They did not fight, by their definition, but there was an unacknowledged substructure of rage, which the anorexic daughter was acting out in her self-destructive behavior.

SYMPTOMS HAVE A CROSS-GENERATIONAL BASIS

Living patterns are passed from generation to generation. Each generation learns how to live from parents who learned from their parents. The learning includes coping styles, marriage styles, child-rearing styles, and illness styles. Symbols are social genes, that is to say, the symbolic meaning given to an experience is inherited and idiosyncratic to a family. The mode of transmission for symbolic patterns is not clear and, perhaps, like personality, is more biological than has been thought. The following cases may help to clarify this idea.

The Bollers: A Family in Confusion

The Bollers were referred to a nurse psychologist by their family doctor because Kim, 17, the oldest of three children, had a series of illnesses that interrupted her school attendance. Mononucleosis was ruled out and the doctor thought she might be depressed; however, Kim was not so much depressed as she was confused by the changes that were occurring in her family.

One of the more difficult years in the life of a family is the year before the first child leaves home, when the fantasies of what will happen next are in the air. Kim was a senior in high school. Her father, a successful salesman, had recently begun to experience a dropoff in his real-estate business and, thus, a decline in income. Because his own family of origin had never allowed depression, he continued to maintain a cheerful, though inappropriate, mood (repressed affect). Kim's mother was subtly pressuring her husband about his long working hours while trying to get her midlife self in focus (a change in the marital relationship was in the works). The entire family seemed slightly depressed and confused.

Kim's mother had been viewed by her family of origin as sickly during her adolescent years, although no syndrome had ever been defined. Recently she began to frequently excuse herself from family activities because she was "too tired" (probably a sign of the family's cautiousness with affect). Her lack of energy was a constant source of irritation to her husband. In addition, the maternal grandmother had been viewed as in poor health for many years, although, again, there was never a defined illness. Thus Kim entered her adolescent identity crisis at a time when her *family* was entering a crisis period. Her mother was attempting to increase the intimacy in her marriage, so her role in the family was changing. In the process, her chronic fatigue was becoming less of a problem. But now, she began to worry about her daughter's illness. This was the same way that *her* mother had shepherded her through adolescence. Thus, Kim, in the third generation, was being groomed to use illness to manage interpersonal difficulties.

Andy: An Encopretic Child

Andy, age 5, was encopretic (chronically constipated and frequently incontinent) and his parents were terribly upset about it. The usual pediatric treatment (which involved treating the constipation and instituting a positive-reinforcement program for having regular bowel movements in the preferred place) was not successful, so they were referred to a child psychiatrist who was a family therapist. In arranging the first interview, she urged the family to include the grandparents. Then, with all three generations present, the therapist gathered information from the parents. After about thirty-five minutes, she focused the interview on the grandparents. The maternal grandmother confessed that, as a child, she had been encopretic until age eight. No one else in the family knew anything about this. She went on to recall some of her experiences, for example, her embarrassment and her parents' frustration. Over the next three weeks, Andy's toileting behavior improved steadily. By the second therapy session, it seemed that the whole family had "loosened up."

In both cases, it is possible to see how *patterns* of dysfunction are repeated. It is hard for the family to see the repetition; when it comes up in the course of family therapy, it is experienced as surprising and often denied. In short, until proven otherwise, every symptom picture and the surrounding pattern can be assumed to have a three-generation basis. It may not be initially obvious (especially if we do not look); sometimes the situation has to unravel a bit before the pattern becomes clear.

FAMILY THERAPY

Family therapy represents a multitude of methods and philosophies for working with families. One type of work aims at helping the family to develop enough administrative power and effectiveness to deal with the community (the school, the neighborhood, the health care system, the court, and so forth), whether these problems are related to an individual family member or to the whole family. Another important aim is to help the family find a way to let individual members both belong to the family and be separate from it without disrupting the family as a whole. In the process, ideally, the family gains an appreciation of the way in which it is a masterpiece.

The family therapist functions something like the coach of a baseball team. The coach wants the team to win, but he cannot play in the game. He works from the sidelines. The patterns of effective coaching are infinite. A team requires high morale to win games, and winning fosters high morale. A team does well when each member plays his own position well. If a player is injured, the team has to find ways to compensate.

Sometimes clinical situations are easy to resolve. For example, a 28-year-old man with cardiac palpitations of unknown etiology, thought to be anxiety-induced, was discovered by the psychiatric consultant to have had two one-night stands with the next-door neighbor. He was afraid that his wife would kill him if she found out about the affair. When he followed the consultant's suggestion and disclosed the matter to his wife, the palpitations ended and marital therapy began.

Family pathology may be characterized as a distortion of reality. The distortions are not always obvious, however, and identifying them requires that the therapist feel free to use his or her imagination in thinking about the family as the therapy process unfolds.

Tom and Mary Clancy: Shifting Family Dynamics

Tom and Mary Clancy were referred because of marital pressures. They were in their mid-30s and had two young children, ages 7 and 5. The overt complaints were standard. Mary was angry at Tom because he seemed so bland and uninteresting. Tom was exasperated by Mary's pushing him and trying to make him over to fit her idea of how he should be, which was based on her family of origin. However, Tom and Mary's background dynamics were unusual.

He had built up a successful dental practice with two separate offices and five associates. Two years prior to the referral he was involved in a serious head-on automobile accident and was in a coma for eight weeks. Mary had been told by the neurologists that Tom would die soon; or, if he did not die, he would live the rest of his life with little to no social and intellectual capability. She began to grieve over the loss of the man she had married. Then she took over administration of his dental clinics; because of her business administration experience, Mary was able to improve the clinic management and increase the efficiency of the business.

But Tom surprised her. He not only survived, he regained his full social, professional, and intellectual capabilities. They never discussed it, but Mary was angry with Tom not only for surviving, but for fully recovering so that he was able to carry a full practice load again (see Chapter 26 on death). She was relegated to the sidelines once again. Tom had confused the family dynamics by surviving and recovering. The system had accommodated to his "death," but shifting again, to adjust to his recovery, proved stressful. It occurred to the therapist that it might have been better (less upsetting to Mary) if Tom had acted as if he were in a coma, and she said so.

Such an interpretation, or diagnosis, of the family situation, that the father should behave as if in a coma, may sound absurd, but it contains slivers of truth and so can broaden the family's perspective in a potentially useful way. The therapist cannot count on facts alone to reach a conclusion; imagination and a sense of humor also can be used therapeutically.

The Johnsons: An Example of Productive Family Therapy

Rob and Betty Johnson, a couple in their late 30s, and their two daughters, Susan, 16, and Lisa, 11, sought family therapy because Susan had become inordinately hostile and hard to live with. She fought her parents on everything. With each skirmish, Betty became increasingly depressed. Susan had done some mild acting out (getting drunk and coming in late once). She was doing well in school and had many friends, however, and did not meet the criteria for any psychiatric diagnosis. Rob and Betty were furious with Susan; the first interview ended in a standoff. The therapists learned that part of the trouble was the fact that Rob owned a small business and worked long hours seven days a week, leaving Betty to deal with the children on her own.

In the second interview, the family reported a shoving match between Susan and her mother on

Sunday morning while getting ready for church. Rob was outraged at his daughter's insolence. The fight ended when he physically shook her, and his action frightened everyone in the family, including him. As they talked about the fight in the interview, there was a new sense of unity, as if Rob's strong action had brought the family together. Midway through the interview, all were in tears. Then Betty began to talk about how depressed she had been feeling. She had been thinking of changing her identity (name and social security number) and leaving the family. The co-therapy team assumed her depression was related to her daughter's anger and her husband's lack of attention.

At the third interview, the therapists found that they were on the wrong track. During the first interview, the therapists had learned that Betty was in conflict with her own mother, Helen. Earlier, the therapy team was unable to explore this fully because of the tension around Susan's behavior. Now it became important to discuss the mother's family history.

Betty's father left the family when she was three, and she did not remember him. She was raised by a stepfather and her mother. In the family's "official" (altered but less complicated) history, Betty's biological father did not exist. He was viewed as disreputable so Helen had declared that he was never to be mentioned. One year prior to the first interview, Betty had located her father in another state and went to visit him. She was surprised by her deep feelings for him and found him to be a delightful person, contrary to family myth. When Betty's mother found out about the reunion, she was outraged. She had Betty, her oldest daughter, removed from her will. In addition, she decreed that no one in the family was allowed to speak to Betty. It was as if she was a magician who could make people disappear. Betty was devastated, but like the rest of her family of origin, accepted her mother's decree. The family members were in tears again as Betty described her distress. It was as if she were under a "spell." Betty seemed to have lost her identity as Susan was fighting to gain hers. Asked what she feared most, Susan said, "That my mother will hate me as much as my grandmother hates her." Betty was deeply ashamed of herself for betraying her mother. The therapist suggested she was doing the right thing by visiting her father. She had done it as a way to know more about herself and escape the domination of her mother's enforced delusion that her father did not exist.

Everyone was in a good mood when the family arrived for the fourth interview. There was no dissension and the family morale was high. The therapy team suggested that Betty arrange for her parents and siblings to come in for an interview. Rob said that he was feeling good about the state of affairs and wondered if it would be all right if he talked some about his family of origin. When it came time to schedule the next interview, Lisa stated that she did not want to return. The therapists said that they wanted her to come back, and with tongue in cheek, suggested that she write a story entitled, "The Advantages of Growing Up in a Crazy Family."

The family returned four more times. Betty made a serious attempt to get her family to come in for a session, but they refused. She was disappointed by their refusal, but not hurt. In fact, she was amused by the flurry her suggestion created in her family of origin. At the second-to-last interview, Lisa brought in her story, a delightful tale about a family that went to see a psychiatrist.

That was the conclusion of a productive course of family therapy. It was productive because it enriched the family's life experience and contributed to the professional growth of the therapists as well.

Sometimes, when we talk about families in relation to clinical problems, we talk about family therapy as an *alternative* treatment modality. This line of thinking leads to the question, "What are the indications and contraindications for family therapy?" In this chapter the focus is not about a treatment modality so much as a clinical orientation in which individuals do not exist, only fragments of families. See Box 21–3 for more on family therapy.

NURSING AND FAMILIES

Physicians typically set the tone in clinical situations for how patients and illness will be viewed. Traditionally, nurses have followed along. But nurses have the opportunity to take a more significant role with families in relation to patient care. Nurses usually have a more intuitive understanding of family dynamics than do physicians, because of their educational background and broader contact with families. The nurse has a better sense of what goes on in the relationship system *around* the patient. Physicians, on the other hand, seem to be best at using the high-power microscope; they pay little attention to what they see in the low-power field. Physicians are also often likely to avoid situations in which they feel confused or inadequate. By learning to talk and think "family," the nurse becomes more thoughtful, creative, and effective in dealing with clinical situations.

A family perspective on health and illness makes intuitive sense, but it is difficult to institute a family perspective clinically. Every nurse cannot be a family therapist. But nurses can learn to pay attention to the

Box 21–3 • Family Therapy

Mental health professionals have always understood that the problems they deal with arise largely in families and take their form from family relationships. Marriage and family problems account for about half of all visits to psychotherapists. Families also play the decisive role in most non-biological explanations of emotional disturbances and mental illness. Psychodynamic psychotherapists are concerned with childhood conflicts between instinctual drives and family prohibitions. Behaviorists and cognitive psychotherapists emphasize social learning, which also occurs mainly in the family. Yet for many years mental health professionals tended to ignore the patients' families. They were often seen mainly as an obstacle to treatment, although they were often called on to care for the patient and of course to pay the bills. More recently, the dominance of biological explanations for some severe forms of mental illness has also reduced emphasis on the family's influence.

A major variation in this pattern is represented by family therapy, which is now about 40 years old. It regards individual symptoms as family problems and treats the family rather than the individual. It is not distinguished by any definite set of ideas about the causes and treatment of emotional disturbances and mental illness. Some of its concepts and techniques are new, some are borrowed, and some are unfamiliar outside the field. There are many varieties of family therapy which may be combined in different ways with one another and with other types of therapy.

Family therapists think of families as having stages of development, like individuals. A couple forms and the partners separate themselves from their original families. The children arrive, introducing new subsystems and the need to exercise a new kind of authority. School-age children learn how other families are run and may demand changes in their own.

Adolescents develop competing social ties and begin in turn to separate themselves from the family. Eventually the couple is alone again.

Each stage has its normal problems and crises and each also produces typical pathological disturbances. While the couple is becoming established, one partner may form an alliance with his or her family of origin against the other partner, or, on the contrary, one set of in-laws may be cut off entirely. As the children grow up, parents may be unwilling to renegotiate family rules or permit them a separate identity; for example, a child develops a school phobia because a parent feels abandoned when the child leaves the house. Teenagers may be unable to achieve independence because their emotional problems serve to keep a troubled family together.

Family therapists may interpret such situations psychoanalytically, assign tasks like behavior therapists, challenge beliefs like cognitive therapists, offer practical advice, support and reassurance, teach social skills, set authoritative limits, or direct the dramatic reenactment of typical family situations. Some family therapists remain almost as neutral as psychoanalysts, and others become intensely involved, trying to sympathize with each member of the family in turn.

Treatment of Schizophrenia

Many experts once thought that the family environment caused schizophrenia; now almost all believe that its roots are biological and partly hereditary. Nevertheless, recent studies have shown that family therapy or family management improves the symptoms and reduces the burden substantially. Families can be educated about the illness without being blamed for it. They are taught to communicate better with schizophrenic patients, to reduce their expectations and temper their criticisms of the patient in recognition of the illness. They can be encouraged to watch for signs of relapse and hold meetings to discuss serious problems. Mutual support and advice may be provided through multiple family groups. Parents can be taught how to enforce rules of behavior for schizophrenic adolescents.

The popularity of family therapy has grown greatly in the last twenty years, but those same years have seen the rise of biological psychiatry, new developments in individual psychology, and increased social criticism of all forms of psychotherapy. Meanwhile, larger historical trends have been changing families in unpredictable ways. The relative influence of all these forces will determine how important family therapy becomes and what forms it takes in the future.

Source: *The Harvard Medical School Mental Health Letter.* "Family Therapy, Parts I and II." Vol. 4 Numbers 10 and 11. 1988. Lester Grinspoon, editor.

family context surrounding their patients. Nurses, by their broader and more personal contact with patients, can take a leadership role among health care professionals in acknowledging the presence of the family and in increasing sensitivity to family dynamics in relation to health.

The first interview of any family therapy effort is analogous to a physical examination. *The goal is not to change anything but to discover what is there.* The therapeutic effort is aimed at helping families develop growthfully with the help of crises. Family repair is complex terrain and requires extensive training and experience.

Nurses can also be effective by teaching families how to participate in the care of a family member who is a patient, and by demanding that family members take an active role in the care of their members. Accomplishing this requires acknowledging the associated tension and growth-obstructing conflicts from the systems perspective.

Case Study: Nonpsychiatric Setting

At age 10, Lewis was found to have a rhabdomyosarcoma, and his leg was amputated at the hip. The subsequent chemotherapy successfully suppressed the cancer, and he did well until the cancer reappeared when he was 15. He rapidly deteriorated during his sophomore year in high school. As he became more and more debilitated, attending school was too taxing, and hospitalizations were more frequent. The nursing staff was aware of tension in the family during the hospitalizations. Lewis seemed angry with his family. His father's visits were infrequent and Lewis did not talk to him when he was there. He attended the group therapy sessions on the ward, but said little. One day he told one of the nurses that he thought his family would be glad when he died because they were sick of him. Lewis did not want to stay in the hospital; he wanted to go home. His family did not want to take him home because they felt that he was too ill for them to take care of him. Something the mother said suggested that Lewis was constantly upset by the way the family took care of him. Lewis asked his primary nurse, Peter Tingley, if the hospital staff felt that his parents would neglect him at home, so that he would die.

Peter suggested to Lewis's physician, a pediatric oncologist, that she request a psychiatric consultation, preferably with a family therapist. She was opposed to the idea, however. Peter expressed concern about what he saw developing in the family. The oncologist said it was normal for a family to have tension around terminal illness and could see no reason to upset the family more by bringing in a psychiatrist. Peter held to his position, but to no avail. The next day, on rounds, the oncologist said that she wanted Lewis to go home, and the issue erupted again. The parents did not want Lewis to come home. The oncologist came back to the ward to talk to Lewis's father. She got no further with him than had Peter or any of the nursing staff, and agreed to a psychiatric consultation with a family therapist. Peter asked that the oncologist join the conference; she appointed the chief resident to represent her.

The family therapist asked that the older sister, Bonnie, age 17, and the younger brother, Dick, age 8, attend the consultation, along with Lewis's parents, his primary nurse, and the chief resident. They discussed what the family was like, told stories related to Lewis's struggle with cancer, how the family had been affected by his illness, and what would happen to the family after Lewis's death. The consultant asked Lewis if he had told his family what things of his he wanted them to be certain to keep. The mother said, "That is the whole problem with Lewis coming home. He won't talk to us about anything. He only gives orders and complains. We need to talk about these things, but he won't." Lewis and his mother cried silently. When the therapist concluded the interview, Lewis's father asked if they could meet again, and another interview was scheduled three days hence. In the interim the nursing staff reported an apparent rapprochement between Lewis and his family. However, his physical condition became somewhat worse.

An interesting thing happened at the second meeting. The parents came without Dick, the 8-year-old brother. They said he was too tired to come. Ten minutes after the beginning of the interview, there was a knock on the door; it was Dick. He was upset that the family had left without him. Apparently, they had tried to protect Dick by leaving him at home, but he wanted to be involved. As the session continued, it was obvious that family unity had been restored. The oncologist was partly right. The consultation had been upsetting, but the upset released the strong feelings that had been hidden, and restored the broken family morale.

The family scheduled a third session. Lewis's condition continued to deteriorate, however, and he died at 1 A.M. the day it was to take place. His whole family was with him when he died. Later, when the family was about to leave the hospital, the question came up about whether they would plan to have the family session as scheduled. Dick insisted that they keep the appointment, and they did. They spent the hour reminiscing about times they all were together before Lewis became ill.

This illustration gives an example of family psychopathology in relation to a physical illness. It also highlights, in an important way, how the nurse can take a leadership role in including the family in the care of the patient. What would have happened if Lewis had been interviewed alone by the psychiatrist? The crucial interaction between mother and son could not have occurred. The family as a whole was needed to make this valuable experience possible. The younger brother's effort to be involved with the family had the effect of giving all members a way to reawaken their dormant emotions. The conflict had developed around their unexpressed sadness. As a result, they had experienced only tension and increasing anger.

There were many unaddressed issues in the family. The marriage was not in good condition. Lewis's mother seemed emotionally closer to him than she was to his father. The older sister was emotionally flat and gave the appearance of someone who was very depressed. Although she was present at all the interviews, she rarely said anything. The apparent explanation was that during Lewis's extensive treatment programs, the parents were constantly preoccupied and had not been very available, physically or emotionally, to her. Dick, on the other hand, was the embodiment of life and fun in the family. He, more than anyone else, kept the family together. The family, however, never sought further treatment.

Nursing Diagnoses

Ineffective family coping: disabling
Altered family processes

Nursing Care Plan for Lewis

Nursing Diagnosis	Desired Outcomes	Interventions	Rationale
1. Ineffective family coping: disabling	Lewis and his family will begin to identify feelings regarding Lewis's illness and hospitalization; they will begin to understand the potential benefits of better communication about those feelings in the family.	Talk with Lewis and his family about their feelings about Lewis's illness and its treatment. Acknowledge what they seem to be feeling, such as anxiety, anger, sadness, labeling these feelings as understandable responses in the situation.	Talking with Lewis and his family separately makes it possible to give full attention to their different (and at times conflicting) needs. The family as well as Lewis needs to know what it is that they are feeling before they can begin to deal with it.
		Suggest that a family therapist might be able to help them talk to each other about these things, pointing out the potential advantages; encourage them to think about this.	Many people don't know what family therapy is or how it can help them.
2. Altered family processes	Lewis and family will begin to talk honestly with each other about feelings regarding Lewis's illness and hospitalization.	Confer with Lewis's doctor about potential benefits of psychiatric consultation by a family therapist; point out indications for consultation, what would be involved, and how it can facilitate medical treatment.	All members of the treatment team need to be involved in the psychiatric aspects of Lewis's care, as they are in its other aspects. The physician may not understand the relationship between this family's dynamics and Lewis's treatment and response to that treatment.
		Talk with consulting psychotherapist (with Lewis's and his family's permission) about own observations and	The nurse can be an excellent data source because of his or her position on the treatment team and access to the patient.

Nursing Diagnosis	Desired Outcomes	Interventions	Rationale
		feelings about this family, focusing on what family dynamics you have observed and the effects they seem to be having on patient, staff, and the course of treatment.	
		With the family's permission, join psychotherapist in treatment sessions. Allow yourself to experience the family without bias or judgment. Focus on *process* and *content* during the session, also on own response to the family. Try to imagine what it is like for Lewis to be in this family now. Express what *you* feel about all this when your feelings might intensify what is occurring in the session, and/or when they might broaden the family's perspective on themselves.	The more the nurse understands Lewis's family's dynamics, and what *his* experience in his family is, the better able he or she will be to identify his needs and begin a nursing care plan to meet them. The nurse's expression of his or her feelings within the family is a model the family can utilize in therapy and with each other.

Case Study: Psychiatric Setting

Ellen, age 12, was admitted to the adolescent inpatient psychiatric unit following an aspirin overdose, which led to a dangerous electrolyte imbalance. She had been feeling despondent for three months. Since she had lost weight and seemed to have stopped eating entirely, her mother had taken her to a nurse therapist at an eating-disorders clinic. Although she did not have a clearly defined eating disorder, Ellen's focus on food and weight was a medium to act out her unhappiness, a jumping off point for talking about it.

In addition to Ellen the family consisted of her brother, Will, age 16, and her parents, who were in their mid-40s. Her father was president of a small but successful corporation. Her mother was chair of the educational psychology department at a local university. The parents had been divorced for five years, after ten painfully disappointing years of marriage. The children lived with their mother, who tended to be tyrannical, given to cold anger and strict moralism. The father, on the other hand, was sheepish and unusually naive about personal relationships. The parents wanted nothing to do with one another.

Family therapy sessions were held once or twice per week during Ellen's six-week hospitalization. The sessions were complex and filled with animosity. The mother did not want the father involved. Initially, Ellen did not want him involved either and tried to run away from the ward. The nursing staff had to provide both support and limits for her. The family was told that Ellen's father's involvement in her treatment was crucial so it continued. This resulted in the airing of many pain-filled issues pertinent to what Ellen and her brother were going through. Their mother reacted intensely to the therapy, would visit Ellen at inappropriate times, and would call nursing staff to complain about her treatment. For example, the ward has a sex-education program for adolescent patients to which she objected. Initially, the staff responded politely to her complaints and tried to find a way to make her more comfortable with the difficult situation. Her anger only escalated. It became clear that she was reacting to the emotionally charged experience of family therapy. Because Ellen's primary nurse or another member of the nursing staff was present at every family interview, they all were aware of the issues and feelings in the family, the context of Ellen's suicidality. Because of the close connection Ellen's primary nurse had with her, she sat next to Ellen during the sessions, and experienced with her what it was like to be a member of her family. The adolescent children wanted to live with their father, but the treatment team was dubious about this. His demeanor was less toxic than their mother's, but he was so dependent himself that it seemed he would be unable to provide a satisfactory home for two teenagers who were stumbling through a difficult time in their lives.

During the hospitalization, as the anger between the parents resurfaced and Ellen and her brother tried to sort out a way to be connected to both of them, Ellen's eating problems were reactivated. She began losing weight, partly because of distress over her family, and partly over her problems with accepting the milieu program of the ward. Here again, the nursing staff, especially her primary nurse, provided Ellen with support and limits.

Near the end of Ellen's six weeks in the hospital, a crucial turning point in the family therapy came when the brother began to talk about how lonely he had been feeling. As his feelings of despondency became clearer, Ellen seemed to feel less burdened. Instead of being so negative about the hospital and her treatment program, she began to enjoy the nurturing she received from the nursing staff. She also began to look forward to the family sessions. During one, Will told how he had had an appendectomy six months prior to his sister's suicide attempt. When he came home from the hospital, he was frightened to talk about some of his experiences there. He had felt detached from his body, and worried that, internally, he was slowly bleeding to death. The only person he dared share these feelings with was Ellen. She was frightened, too, but she took care of him, and talked with him and played music for him. It was the therapists' impression that Will had had a subclinical postsurgery psychotic episode, and that Ellen's eating troubles began at this time.

Ellen was discharged and went to live with her father. Will stayed with his mother, and they all continued therapy in the outpatient clinic. The treatment was successful insofar as Ellen was concerned. Will, whose loneliness and feelings of alienation were prominent in the therapy, experienced much distress, but all in all seemed to get a lot from the family sessions. Ellen's and Will's father became more responsive to his children; however, the treatment was a failure in that their mother's anger at the therapists continued. As a result, she gradually became less and less involved in the family therapy.

This was a very difficult case, and one in which the danger of suicide remained prominent. Psychiatric hospitalization is less frequent in work with families, but in this case, the family was not able to provide a safe "holding environment" for Ellen as her treatment got under way. At the outset, both parents were so emotionally impoverished that neither was able to provide the nurturing that Ellen and Will required.

This is also a case which exemplifies how the nursing staff on an inpatient psychiatric unit is involved in family therapy. The above narrative does not, however, adequately describe how this family pressured the relationship between the nursing staff and the psychiatrist/family therapist, and nearly caused a "split" (see Chapter 12 on personality disorders) between them. Family therapy often disturbs a family, and members are apt to seek solace from the nursing staff. All members of the treatment team need to beware of impulses to help the family be angry at the staff rather than at one another.

Nursing Diagnoses

Ineffective family coping: disabling
Altered parenting

Nursing Care Plan for Ellen

Nursing Diagnosis	Desired Outcomes	Interventions	Rationale
1. Ineffective family coping: disabling	Ellen and her family will begin to verbalize rather than act out strong feelings about one another.	Talk with Ellen and mother separately about their feelings about Ellen's illness, its treatment, and dad's involvement in treatment. Acknowledge feelings of anger, anxiety, and so on that seem to be acted out, and empathize with them.	Talking with Ellen and her mother separately makes it possible to attend fully to the needs of both and respects Ellen's adolescent need for privacy.
		Point out possible consequences of *not* involving father in Ellen's treatment (that is, family therapy, which can be very effective in the treatment of eating disorders and suicidality in an adolescent), namely, that success is unlikely.	Families don't always feel as powerful as they are, or understand how important they are in the treatment program of the eating disorders patient. (Also see Chapter 14 on eating disorders.)
		Point out potential benefits of family therapy (effective treatment of patient, help for family members with *their* feelings); explain what is involved.	People fear what they don't understand.

Nursing Diagnosis	Desired Outcomes	Interventions	Rationale
		Ask what might be done to make dad's involvement less traumatic for Ellen and mother.	Empathy regarding feelings about dad is likely to help Ellen and her mother feel listened to and understood, important to the development of a therapeutic relationship with the nurse as well as with the treatment team.
2. Altered parenting	Ellen's mother and father will resume or begin appropriate and potentially effective parenting of their children.	Label parents' feelings, accepting them and empathizing with them. Separate feelings from behavior, pointing out what behavior is needed now to facilitate Ellen's treatment and recovery, and model it in Ellen's treatment program. Identify where parents can get support and help them to mobilize these resources.	Identifying and empathizing with parents' feelings and needs will facilitate the development of a therapeutic relationship which will lead to more disclosure of feelings that need to be dealt with. Separating feelings from behavior and dealing with them separately can make a situation less overwhelming.

SUMMARY

At the end of *Alice in Wonderland*, Alice wakes up and leaves the dream world behind. Fragments linger. Wonderland was a confusing dream filled with unpredictable experiences. Anything was possible, but all the craziness occurred against a background of normal social living. Characters changed. Their language gave the appearance of sense, but often made no sense. Animals and flowers appeared as people. Similarly, families cannot be appreciated unless we allow ourselves to use images from the nonrational world of dreams. This chapter does not lead to crystal-clear understanding of families or psychopathology. Its aim has been to stimulate thinking more broadly about the question of psychopathology and to point out that any descriptive system of psychopathology is only a guide to understanding; it is not an end in itself. This chapter is an effort to introduce the reader to systems thinking and to the notion that patients come out of a context. It has attempted to show that family living is psychosomatic; there is no difference between mind and body for the family.

Pathology has something to do with pathos, which leads to the neologism, "biopsychopathology." Through the use of clinical examples, this chapter has provided a framework for understanding how clinical symptoms fit into the family system.

It is important not to be entirely dependent on DSM-III-R. To view the psychological dimension of patients only or predominantly through its "lens" would be to take a very narrow view of human experience, including the experience of emotional distress (Faust & Miner, 1986). Any theoretical pattern, including systems theory, induces partial blindness (Whitaker, 1977). To compensate, it is important to keep our creativity alive so as to maintain an intuitive responsiveness to the needs of our patients (Keith, 1987).

KEY TERMS

family system

homeostasis

family phobia systems

STUDY QUESTIONS

1. What are family systems?

2. Describe the concept of psychopathology in families.

3. Discuss a framework for understanding psychopathology in the family, including family morale, the most disturbed family member, anxiety increasing as symptoms diminish, and mislabeled feelings.

4. Identify the major tenets of family therapy.

5. Describe the role of the nurse in working with families.

REFERENCES

Anthony, E. J. (1957). An experimental approach to the psychopathology of children: Encopresis. *British Medical Journal* 30; 146–175.

de Schazer, S. (1983). Diagnosis = researching + doing therapy. In J. C. Hansen & B. P. Keeney (Eds.), *Diagnosis and assessment in family therapy*. Rockville: Aspen Systems Corporation, pp. 123–132.

Faust, D., & Miner, R. A. (1986, August). The empiricist and his new clothes: DSM III in perspective. *American Journal of Psychiatry, 143*, 962–967.

Kavanagh, C. K. (1988). Personal communication.

Keeney, B. P. (1983). *Aesthetics of change*. New York: Guilford Press.

Keith, D. V. (1987, Spring/Summer). Intuition in family therapy: A short manual on post-modern witchcraft. *Contemporary Family Therapy, 9*, 11–22.

Keith, D. V., & Whitaker, C. A. (1988). *The presence of the past. Family transitions*. NY: Guildford Press, pp. 431–448.

Kramer, D. A. (1985, October). Three generations of experiential psychotherapy. Workshop presented at 43rd Annual Conference, American Association of Marital and Family Therapists, New York.

Meyer, A. (1908). *The collected papers of Adolf Meyer, Volume III: Psychiatry*, (Ed.) E. Q. Winters. Baltimore: Johns Hopkins Press.

Rosten, L. (1968). *The joys of Yiddish*. New York: McGraw-Hill.

Warkentin, J. (1972). Personal communication.

Whitaker, C. A. (1976). The hindrance of theory in clinical work. In P. J. Guerin, (Ed.), *Family therapy: Theory and practice*. New York: Gardner Press, pp. 154–164.

Whitaker, C. A. (1978). Cotherapy of chronic schizophrenia. In M. Berger (Ed.), *Beyond the double bind*. New York: Bruner/Mazel, pp. 155–175.

Wright, R. (1988, April). Did the universe just happen? *The Atlantic Monthly*, 38.

22

PSYCHIATRIC MENTAL HEALTH NURSING WITH CHILDREN

RICHARD BARTHEL
CHRISTINE HERRMAN

LEARNING OBJECTIVES
After studying this chapter, the student will be able to:

- Identify theories of emotional growth and development and discuss their application to nursing practice.
- Assess a child for possible psychopathology.
- Describe the common psychopathologies of childhood and adolescence.
- Discuss the needs of the hospitalized child.
- Develop nursing interventions to help the child cope with simple fears of hospitalization and true mental disorders.

INTRODUCTION

All nurses, whether they are generalist nurses or psychiatric nurses, at some point become involved in the treatment of children with emotional problems. Nurses need to appreciate their position as health-care professionals who can do much to prevent children and families from becoming dysfunctional. In doing so, nurses may be at the heart of primary prevention.

The nurse with a developmental and systems focus makes accurate and timely observations in a variety of health-care settings, providing education and anticipatory guidance to families as necessary. Prior to the birth of an infant, for example, she can provide information on growth and development and assess parents' readiness through prenatal classes offered by a hospital or clinic. Public health, obstetrical, pediatric, and many clinic nurses have the opportunity to continue to educate parents in fostering the physical and mental health of their children.

Since nurses are often involved in the care of children and families experiencing situational or developmental crises, they can be at the heart of secondary prevention as well. Secondary prevention activities reduce morbidity in mental illness through early case finding and rapid initiation of effective treatment. The nurse who recognizes a family in crisis (for example, as a result of parental illness) and who appreciates the impact it has on the children is involved in early case finding. This is especially important when young children are involved and when parents are acutely or chronically unable to determine and meet the needs of their children.

The case of Peter illustrates a nurse's contribution to secondary prevention. Without her attention to the subtleties of this family's crisis and recognition of a dysfunctional child, Peter's "problem behavior" could have led to mental illness and increasing family dysfunction.

Peter: A Child Confused by His Brother's Illness

John, age 14, had recently been admitted to the pediatric ICU with encephalitis of unknown etiology. He was comatose and his prognosis was guarded. His parents spent nearly all their time at the hospital. In speaking with them, the nurse discovered that John's 5-year-old brother, Peter, who was staying with his grandmother, had been having nightmares since John's admission. The nurse encouraged John's parents to bring Peter in to see his brother, but they did not want him "to see John this way."

John's mother said, "I know that Peter's routines are all changed and that he is probably angry with us, but he has to understand that we need to be here with John." Additional history revealed that Peter was not minding his grandmother, which was unusual for him, and that he seemed irritable much of the time. The nurse knew that, at his age, egocentrism and magical thinking made him vulnerable to misinterpreting events and being overwhelmed by them, especially because he was separated from his immediate family. She shared this information with the family and offered to help them support Peter during his visits to his brother.

The next day Peter began regular visiting. He had many questions that his parents and the nurse attempted to answer as simply and as honestly as possible. They encouraged Peter to take care of his brother in small ways, for example, by bringing in and playing tapes with messages from family and friends for his brother, and drawing pictures of him to hang in his hospital room. Peter's parents began spending "special time" alone with him. The result was that his nightmares stopped soon after his first hospital visit, and his mood began to improve.

In her early identification of a problem and developmentally focused intervention, the nurse helped this family cope with a crisis more adaptively and resume healthy functioning.

The nurse occasionally comes in contact with children who are severely dysfunctional. It is important that she be able to recognize pathology when it occurs and appropriately refer the child and his family to a competent mental health professional for evaluation and treatment. Her perspective regarding what is going on, and what isn't but should be, will be needed in the multidisciplinary assessment of the child and/or family. Her support of the child and his family as they go through assessment and treatment is important as well.

This chapter is designed to give the nurse information about childhood psychopathology. It should help to bridge the gap between knowledge of normal growth and development and the important work of assessing psychological problems in children and promoting their mental health.

DEVELOPMENTAL THEORIES AND THEIR APPLICATION TO NURSING PRACTICE

Childhood psychopathology needs to be discussed in the context of developmental theory because the child moves along a developmental continuum from birth through adolescence. How his personality unfolds, what his potential is, and how he grows and develops are all influenced by many factors, such as genetic endowment and environmental experiences in the family, culture, and community. The child's personality is made up of many interrelated lines of development. These include, but are not limited to, physical, cognitive, emotional, and social development. To understand and work effectively with children in inpatient and outpatient settings, the nurse must be familiar with these lines of development from infancy through adolescence, and how they affect and are affected by illness, injury, trauma, and so forth.

PSYCHOSEXUAL DEVELOPMENT AND PSYCHOANALYTIC THEORY

Freud did not set out to construct a theory of child development, but theoretical principles of child development have emerged from successive reformulations and expansions of his basic theory (Chess & Hassibi, 1978). There are three basic components to Freud's (1905) structural view of personality development. The **id** is composed of instinctual drives; they motivate the individual to seek gratification at any cost. The hungry newborn who cries until he is fed is one example of the id in operation.

As the infant matures, he becomes more aware of reality. The **ego,** which mediates between the outside world and the demands of the id, develops. The child becomes more equipped to delay need gratification, develop problem-solving skills, and operate under the reality principle.

Finally, the **superego,** the result of the child's identification with parental authority, their praise for doing "well," and the punishment they deliver for doing "badly," begins to develop. The superego contains the moral standards, beliefs, and values incorporated from significant others in the environment.

TABLE 22—1 Early theories of normal growth and development

	Psychosocial Development (Erikson)	Psychosexual Development (Freud)		Cognitive Development (Piaget)
		Area of gratification	Social/emotional development	
1st Year *INFANT* "I am."	*TRUST vs. MISTRUST* Sense of trust or security derived from affection and gratification of needs	*ORAL PHASE* 0–12 months Mouth Sensory	"Id" "Pleasure Principle"	*SENSORIMOTOR STAGE* (0–3 years) "Neonatal reflex": Complete self-world undifferentiation
		Oral dependent 0–6 months Passive, "takes in"	Omnipotent, total dependence, narcissistic	"Primary circular": Simple acts repeated
		Oral aggressive 6–12 months Biting	Beginning awareness of self as an individual "EGO" begins to develop	"Secondary circular": Repetition of acts that affect object. Activities become committed to memory. Learns when he does something, something else will happen
2–3 Years *TODDLER* "I am what I imagine I can be."	*AUTONOMY vs. SHAME and DOUBT* Child viewing self as an individual apart from parents, although dependent on them	*ANAL PHASE* 1–3 Years	Continued growth of ego. Beginning growth of "SUPEREGO." Begins to modify demands. Can postpone need gratification	Trial and error: Actions have specific effect on the environment Decides to do something. Beginning of symbolic activity Recognition of constancy. Egocentric thinking continues to predominate
		Anus Body excretions	Learns to manipulate environment. Begins to learn reality, negativism, rebellion, hostility	

TABLE 22–1 continued

4–5 Years *PRESCHOOL* "I am like others."	*INITIATIVE vs. GUILT* Sense of initiative gained easily if trust and autonomy attained. Period of vigorous reality testing, imagination, fantasy, imitation of adult behaviors	*PHALLIC PHASE* 3–6 Years Genital	Awareness of physical differences between the sexes Oedipal and Electra complexes. Plays cooperatively, needs socialization, curious Superego is strengthened as a result of resolution of Oedipal and Electra complexes.	*PREOPERATIONAL or PRECONCEPTUAL STAGE* (3–7 years) Thought intuitive and prelogical. Magical thinking Thinking still egocentric
6–12 Years *SCHOOL-AGE* "I am what I learn."	*INDUSTRY vs. INFERIORITY* Sense of duty and accomplishment. Laying aside of fantasy play. Undertaking real tasks, developing academic and social competencies	*LATENCY* Sexual drive controlled and repressed. Identifies with members of the same sex	Emotional turmoil quieted. Intellectual curiosity Society forms part of superego Friendships, gangs and cliques Parents are dethroned	*CONCRETE-OPERATIONAL STAGE* (7–12 years) Rational, well organized adaptations. Physical qualities are seen as constant despite changes in size, shape, weight and volume
12–18 Years *ADOLES-CENCE* "I know who I am."	*IDENTITY vs. ROLE DIFFUSION* Sense of identity, clarification of who one is and what one's role is. Predominant values are those of peers *INTIMACY vs. ISOLATION* Fidelity, friendship and cooperation	*ADOLESCENCE* Identifies with the opposite sex, first in group activity, then establishes close personal relationship with opposite sex. Ability to love and work	Resurgence of instinctual drives Two factors must be completed: 1) Emancipation from emotional ties at home 2) Heterosexual adjustment	*FORMAL-OPERATIONAL STAGE* (12–18 years) Deals with reality, abstract thoughts and the world of possibilities Deductive reasoning developed

In addition to this emphasis on a line of cognitive development, Freud described five stages of psychosexual development that reflect the impact of other socialization experiences. Each stage is related to the body part that is the greatest source of gratification during a particular phase of growth and development (see Table 22–1). For example, children in the phallic-oedipal stage (three to six years) typically develop a strong love for the parent of the opposite sex, along with a strong desire to do away with the parent of the same sex. A five-year-old boy whose fa-ther dies might thus be identified as a child at risk for possible emotional problems, since, according to Freud's theory, his wish to eliminate his father, along with his magical thinking that he could kill his father by wishing it so, is likely to make him feel extremely guilty. The adults in his world should be encouraged to listen to his concerns and reassure him that his father's death was not his fault. The surviving parent, because of her own grief, may not be available in such an objective/supportive way to a child at risk. The nurse needs to be sensitive to this and find other resources for the child as well as support for his mother.

Anna Freud and other ego psychologists have focused primarily on the ego and its development as a separate structure of the *personality as evidenced in the observation of children*. Her book, *Normality and Pathology in Childhood* (Freud, 1967) describes developmental lines or tracks, a concept useful to the understanding of child development (see Table 22–2). Her schema for special focus evaluations is a good resource for the nurse working in pediatrics.

Anna Freud's lines of development follow the child's movement from dependence on the irrational id and gratification-determined attitudes to a growing ego mastery over his internal and external worlds. There should be a close correspondence between growth on the various developmental lines (see Table 22–3).

Some children do show irregularities in their development; for example, the school-age child who is still soiling his pants or the preschool child who does not want to play with other children and continues to cling to his mother. Such an imbalance justifies an evaluation to determine whether there are physiological or environmental factors having an impact on the child's development.

PSYCHOSOCIAL DEVELOPMENT AND THE THEORY OF ERIK ERIKSON

Erikson (1963) emphasized the role that sociocultural aspects of the environment play in the development of the child's personality. He built on Freud's observations, expanding Freud's theory. He described development as a continuous process with distinct stages, each characterized by the achievement of particular developmental goals. Each stage presents a developmental task or crisis to be mastered (see Table 22–1). If the child succeeds in mastering a task, he grows and prepares to meet and master the next stage. Inability to master a developmental task results in frustration and difficulty in coping with subsequent stages. Mastery may ultimately be obtained but at a delayed rate, since difficulty at one stage slows progress through others.

Family, school, and peers all play important roles in assisting the child to master each developmental stage. The parents are the key individuals in the first stage, which has been called *trust versus mistrust*. If they respond in ways that are inconsistent and unpredictable and the infant's needs are not met, trust does not develop. The infant is unable to feel that the world is a safe and reliable place and that his instincts

TABLE 22–2 Developmental lines of Anna Freud

Developmental Lines	Infant	Toddler	Preschool	School-Age	Adolescent
Body to toy	Own body source of play and orientation	Transitional objects to symbolic objects	Utilizes play material	Pleasure in finished products of activity/creativity	
Play to work	Autoerotic play	Parallel play	Constructive play	Task completion and problem solving	Ability to love and to work
Egocentricity to Companionship	Others seen as *disturbances* in mother-child relationship	Other children related to as *lifeless objects*	Other children related to as *helpmates*	Other children related to as partners and people in their own right, as *friends*	
Wetting and soiling to Bowel and bladder control	Complete freedom	Ambivalence about body products and external control imposed by mother	Identification with others and autonomous, internalized control		

TABLE 22–3 Normal standard used with behavior-rating instrument for autistic and atypical children

	3 months	6 Months	9 Months	12 Months
Relationship	Infant shows sporadic attending to primary adult. Is capable of recurring eye contact.	Beginning of a regular response to adult. Will give eye contact and smile.	Infant now is interested in adult's coming and going. Begins to initiate contact with adult.	Infant begins to search out primary adult for help. Beginning of give and take in play.
Communication	Infant has undirected vocalizations, increased exertion level. Will cry when frustrated or smile when content.	Infant increases exertion level when feeding. First signs of directing protest to a person appear.	Undirected signs are still present. Subtle directed signs of need are now beginning to appear such as glancing at or reaching for an object.	Mostly subtle signs are present such as directed smiling. Simple and limited communicative signs appear such as pointing to objects wanted.
Drive for mastery	Not appropriate with this age group due to infant's inability to mobilize body to respond to objects.	Some stereotypic response to objects such as banging, shaking, mouthing. Will briefly explore objects presented by others.	Can now sustain some activity with presented objects, but shows little interest.	Infant is beginning to initiate exploration by picking up objects on his own.
Vocalization	Infant may be generally nonvocal. Exhibits cooing, vowel sounds, gurgling, and crying.	Gutteral and vowel sounds continue. Begins babbling in form of vowel/ consonant combination. May laugh.	Vowel/consonant babbling continues. Musical babbling with a greater variety of sounds begins.	Musical babbling continues. Jargon first appears.
Sound/speech reception	Infant has a reflexive response to sound. Does not show real interest in sound.	Infant has inconsistent reactions to sound; may ignore sound. Interest in sound toys begins.	Infant is aware of sound; turns head toward source. Real interest in sound is developing.	Localizes and seeks source of sound.
Social responsiveness	Infant is totally dependent on primary adult for meeting basic needs.	Infant has stereotypic response to self-help objects such as banging a spoon. Beginning response to feeding by trying to grab spoon.	Shows resistance to having face cleaned. Has some sustained response to feeding such as holding own bottle.	Infant may still show resistance to face-cleaning. May feed self, but needs monitoring in self-help functions.
Body movement	Infant has simple, tense, and repetitive gestural movements. Holds parts of body such as toes rigid and shows facial grimacing.	Infant has simple repetitive movements. Eyes now follow movement some of the time. Shows beginning awareness of space.	Tension shifts to different parts of body. Has beginning awareness of own movements. Some jerkiness develops.	Infant has quick and jerky movements. Uses movements to tease. Rigidity and limpness are appropriate to affective state.

	3 Months	6 Months	9 Months	12 Months
Psychobiological	Infant is involved in proprioceptive/kinesthetic stimulation such as leg-kicking. Oral behaviors such as mouthing are also present.	Proprioceptive/kinesthetic self-stimulation such as arm-flailing, nonspeech vocalization, and perseverative grasping continues, as do oral mouthing behaviors.	Proprioceptive/kinesthetic and oral behaviors continue, and are beginning to be incorporated into social interaction.	Direct oral behaviors such as biting still are present. Infant is beginning to replace oral direct drive discharge with personality trait equivalents such as curiosity and visually taking in the environment. He is interested and involved.

	15 Months	18 Months	21 Months	24 Months
Relationship	Infant continues to seek out adult for help, comfort, and play.	Active relationship is established with the primary adult. Infant consistently seeks out adult and directs vocalizations to the adult.	Infant now begins to tease adults, though on own terms. He will resist through distracting behavior.	Infant still relates on own terms. Teasing is pleasurable. There is a regular response to adult's requests.
Communication	Some subtle communicative signs are still present. Infant now uses mostly simple and direct methods such as pointing and vocalizing.	Infant continues both subtle and simple and limited direct methods. Needful self is developing. He knows what and who he wants.	A wide range of communication modes is present. Infant is now developing more varied ways of approaching others.	The needful self is established. A quality of mutuality is beginning to emerge.
Drive for mastery	Initiation continues. The infant now explores objects in a variety of ways, but attention is tenuous.	Infant seeks new toys and new ways of dealing with familiar objects.	Attention span is still short, but objects are explored and manipulated in a variety of ways.	Infant spontaneously hunts for new objects. Varied activity with toys continues.
Vocalization	Infant still babbles and uses jargon. One-word vocalizations begin.	There is still some babbling and jargon. Infant now spontaneously names things and repeats single words.	Jargon and cooperative naming continue. Ungrammatical 2–3 word phrases appear.	Jargon persists. Cooperative and spontaneous naming expands. Phrases begin to enlarge to sentences of 3 or more words.
Sound/speech reception	Infant repeats sound and makes own noises. Words seem meaningful, but he does not know specific meaning.	Infant understands familiar words and commands when accompanied by gestures.	Infant begins to understand words out of context and without gestures.	Individual words regularly have meaning. Teasing may be related to what was heard.

TABLE 22—3 continued

Social responsiveness	Infant is aware of feeding routine and can perform limited behaviors on his own with verbal reminders. He still needs monitoring.	Infant may still show some resistance, but he generally accepts feeding requirements and will perform social behaviors on his own. However, he may still need some reminding.	Infant can carry out behaviors on his own and has a growing repertoire of social behaviors.	Child shows a growing desire to function autonomously and can consistently imitate others. May have pleasure in opposition.
Body movement	Infant beginning to define kinesphere. He will repeat movements of others.	Infant now has a variety of movements, which are still somewhat jerky. Conscious imitation is beginning.	Infant responds to movement in environment and will show a body change when a stranger enters the room.	Toddler's movements are less jerky and seem to move from the joints. There is beginning ability to incorporate fantasy into action.
Psychobiological	Infant enjoys games involving proprioceptive/ kinesthetic stimulation. Enjoys being tickled and tossed in the air. Oral behaviors are still present.	Infant enjoys proprioceptive and oral stimulation. Continues to attend to environment. Beginning to develop gross temper tantrums when frustrated.	Infant is more firmly established in oral-trait behaviors. Development of anal-drive behaviors continues such as stubbornness, smearing, dumping, and gross motor discharge.	Kinesthetic and oral traits continue. Anal traits beginning to develop such as possessiveness and beginning of climbing, piling, and building. Ambivalence, selective resistance, and controlled tantrums, bowel-retention and toilet-training conflicts appear.

Note: This is the normal standard used with BRIAAC: Behavior-Rating Instrument for Autistic and Atypical Children; for early infant psychological assessment, using *minimal* expectations as the "norm." (Adapted from *Frontiers of Infant Psychiatry,* (1983). New York: Basic Books, Inc.)

are accurate. A child who is unable to develop a sense of trust in himself and his world is likely to have difficulty as he grows and faces additional developmental tasks.

In Erikson's second stage, *autonomy versus shame and doubt,* independence develops as the toddler masters new tasks. Shame and doubt win out when parents either do everything *for* him (never allowing autonomous problem solving), or are overly critical and expect perfection. If the nurse observes such parental behavior, she may discuss alternatives with them, or less traumatic ways to deal with children.

Similarly, the preschooler in Erikson's third stage, *initiative versus guilt,* will develop guilt feelings if his activity is unduly restricted and his curiosity belittled or inappropriately punished. In contrast, the child who is allowed to explore safely and investigate will develop a style of assertive initiative.

If the child enters the fourth stage, *industry versus inferiority,* and has difficulty measuring up to adult expectations, or if he is made fun of by peers, he is likely to develop a sense of inadequacy. In contrast, the child who feels good about himself and his abilities develops a sense of duty and accomplishment. School and peers become important, and a sense of pride inside and outside of the family develops.

The fifth of Erikson's eight stages, *identity versus role confusion,* involves the adolescent's task of developing a sense of identity, a culmination of physical and sexual development and his reaching out, with family and societal support, to the world.

A more complete description of Erikson's view of human development can be found in *Childhood and Society* (Erikson, 1963) and *Identity and the Life Cycle* (Erikson, 1954). His developmental theory, one of the most comprehensive, extends into adulthood and has provided the framework for much of the current thinking on self-actualization.

COGNITIVE DEVELOPMENT AS DEFINED BY JEAN PIAGET

Jean Piaget (Piaget & Inhelder, 1969) focused on the cognitive development of the child. His theory, a result of experiential work with children at various ages, provided the basis for other theories, such as Kohlberg's (1976) theory of moral development and Fowler's (Fowler & Keen, 1978) theory of faith development in children. Piaget found that children learn by assimilation, a process by which they integrate new experiences into already existing cognitive structures or "schemes." When a child is confronted with a new experience and is unable to fit it into an existing scheme, he either modifies that scheme or creates a new one. Piaget labeled this process **accommodation.**

Like Erikson, Piaget felt that development proceeds through a series of phases, from simple to complex, concrete to abstract, and egocentric to reality oriented. For a person to develop fully in a Piagetian sense, he must have contact with the physical world, the social world, and the world of ideas. According to Piaget, intellectual behavior begins with motor activity in the world, progresses to activity with thought, and finally, to thought with minimal motor activity. Thus, in order to proceed with cognitive development, the child must mature physically to be able to interact with his environment. Children with physical handicaps and chronically ill children are at a disadvantage and must be helped to find ways to influence and be influenced by their world and continue to develop cognitively. Nurses who work with children and their families in specialty rehabilitation clinics and inpatient units are in an excellent position both to evaluate and to promote the cognitive development of these special-needs children. The case study about Amber is an illustration.

Jean Piaget has often been called the father of child psychology.

Amber: A Child with Many Hospitalizations

Amber, age 16 months, was hospitalized in the pediatric intensive care unit for treatment of bronchitis and pneumonia. Amber was well-known to the staff, who had cared for her from birth to age ten months. Amber had been born three months prematurely, and was initially treated for respiratory distress syndrome and its complications. She had been on a respirator since the newborn period; she was tracheotomized at age six months.

During her first ten months of life, Amber was restricted to her crib, the arms of her caretaker, or a play mat on the floor next to her crib. She engaged in little spontaneous exploration of her very small world, but was responsive to toys offered and to people, especially those most familiar to her—her parents and nurses. Amber smiled and laughed when people paid attention to her; but she looked sad or apathetic when left unattended in her crib, even though she was surrounded by toys and other patients. (She was kept in the ward area in order to increase her sensory stimulation.) At the time of her discharge, Amber was developmentally three to four months old. ICU staff talked extensively with her family about her social and emotional needs and how they could be met. It was going to be a challenge as Amber was going home on a portable respirator.

Box 22–1 ● Bruno Bettelheim on Play, Including Play with Toy Guns

According to child psychologist Bruno Bettelheim, "play is the royal road" to the child's conscious and unconscious inner world. If we want to understand and help the child with his inner world, we must learn to walk this road. From a child's play we can gain understanding of how he sees and construes the world. Through his play, the child expresses what he is as yet unable to put into words.

Besides being a means of coping with past and present concerns, play is the child's most useful tool for preparing himself for the future. Play teaches the child the habits most needed for intellectual growth. For example, perseverance is easily acquired around enjoyable activities such as chosen play. If it is not developed through what is enjoyable, it is not likely to develop through an endeavor like schoolwork.

Developing an inner life, including fantasies and daydreams, is one of the most constructive things a growing child can do. Today's middle-class children, however, spend most of their days in scheduled activities such as scouts, music lessons, orga-

nized sports, and so forth. There is little time left for just being themselves. The resulting lack of sufficient leisure to develop a rich inner life is a large part of the reason why a child will pressure his parents to entertain him or will turn on the television set.

When thinking about organized sports for children, we need to keep in mind that the most important function of games and play for the well-being of the child is to offer him a chance to work through unresolved problems of the past, deal with pressures of the moment, and experiment with various roles and forms of social interaction in order to determine their suitability for himself. When children are in charge of an organized ball game, there are interruptions for displays of temper, digressions for talking things over or to pursue a parallel line of play for a time, and surprising acts of compassion (such as giving the "little guys" an extra turn). If adults want to see a polished game of baseball according to the rule books, they should turn on their television sets.

It is unfortunate that boys in our culture are rarely encouraged to play

---

Despite her continuing physical restrictions, particularly being leashed to her respirator, the change of environment and daily attention of her family and home-care nurses made a tremendous difference in Amber's life.

Despite her illness at the time of rehospitalization at age 16 months, the staff found Amber to be much more active and social than she had previously been. She no longer stayed in the place where she was put, but explored every inch she could comfortably get to. She seemed to know her limits and didn't challenge them. Amber also knew a few hand signs, which helped her communicate. Between signing and pointing, she was now initiating most of her own social interactions. The staff, of course, was very responsive and enthusiastically arranged her environment and life to be as homelike as possible. Amber's mother gave them the following daily schedule, which they tried to integrate into her nursing-care plan as much as possible:

7 A.M.—Bottle. Can hold it herself, but this is a chance for some quiet time together, so I usually hold her and talk to her.

8 A.M.—Breakfast. Amber feeds herself finger foods and is attempting to master spoon feeding. It's a mess, but she eats about one-half of her daily cereal this way.

10 A.M.—Six ounces of juice from a cup. Nap. Amber likes to have her special blanket ("security blanket") for all crib time.

11 A.M.—Playtime. Someone plays with Amber on her floor mat for thirty to forty minutes three times a day: her 5-year-old sister, 8-year-old brother, me or my husband, or her nurse. She enjoys building towers of blocks (with help) and knocking them down (without!). She also has a box of "stuff" which she enjoys emptying and refilling. It is a collection of objects of different textures (furry, hard, squishy) and sizes and things that make noise (bells,

with dolls. Perhaps if parents (and health-care professionals) could see how eagerly boys use dolls and doll houses in psychoanalytic treatment to work out family problems and anxieties about themselves, they would be more ready to recognize the importance of doll play for both sexes. For example, in doll-house play, girls *and* boys put a figure representing an ambivalently regarded sibling out of the house, put a figure representing a parent on the roof or lock it in the basement, place both parents together in bed (or separate them), seat a figure representing themselves on the toilet or have it mess up (even totally destroy) the house, and in countless other ways visualize and act out, and thus become better able to deal with, pressing family problems.

Some adults overreact to shooting play. Parents who do so usually are more concerned with their own feelings about aggression than with helping a child to master rather than merely repress his aggression through play. Some parents, out of their abhorrence of war and violence, try to control, or forbid altogether, any play with toy guns, soldiers, tanks, or other toys suggestive of war. Some parents even fear that such play may make a future killer of the child who enjoys it. In reality, just as playing with blocks doesn't indicate that a child will grow up to be a builder or an architect, playing with toy guns tells nothing about what a child will do or be in later life. Gun play does give a child an opportunity to discharge his aggressive tendencies in the context of fantasy play while parental prohibition of it can lead to real-life frustration and anger about being prevented from using an outlet he sees made available to other children and that is suggested to him by the mass media.

Perhaps the most pernicious attitude prohibition of aggressive play conveys is the parental fear that the child may become a violent person. This thought is far more damaging to the child's emotional well-being and his sense of self-worth than any play with guns can possibly be. A child gains a view of himself primarily from his parents. If they seem to hold such a low opinion of him, he is likely to feel angry at them and at the world, and *this* increases his propensity to act out his anger, not just in symbolic play, but in reality, once he has outgrown parental control.

If one watches the progress of aggressive activity in the child one can gradually discern a developmental move from free play, which permits direct Id expression and satisfaction (for example, an unstructured free-for-all shooting match) to a more structured game setting (such as "Dungeons and Dragons"), in which not mere discharge of aggression, but a higher integration—the ascendancy of good over evil—is the goal. Our children *want* to believe that good wins out, and they *need* that for their own well-being, so that they can turn into good people. It serves their developing humanity to repeat the external conflict of good and evil in a primitive form understandable to them, and to see that good triumphs in the end.

The Atlantic, "The Importance of Play," March, 1987 by Bruno Bettelheim, pp. 35–46.

---

music, rattle). She has become interested in her picture books, but tends to tear the pages if she gets the chance.

12 A.M.—Lunch. All finger foods; milk by cup.

12:30 to 1:30 P.M.—Playtime by herself. Amber likes to be in her walker and will amuse herself for thirty minutes or so. She then drinks another six ounces of juice while someone holds her and reads a story.

1:30 to 3 or 3:30 P.M.—Nap.

3:30 to 5 P.M.—Playtime; milk in a cup and fruit.

5 to 6 P.M.—Amber sits in her walker in the kitchen or living room and watches and interacts with the family as they arrive home. She especially likes to be with her brother and sister.

6 to 7 P.M.—Dinner with family (finger foods by herself, milk in cup, and other things with help).

7 to 8 P.M.—Playtime.

8 to 9 P.M.—Quiet time with mom or dad. Evening bottle. Bed.

Amber sleeps through the night except for needing occasional tracheal suctioning and a drink of juice. At home, her night nurse attends to these things so we can sleep. Sometimes she asks for me, but her nurse tells her I'm asleep and will be back in the morning. Unless she's sick, she is able to wait. In the hospital, she may have trouble. If you talk with her about me and where I am, and that I will come get her when she is well, while you comfort her, and give her her blanket, she should be okay.

Amber's primary nurse, Ann, was anxious to continue to support Amber's cognitive and emotional development during her hospital stay. She felt it would be possible to adhere to her home schedule in the hospital. Her respiratory care and medication administration could easily be worked in during playtime and/or before meals and bedtime. Ann worked with the head nurse to keep the number of nursing staff working with Amber to a minimum, for the sake of

Box 22–2 • Children Learn What They Live

If a child lives with criticism,
   He learns to condemn.
If a child lives with hostility,
   He learns to fight.
If a child lives with ridicule,
   He learns to be shy.
If a child lives with shame,
   He learns to feel guilty.
If a child lives with tolerance,
   He learns to be patient.
If a child lives with encouragement,
   He learns confidence.
If a child lives with praise,
   He learns to appreciate.

If a child lives with fairness,
   He learns justice.
If a child lives with security,
   He learns to have faith.
If a child lives with approval,
   He learns to like himself.
If a child lives with acceptance and friendship,
   He learns to find love in the world.

Dorothy Law Nolte

---

consistency and predictability. In addition to staff, playmates for Amber could be recruited from the occupational therapy and recreational therapy departments with the help of consultation requests.

Despite the two-week separation from her family, Amber's hospitalization was a positive experience. Her fine-motor skills improved and she learned a few new signs, thanks to the help of the communication disorders therapist and interested nursing staff. While Amber had some trouble with the separation from her family, occasionally looking sad and asking for "Mommy," she did not become depressed and had no difficulty returning to life at home after discharge. The child psychiatrist credited the nursing staff with this achievement, since it was their effort to replace what Amber had temporarily lost that probably made the difference.

Piaget has described a sequence of cognitive developmental phases and related subphases (see Table 22–1). An understanding of his theory is invaluable for the nurse involved in pediatric-patient teaching or the development of any patient-teaching tools. It can also be useful when talking with children about their own illness or possible death or their parents' illnesses or impending death (see Table 22–4).

Piaget's theory of cognitive development has formed the cornerstone for much of the current thinking about psychopathology as an interweaving of biological vulnerability and behavioral expression of cognitive distortions. The current work of Greenspan (1981) on the infant's progression from biosocial to psychological symbiosis, Stern (1985) on early communication of affect and affect attunement, and Kagen (1984) on the importance of maturation and

the primacy of biological change in development, all reflect the focus of today's developmental clinicians and theorists built on Piaget's thinking. All involve an exciting fusion of Piagetian concepts with the recent explosion of knowledge resulting from clinical observational research in infant and child development. (See Table 22–3 for summary of current expanded views of infant development.)

THE CONTRIBUTION OF PSYCHOSOCIAL RESEARCH TO DEVELOPMENTAL THEORY AND ITS APPLICATION TO NURSING PRACTICE

ATTACHMENT AND DEVELOPMENT

John Bowlby's (1969; 1973; 1980) work on attachment and the child's response to separation and loss is another framework for understanding normal and pathological development in children. Margaret Mahler (Mahler, Pine, & Bergman, 1975) has also described how the developing infant gradually separates psychologically from his mother and becomes independent (see Table 22–5). Both theorists have made invaluable contributions to the understanding of separation anxiety and its relevance to the young child.

Bowlby has said that if **attachment** does not take place, the relationship between parent and child will forever be vulnerable. Similarly, Mahler and her colleagues have shown how missteps in the progression

TABLE 22—4 Children's cognitive discovery of death

Piaget's Stages of Cognitive Development		Children's Concepts of Death
Sensorimotor infant/toddler	World of here and now. Complete self-world. Experiences through senses and motor movements. No notion of object permanence.[1]	Virtually no understanding of death. Fear and anxiety related to separation and abandonment.
Preoperational preschooler	Language ability develops. Symbolic play. Animistic thinking. (Inanimate objects have motives and intentions.) Phenomenalistic causality. Magical thinking. Egocentric thought.	Concept of death still vague. Curious. Play may show early attempts to conceptualize death. Conceives of dead things as having biological functions. Sees death as reversible. May feel they caused death because of a wish or word that preceded death.
Concrete operations school-ager	Begins to grasp concepts of reversibility, classification, and number. Developing basic concepts of time, space, quantity, and causality. Concrete thinking still predominates.	Understands finality of death. Knows the major difference between going away for a week and going away "forever." "Probably won't happen to me . . . at least not until I'm older." Personifies death; tells scary stories in an attempt to deal with feelings and questions.
Formal operations adolescence	Abstract thought. Generality of thought. Propositional thinking. Hypothetical thinking. Strong idealism.	Death can happen to anybody, anytime. Death can happen to me. Death is universal and permanent. Death is a natural phenomenon. Has the adult's concepts of life and death.

[1]Infant is capable of maintaining the mother's mental representation even in her absence for increasingly longer periods of time (Hartmann, 1939).
Source: Adapted from Ferguson, F. "Children's Cognitive Discovery of Death." *Journal of the Association for the Care of Children's Health,* Vol. 7(1), Summer, 1978, pp. 8–14.

from dependence to stable independence through the toddler years can lead to significant psychological problems. They can occur in childhood (as severe regression or separation-anxiety disorders) or remain dormant only to be rekindled when moves toward independence are called for, for example, at the beginning of school or in adolescence. Both Bowlby and Mahler feel that broken or lost attachments (for example, through death, separation, or divorce) predispose children to the development of psychopathology.

This perspective on child development is relevant for any nurse who works with hospitalized children. **Separation anxiety,** or panic on separation from home and/or parent, is a major problem for the hospitalized child from age six months to approximately three to four years. It can also occur in older children who are vulnerable, as in the case of Peter. Support during separations, for example, by a primary nurse and a minimal number of other nursing staff, which provides empathy and verbal and physical reassurance, can be enormously helpful. The nurse's respect

TABLE 22–5 Margaret Mahler's separation-individuation theory

I. Undifferentiated matrix

A. Normal autism
0–1 Month

During the first weeks of life "absolute primary narcissism" exists. Infant is unaware of mothering agent. Physiological rather than psychological processes are dominant. Minimal responses to external events. Energies focus toward physiological need satisfaction and maintenance of homeostasis.

B. Normal symbiosis
1–5 Months

Mother seen as part of self. Infant gradually perceives need satisfaction as coming from some need satisfying "part object." "Secondary narcissism" develops. Mother's body as well as infant's body is object of infant's narcissism. Unable to differentiate between internal and external experiences. Infant familiarizes self with the mother half of the symbiotic self. Infant molds to mother's body. Social smile response.

II. Separation-individuation

A. Differentiation
5–9 Months

"Hatching," the process of emerging from the symbiotic state of oneness with the mother. More permanent alert sensorium when awake. Infant begins to differentiate his own from mother's body. Visual and tactile exploration of mother: pulls hair and puts food in her mouth. Curiosity of infant to explore "other-than-mother" world, but has strong need for "checking back with mother." Seven–nine months stranger reaction: anxiety, interest, curiosity.

B. Practicing
9–14 Months

Spurt in autonomous functioning. New locomotion helps toddler to go exploring. "Love affair with the world." Mother still viewed as "home base." Infant absorbed in own activities for long periods of time. He appears oblivious to mother's presence. However, returns periodically to her seeming to need physical proximity from time to time, or "refueling."

C. Rapprochement
14–24 Months +

Rediscovery of mother, now as separate individual, yet extension of self. Loves to share experiences with mother. Wishes for reunion with the love object. Follows his mother's every move, "shadowing." At other times we view the opposite behavior. The child "darts away," fearing that he might be engulfed and undo the separateness.

Becomes more aware of separateness and vulnerability. "Rapprochement crisis"—realization of separateness acute. "Ambitendency"—rapidly alternating desire to push mother away and to cling to her. Children can be demanding, clingy, whining, have temper tantrums. Powerful resurgence of stranger reaction. Important for mother to accept ambivalence and love toddler unconditionally during this stressful time.

D. Consolidation
24–36 Months +

Degree of object constancy achieved. Separation of self and object representation is sufficiently established. Mother during her absences can be substituted for, at least in part, by the presence of a reliable internal image that remains relatively stable irrespective of the state of instinctual need or inner discomfort.

E. Object constancy
36 months +

Capacity to perceive and emotionally invest a person as a whole, both good and bad, to retain the investment despite frustration, and to retain the unified mental representation of the person (or love object, e.g. the mother), resulting in the sense that she is available and dependable even when she is physically absent, when child is angry with her, and when she is not providing satisfaction (Edward et al., 1981).

Source: Adapted from Mahler, M., Pine, F. & Bergman, A. (1975). *The psychological birth of the human infant.* New York: Basic Books, Inc., Publishers.

for the child's normal routine, preferences, and coping style, along with familiar toys or pictures from home, can go a long way toward reducing the trauma of hospitalization. If the parents cannot be with their child, they or the child's siblings can make tapes of their voices, reading a favorite story or just talking soothingly. (See Box 22–3.)

Young children usually react to separation from their families by going through stages of protest, despair, and denial. During the protest stage, the child cries and screams for his parents, sometimes for hours, and may be inconsolable (Robertson & Robertson, 1971). Here, the consistent caretaker, preferably a nurse who was there when the child's parents

Box 22–3 ● Day Care In The First Year of Life: A Controversy

Few subjects capture the attention of today's busy working mother like professional viewpoints and recommendations about day care, especially day care in the first year of life. Recently, a national conference on this topic generated a heated debate among specialists in child development and mental health about the risks of full-time (more than 20 hours per week) day care in infancy, some of which was picked up by the lay press and sensationally reported. As a result, it is likely that many parents are feeling alarmed, guilty, and confused about what to do about the situation and who to ask for advice. While concern is appropriate and discussion healthy, alarm and guilt are neither, and can only make problems that do exist worse. It is very important that health-care professionals, including nurses, understand what *is* known about the effects of day care, especially for the very young child, what constitutes "good day care," and how to help parents evaluate the options available to them.

Belsky (1986, 1987) has reviewed the research on full-time, non-maternal day care in infancy and has concluded that there is an "emerging pattern" (1986, p. 4) in research findings which includes the following:

1. Whether day care is in the home or in a day care center, it has been associated with a tendency in the infant to avoid or maintain a distance from the mother following a series of brief separations (specifically, those involved in the Ainsworth Strange-Situation paradigm described in this chapter on p. 821). Some professionals contend that this response to separation reflects underlying doubt or mistrust about the availability of the mother to meet the baby's needs and, thus, ensure attachment. This avoidant response has also been shown to be associated with developmental outcomes such as noncompliance and low frustration tolerance.

Belsky points out that other scientists "read the very same evidence in a very different way" (p. 5), viewing the avoidant response as adaptive or precocious behavior: "In children receiving care exclusively from mother, avoidance may be a pathological response reflecting an interactive history with a rejecting mother, while for children in day care greater distance from, or ignoring of, mother at reunion may be an adaptive response reflecting a habitual reaction to repeated daily separations and reunions. In these latter children, greater physical distance from mother and apparent avoidance may, in fact, signal a "precocious independence" (Clarke-Stewart and Fein, 1986, p. 949).

2. When compared to a group of children reared exclusively at home until entering a preschool day care program, those with histories of infant day care were found, four months after entering preschool, to be more physically and verbally aggressive with adults and peers, less cooperative with grown-ups and less tolerant of frustration. Children from the studies which associated insecure-avoidant attachment with day care early in life, reevaluated at age two, present a similar picture. In addition, these toddlers displayed significantly less enthusiasm in confronting a challenging task than did children who had no day care experience, but it was also the case that these day care-reared infants tended to be less compliant in following their mothers' instructions, less persistent in dealing with a difficult problem, and more negative in their affect. Additional analysis of these same data revealed that although 18-month attachment security was a significant advantage to the children who were home-reared as infants, when studied at 24 months, the securely attached infants who had entered day care in their first year looked more like toddlers with insecure attachment histories (from home and day care groups) than like home-reared children with secure infant-mother relationships.

continued

3. When five– and six-year-olds who had been reared in a high-quality day care center since 3 months of age were compared to children who received non-maternal care of a variety of kinds beginning *after* the first year of life, they were rated ". . . as more likely to use the aggressive acts hit, kick, and push than children in the control group. Second, they were more likely to threaten, swear, and argue. Third, they demonstrated those propensities in several school settings—the playground, the hallway, the lunchroom, and the classroom. Fourth, teachers were more likely to rate these children as having aggressiveness as a serious deficit in social behavior. Fifth, teachers viewed these children as less likely to use such strategies as walking away or discussion to avoid or extract themselves from situations that could lead to aggression" (p. 6).

There has been much criticism of Belsky's conclusions and position that "entry into non-maternal care in the first year of life is a 'risk factor' for the development of insecure-avoidant attachments in infancy and heightened aggressiveness, noncompliance, and withdrawal in the preschool and early school years" (p. 7), some of it by child development experts as accomplished as Dr. Stella Chess of the New York University Department of Psychiatry (1987). Most of the criticism focuses on what is judged to be inadequate research methodology in the studies Belsky bases his conclusions on. For example, it has been charged that variables such as psychosocial stress due to poverty or psychopathology in the parent, instability of child care, and type and quality of day care were not adequately controlled for in these studies, and could account for bad outcomes attributed to *early entry* alone. Belsky's critics have also accused him of "selective review" and have pointed out other studies which associate early entry into day care with more positive outcomes such as

"less tension" and "higher social interaction scores" (Phillips et al., 1987, p. 20). Finally, they advocate responding to questions about the long-term effects of day care on children with "We don't know. The evidence is inconclusive" (p. 20).

Belsky (1987) has responded with the following: "The essay I wrote reflected my desire to bring to the attention of child care professionals the fact that, in contrast to just five or ten years ago, there exists now a sizeable body of evidence linking care initiated in the first year of life with patterns of child functioning that ought to be a cause for concern. This is not to say that benefits do not arise from non-maternal care or that such disconcerting correlates of early care are found in every study, characterize every child, are inevitable or even are caused by experience in infant day care arrangements as routinely experienced in the United States today. In view of the fact that it remains unclear, given the current state of the evidence, under which conditions these correlates of care are most likely and most unlikely, it seems appropriate to characterize infant day care as a risk factor. This phrase does not imply that risk is inevitable, only heightened. Future research, we must hope, will illuminate these very conditions. Future policy, we must further hope, will enable families to maximize their choices, with affordable and quality infant care being one of them" (p. 24).

Belsky and three of his critics, Howes, Phillips, and Scarr, and twelve other leading child care researchers *have* reached a consensus regarding the characteristics of high quality infant-toddler care, whether it occurs in or outside the home and whether the child's parents or other adults provide it. They have recommended that the child care environment provide the infant or toddler with:

— physical protection and attention to health and nutrition;

— awareness of and respect for individual differences in infants and toddlers;

— sensitivity to the infant's cues and communication;

— a capacity to shift caregiving practices as the infant develops and changes; and,

— warm, loving human relationships based on constancy of care.

Child care, the researchers have stated, must be viewed as a support to the whole family. A comfortable "blend" and close collaboration between parents and caregivers are important to the well-being and the development of both children and parents. Since the sensitivity, skills and commitment of the caregiver determine to such a large extent the quality of the child's experience in supplemental care, the researchers have pointed out the urgent need to improve salaries, working conditions, and training for child–care providers, whether in center-based or family day care settings (Schrag, 1988).

Belsky, J. (1986). Infant day care: a cause for concern? *Zero to three*, Vol. 6 (5), pp. 1–9.

Belsky, J. (1987). Risks remain. *Zero to three*, special reprint: infant day care: a continuing dialogue, February, pp. 22–24.

Chess, S. (1987). Comments: infant day care: a cause for concern. *Zero to three*, special reprint: infant day care: a continuing dialogue, February, pp. 24–25.

Clarke-Stewart, K. A., & Fein, G. (1983). Early childhood programs. In M. M. Maith & J. J. Campos (eds.), P. H. Mussen (Series Ed.), *Handbook of childhood psychology:* Vol 2. *Infancy and developmental psychobiology*. New York: Wiley.

Phillips, D., McCartney, K., Scarr, S., & Howes, C. (1987). Selective review of infant day care research: a cause for concern! *Zero to Three*, special reprint: infant day care: a continuing dialogue, February, pp. 18–21.

Schrag, E. (1988). National Center for Clinical Infant Programs press release.

were present, may be most able to calm and reassure him. She or another consistent caretaker should always be with the child when the parents leave the hospital. The parents should be encouraged to tell the child when they are leaving and not "sneak away." Such unclear leave takings will only make the child more fearful, thus undermining trust in his parents and discouraging development of trust in the nurse.

During the second stage, despair, the child may become passive or withdrawn and ignore his parents or act angry when they return to the hospital. Parents must be helped to understand what is happening so they continue to visit, interact with, and reassure their child. The parents will need much reassurance and support themselves during this stage because the intensity of their child's despair or anger can add to their own feelings of helplessness and guilt. This can result in *their* withdrawal from the child, increasing the intensity of the child's feelings of abandonment.

During the final stage, denial, the child may appear to be adjusting well to the hospital environment. In fact, he may be resigning himself to what he feels is total abandonment. An inexperienced nurse, or the experienced one on a busy day, seeing that the child is a "good patient" (passive and quiet) when the parents are gone, and that the parents' presence upsets the child, may consciously or unconsciously discourage the parents from visiting. This perpetuates the problem because the lack of contact with his parents will intensify the child's feelings of abandonment.

In addition to encouraging and supporting the parents' visits and overnight stays, the nurse, if possible, should offer the child realistic reassurance. This includes telling the child where the parents are and when they will return. Labeling the child's anxiety, sadness, and/or anger as these feelings surface, providing opportunities for the child to master these feelings and fantasies through play, and keeping the parents informed of these interactions are additional important nursing interventions.

The older child or adolescent is also vulnerable to separation anxiety. This includes feelings related to separation from peers. The older child's distress may not be as obvious or overwhelming as it is for the younger patient. For this older age group, phone calls, cards, tapes, and regular planned visits from family and friends are helpful. The nurse should encourage these and other creative ways of maintaining the child's contact with his world.

Finally, at the time of his discharge, the child who has forged attachments and relationships during his hospital stay must be helped to separate from the hospital via a thoughtful plan. This may include calls or visits to his hospital unit at the time of followup appointments or at other times when his primary nurse and other special people are available. Cards or calls from the nurse also can facilitate a child's adjustment upon returning home as well as remind the parents of a valuable resource for help with dealing with any negative reactions or regressions the child may have at home. A referral to a public health or home nursing agency may provide useful backup. It is imperative to have a coordinated discharge and followup plan for the chronically physically or emotionally ill child.

BEHAVIORAL THEORY AND DEVELOPMENT

Watson's (Watson & Rayner, 1929) work on the conditioned response of children to stressors and their subsequent formation of behavioral pathology, and Jones' (1924) remediation of such pathology with behavioral methods, led to the development of today's clinical behavior therapies. The behavioral framework of reward for desired behavior and ignoring or punishment for unwanted behavior is central to current everyday child-rearing techniques and is a common expression of behavioral learning theory.

Seligman's (1975) **learned-helplessness theory** and related research is another behavioral framework important to the prevention, identification, and treatment of psychopathology in childhood. Seligman defines *helplessness* as the psychological state that results when events are uncontrollable. For example, if an infant attempting to elicit a response from his mother does not get a response, or gets an inconsistent one no matter what he does, he will learn that outcome is independent of his actions, that he does not affect the world he lives in, and that he is helpless. Infants or children who are continually exposed to situations in which they have no control, for example, parental abuse, become depressed and eventually lose all motivation to keep on trying. They become passive and have trouble changing their behavior when control *is* possible, that is, in school and with peers. Hospitalization is overwhelming for such a child and may result in intense anxiety and severe depression.

Seligman believes that if an individual can learn helplessness he can also learn how *not* to be helpless. As children grow and develop there are many opportunities to "immunize" them against helplessness.

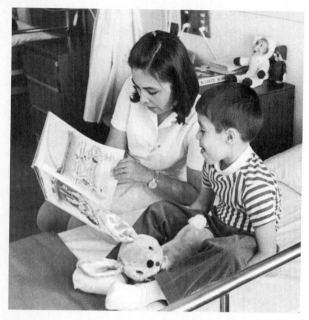

What the hospitalized child misses most is home. Even his favorite toy and the nurse reading his favorite book to him doesn't make up for the fact that he isn't home. It is important that these feelings be understood and acknowledged, even if they sadden him. The nurse needs to encourage the child to share his feelings with her so together they can work on some of his problems, such as his loneliness.

The nurse has the opportunity to do so by teaching parents the importance of contingency and control in a child's life, and by identifying those children who are at risk for developing helplessness as well as those who are already demonstrating helpless behaviors. Thus, the chronically ill child, and the child in crisis, as well as the vulnerable hospitalized child, should be an important focus for all nurses working with children. (For more on learned helplessness, see Chapter 9 on mood disorders and Chapter 25 on the ICU patient.)

FAMILY SYSTEMS THEORY AND DEVELOPMENT

The nurse should be familiar with the characteristics of the normal and pathological family (see Chapter 21 on psychiatric mental health nursing with families), and how they affect a child's development of psychopathology. Especially relevant to the nurse, because of its blend of family psychology and biological issues, is Minuchin et al.'s (1975) work on the family-systems model of and approach to psychosomatic illness, specifically, anorexia nervosa, diabetes,

and asthma (see Chapter 13 on psychophysiological disorders).

The models and theories we use to understand and deal with emotions and behavior in children overlap and reinforce each other. They offer a wealth of information essential to working effectively with children and families during the crisis of illness. They also provide a conceptual framework from which the nurse can assess a child in any context. However, it is extremely important to remember that each child is unique. We must not lose sight of the differences and life experiences that contribute to an individual child's situation. There are multiple determinants of psychopathology just as there are of psychological health, and multiple options for therapeutic intervention.

ASSESSMENT OF THE CHILD

The mentally healthy child has successfully mastered the tasks required at each stage of his development. He has developed an ability to trust adults and feels safe and secure. He likes himself and utilizes adaptive coping mechanisms to deal with stress. He gets along well with his family and peers and has a realistic view of the world and his place in it. He has hope, pride, and a drive to accomplish his goals.

However, not all children function in such a healthy manner. The appearance and behavior of some children elicit concern in those around them. If the concern is serious enough, children are brought by a responsible adult for assessment of emotional and/or behavioral problems at home, in school, or in the community. Sometimes either the child or parent feels guilty about asking for help, or may be angry if they have been coerced into seeking it, for example, by child-protective services. These factors can be unconsciously influential in the assessment process unless the clinician is sensitive to them. Empathic listening by the clinician and awareness of her own reaction (countertransference) to the presenting parent-child dyad, especially as it is influenced by her personal experience, is essential.

The diagnostic evaluation involves collecting subjective and objective data that will help to explain the presenting problem and its possible etiology. The diagnostic impression (assessment) that the clinician forms as she collects and analyzes this data also provides the basis for the development of a treatment plan. The plan includes attention to symptoms contributing to the child's dysfunction (such as temper displays and aggression when demands are made), and recommended interventions designed to remove or control symptoms (such as clear warnings and consistent consequences). These recommendations, as well as those that focus on possible causes of the symptoms, (such as the child's sense of incompetence and parents' inconsistent expectations), should be linked to growth-promoting factors in the child and his environment, for example, a child's strong attachment to his father and their active involvement together. This will result in a family that feels understood and ready to trust the health-care professional rather than one that feels blamed and defensive.

The process of evaluation varies depending on the age and developmental level of the child, the clinician's skills and sphere of influence, and the clinical setting. It is always important to spend time alone with the child during the evaluation. However, because the child is part of the family system, it is imperative that observations also be made of the child in the family context. This can be accomplished by seeing the child with the parents and/or by arranging an extended family interview that includes the siblings and/or, possibly, grandparents or others.

Even if the nurse is not responsible for the complete psychiatric assessment, she can identify an emotional problem or an "at risk" situation. When she sees such a situation, she can gather further data (see Table 22–6) and focus her colleagues as well as the child's parents on the need for further evaluation and, possibly, treatment. (Also see Chapter 18 on crisis for the example of assessment of "at risk for child abuse" and its prevention.)

Jamie: A Child's Reaction to Divorce

The school nurse noted that Jamie, a child who complained of stomachaches and headaches, made frequent visits to her office. In speaking with the child's teacher she discovered that Jamie had had increasing difficulty concentrating in class and seemed to be withdrawing socially. Thus, the nurse asked herself:

- Is this a medical problem?
- Are these psychosomatic symptoms of an underlying emotional problem?
- Is this a medical problem in a child with undetected developmental or emotional difficulties?

The nurse called Jamie's mother and shared her observations and concerns. Jamie's mother explained that she and her husband were divorced one month ago. Jamie's headaches and stomachaches began occuring around that time at home. His mother had not

been aware that his school performance had deteriorated, but had noticed that he had become "quiet." As a result of her conversation with the nurse, she made an appointment with the child's pediatrician.

Jamie's mother gave the school nurse permission to contact the pediatrician in order to share her concerns. When Jamie's medical workup was negative, the pediatrician recommended psychiatric evaluation. The school nurse then focused on helping mother and child accept the need for referral to the school psychologist for a complete psychological evaluation and treatment recommendations.

Marshall: A Child's Reaction to the Death of a Parent

A clinic nurse working with asthmatic children observed Marshall, a school-age child, in the waiting room swearing at his mother and fighting with another child. As she obtained Marshall's history from his mother, she discovered that the child had recently become a behavior problem at school. His mother was extremely frustrated by her apparent inability to get him to listen to her, especially about taking his medication. Marshall was the youngest of five children whose father had been killed in an automobile accident the year before.

Identifying this child as "at risk" for development of serious physical problems and psychosocial dysfunction, the nurse talked with Marshall's mother about a referral to the clinic's consulting child psychiatrist; she readily accepted this suggestion and an appointment was arranged. With the mother's permission, the clinic nurse contacted the child psychiatrist and shared her impression of the child and the information she had obtained from his mother.

TABLE 22–6 Areas of beginning investigation of childhood psychopathology

1. Presenting problem (What is going on?)
2. The presumed reason for its appearance (Why now?)
3. Pertinent past history of the child (What was he/she like before?)
4. School and social history of the child
5. Developmental history of the child (How was she/he while growing up?)
6. Family history and current family functioning (How does all of this affect the rest of you?)

Identifying a Child at Risk for Physical Abuse

A nurse in a well-baby clinic obtained a history from a young, single mother who seemed depressed and complained of "feeding problems" with her six-week-old baby. In the process, the nurse became concerned about the "out of sync" mother-infant interactions she observed. For example, the mother continued to feed the baby though it was clear that he didn't want any more of his bottle. She also made several negative remarks about him and handled him so roughly that he vomited about half the feeding. The nurse modeled appropriate interaction with and handling of the infant, and expressed empathy for the mother who admitted to feeling depressed and angry about how much work the baby demanded and how expensive it was to feed him. The nurse suggested a public health nursing referral as well as a return appointment in one week to further assess the feeding problems and evaluate the mother's depression. In addition, she brought all this to the attention of the pediatrician who, after speaking with the mother, also made a referral to social services.

All the children mentioned in the cases above could have been referred to a child psychiatry outpatient facility. There a nurse with experience and advanced training in child psychiatry might do the complete diagnostic evaluation. This nurse would be responsible for obtaining all the information in Tables 22–6, 22–7, and 22–8. She would also obtain collateral information from the child's parents as well as his pediatrician and teachers, with the parents' permission. In the process, she may identify the need to consult with other professionals (for example, a child psychologist, neurologist, or child psychiatrist) to facilitate or complete the assessment process and begin to develop a treatment plan.

Although there are no truly unique skills necessary to assess a child, the usual modes of observation and history taking need to be adapted for children at various ages and stages of development. The language and interactional methods employed (for example, play and drawing) require that the clinician be comfortable working with children and families, and knowledgeable about child development and psychopathology.

ASSESSING THE INFANT/TODDLER

The prenatal period is an ideal time to begin collecting information necessary to assess the potential for

TABLE 22–7 Guidelines for developmental history: areas of investigation

1. Pregnancy: planning, desire for, parents' feelings regarding pregnancy
2. Delivery and perinatal: premature or normal delivery, medical problems, mother's initial impression, history of "bonding"
3. Feeding: breast or bottle, colic or feeding problems, weaning
4. Sleep: sleep patterns, sleep disturbances (nightmares, night terrors,* night waking) and their management
5. Bladder and bowel: age training began and ended, problems, current functioning
6. Motor development: age child sat/crawled/walked, parental and child affective response
7. Language development: age child began to talk, use of language skills, compliance
8. Self-care skills and play patterns: bathing, teeth brushing, dressing, shoe tying; solitary play, peer play
9. Medical history: trauma, operations, hospitalizations and affective response; past or current medications
10. Separations: age of child, duration, reason, affective response
11. Significant family historical events: divorce, deaths and other losses, family moves, child's affective response

*Sleep state which, unlike nightmares, arises out of non-REM sleep and is characterized by disorientation, automatic behavior, diminished responsiveness to external stimuli, difficulty in being aroused to full alertness, amnesia for events during the episode, and minimal (or no) recall of dreams; associated with immature nervous system and developmentally self-limiting (Herskowitz & Rosman, 1982).

problems in parenting. Additional information can be gathered during the labor, delivery, and neonatal period. Gray et al. (1976) demonstrated that observations of the mother's reaction to her infant in the delivery room offer the most accurate predictive information regarding high-risk for abuse situations. They concluded that "perinatal assessment and early, consistent intervention with families identified as at high risk for abnormal parenting significantly improves the infant's chances of escaping serious physical injury" (p. 389).

Ideally, the child should be assessed for temperament and attachment during the first thirty-six months of his life. These two factors are thought to be critical predictors of later development by most

TABLE 22–8 Guidelines for the mental health interview of the child

Observational data

General appearance:	height, weight, grooming and hygiene, nutrition, physical health, distinguishing features (deformities, tics), maturity level
Motor behaviors:	fine and gross, balance, bizarre motor activity
Speech and language:	receptive, expressive, content, tone, and articulation
Affect:	range of emotion, predominant emotion (depressed, angry, anxious, happy, irritable, labile); emotional reactions to process and/or content of interview (appropriate, inappropriate)
Thought process:	estimated intellectual level via language and knowledge base, orientation (to person, place, time), perceptual distortions (hallucinations, illusions, tangentiality, obsessions?), attention span
Ability to relate to evaluator:	eye contact, attitude toward interviewer (negative, positive, shy, suspicious, withdrawn, friendly, self-centered)

Behaviors displayed during interview:	impulsivity, aggression, inhibited, low frustration tolerance, ability to have fun, sense of humor, creativity

Interactional data

Interpersonal relationships:	attitudes toward and perceptions of family and peers, transitional objects,* pets; social skills with peers, best friend.
Self-concept and image:	self-appraisal (does child like self?), comparison of self with others (sibling, peers), what does he like most about self? what would he like to change about self? sense of pride in accomplishments, sex role and gender identity
Conscience:	Sense of right and wrong, acceptance of guilt, ability to accept limits in the evaluation

*Inanimate objects invested with ability to allay anxiety and tension in lieu of human relationships, especially the mother-child relationship.

infant mental health workers. Temperament, a concept researched and popularized by Chess and Thomas (1984), is best understood as a genetically determined style of response to and engagement with the inner and outer world. Temperament is readily assessed by the use of parent report rating scales or behavioral observations during the first months of life (Carey, 1970).

Chess and Thomas have done longitudinal studies on a variety of infant-parent populations. Their work has shown that anticipatory guidance for parents of the developmentally "difficult" child, counseling regarding the "goodness of fit" between the temperamental styles of infants and their parents, and other early interventions can significantly improve a child's developmental outcome. Often, sim-

ple education and validation of the child's temperament style is enough to allow parents to relax and use their instinctive parenting skills.

An assessment of behavioral indicators of the infant/toddler's attachment to his parents can also be done at an early age. The Massie-Campbell AIDS Scale (Attachment Indicator During Stress) (Massie & Rosenthal, 1984) is a screening tool that can be used in clinical pediatric settings to identify early signs of aberrant infant-parent interaction. Although the predictive value of such screening is not clear, there is evidence that early identification of significant problems leads to the chance for early intervention (Fraiberg, 1980; Greenspan, 1981).

Ainsworth and colleagues (Ainsworth et al., 1978) developed the **Strange-Situation Assessment** as a method of judging attachment in the older toddler. This technique involves observation of the toddler's affect and behavior when separated from and reunited with his mother. The quality of the young child's response to this stress provides insight into the type and intensity of the parent-child attachment that has developed in the context (family environment) these individuals share. As clinical modifications of this assessment tool and others are developed and made available to the nurse, she will be able to use them to corroborate objectively her probably accurate feelings about the distressed parent-infant interactions she sees in the well-baby, preschool, and pediatric clinics.

The Brazelton Neonatal Assessment Scale (1973) was developed to assess the newborn's integrative behavioral processes in response to a variety of stimuli. The nurse who utilizes this instrument has a unique opportunity to interact with the infant and gain an understanding of how he responds to stimuli, interacts with others, and soothes himself when in distress. The Brazelton assessment process can also provide a structure in which the nurse can teach parents how to identify their infant's cues, and demonstrate to them how best to meet his needs. It can be used also to assess parent-infant interactions and attempt to affectively connect parents with their baby by pointing out his unique responsiveness to them, as well as facilitate anticipatory guidance regarding potential problems (Gibes, 1981). Clinical modifications of the scale (Berger, 1981) and standardization of a scale for premature infants are in progress.

The Denver Developmental Screening Test (Frankenburg et al., 1971) is the most commonly used screening instrument in the United States. Able to be administered quickly and with minimal training, it is used to identify developmental delays in children who can then be referred for more thorough

assessment (see Figure 22–1). Clinical revision and modifications continue to make this a very useful instrument.

ASSESSING THE PRESCHOOLER

Assessment of the preschooler (ages three to five) demands a particularly skillful examiner who is comfortable with play techniques and able to use concrete language skills. Paper and crayons, dolls, clay, and puppets are useful equipment. The nurse must have a sense of openness toward a child's startling revelations about family "secrets" and his candid observations of her personal appearance and style. For this age group, the importance of the developmental history cannot be overstated. The parental responses to the questions outlined in Table 22–6 are a means of assessing the child's movement along developmental pathways. They also provide a way to distill parental concerns about the preschool child and their relationship to any symptoms of dysfunction. This information can be obtained through the use of a questionnaire (Garrison & Earls, 1985) or in a parent or family interview. (See Figure 22–2.)

ASSESSING THE SCHOOL-AGE CHILD

The child between the ages of six and twelve will bring to the assessment not only a rich developmental history but also a well-developed interactional style. The child of this age typically presents with a wariness about the assessment process and an ambivalent wish for help due to fear of reprisal. The standard talking session utilized with adults will not be sufficient with this child. Although he will be better able to verbalize than the preschooler, the school-age child may still feel more comfortable engaged in an

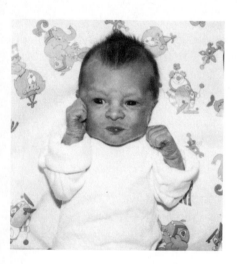

What we see in this photo at left is a "quiet alert" infant. He seems to have been quietly exploring the world with his eyes. It's been such fun that he seems to resist closing them despite the fact that sleep is setting in.

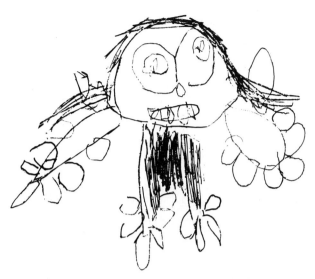

FIGURE 22–1 A Five-Year-Old's Version of Edvard Munch's *The Scream*

activity (for example, a board game or clay molding) as he talks. In addition, this child, like the preschooler, often reveals his personality structure, his conflicts, and his feelings through play, drawings, and story telling as well as verbally (see Figure 22–3). Thus, the clinician must be a flexible and skilled observer—hearing, seeing, and sensing all the data available in each interaction with the school-age child. She must pay attention to what the child is saying (content), as well as how he is saying it and what he is doing while this is going on (process).

> Children communicate through the way they look at, or avoid looking at, the clinician, the style and depth of their personal relatedness, their mood, the variety and types of emotions they manifest, the way they negotiate the space of the interview setting, the themes they develop in talk and play, and in many other ways as well. The organization, depth, age-appropriate relevance and sequence of the child's affect and themes are all vehicles for sharing the structure, character, and content of his or her experience (Greenspan, 1981, pg. 2).

The assessment of the school-age child should always include a respectful and confidential interview and mental-status examination. Table 22–8 outlines the areas of observation and inquiry.[1] School-age children may not be responsive to direct questions, though they should be asked. For example, "Do you feel that the divorce was your fault?" might be met with silence, a shrug, or "No." Moving on to: "I've talked with a lot of kids your age whose parents have divorced and a lot of them feel that it was their fault. What do you think about that?" may elicit a more revealing response. Displacement of feelings onto

[1]See also Cohen, 1979; Looff, 1976; or Simmons, 1987, for elaboration of assessment styles for school-age and older children.

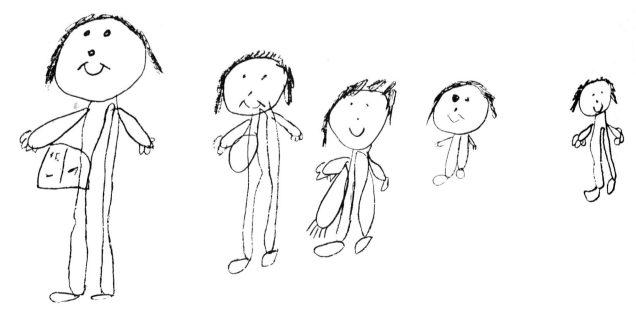

FIGURE 22–2 An Eight-Year-Old's Version of Her Family

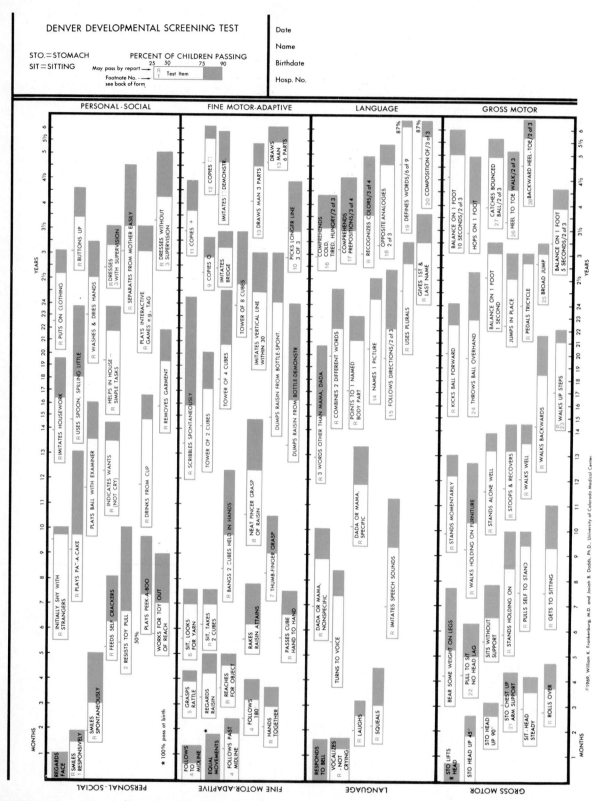

FIGURE 22–3 The Denver Developmental Screen Test The Denver Developmental Screening Test (DDST) was devised to provide a simple method of screening for evidences of slow development in infants and preschool children. The test covers four functions: gross motor, language, fine motor-adaptive, and personal-social. It has been standardized on 1,036 presumably normal children (two weeks to six years of age) whose families reflect the occupational and ethnic characteristics of the population of Denver.

```
                                    DATE
                                    NAME
              DIRECTIONS            BIRTHDATE
                                    HOSP. NO.
```

1. Try to get child to smile by smiling, talking or waving to him. Do not touch him.
2. When child is playing with toy, pull it away from him. Pass if he resists.
3. Child does not have to be able to tie shoes or button in the back.
4. Move yarn slowly in an arc from one side to the other, about 6" above child's face.
   Pass if eyes follow 90° to midline. (Past midline; 180°)
5. Pass if child grasps rattle when it is touched to the backs or tips of fingers.
6. Pass if child continues to look where yarn disappeared or tries to see where it went. Yarn
   should be dropped quickly from sight from tester's hand without arm movement.
7. Pass if child picks up raisin with any part of thumb and a finger.
8. Pass if child picks up raisin with the ends of thumb and index finger using an over hand
   approach.

  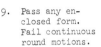

9. Pass any en-   10. Which line is longer?   11. Pass any   12. Have child copy
   closed form.   (Not bigger.) Turn   crossing   first. If failed,
   Fail continuous   paper upside down and   lines.   demonstrate
   round motions.   repeat. (3/3 or 5/6)

   When giving items 9, 11 and 12, do not name the forms. Do not demonstrate 9 and 11.

13. When scoring, each pair (2 arms, 2 legs, etc.) counts as one part.
14. Point to picture and have child name it. (No credit is given for sounds only.)

    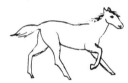   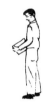

15. Tell child to: Give block to Mommie; put block on table; put block on floor. Pass 2 of 3.
    (Do not help child by pointing, moving head or eyes.)
16. Ask child: What do you do when you are cold? ..hungry? ..tired? Pass 2 of 3.
17. Tell child to: Put block on table; under table; in front of chair, behind chair.
    Pass 3 of 4. (Do not help child by pointing, moving head or eyes.)
18. Ask child: If fire is hot, ice is ?; Mother is a woman, Dad is a ?; a horse is big, a
    mouse is ?. Pass 2 of 3.
19. Ask child: What is a ball? ..lake? ..desk? ..house? ..banana? ..curtain? ..ceiling?
    ..hedge? ..pavement? Pass if defined in terms of use, shape, what it is made of or general
    category (such as banana is fruit, not just yellow). Pass 6 of 9.
20. Ask child: What is a spoon made of? ..a shoe made of? ..a door made of? (No other objects
    may be substituted.) Pass 3 of 3.
21. When placed on stomach, child lifts chest off table with support of forearms and/or hands.
22. When child is on back, grasp his hands and pull him to sitting. Pass if head does not hang back.
23. Child may use wall or rail only, not person. May not crawl.
24. Child must throw ball overhand 3 feet to within arm's reach of tester.
25. Child must perform standing broad jump over width of test sheet. (8-1/2 inches)
26. Tell child to walk forward, ⬯⬯⬯⬯⟶ heel within 1 inch of toe.
    Tester may demonstrate. Child must walk 4 consecutive steps, 2 out of 3 trials.
27. Bounce ball to child who should stand 3 feet away from tester. Child must catch ball with
    hands, not arms, 2 out of 3 trials.
28. Tell child to walk backward, ⟵⬯⬯⬯⬯ toe within 1 inch of heel.
    Tester may demonstrate. Child must walk 4 consecutive steps, 2 out of 3 trials.
```

DATE AND BEHAVIORAL OBSERVATIONS (how child feels at time of test, relation to tester, attention span, verbal behavior, self-confidence, etc,):

## FIGURE 22–3 continued DDST INTERPRETATION

A DELAY is any item failed which falls completely to the left of the age line.

ABNORMAL—2 or more sectors with 2 or more delays.

ABNORMAL—1 sector with 2 or more delays *plus* 1 or more sectors with 1 delay and *in that same sector*, no passes thru the age line.

QUESTIONABLE—1 sector with 2 or more delays.

QUESTIONABLE—1 or more sectors with 1 delay and *in that same sector*, no passes thru the age line.

UNTESTABLE—When REFUSALS occur in numbers large enough to cause the test results to be questionable or abnormal IF they were scored as failures.

NORMAL—Any condition not otherwise listed.

Source: The Journal of Pediatrics, St. Louis Vol. 71, No. 2, Pages 181–191, August, 1967. (Printed in the U.S.A.) (Copyright © 1967 by The C. V. Mosby Company)
```

Box 22–4 ●
Hallucinating Children

Many children have imaginary friends who become the center of an elaborate fantasy life. Although these might be regarded as hallucinations, the child is not considered psychotic if he or she is functioning well. Some children, however, report more troubling hallucinations; researchers in Ottawa have recently considered whether these symptoms represent a psychosis or early signs of schizophrenia.

The subjects of the study were eight boys and three girls aged seven to twelve who were referred to an outpatient clinic—five specifically for hallucinations, and six for other psychiatric symptoms with associated hallucinations. All heard voices or other sounds, and five also had visual hallucinations. The voices often commanded them to harm themselves or someone familiar to them. These episodes usually occurred while the child was lying in bed at night, but they were not hypnagogic phenomena, that is, the quasi-dreamlike experiences which are a common feature of the transition from waking to sleeping. In most cases the hallucinations had persisted for weeks to months. None of the children came from families with histories of psychotic illness.

The authors found that the children were not psychotic. The hallucinations were mostly coherent and intelligible in the light of their situations, unlike the more bizarre and confused hallucinations of schizophrenic children. Seven were having problems in adjusting to a change in their lives, three were suffering from an anxiety disorder, and one had the syndrome known as schizoid disorder of childhood (social withdrawal and emotional detachment). Most of the children were somewhat anxious and socially inept, and they were getting insufficient support from their parents.

The prognosis was generally good. In six cases the hallucinations began to fade soon after the start of psychotherapy and ceased entirely in one to five weeks—usually before underlying psychiatric difficulties were resolved. Symptoms persisted in two children: the one who had been diagnosed as schizoid, and one who had been hallucinating continuously for a year and a half.

Source: *Harvard Mental Health Letter,* 4(6), Dec. 1987, p. 7. Sotiris Kotsopoulos, Joel Kanigsberg, Andre Cote, and Christina Fiedorowicz. Hallucinatory experiences in nonpsychotic children. *Journal of the American Academy of Child and Adolescent Psychiatry,* 26:375-380 (May/June 1987).

other children, toys, or pretend characters can enable the child gradually to move from playing to talking, and from general to personal. It is important to reflect back to the child what his play or words have revealed in order to get verification or clarification. For example: "When I asked about your mother's being in the hospital, you smashed up the house you were building. You must be feeling pretty upset."

Active listening is another invaluable technique when working with the school-age child. As usual, the clinician must guard against allowing her own responses to the child to overshadow the child's material. However, she should not minimize their importance. **Countertransference,** or the *feelings* the child stirs up in the nurse, is as important here as it is with the adult patient. It may reflect the child's conflict or the situation in which he finds himself.

Lisa: A Child's Reaction to Hospitalization

Lisa, a six-year-old girl with severe combined immune deficiency syndrome, allowed the nurse therapist into her life when she agreed to a play session, and then proceeded to isolate her from her emotional world by refusing to talk about feelings. This reflected Lisa's situation of being isolated in a hospital room for several months. As a result, the nurse therapist's feelings of being shut out mirrored Lisa's. Once the nurse therapist recognized this, she became more sensitive to Lisa's feelings about being so isolated, something everyone had begun to take for granted (Kavanagh, 1986).

Despite how revealing it may appear, a single observation of a child is not enough. Children must be observed over time while the clinician formulates and tests hypotheses regarding the origins and meaning of the presenting problem, conflicts, or deficits, in family sessions and alone with the child. Collaborative data from the school are especially important because the school is the most important arbiter of social boundaries and functions for most children. It must also be remembered that the adequacy, reliability, safety, and supportiveness of the school is more accurately judged by personal inquiry rather than by accepting at face value parental perceptions of school staff and the child's functioning there.

With children of all ages, contact with the family physician or pediatrician and review of prior hospital records may be useful. Extending the information net to other family resources (for example, grandparents, noncustodial parents), nonfamily resources (for example, clergy, coaches, and scout leaders), and other agencies may also be appropriate. The child's agreement and parents' informed consent are required before such contacts can be made.

ASSESSING THE ADOLESCENT

It is tempting to deem the child over age fourteen appropriate for independent assessment. Indeed, the child may demand this and accuse the evaluator of collusion with parents if such autonomy is not granted. In addition, it is clear that certain ethical dilemmas, for example, confidentiality, are never more complex than they are in working with adolescents (Miller, 1977). Successful completion of the assessment, appropriate involvement of the parents, and development of a therapeutic alliance with the teenager all depend on the sensitive handling of these issues. Consultation may be necessary, even for the most skilled clinician. This may be especially true if the clinician has teenage children herself, as intense countertransference is likely.

Assessment of the adolescent demands skills in family interaction assessment. Some parents have difficulty focusing on their adolescent due to a need to talk about their own conflicts. In fact, the parental request for evaluation of the adolescent may unconsciously be an attempt to get help for themselves.

While the family interview can be useful in the assessment of a child of any age, it is particularly important to experience the affective tone of parent/adolescent interactions. For example, feelings about issues such as sexuality can often only be accurately assessed in a family session.

CHILDHOOD PATHOLOGY

All DSM-III-R (American Psychiatric Association, 1987) diagnoses, with the exception of some of the personality disorders, can be used with children.[1] All of the axes are designed to be applicable to adolescents and children. A few diagnoses have variant criteria for children, for example, major depressive episode. Others are specifically targeted to issues which, at first glance, may seem inappropriate for children, for example, psychosexual disorders. Finally, though there has been significant dispute about the validity of the DSM-III diagnoses for children (Werry, 1985), there is general agreement that they are a vast improvement over DSM-II. The process of DSM-III-R (Revised) formation involved reviewing a number of disorders as they apply to children, for example, the conduct disorders (see Table 22–9).

DSM-III-R highlights a number of disorders as those first evident in infancy, childhood, or adolescence (see Table 22–9). For discussion in this chapter, we have grouped them into Axis I disorders, some of which will receive special attention, and Axis II disorders.

The Axis II disorders include academic skills, language and speech, and motor skills disorders. A discussion of these is beyond the scope of this chapter. The reader is referred to Dworkin (1985) and Bryan and Bryan (1975) who have addressed these disorders in depth. The nurse will generally not be involved in either the assessment or remediation of these disorders except as they coexist with other pathology, unless she works in a learning disorders clinic.

DISORDERS FIRST EVIDENT IN INFANCY

Psychopathology that is evident in the first year of life usually falls into the category of mental retarda-

---

[1] Antisocial personality disorder is restricted to age eighteen and older in DSM-III-R. Avoidant, borderline, passive-aggressive, and schizoid personality disorders criteria are suggested for use with individuals over eighteen.

Box 22–5 ● Teenage Pregnancy

One of several organizations for pregnant teenagers in Madison, Wisconsin is the School-Age Maternity (SAM) Program. For fathers as well as mothers, its focus is to encourage young, single mothers to finish high school. Even with such programs, over half of the girls do not graduate. Carol McQuaid, a nurse who is part of SAM, suggests that school counselors, nurses, and social workers need to offer support to pregnant teens. Child care in high schools would also help teenage mothers stay in school. The same can be said for teen-parent support groups.

The biggest obstacle programs like SAM face is money. Federal spending cuts for such community services have continued over the past several years despite the parallel decline of the average age of a single mother. (In Wisconsin, a state nearly devoid of large urban areas and associated social problems, in 1986, one of every fourteen children was born to a single mother between the age of ten and nineteen.) Cuts in family planning programs and welfare money for Aid to Families with Dependent Children (AFDC) compound the problem.

According to McQuaid, more than half the mothers in SAM are under fifteen, evidence that teenagers are sexually active at a younger age and older teens are more likely to use contraceptives or choose abortion. She feels that teen pregnancies will decline in time if the state is willing to put enough money in prevention programs which begin education about sex and responsible decision making in kindergarten.

Hannah Rosenthal, chair of the Adolescent Pregnancy Prevention Board in Madison, says that the solution to the problem of teenage pregnancy is not only in the provision of information, but in how it is presented. " 'Just say no' doesn't face the real problem. Kids need to feel good enough about themselves to say no."

The Wisconsin State Journal, Single Teenage Mothers by Renee Botta, Sunday, April 24, 1988, pp. 16 and 56.

---

tion and other "developmental disorders." Included in this grouping, by law in most states, are autism and other pervasive developmental disorders. These disorders range in incidence from unusual (about 0.05 percent for autism) to fairly common (one to three per cent for mental retardation, depending on criteria).

MENTAL RETARDATION. The extent of pathology and need for remediation in the retardation syndromes is variable and often shifting on the basis of social policy and current social expectations of family functioning. For example, two decades ago institutional placement from birth and/or denial of medical treatment to sustain life were commonly accepted practices in the care of children with **trisomy 21 (Down's syndrome).** There is now increasing consensus that such practices are morally and medically reprehensible (American Academy of Pediatrics, 1983).

The impact of retardation disorders on children and families is significant, almost always leading to varying degrees of dysfunction. One reason for this

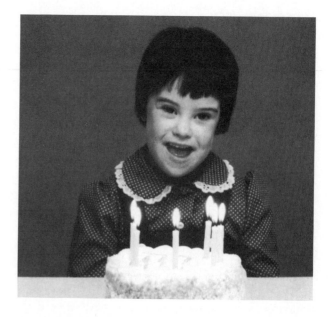

Early identification of mental retardation, in this case Down's Syndrome, is important in order to provide the family and the child with much needed information and emotional support.

TABLE 22–9 Disorders usually first evident in infancy, childhood, or adolescence

DEVELOPMENTAL DISORDERS

Note: These are coded on Axis II.

Mental Retardation

317.00	Mild mental retardation
318.00	Moderate mental retardation
318.10	Severe mental retardation
318.20	Profound mental retardation
319.00	Unspecified mental retardation

Pervasive Developmental Disorders

299.00	Autistic disorder
	Specify if childhood onset
299.80	Pervasive developmental disorder NOS

Specific Developmental Disorders

Academic skills disorders
315.10	Developmental arithmetic disorder
315.80	Developmental expressive writing disorder
315.00	Developmental reading disorder

Language and speech disorders
315.39	Developmental articulation disorder
315.31	Developmental expressive language disorder
315.31	Developmental receptive language disorder

Motor skills disorder
315.40	Developmental coordination disorder
315.90	Specific developmental disorder NOS

Other Developmental Disorders

315.90	Developmental disorder NOS

Disruptive Behavior Disorders

314.01	Attention-deficit hyperactivity disorder
	Conduct disorder,
312.20	group type
312.00	solitary aggressive type
312.90	undifferentiated type
313.81	Oppositional defiant disorder

Anxiety Disorders of Childhood or Adolescence

309.21	Separation anxiety disorder
313.21	Avoidant disorder of childhood or adolescence
313.00	Overanxious disorder

Eating Disorders

307.10	Anorexia nervosa
307.51	Bulimia nervosa
307.52	Pica
307.53	Rumination disorder of infancy
307.50	Eating disorder NOS

Gender Identity Disorders

302.60	Gender identity disorder of childhood
302.50	Transsexualism
	Specify sexual history: asexual, homosexual, heterosexual, unspecified
302.85	Gender identity disorder of adolescence or adulthood, nontranssexual type
	Specify sexual history: asexual, homosexual, heterosexual, unspecified
302.85	Gender identity disorder NOS

Tic Disorders

307.23	Tourette's disorder
307.22	Chronic motor or vocal tic disorder
307.21	Transient tic disorder
	Specify: single episode or recurrent
307.20	Tic disorder NOS

Elimination Disorders

307.70	Functional encopresis
	Specify: primary or secondary type
307.60	Functional enuresis
	Specify: primary or secondary type
	Specify: nocturnal only, diurnal only, nocturnal and diurnal

Speech Disorders Not Elsewhere Classified

307.00	Cluttering
307.00	Stuttering

Disorders of Infancy, Childhood, or Adolescence

313.23	Elective mutism
313.82	Identity disorder
313.89	Reactive attachment disorder of infancy or early childhood
307.30	Stereotypy/habit disorder
314.00	Undifferentiated attention-deficit disorder

is that the etiology of mental retardation is usually not clear, and even when it is, the predictability of outcome is uncertain at best. Nevertheless, early identification and intervention is extremely important, even if its only achievement is the amelioration of the family members' stress (Bradley & Tedesco, 1982).

The nurse needs to understand that because early identification can be emotionally painful for all concerned, it may be unconsciously avoided by both professionals and family. Parents are invariably concerned about evidence of delayed development, but their ambivalence and emotional involvement makes them vulnerable to looking and finding support for their "Oh, he'll be okay" thinking. Thus the nurse's responsibilities in the area of clinical mental retardation include:

1. Knowing the local resources for screening and assessment;

2. Supporting the goal of early and accurate assessment;

3. Providing information and emotional support for child and parents before, during, and after diagnosis;

4. Advocating for community services for the developmentally disabled of all ages.

Additional psychopathology (that is, "dual" or secondary diagnosis) is often evident in the developmentally disabled individual. Since the expression of such pathology is influenced by the degree of retardation, the accuracy of the secondary diagnosis hinges on the clinician's ability to adapt her evaluation techniques to the child's, or young adults's, developmental level. Even with these adjustments, the patience and persistence of the most skilled clinician may be taxed.[1]

All modes of intervention can be used with a developmentally disabled/emotionally disturbed child or adolescent, including the psychodynamic therapies. Response is usually not primarily related to the degree of retardation, but rather to the treatability of the disorder and whether or not parental and/or institutional and societal support for such treatment is available.

Significant bias against and barriers to psychiatric treatment of the developmentally disabled continue to exist. As a result, the nursing responsibilities listed above become more difficult to carry out. Parents are often surprised by the lack of skilled mental-health services for their developmentally disabled child who has coexisting psychopathology. This can be the case especially if the usually helpful and supportive school has been overwhelmed with the psychosocial problems of their students, more likely in these days of decreased financial support for special services.

Suzanne: A Child with Down's Syndrome

Suzanne, age 21, was seen by the nurse at a school for the developmentally disabled because of her teacher's concerns about Suzanne's dizziness. Suzanne had a chronic heart problem and Down's syndrome. Her heart lesion was never repaired in childhood because her parents were told that such surgery was not done on the developmentally disabled. They were advised to place Suzanne in an institution.

Suzanne's parents rejected this advice and became strong advocates for Suzanne and her educational needs. She did well, though her heart disease progressed and she developed the complication of pulmonary hypertension as she grew older. These complications presaged surgical repair when treatment philosophies changed.

The nurse found Suzanne agitated and seated on the floor of the classroom. She refused to rise, complaining that she would get dizzy. She had audible bruxism (teeth grinding) which the nurse recognized as a sign of distress in Suzanne. Suzanne was also mildly cyanotic, but this was not unusual for her. The nurse's concerns included:

1. Are Suzanne's symptoms evidence of heart disease and nothing else?

2. Could Suzanne's symptoms be evidence of anxiety disorder alone?

3. Are Suzanne's symptoms evidence of heart disease and psychopathology, for example, some type of anxiety disorder?

In questioning the teacher, the nurse learned that Suzanne had become more and more anxious during the past three weeks. School was almost over for the year and Suzanne was being evaluated for a job at a sheltered workshop. This had required her to be out of class and to miss some of the special activities planned around graduation.

The teacher also reported that Suzanne's mother recently told her that Suzanne had been refusing to go out with the family and was having problems sleeping. "She always wants to sleep with us, something she hasn't done since she was a child."

The nurse felt that there was evidence of a cardiorespiratory problem and a possible coexisting anxiety disorder with both panic and separation-anxiety features. She suggested that Suzanne and her parents first see Suzanne's cardiologist. Once Suzanne's medical condition was cleared, the nurse suggested that they see a psychiatrist or psychologist as a family.

Suzanne's cardiologist found her physical status to be unchanged from the previous assessment. The cardiac clinic nurse, too, supported a psychiatric evaluation and helped arrange it. Ultimately, a diagnosis of adjustment disorder with anxious mood was made. Supported exposure to feared stimuli (such as the sheltered workshop) for Suzanne and brief use of anti-anxiety medications to control initial anxiety with exposure, were recommended and implemented (see Chapter 8, on anxiety and anxiety disorders). Supportive psychotherapy for the family was also done.

---

[1]See Menolascino (1971) for further information.

Within a month Suzanne had made a successful transition to the sheltered workshop and had tapered off her anti-anxiety medication without a recurrence of symptoms.

Recent studies have shown that psychotropics, especially neuroleptics, are often used inappropriately on the developmentally disabled population (Gualtieri et al., 1982). When expectations are low for the developmentally disabled child, or easy "control" of his behavior is the primary goal of caretakers (parents, school, or institution), treatment may be limited to drug therapy alone. The conscientious nurse will see herself as the patient's advocate and do what she can to prevent this from happening. This includes taking the position that the developmentally disabled have the right to mental-health care and access to a full range of treatment possibilities.

AUTISM. Autism, first described as a clinical syndrome by Kanner (1943) was reclassified in DSM III and DSM-III-R as pervasive developmental disorder—autistic type. This has allowed for grouping of the more severe pathologies in childhood. Disorders previously labeled childhood psychosis are now subgrouped by age of onset and degree of severity. Although controversy exists about the new classification (Tanguay, 1984), the features of autism have been stable since Kanner's first description of them.

Massie and Rosenthal (1984), researchers who have advocated early identification of autism, have maintained that if identified and treated early, a significant number of autistic children will improve.* While many say that this is overly optimistic, the importance of early educational planning and support for the parents of the child with autism has been well documented (Russo & Newson, 1982).

The case of Paul, an autistic child, demonstrates case finding and intervention on behalf of a seriously emotionally handicapped autistic child by nurses who are not psychiatric specialists.

Paul: An Autistic Child

Paul was first seen by a public health nurse visiting his family after the birth of his brother. She noted

---

*Massie and Rosenthal (1984, pg. 251) indicate that forty-two months is "the upper limit of the age when an autistic syndrome can be aborted or resolved."

DSM-III-R
Diagnostic Criteria for Autistic Disorder

At least eight of the following sixteen items are present, these to include at least two items from A, one from B, and one from C.

Note: Consider a criterion to be met *only* if the behavior is abnormal for the person's developmental level.

A. Qualitative impairment in reciprocal social interaction as manifested by the following:

(The examples within parentheses are arranged so that those first mentioned are more likely to apply to younger or more handicapped, and the later ones, to older or less handicapped, persons with this disorder.)

1) marked lack of awareness of the existence or feelings of others (e.g., treats a person as if he or she were a piece of furniture; does not notice another person's distress; apparently has no concept of the need of others for privacy)

2) no or abnormal seeking of comfort at times of distress (e.g., does not come for comfort even when ill, hurt, or tired; seeks comfort in a stereotyped way, e.g., says "cheese, cheese, cheese" whenever hurt)

3) no or impaired imitation (e.g., does not wave bye-bye; does not copy mother's domestic activities; mechanical imitation of others' actions out of context)

4) no or abnormal social play (e.g., does not actively participate in simple games; prefers solitary play activities; involves other children in play only as "mechanical aids")

continued

5) gross impairment in ability to make peer friendships (e.g., no interest in making peer friendships; despite interest in making friends, demonstrates lack of understanding of conventions of social interaction, for example, reads phone book to uninterested peer)

B. Qualitative impairment in verbal and nonverbal communication, and in imaginative activity, as manifested by the following:
(The numbered items are arranged so that those first listed are more likely to apply to younger or more handicapped, and the later ones, to older or less handicapped, persons with this disorder.)

1) no mode of communication, such as communicative babbling, facial expression, gesture, mime, or spoken language

2) markedly abnormal nonverbal communication, as in the use of eye-to-eye gaze, facial expression, body posture, or gestures to initiate or modulate social interaction (e.g., does not anticipate being held, stiffens when held, does not look at the person or smile when making a social approach, does not greet parents or visitors, has a fixed stare in social situations)

3) absence of imaginative activity, such as playacting of adult roles, fantasy characters, or animals; lack of interest in stories about imaginary events

4) marked abnormalities in the production of speech, including volume, pitch, stress, rate, rhythm, and intonation (e.g., monotonous tone, question-like melody, or high pitch)

5) marked abnormalities in the form or content of speech, including stereotyped and repetitive use of speech (e.g., immediate echolalia or mechanical repetition of television commercial); use of "you" when "I" is meant (e.g., using "You want cookie?" to mean "I want a cookie"); idiosyncratic use of words or phrases (e.g., "Go on green riding" to mean "I want to go on the swing"); or frequent irrelevant remarks (e.g., starts talking about train schedules during a conversation about sports)

6) marked impairment in the ability to initiate or sustain a conversation with others, despite adequate speech (e.g., indulging in lengthy monologues on one subject regardless of interjections from others)

C. Markedly restricted repertoire of activities and interests, as manifested by the following:

1) stereotyped body movements, e.g., hand-flicking or -twisting, spinning, head-banging, complex whole-body movements

2) persistent preoccupation with parts of objects (e.g., sniffing or smelling objects, repetitive feeling of texture of materials, spinning wheels of toy cars) or attachment to unusual objects (e.g., insists on carrying around a piece of string)

3) marked distress over changes in trivial aspects of environment, e.g., when a vase is moved from usual position

4) unreasonable insistence on following routines in precise detail, e.g., insisting that exactly the same route always be followed when shopping

5) markedly restricted range of interests and a preoccupation with one narrow interest, e.g., interested only in lining up objects, in amassing facts about meteorology, or in pretending to be a fantasy character

D. Onset during infancy or childhood.

Specify if childhood onset (after 36 months of age).

**DSM-III-R
Diagnostic Criteria for
Reactive Attachment
Disorder of Infancy or
Early Childhood**

A. Markedly disturbed social relatedness in most contexts, beginning before the age of five, as evidenced by either (1) or (2):

1) persistent failure to initiate or respond to most social interactions (e.g., in infants, absence of visual tracking and reciprocal play, lack of vocal imitation or playfulness, apathy, little or no spontaneity; at later ages, lack of or little curiosity and social interest)

2) indiscriminate sociability, e.g., excessive familiarity with relative strangers by making requests and displaying affection

B. The disturbance in A is not a symptom of either mental retardation or a pervasive developmental disorder, such as autistic disorder.

C. Grossly pathogenic care, as evidenced by at least one of the following:

1) persistent disregard of the child's basic emotional needs for comfort, stimulation, and affection. *Examples:* overly harsh punishment by caregiver; consistent neglect by caregiver.

2) persistent disregard of the child's basic physical needs, including nutrition, adequate housing, and protection from physical danger and assault (including sexual abuse)

3) repeated change of primary caregiver so that stable attachments are not possible, e.g., frequent changes in foster parents

D. There is a presumption that the care described in C is responsible for the disturbed behavior in A; this presumption is warranted if the disturbance in A began following the pathogenic care in C.

---

that Paul, age two, sat by himself in a corner of the room, rocking back and forth. Periodically, he stopped to spin the toys he had near him. He appeared to be uninterested in, or unaware of, what was going on around him.

After checking the baby, the nurse gradually approached Paul to see if she could engage him in social interaction. He ignored her. When she touched him, he jumped up, shrieked, and ran off on tiptoes while flapping his arms. Aware that these are not typical behaviors of a two-year-old, the nurse attempted further assessment by asking the mother if she had any concerns regarding Paul and by obtaining a developmental history from her.

Paul's mother readily shared her concerns and frustrations about her son's behavior and the effect it was having on the family. He was never a cuddly baby and breast fed poorly. He was not as responsive to her as her first child had been. He walked at fourteen months but had no speech at two years. She felt that he did not play with toys appropriately and did not interact with other members of the family. When he last saw Paul at eighteen months, Paul's pediatrician told her that he would "outgrow" these things. Since then, Paul's mother had begun to wonder if Paul might have a hearing problem.

Paul's mother said that she and her husband argued frequently about how to manage Paul. She felt her husband was too strict and punished him too severely. No extended family support was available as the family had recently moved to the area.

While the nurse, too, felt that Paul might be deaf, her greatest concern was that Paul might be autistic. She initiated the following care plan.

Nursing Care Plan for Paul

Nursing Diagnosis	Desired Outcomes	Interventions	Rationale
1. Impaired verbal communication	Paul will receive an extensive evaluation.	Encourage the mother to take Paul to his pediatrician.	An accurate diagnosis is the first step toward effective treatment, and the child's pediatrician's

Nursing Diagnosis	Desired Outcomes	Interventions	Rationale
		Contact the pediatrician and share observations and concerns.	office is the appropriate place to continue the evaluation process. The pediatrician will consult a child psychiatrist or psychologist if he or she also suspects autism.
2. Potential altered parenting	Parents will cope adequately with frustrations with child's unresponsiveness. Parents will develop appropriate support systems.	Followup home visits weekly until support systems are in place. Ongoing evaluation of the parents' ability to cope with having an autistic child. Refer for counseling if necessary.	The pediatric or community nurse can play an important role in the family support system, especially during the evaluation process when psychiatric referral can be very anxiety producing. She can begin to help family members focus on their own emotional needs as well as those of their autistic child, and encourage them to get the help they need.

At age 4½, Paul was admitted to a pediatric hospital for abdominal surgery. He had been diagnosed as having infantile autism and was enrolled in a special school that focused on education and training as well as behavioral management. His parents had identified support systems, including a parent support group and respite care, and were coping reasonably well with having a handicapped child.

Paul continued to walk on his tiptoes and flap his arms when he was stressed. However, his receptive language appeared to be improving; for example, he now responded to simple commands. He had developed some speech but did not utilize it reliably to communicate his needs. Rather, he usually echoed what others said to him ("immediate echolalia") or repeated over and over something he had heard on TV. Paul listened to records for hours at a time; in fact, since Paul liked music so much, his parents had begun to use it to calm him when he became upset.

Paul continued to be responsive only to his parents, and then, not consistently. Their greatest concern at this time was how Paul would react to hospitalization because he was very resistant to change. He was to have a nasogastric tube and IV feeding for three to four days after his surgery, with restraints as necessary to prevent disruption to his incision, all of which were sure to be traumatic for him.

Prior to his admission to the hospital, Paul's pediatrician had enlisted the help of the child psychiatrist and pediatric clinical nurse specialist at the hospital. It was decided that the child psychiatrist would assist in pain management and treatment of agitation (for example, with tranquilizing medication). The clinical nurse specialist helped Paul's primary nurse develop a nursing care plan for Paul during his short hospitalization. After a comprehensive history was taken, a nursing diagnosis was made, and a nursing care plan was begun.

Nursing Care Plan for Paul

Nursing Diagnosis	Desired Outcome	Interventions	Rationale
1. Anxiety associated with perceived threat to self and environmental change.	Paul will use available resources to cope with hospitalization and associated anxiety.	Adhere to daily routine (as outlined in schedule at bedside) as much as possible.	Predictability can reduce anxiety. Despite the autistic child's apparent preference for "his own world," he is likely to

Nursing Diagnosis	Desired Outcomes	Interventions	Rationale
		Encourage the parents to stay with Paul through his hospital stay and offer support as necessary.	experience the stress of separation anxiety during hospitalization.
		Have the parents bring in familiar toys, record player, and favorite music.	Paul is also subject to the hospitalization problems of overstimulation, for example during invasive procedures, and understimulation as a result of being removed from his familiar environment, and associated activities and experiences.
		Limit the number of staff involved with Paul to avoid overstimulation.	
		Have the parents explain unfamiliar sounds and activities to Paul before they occur as much as possible.	
		Use soft restraints and tranquilizing medication as necessary to manage agitation.	At times such nursing interventions are not sufficient to reduce anxiety, and additional means to prevent a child from hurting himself need to be employed. One-on-one nursing care in this situation is also desirable.

As expected, the multidisciplinary approach, advance preparation, and family involvement during Paul's short hospitalization all seemed to contribute to the positive outcome: Paul and his parents maintained an optimal level of functioning during a period of stress.

The case of Paul illustrates the full-blown autistic syndrome, which is rarely mistaken for other disorders. Massie and Rosenthal's (1984) observations, based on viewing home movies of infants later diagnosed autistic, led to their assertion that signs of autism can be identified as early as six to twelve months of age. Their diagnostic criteria are based on the infant's: 1) somber mood, 2) avoidance of parental gaze, 3) resistance to being held, 4) stereotypical behavior, and 5) emotional distancing from parents. While more research is needed, Massie and Rosenthal's work has been a significant contribution to the growing ability to identify autism at an early age

when intervention will be most likely to be successful. Individual and family psychotherapy, pharmacotherapy (of both a general and an assumedly specific nature), and behavioral intervention have all had limited treatment success. Significant successes in individual cases, however, seem to depend on early referral of parents of children with autism to the local developmental disabilities specialist or the national support group.*

REACTIVE ATTACHMENT DISORDER OF INFANCY (NONORGANIC FAILURE TO THRIVE). The diagnosis of other types of psychopathology in infancy is difficult because it depends on behavioral observations of both infant and parents. In addition, there is continued controversy regarding affective development in infancy. Emde (1984) has discussed

*National Society for Children and Adults with Autism, 1234 Massachusetts Avenue Northwest, Suite 1017, Washington, D.C. 20005.

these issues and emphasized the complexity of unraveling physical and developmental concerns of parents, the actual problems of the infant, and the influences of parental psychopathology.

Typical problems involved in diagnosing psychopathology in infancy are best illustrated by reviewing the criteria for reactive attachment disorder in DSM-III-R. First, some of the very particular criteria for this disorder depend heavily on the age and developmental intactness of the infant for their assessment. The criterion "grossly pathogenic care" and examples is an improvement over the DSM-III criterion "adequate caretaking," which is too vague to be useful. Unique to this disorder is the DSM-III-R criterion D which makes its "cause" (the "grossly pathogenic care") part of the diagnostic criteria.

Reactive attachment disorder of infancy is often informally referred to as "nonorganic failure to thrive" (Spitzer & Williams, 1980); however, there is still little support in pediatric or psychiatric research for any significant association between attachment disturbance and failure to thrive (Gordon & Jameson, 1979). This disorder was originally touted as a "new category by popular demand" during the early development of DSM-III. Though it is often diagnosed, especially in cases involving child neglect, a scientific basis for the disorder as described by DSM-III-R criteria is as yet lacking. Further assessment of the relationship of attachment to physiological and behavioral symptoms is needed.

DISORDERS FIRST EVIDENT IN CHILDHOOD

Disorders of conduct and affect do occur in infants and preschoolers; however, they too are difficult to categorize. One problem is that symptoms are often not stable over time. Current research attempting to extend affective diagnostic boundaries to these younger age groups includes the work of Gaensbauer et al. (1984) and Zahn-Wexler et al. (1984), who have studied the children of manic-depressive parents. Campbell et al. (1984) have looked at the diagnostic stability of behavior disorders in preschoolers as well as their relationship to conduct disorders in older children.

ATTENTION DEFICIT DISORDER WITH OR WITHOUT HYPERACTIVITY. Unfortunately, controversy about the validity of psychiatric diagnoses is not limited to disorders identified in young children. Currently, significant controversy also exists regarding the diagnosis and treatment of **attention deficit hyperactivity disorder,** which occurs in school-age children.

One of the most extensively studied diagnoses in child psychiatry, attention deficit disorder, formerly called hyperactivity, is a commonly diagnosed problem in the United States, occurring in five to ten percent of school-age children (Edelbrock, 1985). The agreed upon criteria for attention deficit hyperactivity disorder (ADD) are those required by DSM-III-R. How these symptoms should be assessed is controversial, and agreement regarding the validity of attention deficit disorder as a diagnostic category is lacking. Edelbrock (1985) and Quay (1985) have addressed this issue and have pointed out that there is significant overlap among symptoms of ADD and those of other clinical disorders, for example, mood disorders and conduct disorders. The variability of attention deficits, affective symptoms, and behavior problems (including impulsive, hyperactive, and aggressive behavior) in the individual child makes dissecting the core problem a formidable, if not impossible, task.

Despite extensive research on the possible biochemical etiology of ADD (Brown, et al., 1985), none has been found.* This is the case despite strong evidence for the successful management of many core features of the disorder, including attentional, behavioral, and social deficits, with stimulant medications (Cantwell, 1980). There is evidence for psychosocial etiology in the responsiveness of the behavioral difficulties associated with ADD to treatment based on learning theory. Parent and child training in methods of delivering positive reinforcement (for example, token systems) and mildly aversive consequences (for example, a "time out") as an intervention strategy has been especially useful in the school setting.

The nurse may come in contact with children with ADD in a variety of clinical settings. She should always seek the parents' input regarding their usual management methods as the starting point for dealing with any child with ADD in a new environment. She should continue to give the child prompt and reliable praise for appropriate behaviors and consistently implement familiar negative consequences when undesirable behaviors occur. Since the child's self-maintenance skills may dissipate during illness and/or hospitalization, empathic support of nursing and medical staff is needed for him to cope adap-

---

*Earlier formulations that focused on "minimal brain dysfunction" have also not been sustained; hence, this label has been discarded.

DSM-III-R Diagnostic Criteria for Attention-deficit Hyperactivity Disorder

Note: Consider a criterion met only if the behavior is considerably more frequent than that of most people of the same mental age.

A. A disturbance of at least six months during which at least eight of the following are present:

1) often fidgets with hands or feet or squirms in seat (in adolescents, may be limited to subjective feelings of restlessness)

2) has difficulty remaining seated when required to do so

3) is easily distracted by extraneous stimuli

4) has difficulty awaiting turn in games or group situations

5) often blurts out answers to questions before they have been completed

6) has difficulty following through on instructions from others (not due to oppositional behavior or failure of comprehension), e.g., fails to finish chores

7) has difficulty sustaining attention in tasks or play activities

8) often shifts from one uncompleted activity to another

9) has difficulty playing quietly

10) often talks excessively

11) often interrupts or intrudes on others, e.g., butts into other children's games

12) often does not seem to listen to what is being said to him or her

13) often loses things necessary for tasks or activities at school or at home (e.g., toys, pencils, books, assignments)

14) often engages in physically dangerous activities without considering possible consequences (not for the purpose of thrill-seeking), e.g., runs into street without looking

Note: The above items are listed in descending order of discriminating power based on data from a national field trial of the DSM-III-R criteria for disruptive behavior disorders.

B. Onset before the age of seven.

C. Does not meet the criteria for a pervasive developmental disorder.

---

tively. This is especially true if the child's stimulant medication must be discontinued. The child who remains on medication through illness and hospitalization needs to be monitored carefully for physiological consequences of drug interactions, or if necessary, abrupt withdrawal.

Previously, it was thought that ADD was likely to remit as the child grew older. However, extensive followup research has led to the recognition that adolescents and even adults may continue to benefit from treatment (Wender et al., 1984). These individuals must continue development of coping strategies to deal with their impulsiveness in new or changing situations, for example, the work place. There is controversy about the possible increased vulnerability of

hyperactive individuals to drug and alcohol abuse and other psychopathology (Weiss & Hechtman, 1986).

THE CONDUCT DISORDERS. The child or adolescent with the diagnosis of **conduct disorder** will, in most cases, need intensive support when he is in the hospital setting. This angry and aggressive child, whose usual stance is to be alert for threat and expect assault, will find both in even the least invasive medical and nursing procedures. The cognitive distortions that can arise in response to shots, surgery, restraints, and traction are numerous. Thus this child is likely to benefit from an integrated short-term treatment plan developed with the help of consulting

DSM-III-R Diagnostic Criteria for Conduct Disorder

A. A disturbance of conduct lasting at least six months, during which at least three of the following have been present:

    1) has stolen without confrontation of a victim on more than one occasion (including forgery)

    2) has run away from home overnight at least twice while living in parental or parental surrogate home (or once without returning)

    3) often lies (other than to avoid physical or sexual abuse)

    4) has deliberately engaged in fire-setting

    5) is often truant from school (for older person, absent from work)

    6) has broken into someone else's house, building, or car

    7) has deliberately destroyed others' property (other than by fire-setting)

    8) has been physically cruel to animals

    9) has forced someone into sexual activity with him or her

    10) has used a weapon in more than one fight

    11) often initiates physical fights

    12) has stolen with confrontation of a victim (e.g., mugging, purse-snatching, extortion, armed robbery)

    13) has been physically cruel to people

Note: The above items are listed in descending order of discriminating power based on data from a national field trial of the DSM-III-R criteria for disruptive behavior disorders.

B. If 18 or older, does not meet criteria for antisocial personality disorder.

Types

312.20 group type

The essential feature is the predominance of conduct problems occurring mainly as a group activity with peers. Aggressive physical behavior may or may not be present.

312.00 solitary aggressive type

The essential feature is the predominance of aggressive physical behavior, usually toward both adults and peers, initiated by the person (not as a group activity).

312.90 undifferentiated type

This a subtype for children or adolescents with conduct disorder with a mixture of clinical features that cannot be classified as either solitary aggressive type or group type.

---

nurses, a psychologist, and/or a child psychiatrist. The treatment team should set realistic goals (for example, maintenance of baseline behavior rather than improvement) for the child. If the parents seem to be unsupportive of the child, it is important for the nurse and staff to understand that this is a common response to disorders that are so difficult to treat and to live with. The nurse must present to the parents and the child the possibility that tranquilization and restraint may be necessary if the child becomes violent. Countertransference is likely and needs to be monitored by the clinician in order to avoid the development of an angry, punitive approach to the child or family.

Although considerable effort has been expended in the search for the etiology of conduct disorders within several theoretical frameworks, no consensus has emerged.

Jeff: A Difficult Child

Jeff, age 8, was admitted to the orthopedic unit of a pediatric hospital for osteomyelitis of his left index finger; he had reportedly stapled his finger at school. The nursing history obtained from Jeff's foster mother on admission indicated that he was a difficult child to manage. Jeff had been with her only a few months, and had had numerous unsuccessful foster placements before this one. His history also included physical abuse as a young child.

Jeff was initially admitted to a five-bed room, but his abrasive language and inappropriate behavior necessitated a move to a private one. When he was told he needed an IV for antibiotics, Jeff became extremely combative. Despite restraints, he pulled out the first IV. He left the second one alone; however, upon returning to his room after its placement, he tore the bed apart and began throwing things.

The child psychiatrist was consulted. He believed that Jeff was displaying symptoms of a conduct disorder of the unsocialized, aggressive type. There was no evidence of attention deficit disorder. He prescribed tranquilizing medication to help Jeff manage his behavior and anxiety. Jeff took it orally after he was told he would get a shot if necessary to help him "calm down" and allow the staff to take care of the injured finger.

The psychiatrist recommended that the clinical nurse specialist in child psychiatry work with the pediatric nursing staff caring for Jeff. They had expressed their anger and frustration with Jeff and his behavior. However, as they attempted to understand the dynamics of the behavior, they became aware of his need for attention, even if it was negative. After verbalizing their anger and identifying the other feelings Jeff elicited in them, they were able to begin a new care plan.

Nursing Care Plan for Jeff

Nursing Diagnosis	Desired Outcomes	Interventions	Rationale
1. Noncompliance with nursing care 2. Potential for violence: self-directed or directed at others	Jeff will display age-appropriate behavior and not jeopardize his own safety or that of others.	Communicate expected behavior to Jeff; state limits firmly; offer substitute behaviors (for example, "It is time to soak your finger. You may not throw things. If you cannot control yourself you may get hurt or you may hurt someone else. If you are angry, you may punch your pillow and tell me how you feel in angry words and in an angry voice.").	Clearly stated behavioral expectations and limit setting, along with suggestion of alternative behaviors, are essential to eliciting desired behaviors.
		Explain the consequences of unacceptable behaviors (for example, "If you cannot control yourself, I'll have to restrict you to your room, have a staff member or someone from your family be with you at all times, and take away your TV.").	Mild aversives for undesirable behaviors, as well as positive reinforcement for desirable behaviors, are usually needed in working with the child with serious behavior problems.

Nursing Diagnosis	Desired Outcomes	Interventions	Rationale
		State reasons for limits (for example, "Your finger needs to be soaked so it can get better. If you don't soak it you'll have to stay in the hospital longer.").	Presenting behavioral expectations in a context that is clearly in what Jeff would feel is *his* best interest can make them appealing to him.
		Avoid power struggles. Set limits that are not negotiable to ensure safety.	To be effective, behavioral limits need to be nonnegotiable, and consistent from nurse to nurse and shift to shift.
		Be consistent. Deliver positive reinforcement for cooperative self-care behaviors, with praise and small rewards (stickers, a walk) especially when self-initiated. Small rewards, if there are many, can be exchanged for a large reward (a toy) at the end of a 3–7 day period.	
		Develop a daily schedule with Jeff and see that staff as well as Jeff adhere to it.	Predictability decreases anxiety, often the basis of noncompliance or acting-out.
		Provide Jeff with opportunities to make choices and have freedom whenever safely possible, for example, where to have his IV placed; when during the shift to have his finger soaked and dressing changed; and when to have the opportunity to do as much of his dressing change as possible by himself with supervision (from the beginning if possible).	Giving Jeff increased controllability, especially of therapeutic aversives like dressing change, is likely to increase his cooperation with them.
		Encourage Jeff to express his feelings, fears, and concerns verbally rather than behaviorally. Correct cognitive distortions when they occur. Help him find words for feelings when he is upset.	Verbalization of feelings can decrease the likelihood that Jeff will act them out; it can also afford the nurse the opportunity to pick up any cognitive distortions Jeff's feelings might be associated with.

Nursing Diagnosis	Desired Outcomes	Interventions	Rationale
		Assist Jeff in channeling his feelings into his play. Allowing him to use a shark puppet, guns that shoot rubber darts, or squirt-guns in fantasy play, under adult supervision, is extremely effective in surfacing unconscious anger and aggression (stimulated by perceived threat and attack by medical and nursing staff), and neutralizing it in a structured, safe setting with an empathic adult who can help him understand why he feels the way he does.	
		Praise Jeff consistently for appropriate behavior and observation of limits.	Positive reinforcement increases the desired behavior.
		Encourage Jeff to spend time in the playroom with other patients or recreation staff so he can have experiences of positive attention.	
		Plan Jeff's care so that his appointments with the child psychiatrist occur at a time when Jeff is likely to want to talk and play, for example, late morning or after his treatment.	Treatment-related anxiety may interfere with exploration of other feelings.

Jeff began to trust the staff and seemed to feel a sense of security in knowing what his limits were and that staff would help him to control his behavior if he could not. The nursing care plan provided the nursing staff with the structure they needed to help Jeff. The rest of his hospital stay was uneventful. The nurses were rewarded for their efforts when they began to see a definite change in Jeff. They started to see his good points and began to feel good about spending time with him. After his discharge Jeff returned to the unit several times to say "hello" before appointments to see his therapist for outpatient psychotherapy. It was, understandably, hard for him to say good-bye to his new friends.

CHILDHOOD DEPRESSION. Views on **childhood depression** have changed dramatically in recent years. Prior to the 1970s, it was felt that children were not capable of becoming depressed in the adult fashion, despite reports of depressive syndromes in infants and children (Levy 1937, Freud & Burlingham, 1944, Spitz, 1946). The myth of childhood being a happy, carefree time was perpetuated.

Currently, childhood depression is a recognized disorder. Professionals now believe that children do get depressed in ways that do not reflect normal developmental phenomena. The increasing suicide rate among children and adolescents and its relationship to depression is considered a major mental-health

DSM-III-R Diagnostic Criteria for Major Depressive Episode

Note: A "Major Depressive Syndrome" is defined as criterion A below.

A. At least five of the following symptoms have been present during the same two-week period and represent a change from previous functioning; at least one of the symptoms is either (1) depressed mood, or (2) loss of interest or pleasure. (Do not include symptoms that are clearly due to a physical condition, mood-incongruent delusions or hallucinations, incoherence, or marked loosening of associations.)

1) depressed mood (or can be irritable mood in children and adolescents) most of the day, nearly every day, as indicated either by subjective account or observation by others

2) markedly diminished interest or pleasure in all, or almost all, activities most of the day, nearly every day (as indicated either by subjective account or observation by others of apathy most of the time)

3) significant weight loss or weight gain when not dieting (e.g., more than 5% of body weight in a month), or decrease or increase in appetite nearly every day (in children, consider failure to make expected weight gains)

4) insomnia or hypersomnia nearly every day

5) psychomotor agitation or retardation nearly every day (observable by others, not merely subjective feelings of restlessness or being slowed down)

6) fatigue or loss of energy nearly every day

7) feelings of worthlessness or excessive or inappropriate guilt (which may be delusional) nearly every day (not merely self-reproach or guilt about being sick)

8) diminished ability to think or concentrate, or indecisiveness, nearly every day (either by subjective account or as observed by others)

9) recurrent thoughts of death (not just fear of dying), recurrent suicidal ideation without a specific plan, or a suicide attempt or a specific plan for committing suicide

B. 1) It cannot be established that an organic factor initiated and maintained the disturbance

2) The disturbance is not a normal reaction to the death of a loved one (Uncomplicated Bereavement)

Note: Morbid preoccupation with worthlessness, suicidal ideation, marked functional impairment or psychomotor retardation, or prolonged duration suggest bereavement complicated by Major Depression.

C. At no time during the disturbance have there been delusions or hallucinations for as long as two weeks in the absence of prominent mood symptoms (i.e., before the mood symptoms developed or after they have remitted).

D. Not superimposed on Schizophrenia, Schizophreniform Disorder, Delusional Disorder, or Psychotic Disorder NOS.

Major depressive episode codes: fifth-digit code numbers and criteria for severity of current state of Bipolar Disorder, Depressed, or Major Depression:
1–Mild: Few, if any, symptoms in excess of those required to make the diagnosis, **and** symptoms result in only minor impairment in occupational functioning or in usual social activities or relationships with others.

problem (see Chapter 18 on psychological crises). As a result there has been a dramatic increase in clinical work and research related to childhood depression (Carlson & Cantwell, 1980; Kovacs, 1984; Poznanski & Zrull, 1970, 1976; Poznanski et al., 1982; Robbins et al., 1982).

When should the nurse observing the "sad" child become concerned that she is dealing with a child who is experiencing a major depressive episode? Depressed children have sad feelings that persist for extended periods of time (most of the day and for weeks). They have great difficulty remembering the last time they felt happy or had a good time. This inability to have fun, called **anhedonia,** when present, is striking, since having fun is an integral part of a child's life and a necessary ingredient for learning and playing (Poznanski, 1986). Persistently depressed

affect or inability to play are key criteria for diagnosing a major depressive episode among children, according to the DSM-III-R. Other signs and symptoms that may indicate that a child is depressed and in need of further assessment include: 1) inability to concentrate, which leads to decreased performance in school; 2) signs of apathy, loss of interest in school activities, social isolation, and/or boredom; 3) lowered self-esteem, feelings of worthlessness, self-reproach, or pathological guilt; 4) complaints of fatigue; 5) psychomotor retardation (for example, a severely depressed child may sit in a slumped position staring at the floor for long periods of time, have slowed, monotone speech, and give short two-word responses); 6) sleep difficulties (for example, the child may report difficulty falling asleep or talk about waking up in the middle of the night or too

Box 22–6 ● Could Suicide Be Contagious?

Cheerleaders wearing the school's gold-and-green colors led the emotional pep rally. More than a thousand pupils—almost the entire student body—assembled, many of them wearing paper hearts with the words CHOOSE LIFE. They hugged one another, cheered their athletic teams and sang *We Are the World*. The lyric "We're saving our own lives" understandably brought many to tears: the rally had been called to calm the student body after three youths at Bryan High School on the outskirts of Omaha committed suicide within five days.

The three knew one another only vaguely. They were ordinary youngsters with no apparent problems who lived in a predominantly Roman Catholic, blue-collar community. Michele Money, 16, described by friends as a positive, dependable person, had had problems with her boyfriend and talked about dropping out of school. She died of an overdose of Elavil, her mother's antidepressant. Mark Walpus, 15, was a popular, athletic youngster

who had recently spent a lot of time by himself building a drill press. He shot himself in the chest. Tom Wacha, 18, a loner who planned to go to trade school, also shot himself. According to police, he had told a friend that he was "disgusted with life." In addition to these three, four other Bryan students tried to kill themselves in the past three weeks but failed.

The spree of self-destruction sent a shock wave through the school, which was locally branded "Suicide High." Counselors reported that some students dreaded going to class, fearing that another classmate would be dead. "Some of the youngsters are terribly upset and can't seem to control themselves," observed Guidance counselor Nancy Bednar. "It's a sense of 'Who will be next?'" Teachers urged students to take a pledge not to make "any big decisions . . . without taking a day to think it over." At a forum on the suicides, parents and others shouted down psychiatrist John Florian Riedler with such comments as "I once

continued

tried to commit suicide, years ago. No one ever tried to help me." Said Riedler: "Hysteria swept over this part of town last week."

The Omaha deaths raise an obvious question: Is suicide contagious? Recent clusters of adolescent suicides suggest that the answer is yes. In a twelve-month period beginning in February 1983, seven teenagers in Plano, Texas, committed suicide, four by carbon-monoxide poisoning, three by guns. Five boys in New York's Westchester and Putnam counties died by their own hand in February 1984, four of them by hanging. Within the past two weeks, one student at David Prouty High School in Spencer, Mass., committed suicide; at least two schoolmates, possibly four, tried to kill themselves and failed.

Researchers know very little about cluster suicides. Some may be merely coincidences; others may be self-dramatizing efforts to capture the same outpouring of sympathy that surrounded an earlier death. According to Dr. Mark Rosenberg of Atlanta's Center for Disease Control, clusters probably occur "much more frequently than we find out about." Suicides generally tend to be underreported, he notes, in part because of concern about stigmatizing the deceased. Nevertheless, suicide is the

third leading cause of death in adolescents and young adults. In the 15-to-19-year age group, the suicide rate has almost tripled since 1958. However, since 1981, the rate has begun to level off.

Various researchers have blamed youth suicides on such disparate causes as the Viet Nam War, television, the drug culture and stress generated by the sheer number of baby boomers. Los Angeles clinical psychologist Michael Peck suggests that in today's highly mobile families, the high rate of divorce and generally "less available parenting" have left adolescents with little emotional backup.

Even so, specialists in adolescent development argue that these factors merely add to the normal turbulence of adolescent identity crisis and separation from parents. Harvard psychiatrist Douglas Jacobs says that "certain teens reach the point where they feel they are not going to achieve an identity. They don't see a future. For a moment in time, suicide seems to be the only way to get relief."

Louise Kaplan, a New York psychologist specializing in childhood and adolescence, says teenagers go through a normal period of depression and mourning for the loss of childhood attachment. The job of parents, she says, is to help young-

sters remove their passions from the family and place them in the outside community. "That's one reason why so many boys seem to kill themselves after breaking up with a girlfriend," she says. "The breakup is felt as a failure to break out of the family orbit."

In Omaha last week, parents, students and community leaders struggled to come to their own understanding of the sad epidemic. Barbara Wheeler, a store manager who works with the city's "personal crisis" hot line, thought that the Midwest's economic plight places a great burden on status-conscious teens. "Peer pressure about images is worse than ever," she said. Bryan students talked about heavy pressure for good grades and social success. Said Chris Longacre, 17: "You feel like if you make one mistake, your future is gone." Bryan's principal, John McQuinn, pointed to pro-suicide rock lyrics, complaining that "we have a 'life is cheap' philosophy fed to young people." Others expressed the wistful hope that somewhere in the seemingly pointless deaths lay a lesson for the community. Said Assistant School Superintendent Rene Hlavac: "The three young people left us a message and we need to search and find it."

Source: *Time* Feb. 24, 1986, p. 59.

---

early in the morning and being unable to go back to sleep); 7) change in eating habits indicated by weight loss or gain; and 8) recurrent thoughts of death, suicidal ideation, wishes to be dead, or a suicide attempt.

These behaviors are the central symptoms of the depressive syndrome in children. Poznanski (1986) described additional behaviors that may be present; these include irritability, weeping or feeling the desire to cry, and somatic complaints. The most common somatic complaints are stomachaches, headaches, and leg pains. Whenever organic causes for such symptoms cannot be found, the possibility of depression should be considered.

Theories of Etiology. All psychiatric disorders in childhood probably have a multifactorial etiology, and depression is no exception (Cantwell & Carlson, 1983). Theories of the etiology of depression include psychoanalytic, behavioral, sociological, existential, and biological (see Chapter 9 on mood disorders for an in-depth discussion of the etiology of depression. In this chapter only a few of the more common causes of depression in childhood will be mentioned).

Children who are physically or sexually abused are at risk for developing depression. Kazdin et al. (1985), in their research on physically abused children, found that physically abused child psychiatric

Box 22–7 ● Impact of Sexual Abuse on the Child

Many professionals believe that sexual abuse is nearly always a profoundly disruptive, disorienting, and destructive experience for the child. Abuse provides a degree of stimulation that is far beyond the child's capacity to encompass and assimilate. Consequently, there is interference with the accomplishment of normal developmental tasks. The progression of the child's mastery of self, environment, and relationship with others is significantly disrupted by his or her permanently altered awareness and new role, vis-à-vis the perpetrator.

Child sexual abuse is disorienting because profound blurring of boundaries inevitably follows when someone in a power position exploits the child by making him or her a sexual partner. Sexually abused children cannot avoid questioning limits set for them for others. They are confused about appropriate uses of power and authority. Their identities are at issue as they ask: "Who am I, that I am both a child and a sexual partner of someone who is supposed to be parenting or nurturing or protecting me?"

Destructive effects of sexual abuse are readily identifiable. Most sexually abused children encountered by professionals have a very poor self-image. Strikingly attractive youngsters describe themselves as ugly and express great doubt that they could appear attractive or appealing to others. Although some of the children display pseudomaturity[1], they typically possess very poor social skills. Seductiveness is often displayed inappropriately and as a sub-stitute for other social skills that are lacking. Victims tend to be isolated socially with poor peer relationships as well as unsatisfying social relationships. Many are hostile or depressed; some are suicidal. They are often reluctant or unable to trust other human beings.

Data on the long-term impact of child sexual abuse are sadly lacking. Some individuals only disclose the secret after reaching adulthood years later. Many such individuals describe serious difficulty in attaining a satisfactory level of emotional self-sufficiency or independence as adults. Nearly all attribute a poor self-image and lack of confidence to their childhood victimization. Some are plagued by multiple phobic or psychosomatic problems resulting in serious dysfunction or disability. Few incest victims report satisfactory interpersonal relationships with others. Sexual dysfunction is commonly reported.

It is known that a significant proportion of parents in incestuous families report that they themselves have been sexually abused in childhood. Thus, childhood sexual victimization may increase the likelihood that an individual will become a perpetrator later on. There is also an apparent tendency of women who were sexually victimized in childhood to select mates who, in turn, are likely to abuse them and sexually exploit their children. Prospective longitudinal studies are needed to determine the long-term impact of child sexual abuse (pp. 35–36).

Source: Sgroi, S. M., Blick, L. C., and Porter, F. S. (1982). A conceptual framework for child sexual abuse. In S. M. Sgroi (Ed.) *Handbook of Clinical Intervention in Child Sexual Abuse.* Lexington, Mass: Lexington Books, pp. 9–37.

[1]Refers to the abused child's quality of being "old for his or her years," rather than "childlike," i.e. playful, dependent, naive, and so forth. The pseudomature child seems to be on his or her own, and has left the world of the child for that of the adult, with its associated responsibilities, concerns, and, possibly, sexual relationships (Martin, 1976).

inpatients evidenced higher levels of depression, hopelessness, and lower self-esteem than did non-abused inpatients. Barahal, Waterman, and Martin (1981) demonstrated that abused children believe they have little control over their environment, recalling Seligman's (1975) description of learned helplessness as the psychological state that results when events are uncontrollable and unpredictable especially in the context of traumatic experience. Remembering the parallels between learned helplessness and depression, it becomes easy to see why the abused child, who typically can do nothing to control his parents' unpredictable abusive behavior, becomes depressed. (See Figure 22–4.)

Additional evidence for the relevance of the learned-helplessness model of depression to the study of depression in children is found in Seligman and Peterson's (1986) recent work on attributional style of depressed versus nondepressed child subjects. They have reported that attributional style correlates highly with depression in children as it does in adults. Compared to nondepressed children, children with depressive symptoms make more internal, stable, and global attributions for bad events and more external, unstable, and specific attributions for good events (Seligman & Peterson, 1986, p. 239).

Separation and loss, whether actual or perceived, increase the risk of childhood and adolescent depression. Examples of loss include parental separation or divorce, death of a parent, and psychological withdrawal of a parent from the child. The death of a pet can be a significant loss for a young child, while a friend's moving out of state, or breaking up with a girlfriend, may qualify as significant trauma in older children and adolescents.

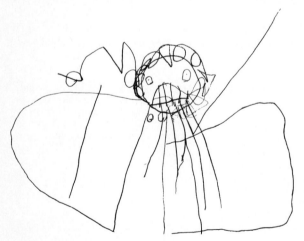

FIGURE 22–4 A Five-Year-Old's View of Helplessness Due to Total Loss of Control

The seriously ill, hospitalized child's separation from family and peers, coupled with loss of control and independence, puts him at great risk for developing depression. Nurses should be alert for depressive symptomatology in their work with pediatric patients, and make referrals for treatment as necessary.

Treatment for Depression. Treatment controversies center on the indications for and therapeutic value of medication and/or psychotherapy in working with depressed children and adolescents. Though the use of drugs for the treatment of depression in children has not been approved by the FDA, major investigators have advocated the use of tricyclic antidepressants (Weller & Weller, 1984). In fact, some clinicians as well as researchers no longer advocate talking therapy alone as the cornerstone of the treatment of depression in children, but rather, individual and/or family therapy, along with a gradual increase in antidepressant medication to specified serum levels, are indicated (Ambrosini et al., 1984). They caution the clinician to be alert for the appearance of any nontherapeutic effects of the drug, for example, sedation, headaches, and dizziness (Preskorn, et al., 1983). (Also see Chapter 9 on mood disorders and Appendix on the use of psychotropic medications in children.)

The majority of mental-health care professionals do rely on psychotherapy of various types (individual, group, family) and orientations (psychoanalytic, behavioral, cognitive) in combination with pharmacotherapy for the treatment of the clinically depressed child. The consensus seems to be that multi-modal treatment directed at the total life of the depressed child, not just his depressive symptomatology, is essential to his treatment. This is especially the case in the treatment of the depressed child who is also suicidal.

The next decade is likely to bring additional clarification of the etiologies of depression in children and adolescents. The search for psychobiological markers of depression (for example, the sleep EEG and neuroendocrine changes), and when over the life span they occur, is especially promising, and likely to shed some light on the etiology and treatment of adult depression as well as that which occurs in childhood (Carlson & Garber, 1986). Currently, clinicians working with children in inpatient or outpatient health-care settings need to be familiar with diagnostic criteria for depression and treatment methods now in use in order to identify and refer affected children and/or participate in their treatment. Primary prevention is even more desirable.

Janet: A Depressed Child

Janet, age 10, is the oldest of five children in her family. Six months ago, her 8-year-old brother was diagnosed as having leukemia. Recently, Janet's parents noted changes in her behavior. Janet, who had always been an outgoing child, was withdrawing from family and friends. In addition, her teacher reported that her school performance was dropping and that she appeared to have great difficulty concentrating.

Janet's mother shared these concerns with the oncology clinic nurse during an outpatient visit with Janet's brother. The nurse observed Janet sitting in a chair looking very sad. Further assessment by the nurse revealed that Janet was eating more "junk food" than usual and had gained six pounds in the past two weeks. She was also having difficulty falling asleep at night.

The clinic nurse was concerned that Janet might be depressed, so she consulted the clinical nurse specialist in child psychiatry. When the clinical nurse specialist met with Janet, she, too, noted her sad affect. Janet could not identify anything that she had done recently that was fun. She said she felt like crying a lot and that she felt it was her fault that her brother was sick.

In talking with Janet's mother, it became clear that Janet had been experiencing depressive symptomatology for at least three weeks. There was a family history of depression; Janet's father had been hospitalized for depression eight years ago. The clinical nurse specialist felt Janet was suffering from a major depressive episode and made an appointment to see her and her family in the psychiatric clinic. She also consulted a child psychiatrist regarding antidepressant medication, and he agreed to see the family with her.

(For more on depression, see Chapter 9 on mood disorders.)

DISORDERS FIRST EVIDENT IN ADOLESCENCE

It was formerly thought that certain psychopathologies first appeared in adolescence because of the unique stresses of that developmental stage. For example, psychoanalytic formulations of the onset of schizophrenia in late adolescence tied it to the maturing individual's struggle with independence. It was felt that exhausted coping mechanisms led to regression to infantile defenses. Similarly, anorexia nervosa was thought to be a response of the young adolescent to fears of sexual maturity and regressive fantasies about oral pregnancy. Currently, only the diagnosis of identity disorder is specifically associated with "normal" conflicts associated with maturing.

Though it is true that the normal developmental struggles of adolescence, including physical maturation, are often associated with disruption in the family system, Offer (1969) has shown that most adolescents do not have difficulties requiring professional intervention. This is not to belie the many and important problems that affect other adolescents, for example, suicide and the epidemic use of alcohol and drugs. The poignancy of adolescent psychosexual conflicts (especially those complicated by teenage pregnancy), including the struggles adolescents often have with gender identity, are also well known to the clinician who deals with this age group.

It is important that the clinician working with adolescents monitor her countertransference because it can be intense, especially if her adolescence was a stormy one or not that long ago. For example, overidentification with the adolescent's rebellion against "authority," or anxiety in response to his or her preoccupation with sexual impulses needs to be understood. Equally troublesome may be the clinician's impulse to abandon the adolescent who resists developing a counselling or therapy relationship with her because of a fear of dependence, which can be overwhelming for the young person struggling for self-identity.

In summary, adolescent psychopathology is unique, not because of the disorders involved, but because of the disturbances present in the context of the developmental conflicts specific to the adolescent and his family. Especially important is the adolescent's struggle with separation and individuation. For further reading, see Chapter 14, on eating disorders, and Chapter 15, on substance abuse. See also specialized resources such as *Adolescent Psychiatry,* the official publication of the American Society of Adolescent Psychiatry for further discussion of these issues.

SEPARATION ANXIETY DISORDER AND TOURETTE SYNDROME. Two disorders of special interest in childhood and adolescence are **separation anxiety disorder** and **Tourette syndrome.** Each is currently being treated psychopharmacologically with apparent success. This follows a long history of focus on psychosocial interventions as the primary therapy for these disorders. Since the symptoms of these disorders seem to show definite stability through the lifespan (though, perhaps, attracting different diagnostic labels), they have become a focus for special study.

Separation Anxiety Disorder. Separation anxiety disorder recognizes the specific trauma of separation from an attachment figure (usually the mother) leading to significant distress and dysfunction due to the associated anxiety. Classically, **school phobia** (or school refusal) has been thought to be the most common manifestation of this disorder.

Current attention to adult anxiety disorders, the panic disorders in particular, has resulted in a reassessment of separation anxiety disorder in children of all ages. Manifestations of anxiety in children, both behavioral (obsessive fear, protest, avoidance) and affective, are similar to those of adults. These symptoms in children respond to behavioral approaches, including a variety of exposure methods to the anxiety-provoking object or event (see Chapter 8 on anxiety and anxiety disorders). The effectiveness of tem-

porary use of anti-anxiety medications has been reported, as well as a therapeutic response to the tricyclic antidepressants, though this is as controversial with adolescent patients as it is with adult patients. Family therapy, in addition to behavioral therapy and psychotropic medication, is also often part of the treatment program. Its purpose is to ferret out family dynamics contributing to the child's anxiety, and attend to other needy family members (e.g. a depressed mother), or previously unacknowledged family issues (e.g. a dying marriage).

How do these problems relate to the adult disorders? Are the manifestations of anxiety associated with the real or threatened loss of the primary caretaker only a normal developmental phenomenon? Will children with severe separation anxiety inevitably develop anxiety disorders as adults? When does

DSM-III-R Diagnostic Criteria for Separation Anxiety Disorder

A. Excessive anxiety concerning separation from those to whom the child is attached, as evidenced by at least three of the following:

1) unrealistic and persistent worry about possible harm befalling major attachment figures or fear that they will leave and not return

2) unrealistic and persistent worry that an untoward calamitous event will separate the child from a major attachment figure, e.g., the child will be lost, kidnapped, killed, or be the victim of an accident

3) persistent reluctance or refusal to go to school in order to stay with major attachment figures or at home

4) persistent reluctance or refusal to go to sleep without being near a major attachment figure or to go to sleep away from home

5) persistent avoidance of being alone, including "clinging" to and "shadowing" major attachment figures

6) repeated nightmares involving the theme of separation

7) complaints of physical symptoms, e.g., headaches, stomachaches, nausea, or vomiting, on many school days or on other occasions when anticipating separation from major attachment figures

8) recurrent signs or complaints of excessive distress in anticipation of separation from home or major attachment figures, e.g., temper tantrums or crying, pleading with parents not to leave

9) recurrent signs of complaints of excessive distress when separated from home or major attachment figures, e.g., wants to return home, needs to call parents when they are absent or when child is away from home

B. Duration of disturbance of at least two weeks.

C. Onset before the age of 18.

D. Occurrence not exclusively during the course of a pervasive developmental disorder, schizophrenia, or any other psychotic disorder.

developmentally appropriate ("normal") separation anxiety become a disorder?

There is no unidimensional framework for understanding or predicting normal versus pathological development. While *high-risk factors* such as parental conflict and difficult temperament in early childhood, a strong family history of depression, and brain damage (especially if associated behavior has impulsive and aggressive components) have been identified, there is no explanation, for example, for the "defiers of negative prediction"—the high-risk children who ultimately do *better* than the low-risk children. No theory attempts to account for this or the variability of outcome in general. However, theory building has not been given up, and "benign neglect" has not replaced aggressive attempts to intervene in high-risk situations. Clinicians and researchers are continuing to ask questions and look for their answers, though in a different investigative climate. As Chess and Thomas (1984), the researchers responsible for the only prospective long-term study of human development, known for their "goodness of fit" model which involves looking at the *interaction* of the child with his environment, have stated:

> As the field of developmental studies has matured, we now have to give up the illusion that once we know the young child's psychological history, subsequent personality and functioning are ipso facto predictable. On the other hand, we now have a much more optimistic vision of human development. The emotionally traumatized child is not doomed, the parents' early mistakes are not irrevocable, and our preventative and therapeutic intervention can make a difference at all age periods (p. 293).

Tourette Syndrome. In contrast, it is clear from current research (Cohen et al., 1984) that Tourette syndrome is probably the same in adults as it is in children. Though its etiology is still unclear, the good response of the motor symptoms to psychopharmacological treatment, and the overlap between attention deficit disorder with hyperactivity, obsessive-compulsive disorder, and Tourette syndrome, make it very likely that a genetic, neurobiochemical vulnerability exists in affected individuals. This vulnerability will be expressed in a variety of ways from early in the child's life. The most common manifestations are problems with attention span, obsessive thoughts, or recurrent tics. The recurrent tics of Tourette syndrome increase and decrease, especially in response to stress.

Though tic patterns that are short lived (days to weeks) are common in preschool and early school-aged children, the true Tourette syndrome is considered rare, as it occurs only in five in 10,000 children. Vocal phenomena, for example, uncontrolled swearing **(coprolalia),** are the hallmark of the current diagnostic criteria.

As a visible behavioral "marker," tics should be an easy sign for health-care professionals in all areas of practice to note and inquire about. However, since tics can frequently be controlled to some degree by the child, the clinician may need to develop a safe relationship with the child for him to reveal his tics. For this reason, the nurse at school, or the clinic nurse able to observe unobtrusively the child in the waiting area, may be more likely to be the first to recognize these symptoms. Recent public-education campaigns by the national support group for Tourette syndrome patients and families* has made this a disorder often first diagnosed by parents.

Once diagnosed, the child with Tourette syndrome and his family need sensitive health care that focuses on the disruptive effects of this disease on their world. Family and peer relationships can deteriorate as a result of the stress of Tourette syndrome, and the affected child may suffer significant blows to his self-esteem (Holder & Cohen, 1983). The clinic nurse is in a good position to provide support to the family. She can also do an ongoing psychological assessment of this child and his family while they are in treatment, and refer them to a mental-health professional if anyone becomes dysfunctional.

Important questions still unanswered about this disorder include those about the efficacy and safety of treatment with medications (usually high-potency neuroleptics such as haloperidol), the use of alternative therapies (behavioral and psychoanalytic psychotherapy), and the overlap of other disorders in the child and the family's history (Barabas & Mathews, 1985). Since symptoms associated with Tourette syndrome include such common problems as attentional symptoms and such "unique" symptoms as severe obsessive-compulsive states, it is a disease that is likely to be instructive as a model of childhood psychopathology.

Tourette syndrome has also become a model in a different arena, that of "orphan" drug development. An "orphan" drug is one that is recognized as having

*Tourette Syndrome Association, 41–02 Bell Boulevard, Bayside, N.Y. 11361.

**DSM-III-R
Diagnostic Criteria for
Tourette Disorder**

A. Both multiple motor and one or more vocal tics have been present at some time during the illness, although not necessarily concurrently.

B. The tics occur many times a day (usually in bouts), nearly every day or intermittently throughout a period of more than one year.

C. The anatomic location, number, frequency, complexity, and severity of the tics change over time.

D. Onset before age 21.

E. Occurrence not exclusively during psychoactive substance intoxication or known central nervous system disease, such as Huntington's chorea and postviral encephalitis.

such a small market (i.e. few individuals will purchase it because of the rarity of the disorder it treats), that it has no one to "parent" it through the Federal Drug Administration licensing process. The success of the Tourette Syndrome Association in influencing the United States federal government to modify its standards for approval of drugs for this uncommon disease demonstrates that advocacy for special patients can be effective.

PSYCHOLOGICAL NEEDS OF THE HOSPITALIZED CHILD

When a child is hospitalized, even for a minor illness, it is a stressful event for both the child and his family. While all health care professionals need to be sensitive to the needs of the hospitalized child, it is for the most part up to the nurse to mitigate this potentially traumatic experience.

It is beyond the scope of this chapter to discuss in depth how and why hospitalization can be harmful to children, especially young children, and how this can be prevented. Several key issues, in addition to separation anxiety and depression, are discussed here.

IMMOBILITY

Although immobility affects people of all age groups adversely, psychologically as well as physiologically, it is particularly difficult for the hospitalized toddler (age eight months to thirty-six months). During this stage of development, locomotion is an important means of demonstrating independence and autonomy as well as the predominant method of learning about the world.

Use of restraints on a child of this age should be avoided whenever possible. Simple statements about

not touching the intravenous or nasogastric tubes *while distracting the child with other activities,* such as reading a story, watching cartoons, or playing with a toy, are often enough. Providing children with activities and toys that demonstrate motion is helpful. For example, younger children like mobiles, balls, and bubbles; older children might like a foam basketball with a hoop (and a playmate who can retrieve the ball) or a remote-control TV with access to action-oriented video games such as "Ninja Turtle." If the child is unable to move at all, the adults around him may play *for* him. Whenever possible, children who are on bed rest should be up in strollers, buggies, wagons, wheelchairs, or carts, and taken around the unit or the hospital to get a sense of mobility. It takes a creative nurse to deal with the immobilized child.

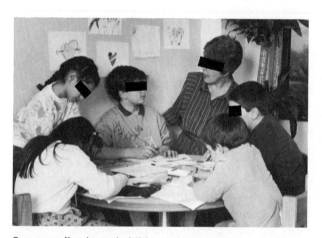

Some pediatric and child psychiatry inpatient units provide school for the patients during their hospital stay. This is very helpful for the student who worries about being "held back" and is also a way to provide a sense of normalcy for the chronically ill or dying child.

FEAR OF PUNISHMENT AND MUTILATION

The hospitalized preschool child is especially vulnerable to fears regarding punishment and mutilation. For the child between the ages of three and six, magical thinking predominates. He is involved in vigorous reality testing, imagination, and fantasy. Because of the developing superego or conscience, the preschooler is, in addition, vulnerable to interpreting aversive experiences as punishment. The child feels he must have done something bad, and that is why he is getting poked with needles and has been left in the hospital. Preschoolers, like toddlers, need frequent reassurance that what is happening to them in the hospital is not happening because they have been "bad."

This age group is also very fearful of mutilation. Simple, accurate explanations are essential. If a child is to have surgery, he and his siblings need to understand what will happen and what won't. A common fear is that other parts of his body will be cut or taken off. The young child needs reassurance that when bandages or sutures are removed, his body will not fall apart. Because of the predominance of concrete thinking, words will be taken literally, so care must be taken when talking to a young child. Referring to the suture line as a "zipper" may increase rather than decrease the child's anxiety because zippers can get unzipped. The young child should also not be told he will be "put to sleep" because the family's dog may have been "put to sleep," that is, destroyed. Regardless of what he is told, the young child's perception of the situation should be assessed and distortions corrected as necessary.

LOSS OF CONTROL

As has been mentioned, loss of control is as traumatic for the toddler, preschooler, school-age child, and adolescent as it is for the adult. While the sense of accomplishment and mastery varies with the individual, it is no less important, especially during hospitalization, for the two-year-old than it is for a twenty-two-year-old. Both will be traumatized if their need for control is not appreciated and dealt with seriously. The nurse can, at least, offer the child choices whenever possible. However, there is often much potential in the environment for increasing the child's sense of control if the nurse is creative and persistent. For example, she can have the child participate in much, if not all, of his nursing care. (Also see Chapter 25 on the intensive care patient.) Some children need much encouragement to regain control once it has been lost. They have begun to feel helpless and need to regain power. School-age and adolescent patients may benefit from diagrams and models of the human body in order to better understand their own and what is happening to it. Increasing the predictability of their physical sensations, for example, by telling them what they are likely to feel (pulling, pressure, cold) prior to upcoming procedures, is especially helpful to children as they work to master anxiety, depression, and anger about illness or injury and its treatment. This is particularly true when giving them actual control of aversive procedures is not possible.

FEAR OF DISFIGUREMENT AND LOSS OF INDEPENDENCE

For the adolescent in the hospital, fear of disfigurement and loss of independence become major concerns. Also, the adolescent's achievement of separation and individuation from parents may be threatened when faced with illness and injury and associated hospitalization and dependency needs. In addition, because the adolescent does not want to be seen as "different" from his peers, he may not comply with medical or nursing orders, for example, medication and dietary restrictions in the case of diabetes. While limit setting, positive reinforcement, opportunities to express the grief and anger associated with illness, especially when chronic, and family involvement may help, a psychiatric referral is necessary if noncompliance continues or is life-threatening.

If the adolescent is hospitalized for surgery or because of a disfiguring accident, special attention should be paid to his already complex feelings regarding his changing body-image and self-esteem. The adolescent should be encouraged to express his feelings and begin to deal with the new situation, for example, his feelings about himself, and questions and reactions from peers. Finally, the adolescent as well as the school-age child's need for privacy should be acknowledged whether or not it can be honored.

It is essential that, in addition to these developmental considerations, the nurse keep in mind that children of all ages must be dealt with honestly. Clear, enforced limits help the child know what is expected of him and at what point the nurse will take control. This is essential for the child to feel safe and secure in the hospital environment. In addition, since the anxiety level of the child is directly related to the anxiety level of his parents, the nurse should determine the parents' perception of the child's illness or injury and its treatment, and correct any distortions. She should assess the family's support system and coping mechanisms and intervene as necessary. Par-

Box 22–8 • Families of Children with Chronic Illness

In order to find out the specific needs of parents of chronically ill or handicapped children, three nurses in Wichita, Kansas conducted a survey of such parents. A questionnaire was mailed to a convenience sample of 493 families in a midwestern city. The major findings follow.

It is not always easy to tell when chronic stress causes psychiatric disorders in children, because family stress often results from a parent's psychiatric disorder, which may produce effects on the children independently through heredity. This is not a problem in families where one child has a severe physical handicap such as cystic fibrosis or cerebral palsy—a source of stress unrelated to any previous emotional mental disturbance in the parents. Researchers have recently completed a study comparing

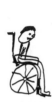
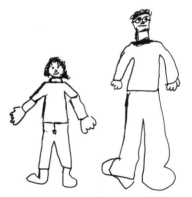
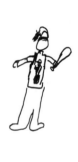

(a) A significant difference in a brother and sister's view of their family—their father with terminal cancer—is evident in these two drawings. The first is the 8-year-old boy's view. He sees his father as much smaller in size (powerless) and separate. His mother is the family's center and source of stability; his sister is by her side, while the boy is on the opposite periphery—faceless.

ents should also be encouraged to deal with the impact of their child's hospitalization on the rest of the family and to discuss this with a mental-health professional if it seems to be more than they can manage on their own. Parents should be encouraged to participate in their child's nursing and medical care as much as they and the child can comfortably allow. They need information about and sometimes help with managing the child's emotional reactions in the hospital as well as when he returns home. Psychiatric referral is appropriate if the parents and/or the child feel overwhelmed and unable to manage with anticipatory guidance and nursing support alone.

Based on their research on the interaction patterns among nurses, hospitalized children, and their families, Knafl, Cavallari, and Dixon (1988) have proposed a negotiative model of family-centered care to help promote a collaborative working relationship

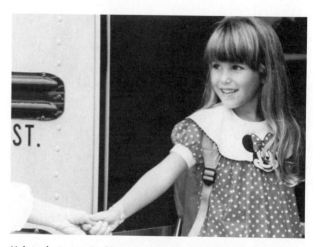

Kristy has cystic fibrosis and since age 2 has been hospitalized many times. She is proof that chronic illness and hospitalization don't have to be "damaging" or developmentally disabling.

284 children in normal families with 192 brothers and sisters of physically handicapped children. Twice, at five-year intervals, the mothers were asked to fill out a questionnaire identifying psychiatric symptoms in their children: self-destructive behavior, anxiety, fighting, social isolation, and so on. At the follow-up, the children themselves were also given a standard diagnostic interview.

At the beginning of the study, brothers and sisters of handicapped children showed more impulsive and aggressive behavior, conflict with parents, anxiety, depressive symptoms, and psychiatric symptoms in general. Both groups of children had the same levels of self-destructive behavior, cognitive problems, social isolation, and severe psychiatric impairment, including severe depres-

sion. These results were unchanged when the researchers corrected for the mother's level of education, which they used as one indication of social class.

There were a few changes during the five years. On the average, children with a handicapped brother or sister became somewhat more isolated, depressed, and self-destructive, although not more aggressive. The youngest children (ages 6 to 9 at the beginning of the study) and children of lower social classes were most likely to become isolated.

Isolation developed especially when the mother's level of distress was high; it did not result from restricted family activities, a heavier burden of care for the handicapped child, or disruption of the family by divorce. The authors conclude that the strain on mothers was the main cause of emotional disturbances in children with handicapped brothers and sisters.

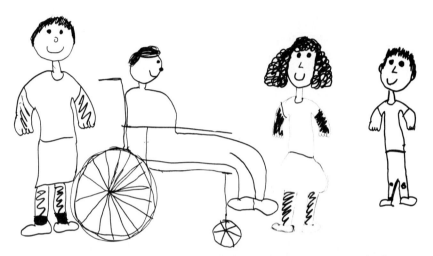

(b) The second drawing, done by the boy's 12-year-old sister, depicts the family differently. Everyone is smiling (denial). Her father is shown without arms (helpless) while she and her mom are by his side. Her brother is seen standing back and watching, feeling as helpless as his father with whom he strongly identifies.

Source: *Harvard Mental Health Letter,* 4(12), June 1988, p. 6. *Naomi Breslau and Kenneth Prabucki.* Siblings of disabled children: effects of chronic stress in the family. *Archives of General Psychiatry, 44:1040–1046 (December 1987).* (Also see Chapter 19 on women for more information on women and stress.)

---

between parents and nurses. The authors recommend that nurses:

1. elicit family members' views, preferences, and needs:

2. communicate to families what the nurse's role in the care of their child entails; and

3. negotiate with family members to reach a mutually satisfactory understanding of how the child's care is going to be managed.

(Also see Chapter 21 on Families.)

In summary, hospitalization of a child does not have to be traumatic for the child or the parents. The nurse is in a key position to assist the child and his family to cope adaptively with the situation, even make it a positive, growth promoting experience for all.

Case Study: Nonpsychiatric Setting

Diane Taylor took her 14-year-old daughter, Carolyn, a freshman in high school, to see her pediatrician, Dr. Rob Anderson, for the third time in two weeks. Carolyn had been experiencing a variety of vague physical problems including nausea with vomiting, low back pain, diarrhea, headaches, dizziness, and photophobia. The symptoms had been varying in intensity, and occurring in different combinations over the past two weeks, and Carolyn hadn't been in school because of them. She was spending most of her time in bed or on the living room sofa watching television and sleeping intermittently.

At this appointment, as at the past two, Carolyn had a normal physical exam. She reported an additional symptom at this time, however—a sleep disturbance which involved sleeping only two to three hours at night because of frequent waking with a sensation of "choking" or a sore throat. Dr. Anderson told Carolyn to continue the antacids he prescribed the week before as well as Tylenol for pain. He told her she should try to attend school since it appeared that there was nothing seriously wrong with her. Carolyn said she would try, but if she felt the next morning the way she did then, she "couldn't imagine going to school."

Diane took Carolyn in to see Dr. Anderson again three days later. She had called his office twice per day since their last visit with questions about Carolyn's changing symptoms and the over-the-counter medication she was taking. Carolyn had not been to school yet, though she reported that her gastrointestinal distress was better. She still "vomited small amounts occasionally," however, and her headaches and dizziness when upright had worsened. Carolyn's physical exam was again normal. Dr. Anderson expressed his frustration about the situation as well as concern that Carolyn's continuing symptoms were making her miss a lot of school, which was also a problem. He told Carolyn and her mother that sometimes psychological distress can cause physical problems such as the ones Carolyn had been experiencing. For this reason, he told them that he wanted to refer Carolyn to a nurse psychologist in private practice for evaluation and possible treatment of her unremitting physical distress. Carolyn denied feeling depressed, or anxious, including about missing so much school. Her mother, on the other hand, was very concerned about both. Diane also felt guilty since the family had moved four times in the past five years (with Carolyn and her brother transferring schools with each move) as a result of her divorce from Carolyn's father and her employment difficulties. She said that life had been fairly stressful in the past few years, and the idea that Carolyn might be suffering from some kind of psychosomatic illness as a result made sense to her. They agreed to the referral.

Diane and Carolyn saw the nurse psychologist, Dr. Kelly Wagner, the next afternoon. Carolyn had again stayed home from school due to her gastrointestinal and other symptoms. Dr. Wagner saw Carolyn and her mother separately and together. As with Dr. Anderson, Diane seemed much more concerned about Carolyn's physical problems and absence from school than did her daughter. Both denied experiencing any significant emotional problems over the last few years; however, the family history was positive for psychiatric illness in Diane's family. Her father was alcoholic and homicidal, and committed suicide after beating his wife (Diane's stepmother) to death. This occurred when Diane was pregnant with Carolyn. Diane's paternal grandfather also had a history of depression and committed suicide. Diane reported that Carolyn's father and his family had no history of psychiatric illness as far as she knew. The same was true for Carolyn and her brother Alan.

In the interview with Carolyn, Dr. Wagner determined that her mood had been somewhat "irritable" over the past three weeks. Her sleep disturbance was preexisting ("I've always had trouble falling asleep and I sleep restlessly") but it had worsened over the past two weeks. Carolyn seemed apathetic and uninterested in her illness, school, friends, and social activities. She had no feelings about her parents' divorce despite the fact that her contact with her father had steadily decreased over the past four years. Currently he was remarried and the father of a six-month-old daughter. Carolyn was hoping to visit her father in California over her Christmas vacation. She hadn't considered the fact that she might not be able to go if she were ill.

Diane told Dr. Wagner in her interview that she had been worried about Carolyn for some time. She felt that she had been withdrawing socially before they moved from Utah to Ohio, but didn't know what to do about it. She had hoped the move would mean a fresh start for her daughter.

Carolyn denied having any problems with her peers in Utah. Similarly, she denied having any feelings about not making the cheerleading squad at her new school, something she had accomplished in Utah. She also had had to give up dance lessons after the move, as the dance facilities in their new neighborhood were not convenient. Diane, however, wondered if these disappointments could have something to do with her current problems.

Dr. Wagner suggested a trial of family therapy which would include Alan and, possibly, a conference call to their father. Diane and Carolyn were agreeable. Dr. Wagner urged Carolyn to try going to school the next day, even if she was not feeling her best. Carolyn said she would try; Diane rolled her eyes and said "I hope *this* helps."

Diane called Dr. Wagner about two hours after their appointment with questions about Carolyn's activity level and how forceful Diane should be in getting her to go to school. She also had questions about Carolyn's continuing dizziness. Dr. Wagner empathized with Diane's anxiety and frustration, but suggested she call Dr. Anderson about the dizziness.

Over the next five days, the first family session was held and went well, though nothing of significance emerged or was discussed. Diane had continued to call Dr. Wagner and Dr. Anderson on the average of twice per day, and Carolyn still had not attended school. As a result, after consultation with Dr. Anderson, Dr. Wagner hospitalized Carolyn at University Hospital on the pediatric unit. The rationale was that hospitalization would allow: (1) observation of Carolyn by nursing staff in a neutral setting in order to gather objective data about her physical problems; (2) a separation between Carolyn and her mother (though it was likely that anxiety in the system would increase as a result); (3) medical and psychiatric consultation; and (4) return to school since the hospital had a high school teacher on the premises who worked with the pediatric patients who could attend the hospital school for up to four hours each day. Dr. Wagner hoped that the outcome of the hospitalization would be a better sense of Carolyn's diagnosis (atypical depression? psychophysiological disorder?). She also hoped that the family dynamics would become clearer as a result of the increase in the anxiety in the system. In addition, she and Dr. Anderson felt that Diane and Carolyn would experience hospitalization as acknowledgement of the severity of Carolyn's physical distress and the associated anxiety in Diane, and so be supportive. They did.

Carolyn was hospitalized for five days. She continued to have a normal physical exam each day though her complaint of symptoms "in *every* organ system" continued as before. After two days, the pediatric staff felt that there was no reason to keep Carolyn in the hospital. However, since the consulting psychiatrist and Dr. Wagner now agreed that Carolyn was depressed and school phobic, they worked out the following program for the last three days of Carolyn's hospitalization. Carolyn was to attend the hospital school daily despite any physical distress. She was also to participate in the recreational therapy program on the unit, and begin a trial of an antidepressant, Nortriptyline (50 mg at bedtime to start). If Carolyn was able to attend the hospital school for at least two hours per day over the next three days, she could be discharged. After discharge, Carolyn was to return to school. If she felt too ill to go to school in the morning, she was to call Dr. Wagner who would assess the situation and refer her to Dr. Anderson if medical consultation was warranted. In that event, Diane would take Carolyn immediately to Dr. Anderson's office for a physical exam. If he diagnosed her as ill enough to stay home from school, she could stay home; if he felt she was up to going to school, she would go to school. If, when at school, she was unable to function in class, she was to go to the nurse's office until she felt better, and then try again. Under no circumstances was Carolyn to call her mother or leave school before 3:15 P.M. It was also recommended that Carolyn plan to visit her father in California over the Christmas holiday (which was to begin the following week) unless she felt too ill to travel.

On her first morning at home, Carolyn got up, got ready for school, but then became light-headed and collapsed in the bathroom, hitting her head on the sink as she fell. Carolyn's mother had already left for work, thinking that Carolyn would walk to school as it was only two blocks away. Carolyn was still lying on the bathroom floor in a semiconscious state when her brother got home after school. He called Diane at work and told her about the situation. She came home immediately and found her daughter shaken but okay. She called both Dr. Anderson and Dr. Wagner. They suggested that the program be started again the next day.

The next morning, Diane called Dr. Wagner at 7:45 A.M. She said she was "unable to get Carolyn off the toilet." Her diarrhea had, apparently, worsened. Dr. Wagner reminded her that, according to the program, she needed to take Carolyn to Dr. Anderson's office. Diane replied, "What if I can't get her off the toilet?" Dr. Wagner said that in that case Carolyn should wear some kind of protective garment for the trip to the doctor's office. Later that afternoon, Dr. Wagner received a call from Diane who said that after their phone conversation, she and Carolyn decided that Carolyn would go directly to school since they were fairly certain that Dr. Anderson would tell them to do that. Once at school, Carolyn spent the day in the nurse's office as a result of continuing "vomiting and diarrhea." Dr. Wagner obtained permission from Diane and Carolyn to phone the school nurse, Sara Miller, who told her that though Carolyn spent most of the day in the bathroom, she "never heard anything but the flushing of the toilet." Dr. Wagner told Ms. Miller about the tentative diagnosis of depression and school phobia, as well as about the treatment plan and asked for her help with it. The nurse suggested that she instruct Carolyn to not flush the toilet after vomiting or having diarrhea so that she could determine how serious Carolyn's symptoms were.

Carolyn attended school the next day, spending half of it in the nurse's office with complaints of headache and dizziness. She was able to stay in class for most of the following two days, however, and though her vomiting and diarrhea returned over the weekend, she decided to visit her father the following week as planned. She returned from her Christmas visit with her father and his family feeling much improved. In fact, all of her physical symptoms had remitted. Carolyn was taking her antidepressant medication which had been gradually increased to 100 mg. She reported that she was sleeping well and feeling happier and was looking forward to returning to school.

The following is a nursing care plan developed by Carolyn's primary nurse for her hospital stay on the pediatric unit.

Nursing Diagnoses

Activity intolerance
Ineffective individual coping
Ineffective family coping
Altered parenting

Nursing Care Plan for Carolyn

Nursing Diagnosis	Desired Outcomes	Interventions	Rationale
1. Activity intolerance	Carolyn will begin to tolerate normal activities of daily living, first in the hospital, then at home, then at school.	Set expectation that Carolyn will be up and take part in unit activities including the school program despite physical complaints. If her physical distress causes a disturbance in the group, or if she becomes unable to continue an activity, she will be examined by a physician and advised to stay up or be on bedrest without television privileges.	Carolyn needs limit setting, emotional support, positive reinforcement for desirable behavior, and negative consequences for undesirable behavior in order to come out of her depression and overcome her school avoidance.
2. Ineffective individual coping; ineffective family coping; altered parenting	Carolyn and her family will begin to acknowledge their feelings about the recent major changes in their lives, and begin the process of working those feelings through and adapting to the changes. Carolyn will return to normal adolescent developmental progress and associated activities such as school with enthusiasm. Diane will begin to pull back from her daughter's life, especially its physical aspects, and Carolyn's father will become more involved with her.	Talk with Carolyn and her family about their concerns and anxieties. Label and empathize with their feelings, while setting behavioral expectations for all family members. For example, Carolyn will attend the hospital school program; Diane will visit her daughter for only two hours in the evening after dinner; Carolyn's father will be apprised of the situation and included in his daughter's treatment program via conference calls.	Feelings as well as behavior must be attended to in order to successfully treat depression and school phobia. The treatment of school phobia in the adolescent demands a family-centered approach and a team of health-care professionals during inpatient and outpatient programming.

Nursing Diagnosis	Desired Outcomes	Interventions	Rationale
		Confer with Dr. Wagner and the consulting psychiatrist regarding their treatment goals and approaches so that the nursing care plan is consistent with them; share your observations and feelings about Carolyn and her family with these members of the treatment team.	The hospital program is the first step in the treatment of Carolyn's depression and school phobia; an outpatient program will be essential to maintaining any treatment gains achieved in the hospital.
		With the family's permission, confer with the school and clinic nurses working with Carolyn about the outcome of hospitalization and the ongoing treatment plan at time of discharge.	Outpatient treatment programming is essential to maintaining gains achieved in the hospital, and to preventing behavioral regression or a return to maladaptive coping.

SUMMARY

The nurse who works with children, either primarily or secondarily, must be as informed in the areas of mental health and mental illness as she is in the areas of physical growth and development, if she is to function effectively.

The nurse must assess continually mental health needs and intervene appropriately in a timely fashion. When she feels she has identified a serious psychiatric problem in a child, or when she does not feel she is capable of or does not have the time to handle a problem which could turn into a crisis, she should refer the child and family to a mental health professional for evaluation and treatment.

The nurse enters the lives of children in many different roles: advocate, teacher, support person, caregiver, and friend. In these different roles the nurse must make dynamic use of herself if she is to be successful in helping children and families. Countertransference is often intense and is especially important when working with children. It *can* be used to better understand what the child or parent may be experiencing. When working with children, the nurse needs to know about physical and psychological development, psychopathology, and the principles of effective communication, and she needs to know herself, including the "child" within her.

KEY TERMS

id
ego
superego
accommodation
attachment
separation anxiety
learned helplessness theory
Strange-Situation Assessment
Brazelton Neonatal Assessment Scale
Denver Developmental Screening Test
countertransference

trisomy 21 (Down's syndrome)
autism
reactive attachment disorder of infancy
attention deficit disorder
conduct disorder
childhood depression
anhedonia
separation anxiety disorder
Tourette syndrome
coprolalia

STUDY QUESTIONS

1. Identify and describe briefly each of the three major developmental theories and the people who developed those theories.

2. Name and describe three methods for assessing the infant/toddler for psychopathology.

3. Discuss how a school-age child should be assessed for psychopathology.

4. Define and describe childhood depression.

5. Name and describe the major fears of the hospitalized child. In what ways can the nurse help the child cope with his or her situation?

REFERENCES

Ainsworth, M. D. S., Blehar, M. C., Waters, E., & Wall, S. (1978). *Patterns of attachment*. Hillsdale, N.J.: Lawrence Elsbaum Associates.

Als, H., Lester, B. M., & Tronick, E. Z. (1982). Manual for the assessment of preterm infants' behavior (APIB). In Fitzgerald, H. E., Lester, B. M., and Yogman, M. D. (Eds.) *Theory and research in behavioral pediatrics Vol. 1*. New York: Plenum.

Ambrosini, P. J., Harris, R., & Puig-Antich, J. (1984). *Biological factors and pharmacological treatment in major depressive disorder in children and adolescents*. Sudek, H. S., Ford, A. B., & Rushforth, N. B. (Eds.) *Suicide in the young*. Boston: Wright/DSG.

American Academy of Pediatrics, Committee on Bioethics (1983). Treatment of critically-ill newborns. *Pediatrics*, Vol. 72, 565–566.

American Psychiatric Association (1987). *Diagnostic and statistical manual of mental disorders*, 3rd Edition, revised. New York: American Psychiatric Association Press.

Barabas, G., & Mathews, W. S. (1985). Homogeneous clinical subgroup in children with Tourette syndrome. *Pediatrics, 75*, 73–75.

Barahal, R. M., Waterman, J., & Martin, H. P. (1981). The social-cognitive development of abused children. *Journal of Consulting and Clinical Psychology, 49*, 508–516.

Berger, L. R. (1981). Newborns are people too: An abbreviated Brazelton assessment for clinical use. *Developmental and Behavioral Pediatrics, 2*, 109–111.

Bowlby, J. (1969). *Attachment and loss. Volume I: Attachment*. New York: Basic Books.

Bowlby, J. (1973). *Attachment and loss. Volume II: Separation*. New York: Basic Books.

Bowlby, J. (1980). *Attachment and loss. Volume III: Loss*. New York: Basic Books.

Bradley, R. H., & Tedesco, L. A. (1982). Environmental correlates of mental retardation. In J. R. Lachenmeyer & M. S. Gibbs (Eds.), *Psychopathology in childhood*. New York: Gardner Press.

Brazelton, T. B. (1973). *Neonatal behavioral assessment*. National Spastics Society Monograph, Clinics in Developmental Medicine #50. London: William Heinemann and sons.

Brown, G. L., Ebert, M. H., & Minichiello, M. D. (1985). Biochemical and pharmacological aspects of attention deficit disorder. In L. M. Bloomingdale (Ed.), *Attention deficit disorder: Identification, course and rationale*. New York: Spectrum.

Bryan, T. H., & Bryan, J. H. (1975). *Understanding learning disabilities*. Port Washington, N. Y.: Alfred Publishing Co.

Call, J. D. (1983). Toward a nosology of psychiatric disorders in infancy. In J. D. Call, E. Galenson, & R. L. Tyson (Eds.) *Frontiers of infant psychiatry Volume I*. New York: Basic Books.

Campbell, S. B., Breaux, A. M., Ewing, L. J., & Szumowski, E. K. (1984). A one year follow-up study of parent-referred hyperactive preschool children. *JAACP, 23*, 243–249.

Cantwell, D. P. (1980). A clinician's guide to the use of stimulant medication for the psychiatric disorders of children. *Developmental and behavioral pediatrics, 1*, 133–140.

Cantwell, D., & Carlson, G. (1983). *Affective disorders in childhood and adolescence: an update*. New York: SP Medical & Scientific Books.

Carey, W. B. (1970). A simplified method of measuring infant temperament. *Journal of Pediatrics, 77*, 188–194.

Carlson, G. A., & Cantwell, D. P. (1980). A survey of depressive symptoms, syndrome and disorder in a child psychiatric population. *Journal of Child Psychology and Psychiatry, 21*, 19–25.

Carlson, G., & Garber, J. (1986). Developmental issues in the classification of depression in children. In M. Rutter, C. Izard, P. Read (Eds.), *Depression in young people, developmental and clinical perspectives*. Guilford, N.Y.: p. 399–434.

Chess, S., & Hassibi, M. (1978). *Principles and practice of child psychiatry*. New York: Plenum Press.

Chess, S., & Thomas, A. (1984). *Origin and evolution of behavior disorders from infancy to early adult life*. New York: Brumer/Mazel.

Cohen, D. J., Riddle, M. A., Leckman, J. F., Ott, S., & Shaywitz, B. A. (1984). Tourette's syndrome. In D. V. Jeste & R. J. Wyatt (Eds.), *Neuro-psychiatric movement disorders*. New York: American Psychiatric Association Press.

Cohen, R. L. (1979). Assessment. In J. L. Noshpitz (Ed.), *Basic handbook of child psychiatry*, Vol. 1, Section 3. New York: Basic Books.

Dworkin, P. H. (1985). *Learning and behavior problems of school children*, Volume 27 of *Major problems in clinical pediatrics*. Philadelphia: W. B. Saunders.

Edelbrock, C. (1985). Identifying the attention deficit syndrome. In L. M. Bloomingdale (Ed.), *Attention Deficit Disorder: Identification, Course and Rationale*. New York: Spectrum.

Edward, J., Ruskin, N., & Furrini, P. (1981). *Separation-individuation: Theory and application*. New York: Gardner Press.

Emde, R. (1984). Infant psychiatry in a changing world: Optimism and paradox. In J. D. Call, E. L. Alenson, & R. L. Tyson (Eds.) *Frontiers of infant psychiatry Volume II*. New York: Basic Books.

Erikson, E, (1954). *Identity and the Life cycle. Psychological issues* Vol. 1. Monograph #1. New York: International Universities Press.

Erikson, E. (1963). *Childhood and society*. New York: W. W. Norton.

Fowler, J., & Keen, S. (1978). *Life maps: Conversations in the journey of faith*. Waco, Texas: Word Books.

Fraiberg, S., Ed. (1980). *Clinical studies in infant mental health*. New York: Basic Books.

Frankenburg, W. K., Goldstein, A. D., & Camp, B. W. (1971). The revised Denver Developmental Screening Test. *Journal of Pediatrics, 79,* 988–995.

Freud, A. (1967). *Normality and pathology in childhood.* New York: International Universities Press.

Freud, A., & Burlingham, D. (1944). *Infants without families.* New York: International Universities Press.

Freud, S. (1905). *Three essays on the theory of sexuality in children,* Standard Edition, vol. 7, J. Strachey (Ed.). London: Hogarth Press, 1953, pp. 135–243.

Gaensbauer, T. J., Harmon, R., Cytryn, L., & McKnew, D. (1984). Social and affective development in infants with a manic-depressive parent. *American Journal of Psychiatry, 141,* 223–229.

Garrison, W. T., & Earls, F. (1985). The child behavior checklist as a screening instrument for young children. *JAACP, 24,* 76–80.

Gibes, R. (1981, May/June). Clinical uses of the Brazelton Neonatal Behavioral Assessment Scale in nursing practice. *Pediatric Nursing,* 23–26.

Gordon, A. H., & Jameson, J. C. (1979). Infant mother attachment patterns in patients with nonorganic failure to thrive syndrome. *JAACP, 18,* 251–259.

Greenspan, S. I. (1981). *The clinical interview of the child.* New York: McGraw Hill.

Greenspan, S. I. (Ed.). (1986). *Infants in multirisk families: Case studies in preventive intervention.* New York: International Universities Press.

Gray, J., Cuther, C., Dean, J., & Kempe, C. H. (1976). Perinatal assessment of mother-baby interactions. In R. Helfer & C. H. Kemp (Eds.), *Child abuse and neglect: The family and the community.* Cambridge, Mass.: D. Ballinger Publishing Company.

Gualtieri, C. T., Breuning, S. E., Schroeder, S. R., & Quade, D. (1982). Tardive dyskinesia in mentally retarded children, adolescents, and young adults. *Psychopharmacology bulletin,* 18; 62–65.

Hartmann, H. (1939). *Ego psychology and the problem of adaptation.* New York: International Universities Press.

Herskowitz, J., & Rosman, N. (1982). Sleep disorders: nightmares, night terrors, and hypersomniacs. In *Pediatrics, neurology, and psychiatry: Common ground.* New York: Macmillan, pp. 195–226.

Holder, E., & Cohen, D. (1983). Repetitive behavior patterns of childhood. In M. Levine, W., Carey, A. Crocker, & R. Gross (Eds.). *Developmental behavioral pediatrics.* W. B. Saunders, Philadelphia: pp. 618–620.

Jones, M. C. (1924). The elimination of children's fears. *Journal of Experimental Psychology, 7,* 382–390.

Kagen, J. (1984). *The nature of the child.* New York: Basic Books.

Kanner, L. (1943). Autistic disturbances of affective contact. *Nervous Child, 2,* 217–250.

Kavanagh, C. K. (1986). Personal communication.

Kazdin, A. E., Moser, J., Colbus, D., & Bell, R. (1985). Depressive symptoms among physically abused and psychiatrically disturbed children. *Jounral of Abnormal Psychology, 94,* 298–307.

Knafl, K. A., Cavallari, K. A., & Dixon, D. M. (1988). *Pediatric hospitalization.* Glenview, IL: Scott, Foresman. p. 299.

Kohlberg, L. (1976). Moral stages and moralization: The cognitive developmental approach. In T. Likona (Ed.), *Moral development and behavior,* New York: Holt, Rinehart & Winston.

Kovacs, M. (1984). Depressive disorders in childhood: A longitudinal prospective study of characteristics and recovery. *Archives of General Psychiatry, 41,* 229–237.

Levy, D. M. (1937). Primary affect hunger. *American Jounral of Psychiatry, 94,* 643–652.

Looff, D. H. (1976). *Getting to know the troubled child.* Knoxville: University of Tennessee Press.

Mahler, M., Pine, F., & Bergman, A. (1975). *Psychological birth of the human infant.* New York: Basic Books.

Massie, H., & Rosenthal, J. (1984). *Childhood psychosis in the first four years of life.* New York: McGraw Hill.

Menolascino, F. (1971). *Psychiatric aspects of the diagnosis and treatment of mental retardation.* Seattle: Special Child Publications.

Miller, D. (1977). The ethics of practice in adolescent psychiatry. *American Journal of Psychiatry, 134,* 420–424.

Minuchin, S., Baker, L., Rosman, B., Liebman, R., Milman, L., & Todd, T. (1975). A conceptual model of psychosomatic illness in children. *Archives of General Psychiatry, 32,* 1031–1038.

Offer, D. (1969). *The psychological world of the teenager.* New York: Basic Books.

Piaget, J., & Inhelder, B. (1969). *The psychology of the child.* New York: Basic Books.

Poznanski, E. O. (1986). Childhood depression. In C. Kelley (Ed.), *Practice of pediatrics,* revised edition. New York: Harper & Row, chapter 54.

Poznanski, E. O., & Zrull, J. R. (1970). Childhood depression. *Archives of General Psychiatry, 23,* 8–15.

Poznanski, E. O., & Zrull, J. P. (1976). Childhood depression: A longitudinal perspective. *JAACP, 15,* 491–501.

Poznanski, E. O., Carroll, B. J., Banegas, M. C., Cook, S. C., & Grossmann, J. A. (1982). The dexamethasone suppression test in prepubertal depressed children. *American Journal of Psychiatry, 139,* 321–324.

Preskorn, S. H., Weller, E. B., Weller, R. A., & Glotzbach, E. (1983). Plasma levels of imipramine and adverse effects in children. *American Journal of Psychiatry, 140,* 1332–1335.

Quay, H. C. (1985). Agression, conduct disorder and attention problems. In L. M. Bloomingdale (Ed.), *Attention deficit disorder: Identification, course and rationale.* New York: Spectrum.

Robbins, D. R., Alessi, N., Yanchyshyn, G., & Colfer, M. (1982). Preliminary report on the dexamethasone suppression test in adolescents. *American Journal of Psychiatry, 139,* 942–943.

Robertson, J., & Robertson, J. (1971). Young children in brief separations: A fresh look. In Eissler, R. S., Freud, A., Kris, M., Lustman, S. L., & Solnit, A. J. (Eds.) *Psychoanalytic study of the child,* Vol. 26. New York: Quadrangle Books.

Russo, D. C., & Newson, C. D. (1982). Psychotic disorders of childhood. In J. R. Lachenmeyer & M. S. Gibbs (Eds.), *Psychopathology in childhood.* New York: Gardner Press.

Seligman, M. (1975). *Helplessness; On depression, development and death*. San Francisco: W. H. Freeman.

Seligman, M., & Peterson, C. (1986). A learned helplessness perspective on childhood depression: theory and research. In M. Rutter, C. Izard, & P. Read (Eds.). *Depression in young people*. New York: Guilford Press, pp. 223–249.

Simmons, J. E. (1987). *Psychiatric examination of the child*, 4th ed. Philadelphia: Lea and Febiger.

Spitz, R. (1946). Anaclitic depression. *Psychoanalytical Study of the Child, 2*, 113–117.

Spitzer, R. L., & Williams, J. B. (1979). *DSM-III "Micro-D"*. DSM-III Field Trial Materials.

Spitzer, R. L., & Williams, J. B. W. (1980). *DSM-III classification: With annotations*. Roering/Pfizer Pamphlet. American Psychiatric Association, Washington, D. C.

Stern, D. N. (1985); *The interpersonal world of the infant— A view from psychoanalysis and developmental psychology*. New York: Basic Books.

Tanguay, P. E. (1984). Towards a new classification of serious psychopathology in children. *JAACP, 23*, 373–384.

Thomas, A., & Chess, S. (1977). *Temperament and development*. New York: Brunner/Mazel.

Watson, J. B., & Rayner, R. (1920). Conditioned emotional reactions. *Journal of Experimental Psychology, 3*, 1–14.

Weiss, G., & Hechtman, L. T. (1986). *Hyperactive children grow up*. New York: Guilford Press.

Weller, E. B., & Weller, R. A. (Eds.) (1984). *Current perspectives on major depressive disorders in children*. Washington, D.C.: American Psychiatric Association Press.

Wender, P. H., Wood, D., & Reimherr, F. (1984). Studies in attention deficit disorder—residual type (minimal brain dysfunction in adults). *Psychopharmacology Bulletin, 20*, 18–20.

Werry, J. S. (1985). ICD 9 and DSM-III classification for the clinician. *Journal of Child Psychology and Psychiatry, 26*, 1–6.

Work, H., (1979). Mental retardation. In J. L. Noshpitz (Ed.), *Basic handbook of child psychiatry*, Volume II. New York: Basic Books, p. 404.

Zahn-Waxler, C., McKnew, D., Cummings, E., Davenport, Y., & Radke-Yarrow, M. (1984). Problem behavior and peer interactions of young children with a manic-depressive parent. *American Journal of Psychiatry, 141*, 236–240.

23

PSYCHIATRIC MENTAL HEALTH NURSING WITH THE ELDERLY

LOIS GRAU

LEARNING OBJECTIVES

After studying this chapter, the student will be able to:

- Describe the different theories of aging.
- Recognize disorders specific to the elderly.
- Assess the elderly patient for mental disorders.
- Develop a nursing care plan for the elderly patient with a mental disorder.
- Identify community resources for the elderly patient with a mental disorder.

INTRODUCTION

The field of geriatric mental health, relative to other mental health specialty areas, is in its infancy. Its emergence as a rapidly growing area of research and clinical interest is the consequence of various factors, the most important of which is the aging of the population. The rapid growth in the number of elderly (people over age 65), both in the United States and throughout the world, has expanded knowledge of older people and the aging process. This knowledge reinforces the commonsense notion that older people are, in many ways, different from their younger counterparts. And it is these differences—biological, social, economic, and psychological—that justify the field of specialized research inquiry and clinical practice that has come to be known as **geriatric mental health.**

The role of nursing in geriatric mental health is multifaceted. The inclusion of geriatric/gerontological content in undergraduate, graduate, and continuing education curricula has resulted in rapid advancements in geriatric mental health nursing research and practice. However, despite these achievements, many important issues remain unresolved, such as distinguishing the normal aging process from disease, understanding the influence of cohort and ethnic background on the expression of illness, and untangling the interplay of physical and mental illness among the elderly. The delivery of mental health services to older persons is also of vital importance. Current health care policies and financing mechanisms limit the elderly's access to mental health services, with the result that they are underserved relative to other middle-class/nonminority groups.

These problems present challenges and opportunities for nurses, whether their interests lie in clinical practice, administration, research, or education. This chapter provides an overview of the elderly population with a focus on mental health and related issues.

Its purpose is to touch on a variety of topics—sociodemographic characteristics, theories of aging, sources of diversity within the geriatric population, and mental health service issues—that create the context for understanding the mental health needs of older persons. The chapter focuses on geriatric mental health problems and associated issues, including patient assessment and nursing interventions. (Detailed clinical information on specific types of psychiatric and organic disorders is provided in other chapters.)

THE AGING OF SOCIETY

During this century, the number and proportion of elderly persons in the world's population has increased dramatically. Never before in history have so many persons lived for so long. Between 1900 and 1980, the number of older persons in the U.S. increased eightfold, from 3.1 million to 26 million people. During this same time period, the proportion of the elderly rose from 4.1 percent to 11 percent of the population (Brody, 1984). The U.S. Bureau of the Census projects that in the year 2000, 13 percent of the population will be over age 65 and this figure will rise to 20 percent by the year 2025 (U.S. Bureau of the Census, 1984). (See Fig. 23–1.)

Older people are classified into three subgroups—the "young old," those between ages 65 and 75; the "middle old," those between ages 75 and 85; and the "old old," those over 85 years of age. The majority of the elderly, roughly 60 percent, are the "young old." Thirty percent of older people fall into the "middle old" category and the remaining 9 percent are 85 years of age or older. This latter group, the "old old," are increasing in number more rapidly than the "young old" persons. By the year 2020, it is projected that the "old old" will triple in

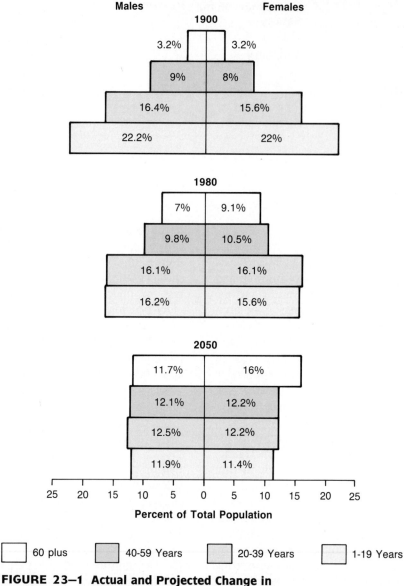

FIGURE 23–1 Actual and Projected Change in Population Distribution between 1950 and 2000.

Note: Projections are middle series. Source: From U.S. Bureau of the Census, 1982. Decennial census of population, 1900–1980 and projections of the population of the United States, 1982 to 2050, Current population reports, Series P-25, No. 922, U.S. Government Printing Office, Washington, D.C.

number to nearly 8.6 million persons, and will double again by the year 2040 (U.S. Bureau of the Census, 1984). This is important because the "old old" are more likely than the "young old" to be poor, widowed, and suffering from physical and mental illnesses and hence require significant amounts and types of health care.

WHO ARE THE ELDERLY?

Because women live, on average, seven years longer than men, they comprise the bulk of the elderly population. Sixty percent of all older persons, and 70 percent of those over age 85, are women. Slightly more than 50 percent of all older women are widowed.

Most older Americans—91 percent—are white. However, higher nonwhite fertility rates and more rapid gains in life expectancy among blacks has resulted in a more rapid growth among nonwhites than whites in the last decade (U.S. Senate Special Committee on Aging, 1984). Furthermore, it is anticipated that nonwhite persons will comprise 18 percent of the older population by 2050 (U.S. Senate Special Committee on Aging, 1985).

Currently, 50 percent of all older people are married and live with their spouses. Roughly 15 percent live with children or other relatives, and 2 percent with friends. However, 30 percent of the aged live alone: 41 percent of all older women, and 15 percent of elderly men (Cantor, 1986).

Although today's elderly are economically advantaged as compared to their predecessors, 13 percent fall below the poverty line. Women are more likely than men to be poor: women make up 60 percent of the elderly population but comprise 72 percent of the aged poor. Older women have lower incomes than older men; for example, in 1985 the average monthly social security benefit for women was $399 per month as compared to $521 for men (U.S. Dept. of Health & Human Services, 1985). Women are also disadvantaged by their minimal participation in job-related pension plans. Only 20 percent of elderly women receive pension benefits as compared to 43 percent of aged men, and those who do qualify receive only one-half the pension income of men (Congressional Clearinghouse of the Future, 1985). There are several reasons for this: women have traditionally been involved in lower paying jobs, women have had their careers interrupted because of child bearing, and pension benefits for widows are lower. For women, long-term planning for retirement is a relatively new way of thinking.

Minority membership increases the risk of poverty in old age. Blacks and Hispanics represent the poorest group of aged Americans. Thirty-six percent of aged blacks and 38 percent of elderly Hispanics lived in extreme poverty in 1982 (U.S. Congress, Senate Special Committee on Aging, 1983). Minority women fare even worse than all other aged persons. In 1981, 80 percent of black women (Women's Equity Action League, 1985) and 50 percent of Hispanic women lived in poverty (Berger, 1983).

Although most aged persons suffer from at least one chronic illness, the majority are independent with respect to carrying out routine activities of daily living. It has been estimated that 10 percent of the total elderly population are extremely impaired and dependent on the help of others. Of this group, only 37 percent reside in institutions (U.S. General Accounting Office, 1977). There are twice as many homebound or bedfast elderly persons (10 percent) in the community as these are in institutions (4–5 percent) (Shanas, 1977). Prevalence rates of mental disorder are higher in the elderly than in other populations. It has been estimated that 25 percent of the elderly who live in the community and more than 70 percent of those who live in institutions suffer from some type of mental disorder (Gurland, 1980).

This brief sociodemographic profile of older persons underscores the need for nursing and other human-service workers to direct their attention to the life circumstances of older persons. The poor, along with those on the edge of poverty, may not be able to afford needed care and services, particularly community services such as nursing and medical psychiatric care, long-term personal care, and household assistance, services that are only minimally covered or are excluded by Medicare. Life change events, such as widowhood, the death of friends, the onset of chronic physical illness, and subsequent limitations on mobility and social involvement, are risk factors for mental disorders thought to be stress-induced, such as some of the anxiety disorders. Because these events are associated with advancing chronological age, they are considered to be, in a statistical sense, "normal" age-related occurrences. As such, it is some-

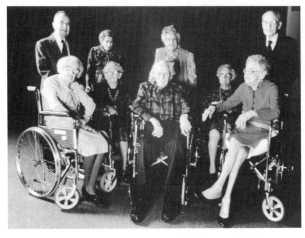

Experts believe that people who live long lives, like these centenarians, have habits like those that health groups advise us all to live by. In this country, women outlive men by approximately seven years, and consequently comprise the majority of older Americans in contemporary society.

times assumed that the death of a friend or the experience of a debilitating chronic illness is less stressful for older than for younger persons. This is not the case.

THEORIES OF AGING

Sociodemographic data provide a snapshot or cross-sectional view of some of the characteristics of today's elderly population. Although helpful for descriptive purposes, such data do not provide information about the dynamics of the aging process. Gerontologists and social scientists have attempted to understand what aging means to the individual and society through the development of a range of theories and theoretical frameworks. These formulations have in common the goal of explanation and prediction, but their focal points of interest vary widely. Some attempt to explain and predict attitudes and behaviors on the basis of their association with normal aging; others predict the individual's response to aging in terms of the individual's unique life history; others view older persons in terms of their relationship to the larger society and/or to cultural values and expectations. An overview of some of these views follows. The purpose is to provide examples of some of the approaches employed in an attempt to understand both the process of aging and the place of older persons in society.

DISENGAGEMENT THEORY AND ACTIVITY THEORY

Disengagement theory is one of the earliest and most influential theoretical approaches (Cumming & Henry, 1961). This theory states that aging entails an inevitable withdrawal of the individual from society, and of society from the individual, during the later years of life. The theory implies that older people gradually prepare, through various disengagement processes, for the final disengagement of death. Society "gains" because the withdrawal of older persons creates room for younger individuals to fill societal roles.

Disengagement theory has been sharply and persistently criticized. The presumed inevitability of disengagement and its positive functional consequences for both the individual and society have been questioned. Maddox (1964) has pointed out the importance of personality factors that make the individual more or less amenable to disengagement and the need to recognize these differences in theory devel-

opment. Others are concerned about the way in which disengagement theory might be used to justify public policies and social actions that limit access by the elderly to valued social roles and resources (for example, mandatory retirement based on the false belief that withdrawal from the work force is a "natural" concomitant of growing old).

A direct retort to disengagement theory is **activity theory,** formulated by Robert Havighurst (1963), which posits that the relationship between the individual and society in old age is little different than that during the younger, productive years of life. Middle-age social norms and expectations of involvement in work, family, and the community are carried into the later years and the behavior of older persons should be evaluated on the same terms as for younger individuals.

Like disengagement theory, activity theory assumes that older people are all similar in their response to the aging process. Personal preferences for social involvement based on individual ability and inclination are minimized. Activity theory has been criticized for its assumption that the societal roles of older persons differ little from those of younger persons. If taken literally, this assumption could be used to deny the need for structured alternatives to compensate for losses, both physical and social, that individuals experience as a part of the aging process.

Interest in the validity of disengagement theory versus activity theory has spawned a number of studies to test the effects of social participation on well-being. The findings of these studies are mixed. Some research demonstrates a positive relationship between activity and life satisfaction or morale (Havighurst & Albrecht, 1953; Graney, 1975); other studies indicate that mediating factors, such as health and socioeconomic status, are more important than social involvement (Bull & Aucoin, 1975). One study, undertaken by the authors of disengagement theory, found no relationship between social activity and well-being (Cumming & Henry, 1961). There is a range of potential explanations for these discrepancies. It may be that the use of different definitions and measures of social activity is a confounding variable. For example, some researchers have focused on social networks; that is, the number and configuration of social ties. Other studies have looked at both the quantity of social contacts and their quality as perceived by the individual. Still other studies were concerned with various types of social activity or contact.

Although disengagement and activity theory are based on opposite assumptions about the normal aging process, they are alike in their tendency to treat all older persons as having similar needs with respect to social involvement. More recent thinking emphasizes life-cycle and human-development approaches. They emphasize individual psychosocial processes and dynamics rather than the expression of specific types of behavior in old age.

CONTINUITY THEORY

Continuity theory emphasizes the uniqueness of the individual's response to the aging process, which is based on the complex interplay between biological, psychological, and social characteristics and experiences that result in certain habits, preferences, and activities which remain relatively stable over time (Cox, 1988). Hence, the extent to which older people relinquish social roles or maintain earlier levels of social involvement is an individual matter. When ill health or age-related losses result in the need for adaptation, individuals tend to maintain roles that were valued by society and themselves, and which conferred the greatest status, leaving behind those that held less personal importance.

Life-cycle theoretical orientations appear in sharp contrast to disengagement and activity theory. They represent a psychological approach in which the focus is on the individual, and the influence that personality, behavior, and experience have on the person's response to old age. This orientation underscores the nurse's traditional concern for individualizing patient care on the basis of ongoing individual patient assessment, which necessarily includes pertinent life history data. Disengagement and activity theory, in contrast, hypothesize that certain behaviors are "normal" because they are associated in a statistically significant way with positive outcomes such as high morale or well-being. When such theories are substantiated through valid and reliable studies, they provide important information about aging that can be used to guide, *in general only,* nursing care planning and intervention. Statistical data provide important information about predominant behaviors, beliefs, and attitudes that can serve as a useful guide for nurses. Still, the findings of even the most methodologically sound social science studies contain some degree of sampling error. As a result, while study findings can be generalized to the population from which the sample was drawn with a known degree of confidence, generalization to a specific individual is far more risky and should not be undertaken without relevant, substantiating patient information.

AGE-STRATIFICATION THEORY

Theories of individual and group behavior are complemented by sociological approaches that view older persons in terms of their social roles and societal expectations. **Age-stratification theory** conceptualizes society as comprised of strata based on age (Riley, Johnson & Foner, 1972). Persons of different ages have open to them different opportunities to engage in social roles. Age influences how persons are evaluated and treated by both their agemates and younger and older individuals. Theories such as age stratification have helped us understand why societies respond as they do to older people. For example, more traditional societies such as Japan and some developing countries usually accord high status to older persons because of their role as interpreters and translators of cultural tradition and wisdom. In societies such as our own, technical information collection and dissemination systems have taken over these functions. Cross-cultural comparisons can assist in identifying factors associated with age-related discrimination and, in turn, enhance social awareness.

THE ELDERLY AS A SUBCULTURAL GROUP

Theorists have also suggested that the elderly be viewed as a distinct subcultural group. This theoretical orientation is based on the belief that older persons, like minority group members, have interpersonal affinity among themselves and suffer from various forms of discrimination at the hands of majority members of society (Rose & Peterson, 1965). The problem of discrimination against older persons led Robert Butler (1969) to coin the term **ageism** as an analogue to racism in our society. Ageism refers to the tendency of society to stereotype all older people in negative terms that have little or no basis in reality. The findings of multiple studies attest to the reality of ageism. Both lay persons and health professionals have been found to perceive the elderly in negative terms; for example, as "stubborn," "touchy," and likely to "complain" and as "rigid," "irritable," and set in their ways (McTavish, 1971; Branco & Williamson, 1982). Ageism may influence the attitudes of health professionals toward geriatrics as a specialty field. Working with the elderly often involves facing one's own, sometimes frightening, feelings about aging, including:

1. thoughts about one's own age and inevitable death;

2. awakening of adult-child conflicts between the professional and the patient;

3. the feeling that despite treatment the elderly are likely to die (Poggi & Berland, 1985).

Although ample evidence attests to the negative stereotyping of older persons in our society, that they comprise a distinct subcultural group has been questioned on the basis that such a definition fails to recognize that the elderly themselves vary in ethnic, racial, and social class background and, hence, represent heterogeneous cultural traditions, ethos, and values. In addition, Streib (1968) notes that the aged do not represent an exclusive or permanent group. All persons will become elderly if they live long enough.

AGE, SOCIAL CLASS, AND COHORT

Although old age is considered to be age 65 and over, 65 is not a magic number that transforms middle-aged adults into old people overnight. The use of age 65 as an entry point into old age is an arbitrary marker, an artifact of early social welfare legislation. People over age 65 are not a homogeneous group, somehow made alike by virtue of age alone. Chronological age, in and of itself, differentiates subgroups of older persons. Because advancing age is associated with risk of illness and disability, the social roles and responsibilities of the "young old" are likely to differ

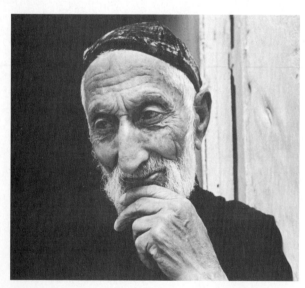

Older Americans are stereotypically clumped together as "senior citizens," and are often considered to be devoid of any cultural, ethnic, or social heritage.

from those who have reached more advanced years. It has become increasingly common for "young old" women to be responsible for the care of frail parents who are in their eighties or nineties. Despite the fact that both "old" children and their "old old" parents are entitled to the same age-categorical benefits, such as Medicare, it is likely that their health status and need for nursing and other health and social services will differ dramatically.

A second factor that differentiates among older persons is social class and ethnic membership. Social class influences life opportunities which, in turn, affect attitudes, expectations, and behavior in old age. Membership in a particular ethnic or racial group provides a subgroup identity on the basis of cultural values and traditions. Minority membership is generally associated with lower socioeconomic class membership and societal discrimination leading to limited access to societal resources. Aged members of minority groups have been described as being in "double jeopardy" (Talley & Kaplan, 1956) on the basis of poverty and discrimination, factors associated with higher morbidity and earlier mortality among the elderly. On the other hand, there is some evidence that minority elderly have the advantages of greater family support than their majority counterparts as a result of traditional extended family relationships (Jackson, 1980).

Lastly, the elderly are differentiated on the basis of their membership in a particular cohort group. Cohort membership is based on the year of birth and subsequent exposure to historical events throughout the life span. Typically, cohorts are defined in terms of generational membership with respect to major historical occurrences; for example, persons born into the post-World War II "baby boom" generation, or "children of the Depression." Today's "young old" population experienced World War II as young adults and were economically advantaged by postwar educational opportunities and economic expansion. In contrast, persons in their 80s experienced World War I as young children and entered adulthood during the Depression. These differences in the timing of exposure to historical events affect life opportunities and experiences, the results of which are carried into old age. The elderly of the future may differ significantly from their predecessors as a result of social and demographic changes. Tomorrow's elderly will probably be better off economically and educationally, will experience better health, be more socially and politically involved, and have higher expectations and greater self-respect.

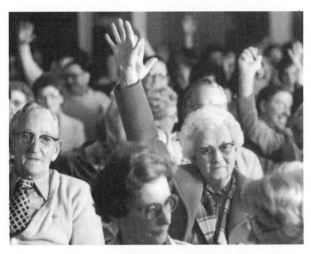

As the numbers of older Americans increase . . .

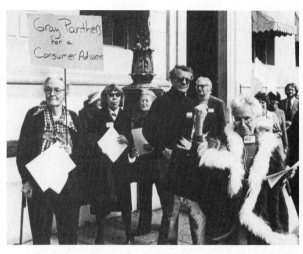

. . . so will their impact on various social and political institutions.

MENTAL HEALTH AND OLDER PERSONS

Recent research in geriatric mental health focuses on the prevalence, course, and treatment of specific organic and psychiatric disorders. Earlier studies of older persons focused on the more general concept of "life satisfaction" or "morale." This construct of life satisfaction, which rarely comes into play in the mental health literature of younger populations, reflects the long-standing emphasis in gerontology on various domains of quality of life. During the 1960s and 1970s, the elderly were often portrayed by society as disenfranchised citizens, abandoned by their families and society. This negative stereotype directed research interests toward the investigation of the well-being of older persons and the extent to which they were satisfied or dissatisfied with their current lives. Such studies were motivated by the relevance of life-satisfaction findings for public policy, as well as by interest in theoretical factors associated with subjective well-being.

Although the findings of these studies are not clear cut (because of problems of measurement such as the validity and reliability of measures of life satisfaction and the use of nonprobability samples), it appears that the most important factor associated with positive evaluations of life satisfaction is physical health (Cutler, 1972; Thompson, 1973; Palmore & Kivett, 1977). That health is associated with morale and life satisfaction is not surprising in view of the fact that most illnesses of older people are chronic and disabling, resulting in a loss of independence and in a continual decline toward death. Employment, income, housing arrangements, and marital status have also been studied for their relationship to life satisfaction, but their results are somewhat ambiguous. Most studies of retirees find that nonretired persons are more satisfied with their lives than retirees (Edwards & Klemmack, 1973; Thompson, 1973; Harris & Associates, 1975). Other research indicates that socioeconomic status is as important as employment status in accounting for life satisfaction; that is, when socioeconomic status is controlled for in the statistical analysis, the influence of employment disappears except among those in the lowest income groups (Chatfield, 1977). Also, the reasons for retirement, rather than retirement itself, may account for lower satisfaction. A study by Thompson (1973) concluded that retired persons had lower morale because they experienced poorer health, were more functionally impaired, poorer, and older than those who were still employed.

A major policy issue among the elderly, professionals, and legislators has been the role that age-segregated housing plays in the well-being of older persons. Age-segregated living arrangements, such as public housing projects, retirement villages, and age-segregated life-care communities, operate on the assumption that older people prefer to live among their own kind. However, this assumption has not been consistently supported in the findings of empirical studies. Some studies have found that persons in an age-segregated environment have high morale (Carp,

1967; Teaff et al. 1978), while others have found the opposite (Gubrium, 1978; Poorkaj, 1967). Older people vary in their preference for housing as they vary in other areas of life. Moreover, age composition is but one aspect of a living situation, and it may be less important than other factors such as physical location, affordability, and proximity to children and friends. Nor is it possible to generalize among different types of age-segregated arrangements. Residence in a luxury retirement community, with a golf course and pool, is a far cry from survival in a state or county institution.

Life-satisfaction research set the groundwork for identifying risk factors for low morale and dissatisfaction with life. More recent studies are epidemiological and use data-collection techniques (screening and diagnostic interviews) patterned after criteria specified in DSM-III-R.

SPECIFIC MENTAL DISORDERS AND MENTAL HEALTH PROBLEMS AMONG THE ELDERLY

Epidemiological studies of the general population consistently suggest that approximately 10 percent of all persons residing in a given community require some type of mental health care. This rate is higher among the elderly (Redick & Taub, 1980; Romaniuk, McAuley, & Arling, 1983). A review of associated studies by Finkel (1981) concludes that between 15 and 25 percent of the elderly display significant symptoms of mental illness.

DEPRESSION

Depression is a major problem for older persons. Roughly 13 percent of the elderly in a community evidence symptoms of depression (Gurland, Dean, Cross, & Golden 1980), and estimates suggest that between 21 and 54 percent of all elderly psychiatric patients are depressed (Peak, 1973; Vickers, 1976; Redick & Taub, 1980). However, the determination of the prevalence of depression is complicated by the use of different definitions and methods of assessment. Gurland (1976) notes that when psychiatrists define cases of depression, milder depressions have their greatest incidence between the ages of 35 and 45, while psychotic depressions manifest themselves for the first time most frequently among those between the ages of 55 and 65. After that age, depres-

sion becomes infrequent. On the other hand, when depression is assessed on the basis of survey instruments in community studies, the highest prevalence has been found among persons over age 65. But even community studies vary in their findings from prevalence rates of 30 percent to less than 5 percent because of the use of different assessment instruments and scoring procedures (Gianturco & Busse, 1978; Gurland & Toner, 1982). A recent community study by Blazer, Hughes, and George (1987) attempted to address this problem by assessing various subtypes of depressive disorders. They found that 8 percent of elderly persons living in the community suffered from various forms of severe or moderate depression. Nearly 19 percent had less severe dysphoric symptomatology. They point out that there are relatively large numbers of older persons in the community who suffer from clinically significant depressive symptoms who do not meet the DSM-III-R criteria for a major depressive episode or dysthmia.

BIOLOGICAL THEORY OF DEPRESSION. The catecholamine or indoleamine hypothesis of mood disorders asserts that many, if not all, depressions are linked to a deficiency in catecholamines or a change in their metabolism. A lack of either norepinephrine or serotonin at critical receptor sites is believed to be of major significance in depression (Zis & Goodwin, 1982; Lipton, DiMascio, & Killam, 1978). The following reports represent selected components of research attempting to confirm the catecholamine hypothesis in mood disorders among the elderly.

MHPG in Urine. 3-methoxy-4-hydroxyphenylglycol (MHPG) is a metabolite of norepinephrine found in the brain and the peripheral sympathetic nervous system. Research studies have found that MHPG in the urine is lower in depressed patients and higher in nondepressed and manic patients. When depressed patients received electroshock therapy, the MHPG levels normalized (Lipton, DiMascio, & Killam, 1978; Renner & Birren, 1980).

MHPG in the Cerebrospinal Fluid. MHPG levels in the lumbar cerebrospinal fluid among depressed patients is lower when compared to nondepressed and manic patients. These levels reflect norepinephrine metabolism that occurs in the brain and spinal cord (Lipton, DiMascio, & Killam, 1978; Renner & Birren, 1980).

Homovanillic Acid (HVA). Homovanillic acid is derived (metabolized) from dopamine and can be measured in the cerebrospinal fluid. Baseline HVA levels are often lower in depressed patients than in nondepressed patients.

Monoamine oxidase (MAO) platelet activity is considered to be lower in depressed patients than in patients with bipolar and other types of illnesses. Also, catechol-o-methyltransferase (COMT) in red blood cells and dopamine-beta-hydroxylase (DBH) serum activity tend to be reduced in depressed patients (Renner & Birren, 1980).

Indoleamines. Further research has examined the role of indoleamines in depression in the elderly. Levels of serotonin (found in the midbrain, hypothalamus, and the limbic system) have been found by some to be reduced.

This has supported the administration of tryptophan to patients to increase brain serotonin. It is well established that tricyclic antidepressants act on both serotonin and norepinephrine in the brain.

It is believed that serotonin is involved in sleep, eating, sex behaviors, and psychomotor activity. It is also assumed that serotonin deficits can be corrected to relieve the depression experienced by older people. Whether or not the effective antidepressant drugs correct deficits in serotonin or norepinephrine is not currently known.

Taken together, these findings are suggestive of central nervous system pathology in the mood disorder. These hypotheses are in need of further scientific explanation but have promise for advancing the understanding of neurochemistry of the central nervous system and its relationship to depression in the elderly (Lipton, DiMascio, & Killam, 1978; Renner & Birren, 1980; Schoonover, 1983).

PSYCHOANALYTIC THEORY OF DEPRESSION. When applying the psychoanalytic model in explaining depression among the elderly, one needs to consider that depression frequently develops within a few months after a real or perceived object loss. These losses can be numerous: death of a loved one; separation from family and friends; retirement and loss of job and companionship; gradual loss of health and diminished bodily functions; and so forth (Engel, 1962; Zung, 1980).

Eric Erikson (1950) developed the terms ego integrity versus despair to describe the developmental stage of old age. With integrity, the individual can examine his life and determine that it has been satisfying, useful, and goal attaining and has provided the type of recognition and status that one desires. However, if one's goals and aspirations have not been realized, one may experience despair, anxiety, depression, bitterness, and so forth (Erikson, 1950; Birren & Renner, 1980).

The ideal self (a part of the superego structure) can indeed be punitive to the ego if one has conflicts with what should have been and what, in reality, was (Birren & Renner, 1980; Erikson, 1950). As unresolved conflicts surface, they can be identified and addressed through psychoanalytically oriented individual, group, and family therapies.

BEHAVIORAL THEORY OF DEPRESSION. The depressed elderly person can be in an untenable situation; failing health, numerous losses, and so forth can lead to the development of a perception that their situation is uncontrollable. Learned helplessness is frequently a response to this plight. However, social support and social interactions are important in reinforcing self-care skills. For example, self-care can, in some instances, be maintained in older people if there are others in the environment who reinforce specific habits, beliefs, and behaviors (Davis, 1986; Dolphin, 1986).

The reinforcement of self-care skills, independence, interpersonal relationships, close family contacts, and so forth, can facilitate longevity in the community and avoid institutionalization (Gaitz & Varner, 1980; Greenblatt & Chein, 1983).

The cumulative-losses concept suggests that a person begins to experience losses in midlife; the frequencies of losses continue into old age where they increase (Gaitz & Varner, 1980). The cumulative effect of these losses results in a tremendous decrease in positive reinforcement that leads to sadness and depression. Positive-reinforcement methods, in the form of token economy programs where positive behaviors are rewarded, have revealed some success in the treatment of the elderly (Ullman & Krasner, 1965).

In summary, Wang (1977) purports that there is a dynamic interplay among the biological, psychological, and environmental systems which interact and help to intensify the effects of each loss that the individual experiences during the latter years.

DEMENTIA

Estimates of the prevalence of **dementia** among elderly in the United States range from 2 percent to nearly 7 percent (Cross & Gurland, n.d.). Epidemiological studies in Europe have similar findings, with prevalence rates varying from 1 percent to 8 percent. The range in figures is due to differences in the type of assessment instruments used and the populations studied. For example, some studies do not include persons in institutions such as nursing homes. Because more than 50 percent of nursing home residents and two-thirds of patients in state and county mental hospitals have a diagnosis of "senility" or "chronic organic brain syndrome" (Milazzo-Sayre, 1978; Meyer, 1977), their inclusion in or deletion from samples is important.

Alzheimer's disease and related disorders account for roughly 50 percent of all dementias among the elderly, followed by multi-infarct dementia, which is estimated to represent between 13 and 50 percent of cases of dementia (Cross & Gurland, n.d.).

The risk of dementia increases with age. About 1 percent of those between the ages of 65 and 74 suffer from dementia. This figure increases to 7 percent for those between age 75 and 85, and to 25 percent for persons over age 85. If these age-specific rates remain unchanged, the growth in the number of older persons will result in a fourfold increase in cases of dementia by the year 2040 (Cross & Gurland, n.d.).

ACUTE CONFUSIONAL STATES

Acute confusional states occur in approximately 30 to 50 percent of hospitalized elderly patients (Foreman, 1984). Despite this high prevalence, relatively little is known about this disorder.

This form of organic brain dysfunction is characterized by abrupt onset and is of relatively brief duration. The individual experiences numerous psychobiological disturbances involving sleep-wake cycle, psychomotor behaviors, emotional responses, and attention span (Foreman, 1984). The disorder occurs more frequently among elderly hospitalized patients than among younger patients. Older persons may be more vulnerable to these states due to altered physiology, the presence of chronic physical illness and sensory impairments, depression, malnutrition, or polypharmacy.

SUNDOWN SYNDROME

Sundown syndrome among the elderly is another condition about which relatively little is known. It tends to occur among the institutionalized elderly and its symptoms are similar to acute confusional states—disordered cognition, disturbed sleep-wake cycle, and disturbed psychomotor behavior. However, the symptoms of sundown syndrome tend to be exacerbated during the late day or evening hours and it tends to be a long-term rather than a self-limiting problem (Evans, 1987).

Little is known about the cause of the disorder. One study found that persons affected by sundown syndrome were more likely than others to suffer from dementia, to have fewer prescribed therapeutic activities, to be socially isolated, and to have experienced some type of major stress or life change in the recent past (Evans, 1987).

SUICIDE

Suicide is a serious problem among the elderly, particularly men. At younger ages the ratio of successful suicides to attempts is 1:10; among the elderly, this ratio is reversed (National Center for Health Statistics, 1985). Older persons make few suicidal "gestures"; they seek fatal outcomes. White males are at highest risk and this risk increases with age (Gurland, et al., 1980). Other high-risk groups include widows, persons who have experienced recent losses, those with terminal physical illnesses and intractable pain, and individuals who have undergone status changes such as retirement.

In 1980, suicide rates were 11.9 per 100,000 for the nation as a whole; 12.3 per 100,000 for persons between the ages of 15 and 24; and 17.7 per 100,000 for persons over 65 (Gurland et al., 1980; Templer & Cappelletty, 1986). Despite this high rate, suicides among the elderly have actually decreased in recent decades, although why this is the case is not clear. The presence of an increasing proportion of women in the elderly population may be responsible because women are at lower risk of suicide then men at all ages (Manton, Blazer, & Woodbury, 1987). The improved economic status of older men may also be a factor.

ELDER ABUSE

Elder abuse, although not a mental disorder itself, has mental health implications for both its victims and its perpetrators. "Granny bashing," as it is called in England, has increased in prevalence with the aging of the population. Like child abuse, the problem is not one of the individual but of the family unit in which the older person lives.

The elderly who experience abuse are likely to be dependent women, over age 75, who have physical and/or mental limitations. In most instances, abuse of the elderly includes: neglect (74 percent), physical abuse (15 percent), exploitation (10 percent), and abandonment (3 percent) (Pagelow, 1984). Pagelow also points out that this abuse is not necessarily deliberate, but can be a result of extreme frustration, fatigue, stress, and the responsibility of daily care for these frail and vulnerable individuals.

The public attention and concern given to the problem of elder abuse has not been matched by methodologically sound investigations of the problem (Kosberg, 1983). A clear picture is blurred by the fact that researchers define elder abuse in different ways. For example, Lau and Kosberg (1979) found that 9.6 percent of admissions to a chronic care facility were defined as abuse cases, with 74 percent of the group evidencing signs of physical abuse and neglect. Psychological and material abuse and violation of rights were less common. Another evaluation of case study data from state social and legal welfare agencies in Maryland defined abuse in terms of physical, psychological, material, and neglect (Block & Sinnott, 1979). The prevalence of abuse was far lower than in the Kosberg study, and psychological abuse prevailed over the other types.

Although study findings are difficult to compare and interpret, abuse seems to occur more frequently to elderly women who are physically or mentally frail, who live with relatives, and who are dependent on them to meet their daily needs. Also, one incident of abuse tends to lead to others, and one type of abuse is often followed by another type (Zdorkowski & Galbraith, 1985). Study findings suggest that a significant number of abusers are themselves elderly (Walker, 1985). However, abuse and neglect appear to stop when the caregiving burden is reduced by the introduction of formal services. This suggests that, in many cases, elder abuse is a symptom of family stress and strain.

The nurse can intervene by assessing the degree of stress that the family experiences when providing care to the elderly. The nurse should be alert to: 1) limited financial resources available for care; 2) the type of relationship that the adult child has with the elderly parent (patient); 3) the type of communication used and its effectiveness; 4) the type of expectations the caregiver has about the elderly person; 5) the degree of knowledge the caregiver possesses about illness, disabilities, outcome, and so forth; and 6) the type of coping mechanisms available to the caretaker.

The nurse is in a unique position to provide support, health information, referrals, and demonstrations of specific skills and to facilitate effective coping strategies (Hirst & Miller, 1986).

PSYCHIATRIC MENTAL HEALTH NURSING CARE OF THE ELDERLY

Although older persons are like younger adults in many ways, they are more likely to experience certain kinds of disorders such as dementia, to face age-related stressful events such as widowhood, and to contend with debilitating and chronic physical illness. In addition, older persons may express mental disorders in terms that are somewhat different from younger persons. Hence nursing assessment, diagnosis and intervention raise issues that, while important in the nursing care of all age groups, take on particular significance for the elderly.

NURSING ASSESSMENT

Nursing assessment of the elderly patient is complex. Like assessment of other types of patients, it includes a health and social history, plus data on current physical, mental health, and socioenvironmental status. Older persons frequently suffer from multiple health problems, are at risk for age-related stressful events, and bring into the clinical situation their own unique fears, hopes, and expectations based on more than six decades of life experiences. A limited assessment consisting of, for example, only mental status, can result in inappropriate problem identification and plans for nursing care. While this would be the case in any assessment, it's even more of a problem with the elderly because of the impact of long life on current health needs and expectations. The patient's needs and expectations can only be understood in the context of his past and current life situation (see Box 23–1).

A number of areas are particularly problematic with respect to nursing assessment of older persons. These are summarized below to underscore potential pitfalls in the assessment process. The next section gives descriptions of some of the more common mental disorders of the elderly and associated assessment issues.

DIFFERENTIATING NORMAL FROM ABNORMAL PROCESSES OF AGING. Distinctions between normal age-related biophysiological changes and pathological processes have been made in some

Box 23–1 ●
Communicating With Older Adults

Barriers to Communication with Older Adults

Barriers in Older Adults

- Sensory impairments
- Physical discomfort (e.g., pain, thirst, hunger)
- Effects of medications or pathological conditions
- Impaired psychosocial functioning secondary to dementia or depression
- Diminished contact with reality

Barriers in the Interview Atmosphere

- Environmental noise and distractions
- Too much information at one time
- Too many people involved in the interview
- Cultural differences
- Language differences
- Prejudices and stereotypes

Barriers in the Interviewer

- Insensitivity
- Poor listening skills
- Trite remarks
- False reassurance
- Judgmental attitudes
- Use of inappropriate or unacceptable names
- Inarticulate speech
- Obstructive mannerisms

Techniques to Enhance Communication with Older Adults

Verbal and Nonverbal Communication

- Begin contacts with an exchange of names and a handshake.
- Use touch purposefully to reinforce verbal messages and as a primary method of nonverbal communication.
- Explain the purpose of the interview in relation to a nursing goal.
- Begin with questions about more remote, less threatening topics.
- Use open-ended questions, and learn to use silence effectively and comfortably.
- Periodically clarify the messages.
- Maintain good eye contact, use attentive listening, and encourage the person to elaborate on information.
- Remain nonjudgmental in responses, but show appropriate empathy.
- Ask the formal mental status questions, or the most threatening questions, toward the end of the interview.
- Gain the person's permission before asking formal assessment questions regarding memory and other cognitive abilities.

The Interview Environment

- Sit in a face-to-face position.
- Ensure as much privacy as possible.
- Provide good lighting, and avoid background glare.
- Eliminate as much background noise as possible.

Source: Miller, C. A. (1990). *Nursing care of older adults: Theory and Practice.* Glenview, IL: Scott, Foresman, pp. 128, 133.

---

areas but remain problematic in others. For example, until fairly recently, senility was viewed as part of the normal process of growing old. Today the organic basis of dementia is recognized, despite the fact that its etiology remains uncertain.

Manifestations of aging have been defined as biological processes that are time related, irreversible, and deleterious. Illness, on the other hand, is assumed to be time related, deleterious, but possibly reversible (Chebotareu, 1979). It is clear this distinction is not satisfactory. Dementia, for example, is time related, irreversible, and deleterious but is not a normal part of aging. Nor does this definition apply to other chronic and irreversible conditions. Hence, biological definitions are not, at least at present, satisfactory.

From the perspective of nursing assessment, it is more helpful to focus on the severity and characteristics of symptoms and the broader biological and psychosocial context in which they occur. Data on the onset of occurrence, history of past episodes, and the frequency and severity of current symptoms should be assessed along with data on medication usage and social history.

DIFFERENTIATING PHYSICAL FROM MENTAL DISORDERS. A critical dimension of assessment is the accurate determination of the primary source of pathological symptoms. Depression is frequently expressed through somatic symptoms rather than through self-reports of mood disturbances such as dysphoria. In such situations, symptoms can be attributed inaccurately to physical illness or to hypochondriasis leading to inadequate problem identification and intervention.

Conversely, physical problems such as hearing loss can result in pseudoschizoid symptoms of paranoid behavior because of the individual's misconstruction of reality due to limited sensory input. Metabolic disturbances can create symptoms of pseudodementia, such as confusion, withdrawal, and memory loss.

It is also important to recognize the possibility that physical and mental disorders may *coexist*. The majority of older persons suffer from at least one chronic physical illness. Too often, attention is directed exclusively at minimizing or controlling physical symptoms and disability, ignoring the possibility of a coexisting depression or other treatable psychological disturbances (see Table 23–1).

DIFFERENTIATING ACUTE FROM CHRONIC MENTAL DISORDERS. Because the manifestations of psychotic disorders, transitory abnormal states, and organic brain disorders can be similar, it is easy to confuse one for the other. For example, the transitory confusional states experienced by many elderly hospitalized patients may mimic the symptoms of cognitive impairment associated with dementia. Likewise, depressive symptoms can include diminished cognitive ability, falsely suggesting an organic brain disorder (see Table 23–1).

ASSESSMENT OF DEMENTIA

DSM-III (American Psychiatric Association, 1987) describes Alzheimer's disease as consisting of three

TABLE 23–1 Normal physical and cognitive effects of human aging

1. Decreased basal metabolic rate
2. Reduced oxygen uptake in the brain due to insufficient cerebral circulation
3. Reduced visual acuity
4. Reduced auditory acuity, especially for higher frequencies
5. Decreased sensitivity to taste and smell
6. Decreased sensitivity to pain and vibration
7. Increased susceptibility to changes in temperature
8. Digestive problems, including difficulties in elimination, as well as upper gastrointestinal tract symptoms
9. Increased decay and loss of teeth
10. Loss or graying of hair
11. Drying, thinning, and wrinkling of skin, increased pigmentation and loss of skin turgor
12. Loss of muscle tone and atrophic changes in muscle
13. Skeletal changes due to osteoporosis
14. Decreased kidney function
15. Decreased cardiac output
16. Loss of elasticity of connective tissue
17. Loss of neurons within the central nervous system

Source: Berezin, M.A. & Stotsky B.A. (1970). The geriatric patient. In H. Grunebazem (Ed.), *The practice of community mental health*. Boston: Little, Brown.

components: 1) memory and other cognitive impairment; 2) functional and structural impairment of the brain; and 3) behavioral manifestations that affect the ability for self-care, interpersonal relationships, and life in the community. As of yet, there are no diagnostic tests specific to Alzheimer's disease and related dementias. The existence of the disease can only be determined definitively on the basis of autopsy or biopsy of large numbers of neurofibrillary tangles and senile plaques in the cerebral cortex of clinically demented individuals (U.S.D.H.H.S., 1984). Hence, clinical diagnosis is based on the elimination of other known causes of cognitive impairment based on the patient's history, physical assessment, neurological and psychiatric evaluations, mental-status examinations and psychometric tests, as well as by laboratory studies and computerized axial tomography (CT).

Early symptoms of Alzheimer's disease include short-term memory loss, such as forgetting familiar names or where objects were placed. However, the clinical interview may fail to reveal objective evidence of memory impairment. As the disease progresses, the patient encounters problems with retaining information and recalling recent events. The individual is unable to recall the *context* of forgotten events so cues that normally trigger recall fail to work. Memory loss is accompanied by a decline in the performance of routine activities, accompanied by social withdrawal, loss of initiative, impaired judgment, and inappropriate social behavior.

Eventually, the patient is no longer able to live without assistance in activities such as bathing and dressing, although toileting and eating often remain intact. The latter stage of the disease is characterized by a lack of awareness of time and place, the inability to recognize family members and friends, and personality and emotional changes (including delusional, paranoid, and obsessive behavior and agitation). Finally, the patient loses most communication skills, is incontinent, and requires total assistance in personal care.

Possibly the two most difficult problems associated with the assessment of Alzheimer's disease are distinguishing between Alzheimer's and normal benign senescence, and distinguishing Alzheimer's from other types of dementia and pseudodementias.

Diagnosis is particularly difficult during the early stage of the disease because symptoms of memory loss may mimic the benign loss associated with normal senescent forgetfulness (U.S.D.H.H.S., 1984). The publicity accorded to Alzheimer's disease and its progressive tragic course have created the fear in many elderly that they have it or will become its victims. As a result, they may focus on situations of short-term memory failure, exaggerating its severity and frequency of occurrence. Assessment of the onset, type, context, and frequency of memory loss can aid in diagnosis. The memory loss associated with Alzheimer's disease tends to be gradual in onset and progression, and the individual has difficulty recalling forgotten events even with prompting. The use of psychometric tests, coupled with clinical evidence of cognitive impairment, may be instructive, but not indicative, of the presence of organic brain disease. In brief, the diagnosis of the disease in its early stages can never be made with complete certainty.

Another critical issue is distinguishing Alzheimer's disease and related disorders from other organic dementias and from psuedodementia. Multiinfarct or arteriosclerotic dementia is the result of small strokes that cumulatively lead to progressive dementia. Whereas the symptoms of Alzheimer's disease tend to have a gradual onset and generally progress slowly, arteriosclerotic dementia is characterized by an abrupt onset, sudden deterioration with stable intervals between, emotional lability, and evidence of ateriosclerotic disease. The distinction between Alzheimer's disease and multiinfarct dementia is important because the causes of the latter are similar to those for major strokes (hypertension, high blood cholesterol, obesity, and smoking) and may be ameliorated by preventive measures.

Global cognitive impairment may be the result of self-limiting or treatable disorders such as depressive psuedodementia and acute confusional states or deliria (Kral, 1962). The term **pseudodementia** has been applied to elderly persons who complain both of depression and of memory and other cognitive problems. It has been estimated by Post (1962) that between 7 and 19 percent of dementias are, in fact, pseudodementias. However, Post points out that it is difficult to determine whether memory deficits are concomitants of depression, or whether depression occurs as a result of memory loss in the early stages of organic dementia. This problem is complicated by the fact that psychomotor slowing or agitation, labile affect, decreased libido, constipation, and paranoid ideation may be features common to both depression and organic brain syndrome (Zung & Green, 1972). However, other symptoms appear to differ between the two disorders. Symptoms of depression usually occur with a clearly defined onset and without progressive deterioration, while patients with dementia are characterized by an insidious onset with progressive failure at work and in routine activities. Depressed patients have difficulty concentrating, learning new information, and remembering recent events while demented patients have decreased attention, engage in confabulation and perseverate. (See Table 23–2, Box 23–2.) Still, there is some evidence that depressed patients usually perform better on memory tests than those who are demented; however, depressed patients complain more than their demented counterparts about memory problems (Miller, 1980). For a further discussion of assessment of dementia, see Chapter 11.

Problems of differential diagnosis between organic brain dementia and other nonorganic problems are attested to by the fact that somewhere between 10 and 20 percent of cases diagnosed as dementia actually represent other, treatable conditions such as hyperthyroidism, depression, or untoward drug reactions (Gurland et al. 1980). This problem is crucial because misdiagnosis can lead to unnecessary despair and anguish for the patient and his family. In addi-

TABLE 23–2 Differential diagnosis between dementia and depression

Dementia	Depression
1. AFFECT: Labile, fluctuating from tears to laughter, not consistent or sustained; may show apathy, depression, irritability, euphoria, or inappropriate affect. Normal control impaired, can be influenced by suggestions.	1. Depressed, feelings of despair which are pervasive, persistent. Anxious, hypomanic. Affect not influenced by suggestion.
2. MEMORY Decreased attention. Decreased for recent events. Confabulation. Perseveration.	2. Difficulty in concentration. Impaired learning of new knowledge. Decreased attention, with secondary decrease in recent memory.
3. INTELLECT: Impaired, decreased, as tested by: serial 7's, similarities, recent events.	3. Impaired, but can perform serial 7's, remember recent events.
4. ORIENTATION: Fluctuating with varying levels of awareness. May be disoriented for time, place.	4. May have some confusion, not as profound as in dementia.
5. JUDGMENT: Poor judgment with inappropriate behavior, dress. Deterioration of personal habits, and personal hygiene. Loss of bladder and bowel control.	5. May be poor.
6. SOMATIC COMPLAINTS: Fatigue. Failing health complaints, with vague complaints of pain in head, neck, back.	6. Typical complaints as: decreased sleep decreased appetite decreased weight decreased libido decreased energy constipation.
7. PSYCHOTIC BEHAVIOR: Mainly visual, hallucinations, delusions.	7. May occur in psychotic depressions, with mainly auditory hallucination; delusions.
8. NEUROLOGICAL SYMPTOMS: Dysphasia, apraxia, agnosia.	8. Not present.

Source: Zung, W. (1980). Affective disorders. In E. Busse and D. Blazer (Eds.), *Handbook of geriatric psychiatry*. New York: Van Nostrand Reinhold, p. 357.

tion, the irreversible and progressive nature of dementia can result in labeling patients as "untreatable" when, in fact, treatment may result in cure or improvement.

Nursing assessment can contribute to diagnostic accuracy by providing in-depth information on patterns of a patient's behavior and stability over time. In addition to assessing subjective complaints of cognitive impairment, it is important to assess the patient's functional status through evaluation of his ability to perform the activities of daily living (ADL) such as bathing, dressing, and preparing meals, as well as instrumental activities of daily living (IADL), for example, shopping, cooking, and household chores. The identification of changes in functional status over time, and factors that may be associated with such changes (for example, physical illness, exacerbation of a chronic illness, changes in living environment, or some type of personal loss) provide important information about symptom progression and disease etiology.

The nurse collects assessment data from the patient and, when possible, from the "primary family caregiver" (the family member who has assumed the

Box 23–2 • Terms Used to Describe Neurological Deficits

Agnosia: Inability to recognize objects.

Aphasia: Loss of a previously possessed ability to comprehend or use words.

Apraxia: Loss of previously possessed ability to perform skilled motor tasks; often seen with parietal lobe damage.

Confabulation: Spontaneous and unconscious fabrication of stories in response to questions about experiences that cannot be recalled, in order to hide memory loss.

Dysphasia: A form of aphasia which involves difficulty understanding language.

Perseveration: Tendency to talk about the same things over and over again or use one word to the exclusion of all others.

greatest responsibility for the care and well-being of the patient). Patients who are in the early stages of dementia often compensate for cognitive impairment by employing firmly entrenched social skills, such as table manners or common courtesies, that smooth over or detract from memory slips or inappropriate remarks. Family members are often aware of such compensatory behavior and other behavioral changes; thus their participation in the assessment process is invaluable.

ASSESSMENT OF DEPRESSION

Depression is characterized by a persistently **dysphoric** or sad mood with loss of pleasure in usual pastimes (see Chapter 9 on mood disorders). The symptoms are physical as well as behavioral and emotional, and might include appetite and weight changes, and sleep disturbances. Frequently, the individual will complain of limited energy and hampered ability to think and concentrate. Suicidal ideation, gestures, and attempts might also be present (American Psychiatric Association, 1987). Depression among older persons may not always include dysphoria as it does in younger patients. Epstein (1976) found that older depressed patients are more likely to experience apathy, listlessness, and self-deprecation than younger depressed persons. Worry, feelings of uselessness, sadness, pessimism, fatigue, inability to sleep, and volitional difficulties also tend to be somewhat more common among older patients (Blazer, 1982).

Another important difference is the tendency of the elderly depressed patient to express his symptoms in somatic, rather than psychological, terms (Blumen-

thal, 1975a, 1980b; Card & Judge, 1974; Goldstein, 1979; Auso-Gutierrez, 1983; Pfeiffer & Busse, 1973; Klerman, 1983), and to deny the existence of dysphoria or sadness, the linchpin of DSM-III-R criteria. Common somatic complaints include constipation, insomnia, anorexia, fatigue, and decrease in libido (Pfeiffer, 1970). Despite the denial of psychological symptoms, these individuals are as likely as those with psychological complaints to respond to treatment.

The elderly person's preoccupation with his body (somatization)—appetite, bowel movements, sleep, etc.—can result in the health care professional's pursuing organicity rather than asking about mood, recent losses, history of depression, etc. This situation, a common one, has lead some gero-psychiatrists (Fogel & Fretwell, 1985) to suggest that a new subtype of geriatric depression be included in the DSM-III-R classification system in order to prevent inappropriate health-service utilization (Waxman, Carner, & Blum, 1983), diagnostic uncertainties (Salzman & Shader, 1979), and misdiagnosis by primary care physicians (Levin, 1965; Fogel & Fretwell, 1985). Not surprisingly, somatization can also result in erroneous problem identification for the elderly among nurses if somatic symptoms are always assumed to be the result of physical illness. Differential diagnosis is a complex problem with which the nurse and physician must grapple.

It is important to note that work in cross-cultural psychiatric epidemiology indicates that an organic focus has been found to be the most prevalent symptomatic expression of depression among adults in most non-Western countries (Kleinman & Kleinman, 1985; Marsella, 1980). Also, adults in developed countries who are of a lower socioeconomic class, reside in rural areas, or maintain traditional religious or ethnic lifestyles are more likely to somatize than their more affluent counterparts (Kleinman & Good, 1985). This aside is made to underscore the importance that membership in a particular socioeconomic and ethnic group may have on the ways in which mental disorders are manifested.

In addition to being sensitive to depression that is manifested somatically, the nurse must also be sensitive to the fact that depression can accompany physical disorders. For example, the early stages of dementia are associated with depression. Persons with Parkinson's disease are also vulnerable to depression, although it is not known whether this is a reaction to disability or biochemically related to the disease process itself (Assnis, 1977). Endocrine disorders also place the individual at high risk for depression; hypothyroidism is particularly notable, with an 80 percent incidence of depression (Addington & Fry, 1986).

Because physical illness can trigger depressive reactions among the elderly (Pfeiffer, 1970), Verwoerdt (1981) contends that the magnitude of the depressive response is associated with the severity, rate of progression, and duration of the illness. Some conditions likely to result in depressive reactions include cardiovascular disease and cancer, as well as vision and hearing losses.

Lastly, certain medications can aggravate preexisting depression or trigger depressive-like symptoms such as sedation, apathy, and lethargy (Blazer, 1982). These medications include digitalis, antihypertensives, antiparkinson drugs, and anticancer drugs (Brody, 1985).

The assessment of depression is complex and difficult because its manifestations may mimic those of physical illness and dementia or it may coexist with these disorders. The recognition of the potential for the coexistence of and interaction among social, physical, psychological, and organic brain problems is crucial to assessment. Health and functional status are often influenced by multiple factors so that the assignment of cause and effect is difficult and sometimes even impossible. One approach to the problem of accurate identification and diagnosis is the use of multidisciplinary assessment teams that ideally include nurses, psychologists, physicians, geriatric psychiatrists and social workers. This approach increases the opportunity to identify contributing factors and to develop an integrated plan of care with the patient and his family (see Table 23–3). For more discussion of the assessment of depression, see Chapter 9 on mood disorders.

NURSING INTERVENTIONS FOR THE ELDERLY

The psychotherapeutic and psychopharmacological interventions developed for the treatment of younger persons serve as the basis for psychiatric mental health care of the elderly. However, many treatment modalities have required modification in response to the unique biophysiological and psychosocial needs of older persons. Some important aspects of intervention are described below.

1. *The use of psychopharmacological agents.* The presence of chronic or multi-system pathology, in addition to organic brain or functional psychiatric disorder, requires lower or modified doses of many medications. Effectiveness and manifestations of side effects may vary due to dysfunction of the cardiovascular, gastrointestinal, or endocrine and/or central nervous system.

2. *Modified psychotherapeutic approaches.* Although traditional psychotherapeutic approaches are efficacious for many older persons, modified approaches may be required in the treatment of depressive illness depending on the patient's cognitive and physical status. In addition, nursing interventions have been developed to respond to specific cognitive, psychological, and behavioral problems of the **mentally frail elderly,** usually, but not always, those elderly over the age of 75, who because of the accumulation of various continuing problems often require one or several supportive services in order to cope with daily life. Factors such as ethnicity (Black, American Indian, Hispanic) and gender (female) may increase a person's likelihood of becoming frail (Perlmutter & Hall, 1985; Butler & Lewis, 1982). This population is the fastest growing segment of our society; it is also considered the most vulnerable to physical and mental illness (Butler & Lewis, 1982; Perlmutter & Hall, 1985).

3. *Environment interventions.* A range of interventions designed to modify both the physical and interpersonal environments of the mentally frail elderly have been, and are continuing to be, developed. They include modification of the physical environment and control of level of sensory stimuli.

4. *The involvement of family members and significant others.* An important dimension of gero-psychiatric mental health nursing is its focus on the patient/family system as the primary unit of care. Despite myths to the contrary, the elderly are not always abandoned by their families. In fact, families provide more than 70 percent of all the care received by older persons (Brody, 1985). This is underscored by the fact that,

TABLE 23—3 Short psychiatric evaluation schedule

Please answer the following questions *Yes* or *No* as they apply to you now. Do not skip any questions. Occasionally a question may not seem to apply to you, but please *circle* either Yes or No, whichever is more nearly correct for you. (No = 0, Yes = 1)

1. Do you wake up fresh and rested most mornings?	yes	no
2. Is your daily life full of things that keep you interested?	yes	no
3. Have you, at times, very much wanted to leave home?	yes	no
4. Does it seem that no one understands you?	yes	no
5. Have you had periods of days, weeks or months when you couldn't take care of things because you couldn't "get going?"	yes	no
6. Is your sleep fitful and disturbed?	yes	no
7. Are you happy most of the time?	yes	no
8. Are you being plotted against?	yes	no
9. Do you certainly feel useless at times?	yes	no
10. During the past few years, have you been well most of the time?	yes	no
11. Do you feel weak all over much of the time?	yes	no
12. Are you troubled by headaches?	yes	no
13. Have you had difficulty in keeping your balance in walking?	yes	no
14. Are you troubled by your heart pounding and by a shortness of breath?	yes	no
15. Even when you are with people, do you feel lonely much of the time?	yes	no
TOTAL SCORE		

To Be Completed by Interviewer

Patient's Name:_____Date_____

      Sex: 1. Male   Race: 1. White
          2. Female   2. Black
                    3. Other

Years of Education:_____1. Grade School
                          2. High School
                          3. Beyond High School

Interviewer's Name: _____

Source: Pfeiffer, E. (1980). The psychosocial evaluation of the elderly patient. In Busse, E., & Blazer, D. (Eds.) (1980) *Handbook of geriatric psychiatry*. New York: Van Nostrand Reinhold Co., p. 280.

for every disabled older person who lives in a nursing home, two or more equally impaired elderly live with and are cared for by family members. An even greater number of family members provide instrumental support and assistance to elderly parents who continue to reside in their own homes (Brody, 1985).

The family may be described as individuals who are related genetically or through marriage or it may consist of unrelated individuals who live together or rely on each other for mutual support. Family members and significant others make up the "informal system" of care.

PSYCHOPHARMACOLOGICAL APPROACHES. Although investigations have been undertaken in the hope of finding pharmacologic agents that improve or arrest cognitive impairment in persons with irreversible organic dementia, at present no clinically effective agents have been identified. Hence, therapeutic modalities are geared to the relief of accompanying depression and anxiety, to efforts designed to compensate for cognitive losses, and to the relief of specific symptoms.

Unfortunately, the major antipsychotic drugs are often used and abused in the symptomatic treatment of the demented elderly. The risk of adverse drug reactions are more often associated with these types of drugs than with any other, especially when anticholinergic and sedative drugs are prescribed concurrently (Segal, Thompson & Floyd, 1979).

When aggressive, agitated, or paranoid behavior cannot be relieved through reassurance or the introduction of structured activities, small doses of Valium (2 mg t.i.d.) may help.

Haloperidol (Haldol), thioridazone (Mellaril), and other antipsychotic agents may cause severe side effects and should only be used when other interventions fail. Too often, nursing home residents are unnecessarily medicated because the sedative effects of psychotropic agents reduce the patient-care burden of the nursing staff.

Alzheimer's patients commonly suffer from sleep disturbances, particularly in the later stages of the disease. Triazolam (Halcion), chloral hydrate, and diphenhydramine (Benadryl) are often used to promote nighttime sleep. While the judicious use of these medications can be helpful, it is important to recognize that many soporifics have long metabolic half-lives among the elderly and, as a result, impair daytime functioning by reducing alertness and altering cardiopulmonary functions (Thompson, Moran, & Nies, 1983). Nonpharmacological interventions to promote nighttime sleep, such as encouraging daytime activities and offering warm milk at bedtime are interventions of choice.

For too long, it was assumed that depression among the elderly was an untreatable disorder. Today, researchers recognize that the treatment response rates of older persons are similar to those of younger individuals. However, there are special concerns about pharmacological treatment for the elderly. The tricyclic antidepressants have prominent anticholinergic side effects that can cause serious problems related to brain functioning in an elderly person, who may be already deficient in cholinergic function. In addition, the half-life of these drugs is increased in older persons, which contributes to the sedative and hypotensive side effects. Hence, dosage is generally reduced by about one-half to two-thirds of that recommended for younger patients. Desipramine hydrochloride, which has low anticholinergic and sedating effects,

may prove to be the drug of choice for elderly depressed (Robinson, Davis, & Nies, 1971). Monoamine-oxidase inhibitors are also used, based on the association between decreased enzyme activity with age and associated risk of depression (Robinson, Davis, & Nies, 1971). However, these agents increase risk of hypertensive crisis and must be used with caution in patients with hypertension.

Nursing intervention must include ongoing assessment of the type, dosage, and potential interaction of medications. Polypharmacy, both as a result of prescription drugs and over-the-counter medications, is a common and preventable problem among older institutionalized persons as well as among those who live at home. Changes in metabolic function extend the half-life of many drugs, warranting reduced dosage. The presence of physical illness can also alter medication response. Careful monitoring of medication intake and observation for untoward responses is a critical nursing function.

ELECTROCONVULSIVE THERAPY (ECT). It is a myth that electroconvulsive therapy (ECT) is both dangerous and ineffective for older persons. Actually it has been demonstrated to be an effective treatment modality, particularly for persons with multiple medical problems (Gerring & Shields, 1982). However, treatment is not without risk. Tachycardia and bradycardia may present complications (Gerring & Shields, 1982). Memory loss following treatment is a common problem, but is generally recoverable within two to three months. Lowering the dosage of electrical stimulation and placing electrodes on the nondominant hemisphere of the brain may reduce memory loss, but persistent mild memory dysfunction may remain a problem (Kiloh, 1982).

Nursing care includes making sure that the patient or responsible family member has given full and informed consent for the procedure after all risks have been discussed and understood. This is particularly important with older persons whose judgment may be impaired due to depression or cognitive impairment. Regardless of whether the patient or a family member provides consent, it is important that the patient understand that memory impairment is a normal and relatively short-term response to treatment that might persist for varying periods of time. Following treatment, the patient should not be tested repeatedly for the degree of memory loss or encouraged to "try to remember." Such tactics will not hasten memory return; they will only increase the patient's anxiety.

PSYCHOSOCIAL INTERVENTIONS. Nurses, social workers, and psychiatrists have developed a range of psychosocial interventions to increase patients' attention and social interaction, and to improve cognitive function. Most were developed and implemented in institutional settings, although many of these interventions can be modified for use in the home or in community programs.

Some psychosocial interventions are geared toward persons with cognitive impairment, while others are designed to improve the functioning and well-being of the elderly who are socially isolated or withdrawn, or who manifest behavioral problems.

Remotivation therapy is based on the assumption that many symptoms of confusion are iatrogenic consequences of institutional living (Dennis, 1978). This therapy is designed to treat symptoms of mild confusion, apathy, withdrawal, and inactivity, through group sessions conducted by a nurse, psychologist, or social worker trained in this technique. Typically, sessions are held once or twice a week for a period of four to six weeks, with a focus on the discussion of topics that create interest in the world outside of the nursing home.

Reality orientation and its many versions is one of the better known and most debated strategies used to deal with impaired cognition. It is designed to relieve disorientation by increasing the patient's awareness of himself and his relationship to his immediate environment (Taulbee & Folsom, 1966). Sessions usually consist of small and relatively short group meetings led by a nurse or other professional trained in reality orientation. The approach is educational, designed to inform and reinforce knowledge of time, persons, and places and the relationships among them. Repetitive question/answer sessions with visual guides are used to establish the current day and month, the names of group participants, and other here-and-now aspects of the situation.

Although neither remotivation therapy nor reality orientation have been demonstrated definitively to improve cognition or social impairment (Brook, Degun & Mather, 1975) they do provide an opportunity for social interaction with other elderly persons and with staff members. Hence, their potential contribution to the quality of life of the elderly in institutions should not be underestimated. In addition, such programs can provide additional purpose and reward for involved paraprofessionals such as nursing assistants. At the same time, remotivation therapy

and reality orientation can be misused when excessive pressure is placed on residents for improved performance.

BEHAVIORAL AND ENVIRONMENTAL APPROACHES. Recently, attention has been directed to the "difficult to manage" or "senile" (Blazer, 1986, pp. 593, 594) elderly person with dementia. The development of new or exaggerated personality traits, along with diminished spontaneity and a narrowing of the emotional response range, may give rise to irritability, wandering, agitation, suspiciousness, accusations, complaints, demands, and poor judgment.

Behavior modification is based on application of operant conditioning and includes the use of various rewards to reinforce desired behavior and aversion techniques to reduce undesired behavior. The effectiveness of this approach for the elderly has not been studied. Although the use of various types of rewards, such as praise, is inherent to many group and individual psychosocial interventions, as well as a part of humanistic nursing care, employment of aversion techniques is at best risky, particularly when the patient is not aware of or unable to control his actions.

Environmental techniques are effective in controlling some types of unsafe or undesirable behavior and in providing cues that encourage independence in the patient's home or in an institution. For example, wandering outside or into unsafe areas can be prevented with physical barriers. Stoves can be made temporarily inoperable and bathrooms made safe through the installment of safety devices that control water temperature. Rocking chairs can release tension and reduce anxiety (unlike geri-chairs, which immobilize the patient) (Earl, 1988). In addition, the physical environment can be marked with cues to trigger memory. The contents of drawers can be labeled, alarms used as a reminder of mealtimes, and time-locked medication containers can be purchased to prevent under- or overmedication. A full review of interventions is beyond the scope of this chapter, but the student should be aware of the range of technological devices that are available or being developed. They include a computerized in-home system that "calls" patients and instructs them in activities throughout the day (Holmes, 1988).

PSYCHOTHERAPEUTIC INTERVENTIONS. Psychotherapeutic interventions are used to treat depression as well as to improve the well-being and quality of life of older persons.

Depression is probably the most treatable aspect of dementia. Treatment methods are similar to those used for depressed older persons without dementia. Although some would argue that the demented elderly person cannot be assisted by therapy, others claim that behavior problems and anxiety can be reduced with the use of modified psychotherapeutic interventions that limit treatment goals to improving well-being and social behavior rather than addressing personality change (Steury & Blank, 1977).

Group therapy has been used with the elderly with cognitive impairment to enhance functioning and reduce depression and anxiety. Techniques range widely, borrowing from remotivation therapy, reality orientation, and psychoanalytic approaches among others. Focusing on affective issues such as maintaining self-esteem and providing support is more effective than focusing on behavioral change. (Butler & Lewis, 1982; Zarit, 1980). Lazarus and Weinberg (1980) suggest that therapeutic goals should be geared toward helping the patient: 1) work through grief and mourn losses, 2) find realistic substitutes for lost sources of gratification, and 3) revise goals to accord with diminished capacities.

Cognitive therapy has been used with older persons to relieve depressive symptoms and improve functioning. This approach involves collaboration between the therapist and the patient. Sessions generally last 15 to 20 minutes and are structured by an agenda that is set at the beginning of each session (Young & Beck, 1980). The purpose of the therapy is to pinpoint problems and elicit the "automatic thoughts" of the patient. The therapist compares these thoughts with objective information from the environment to point out the irrationality of the patient's negative beliefs. Behavioral strategies provide evidence about unfounded assumptions. When a patient's negative beliefs are based, at least in part, on reality, problem-solving methods may alter the situation or help the patient cope with the problem.

Psychodynamic approaches assist older persons in dealing with grief over the loss of loved ones, fear of physical illness and death, and guilt and despair over the past. Studies indicate that insight-oriented psychotherapy is effective for older persons. The criteria for selecting this type of therapy include the patient's diagnosis, personality structure, cognitive resources, "psychological mindedness," introspective ability, and willingness to establish a therapeutic relationship (Cath, 1982). Treatment objectives are based on similar criteria and include the development of more mature defense mechanisms and alterations in personality structure.

Supportive psychotherapy may be helpful for elderly persons who are psychologically regressed or suffer from organic brain disorders. Therapeutic goals include shoring up defensive mechanisms, compensating for failing ego functions, and providing reconfirmation of the patient's strengths in the face of age-related social and physical losses (Meerloo, 1961). The therapist must pay attention to the possibility of sensory and perceptual problems, the slowing of cognitive processes, and decreased ability to retain information. Flexibility is required in the structure of sessions and their content.

Therapists have advocated reminiscence as a part of work with the elderly because of its ability to enhance self-worth and the continuity of the self over time. Butler and Lewis (1982) describe life review as the verbal expression of an extensive autobiography that includes crucial memories and understanding of life events. A reexamination of life serves to expiate guilt, resolve intrapsychic conflicts and understand family relationships, as well as to transmit one's personal history to those who follow. The review process assists in reclaiming and mastering the past and enables the individual to cope more freely and effectively with the present and the future.

FAMILY THERAPY. As noted earlier, family members are the primary caretakers of the elderly. When family members are involved with a mentally frail elderly relative they often contend with complex issues, such as the provision of care, feelings of guilt and burden, the revisiting of old family conflicts, and an uncertain future in which more and more of their time may be occupied by the needs of their elderly relative. Hence, it is not unusual to find that family members require as much or more nursing care as the elderly patient.

Family therapy can be of help to both the elderly person's functional status and the family system. Assessment and intervention must recognize the interdependency of family members in terms of both the past and the present. Family problems often result from a change in the functional status of an elderly member and its effect on family functioning. The type and intensity of intervention is based on the severity of the problem and the ability of individual family members as well as the family unit to cope. Sometimes the provision of information, guidance, and support to a primary family caregiver is adequate. In other situations, however, intergenerational therapy may be necessary to deal with maladaptive patterns that have been in the family for generations.

Duffy (1986) reviews a number of therapeutic strategies that help clarify family tension and increase adjustment. Adult children may bring to the caregiving situation unresolved anger that results in guilt and resentment over their parent's dependency on them. One approach is to have the adult child compose a written communication of his feelings to which the therapist reacts from the parent's perspective. This helps the adult child recognize and appreciate the parent's stance and dilemma. It also provides the opportunity to clarify feelings by venting them openly.

Intergenerational sessions may be appropriate to clarify feelings, reveal misunderstandings, and serve as a vehicle for problem solving. However, this approach is difficult, requiring sophisticated skills and maturity on the part of the therapist. Intergenerational therapy requires that the therapist direct her alliance to the family unit rather than an individual family member (Duffy, 1986).

EVALUATION OF NURSING CARE

As with assessment and intervention, evaluation of nursing care is often complicated by coexisting physical and mental disorders and the variable life circumstances of the older patient. A number of these issues are described below.

THE PHYSICAL HEALTH STATUS OF THE PATIENT. As described earlier, the interplay between physical and mental disorders makes care of the elderly complex. Evaluation must be based on nursing care goals that take into account the existence and prognosis of physical disease as it affects and is affected by mental health status. Exacerbation of a chronic illness, or the diagnosis of a physical illness, can result in new or magnified mental health problems requiring modification of nursing care goals. Also, increasing disability can result in hospitalization or placement in a nursing home.

THE EXPECTATIONS OF THE PATIENT AND HIS FAMILY. Both the process of nursing care and its anticipated outcomes must take into account the desires and expectations of patients and their families. This requires recognition of the family's value system with respect to the provision of specific nursing care interventions. At the same time, the nurse must also deal with the sometimes difficult issues of a patient's mental competence in terms of his decision-making ability. Determining who has the right to make decisions—the patient or a family member—can cause much tension when the two parties disagree. Although psychiatric assessment can determine whether the patient is mentally competent in the eyes of the law, it does not negate the patient's right to continue to participate, whenever possible, in decisions about care.

EVALUATION OF STRUCTURE, PROCESS, AND OUTCOME GOALS. Ideally, the outcomes of nursing care should be predictable, based on knowledge of the relationship between interventions and outcomes. However, patient care outcomes among the elderly are vulnerable to unpredictable factors or those over which there is no control. Hence, evaluation should be ongoing and include structure and process, as well as outcome goals. That is, it should include the adequacy and appropriateness of human and material resources (structural charcteristics) and caregiving activities and interventions (process characteristics) in addition to the extent to which nursing care goals are accomplished.

THE PROVISION OF CARE TO THE MENTALLY FRAIL

The opportunities for geropsychiatric mental health nursing are underscored by a review of the current status of mental health care of the elderly. Probably the most significant and shocking aspect of care delivery is that the **mentally frail,** with few exceptions, are cared for by non–mental health workers. The reasons for this are complex. First, there is the issue of access to care. Economic barriers to care exist as a result of limited payment by Medicare for outpatient mental health services, the relatively small proportion of older persons who carry private health care insurance, and the high costs of mental health treatment. Second, there is a shortage of mental health providers available to older persons. Mental health providers, including psychiatric mental health nurses, tend to cluster in areas where the vast majority of the population is comprised of young and middle-aged adults. In the United States there are more counties in the country *without* any licensed mental health providers than there are *with* providers. Third, the elderly themselves are often reluctant to seek mental health care. Many understand psychiatric illness only in terms of "going crazy." The stigma of mental illness places mental health care outside of psychological reach.

What, then, are the consequences of these problems for service utilization? Although approximately 25 percent of the elderly living in the community suffer from symptoms of mental disorder, only .6 percent to 2.7 percent of patients treated by private mental health practitioners are older adults (Butler & Lewis, 1982). And, while the elderly comprise over 11 percent of the population, only 6 percent of the patients of community mental health centers are 65 years of age or older (Redick & Taub, 1980). Elderly people who are members of minority racial and ethnic groups fare even worse. The community mental health movement of the 1960s and 1970s failed to assess adequately their needs, and treatment programs were not designed to deal with their particular problems. As a result, the minority elderly continue to be significantly underrepresented in the utilization of mental health services (Kobata, Lockery & Morlwaki, 1980).

Who, then, provides care and services to the "mentally frail" elderly? As noted earlier, the foremost caretakers of the elderly are the family. This informal system of care is often augmented by formal care and services, many of which are community-based programs targeted to older persons. It is only when the resources of these informal and formal systems are inadequate to meet the care needs of the frail elderly that these individuals are likely to enter institutions. Approximately 5 percent of older persons are in nursing homes at any given time; however, about 25 percent of the elderly population will, before they die, have entered a nursing home (Kastenbaum & Candy, 1973).

FORMAL COMMUNITY-BASED SERVICES

The availability of community-based geriatric services varies from one geographic region to the next. Unlike the western European countries, the United States does not have a national policy or system of care for the aged. Because of this, community care resources vary, depending on state and local legislation, level of economic resources, and the extent and type of philanthropic or voluntary organizations and services. Hence, what may be true for one city or part of the country is not necessarily true for another.

Despite these differences, there are national trends in service delivery. One of the most important is in the development of daycare centers for the elderly. In 1980, there were fewer than 600 such programs in the country. Today there is a vastly greater number, and their growth continues. Some programs are medical; that is, they provide health assessment, rehabilitation, and other health-related services. The majority of centers draw on a social model of care,

emphasizing group activities and outings, but also offering programs such as reality orientation. Day centers serve another critical function—they provide respite to family caregivers by giving them time during the day to work outside of the home, to do chores, or to socialize with friends. The major complaint of family caregivers is that most centers can provide only limited service, 4 to 6 hours a day for two to five days of the week. Another barrier is cost. Some programs are funded by public monies and charge limited or no fees, but others are private and may charge more than many families can afford.

Another form of community-based care is **case management.** Case-management functions vary, but their major role is to tie together packages of services to meet the individual needs of clients. Case management has been the core of a number of federal demonstration projects that provide Medicare or Medicaid waivers enabling patients to have access to services that are otherwise not reimbursed by public dollars. In some parts of the country private enterprises are going into the case-management business. As nursing homes become multipurpose "geriatric centers" offering day care, meals on wheels, home care, and respite care, case managers are needed to coordinate and monitor service delivery.

Some nursing homes are beginning to offer inpatient respite services. Beds are set aside for short-term stays of a few days to two weeks to enable family caregivers to vacation or be temporarily relieved of caretaking responsibilities. Community agencies and private entrepreneurs are beginning to offer a range of various types of in-home "sitting" services for the same purpose. With rare exceptions, respite care is private and not reimbursed by Medicaid, Medicare, or other government programs.

A major source of home care for the mentally frail elderly living in the community are nonprofessional home-care workers. Home-care workers are comprised of a variety of subgroups—home health aides, home attendants, and personal-care workers—based on level of training and funding source (Medicaid, Medicare, or private pay). Although different in title, they have in common low wages and minimal training, despite the high level of responsibility they assume on the job. This situation has resulted in public scandals of cases of elder abuse and neglect by home-care workers. The actual incidence of such cases is unknown, but it appears to be relatively low. However, the potential for abuse and neglect remains high. Home-care workers may operate with little or no supervision, and attempts at quality assurance techniques are in their infancy. On the other hand, home-care workers have reported abuse from patients and from their families. Hence, the problem is complex. The growing numbers and frailty of the elderly in the community indicate that the demand for non-professional workers will increase. Clearly, nursing must assume a larger role in this aspect of home care. With the exception of Medicare-sponsored home care, which mandates nursing visits, nonprofessional home care is conducted with minimal to no nursing intervention.

Community-based nursing care is available to older persons under the Medicare program. Patients must qualify as needing "skilled" and "intermittent" care under the order of a physician. As will be discussed, the Medicare program is geared toward acute care needs so that home-care services are limited. Nursing care may also be obtained for a fee from the private sector, but costs are high and generally not covered by public programs or private insurance.

INSTITUTIONAL CARE

Today, the nursing home is the foremost source of institutional care for the elderly with psychiatric and organic mental disorders. It is estimated that between 50 and 66 percent of all nursing-home residents suffer from depression or some type of organic brain disorder (National Center for Health Statistics, 1981; Cross, Gurland & Mann, 1983). The evolution of the nursing home into a mental health institution is the result of a number of factors, including the enormous growth in the private nursing-home industry since the 1950s; the rapid rise in the number of elderly and the concomitant increase in the prevalence of dementia; and the failure of public policy to finance and regulate institutions designed to care for the elderly mentally ill.

Nursing homes are not financed, regulated, or staffed as mental health institutions. As a result, most facilities do not have professional personnel trained in psychiatry or mental health, let alone in geriatric psychiatry. Although some institutions use psychiatrists on a consultant basis, such persons may or may not have the training and experience necessary to deal appropriately with the complex diagnostic and treatment issues that are presented by the elderly suffering from multiple physical and mental disorders.

MEDICARE AND MEDICAID

One difficulty in dealing with the mental health problems of the elderly is the coexistence of mental illness and physical disability. As a result, services cannot be provided on a piecemeal basis. This problem is compounded by Medicare and Medicaid, the major sources of payment of health care for the elderly. Each program has its own focus and goals, making it difficult to bring together services that address mental and physical health-care needs.

Medicare is a health insurance program that pays a substantial portion of the costs of hospital and physician services for individuals aged 65 and over, for certain disabled persons under age 65, and for persons with end-stage renal disease. The program was designed to assist the elderly in obtaining acute medical care services rather than long-term home care or institutional care. This limited focus is the program's major deficit. The types of care and assistance the elderly are most likely to require—dentures, hearing aids, and community or institutional long-term care—are not covered by the program. Nor does Medicare cover, except in a very limited way, outpatient psychiatric or mental health care. These failures of the program necessitate high out-of-pocket expenditures and, for some, eventual reliance on welfare.

The aged who are not covered by supplemental **Medigap** insurance—and this is the majority of the poor and near-poor—face growing out-of-pocket payments for hospital care and possible destitution should they experience a catastrophic illness. The supposed safety net for persons unable to pay for needed health care not reimbursed by Medicare is the **Medicaid** program. Medicaid is a federal/state welfare program designed to provide medical care to the poor of all ages. Although participating states are required under federal guidelines to provide a minimal set of services, states have wide discretionary power over eligibility criteria and access to and utilization of funded services. This discretionary power underlies the wide variation among states in expenditures (Harrington, et al., 1986).

One of the major problems facing mentally frail persons and their families is the cost entailed in providing home care. Rarely can children or spouses provide the intensive round-the-clock care required by older persons with advanced dementia. Medicare will not pay for long-term home care and only a few states offer this service under their Medicaid programs. As a result, families are faced with the choice of managing on their own with whatever relief they can afford to purchase, or "spending down" to Medicaid eligibility levels. In most states, *Medicaid eligibility is determined by complex formulas of such strictness that almost one-half of the nation's poor do not qualify for the program.* Another paradox of the Medicaid program is the fact that eligibility requirements are tied to other welfare benefits—in the case of the elderly, to Supplemental Security income (Joe, Meltzer & Yu, 1985). As a result, while individuals may qualify for Medicaid supported services, their welfare income may be inadequate to support continued residence in the community. The result is an institutional bias in which individuals may have no choice but to accept nursing-home placement because of inadequate expendable income and inadequate Medicaid-supported community-based care. Although some states do provide comprehensive community programs, these are rare and qualification may require impoverishment.

OPPORTUNITIES FOR NURSES IN GERIATRIC MENTAL HEALTH CARE

This chapter has only touched on the many issues facing people working in the field of geriatric mental health. Clearly, the opportunities for nurses are great. The recognition by the ANA of the importance of this specialty area, and the unique role nurses can play within it, is but one sign of the future growth of geriatric mental health nursing practice and research.

The care of older persons is filled with challenges, opportunities, and rewards. Clinical practice demands sophisticated knowledge of both normal aging and disease, as well as the complex interplay of physical and mental problems and socioenvironmental factors. Nursing care of the elderly focuses on the family. Because spouses and adult children provide the majority of care and support to older persons, their inclusion in nursing-care assessment, intervention, and evaluation is critical.

Although the research base of geriatric mental health is growing, a great deal is yet to be learned. Nurses have become increasingly skilled and productive in investigating clinical geriatric problems and in contributing to our knowledge of the health-care delivery system and its role in meeting the needs of the elderly. Research in geriatric mental health affords the opportunity of working collaboratively with nurses prepared in other specialty areas as well as with investigators from other disciplines.

Because there is a shortage of nurses trained to work in long-term nursing care administration, the organization and delivery of health care to the elderly remains fragmented. Nursing's orientation to holistic care can encourage the integration, or enhanced articulation, of physical and mental health services and programs. Administrative opportunities exist in a wide range of settings, including community-based agencies and programs, nursing homes, and hospitals. Lastly, the field of geriatric mental health affords opportunities for nurses to participate in the development of local, state, and national health-care policy.

Case Study: Nonpsychiatric Setting

Demographic Data

Name: Margaret Vezi
Age: 82
Ethnicity: Black
Geography: Chicago
Religion: Holiness
Residence: The Southside Villa
Occupation; Retired social worker

Presenting Problem

Mrs. Vezi had lived with her daughter until she became increasingly difficult to manage. She was admitted to the Southside Villa approximately three months ago. Recently, at the Southside Villa, she has become increasingly agitated, is occasionally helpless, refuses to eat, complains of constipation (occasional incontinence), is withdrawn, and is disinterested in her environment and her personal hygiene, and so forth. She remains awake for long hours during the night. Lately, during the early mornings, she sings quite loudly, "Oh beautiful, for spacious skies . . ."

History of Presenting Problem

(Information obtained from family members.) Mrs. Vezi lived and worked in Chicago for 45 years. She retired at age 68. After retirement, she volunteered at a drug rehabilitation facility, served as chairwoman at the Newcomers Club in her church, and worked in voter registration campaigns sponsored by community agencies. Her activities began to wane at about age 80.

Although Mrs. Vezi remained in her home and managed her activities of daily living, she began to show little interest in social and civic affairs. She constantly complained to her daughter of being tired, unable to sleep, not interested in eating, and not knowing where she was, which was frightening to her.

Her daughter, Dr. Vaughn, reported that her mother began crying and seemed sad and depressed. She took Mrs. Vezi to a physician who found no physical problems. She was prescribed 5 mg. Valium at night for sleep.

Mrs. Vezi moved into her daughter's home, where she remained until she was admitted to Southside Villa.

Psychiatric History

None.

Family History

Mrs. Vezi's father was a career military person. Her mother was a housewife who occasionally worked as a secretary in the various communities where they lived. Mrs. Vezi is an only child.

Social History

Mrs. Vezi had spent some of her formative years with family members in Mississippi and other southern states. She was a high achiever, completed high school with honors, earned a scholarship for undergraduate studies, and again, graduated with honors. She received a Masters of Social Work at about age 30. Mrs. Vezi was employed for the greater part of her career as a social worker in the public schools of Chicago. Her daughter described her as meticulous and somewhat compulsive about her paperwork at school, as well as having a clean and orderly home.

Mrs. Vezi married and is the mother of two daughters. The other daughter resides in San Francisco with her husband and four children. Mrs. Vezi's husband died of cancer approximately eight months ago. After his death, Dr. Vaughn stated, "Mother has declined steadily since his death. She cries, refuses to eat, and is always dysphoric, even when her grandchildren visit, something she used to love."

Medical History

Mrs. Vezi has been relatively healthy during her life. Her daughter stated she had a hysterectomy at about age 56 and an appendectomy at age 61.

She has been taking multivitamins, stool softener, and aspirin for "stiffness in the joints" for several years. Currently, her appetite is poor; fluid intake and physical activity are limited. She has cataracts in both eyes but has refused surgery.

Hobbies

Mrs. Vezi was once an excellent gardener. She grew vegetables (for the people in the church) and flowers. In fact, she had won several "blue ribbons" at the community flower show. She also sang in the church and community choir.

Current Mental Status

General Appearance: Disheveled, poor hygiene, in hospital gown, lying in bed. Quiet.

Sensorium: Difficulty concentrating. Disinterested in interviewer's questions.

Emotions: Tearing/wringing hands; staring at the floor, with an occasional stare at interviewer; mood is that of sadness, loneliness, and hopelessness.

Motoric Behavior: Lying still in bed.

Thought Process: Slow, little concentration, detached.

Thought Content: Vacuous

Medication

Colace for constipation, multivitamin tab.

Summary

Mrs. Margaret Vezi is an 82-year-old black woman who has resided at the Southside Villa nursing home for approximately 45 days. Recently, she has become increasingly confused, manifesting little interest in the environment; she is unable to perform activities of daily living, has limited nutritional intake, cries frequently, and so forth. For several weeks she has had increased difficulties in sleeping, awaking in early morning, singing "Oh beautiful, for spacious skies . . ."

Nursing Diagnoses

Sleep pattern disturbance
Grieving (related to actual loss)
Altered nutrition: less than body requirements
Constipation

Nursing Care Plan for Mrs. Vezi

Nursing Diagnosis	Desired Outcomes	Interventions	Rationale
1. Sleep pattern disturbance.	Mrs. Vezi will experience adequate and restful sleep as evidenced by 1) falling to sleep 20–30 minutes after retirement, and 2) awakening feeling rested after 7–8 hours of sleep.	Determine Mrs. Vezi's sleep pattern before she became depressed by communicating with daughter and reviewing records in the nursing home and communicating with staff.	Baseline data is helpful in determining change in sleep behavior for current goal setting.
		Engage Mrs. Vezi in physical activities in late afternoon. (The recreation therapist and occupational therapist will be asked to assist nursing staff.)	Physical activity will assist in tension release and induce fatigue, which will facilitate rest.
		Limit the amount of time Mrs. Vezi sleeps during the day. Nurse should encourage Mrs. Vezi to stay out of her room during the day.	The room (bed) should be associated only with *sleep* at night.
		Encourage Mrs. Vezi's participation in ward activities such as resocialization, remotivation groups, and ward activities such as social communication and group games (checkers, cards, etc.) with other patients.	Socialization groups and participation in ward activities will give Mrs. Vezi a sense of belonging in a social setting as well as provide her with a reality base.
		Arrange nursing care functions as to alleviate need to awaken Mrs. Vezi during the night (for example, for medications).	Facilitates sleep.
		Employ such measures as closing her door, unplugging her television, providing a night light (but limited use of bright lights during the night), playing soft music for relaxation. (Music with nature sounds is recommended.)	These measures eliminate interruptions and distractions that occur in the environment.

Nursing Diagnosis	Desired Outcomes	Interventions	Rationale
		Provide P.M. care: warm sponge bath, oral hygiene, warm milk, clean and warm bed, proper lighting, and so on.	These are comfort measures that should assist in the inducement of sleep.
2. Grieving (related to actual loss).	Mrs. Vezi will express her grief about her husband's death and discuss the significance of the loss to her.	Encourage Mrs. Vezi to talk about her husband, and assist her in labeling her feelings: shock, anger, disbelief, fear, loneliness, guilt, isolation, depression, giving up, and so on.	The loss (death) must be acknowledged before the grieving process can be effective.
		Assess how Mrs. Vezi has handled losses in the past by communicating with her daughter.	Provides an historical perspective; provides data about strengths and weaknesses and defense mechanisms used for coping.
		Acknowledge Mrs. Vezi's grief: "You look very sad. Are you thinking about your husband? You must be lonely without him."	Communicates empathy, understanding, and caring.
		Focus on emotional responses: denial, anger, anxiety, fear, rejection, isolation, and so on.	These feelings are commonly associated with losses (death) and they need to be verbalized.
		Encourage Mrs. Vezi to participate in a grief group that meets in the facility.	Another modality that encourages expression of feelings among peers who can help each other.
3. Altered Nutrition: Less than body requirements.	Mrs. Vezi will gain weight by increasing the amount of her food intake.	Record Mrs. Vezi's weight. Develop a specific goal for weight gain such as, "Mrs. Vezi will gain 2–3 pounds per week."	Baseline data assists nurse in planning, implementing and evaluating goals.
		Determine if there are physical barriers to Mrs. Vezi's limited food intake such as difficulty swallowing, inadequate dentures, dry mouth, and so on. Provide oral hygiene before each meal is offered.	If patient is on antidepressant medication, side effects may include dry mouth and difficulty swallowing.

Nursing Diagnosis	Desired Outcome	Interventions	Rationale
		Offer liquid supplements such as Instant Breakfast with added ice cream or banana, high calorie/high protein supplement.	Another source of nutritional intake that is convenient and tasty; small, frequent feedings help to stimulate the appetite.
		Assess for Mrs. Vezi's food preferences: determine if foods are prepared the way she prefers (if not harmful to health).	Sociocultural factors must be considered in meal planning.
		Encourage Mrs. Vezi's daughter to bring Mrs. Vezi's favorite foods that are high in protein and calories to residence. Connect with dieticians about specific meals for Mrs. Vezi.	Facilitates family's involvement with Mrs. Vezi; provides her with foods that she likes and is familiar with; increases her attraction to food.
4. Constipation	Mrs. Vezi will be free of constipation and have regular bowel movements.	Determine Mrs. Vezi's previous elimination pattern, and determine if there has been a change.	Assists nurse in planning care.
		Offer water, juices, and foods that stimulate bowel elimination (such as prunes, pear nectar, and so on). Offer foods with high bran/roughage content (fruits, leafy vegetables, nuts, corn bread, grains, and so on).	These foods stimulate peristalsis and bowel evacuation.
		Use mild laxative such as Milk of Magnesia, stool softeners, if necessary, but discontinue use as soon as possible.	Laxatives can be abused by the elderly; frequent use of most laxatives encourages dependency.
		Encourage activities that assist in bowel evacuation, such as: 1) Assist patient to bathroom and encourage use of commode (if possible); 2) Privacy: Close door; do not interrupt. (Instruct patient about how to use the emergency nurse call.); 3) Use deodorizers (if needed); 4) Assist	These activities will facilitate evacuation of bowel.

patient in cleaning self after evacuation. Have on hand toilet paper, warm water, cloth, soap, and so on. 5) Encourage exercise as tolerated to include walks, passive range of motion, "rocking" in rocking chair.

Request consultation from a physician when indicated.

In-depth assessment might be needed if symptoms do not abate.

Assess for laxative use/abuse.

Long-term usage can be dangerous.

SUMMARY

The field of geriatric mental health is still in its infancy, but it is rapidly growing, as is the role of the nurse. Between 1900 and 1980, the population of persons in the United States over age 65 increased eightfold, and by the year 2000, 13 percent of the population will be considered elderly; the need for nurses skilled at geriatric mental health care is evident.

Several theories of aging are debated: disengagement theory, activity theory, continuity theory, and age-stratification theory. These theories can promote ageism, to the extent that they may stereotype or cause discrimination against older persons.

Several specific disorders present problems for elderly patients, including depression and suicidality, dementia (Alzheimer's disease and multi-infarct dementia), acute confusional states, sundown syndrome, and elder abuse. Some of these disorders may coexist and therefore the nurse must assess the patient carefully in order to make an accurate evaluation of his condition. Overall, she must differentiate normal from abnormal processes of aging, physical from mental disorders, and acute from chronic mental disorders.

When planning nursing interventions for an elderly patient, the nurse considers the following: the past and present use of psychopharmacological agents, modified psychotherapeutic approaches, environmental interventions, and the involvement of family members and significant others. Some specific interventions include the use of medication, electroconvulsive therapy for depression; psychosocial interventions, behavioral and environmental techniques (such as providing cues to encourage independence, installing safety devices on dangerous appliances, and using rocking chairs for tension release), psychodynamic and supportive psychotherapy, and family therapy.

Resources of care for the elderly include formal community-based services, institutional care, and Medicare/Medicaid. However, families continue to provide the bulk of care for the elderly.

Finally, the nurse, with her holistic background and perhaps specialized training in geriatric care, is in a unique position to coordinate resources in order to help the elderly patient get the best care possible.

KEY TERMS

geriatric mental health
disengagement theory
activity theory
continuity theory
age-stratification theory
ageism
depression
dementia
Alzheimer's disease
acute confusional states
sundown syndrome
pseudodementia
remotivation therapy
reality orientation
mentally frail elderly
case management
Medigap
Medicaid

Medicare   dysphoria
confabulation   somatization
perseveration

STUDY QUESTIONS

1. Describe disengagement theory and activity theory; explain their relevance to the mental health care needs of the elderly.

2. Why is depression such a common problem for the elderly patient and his nurse?

3. Name and describe briefly the diagnostic differential criteria the nurse must pursue in assessing the elderly patient.

4. Name and describe briefly at least three theoretically different nursing approaches used with the elderly.

5. Name and describe briefly the three major resources (other than family) for care for the elderly patient. Which is the most common? Why?

REFERENCES

Addington, J., & Fry, P. S. (1986). Directions for clinical-psychosocial assessment of depression in the elderly. In T. L. Brink (Ed.), *Clinical gerontology: A guide to assessment and intervention*. New York: The Haworth Press.

American Psychiatric Association (1987). *Diagnostic and statistical manual of mental disorders*, 3rd Ed., Revised. Washington, D.C.: A.P.A.

Assnis, G. (1977). Parkinson's disease, depression and ECT: A review and case study. *American Journal of Psychiatry, 134,* 191–199.

Auso-Gutierrez, L. (1983). Late life depression—clinical and therapeutic aspects. In J. M. Davis and J. W. Mass (Eds.), *The affective disorders*. Washington, D.C.: The American Psychiatric Press.

Berger, P. (1983). The economic well-being of eldery Hispanics. *Journal of Minority Aging, 8,* 36–46.

Birren, J. E. & Renner, V. J. (1980). Concepts and issues of mental health and aging. In J. E. Birren and R. B. Sloane (Eds.), *Handbook of mental health and aging*. Englewood, NJ: Prentice-Hall, Inc., pp. 3–33.

Blazer, D. (1986) Psychiatric disorders. In I. Rossman (Ed.) *Clinical geriatrics*, 3rd ed. Philadelphia: J. B. Lippincott, pp. 593–594.

Blazer, D. G. (1982). *Depression in late life*. St. Louis: C.V. Mosby.

Blazer, D. G., Hughes, D. C., & George, L. K. (1987). The epidemiology of depression in an elderly community population. *The Gerontologist, 27,* 3.

Block, M., & Sinnott, J. D. (Eds.) (1979). *The battered elder syndrome: An exploratory study*. College Park, MD: University of Maryland Center on Aging.

Blumenthal, M. D. (1975) Measuring depressive symptomatology in a general population. *Archives of General Psychiatry, 32;* 971–978.

Blumenthal, M. D. (1980, April). Depressive illness in old age: Getting behind the mask. *Geriatrics,* 34–43.

Branco, K., & Williamson, J. (1982). Stereotyping and the life cycle: Views of aging and the aged. In A. Miller (ed.), *In the eye of the beholder: Contemporary issues in stereotyping*. New York: Praeger.

Brody, E. M. (1985). Parent care as a normative family stress. *The Gerontological Society of America,* Volume 25, No. 1.

Brody, J. A. (1984). The nation grows older. *Health and Medicine, 2,* 6–13.

Brook, P., Degun, G., & Mather, M. (1975). Reality orientation. *British Journal of Psychiatry, 127,* 42–45.

Bull, C., & Aucoin, J. (1975). Voluntary association participation and life satisfaction: A replication note. *Journal of Gerontology, 30,* 73–76.

Busse, E., & Blazer, D. (1980). The future of geriatric psychiatry. In E. Busse and D. Blazer (Eds.), *Handbook of geriatric psychiatry*. New York: Van Nostrand Reinhold Co.

Butler, R. N. (1969). The effects of medical and health progress on the social and economic aspects of the life cycle. *Industrial Gerontology 1,* 1–9.

Butler, R. W., & Lewis, M. I. (1982). *Aging and mental health*, 3rd ed. St. Louis: C.V. Mosby.

Cantor, M. (1986). Patterns of aging and sound supports in the U.S. Paper presented at the International Conference on Aging, Beijing, Peoples Republic of China, May, 1986.

Card, F. I., & Judge, T. C. (1974). *Assessment of the elderly patient*. London: Pitman Medical.

Carp, F. (1967). The impact of environment on old people. *The Gerontologist, 7,* 106–108.

Cath, S. H. (1982). Psychoanalysis and psychoanalytic psychotherapy of the older patient. *Journal of Geriatric Psychiatry, 15,* 43–53.

Chatfield, W. (1977). Economic and sociological factors influencing life satisfaction of the aged. *Journal of Gerontology, 32,* 393–399.

Chebotareu, O. F. (1979). The biology of human aging and disease. In J. Orimo, K. Shimada, M. Iriki, & D. Maeda (Eds.), *Recent advances in gerontology*. Amsterdam: Excerpta Medica.

Congressional Clearinghouse of the Future (1985). *Tomorrow's elderly: Issues for Congress*. Prepared for the House Select Committee on Aging: Congressional Institute for the Future.

Cox, H. (1988). *Later life: The realities of aging*. Englewood Cliffs, New Jersey; Prentice Hall, Inc.

Cross, P. S., & Gurland, B. J. (n.d) *The epidemiology of dementing disorders*. A Report on Work Performed for and Submitted to the United States Congress, Office of Technology Assessment, Washington, D.C.

Cross, P., Gurland, B., & Mann, A. (1983). Long-term institutional care of demented elderly people in New York City and London. *Bulletin of the New York Academy of Medicine, 59,* 267–275.

Cumming, E., & Henry, W. (1961). *Growing old*. New York; Basic Books.

Davis, L. (1986) Health of older adults. In B. P. Logan & C. E. Dawkins (Eds.), *Family-centered nursing in the community*. Menlo Park, CA: Addison-Wesley, pp. 578–607.

Dennis, H. (1978). Remotivation therapy groups. In I. M. Burnside (Ed.), *Working with the elderly: Group processes and techniques*. Boston, Mass.: Duxbury Press.

Dolphin, N. (1986). Rural health. In B. P. Logan & C. E. Dawkins (Eds.), *Family-centered nursing in the community*. Menlo Park, CA: Addison-Wesley, pp. 516–544.

Duffy, M. (1986). The techniques and contexts of multi-generational therapy. In T. Brink (Ed.). *Clinical gerontology: A guide to assessment and intervention*. New York: The Haworth Press.

Earle, A. (1988). Personal communication.

Edwards, J., & Klemmack, D. (1973). Correlates of life satisfaction: A re-examination. *Journal of Gerontology, 28*, 497–502.

Engel, G. (1962). *Psychological Development in Health and Disease*. Philadelphia: W. B. Saunders Co.

Epstein, L. J. (1976). Depression in the elderly. *Journal of Gerontology, 31*, 271–282.

Erikson, E. (1950). *Childhood and society*. New York: W. W. Norton.

Evans, L. K. (1987). Sundown syndrome in institutionalized elderly. *Journal of American Geriatric Society, 35*, No. 2.

Finkel, S. (Ed.) (1981). *Task force on the 1981 White House Conference on Aging of the American Psychiatric Association*. Washington, D.C.: APA Press.

Fogel, B. S., & Fretwell, M. (1985). Reclassification of depression in the mentally ill elderly. *Journal of the American Geriatrics Society, 33*, 446–448.

Foreman, M. C. (1984). Acute confusional states in the elderly: An algorithm. *Dimensions of Critical Care Nursing, 3*, 207–215.

Gaitz, C., & Varner, R. (1980). Preventive aspects of mental illness in late life. In J. Birren & B. Sloanne (Eds.), *Handbook of Mental Health and Aging*. Englewood Cliffs, NJ: Prentice-Hall.

Gerring, J. P., & Shields, H. M. (1982). The identification and management of patients with high risk for cardiac arrhythmias during modified ECT. *Journal of Clinical Psychiatry, 43*(4), 140–143.

Gianturco, D. T., & Busse, E. W. (1978). Psychiatric problems encountered during a long-term study of normal aging volunteers. In A. D. Isaacs and F. Post (Eds.), *Studies in geriatric psychiatry*. New York: John Wiley.

Goldstein, S. E. (1979). Depression in the elderly. *Journal of the American Geriatrics Society, 27*, 38–42.

Graney, M. (1975). Happiness and social participation in aging. *Journal of Gerontology, 30*, 701–706.

Greenblatt, M. & Chein, C. P. (1983). Depression in the elderly: Use of external support systems. In L. D. Breslau & M. R. Haug (Eds.), *Depression and aging: Cause, care, & consequences*. New York: Springer Publishers, pp. 193–207.

Gubrium, J. (1978). Environmental effects on morale in old age and the resources of health and solvency. *The Gerontologist, 10*, 294–297.

Gurland, B. (1980). The assessment of the mental health status of older adults. In J. E. Birren and R. Sloane (Eds.), *Handbook of mental health and aging*. Englewood Cliffs, N.J.: Prentice-Hall, Inc.

Gurland, B. J. (1976). The comparative frequency of depression in various adult age groups. *Journal of Gerontology, 31*, 283–292.

Gurland, B., Dean, L., Cross, P., & Golden, R. (1980). The epidemiology of depression and dementia in the elderly: The use of multiple indicators of those conditions. In J. O. Cole & J. E. Barrett (Eds.), *Psychopathology in the aged*. New York: Raven.

Gurland, B., & Toner, J. A. (1982). Depression in the elderly: A review of recently published studies. In C. Eisdorfer (Ed.), *Annual review of geriatrics and gerontology*, vol. 3, pp. 228–265. New York: Springer Publishing Co.

Harrington, C., Estes, C., Lee, P., & Newcomer, R. (1986). Effects of state Medicaid policies on the aged. *The Gerontologist, 26*, 437–443.

Harris, L., and Associates (1975). *The myth and reality of aging in America*. Washington: National Council on Aging.

Havighurst, R. J. (1963). Successful aging. In R. H. Williams, C. Tibbit, & W. Donahue (Eds.), *Processes of aging*. New York: Lieber-Atherton.

Havighurst, R., & Albrect, R. (1953). *Older people*. New York; Longmans, Green.

Hirst, S. P. & Miller, J. (1986). The abused elderly. *Journal of psychosocial nursing and mental health services, 24*(10), 28–34.

Holmes, D. (1988). Personal communication.

Jackson, J. (1980). *Minorities and aging*. Belmont, CA.: Wadsworth.

Joe, T. C., Meltzer, J., & Yu, P. (1985). Arbitrary access to care: the case for reforming Medicaid. *Health Affairs, 4*, 59–74.

Kastenbaum, R., & Candy, S. (1973). The 4% fallacy: A methodological and empirical critique of extended care facility population statistics. *International Journal of Aging and Human Development, 4*, 15–21.

Kiloh, L. G. (1982). Electroconvulsive therapy. In E. S. Paykel (Ed.), *Handbook of affective disorders*. New York; Guilford Press. pp. 262–275.

Kleinman, A., & Good, B. (Eds.) (1985). *Culture and depression*. Berkeley, CA.: University of California Press.

Kleinman, A., & Kleinman, J. (1985). Somatization: The interconnections in Chinese society among culture, depressive experiences, and meanings of pain. In A. Kleinman & B. Good (Eds.), *Culture and depression*. Berkeley: University of California Press.

Klerman, G. L. (1983). Problems in the definition & diagnosis of depression in the elderly. In L. D. Breslau & Haug (Eds.), *Depression & Aging: Causes, Care, & Consequences*. New York: Springer Publishing Co., pp. 3–19.

Kobata, F. S., Lockery, S. A., & Morlwaki, S. Y. (1980). Minority issues in mental health and aging. In J. E. Birren & R. B. Sloan (Eds.), *Handbook of mental health and aging*. Englewood Cliffs, N.J.: Prentice Hall.

Kosberg, J. I. (Ed.) (1983). *Abuse and maltreatment of the elderly: Causes and interventions*. Littleton, MA: John Wright PSG.

Kral, V. A. (1962). Senescent forgetfulness: Benign and malignant. Canadian Medical Association Journal, 86,

257–260.

Lau, E., & Kosberg, J. (1979). Abuse of the elderly by informal care providers. *Aging,* September-October, 10–15.

Lazarus, L. W., & Weinberg, J. (1980). Treatment in the ambulatory care setting. In E. W. Busse & D. G. Blazer (Eds.), *Handbook of geriatric psychiatry.* New York: Van Nostrand Reinhold, pp. 427–452.

Levin, S. (1965). Depression in the aged. In M. A. Berezin & S. H. Cath (eds.). *Geriatric psychiatry: Grief, loss and emotional disorders in the aging process.* New York: International Universities Press, Inc., pp. 203–245.

Lipton, M. A., DiMascio, A., & Killam, K. F. *Psychopharmacology: A generation of progress.* (1978). New York: Raven Press.

McTavish, O. (1971). Perceptions of old people: A review of research methodologies and findings. *The Gerontologist, 11,* 90–101.

Maddox, G. (1964). Disengagement theory: A critical evaluation. *The Gerontologist, 4,* 80–82.

Manton, K. G., Blazer, D. G., & Woodbury, M. A. (1987). Suicide in middle age and later life: Sex and race specific life table and cohort analysis. *Journal of Gerontology* 42(2), pp. 219–227.

Marsella, A. J. (1980). Depressive experience and disorder across cultures. In H. Triandis & J. Draguns (Eds.), *Handbook of cross-cultural psychology, vol. 6: Psychopathology.* Boston: Allyn and Bacon, Inc., pp. 237–289.

Meerloo, J. M. (1961). Modes of psychotherapy in the aged. *Journal of the American Geriatric Society, 9,* 225–234.

Meyer, N. (1977). Diagnostic distribution of admissions to inpatient services of State and County mental hospitals, United States, 1975. *Mental Health Statistical Notes No. 138.* United States National Institute of Mental Health.

Milazzo-Sayre, L. (1978). Changes in the age, sex, and diagnostic composition of resident populations of State and County mental hospitals, United States, 1965–1973. *Mental Health Statistical Note No. 146.* United States National Institute of Mental Health.

Miller, E. (1980). Cognitive assessment of the older adult. In J. E. Birren and R. B. Sloane (Eds.), *Handbook of mental health and aging.* Englewood Cliffs, NJ: Prentice Hall, pp. 520–536.

National Center for Health Statistics (1981). *Characteristics of Nursing Home Residents, Health Status, and Care Received: National Nursing Home Survey, United States, May–Dec., 1977.* Pub. No. (PHS) 81-1712. U.S. Dept. of Health and Human Services.

National Center for Health Statistics (1985). *Vital Statistics of the United States, 1980, Vol II—Mortality, Part B.* USDHHS, PHS, Hyattsville, MD.

Pagelow, M. D. (1984). *Family violence.* New York: Praeger.

Palmore, E. B., & Kivett, V. (1977). Change in life satisfaction: A longitudinal study of persons aged 46–70. *Journal of Gerontology, 32,* 311–316.

Peak, D. (1973). Psychiatric problems of the elderly seen in an outpatient clinic. In E. Pfeiffer (Ed.), *Alternatives to institutional care for older Americans: Practice and planning.* Durham, NC: Center for the Study of Aging and Human Development.

Perlmutter, M. & Hall, E. (1985). *Adult development & aging.* New York; John Wiley & Sons.

Pfeiffer, E. (1970). *Multidimensional functional assessment: The oars methodology.* Durham, NC: Duke University, Center for the Study of Aging and Human Development.

Pfeiffer, E., & Busse, E. W. (1973). Affective disorders. In E. W. Busse and E. Pfeiffer (Eds.), *Mental illness in later life.* Washington: American Psychiatric Association.

Poggi, R. E., & Berland, D. I. (1985). The therapist's reactions to the elderly. *The Gerontologist, 25*(5), 508–513.

Poorkaj, H. (1967). *Social psychological factors and "successful aging."* Doctoral dissertation. University of Southern California, Dissertation Abstracts International, 28(1A), (No. 306).

Post, F. (1962). *The significance of affective symptoms in old age.* Maudsley Monograph 10. London: Oxford University Press.

Redick, R., & Taub, C. (1980). Demography and mental health care of the aged. In J. E. Birren & R. B. Sloane (Eds.), *Handbook of mental health and aging.* Englewood Cliffs, NJ: Prentice Hall, Inc.

Renner, V. J. & Birren, J. E. (1980). Stress: Physiological and psychological mechanisms. In J. E. Birren & R. B. Sloane (Eds.), *Handbook of mental health and aging.* Englewood, NJ: Prentice-Hall, Inc., pp. 310–336.

Riley, M. W., Johnson, M., & Foner, A. (1972). *Aging and society, Sociology of age stratification,* volume 3. New York: Russell Sage Foundation.

Robinson, D. S., Davis, J. M., & Nies, A. (1971). Relation of sex and age to monoamine oxidase activity of human brain, plasma and platelets. *Arch. General Psychiatry, 24,* 536–539.

Romaniuk, M., McAuley, W., & Arling, G. (1983). An examination of the prevalence of mental disorder among the elderly in the community. *Journal of Abnormal Psychology, 92,* 458–467.

Rose, A. M., & Peterson, W. H. (1965). *Older people and their social world: The sub-culture of aging.* Philadelphia: F. A. Davis.

Salzman, C., & Shader, R. I. (1979). Clinical evaluation of depression in the elderly. In A. Roskin & L. Jarvik (Eds.), *Psychiatric symptoms and cognitive loss in the elderly.* Washington, D.C.: Hemisphere Publishing Corp.

Schoonover, S. C. (1983). Depression. In E. L. Bassuk, S. C. Schoonover, & A. J. Gelenberg (Eds.), *The practitioner's guide to psychoactive drugs,* 2nd ed., New York: Plenum Publishing Co.

Segal, J. L., Thompson, J. F., & Floyd, R. A. (1979). Drug utilization and prescribing patterns in a skilled nursing facility: The need for a rational approach to therapeutics. *Journal of the American Geriatrics Society, 27,* 117–122.

Shanas, E. (1977). *The National Survey of the Aged.* Illinois: University of Illinois at Chicago Circle, A. A. Grant # 90-A-369 Final Report.

Steury, S., & Blank, M. (Eds.) (1977). *Readings in psychotherapy with older people.* SHEW Publication No. (ADM.) 77-409/Maryland.

Streib, G. F. (1968). Are the aged a minority group? In B.

Neugarten (Ed.), *Middle age and aging*. Chicago: The University of Chicago Press.

Talley, T., & Kaplan, J. (1956). The negro aged. *Newsletter*. The Gerontological Society, *3*.

Taulbee, L., & Folsom, J. C. (1966). Reality orientation for geriatric patients. *Hospital and Community Psychiatry, 17*, 133–135.

Teaff, J., Lawton, M., Nahemow, L., & Carolson, D. (1978). Impact of age integration on the well-being of elderly tenants in public housing. *Journal of Gerontology, 33*, 126–133.

Templer, D. I., & Cappelletty, M. A. (1986). Suicide in the elderly. In T. L. Brink (Ed.), *Clinical gerontology*. New York: The Haworth Press.

Thompson, G. (1973). Work versus leisure roles: an investigation of morale among employed and retired men. *Journal of Gerontology, 18*, 339–344.

Thompson, T. L., Moran, M. G., & Nies, A. S. (1983). Psychotropic drug use in the elderly. *New England Journal of Medicine, 308*, 134–138.

Ullman, L. P., & Krasner, L. (1965). *Case studies in behavior modification*. New York: Holt, Rinehart and Winston.

United States Bureau of the Census (1984). Projections of the population of the U.S. by age, sex, and race: 1983 to 2080. *Current population reports*, Series P-25, No. 952. pp. 2–9. Washington, D.C.: U.S. Government Printing Office.

United States Department of Health and Human Services (1984). Alzheimer's Disease: *Report of the Secretary's Task Force on Alzheimer's Disease*. Chapter 3. Washington, D.C.: U.S. Government Printing Office.

United States Department of Health and Human Services (1985). *Monthly benefit statistics program data: Old-age survivors disability and health insurance*. Washington, D.C.: U.S. Government Printing Office.

United States General Accounting Office (1977). *Home health: The need for a national policy to provide for the elderly*. Washington, D.C. Report # HRD 78-19.

United States Senate Special Committee on Aging (1983). *Developments in Aging*. Washington, D.C.: U.S. Government Printing Office.

United States Senate Special Committee on Aging (1985). *America in transition: An aging society* (1984–1985 Edition). Washington, D.C.: U.S. Government Printing Office.

United States Senate Special Committee on Aging in Conjunction with the American Association of Retired Persons (1984). *Aging America: Trends and projections*. Washington, D.C.: U.S. Government Printing Office.

Verwoerdt, A. (1981). *Clinical geropsychiatry* (2nd ed.). Baltimore, MD: Williams and Wilkins.

Vickers, R. V. (1976). The therapeutic milieu and the older depressed patient. *Journal of Gerontology, 31*.

Walker, J. C. (1985). Protective services for the elderly: Connecticut's experience. In J. I. Kosberg (Ed.). *Abuse and maltreatment of the elderly: Causes and interventions*. Littleton, MA: John Wright PSG, pp. 292–301.

Wang, H. S. (1977). Dementia in old age. In C. E. Wells (Ed.), *Dementia*, 2nd edition. Contemporary neurology series, Number 15, Philadelphia: Davis, pp. 15–26.

Waxman, H. M., Carner, E. A., & Blum, A. (1983). Depressive symptoms and health service utilization among the community elderly. *Journal of the American Geriatrics Society, 31*, 417–420.

Women's Equity Action League (WEAL) (1985). *Facts on social security*. Washington, D.C.: U.S. Government Printing Office.

Young, J., & Beck, A. T. (1980). *Cognitive therapy rating manual*. Unpublished manuscript. Center for Cognitive Therapy, University of Pennsylvania, Philadelphia, PA.

Zarit, S. H. (1980). *Aging and mental disorders*. New York: Free Press.

Zdorkowski, R., & Galbraith, M. W. (1985). An inductive approach to the investigation of elderly abuse. *Aging and Society, 5*, 413–429.

Zis, A. P. & Goodwin, F. K. (1982). The amine hypothesis. In E. S. Paykel (Ed.). *Handbook of affective disorders*. New York: The Guilford press, pp. 175–190.

Zung, W. (1980). Affective disorders. In Busse and Blazer (Eds.), *Handbook of Geriatric psychiatry*. New York: Van Nostrand Reinhold.

Zung, W. W. K., & Green, R. C. (1972). Detection of affective disorders in the aged. In C. Eisdorfer & W. E. Fann (Eds.), *Psychopharmacology and Aging*. New York: Plenum, pp. 213–224.

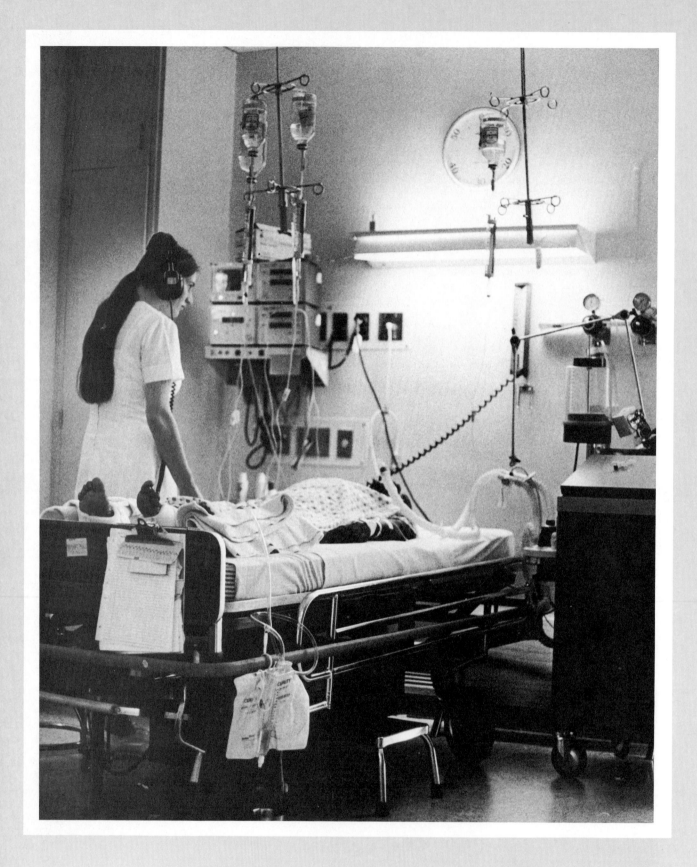

Part Four

PSYCHIATRIC MENTAL HEALTH NURSING WITH SPECIAL POPULATIONS

24

PSYCHIATRIC MENTAL HEALTH NURSING WITH THE VIOLENT PATIENT

BURR EICHELMAN

LEARNING OBJECTIVES

After studying this chapter, the student will be able to:

- Identify and describe the major theories of aggression.
- Assess the violent patient.
- Describe the three means used to control the potentially violent patient.
- Recognize a possible victim of violence and understand victim behavior.
- Describe the role of the nurse with the violent patient, including conflicts and limits in violence intervention.

INTRODUCTION

Interpersonal violence is at an alarming level in our society. Death by homicide was more common than death by bronchitis and emphysema combined (8.6/100,000) in 1986 (U.S. Dept. of Justice, 1987). Battery is the single major cause of injury to women, more significant than automobile accidents, rape, or mugging (O'Reilly, 1983). According to Public Health Reports (1987), an estimated 1.8 million wives and an estimated 6.9 million children are severely assaulted each year, though the number of actual cases reported is way below these figures because of a reluctance to report abuse by family members.

Violence in mental health facilities, which house and care for some of the most troubled members of our society, exists at even higher levels. During the mid-1970s, for instance, a legislative committee in New York reported that there were more than 12,000 violent incidents each year in the twenty-eight psychiatric facilities in New York State (NY State Senate Select Committee, 1976). Aggression can present many formidable challenges for the mental health professional. The term aggression may imply assertive or competitive behaviors or destructive, violent ones. The roles of patient and clinician may become confused with the roles of criminal and law enforcer. Violent behavior permeates clinics and hospitals, where patients are both perpetrators and victims. Consequently, mental health professionals have developed clinical skills that assist in the assessment and management of aggressive, particularly violent, behavior.

A working definition of aggression for this chapter is "behavior that leads to, or appears to an observer to lead to, the damage or destruction of a goal entity" (Moyer, 1968). Violence is defined here as destructive aggression that inflicts physical damage on persons or property.

In addressing the issue of violence, it is more helpful to look at aggressive behavior as a *class* of behaviors and not as a single disease. Both research and treatment of violent behavior have been hampered by a highly variable and poorly developed classification system. According to the DSM-III-R, violent behavior in the adolescent might generate a disruptive behavior disorder diagnosis (conduct disorder group type, solitary aggressive type, or undifferentiated type). (See Chapter 22, Psychiatric Mental Health Nursing with Children.) In the adult, such behavior might be categorized as an intermittent explosive disorder. On the other hand, the behavior might not be classified as a mental disorder at all. (See DSM-III-R

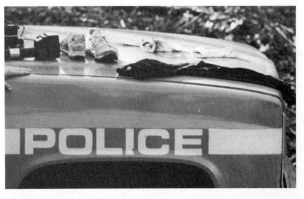

Violence comes in many forms. "Anonymous" urban violence, i.e., violence inflicted on strangers, often receives the most publicity. But violence actually occurs more often between people who know each other.
© Ken Sawchuk/New York Newsday

box.) For example, in certain cases of child abuse, the behavior might be given a DSM-III-R "V" Code of parent-child problem. Violent behavior might also be considered a symptom of other psychiatric disorders including dementia, schizophrenia, alcohol or other drug intoxication, depression, mania, antisocial personality disorder, mental retardation, or attention-deficit hyperactivity disorder.

THEORIES OF AGGRESSION

Several theories have been proposed to explain aggressive behavior. Freud (1958) hypothesized a drive state—thanatos—that was directed toward death and destruction. This **drive theory of aggression** was popularized by Konrad Lorenz in his book *On Aggression* (1966). According to this theory, intervention requires a rechanneling of the release of violent urges in less destructive ways.

A **frustration-aggression theory** proposed by behaviorists Dollard, Miller, and others during the 1930s (Dollard et al., 1939) conceptualized a reservoir of aggressive energy seeking an outlet, (similar to Freud's drive theory). According to this theory, the interruption of goal-directed behavior increases the probability of aggressive behavior. If the goal-directed behavior is repeatedly blocked, the probability of aggression increases proportionately to the frustration. This theory received support from social scientists and has been used to explain ghetto riots and the high incidence of violence among members of the

901

DSM-III-R Diagnostic Criteria for Intermittent Explosive Disorder

A. Several discrete episodes of loss of control of aggressive impulses resulting in serious assaultive acts or destruction of property.

B. The degree of aggressiveness expressed during the episodes is grossly out of proportion to any precipitating psychosocial stressors.

C. There are no signs of generalized impulsiveness or aggressiveness between the episodes.

D. The episodes of loss of control do not occur during the course of a psychotic disorder, organic personality syndrome, antisocial or borderline personality disorder, conduct disorder, or intoxication with a psychoactive substance.

---

disadvantaged portions of society. The social-learning theories (Bandura, 1971) propose that organisms learn violent behavior through modeling or the reinforcement of random activity. Positive reinforcement contingencies maintain violence. For example, the toddler who sees another toddler successfully obtain a dump truck from another child after hitting him tries the same behavior (modeling) and also obtains the truck or other sought-after toy. This success (positive reinforcement) increases the likelihood that the child will try this same strategy in another situation. Such learning-theory techniques as modeling and positive reinforcement can be used to treat violent behavior (Goldstein et al., 1981).

Biological theories also seem to mesh with Freudian drive theory. There appears to be some evidence that antisocial—not necessarily violent—behavior traits can be inherited, having higher-than-chance levels of occurrence even when children from antisocial natural parents are raised by normal foster-parents (Hutchings and Mednick, 1975). Abnormal karyotypes such as XYY have been alleged to be associated with increased violence, but the association remains inconclusively demonstrated (Meyer-Bahlburg, 1981). There is also recent evidence that violent humans with personality disorders may have lowered levels of serotonin metabolites in their spinal fluid and significantly reduced central serotonergic activity (Brown et al., 1979; Linnoila et al., 1983).

ASSESSMENT OF VIOLENT BEHAVIOR

The health professional may be confronted with violent behavior in the emergency room, the admitting area, or the wards of the hospital. He or she may be asked to assess the dangerousness of an individual brought to the medical facility because of his recent violent or threatening behavior. Such an assessment and disposition of the patient involves two areas of expertise: 1) clinical knowledge about the characteristics of violent behavior; and 2) the techniques useful in managing a violent patient. This expertise must be translated into action. Can the patient be assessed alone? Are restraints or hospital security needed? Should the patient be allowed to go home? Should medication be given? Is the risk of harm substantial enough to warn potential victims?

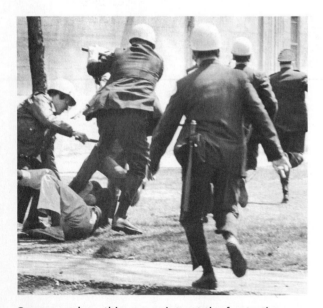

Scenes such as this one point out the frustration-aggression theory. This theory proposes that a reservoir of aggressive energy seeks an outlet and the interruption of goal-directed behavior increases the probability of aggressive behavior.

CHARACTERISTICS OF VIOLENT BEHAVIOR IN THE MEDICAL SETTING

The nurse must be aware that patient violence directed toward health professionals does occur in the hospital setting. Madden, Lion, and Penna (1976) reported results of a survey of psychiatrists that indicated that 48 of 115 respondents had been assaulted. A survey of 31 Los Angeles psychiatry residents noted that 14 had been assaulted (Ruben, Wolkon, & Yamamoto, 1980). Figures for assault in inpatient hospital settings vary widely and probably reflect considerable variability in reporting (Lion & Reid, 1983). However, it is clear that clinicians are at risk for assault and must develop a healthy sense of caution around patients.

There is considerable disagreement in the literature about which patients constitute the greatest risk of assault. Some surveys have reported that schizophrenic patients with either paranoid (Hatti, Dubin, & Weiss, 1982) or schizoaffective characteristics (Shader et al., 1977) are the most violent. Tardiff (1983) found patients with mental retardation, psychotic organic brain syndromes, and nonparanoid schizophrenia more likely to be assaultive in a state hospital setting. Other reports, those with a greater emphasis on outpatients, have described as high-risk patients those with disruptive developmental histories, drug abuse, suicide attempts, and antisocial behavior (Kermani, 1981).

While the prediction of violent behavior is imperfect (Monahan, 1980), most clinicians agree that a constellation of behaviors, present and past, increase the probability of assaultive behavior. These behaviors include agitation, history of suicide attempt or previous assaultive behavior, active resistance to treatment, severe drug intoxication or withdrawal, emotional instability, and threats of violence.

MANAGEMENT OF THE VIOLENT PATIENT

Successful management of the aggressive patient includes the following four steps:

1. Control and stabilize the situation.
2. Make a diagnostic evaluation.
3. Provide the indicated acute treatment.
4. Provide for a longer term treatment plan.

Taking these steps will help the nurse and other health care team members achieve the goals of decreasing tension and preventing the violent episode or its recurrence.

CONTROLLING AND STABILIZING THE SITUATION

During this initial period, the nurse rapidly assesses the presenting circumstances and state of the potentially violent patient. She asks: Is this person armed? Is he or she intoxicated, delusional, or able to maintain some rational dialogue? Since these elements are often very difficult to assess quickly, many health care workers argue for caution and erring on the side of security.

Controlling the patient and situation may simply mean quickly establishing therapeutic rapport, or it may involve the application of restraints and medication. Thus, control may be carried out at three levels: verbal restraint, physical restraint, and chemical restraint.

VERBAL RESTRAINT. Keys to establishing therapeutic rapport and control through verbal restraint include: 1) therapist identification; 2) appropriate physical distance; 3) active listening; 4) paraphrasal; and 5) brief verbal interventions. (See Table 24–1.)

Identifying oneself as a therapist can be as simple as donning a white coat, if dressed in street clothes. The white coat may provide the patient with an inhibition against assault, especially if he is disoriented or delusional. This may also help to distinguish the clinician from the police or complainants (if any) who brought in the individual. When approaching the potentially violent individual, the nurse repeats who she is and why she is there. For example, she may remark to a male patient that his family apparently was concerned that he was going to lose control and hurt someone and that he did seem very angry about something. She now wants to understand what is going on in order to assist him in maintaining con-

---

TABLE 24–1 Keys to establishing therapeutic rapport

1. Identification
2. Appropriate Physical Distance
3. Active Listening
4. Paraphrasal
5. Brief Verbal Interventions

Box 24–1 • Avoiding Murder by a Violent Patient

A gust of December air followed Bill Green into the admitting area of the mental hospital. Dr. White, the resident psychiatrist on duty, looked up, surprised. Only two days before, Bill had declared that he needed to leave the hospital and obtain a gun so that he could kill himself. The staff responded, as they had on many of his other admissions, by beginning antipsychotic medications. This time, however, Bill had escaped before the medications had any chance of helping his paranoid delusions.

Bill walked walked up to the resident and demanded a private talk. Dr. White led him to a small interviewing room and had barely closed the door when Bill suddenly pulled a pistol from his pants pocket. Brandishing it, he angrily stated that he needed to kill the young physician "because you're reading my mind . . . controlling me . . . playing games with my mind . . . messing up my mind with drugs . . . and it's time for a revolution!"

Dr. White tried to calm him, attempting to shift the focus of his rage. After 10 minutes of verbal sparring, both men were sweating, frightened, and under great strain. When the sound of voices in the corridor convinced Dr. White that help was on the way, he lunged for the gun in Bill's hand, grabbing his wrist. The struggle was brief, and the stronger patient overpowered the young physician, who slumped back in his chair. Bill began to rant, alternating threats to the doctor and himself: "I should die! I should end it all right now!" Suddenly, Bill aimed the gun and fired. The bullet smashed into the tiled wall to the right of the physician's head. Another bullet flew past, this time on the other side, and

again the wall exploded with shards of tile. When questioned later, Dr. White reported that Bill had seemed to take "dead aim" at his head, but swerved his hand at the last minute to avoid hurting him. It appeared that, despite his psychosis, the patient's ambivalence prevented him from carrying out the threatened murder.

The shots alerted the ward to the deadly situation. Dr. White now heard raised voices and running feet. Bill appeared stunned, staring at the weapon in his hand, saying nothing. The room filled with acrid smoke and neither man spoke, but a knock at the door made them snap to attention. Bill asked, "Who is it?" and Dr. Black, the senior psychiatrist on the ward, slowly opened the door and peered in. Quickly assessing the crisis, he began to speak from the doorway, attempting to engage Bill as Dr. White had done a few minutes earlier. He asked and received permission to enter the room and sat in the remaining chair.

Now both physicians began to reason with Bill and the debate picked up where it had left off: threats to kill, complaints about people reading his mind and "messing up" his brain. Although the strain was evident in their faces, the psychiatrists worked hard to reason with the agitated man. Unexpectedly, Dr. Black's arm brushed a piece of paper on the desk to the floor. The three men watched it float gently down. Dr. Black slowly picked up the paper, sat back in his chair and began to study it intensely.

A loud gunshot broke the silence and Dr. Black slumped in the chair. Bill looked stunned as he stared at the blood flowing from the

---

trol despite his anger, to prevent injury, and perhaps even to assist in solving the problem that set off the anger. To gain necessary trust in this initial encounter, it is extremely useful for the nurse to make contact with the patient *before* hearing the story from the family, police, or neighbors.

Physical distance is important during verbal intervention. Individuals who are violence prone have been reported to have a larger personal space than their nonviolent counterparts, particularly when approached from behind (Kinzel, 1970). That is, they become anxious (edgy) with the approach of others

wound in the psychiatrist's head. "Please go out," he mumbled to Dr. White without shifting his gaze from his victim. The shaking resident slowly left the room. The ward was quickly evacuated and police called. Bill allowed them to remove Dr. Black and the ambulance could be heard rushing off to the hospital. A four-hour siege ended with Bill's surrender and arrest.

Dr. Black died two days later of a gunshot wound to the head, never having regained consciousness. Bill Green was taken to the state's maximum security mental hospital, where, after an extended period of being declared incompetent, he was able to go to trial. Two-and-a-half years after the murder he was found not guilty by reason of insanity. He remained incarcerated eight years longer, was then transferred to a maximum security hospital in his family's distant home state, and was discharged six months later, as no longer dangerous to himself or others.

Studies of Patient Violence

This tragedy occurred a dozen years ago but the passage of time does not diminish the pain of recalling it. It is frightening to acknowledge the potential dangers of the therapeutic situation, but attempts to understand such events may help to prevent future tragedies.

The most impressive data available today suggest that years of experience correlate with degree of risk. In one study reported in the *American Journal of Psychotherapy* (October, 1981) Bernstein sent questionnaires to 988 therapists in the San Diego area. [While it was found that] 14.2 percent (60 persons) had been as-

saulted on 116 occasions, . . . those with less than 11 years experience [were] assaulted *four* times *more* frequently than those with 11 or more years of experience. Also, [studies show that] there is strong correlation between site of employment and degree of risk; high-risk sites are often training sites and places of first employment for clinicians. Though data are insufficient to determine which factor is more important, it is clear that training in the management of dangerous patients is vital for junior clinicians in high-risk sites.

How can this information be incorporated into day-to-day practice? Note the remarkable parallels between the case of Bill Green and the statistical data:

—The aggressor was a man with a well-documented prior history of both suicidal and assaultive behavior. He had threatened suicide only 48 hours before the actual incident.

—The victim first threatened by the aggressor was a psychiatric resident, clearly in his first years of practice.

—The site of aggression was a high-risk site: the admissions ward of an inner-city mental hospital.

Analysis of interviews with the aggressor and staff at the time of the incident suggests the following issues:

—The availability of a weapon and the aggressor's agitated and confused state created an extremely high risk.

—The attempted struggle over the weapon may have only increased the tension in an already volatile situation.

—The struggle for the weapon shows the therapist's unrealistic sense

of omnipotence in the face of an obviously life-threatening situation.

—Attempts to calmly and rationally defuse the situation through conversation appear to have been a reasonable approach. Although it is impossible to know whether continued discussion might have concluded the crisis nonviolently, experience suggests that such crises are best resolved through skilled negotiation.

—The patient experienced rejection and betrayal when the senior psychiatrist shifted his involvement from him to the paper. The aggressor reports that, from his point of view, the clinician was behaving in a "God-like" manner, showing no fear for his safety. The patient reported that it was his belief that the doctor "wasn't taking me seriously" at that moment.

A clinician confronted with an aggressive patient should treat the situation as realistically as possible. Therapists are as vulnerable to knives and bullets as anyone else. Patients, particularly paranoid and agitated patients, need to know they are cared about and are being taken seriously. It is appropriate to acknowledge fear, a wish to live, and a desire to end the situation without violence. A threat, a weapon, and facial and bodily expressions of rage change the situation significantly. Therapists need to be secure enough to face the reality as they would have their patients face it. Acknowledge vulnerability, deal with the person as a human being of equal value, and show a least as much respect for yourself as for those with whom you interact.

Source: Ebert, R. (1987). "Avoiding murder by a violent patient," *The Psychiatric Times*, Dec., p. 4.

sooner than nonviolent people. Therefore, at first the nurse approaches no closer than twelve feet (four steps), and not from behind. Many clinicians find talking to the patient from an oblique position (45°) the least threatening. It is also helpful to avoid aggressive postures of folded arms or standing above a

seated patient. If rapport develops after perhaps three to five minutes, it may be helpful, for instance, for the nurse to touch the person gently and reassuringly on the forearm, in order to help establish her presence and maintain the reality of the situation.

While obtaining the initial history and establishing rapport, the nurse engages in **active empathic listening**, which includes such body language as eye contact and a sincere, concerned expression as well as questions that signal concern and a desire to clarify the history. The goal of active empathic listening is the conversion of the potentially violent impulses of the patient into verbal, nondestructive output. **Paraphrasal**—that is, the repetition back to the patient in succinct phrases what one understands him to be saying—can be a successful technique of active listening. Examples of paraphrasal include "You are very angry" and "You feel right now that you are angry enough to kill your lover." It is not productive to use only open-ended, neutrally posed, "tell-me-more" kinds of questions when interviewing impulsive, angry individuals in highly charged emotional situations. Violent situations call for greater therapist participation and a more structured interview, which are more likely to decrease rather than increase the patients' agitation or emotionality. Further, the violent patient is often poor at verbal communication skills. It is sometimes this verbal deficit that has prevented him from expressing his rage nonviolently or from correcting the situation that has generated his anger. Finally, as a rule of thumb, it is best to use brief statements in the interchange. The nurse should say what needs to be said in ten seconds, and then allow the patient his chance to ventilate for the next fifty.

Robert: A Violent Patient

Robert was brought to the emergency room in handcuffs by the local police and placed in an examining room. The police told the emergency room clerk that Robert "went berserk" at home and then refused to talk. The emergency room nurse was the first clinician to approach Robert. She observed that he appeared angry and showed signs of arousal (perspiration, flushed face, and rapid pulse noted in his neck). She noted no sign of drug intoxication. He made eye contact and did not appear to be hallucinating. The nurse introduced herself to him as Ms. Seaton, the emergency room nurse; she remained two steps away from him. Ms. Seaton noted to Robert that he looked very angry, but she needed to talk with him because he had been brought in for assessment by the police. She asked Robert, "Would it be safe for me to talk with you with the police outside the room? Would you be able to remain in control if the handcuffs were removed?" (She considered this to be a safe question because no actual assault had been re-

ported.) Robert's affirmative answers to these questions formed the beginning of a "nonviolence contract" between him and Ms. Seaton. In response to Robert's affirmative answers, the police removed the handcuffs and waited across the hall, out of earshot; however, Ms. Seaton left the examining room door open enough so that she and Robert could be observed by the police.

Ms. Seaton began by telling Robert that she knew little about him other than that he was very angry. "What made you so angry?" she queried. At this point, Robert launched into an angry tirade against his best friend whom he just discovered was having an affair with his wife, and stated that he wanted to kill both his wife and friend. Ms. Seaton briefly reiterated this to Robert. As the history taking proceeded she assessed his past history of violence, his access to weapons, and his social-support system to attempt to determine his dangerousness and any necessary acute interventions.

Had Robert been markedly intoxicated or delusional, or unable to make a believable "nonviolence contract" with Ms. Seaton, she could have had the police assist her in transferring Robert to leather restraints prior to her history taking. Even when such a nonviolence contract is elicited initially, it must be reaffirmed during the interview and into the period following the initial therapy contact.

PHYSICAL RESTRAINT. In many cases, the presenting patient is difficult to manage and assess without physically structuring the environment. The most extreme form of physical control is the application of leather restraints; at the other end of the continuum is the use of a restrictive environment. The clinician and patient should be in an area free from excessive stimulation and distractions as well as potential weapons (for example, heavy ashtrays or bottles). The area should be large enough to afford room for additional personnel, and close enough to other staff if additional help is required. Ideally, this area is designed so that the clinician cannot become cornered or locked in by the patient, and open enough that a paranoid patient will not feel trapped.

With very angry, labile, or intoxicated individuals it is often prudent to initiate the intake with a "show of force." This simply means having visible to the patient at least five staff members whose presence reinforces the authority of the clinician who is thus obviously prepared to prevent the patient from going out of control and hurting himself or others. It may be useful to have one or two of these team members be uniformed security personnel. They need not wait within the interview room; they may even be out of earshot of the interview, but they should be visibly present.

Should it become necessary, a five-person team can best immobilize the violent or out-of-control patient. (Some hospitals maintain code teams for behavioral emergencies, much as they do "code blue" resuscitation teams.) The patient is informed by the team that he is going to be immobilized. The team leader assigns a part of the patient's body to each member of the team: his head or an arm or leg. At a prearranged verbal signal, the team moves together, immobilizes the patient, and places him in leather restraints on a litter. During this period of physical restraint, at least one member of the team continues to talk with the patient, attempting to explain why he is being restrained and to reassure him. Some professionals believe that the primary clinician or therapist should, if possible, avoid being a member of the physical restraint team, in order to preserve what might remain of therapeutic rapport. Finally, whenever leather restraints are used, this should be indicated in *the doctor's orders* and a preplanned protocol should be followed to maintain adequate observation and monitoring of the restrained person (see Table 24–2). This will avoid possible complications such as aspiration, if the patient is intoxicated and vomits. The American Psychiatric Association has prepared excellent guidelines concerning restraint (Tardiff, 1984). The use of physical restraints should be considered for patients meeting one or more of the indications in Table 24–3.

CHEMICAL RESTRAINT. Chemical restraint can be useful in decreasing the risk of violence and stabilizing the situation to allow for more complete history-taking and a more thoughtful treatment plan in the case of the individual who is actively violent or who appears to be on the brink of violent behavior. (This is assuming that there are no medical contraindications.) There are three classes of drugs that act rapidly: neuroleptics, benzodiazepines, and barbiturates. Table 24–4 shows examples of treatment doses.

In moderate situational disturbances, 30 mg of oral oxazepam or its equivalent is usually sufficient to defuse the situation. In more volatile situations, or when the violence is associated with schizophrenia or mania, the use of an antipsychotic medication such as haloperidol can be effective. IV medication is usually unnecessary.

STABILIZATION. During the initial period of control and stabilization, the patient's violent behavior

---

TABLE 24–2 Guidelines for care of the patient in leather restraint

1. Restraint use requires a physician's written order at least every 24 hours. (An RN may institute restraints in an emergency situation preceding the written order by no more than one hour.)

2. Reasons for initiating or discontinuing restraints are documented in the progress notes as well as the time applied, the type of restraint, and the patient's response to the restraint.

3. Leather restraints are secured to the bed frame. The restraint key is kept in a nearby, designated location (for example, taped at the foot of the bed under the patient's ID card).

4. Patients in four-point leather restraints are observed every 15 minutes and the observations are documented. Circulation should be assessed as adequate. Bedrails are raised.

5. Patients in restraints must be protected from other patients or dangerous environmental conditions.

6. Restraints are removed and limbs massaged with lotion every two hours. Limbs are exercised at frequent intervals.

7. Patients recently removed from restraints are observed closely for recurrence of the behavior that necessitated restraint.

TABLE 24–3 Indications for considering physical restraint

1. Agitation
2. Suicide attempt
3. History of assaultive behavior
4. Active resistance to emergency treatment
5. Severe drug intoxication or withdrawal
6. Emotional lability
7. Threats of violence

---

should not be allowed to mask life-threatening situations that require immediate intervention. For example, the patient may be suicidal, may have overdosed, and may be acting violently to ward off medical treatment. He may be delirious with encephalitis or meningitis. He may be in shock or in delirium tremens, or may have sustained a subdural he-

TABLE 24—4 Examples of drug doses used in acute modification of behavior

Haloperidol (Haldol)	orally:	5–30 mg	30 min. to 1 hr. for onset
	IM:	5–10 mg	Can be repeated up to every 30 min. barring severe sedation or hypotension; onset in about 20 min.; no marked advantage in IV route of administration
Thiothixene (Navane)	orally:	15–60 mg	
	IM:	10–20 mg	
Oxazepam (Serax)	orally:	15–30 mg	Acutely
Lorazepam (Ativan)	IM:	1–2 mg	Can be repeated IM every 30–60 min., barring severe sedation
Sodium amobarbital (Amytal)	orally:	200–500 mg	
	IM:	200–500 mg	

matoma. Violent behavior in a patient should never become an excuse for failing to check for anisocoria, Babinski reflexes, and fever.

DIAGNOSTIC EVALUATION

Once the situation is stabilized, the clinician moves swiftly to complete the initial diagnostic evaluation, which focuses on psychosocial aspects, disease, and legal issues in order to move toward effective acute treatment and final, long-term treatment planning.

The report of the patient's psychiatric history should include a "present illness," or the facts and circumstances of the immediate precipitants of anger or violence; a past history; a mental-status examination; and a physical examination.

When taking the patient's history, the clinician pays special attention to risk factors that parallel suicide risk factors. Has the patient a specific plan of violence? Is there a named victim? Is there an available weapon? Does the patient have a past history of violent behavior? Is the patient intoxicated or delirious? Is the patient acting on the basis of delusional thinking or command hallucinations (Lion, 1972)?

Since risk to life is often suspected under these circumstances, the clinician obtains as much history and involvement as possible from significant others. He or she does not refrain from calling a spouse or roommate simply because it may be the middle of the night. Failure to follow through with this only denies the gravity of the situation. The involvement of sig-

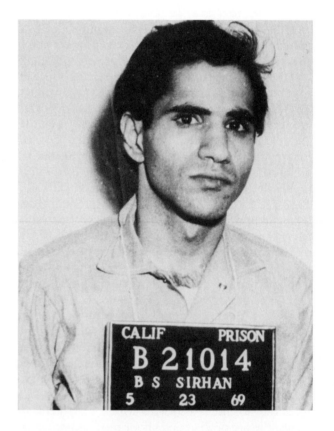

Convicted of the assassination of Robert F. Kennedy, Sirhan Sirhan has been in San Quentin since 1969. He recently requested and was denied parole on the basis of his having made sufficient restitution for his crime, which he says he now sees as heinous and greatly regrets.

nificant others, particularly the potential victim, is often crucial to preventing more violence and/or serious injury.

In addition to understanding the precipitants and assessing the risks of violent behavior, a specific diagnosis is necessary for effective treatment. The intoxicated alcoholic requires an intervention different from the schizophrenic, who requires an intervention different from the patient with a personality disorder.

Finally, the clinician obtains the information that will allow him or her to assess, to the best of their ability, whether there is probable cause that this individual is imminently dangerous to others or to himself. U.S. states differ markedly in the latitude given health professionals in initiating involuntary treatment. For the most part, clinicians are afforded by the law the opportunity, and probably the duty, to detain an individual suspected of being imminently dangerous long enough for an assessment by those responsible for instituting a civil commitment.

In many states, the filing of commitment papers allows the patient to be detained in a designated treatment facility until a probable-cause court hearing is held, often in 48–72 hours. If the court finds probable cause to further detain the individual, a commitment may be instituted or there may follow a further hearing for a final court decision. In some states, treatment is deferred if the patient refuses it until a final hearing (unless the patient exhibits dangerous behavior). It is important for the clinician to be familiar with his or her state commitment laws in order to avoid liability either for failing to intervene in a life-threatening situation or for overreaching the legal limitations and committing battery if the patient refuses voluntary treatment.

In addition to the assessment of the *overtly* violent or threatening patient, there must be a continued inquiry directed to all psychiatric patients regarding their temper, impulse control, and urges to hurt others. The schizophrenic patient who comes to the emergency room seeking a sleeping pill may be—upon closer questioning—experiencing command hallucinations telling him to kill his mother, which he fears he cannot resist any longer. The quiet spouse bringing his wife to the emergency room with a blackened eye "from a door" may only need brief encouragement to affirm his abusive behavior and commit himself to treatment. The mother who brings her toddler with burned buttocks to the emergency room must be questioned regarding child abuse. If the difficult questions are never asked, the critical life-saving interventions may never get a chance to commence.

Notes of a Murderer.

ACUTE AND PROLONGED TREATMENT PLANNING

Keys to successful management of the violent patient lie in making a proper diagnosis as well as attempting to remove the acute precipitants. In general, the rule of thumb for treating violent behavior (once the patient is stabilized) is to treat the underlying condition. Thus treatment of violent behavior that is associated with delusions or hallucinations in schizophrenics requires management of the schizophrenic symptoms with more aggressive neuroleptic and psychotherapeutic interventions. Violent manic patients are treated pharmacologically with neuroleptics and lithium. Depressed patients can be treated with psychotherapy and antidepressants. Patients with acute brain syndromes due to drug intoxication or withdrawal are detoxified in accordance with standard routines. Patients with chronic organic brain syndromes are treated with a more simplified and protective environment and perhaps low doses of a neuroleptic. Patients whose violence stems from a seizure disorder require a diagnostic workup to determine the etiology of the seizures, followed by an effective anticonvulsant regimen.

For impulse-control personality disorders, treatment regimens have included psychotherapy with a reality/consequence base (Goldstein et al., 1981) and occasionally psychopharmacologic treatment with lithium, benzodiazepines, propranolol, or anticonvulsants (Eichelman, 1986). Child- and spouse-abuse therapy programs have made use of group therapy with instruction in new coping strategies and role modeling (Sonkin, Martin, & Walker, 1985). (See Chapter 18 on crisis for more on treatment of abused children.) Programs dealing with sexual violence have attempted therapies based on group and behavior-modification techniques as well as the prescription of "antiandrogen" drugs (Money, 1970). All of these regimens are innovative at best and require substantial efficacy studies. An NIMH monograph (Roth, 1985) provides an in-depth review of the treatment of the violent patient.

The following cases illustrate briefly the differences in treatment regimens for violent behavior.

John: A Violent Patient with Schizophreniform Disorder

John was a 21-year-old, white, single male under commitment following his assault on a community worker. He had been living at home, but was disheveled, eating only sporadically, and was essentially mute. When approached by staff, he would mumble incoherently with occasional outbursts of, "Get away!" If staff continued to approach, he would threaten assault until they backed away. All medical evaluation had to be performed while John was restrained. John's blood chemistries were normal, as were his X-rays, an EEG, and a CT scan. As part of a diagnostic interview sodium amytal was administered (see Eichelman, Estess, & Gonda, 1977) during which John became communicative and presented a marked thought disorder with much delusional thinking. John was diagnosed as having a schizophreniform disorder (see Chapter 10 on Schizophrenia) and was treated with gradually increasing doses of a neuroleptic, following which he became more communicative and socialized without violent outbursts, although he still remained hospitalized.

James: A Violent Patient with Intermittent Explosive Disorder and Alcohol Abuse

James was a 34-year-old, white, married male who worked in a lumberyard. His first marriage ended in divorce because of his serious assaultive behavior. He had been remarried for two years, but once again, his marriage was jeopardized by episodic unpredictable violent outbursts, both verbal and physical. The violence was often but not exclusively associated with his or his wife's drinking. A precipitant often seemed to be the management of the children, ages 6 and 8. There was also a family history of depression, although James did not meet the DSM-III-R criteria for a major depressive episode. Rather, he was diagnosed as having an intermittent explosive disorder and an episodic alcohol-abuse disorder. Treatment interventions required first addressing the drinking problems. Both husband and wife were referred to Alcoholics Anonymous. The issues of coparenting were addressed in a problem-solving couples therapy that taught and encouraged nonviolent coping strategies. The impulsivity and possible affective component in James's history prompted a concurrent trial of lithium. Thus in this case intervention was multifaceted and involved both perpetrator and victim.

Karl: An Abusive Parent

Karl was a 26-year-old, white, pharmacology student living in university married-student housing. His wife, Carol, was employed as a secretary. Their son, two-and-a-half-year old Joshua, was brought to the university hospital emergency room on a Friday morning with burns across his buttocks. Karl claimed that Joshua had backed into a radiator. However, careful physical examination of Joshua revealed bruises on his forearms and buttocks with healing "belt" marks on the back. X-rays of the long bones showed subperiosteal thickening. Joshua was hospitalized and a report of suspected child abuse was filed by the pediatric social worker with the county's child protective services department. Initially, Karl and his wife denied any role in Joshua's injuries. The staff's refusal to accept the explanations offered for the injuries finally prompted Karl's confession to his loss of control and assault upon Joshua during bouts of prolonged crying or toilet training "accidents." With Karl's statement, his wife confirmed her husband's behavior, which she had witnessed, but on which she felt paralyzed to act. After discharge, Joshua was placed in a therapeutic foster home; however, frequent parental visitation was encouraged. Social workers made frequent regular assessments during parental visitation as well as at other times. Karl's sentence for child abuse (sixty days in jail) was suspended by a judge who was convinced that treatment rather than punishment stopped the generational cycle of child abuse. Karl entered and completed treatment in a program for abusive parents that taught alternatives to violence and dispelled some of the associated parental myths that can accompany child abuse. (For example, "He soiled his pants just to get even with me. He knew better.") Karl also became acquainted with a parental hotline he could use once Joshua returned home, if he became angry at Joshua and felt like hurting him.

Box 24–2 ● Domestic Violence: Who is Responsible?

The popular image of the domestic aggressor is a man who abuses his wife and children. A social worker and a teacher of disturbed children have written an article claiming that this image oversimplifies a complicated situation and distorts our understanding of an important social issue.

According to the authors, most studies show that women are not passive victims of family violence. Wives kill their husbands just as often as husbands kill their wives, and surveys suggest that female violence in marriage is about as common as male violence. One survey found that wives struck husbands just as often as husbands struck wives, and women were just as likely as men to initiate violence, although men caused serious injury more often because of their greater strength. A telephone survey found that 19 percent of men and 13 percent of women had been struck by a spouse. Another study found that 5 percent of husbands and 5 percent of wives had been victims of family violence as often as once every two months; 7.5 percent of wives and 2.5 percent of husbands were victimized once a month or more.

In a survey of a representative national sample, women were shown to have committed an average of ten assaults a year against husbands and men an average of eight assaults a year against their wives. In most cases this meant only grabbing, pushing, or slapping, but women were actually more likely to perpetrate some of the more severe forms of violence. They kicked, bit, and hit with fists more often, and they more often threatened to use knives or guns. Men were more likely to beat up women (an average of 1.7 versus 1.4 times a year), and they used guns and knives more. The authors point out that this survey probably underestimated the actual rate of domestic violence because it excluded divorced and separated couples.

The National Crime Survey, which is funded by the Department of Justice and conducted by the Bureau of the Census, revealed that in 6200 cases of domestic assault (some reported to the police and some reported only to interviewers), men were injured more often and more seriously than women, chiefly because women were more likely to attack with something besides their hands.

The authors also point out that the current trend suggests decreasing abuse of women as compared with men. They report a survey showing that in 1975, 12.1 percent of women reported at least one incident of domestic violence; in 1985, 11.3 percent reported an incident. The percent reporting severe violence dropped from 3.8 percent to 3 percent, a 26 percent decrease. Reports of severe violence directed against men also decreased between 1975 and 1985, but reports of less severe

continued

forms of violence actually increased from 11.6 percent to 12.1 percent.

The authors say that the standard picture of domestic violence is derived largely from police reports and interviews in which both spouses are present. They believe that these sources are unreliable because men are hesitant to lodge official complaints and reluctant to admit to an interviewer that they have been abused by their wives, especially when the wives are present. The authors also say that the histories of battered women undergoing psychotherapy or living in shelters create a misleading impression when they are taken as typical of domestic violence in general.

According to the authors, men remain in violent homes for some of the same reasons women do. They may be trying to protect the children from women who are likely to gain custody after divorce. (One survey found that mothers abuse children 62 percent more often than fathers.) Men also stay on for economic reasons; their standard of living is likely to fall when they leave, especially if they pay child support.

Source: *Harvard Medical School Mental Health Letter* (1988) Vol. 4, No. 11, p. 6. R. L. McNeely and Gloria Robinson-Simpson. The truth about domestic violence: a falsely framed issue. *Social Work*, 32:6:485–490 (November/December 1987).

George: A Sexually Abusive Parent

George was a 38-year-old divorced male. He had visitation rights with his 12-year-old daughter and his 11- and 8-year-old sons every other weekend. His ex-wife heard the boys talking about "Daddy's weiner" and its white juice. In talking with her children, she learned that George had been showering with the boys and apparently had them masturbate him to orgasm. When she spoke with her daughter, no episodes of intercourse were described, but she did admit that Daddy had touched her "down there" several times when she had come into his bedroom before going to sleep. George would not fully admit to the alleged behaviors. Nevertheless his ex-wife reported him to the police and filed sexual-abuse charges, of which George was convicted. He was paroled on the condition he participate in a forensically based sexual-abuse program in which he received peer counseling in a group format (see Giaretto, 1982). The children also received counseling and George was subsequently allowed visitation with them, at first under supervised conditions.

THE VICTIM AND VIOLENCE

Often the nurse is presented with the violent individual as the sole identified patient. It is the obligation of the astute clinician to look for and attend to his nonviolent victims. The depressed housewife may be a target for spouse abuse. The child brought to the clinic with nightmares and school problems may be responding to episodes of parental beatings. Unless the nurse asks the key questions, these terrorized individuals may remain silent. Table 24–5 lists physical and behavioral indicators of possible child abuse. Work with hostage victims has revealed a powerful positive attachment that can develop in the victim toward the terrorist (the Stockholm syndrome). This can often impede intervention. Moreover, some vic-

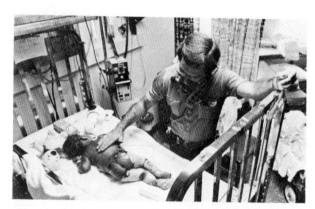

This police officer can't resist comforting the infant, a victim of one of the worst kinds of child abuse—burning. Most child abuse is impulsive and results in bruises, at most broken bones, and is regretted by the parent almost immediately. The child is brought in for medical evaluation and the sharp nurse or physician will put the facts together and come up with a diagnosis of possible child abuse. The child is usually placed in the hospital overnight during which time the Hospital Child Abuse Team will evaluate the situation and determine whether it warrants reporting to the county social services department. (For more on child abuse, see the chapters on crisis, violence, and children.)

TABLE 24–5 Physical and behavioral indicators of child abuse and neglect

Type of CA/N	Physical Indicators	Behavioral Indicators
Physical abuse	Unexplained Bruises and Welts: —on face, lips, mouth —on torso, back, buttocks, thighs —in various stages of healing —clustered, forming regular patterns —reflecting shape of article used to inflict (electric cord, belt buckle) —on several different surface areas —regularly appear after absence, weekend or vacation Unexplained Burns: —cigar, cigarette burns, especially on soles, palms, back or buttocks —immersion burns (sock-like, glove-like, doughnut shaped on buttocks or genitalia) —patterned like electric burner, iron, etc. —rope burns on arms, legs, neck or torso Unexplained Fractures: —to skull, nose, facial structure —in various stages of healing —multiple or spiral fractures Unexplained Lacerations or Abrasions: —to mouth, lips, gums, eyes —to external genitalia	Wary of Adult Contacts Apprehensive When Other Children Cry Behavioral Extremes: —aggressiveness, or —withdrawal Frightened of Parents Afraid to go Home Reports Injury by Parents
Physical neglect	Consistent Hunger, Poor Hygiene, Inappropriate Dress Consistent Lack of Supervision, Especially In Dangerous Activities or Long Periods Constant Fatigue or Listlessness Unattended Physical Problems or Medical Needs Abandonment	Begging, Stealing Food Extended Stays at School (early arrival and late departure) Constantly Falling Asleep in Class Alcohol or Drug Abuse Delinquency (e.g. thefts) States There is No Caretaker
Sexual abuse	Difficulty in Walking or Sitting Torn, Stained or Bloody Underclothing Pain or Itching in Genital Area Bruises or Bleeding in External Genitalia, Vaginal or Anal Areas Venereal Disease, Especially in Pre-teens Excessive Masturbation Pregnancy	Unwilling to Change for Gym or Participate in PE Withdrawal, Fantasy, or Infantile Behavior Bizarre, Sophisticated, or Unusual Sexual Behavior or Knowledge Poor Peer Relationships Delinquent or Run Away Reports Sexual Assault by Caretaker

continued

TABLE 24–5 continued

Type of CA/N	Physical Indicators	Behavioral Indicators
Emotional maltreatment	Habit Disorders (sucking, biting, rocking, etc.) Conduct Disorders (antisocial, destructive, etc.) Neurotic Traits (sleep disorders, speech disorders, inhibition of play) Psychoneurotic Reactions (hysteria, obsession, compulsion, phobias, hypochondria)	Behavior Extremes: —compliant, passive or —aggressive, demanding Overly Adaptive Behavior: —inappropriately adult —inappropriately infantile Developmental Lags (physical, mental, emotional) Attempted Suicide

Source: Adapted from Schmitt, B. D., Bross, D. C., Carroll, C., Gray, J. D., Grosz, C. A., Kempe, C. H., & Lenherr, M. R., (1978). *Guidelines for the hospital and clinic: Management of child abuse and neglect,* DHEW publication no. 79-30167, Washington, D.C.; U.S. Dept. of Health, Education, and Welfare.

tims have limited means to escape and must be educated about community resources such as shelters for battered women.

At times, the victim may be involved in inciting or risk-taking behavior that also requires intervention. It is frequently cited that fifty percent of homicides are committed by persons who have been using alcohol (Wolfgang, 1958). It is less frequently noted that fifty percent of the *victims* are also alcohol users (Wolfgang, 1967). Victims may bait or challenge the aggressor; they may even provide the weapon. Successful intervention should include interacting with a named potential victim, from warning this person to attempting more directly to counsel this person about possible behavior patterns this person is employing that raise the probability of victimization.

THE NURSE AND VIOLENCE

Dealing with violent patients carries some physical risks as outlined earlier in this chapter. These real risks provide the basis for countertransference issues that may impede assessment and treatment or may increase the risk of injury. Peer supervision and/or interdisciplinary consultation is the best prevention for this common problem.

The most frequent reactions to the violent patient include fear and emotional (and sometimes physical) distancing. The nurse may also feel revulsion toward the patient who has been violent. Such emotional distancing can impede sensitive monitoring of the patient necessary to clearly read his degree of anger and potential loss of control. It can also be read as anger by the patient. It blocks the potential for a therapeutic relationship between staff and patient that is often the cornerstone of successful intervention. Distancing can take many forms; it can manifest itself in staff withholding last names and taping over name tags; it can be detected in a diminished number of verbal exchanges or reduced physical contact by nursing staff; and it can be reflected by the staff's agitation for a rapid transfer of the violent patient off the unit, even if the alternative is of low therapeutic merit. All these elements of "fearful distancing" may be underscored with elaborate rationalizations by the staff. Extensive group processing may be necessary to unmask the staff's fear and reduce the rationalizing that can impede the formation of a therapeutic alliance with the patient.

Counterphobic behaviors may also develop (for example, "In order to prove that I'm not afraid, I will take a tough stance"). In this process, the staff may begin to set unreasonable or unenforceable limits. Such behavior can be exceedingly risky. The 4-foot, 6-inch tall nurse telling the 6-foot, 2-inch tall patient that she will prevent him from leaving the unlocked ward is an open invitation for assault. The trembling nurse who stammers that she is not afraid when admitting a violent individual loses credibility; the nurse who honestly replies that loud, agitated behavior is both frightening and distancing increases her credibility. The male nurse who moves rapidly into an agitated patient's personal space may display a lack of fear, but he illustrates poor clinical judgment and increases the risk of assault. It is not only a good clinical move for the nurse to check with the patient about the patient's own sense of potential violence, but such frank dialogue can often pave the way for more honest communication in the future. If limits must be set with the patient to ensure safety, the nurse should set limits that are unequivocally enforceable even if this requires calling for help and a "show of force." Awareness of negative countertransference can aid in reducing "punitive" treatments such as overmedication or refusal of appropriate ward privileges.

CONFLICTS AND LIMITS IN VIOLENCE INTERVENTION

Good clinical care of the violent patient can pose both legal and ethical dilemmas for the nurse. A common example is the conflict between the principles of confidentiality and the duty to warn named victims (also see Chapter 28 on Ethical Issues in Mental Health Practice). This tension is reflected in the Tarasoff decision in California (*Tarasoff* v. *Board of Regents,* 1976) in which the court holds that a therapist should warn a named potential victim. To date, this law has not been tested in most other states; nevertheless, clinicians have been confronted for some time with legal precedent to breach confidentiality and warn potential victims if the threats they hear from patients are convincing.

Tension exists between issues of personal responsibility and biological determinism when the court asks for clinical participation in an assessment of a psychiatric legal defense (that is, not guilty by reason of mental illness), in which mental illness serves as an excusing condition. The clinician is often trapped in the middle: for example, if a patient assaults a nurse on a psychiatric unit, the local district attorney may refuse to prosecute, alleging that the patient is "sick" and not responsible. This, in turn, may serve as a positive reinforcer for the nonpsychotic, violence-prone personality-disordered patient, and lead to more violence. Psychiatric inpatient unit staff themselves often have great difficulty in assigning responsibility for their behavior to their disturbed patients.

Social problems have often generated an overambitious response from the health-care community. We must acknowledge that there is no standard medical treatment for the hired assassin who works just as methodically as if he were an accountant. Even in treating impulse-disordered or sociopathic personality-disordered individuals, most therapists would now affirm that *the disorder is not an excuse for the antisocial behavior* and that the individual must accept the legal consequences of his behavior, which might include fines, jail, or even execution. This is a change from the liberal "Durham rule" applied during the 1960s, which sent personality-disordered individuals to St. Elizabeth's Hospital in Washington, D.C., rather than to jail.

Social problems pose tantalizing areas for mental health clinicians' involvement. At times, these clinicians have been asked to serve as mediators for labor or political disputes or in hostage situations. Success in these ventures probably relates to the interpersonal skills of the mediator or to specialized training in negotiation, rather than to any particular mental health care expertise. Courts often call upon clinicians to offer opinions about whether a person is lying or to predict long-term future dangerousness. *Studies generally confirm that clinical training does not produce special expertise in these areas and the wise clinician will simply acknowledge her inability to offer an informed clinical opinion* (Wiggins, 1973).

Societal interventions can raise difficult ethical issues for the clinician (Eichelman & Lion, 1983). Is the nurse, for example, functioning in the role of a health professional? Or is she working as an agent for social change? In a hostage event, should a health professional ally him or herself with agencies that frequently employ deceit? The clinician should enter these areas with caution, paying attention to the ethics of the situation, the best interests of the "patient," and any specialized training required. The clinician's role should be clearly revealed, particularly if it differs from the traditional role of the health professional as caregiver. (Also see Chapter 28 on ethics in psychiatry.)

Violence is a social problem, but it is also a public health and clinical problem. It presents itself to the health-care professional requiring, even demanding, assessment and intervention. Successful clinical interventions must often utilize a variety of approaches grounded in psychoanalytic, behavioral, and biological theory. The nurse who works with the violent patient must remain compassionate and sensitive but keenly alert to risk. One must be ready to affirm limits but refrain from punitive intervention. The clinician must also avoid grandiose machismo stances, but nevertheless be effective at mobilizing clinical and social resources to block the expression of violence.

Case Study: Psychiatric Setting

Linda was admitted to the psychiatric unit of University Hospital at 8:00 P.M. She was brought there by police who were called to the post-partum unit of a small community hospital after Linda delivered a heavy blow to the jaw of her obstetrician. She had delivered a healthy newborn baby girl about eight hours previously. This was the first child for Linda, who was unmarried and living with the child's father. Linda's mother was available, as she had recently arrived in town for a long visit to help Linda with the baby. It was not clear what elicited Linda's violent behavior. She told a nurse that her doctor "had a foul mouth" and "tried to rape me." While arrangements were being made for Linda's transfer, the community hospital's social worker called the county social services crisis number to report a child (Linda's baby) in need of protective services.

When Linda and her boyfriend were interviewed in the University Hospital emergency room by the psychiatry resident on call, a history of mood swings since adolescence was elicited. While Linda had never been severely depressed, she occasionally became "hyperactive." This involved taking on extra jobs in her landscaping business and working fifteen-hour days, as well as going without sleep for days at a time. Linda would also "party" more than usual during these episodes, wearing out her boyfriend. Linda had no history of previous violent behavior. Her family history was positive for alcoholism and suicide (at age 63 by her maternal grandfather). Linda's recent history, reported by her boyfriend, included three days of heightened activity and little sleep in preparation for the baby's arrival. Linda had painted the nursery, shampooed all the carpets in their apartment, and gone on a shopping spree for baby clothes and equipment. Currently, Linda manifested pressured speech, flight of ideas, distractibility, and delusional thinking. (She told the ER nurse that her doctor raped her after her delivery.) Linda was diagnosed as in a manic episode with psychotic features and involuntarily detained and admitted to the psychiatric unit of University Hospital. She was given 20 mg of Navane IM and started on lithium therapy. Blair Stephenson, who admitted Linda to the psychiatric unit and became her primary nurse, developed the following nursing care plan after spending about an hour with her patient.

DSM III-R Diagnosis

Axis I: Bipolar disorder, manic, with psychotic features (266.44)
Axis II: No diagnosis on Axis II
Axis III: Recent delivery of healthy baby
Axis IV: Psychosocial stressors: birth of first child, living with but not married to father, mother available to help. Severity : 4
Axis V: GAF : 0 (inadequate information)

Nursing Diagnosis

Alteration in thought processes
Potential for injury to self and others
Family coping: potential for growth

Nursing Care Plan for Linda

Nursing Diagnosis	Desired Outcomes	Intervention	Rationale
1. Alteration in thought processes	Effective treatment of Linda's mania	Start Linda on Navane and lithium per medical orders. When Linda settles down and is able to absorb information, explain the purpose of each medication to her and to family members who are present, along with their side effects including the possibility of acute extrapyramidal effects of Navane.	Linda's recent history of injuring her physician whom she thought raped her, and her hypomanic and manic behavior is an indication for acute administration of anti-psychotic medication and beginning treatment with lithium.
2. Potential for injury to self and others	Linda's safety and that of others with whom she comes into contact will be assured.	Maintain a one-to-one nursing contact and/or constant presence of a trusted family member until Linda is no longer acutely psychotic.	Until Linda's paranoia has subsided, she will need close observation and attention and reassurance about her and her child's safety.
3. Family coping: potential for growth	Reunion of Linda and her baby	The treatment plan must take into consideration the need to protect and foster the mother-child relationship. Arrange for gradually increasing supervised visitation for Linda and her baby. The County Social Services Department will need to be contacted due to their current (and likely to be continuing) involvement with this family to help family members (mother and boyfriend) plan for Linda's and her baby's return home. With Social Services, determine if additional support services will be necessary and help to arrange for them.	Frequent, regular contact between Linda and her baby in a safe context is essential to the ongoing process of attachment. Focusing on the return of Linda's baby to her, their beginning relationship, and their return home together will promote Linda's attachment to her baby.
		Help Linda get used to the idea of being a mother by helping to arrange enough visitation time to permit	Since this is Linda's first baby, she will need the usual nursing care given to new mothers on the post-partum unit.

Nursing Diagnosis	Desired Outcome	Interventions	Rationale
		bathing, feeding, and quiet time for Linda and the baby. Involve family members as appropriate.	
		Participate with other members of the health-care team and Social Services in determining when discharge with support services is in the interest of Linda and her baby.	Psychiatric unit nursing staff are in an excellent position to promote and help determine Linda's ability to care for herself and her baby with support, first in the hospital, and then at home with family.

SUMMARY

Violence has reached an alarming level in U.S. society. Violent behavior can be defined as destructive aggression that inflicts physical damage on persons or property; aggression can be behavior that leads to, or appears to lead to, the damage or destruction of a goal entity.

Several theories have been formulated to explain aggressive behavior—Freud's drive theory, Dollard and Miller's frustration-aggression theory, and the various social-learning theories, which incorporate concepts of desensitization and dehumanization of victims.

Violent behavior occurs regularly in mental health care facilities, and the nurse must take great care to protect her own safety as well as the safety of other patients, health care workers, and the violent individual and his family. When the nurse begins assessment of the violent patient, she attempts to answer five critical questions: 1) Can the patient be assessed alone? 2) Are restraints or hospital police needed? 3) Should the patient be allowed to go home? 4) Should medication be given? 5) Is the risk of harm substantial enough to warn potential victims?

There are four steps to successful management of the violent patient: 1) controlling and stabilizing the situation; 2) making a diagnostic evaluation; 3) providing the indicated acute treatment; and 4) providing for a longer term disposition. In managing the patient, the nurse uses several key interventions to establish therapeutic rapport: identification, appropriate physical distance, active listening, paraphrasal, and brief verbal interventions. If the patient must be restrained, the staff can employ verbal, physical, or chemical restraints.

The nurse may be in a position to recognize possible victims of abuse; for example, the depressed housewife or the depressed child with unexplained injuries. The nurse may be able to uncover abusive situations simply by asking key questions of these possible victims.

The nurse is at some physical risk in dealing with the violent patient and may respond to him with fear and distancing; such countertransference may not only impede assessment and treatment, but may increase the nurse's risk of injury. Thus she should be aware of these feelings, attempt to deal with them, and not work with the violent patient *alone,* until she is able to do so safely and therapeutically.

There are some conflicts and limits in violence intervention. A common example of this is the conflict between confidentiality and a duty to warn named potential victims, as illustrated by the *Tarasoff* v. *Board of Regents* decision in 1976. A mental health professional may be called to try to intervene in a hostage event as a mediator rather than a caregiver.

Mental health professionals are often asked by the court to give an informal opinion about whether a person is lying or whether he may be dangerous. Studies have shown that it is difficult, if not impossible, to do either. If the nurse finds herself facing any of these difficult ethical issues she should recognize her role as caregiver, and respond accordingly.

KEY TERMS

aggression

violence

drive theory of
aggression

frustration-aggression
theory

desensitization

dehumanization of
victims

active empathic
listening

paraphrasal

STUDY QUESTIONS

1. Define the terms *aggression* and *violence* as they pertain to mental health nursing.

2. According to social-learning theory, how does an organism learn violent behavior?

3. Name and describe briefly the four steps in successful management of the violent patient.

4. How might the nurse recognize a patient as a possible victim of violence?

5. How does countertransference affect the nurse's effectiveness with a violent patient? Explain.

REFERENCES

American Psychiatric Association (1987). *Diagnostic and statistical manual of mental disorders* (DSM III-R, Third Edition, Revised. Washington, D.C.: American Psychiatric Association.

Bandura, A. (1971). Social learning theory of aggression. In J. F. Knutson (Ed.), *Control of aggression*. Chicago: Aldine, pp. 201–250.

Brown, G. L., Ballanger, J. C., Minichiello, M. D., & Goodwin, F. K. (1979). Human aggression and its relation to cerebrospinal fluid 5-hydroxyindole-acetic acid, 3-methoxy-4-hydroxyphenylglycol, and homovanillic acid. In M. Sandler (Ed.), *Psychopharmacology of aggression*. New York: Raven Press, pp. 131–148.

Dollard, J. C., Doob, L., Miller, N., Mowrer, O., & Sears, R. (1939). *Frustration and aggression*. New Haven: Yale University Press.

Eichelman, B. (1986). The biology and somatic experimental treatment of aggressive disorders. In H. K. H. Brodie & P. A. Berger (Eds.), *American handbook of psychiatry*, vol. VIII. New York: Basic Books.

Eichelman, B., Estess, F. M., & Gonda, T. A. (1977). Hypnotic agents in psychiatric evaluation. In J. D. Barchas, P. A. Berger, R. D. Ciaranello, & G. R. Elliott (Eds.), *Psychopharmacology from theory to practice*. New York: Oxford University Press, pp. 270–275.

Freud, S. (1958, originally published in 1930). Civilization and its discontents. In J. Strachey (Ed.), *The standard edition of the complete works of Sigmund Freud*, vol 21. London: Hogarth Press, pp. 64–145.

Giarretto, H. (1982). Integrated treatment of child sexual abuse: a treatment and training manual. Palo Alto, CA: Science and Behavior Books, Inc.

Goldstein, A. P., Carr, E. G., Davidson, W. S., & Wehr, P. (1981). *In response to aggression: methods of control and prosocial alternatives*. Elmsford, NY: Pergamon Press.

Hatti, S., Dubin, W. R., & Weiss, K. J. (1982). A study of circumstances surrounding patient assaults on psychiatrists. *Hospital & Community Psychiatry, 33*, 660–661.

Hutchings, B., & Mednick, S. A. (1975). Registered criminality in the adoptive and biological parents of registered male criminal adoptees. In R. R. Fieve & B. Rosenthal (Eds.), *Genetic research in psychiatry*. Baltimore: John Hopkins University Press, pp. 105–116.

Kermani, E. J. (1981). Violent psychiatric patients: a study. *American Journal of Psychotherapy, 35*, 215–225.

Kinzel, A. F. (1970). Body-buffer zone in violent prisoners. *American Journal of Psychiatry, 127*, 99–104.

Linnoila, M., Virkkunen, M., Scheinin, M., Nuutila, A., Rimon, R., & Goodwin, F. K. (1983). Low cerebrospinal fluid 5-hydroxyindole acetic acid concentration differentiates impulsive from non-impulsive violent behavior. *Life Sciences, 33*, 2609–2614.

Lion, J. R. (1972). *Evaluation and management of the violent patient*. Springfield: Charles C. Thomas.

Lion, J. R., & Reid, W. H. (Eds.) (1983). *Assaults within psychiatric facilities*. New York: Grune & Stratton.

Lorenz, K. (1966). *On aggression*. New York: Harcourt, Brace, Jovanovich, Inc.

Madden, D. J., Lion, J. R., & Penna, M. (1976). Assaults on psychiatrists by patients. *American Journal of Psychiatry, 133*, 422–425.

Meyer-Bahlburg, H. F. L. (1981). Sex chromosomes and aggression in humans. In P. F. Brain & D. Benton (Eds.), *The biology of aggression*. Rockville: Sijthoff & Noordhoff, pp. 109–123.

Monahan, J. (1980). *The clinical prediction of violent behavior*. D.H.H.S. Pub. No. (ADM) 81–921. Washington, D.C.: U.S. Government Printing Office.

Money, J. (1970). Use of androgen-depleting hormone in the treatment of male sex offenders. *Journal of Sex Research, 6*, 165–172.

Moyer, K. E. (1968). Kinds of aggression and their pathological basis. *Communications in behavioral biology* (Part A), *2*, 65–87.

National Center for Health Statistics, (1987). *Public Health* Report. Washington, D.C.: U.S. Government Printing Office.

New York State Senate Select Committee on Mental and Physical Handicap. Senator James H. Donovan, chairman (1975–1976). *Violence revisited . . . a report on traditional indifference in state mental institutions toward assaultive activity.*

O'Reilly, J. (1983 September 5). Wife beating; the silent crime. *Time*, 23–26.

Roth, L., Ed. (1985). *Clinical treatment of the violent person*. D.H.H.S. Publ. No. (ADM) 85-1425. Washington, D.C.: U.S. Government Printing Office.

Ruben, I., Wolkon, G., & Yamamoto, J. (1980). Physical attacks on psychiatric residents by patients. *Journal of Nervous and Mental Diseases, 168*, 243–245.

Shader, R. I., Jackson, A. H., Harmatz, J. S., & Applebaum, P. S. (1977). Patterns of violent behavior among schizophrenic inpatients. *Diseases of the Nervous System, 38,* 13–16.

Sonkin, D. J., Martin, D., & Walker, L. E. A. (1985). *The male batterer: a treatment approach.* New York: Springer Publishing Co.

Tarasoff v. *Board of Regents* (1976). 17 Cal.3d 425, 131 Cal. Reptr. 14, 551 P.2d 334.

Tardiff, K. (1983). A survey of assault by chronic patients in a state hospital system. In J. R. Lion & W. H. Reid (eds.), *Assaults within psychiatric facilities.* New York: Grune & Stratton, pp. 3–19.

Tardiff, K. (Ed.)(1984). *The psychiatric uses of seclusion and restraint.* Washington, D.C.: American Psychiatric Association Press.

U.S. Department of Justice, Bureau of Justice Statistics. (1987). *Sourcebook of criminal justice statistics.* Washington, D.C.: U.S. Government Printing Office.

Wiggins, J. S. (1973). *Personality and prediction, principles of personality assessment.* Reading, Mass.: Addison-Wesley, pp. 120–180.

Wolfgang, M. E. (1958). *Patterns in criminal homicide.* Philadelphia: University of Pennsylvania Press.

Wolfgang, M. E. (1967). Victim precipitated criminal homicide. In M. E. Wolfgang (Ed.), *Studies in homicide.* New York: Harper & Row, pp. 35–70.

25

PSYCHIATRIC MENTAL HEALTH NURSING WITH THE PATIENT IN INTENSIVE CARE

CHARLENE KATE KAVANAGH

LEARNING OBJECTIVES

After studying this chapter, the student will be able to:

- Describe assessment techniques for individuals in crisis.
- Define the concept of learned helplessness.
- Assess, formulate nursing diagnoses, and develop nursing care plans for ICU patients who are anxious, clinically depressed, or hostile.
- Provide effective environmental interventions for ICU patients who suffer from delirium.
- Help to recognize, prevent, and treat psychiatric problems among ICU staff.

INTRODUCTION

The most likely place to find individuals with psychiatric problems is the inpatient psychiatric unit. The next most likely place is the **intensive care unit.** Patients in medical and surgical intensive care units (ICUs) have a high incidence of psychiatric illness (Cassem & Hackett, 1978). In most cases, the etiology of this psychiatric illness is multi-factorial and includes genetic predisposition as well as physiological events (for example, blood loss, oxygen deprivation, and drugs, particularly anticholinergics such as atropine). However, the patient's emotional response to his or her physical illness and/or injury and the intensive care setting seems to play the greatest role in the development of psychopathology in ICU patients.

Medical and nursing staffs in intensive care units also have a higher incidence of psychiatric illness than their peers in other health care settings. ICU nurses report significantly more depression, feelings of hostility, and anxiety than non-ICU nurses (Cassem & Hackett, 1978). While there are many reasons for this, it is likely that such emotional states are, for the most part, a result of the highly unpredictable and often uncontrollable setting of the ICU. Such an environment is conducive to the development of **learned helplessness** (Seligman, 1968; 1975) in staff as well as patients. Learned helplessness is a recognized phenomenon characterized by anxiety and depression, and, in a sample of pediatric ICU patients, hostility (Kavanagh, 1981; 1983a; 1983b). It

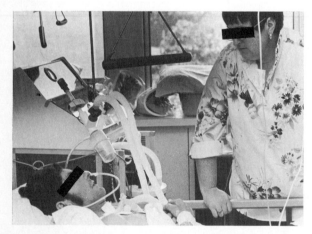

This middle-aged man has recently suffered a massive heart attack. His wife is allowed to be with him 24 hours a day if she desires. She says that she wants nothing less as she feels she can be of help to her husband in maintaining a positive attitude.

will be discussed in detail later in this chapter, and has been described in Chapter 9 on mood disorders. At this point, it is just important to understand that ICU patients and their families experience high levels of anxiety, depression, and, at times, hostility, and to understand why. The patients' fluctuating physiological states are not the sole cause of the "intensity" in ICUs that challenges even the most confident, competent, and psychologically healthy clinician.

Nurses who practice in ICUs must have a working knowledge of psychopathology—its assessment (in patients, their families, staff, and themselves) and its treatment. Efforts at preventing psychiatric complications of physical illness and injury need to be as intense as those that attempt to prevent and treat physiological complications. In addition, principles of crisis intervention have an important place in the framework for nursing intervention in the ICU.

NURSING INTERVENTION IN INDIVIDUAL CRISIS

According to Burgess and Baldwin (1981), the characteristics of an individual in crisis are: 1) decreased ability to maintain perspective; 2) decreased ability to mobilize resources; and 3) decreased ability to solve problems. A nurse who is involved with a patient who has these characteristics is more active, even directive, than she is under other circumstances. The ICU nurse actively confronts emotional and behavioral issues and encourages the patient, the patient's family, and other staff to do the same. It would be inappropriate and possibly catastrophic in some instances to be simply an empathic listener who offers feedback only when invited to do so.

In an active stance, the nurse screens the data available to her and focuses on the most important issues. Suppose a child of two is admitted to the ICU with a severe head injury that the nurse suspects has been inflicted by one of the parents. The nurse faces several pressing issues in addition to the child's physical condition: 1) the state statute requiring that nurses and medical staff report any injury to a child that is suspected of having been inflicted, to the local child protective services agency; 2) the events likely to follow reporting (for example, immediate police investigation and possible arrest of one or both parents); and 3) a myriad of other problems, such as the child's and the family's anxiety. While all these things are important, once the child's physical condition has been stabilized, the most pressing matter is the need to tell the child's parents that the nurse (or hospital) is obligated by law to report the child's injury. Then the nurse and staff must immediately make the report so that investigation and treatment, if indicated, can begin. This increases the chances of the child's being able to live safely with his family in the future.

ASSESSMENT OF INDIVIDUALS IN CRISIS

Whenever acting and, especially, when taking a directive stance, the nurse is as responsible for her actions in the crisis context as she is in other situations. The need to assess, triage, and act as quickly as possible does not relieve the nurse of her responsibility to be accurate in both assessment and intervention. Like the physical assessment, the psychiatric assessment is thorough but does not delay the acute medical intervention that is necessary. The assessment includes a brief medical and psychiatric history and a mental status exam (see Chapter 5 on assessment). The nurse decides, on the basis of the information obtained, whether an immediate psychiatric consultation is necessary, or whether the ICU staff can manage the patient's anxiety and grief on its own. For example, a

patient with a history of bipolar mood disorder (who is delusional and extremely agitated) admitted to the ICU for treatment of injuries sustained in a motor vehicle accident should have immediate psychiatric consultation. A four-year-old child with a serious burn probably will benefit more from the care of an experienced nursing staff, especially if the staff includes nurses who are familiar with the **learned-helplessness model** of depression (see Chapter 9 on mood disorders.)

Whether the nurse works alone or with a mental health professional in caring for the patient in crisis, she needs to identify the most pressing problem and reduce it to manageability by suggesting to the patient and his family an **active and adaptive response,** as well as by offering her support. For example, a young farmer was admitted to the intensive care unit after the traumatic amputation of both his legs in a threshing machine. Soon after his admission, a nurse discovered the farmer's wife crying in the family waiting area; the patient was agitated and asking for her. The nurse in this situation faced the many needs of her patient and his wife. She quickly determined who was the most needy and how the needs could be

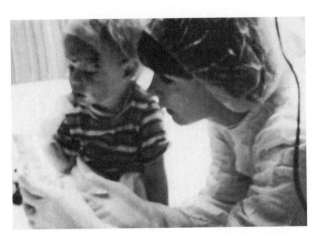

Dr. Kavanagh attempts to get this depressed 2 1/2-year-old burn patient to play prior to burn care. Sadly he says again and again, "I can't do it" in characteristic learned helplessness posture—arms limp at sides. A standard care patient in Kavanagh's et al's research, his burn care has been done with the nurse in control and attempting to distract the patient from her work and his pain. He gets Tylenol and codeine prior to burn care but still experiences it as very painful. He cries and protests throughout procedures, for example, piercing blisters on his forehead sheet graft, at times interfering with them.

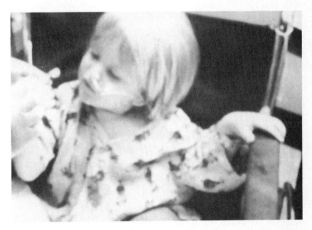

This is a 3-year-old patient in the experimental group who has had maximum predictability and controllability of burn care, with the nurse directing the procedure, since admission. He is an active participant in what would be thought to be a painful procedure (piercing blisters with a needle) without experiencing pain. Kavanagh has hypothesized that this is the result of maintaining endogenous non-opiate analgesics in the CNS by not overwhelming the organism, thus avoiding output of endogenous *opiate* analgesics, those associated with learned helplessness depression. He also shows no indication of depression or learned helplessness. After burn care he requests a ride outside in his wheelchair.

met. She said to the farmer's wife, "How can we help you give your husband the emotional support he needs right now?"

MALADAPTIVE FAMILY RESPONSE

In addition to suggesting adaptive responses to the patient or family member, the nurse needs to label or interpret **maladaptive responses**—those not in the patient's best long-term interest. If the parent of a terminally ill child begins to withdraw from the child, for example, the nurse should gently tell the parent that this response to the situation is a maladaptive one and is likely to make a bad situation worse. Her next intervention will be to help with what *is* needed, in this case, physical and emotional support for the child *and* parents. The case study on Mary illustrates how the nurse might do this.

Mary: An ICU Patient in Crisis with Leukemia

Mary Smith, age 13, was hospitalized in the University Hospital pediatric intensive care unit in septic shock. She was diagnosed as having acute myelogenous leukemia one year ago. She responded to chemotherapy but had a recurrence of her disease shortly after chemotherapy was completed. She was readmitted two weeks ago for another course of chemotherapy and radiotherapy in preparation for a bone-marrow transplant, an experimental treatment that would increase her chance of survival slightly. Mary and her family were informed and assertive consumers, and asked many questions about the rationale for Mary's care. Mary herself was a demanding patient, frequently asking for pain medication and special treatment, for example, to have her mother sleep in her room with her despite the ICU rule that prohibited this because of the safety hazards it would impose. Mary was very close to her mother but seemed estranged from her father, who admitted to being very peripheral in the family because of his busy law practice.

Mary was on a ventilator and was being dialyzed at the bedside. She drifted in and out of consciousness, which limited her ability to communicate. Though Mary's sepsis was being treated vigorously, her prognosis was guarded. Her parents understood this but did not want Mary told how serious the situation was. Mary's nurse noted that her parents were spending much less time with her in the ICU this time than they had in the past. They claimed that they didn't want to disturb Mary or upset her with their sadness, which was difficult to contain when they were with her. Mary's primary nurse noticed that

Mary was not at all demanding during this stay in the ICU, but was very passive, except for requesting pain medication even more often than usual. She seemed depressed and, at times, somewhat anxious.

Based on Mary's and her parents' behavior, Mary's nurse hypothesized that the parents had given up and had begun to grieve the loss of their daughter. Mary's mother, who had been especially devoted to her daughter during the past year, had said that a part of her was dying with Mary. She spent most of her day alone in the parents' lounge, visiting Mary briefly at intervals, often when Mary was sedated. Mary's father spent less time than ever at the hospital, saying that he couldn't take time off from work.

After discussing the situation with Mary's physician, the nurse approached the Smiths and told them what she had observed: their unintentional emotional withdrawal from their daughter in their attempts to cope with an overwhelming situation and to protect her as well as themselves from more emotional pain. She also told them about Mary's withdrawal and suggested that these two things might be related. She explained that while children are normally very resilient physically and emotionally, this situation could change very fast if they begin to feel alone with their pain and anxiety. "As long as Mom and Dad are close by," the nurse said, "children seem to manage just about everything pretty well, even the anticipation of death."

The nurse empathized with the Smiths and their very difficult task, to support their daughter while they themselves needed so much support. She suggested that they meet with the ICU psychiatric social worker or the hospital chaplain about how *they* were feeling and about their needs. Finally, she offered to be there with them when they visited Mary, including at the time of her death, if they felt this might help.

MOBILIZING THE PATIENT'S AND FAMILY'S RESOURCES

The nurse actively mobilizes the patient's and family's resources rather than focuses on their shortcomings. Returning to the case of the possibly abused child, the nurse needs to look for the strengths in what may be a chaotic, multi-problem family. If the young child and parent seem to be emotionally attached to one another and protest separation, the nurse focuses on this strength, interprets it as such, and facilitates its expression. She might say, "I see that Tommy is really hanging on to you. He's understandably afraid of us and the hospital. My guess is that your staying with him now would do more to reassure him than just about anything we could say or do. There really is no substitute for Mom." This intervention is likely to decrease significantly the anxiety in the family system, since in addition to reassuring the child, the nurse's intervention will also reassure the guilty, abusive parent who is likely to be worrying about being judged a "bad" mother or father (rather than one who needs social services) and losing the child.

PROVIDING INFORMATION TO PATIENTS AND THEIR FAMILIES

A crisis is made worse by misinformation or lack of information. However, this problem often is not obvious. A patient or family may not recognize the physical symptoms of anxiety, such as rapid heart rate, hyperventilation, tremor, pallor, and diaphoresis, and may interpret them as signs that the patient's condition is deteriorating. A parent may confuse *feeling* guilty with *being* guilty, that is, responsible for a child's serious injury or illness. The patient or family may not understand that anger (at the staff, each other, or even the patient) is a normal, even positive, response to a crisis, and must be recognized, legitimized, and expressed adaptively (for example, in words rather than destructive actions). Doing so avoids building resentment and/or depression. Thus the nurse stays alert for any evidence of distorted thinking or misinterpretation of events, correcting them with direct, understandable explanations that reflect what is going on, why (if it is known), and what can be done about it.

The case study on Amy exemplifies a crisis in the ICU and the principles of nursing intervention outlined above.

Amy: An Attempted Suicide

At 6:00 A.M., Amy Green, a 14-year-old girl, was admitted to the pediatric intensive care unit at Memorial Hospital after a suicide attempt in which she ingested an unknown amount of automobile antifreeze. Amy was delirious. During Amy's admission to the unit, her mother told the nurse that she hadn't known her daughter was depressed, possibly because she had been depressed herself for quite awhile. Although she had not been in psychiatric treatment, she had visited her family doctor and complained of "nerves," for which he had prescribed the tranquilizer, Ativan (lorazepam). After Amy was settled in bed, the nurse observed Amy's mother pacing at Amy's bedside and in the hall outside Amy's room.

By 10:00 A.M., blood tests indicated that Amy needed to be transferred to the University Hospital for dialysis. When Amy's mother was told this, she had no emotional response. Her affect was flat when she said: "I need to leave now since I have to be at work by noon."

The nurse invited Amy's mother to join her in a quiet corner of the unit. She knew that if Amy responded to the dialysis and her delirium began to lift, she would still be anxious, confused, and possibly still suicidal. The nurse also knew that if Amy did not respond to this treatment, she would die. The nurse took Mrs. Green's hand and, looking directly at her, said, "Mrs. Green, it is not a good idea for you to go to work. Amy is very ill. We hope that she will respond to dialysis, but she may not. In either case, it is very important for you to be with Amy. I understand that all this has been very difficult for you and I am wondering if there is anyone that I can call to be with you and Amy." Mrs. Green replied: "No, no one. My husband is at work. He doesn't even know what has happened, but I can't tell him because he'll be angry with me. He'll blame me. He'll say this is all my fault."

The nurse persisted: "Nevertheless, he must be told what has happened. Like you and Amy, he needs help with his feelings about it, including his anger, which is a normal response in a situation like this. Someone can be with you when you talk with him if you like." Mrs. Green answered, "I suppose he has to be told, but I'm scared and I don't know anyone at the other hospital."

The nurse answered, "Since I've been working with Amy this morning, I'll accompany her to University Hospital. You can ride with us in the ambulance and I'll stay with you and Amy until she is settled there. I'll make sure that the nurse and physician who will be working with Amy there understand the situation. With your permission, I'll also suggest psychiatric consultation. Amy's depression and suicide attempt need to be evaluated by a professional. Also, the family is going to need the support of a mental health professional." Mrs. Green replied, "I don't know. My husband doesn't like psychiatrists."

The nurse answered, "Many people feel that way. Whoever talks with you and your husband may help change his mind about that. We have to leave soon, Mrs. Green. It might be a good idea for you to take some Ativan right now since you seem very anxious. How much do you usually take for your nerves?" Mrs. Green said, "My doctor told me to take one to two tablets three times a day, and two at bedtime if I can't sleep. I usually take one, but sometimes I take two."

The nurse said, "I think you should take your afternoon dose now. You may want to ask the psychiatrist, psychologist, or psychiatric nurse who talks with you later today about taking your Ativan while going through this crisis with Amy. I'm going to get Amy ready for transfer. Why don't you call your husband and tell him to meet us at the pediatric intensive care unit at University Hospital? If he would like to talk with me or Amy's physician here before we leave, let me know."

In the example about Amy, the nurse assessed Mrs. Green to be extremely anxious and, because of her anxiety, unable to determine the seriousness of her daughter's situation and come up with an adaptive response to it. The nurse determined that if she did not intervene, Amy would be without the emotional support she needed, and her mother would be left with what could be overwhelming guilt about not being with her daughter during her crisis (especially if she died). In confronting Mrs. Green with the seriousness of the situation, the nurse defined the most pressing problem—Mrs. Green's difficulty with providing the emotional support her daughter needed. The nurse made it clear to Mrs. Green that she should not leave Amy or avoid telling her husband about Amy's suicide attempt. The nurse also began to mobilize family and professional resources in order to help Mrs. Green support her daughter. Finally, the nurse attempted to educate Mrs. Green about feelings that normally surface in a crisis such as attempted suicide.

ANXIETY IN THE ICU

Regardless of their specialty, intensive care units have an air of urgency, danger, and impending crisis, and ICU patients (whether children or adults) react to the ICU setting in predictable ways. Complex mind-body and body-mind interactions are involved in the patient's presentation at any one time, with psychological responses ranging from moderate anxiety and sadness to psychosis. Understanding this and being able to assess and deal with these responses is essential to delivering nursing care that will maximize physical and psychological recovery.

Anxiety is the most common emotion among ICU patients and staff, but not *all* anxiety is bad. Mild anxiety can be therapeutic. Patients who are mildly anxious about their well-being will be motivated to cooperate with staff in their treatment. Mildly anxious staff will attend to even subtle manifestations of changing physical and/or psychological states in patients.

Anxiety in the ICU typically rises as environmental predictability falls (Seligman, 1968; 1975). Due to the types of illnesses and injuries treated in ICUs, namely those involving multi-system failure, it is difficult to ensure even low levels of predictability. However, since predictability is increased every time a patient is actively involved in his or her care and is focused on treatments, rather than distracted from them, the nurse can significantly decrease the anxiety in the ICU patient (Kavanagh, 1981; 1983a; 1983b; Kavanagh et al., 1990).

PREVENTION AND TREATMENT OF ANXIETY AMONG ICU PATIENTS

The nurse can help prevent and treat anxiety among ICU patients in the following ways:

1. She can encourage the patient to verbalize his anxiety and what he feels are its sources so any erroneous or distorted thinking can be corrected.

2. She can prepare the patient for procedures by telling him what will be done, when, and why, and giving him accurate sensory information about what he can expect to feel (Leventhal, 1979).

3. She can implement supported exposure to feared objects and situations in the case of conditioned anxiety (see Chapter 8 on anxiety and anxiety disorders).

4. She can educate the patient about the normalcy of anxiety in the ICU setting, its physical symptoms, and how it can be prevented or treated.

5. The nurse can teach the patient to use the physical symptoms of anxiety as stimuli to invoke relaxation exercises and positive mental imagery (see Tables 25–1 and 25–2 and Box 25–1).

Sarah: A Trauma Patient with Severe Anxiety

Sarah was a 7-year-old Lebanese child who sustained multiple injuries in a bomb explosion in Beirut. A community organization arranged for Sarah and her mother to travel to the United States so that Sarah could receive medical care. Sarah was in the ICU for one week and her mother remained at her bedside most of the time. Neither Sarah nor her mother spoke English; however, an interpreter was available.

Sarah's injuries resulted in paraplegia, surgical amputation of her left arm, and inhalation injury. Her nursing care was very difficult due to her immobility and the need for frequent painful procedures such as chest percussion, stump dressing change, and physical therapy.

Sarah refused to eat and spat out her medication.

TABLE 25–1 Guidelines for relaxation induction*

1. Allow 5–10 seconds of tension for each muscle group followed by approximately 20 seconds of suggestions to let go. Go through two tension-relaxation cycles for each muscle group.

2. Tell the patient that the tension phase of the procedure will help him become more sensitive to sensations associated with anxiety, and that these sensations will begin to serve as a signal to relax away the tension.

3. Instruct the patient to release a tensed muscle group as suddenly as possible, as if to throw the tensions out of the body.

4. It may be helpful to practice along with the patient as he goes through at least the initial relaxation induction.

5. Attend to the following muscle groups: 1) feet, ankles, and calves; 2) shins, knees, and thighs; 3) buttocks and hips; 4) lower body; 5) stomach, waist, lower back; 6) upper back, chest, and shoulders; 7) upper arms, forearms, and hands to the tips of the fingers; 8) throat and neck muscles; 9) jaw and facial muscles.

The following is a portion of a transcript of tension-relaxation induction.

Now, settle back as comfortably as you can, close your eyes, and listen to what I'm going to be telling you. I'm going to make you aware of certain sensations in your body and then show you how you can reduce these sensations. First, direct your attention to your left arm, your left hand in particular. Clench your left fist. Clench it tightly and study the tension in the hand and in the forearm. Study those sensations of tension. Now, let go. Relax the left hand and let it rest on the arm of the chair. Note the differences between the tension and the relaxation. (10 second pause.) Once again now, clench your left hand into a fist, tightly, noticing the tensions in the hand and in the forearm. Study those tensions, and now, let go. Let your fingers spread out, relax, and note the difference once again between muscular tension and muscular relaxation. (10 second pause.) . . .

Now clench both your hands into fists and bring them towards your shoulders so as to tighten your biceps muscles. Now, relax. Let your arms drop down again to your sides, and note the difference. . . .

Now we can direct our attention to the shoulder area. Shrug your shoulders, bringing both shoulders up towards your ears, as if you wanted to touch your ears with your shoulders. Note the tension in your shoulders and up in your neck . . . etc.

You can also learn to relax more completely the various muscles of the face . . . wrinkle up your forehead and

brow. Wrinkle it until you feel all your forehead very much wrinkled, the muscles tense, and the skin furrowed. Now, relax . . . etc.

Now close your eyes very tightly. Close them tightly so that you can feel tension all around your eyes and the many muscles that control the movements of the eyes . . . etc.

Now purse your lips, press your lips together . . . and feel the tension all around the mouth. And now relax, relax those muscles around the mouth, and just let your chin rest comfortably.

And now, we'll turn our attention to the neck. Press your head back against the surface on which it is resting. Press it back so that you can feel the tension, primarily in the back of the neck and the upper back . . . bring your head forward, and try to bury your chin into your chest. Feel the tension, especially in the front of your neck. And now relax, let go, further and further . . . etc.

Now we can direct our attention to the muscles of the upper back. Arch your back, arch it, sticking out your chest and stomach so that you feel tension in your back, primarily your upper back . . . etc.

Now, take a deep breath, filling your lungs, and hold it. Hold it and study the tension all through your chest and down into your stomach area . . . etc.

Now tighten up the muscles in your stomach. Tense those stomach muscles, hold it. Make the stomach very hard. Now relax. . . .

Now tense both calf muscles by pointing your toes towards your head. If you point your toes upward toward your head, you can feel the pulling, the tension, the contraction in your calf muscles and in your shins as well . . . .

Just as you have been directing your muscles to tense, you've also been directing them to relax or to loosen. You've noted the difference between tension and muscle relaxation. You can notice whether there is any tension in your muscles, and if there is, you can try to concentrate on that part, send messages to that muscle to loosen, to relax. If you think of loosening that muscle, you will in fact be able to do so, even if only a little.

---

*For use with the older child and adolescent as well as the adult patient.
Source: Reproduced by permission of Holt, Rinehart, and Winston from the book *Clinical behavior therapy* by Marvin R. Goldfried and Gerald C. Davison, New York, 1987, pp.86–92.

When staff were not present, she smiled and played with her mother; but as soon as a nurse entered the room, Sarah began to scream and ask her mother to make the nurse go away. Sarah's mother begged her child to "be good" and threatened to leave if she did not behave. However, she never left her child's side.

Sarah's primary nurse formulated the following nursing care plan directed at decreasing Sarah's anxiety and increasing her adaptive coping with her injuries and their treatment.

The nurse might begin to implement this nursing care plan by speaking to Sarah's mother about it and enlisting her support. For example:

Nurse: "Mrs. Shamma, bringing Sarah to a hospital in a foreign country for treatment has been very difficult both for Sarah and for you. We would like to help you and Sarah with your feelings about this, as well as see that Sarah gets the care she needs to recover and return home as soon as possible. We understand that you and Sarah are at times very frightened of the things we must do to help Sarah get well. In order for our care and treatment of Sarah to be most effective, we need to decrease her and your anxiety about it.

"We have developed a plan to do this, and need your help to carry it out. It involves a daily routine, telling Sarah what she will feel before each treatment, and teaching her how to help us take care of her. You can help us keep Sarah on schedule, explain as much as possible to her before each intervention, and reward her for being cooperative. If and when Sarah doesn't cooperate, we will need your support to remind her that she must cooperate, perhaps by taking away television privileges or a favorite toy for a while. We hope that we won't need to do this; we would rather increase her cooperation with us by rewarding her efforts to do so."

Box 25–1
● Therapeutic Benefits of the Relaxation Response

Researchers have now been investigating therapeutic uses of the relaxation response for 15 years. It is likely to be helpful for any problem or disorder caused or made worse by conditions that set off the fight-or-flight response. Recent physiological studies suggest one reason why the relaxation response works. After someone has practiced it regularly for about a month, the body responds less intensely to norepinephrine, one of the major neurotransmitters involved in the fight-or-flight response. As the effects of norepinephrine are partially blocked, symptoms associated with its activity diminish. There is also evidence that the relaxation response allows the right and left hemisphere of the brain to interact more, increasing cognitive receptiveness and making it easier to think innovatively. During the relaxation response, the right and left hemispheres show similar patterns of alpha and theta waves.

Controlled studies have established that regular elicitation of the relaxation response significantly lowers blood pressure in hypertensive patients. On the average, systolic pressure decreases by ten millimeters of mercury and diastolic pressure by five to ten millimeters, even at times when the relaxation response is not being practiced. The National Institutes of Health recommend non-drug therapy, including techniques that elicit the relaxation response, as the first treatment for borderline and mild hypertension and as an adjunct in the treatment of more severe hypertension.

Regular elicitation of the relaxation response also reduces the frequency and intensity of pain. It virtually cures some pain disorders, such as tension headache. Migraine headaches become less severe and much less frequent in about two-thirds of patients. Severe low back pain and cancer pain are still felt but become less bothersome and less physically limiting. In an investigation of patients suffering from chronic pain, two groups were treated for ten weeks. One group, treated with stan-

TABLE 25–2 Use of pleasurable mental imagery*

The following transcript contains the instructions given to a patient who would like to prolong the relaxed state he has achieved with the help of systematic muscle relaxation.

Okay, now just keep relaxing like that, nice and calm and comfortable. You may find it helpful to imagine a scene that is personally calm and relaxing, something that we'll refer to as your pleasant scene . . . fine. Now tell me how relaxed you feel on a scale of 0–100, where 0 indicates complete relaxation and 100 maximum tension. (The goal is usually in the range of 15–25).

Fine. Soon I shall ask you to imagine a scene. (At this point, the patient is presented with a mental image associated with anxiety, for example, the changing of the tracheotomy tube.) After you hear the description of the situation, please imagine it as vividly as you can, through your own eyes, as if you were actually there. Try to include all the details in the scene. While you are visualizing the situation, you may continue feeling as relaxed as you are now. If so, that's good. After 5, 10, or 15 seconds, I'll ask you to stop imagining the scene and return to your pleasant image and to just relax. But, if you begin to feel even the slightest increase in anxiety or tension, please signal this to me by raising your left forefinger. When you do this, I'll step in and ask you to stop imagining the situation and then will help you get relaxed once more. It's important that you indicate tension to me in this way, as we want to maximize your being exposed to fearful situations without feeling anxious.

*For use with the older child and adolescent as well as the adult patient.
Source: Reproduced by permission from Goldfried, M. R., and Davison, G. C. (1978). *Clinical behavior therapy,* New York: Holt, Rinehart, and Winston, p. 124.

dard medical techniques, did not improve. The other group was trained in meditation to induce the relaxation response; pain levels were reduced by more than a third in 72 percent of the patients and by more than half in 61 percent of the patients. The effect lasted for at least 15 months.

The relaxation response also relieves anxiety and the accompanying hostility, anger, short-temperedness, and insomnia, as well as associated physical symptoms such as nausea, diarrhea, and constipation. People who regularly induce the response say they feel calmer and in better control of their lives.

The relaxation response appears to increase the benefits of the poorly understood mind-body interaction known as the placebo effect, in which beliefs and expectations powerfully influence physical and emotional symptoms. The support of personal beliefs contributes to this effect. By allowing feelings to emerge without anxiety, the relaxation response may also improve the effectiveness of psychotherapy. Habits become easier to change, and such disorders as phobias may become curable. Studies also suggest that, in combination with other techniques, the relaxation response can be helpful in treating anxious overeating and in improving job efficiency, business problem-solving, and schoolwork. In one study, elementary school children who were taught meditation techniques scored higher than a comparison group on a standard achievement test.

Use of the relaxation response should be viewed as an adjunct to modern medicine. Our medical practices are probably the best the world has ever known, yet modern remedies are successful in only about 25 percent of illnesses that bring an average patient to an average physician. The other 75 percent of illnesses, when they do not get better by themselves, usually involve the effects of stress and related mind-body interactions. Such interactions are important even in cases where modern medical treatments are useful, since stress may retard the healing effects of a drug or surgery. Elicitation of the relaxation response may reduce dependence on drugs and other sometimes dangerous medical techniques. As a bridge between scientific medicine and older religious practices, the relaxation response is therefore useful in a very wide range of illnesses.

Source: Benson, H. B. (1988). The relaxation response: a bridge between medicine and religion. *The Harvard Medical School Mental Health Letter,* Vol. 4 (9), p. 4–6.

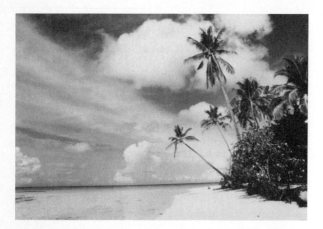

While positive mental imagery can help evoke the relaxation response, simpler interventions are likely to be even more powerful. For example, *abdominal* (rather than *chest*) breathing along with thoughts of being wrapped up, comfortable, safe, and warm will increase body temperature and oxygenation of tissues. Both promote physical and mental relaxation.

The adult ICU patient's behavior also often reflects unsuccessful attempts to cope with anxiety. One of the most common sources of anxiety in the ICU patient, adult or child, is the process of being weaned from a respirator. Patients who have depended on a respirator to breathe for more than a few hours do not give up this means of life support easily. Reassurance about the safety of weaning as well as increased predictability, for example, through sharing the weaning schedule with the patient, is often *not* enough to prevent or manage the patient's anxiety. Gradual exposure to the feared stimulus, in this case, time off the respirator, in a safe, supportive context is the most effective way to reduce weaning-related anxiety (see Chapter 8 on anxiety and anxiety disorders). Guided relaxation and pleasurable mental imagery may also be helpful (see Table 25–1 and Table 25–2).

Nursing Care Plan for Sarah

Nursing Diagnosis	Desired Outcomes	Interventions	Rationale
1. Anxiety	Sarah's anxiety will decrease and she will begin to cooperate with medical and nursing care.	Establish daily routine for meals, treatments, play, and rest. Make pictorial chart that reflects this routine and, with help of interpreter, go over it with Sarah and her mother at beginning of each day.	Predictability decreases anxiety; in the case of a language barrier, a pictorial chart that reflects the daily routine can help to convey predictability.
		Prior to beginning each treatment, for example, stump dressing change, explain to Sarah clearly and simply, through interpreter, what you will be doing and why. Also tell her what she can expect to feel. Avoid using emotionally charged words such as "hurt" and "pain" since they are likely to increase anxiety and, thus, pain; use words that reflect accurately the sensory experience ahead, for example, "pressure," "pulling," or "tingles" (Leventhal, 1979).	If aversive sensations (such as "pulling," or "stinging," or "pressure") have been predicted prior to being experienced, they will be experienced as less painful.

Nursing Diagnosis	Desired Outcomes	Interventions	Rationale
		Teach and encourage Sarah to do as much of her own care as is safely possible, and praise her for her attempts. She can, for example, unwrap the stump dressing and help wash the wound.	Self-care involves increased patient control; increased control of aversive events (like dressing change) results in decreased pain and anxiety.
2. Ineffective individual and family coping.	Sarah and her family will begin to develop positive ways of mastering anxiety associated with injuries and hospitalization.	Talk with Sarah's mother to determine what is a practical and effective reinforcer for Sarah, for example, special playtime with mom. Establish a positive reinforcement program to increase Sarah's incentive to take medication, eat, and cooperate with treatment. Consistently reward all cooperative behavior using the reinforcer.	Positive reinforcement needs to be determined on an individual basis; positively reinforcing behavior will increase the probability of its reoccurrence.
		Offer play therapy that encourages Sarah to master anxiety associated with her injuries and their treatment by allowing her to play out role of nurse or physician performing tasks such as chest percussion or dressing change on a doll or stuffed animal.	Play therapy offers the opportunity to master anxiety by allowing the child to reverse roles, increasing his subjective sense of being in control, and to face or increase exposure to the feared situation in a less threatening context.
		Elicit Sarah's mother's cooperation by being directive but empathic. Define the nursing problems in terms of what medical and nursing care her child needs in order to recover, and how her mother can help. Point out what *only* her mother can do, for example, continue to carry out bedtime ritual established at home, explaining why it is important.	A crisis situation determines a directive approach; if a patient or parent feels understood (as a result of the nurse's empathic stance), she is likely to trust the nurse and follow her direction. In their sometimes over-determined attempts to help their critically ill children, parents become "medical experts" or "nurses" practicing without licenses. They often need to be reminded that they are most valuable to the

Nursing Diagnosis	Desired Outcomes	Interventions	Rationale
			critically ill child as *parents* who continue to comfort, nurture, reassure, and cherish their children. If Sarah's mother can maintain a familiar routine—for example, telling her a bedtime story—Sarah's feelings of trust and security are likely to be strengthened.

It is important that this patient's nurse be competent at caring for the respiratory patient, comfortable with respiratory emergencies, and familiar with the patient being weaned. If she is unsure of herself or is likely to get rattled if a problem occurs or if the patient begins to get upset, she is certain to increase, not decrease, this patient's anxiety. An example of a nursing care plan directed at decreasing the anxiety of a patient, adult or child, being weaned from a respirator is presented below. The goal of this plan is the achievement of a physical state incompatible with the physical manifestations of anxiety. This is important because, in this situation, symptoms of anxiety could trigger a real or imagined respiratory emergency, and set the patient back in the rehabilitation process.

Nursing Care Plan to Decrease Anxiety of Patient Being Weaned from Respirator

Nursing Diagnosis	Desired Outcome	Interventions	Rationale
Anxiety	Decreased anxiety and increased cooperation during process of being weaned from respirator.	Tell the patient he will be started on program of gradual exposure to time off respirator, for example, fifteen minute exposure which is gradually increased to several hours and, ultimately, complete weaning. Explain weaning process and its rationale. Increase predictability by describing to the patient physical sensations he can expect throughout, especially at time of extubation.	Predictability, especially of aversive events (like the process of being weaned from a respirator) and associated physical sensations, decreases anxiety. Gradually increasing supported exposure to a feared stimulus or event is one means of decreasing the anxiety associated with it. (See Chapter 8 on anxiety and anxiety disorders.)

Nursing Diagnosis	Desired Outcomes	Interventions	Rationale
		Have the patient go through steps of systematic deep muscle relaxation (see Table 25–1) and/or encourage him to close his eyes, imagine a pleasant scene, and describe it in detail (see Table 25–2).	One way to decrease anxiety is to use anxiety-associated stimuli as cues to engage in deep muscle relaxation and pleasant mental imagery, a physical state thought to be incompatible with the physical experience of anxiety.
		At bedside, keep a graph or chart that shows clearly the patient's progress toward the goal of independent respiration and show him progress he may deny feeling. This will increase motivation that often wanes during long, complicated stays in the ICU.	Concrete indicators of progress can help to motivate the patient struggling to master anxiety associated with being weaned from a respirator.

DEPRESSION IN THE ICU

Sadness or grief associated with the loss of a significant other, body part, or body function is common among patients in the intensive care unit. When a patient's low mood is associated with symptoms of clinical depression, however, it is likely to be best understood in the context of the learned-helplessness model of depression (see Chapter 9 on mood disorders). Work with the burned child and adolescent has validated the relevance of this model to the nursing care of the ICU patient most vulnerable to the development of depression, the pediatric burn patient. The model primarily involves increasing the predictability and controllability of aversive events in the patient's hospital world. Burn patients as young as two years old have been taught to be involved actively in daily painful treatments. Older children and adolescents have participated in their nursing care by watching and helping with their own dressing changes, for example, by removing adherent dressings and washing and debriding burned tissue (Kavanagh, 1981; 1983a; 1983b; Kavanagh et al., 1990).

Seligman (1968; 1975) was the first to demonstrate that it is not the intensity of an aversive event that determines its stressfulness, but whether or not it is predictable and/or controllable. **Experimental neurosis** (Mineka & Kihlstrom, 1978), a specific type of learned helplessness, is the name given to the collection of cognitive, affective, and somatic disturbances that result from exposure to unpredictable and uncontrollable aversive events, especially those that are intense, frequent, or prolonged (like burn care). It is a phenomenon similar to that observed in the pediatric ICU patient, particularly the toddler-preschooler between the ages of fifteen months and six years hospitalized with severe burns (Kavanagh, 1981; 1983a; 1983b; Kavanagh et al., 1990). The experimental-neurosis symptom picture includes: agitation followed by lethargy and depression, feeding disturbances, decreased ability to learn new associations between responses and outcomes, and chronic anxiety (Mineka & Kihlstrom, 1978). While the older child, due to greater cognitive development, is less vulnerable to these complications of severe illness or injury and its treatment, he or she is not immune to them. Predictability and patient control over aversive events is still warranted.

STRESS ANALGESIA

An especially interesting phenomenon associated with the clinical picture of learned helplessness or experimental neurosis is **stress analgesia,** or passivity and withdrawal (rather than fight or flight) in response to uncontrollable aversive events. One researcher has termed this the experience of "defeat" (Miczek, Thompson, & Shuster, 1982). In animal studies this self-induced analgesia lasts from twenty-four to forty-eight hours and can be reproduced with brief reexposure to the aversive stimulus (Grau et al., 1981; Maier & Jackson, 1979; Maier et al., 1981). These studies suggest that uncontrollable stress not only triggers analgesic withdrawal in an organism but also predisposes it to respond to future stress in the same way.

Why does this reaction to uncontrollable stress occur? Its physiological components suggest adaptation, but the adaptiveness of withdrawal in the face of threat is not readily apparent. Engle and Reichsman (1956), Engle (1962), Engle and Schmale (1972), and Kaufman (1973) hypothesize that passivity or withdrawal results in decreased cost to an organism in a stressful situation that it perceives as unmodifiable. By conserving energy, the organism not only prevents exhaustion but also preserves response capability that might be useful should environmental events change enough to make relief possible. Despite the immediate benefits, however, Maier and Jackson (1979) caution that conservation-withdrawal may be costly in the long run, as the sensitization phenomenon described above has implications for future problem solving. The nutritional and social deprivation that accompany conservation-withdrawal also militate against this response's ultimately being termed "adaptive," especially in the case of the critically ill child.

The likely etiology of stress-induced analgesia is endorphin production in the brain stem (Maier & Jackson, 1979; Maier et al., 1981). Studies have shown that an opiate antagonist can block the analgesia produced via intermittent inescapable stress (Maier et al., 1981; Miller, Dehen, & Cambier, 1981), that cross-tolerance develops between stimulation-produced and synthetic opiate analgesia, and that the opioid peptide concentration in human cerebrospinal fluid is altered by chronic pain and by analgesic central or peripheral stimulation (Lewis,

Cannon, & Liebeskind, 1980). Other studies indicate that there are probably both opioid and nonopioid systems of analgesia. What system is predominantly engaged seems to be a factor of quantitative characteristics of a given stressor, for example, its duration or its pattern (Lewis, Cannon, & Liebeskind, 1980). (See Boxes 25–2 and 25–3.)

TREATMENT OF DEPRESSION IN THE ICU

Increasing the patient's control over aversive events decreases his or her pain and prevents or treats the associated depression. Increasing the patient's general level of activity and "dragging" him or her, if necessary, through experiences set up to be successful are helpful adjuncts. This technique was developed by Seligman (1968; 1975) and initially involved dragging the animal subject, depressed as a result of unpredictable and uncontrollable shock, through an open cage door to safety. Application to humans might involve getting the patient up and out of bed

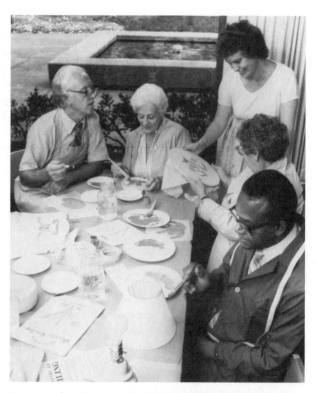

Nurses often have to insist that patients partake in occupational therapy in order for them to realize their own potential for success and mastery as physical problems decrease and functioning returns.

Box 25–2 ● Stress-Analgesia Research

Opioid-Like Analgesia in Defeated Mice

Abstract. *Mice exposed to repeated attacks by other mice showed decreased nociception in response to radiant heat focused on their tails. This form of analgesia was blocked by centrally acting opiate antagonists and was not observed in morphine-tolerant mice: furthermore, mice repeatedly subjected to defeat showed much less analgesia after receiving morphine than mice that were not subjected to defeat. Mice of the CXBK strain, which respond weakly to morphine, displayed only moderate analgesia following defeat. These findings suggest that endogenous opioid-mediated analgesic mechanisms are readily activated by situations involving biologically significant forms of stress, such as defeat.*

Miczek et al.'s research suggests that defeat-induced, naloxone-reversible analgesia is probably not limited to mice, and can be induced over a wide range of experimental parameters. They have concluded that "defeat in a social confrontation is stressful and engenders analgesia" (p. 1522). Because *attacking* mice show no increase in tail-flick (response to hot plate) latencies, even though they receive occasional retaliatory bites by the intruders and experience substantial pituitary-adrenal activation while attacking, it appears that the "special

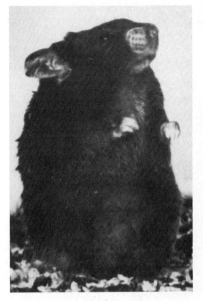

Mouse in characteristic "defeated position."

biological significance of the *defeat* experience, and not simply the experience of being stressed, is critical to the occurrence of opioid-like analgesia" (p. 1522).

Source: Miczek, K., Thompson, M., and Shuster, L. (1982). Opioid-like analgesia in defeated mice. *Science,* Vol. 215, pp. 1520–1522.

or out of the room, gradually increasing the amount of self-care, and insisting that the patient spend time with the occupational or recreational therapist, on their turf if that is medically feasible.

Because of the cognitive distortions associated with learned helplessness (see Chapter 9 on mood disorders), the ICU patient may be unable to recognize when he or she is doing well, or appreciate his or her own potential for success and mastery as physical problems decrease and functioning returns. As a result, the nurse often has to insist that a patient move or participate in some therapeutic activity, such as occupational therapy, despite his or her protest. In short, the nurse may have to insist that a patient do

something, despite his protest, in order to make him realize that he can do it.

In spite of the importance of the learned-helplessness model of depression in understanding and treating depression in the ICU patient, nursing care that springs from psychodynamic and biological models (see Chapter 9 on mood disorders) is also helpful. Specifically, the nurse should encourage the patient to verbalize feelings, especially the anger about what has happened and is happening to him. Antidepressant and/or antipsychotic medication may be necessary in some cases, for example, when the depression has reached psychotic proportions; predictability and controllability are difficult, if not impossible, to implement with the delusional or unresponsive patient.

It is important to remember that learned-helplessness symptomatology may be made worse and/or induced in vulnerable individuals by narcotics (Kavanagh, 1983b; Kavanagh et al., 1990). This may be because narcotics exacerbate endogenous opioid effects or interfere with nonopioid systems of analgesia (Lewis, Cannon, & Liebeskind, 1980). Maier et al. (Maier & Jackson, 1979; Maier et al., 1981)

have shown that giving narcotics to animal subjects in learned-helplessness experiments is comparable to increasing the level of uncontrollability in the environment, and thus increases helplessness and depression. Kavanagh (1983a; 1983b; Kavanagh et al., 1990) has hypothesized that giving the severely burned young child narcotics to control pain may have a similar effect.

Whether the depressive effect of narcotics is the result of altered physiology in the neurotransmitter

Box 25–3 • Learned Helplessness Research

In order to further evaluate a new approach to the dressing change/wound care of the burned child, designed to minimize anxiety and prevent the development of depression, replication of the pilot study was done over a two year period at two burn centers. Thirty-two patients ages 16 months to 16 years with second and third degree burns over 2–58% of body surface were studied. Nursing staff on both burn units were trained in two approaches to dressing change: standard care (which emphasizes staff control and patient distraction) and the experimental approach based on the learned-helplessness model of depression (which emphasizes predictability and patient control of aversive events). The effect of narcotic and non-narcotic medication in combination with both approaches was also examined. Dressing-change

behavior, pre- and post-dressing change serum cortisol and beta-endorphin levels, general behavior, and type of pain medication actually received were the major dependent variables used to evaluate the effect of both approaches. Blind analysis of videotapes of dressing change was used to validate the approach actually used with the study subjects. As in the pilot study, subject receiving the experimental treatment did better on all variables of interest except general behavior, where there were no significant differences between the groups. Most significant is the experimental treatment group's significantly lower post-dressing change serum cortisol ($p < .01$) and beta-endorphin ($p < .05$). Experimental treatment patients also needed less narcotic medication than those in the standard care group ($p < .001$).

Learned Helplessness	Stress-Induced Analgesia	Severely Burned Child
Etiology Loss or absence of predictability and controllability, especially in aversive context	**Etiology** Learning that an aversive event is inescapable	(Typical Situation) Physical and psychological trauma via flame, scald, electrical contact
Symptoms Initial anxiety and fear followed by depressed mood, passivity, withdrawal	**Symptoms** Lack of response to noxious stimuli associated with other symptoms of learned helplessness; reversed by naloxone; can result in sensitization phenomenon: reoccurrence with brief exposure to aversive or exposure to	Hospitalized*: involves painful dressing changes, 30–60″ in length two times daily for weeks, months, often prolonged due to medical complications and patient's protest; dressing change pain increases rather than decreases over time due to regeneration of nerves and creation of donor sites
Disruption of characteristic behavior (eating, sleep, self-protective behavior when threatened, work, play)		

system or the behavioral effects of the drug, namely, drowsiness, changes in mood, and mental clouding (which decreases the ICU patient's already compromised ability to accurately perceive and predict events and control his environment), the clinical evidence is impressive. Not only do narcotics seem ineffective in controlling the pain associated with burn dressing change, especially in the young child, they are associated with especially severe depression that is resistant to treatment in some patients (Kavanagh, 1983b). This may also be the case in other ICU patients, such as the chronic renal patient (Cassem & Hackett, 1978), since many are susceptible to the development of learned helplessness. It follows that all these patients are likely to benefit from a nursing approach that maximizes predictability and controllability from the moment they enter the intensive care unit until discharge. In conjunction with this approach, the effects of narcotic medication on patients should be monitored closely, and the dose decreased

---

Persistent cognitive deficit (inability to learn that escape or control is possible when situation changes)

Gastric ulceration

Weight loss

Endogenous opiate mediated analgesia

Nor-epinephrine depletion

Cortisol increase

Prevention and Treatment
Control especially of aversive events; drag through success if necessary to overcome cognitive deficit

Maximize predictability when opportunities for control are limited

---

neutral events associated with unpredictable, uncontrollable aversive event

Preceded by endogenous non-opioid analgesia (analgesia *not* associated with learned helplessness)

Potentiated, exacerbated, and re-elicited by exogenous opiate administration

Prevention and Treatment
Control, especially of aversive events; drag through success if necessary to overcome cognitive deficit

Maximize predictability when opportunities for control are limited

---

Activity, eating, elimination all painful; nightmares re-traumatize

Protest met with anger from staff and redoubling of their efforts to maintain control during dressing change (second nurse immobilizes patient, pancuronium administered)

(Typical Outcome)
Pan-anxiety, depressed affect, regression, decreased physical activity, behavioral withdrawal, negativism and behavior problems (e.g., lack of cooperation with all care), gastric ulceration, eating and sleep disturbances, decreased interest in social interaction and play, cognitive deficit (e.g., patient protests care of healed skin as if it were new burn), lack of response to noxious stimuli in context of withdrawal and other depressive symptomatology

Prevention and Treatment of Typical Outcome
Maximize predictability and controllability of burn care from first dressing change to discharge

Conservative use of narcotic medication

Drag through success (persist in expectation that patient take control during aversive events) when necessary (e.g., with child who has had previous loss of control of aversive events)

---

*Hospitalization in most cases is modified to normalize environment through parent contact/care; socialization/recreation program; supportive psychotherapy; staff geared to special needs of children.

Source: Kavanagh, C., et al. (1990). Learned helplessness and the pediatric burn patient: dressing change behavior and serum cortisol and beta endorphin. *Advances in Pediatrics, 37,* July.

if it seems to interfere with pain control and the antidepressant effect of increased predictability and controllability. (See Box 25–4.)

Joe: A Depressed Patient in the ICU

Joe was an 18-year-old victim of a car accident in which both his parents and his younger brother were killed. He survived, apparently because he was wearing a seat belt and was sitting in the front passenger seat, the place his mother usually occupied. He was in the ICU for two weeks receiving treatment for multiple injuries, including a crushed right arm and multiply fractured femurs. His arm had been partially repaired with muscle, vein, and skin grafts. Dressing change was done twice daily in his bed, where he was immobilized with traction to his femurs. Joe did not seem to be in pain at times other than during his arm dressing change. He had full use of his left arm.

After several days of hospitalization, Joe began to seem withdrawn. He slept most of the day and refused to eat. He was passive except during his arm dressing change, when he protested with screaming and swearing, despite receiving the maximum dose of morphine. After each dressing change, he asked only to be left alone.

Joe's primary nurse assessed that he had become clinically depressed, probably due to the loss of his family, the temporary loss of his usual sources of positive reinforcement (that is, school, his part-time job, friends, and so forth), and the loss of normal functioning. The absence of predictability and control in his days in the ICU (especially in the case of aversive events like dressing change) and, possibly, the narcotic-induced exaggeration of a subjective sense of helplessness, no doubt, were also contributing factors. Joe's nurse developed the following nursing care plan to treat Joe's depression and prevent it from becoming worse.

Nursing Care Plan for Joe

Nursing Diagnosis	Desired Outcomes	Interventions	Rationale
Powerlessness	Joe will begin to gain a feeling of control over his situation and realize that his own actions can affect his physical improvement.	Do not let Joe withdraw. Provide sensory stimulation, for example, time out of room and one-to-one nursing contact despite his request to be left alone or to sleep.	Withdrawal is associated with feelings of helplessness and defeat. Activity and experiences of success counteract both.
		Encourage Joe to talk about guilt feelings he might have about deaths of parents and brother, pointing out that *feeling* guilty is not evidence of *being* guilty. Label his anger understandable and don't try to talk him out of it. Empathize with his feelings of loss.	Feelings of guilt can lead to self-directed anger and punishment. While they are normal, the patient usually needs help putting them in a realistic perspective. Without intervention, the "guilty" patient is likely to become the depressed patient.

Nursing Diagnosis	Desired Outcomes	Interventions	Rationale
		Encourage Joe to participate actively in his dressing changes. He should be able to at least remove adherent dressings with his left hand, and may gradually be encouraged to cleanse his wounds and skin grafts as appropriate under the nurse's supervision.	Increasing patient control, especially of aversive events, will decrease associated pain and prevent or treat the learned helplessness type of depression. Any physical activity and self-care responsibility contributes to this therapeutic effect and combats helplessness and depression.
		Encourage Joe to do as much as possible with his left arm in order to facilitate activity during all of Joe's day, not just during dressing change.	(Same as above)
		Talk with Joe about trying a lower dose of narcotic medication, or nonnarcotic pain medication, at time of dressing change. With his and physician's permission, set up double blind cross-over trial* of both types of medication in order to determine objectively which medication is best for him.	There is some evidence that narcotics may, in some cases, exacerbate learned helplessness; thus, they should be used with caution in the case of the depressed patient in need of pain control.
		Consult a psychiatrist for help with management of Joe's depression, especially its biological aspects (anorexia, decreased energy) if they are not responsive to the above.	Antidepressant medication has been shown to be especially effective in ameliorating persistent physical symptoms of depression such as anorexia, insomnia, and loss of energy, all of which can interfere with physical recovery in Joe's situation. (See Chapter 9 on mood disorders.)

*An experiment involving drugs A and B or a drug and a placebo. Neither patient nor nurse knows the identity of either medication at the time of its administration. Both are given, and may be repeated, over a specified period of time. For example, first A, then B, or A B A B. Effects are monitored over the duration of the experiment. The identity of the medications is not revealed until the experiment has been completed.

Box 25–4 ● Nursing Interventions to Prevent or Treat Learned Helplessness in Context of Piagetian Theory of Cognitive Development

Preschool (18 mos.–5 years)

Thinking is egocentric and universal. Corrections in thinking made by others can be incorporated into his beliefs, but old ideas are not easily discarded. Focus is on central characteristic of something and categorization is done accordingly; e.g. this child thinks "The nurse hurt me, so all nurses hurt"; or "The nurse will always hurt me."

Understanding is dominated by physical sensation. Inanimate objects are given animate characteristics. Thinking is predominantly pre-causal or "magical," e.g. "The I.V. pump is some kind of monster" "I hurt because I was bad (and am being punished)" "I'm bleeding so I must be in danger."

Preference is to do things himself.

Interventions

Focus simple explanations on concrete events and behavior happening now or in near future. Avoid use of metaphors and be as literal as possible; e.g. avoid saying "Let's cut this arm off now," when what is meant is "Let's cut the bandage off this arm now."

Encourage child to actively participate in all aspects of his care before he develops anxiety about loss of control.

Encourage child to reenact aversive procedures with doll or stuffed animal.

School-Age (5–11 years)

Child begins to encounter conflict as he experiences perspectives different from his own. Able to attribute multiple characteristics to an object but thinking still dominated by concrete reality he understands through his physical senses.

Sees causal relationships between events, but not always correctly. Has ability to internalize another's perspective which enables him to give up cognitive distortions when corrected.

Fascinated with his body and how it works.

Interventions

Talk to child throughout procedures, especially aversive ones, in order to help him develop cognitive control of hospital world. Answer questions simply and concretely including rationale for treatment and sensory information. Correct cognitive distortions as they become apparent. Encourage child to focus on his body and what is happening to it, and to ask questions about what he sees.

HOSTILITY IN THE ICU

Occasionally ICU patients become hostile to their families, other patients, and staff. This hostility probably has its roots in unexpressed anger associated with loss and pain. If the nurse validates the patient's anger (for example, by saying, "You sound angry") and the anger is channeled adaptively (for example, into words or productive activity), it is less likely to result in out-of-control behavior or destructive acting out. Encouraging a patient to tell his doctor that he is angry, for example, about what he feels is inadequate medical attention, may prevent him from acting out his anger by refusing treatment or sabotaging his care in other ways. When this kind of acting out occurs, it is important for the nurse to set and enforce limits; however, the limits must be on the patient's behavior, not on feelings. The angry hematology patient on immunosuppressants should be told

Adolescent (11–17 years)

Thinking much like adult's. Avoids trial-and-error approach to problem solving and plays with hypothetical. Values highly his ability to think abstractly and is insulted by simplistic explanations. Constructs own theories and values about life and society.

Peers very important. Rebellious nature.

Needs to cognitively control and predict events.

Interventions

"What do *you* think about this or that?" Helps to establish working relationship with adolescent, and subtly gives him control.

In teaching, start with theoretical and progress to rationale, ending with concrete behaviors associated with procedures.

Use other adolescent patients as examples and sources of information.

Avoid "you should" or "you must." Assume patient will do the appropriate thing and appeal to his intellect. Offer suggestions including their rationale for what *he* can do to decrease his stress.

Do not get into endless negotiation about who is to do what. Define parameters of what patient can be in control of, and what nurse needs to do. Be clear about what needs to happen and why.

Always give advance warning when patient will have to relinquish control during a procedure, focusing on the rationale for this.

Source: Kavanagh, C. (1988). Concerns, responses, and interventions related to critical illness in the pediatric patient. In B. Riegel and D. Ehrenreich (Eds.), *Psychological aspects of critical care nursing.* Rockville, Md.: Aspen, adapted from "Burn care and the pediatric patient." C. Kavanagh and R. Pressman, *PRN Forum.* Vol. 3, No. 2. May/June, 1984, and from Ginsburg, H., and Opper, S. *Piaget's Theory of Intellectual Development.* New Jersey: Prentice-Hall, Inc., 1969.

that he cannot refuse mouth care or drugs with unpleasant side effects if he wants to stay in treatment. He should *not* be told or subtly given the message that he shouldn't be *angry* about these things. The patient *can* control his behavior; he cannot control his feelings.

Until what is making the patient angry stops or changes appreciably, he will be angry. This can be hard for staff to tolerate. No one likes to bear the brunt of someone's anger. However, telling the pediatric patient or immobilized adult that he or she may not yell, scream, swear, or be rude to you, physicians, and family members leaves the patient with no outlet for the anger. According to psychoanalytic theory, if the patient manages to keep the lid on his anger, he will be more vulnerable to depression. Also, a patient who is unable to control his feelings but controls what he says may be impelled to act out in some way. He may not cooperate with his treatment, sabotage his medical or nursing care, develop psychosomatic symptoms such as vomiting or diarrhea, or be self-destructive in other ways. Ways in which the nurse can help the hostile patient in the ICU are described in the case study on Jane and in the nursing care plan at the end of this chapter.

In summary, when dealing with the hostile patient, the nurse sets clear, achievable expectations for behavior. She positively reinforces desired behaviors consistently and with enthusiasm when they occur. She points out matter of factly the negative consequences of undesirable behavior. She does not set limits on feelings; rather she labels them and helps the patient to channel them in an adaptive way. She understands that anger is always present in the ICU patient, and often in his family. Anger does not need to be destructive to the patient or to others. It can motivate and energize a patient and can help ward off clinical depression. The sooner the anger is recognized and labeled, the less threatening and destructive it is likely to be.

DELIRIUM IN THE ICU

Delirium or **acute organic brain syndrome** is a common problem among patients in the ICU. Delirium is the result of impaired functioning of brain tissues due to metabolic, traumatic, neoplastic, vascular, hematologic, hypoxic, endocrine, or toxic events (Cassem & Hackett, 1978) (see Chapter 11 on organic mental disorders). A drug reaction should also be considered as a cause of delirium, especially in the delirious ICU patient who may recently have received lidocaine or atropine. Alcohol withdrawal and amphetamine or hallucinogen toxicity should also be considered as possible etiologies.

Symptoms of delirium include a disturbance in consciousness and level of arousal; agitation and/or somnolence; impairment of orientation, memory, and other cognitive functioning; misperceptions and paranoia that lead to combativeness; and visual hallucinations.

The reversibility of delirium depends on early recognition and treatment. The longer it goes unrecognized and untreated or the longer it persists despite treatment, the greater the likelihood of irreversible cerebral damage in the patient. Since the etiology of delirium may take time to find, symptom management that involves medication and **environmental intervention** (for example, decreasing the number of staff members involved with a patient) is necessary in

the interim. While some drugs can make delirium worse, the right drug can reduce fear, anxiety, irritability, anger, hallucinations, and delusions without causing undesirable sedation or respiratory depression. This can promote the patient's safety since the agitated patient pulls out tubes, lines, and, in general, resists therapy necessary to sustain life.

Sometimes the problem is not *which* drug to use (though they do differ in their undesirable side effects) but the dose. The goal is symptom control without producing *obtundation,* coma, or respiratory depression. The right drug can quickly get an agitated, uncooperative, panicky patient under control, especially if it is given parenterally. Drugs cannot help disorientation, memory impairment, or other cognitive dysfunctions.

Anti-anxiety medications (for example, the benzodiazepines) and antipsychotics (major tranquilizers) are the drugs most commonly used to treat delirium. Haloperidol is often recommended since it is the least sedating major tranquilizer and has a milder effect on the cardiovascular and respiratory systems than the benzodiazepines (Murray, 1978). Problems associated with haloperidol include decreased seizure threshold, undesirable cardiovascular effects, and extra-pyramidal symptoms. Two to ten milligrams may be ordered by the physician to be injected intravenously every three minutes until sedation is achieved (the drug's peak effect occurs in ten minutes). The half-life of haloperidol is fourteen hours when given intravenously and twenty-four hours when given orally. A maintenance dose is achieved via gradual injection of decreasing amounts until the point of the most sedation for the least drug is achieved. Regardless of which medication is prescribed, the following guidelines should be kept in mind by the nurse administering it:

1. If the patient is unresponsive and more agitated with pharmacotherapy, the delirium may be of anticholinergic drug etiology. If so, it will be responsive to physostigmine, so a physician should be contacted.

2. Occasionally, acute adverse reactions occur with administration of haloperidol, for example, motor restlessness, akathesia, and opisthotonos. If this occurs, the medication should be stopped immediately (Murray, 1978; *Physicians Desk Reference,* 1987).

3. In case of either of the above, the physician may order thiothixene or trifluoperazine, since both are alternatives for the patient who is very ill and whose condition is unstable (Murray, 1978).

Regardless of the therapeutic effect of drug treatment for delirium, environmental intervention is always necessary. The ICU is the worst place for the delirious patient because of the high level of activity. The overstimulation that results is accompanied by the absence of a normal, familiar environment, or understimulation. This parallels the over- and underactivity in the brain responsible for the symptomatology of delirium. As a partial solution to these problems, the nurse may move the delirious patient to a quiet room or cubical in the ICU. Soft lights should be maintained since darkness can precipitate visual hallucinations. The patient should be attended to on a twenty-four-hour basis, preferably by people with whom he or she is familiar. The number of medical and nursing professionals involved with the patient should be kept to as few as is safely possible. Each staff or family member should identify and explain him or herself with each patient contact. Nursing responsibilities include constant attention to the patient's safety, reassurance, and frequent orientation to name, time, and place. Physical restraints may be necessary but should be avoided if possible since they often increase the patient's agitation.

PSYCHIATRIC PROBLEMS AMONG ICU STAFF

Patients are not the only people in the ICU who are beset by anxiety, depression, and hostility. Physicians who may have been working continuously for twenty-four hours or more can become so emotionally drained that they cannot function effectively. They may defensively "attack" the nurse, or even the patient. The nurse must be able to handle this.

One of the greatest emotional burdens that the physician has to bear is a tremendous sense of responsibility. Ideally, an interdisciplinary group, such as a hospital ethics committee, helps the physician to make difficult ethical decisions such as whether to sustain life or let it go (Fost & Cranford, 1985). In current practice, however, physicians often bear this responsibility alone. The burdens of such decision-making and long working hours, and the stress of dealing with critically ill patients and their families, can push even the most competent and experienced physician over the edge (see Box 25–5). The nurse must be able to handle this, too.

Although the burden of ultimate responsibility is not theirs, nurses *are* responsible for everything they do, with or without doctor's orders. ICU nurses typically do not work twenty-four hours or more continuously as the physician sometimes does, but they frequently work overtime due to unpredictable shifts in patient load. In addition, the nurse's close contact with the patient and his family leaves her with a potentially greater emotional burden. It is the nurse who hears the patient's pleas to be left alone and no longer be "tortured." If the patient cannot talk due to intubation, the anguish and anxiety in his eyes tell the story. It is also the nurse who bears the brunt of the patient's or his family's anger, not only because she is *there,* but because she often does things that cause pain and cannot always be counted on to relieve it, despite her best efforts.

It is difficult, nevertheless, to say which is more stressful: taking care of the patient who shows such emotion or the one whose emotions cannot be read at all, such as the patient who is comatose. Due to the sophistication of today's medical technology, even the most critically ill or injured patients can have life sustained, and often do. Thus the indefinitely comatose patient has become a typical ICU patient. This has added tremendously to the psychological burden of the ICU nurse.

Lack of patient feedback is especially difficult for the ICU nurse to cope with when, rather than reflecting a lack of feeling, it reflects an inability to *express* feelings. The patient whose level of consciousness is difficult to assess because of disease process or "paralyzing" medication such as pancuronium* may have a lot of feelings but be unable to express them. One nurse has said about such patients: "Working in the ICU involves taking care of semi-dead people." Perhaps it is easier to think of them that way, as people whose feelings are deadened, rather than as people who are alive psychologically and experiencing anxiety and pain while trapped inside bodies that indicate they are experiencing nothing at all.

Physicians and nurses working in the ICU, like their patients, have to deal with constant unpredictability and uncontrollability. As a result they, like their patients, get anxious and depressed. They may also get angry in a futile attempt to ward off depression, only to be alienated by peers who are, so far, successfully avoiding emotional decompensation. If many staff are angry, anxious, and/or depressed, the esprit de corps in the ICU will fade and be replaced by maladaptive acting out of feelings. Poor communications, resentment of patients and each other, blaming and scapegoating, and low unit self-esteem become the context for patient care. As a result, patients and their families begin to respond in similar ways. Anxiety, depression, and hostility increase. Physical com-

---

*Neuromuscular blocking agent used to prevent physical resistance to mechanical ventilation, procedures, and so on (*Physicians Desk Reference,* 1987).

Box 25–5 ● Making Sure Doctors Get Enough Sleep

It was 4 A.M., nap time for a second-year resident who had been on duty at a Long Island hospital for 20 hours. As she dozed off, her beeper sounded. A patient was having a seizure. She gave him the drug he needed, keeping close watch on his heart monitor. To stay awake, she sang along with the radio in his room.

She finally got to bed at 7 A.M., only to rise at 7:30 for regularly scheduled rounds.

Long hours like those have been a rite of passage for generations of doctors-in-training. New York State will move a step closer to breaking the century-old tradition this week when a committee of the State Hospital Review and Planning Council considers restrictions on hours for interns and residents. A final decision is expected next month, and the Health Commissioner, Dr. David Axelrod, hopes to phase in the rules starting this fall. California, Hawaii, Pennsylvania and Massachusetts are also considering limits on how long residents and interns are scheduled to work.

Under the New York proposal, interns and residents would be restricted to 12-hour emergency room shifts. In other parts of the hospital, they could work for up to 24 hours without time off, but not more than an average of 80 hours a week.

Now 24-hour and even 36-hour shifts are not uncommon. The result, said Dr. Bertrand M. Bell, who headed the committee that drew up the proposals, is that "the least experienced, most stressed person with the least amount of sleep gets the worst work."

A recent Harvard Medical School study found that "a continuous 36-hour span of service impedes participation in educational efforts and detracts from the learning experience." After urging hospitals to limit time on duty to 16 hours at a stretch, the Harvard panel recommended something that unionized workers have enjoyed for generations—at least one day off a week.

plications in patients and delayed recovery are likely to follow since anxious, depressed, and hostile patients do not cooperate with their medical treatment and nursing care. Delayed recovery means a longer stay in the ICU. The staff's workload and associated burdens can multiply rapidly in this situation.

PREVENTION AND TREATMENT OF ICU PSYCHOSIS IN ICU STAFF

Cassem and Hackett (1978) have suggested strategies to prevent psychopathology among ICU staff. These strategies include strong medical and nursing leadership, group meetings and group therapy, a quiet secluded place with a coffee pot for staff, and making allies of families so that they can help with rather than interfere with the care of the patients.

While group therapy or venting sessions are likely to help staff members identify their own feelings and elicit support for themselves when neces-

sary, the most important preventative against the development of emotional or psychological chaos in the ICU is effective leadership. It must be clear to all staff who the medical and nursing leaders are. As the authors of *In Search of Excellence* (Peters & Waterman, 1982) state, the effective leader is "visible when things are going awry and invisible when they are working well" (p. 82). They also say that leadership involves "building a loyal team . . . that speaks more or less with one voice. It's listening carefully much of the time, frequently speaking with encouragement, and reinforcing words with believable action. It's being tough when necessary and it's the occasional naked use of power. . . ." (Peters & Waterman, 1982, p. 83). The ICU head nurse should be willing and able to take patients herself when necessary (that is, never putting "management" duties first) and be in her office only when her nurses are unlikely to be needing her advice and support "on the front lines." She must be sensitive to interpersonal problems

Hospital administrators say that shorter hours would force them to make expensive changes and raise costs. The Greater New York Hospital Association, which represents about 80 private, nonprofit hospitals, estimates that shorter shifts would cost at least $100 million and play havoc with hospital schedules.

"The proposal doesn't address where to find more staff and how to pay for it," said Kenneth E. Raske, the association's president. "It would be a mistake to replace residents who might be tired with nobody at all."

Doctors who see no reason for the changes contend that long hours build stamina. Furthermore, they say, a surgical resident who has checked on a patient throughout the day is more likely to notice post-operative complications that a doctor fresh on the case might miss.

In addition, some medical educators worry that shorter hours would mean that young surgeons would attend fewer operations, taking longer to learn their craft. Other opponents invoke familiar arguments against government intervention in medical matters.

The grueling marathon schedules were called into question after Libby Zion died at New York Hospital in 1984. Miss Zion, the 18-year-old daughter of Sidney E. Zion, the writer, died less than a day after she was hospitalized with an earache and fever. A grand jury later attributed her death to mistakes made by exhausted, unsupervised interns and residents.

Dr. Bell's committee found that residents in New York City averaged 2.4 hours of sleep a night when they were on call. A study by the American Medical Association found that residents in nine major specialties averaged 74-hour workweeks last year.

First-year residents in pediatrics and obstetrics were on the job even longer, averaging 90 hours a week, and 1 in 10 surgical residents worked at least 122 hours a week.

Dr. Bell said he doubted that it would be very difficult for hospitals to recruit enough doctors to make up for shorter schedules. Despite lower salaries at the city-owned hospitals where he has been an administrator, "I never had any trouble recruiting first-rate doctors who were satisfied driving Corollas, not Mercedeses," he said. "With the doctor glut, maybe people who think otherwise need to take another look around."

Dr. Janet E. Freedman, president of the Committee of Interns and Residents, which represents about 5,000 residents in private hospitals in New York, New Jersey, and the District of Columbia, argues that the changes are overdue.

"Residents are severely overworked," she said. "Hospitals have depended on us as a source of cheap labor for a long time, and that's why they've been reluctant to change."

Source: Barron, James. "Making Sure Doctors Get Enough Sleep," *The New York Times*, Sunday, May 22, 1988.

---

among the staff and deal with them directly, before resentment, hostility, and factions begin to form. She sets the example of talking *with* rather than about patients *and* each other, even when the topic of conversation is negative feelings or problems.

Perhaps most important, the head nurse takes the time to listen to the concerns of the staff nurse who feels that the unit is too busy for the nurses scheduled. She documents incidents that indicate the need for more nursing staff, more space, and new or better equipment. She uses her management skills and the authority of her position to convey the professional goals and values and legitimate concerns of her staff to nursing administration (and vice versa) (see Box 25–6).

If this seems to be the description of Super Nurse, that is because it is. Nothing less will suffice. To put it simply, the ICU head nurse cannot serve as a nursing model of sensitivity to mind-body and body-mind connections in those around her, staff as well as patients, unless she is in their midst.

Jean: An ICU Nurse

Jean Pringle was the newest member of the ICU staff. She had been on the unit for only two weeks, but was expected to function independently. The unit was a busy one and the staff seemed to be quite stressed, apparently because of a nursing shortage. As a result, Jean's orientation was cut short.

On one especially busy day, Jean was assigned to an adolescent burn patient and a comatose victim of a motor vehicle accident. Jean was anxious about her workload, since she had not worked with a burn patient for a long time, and worried that she wouldn't be able to manage the comatose patient on her own since he was quite large. As Jean was collecting her thoughts and looking at her patients' charts, she felt angry. She felt that the charge nurse assigned the unit's two most difficult patients to her because she was new.

The burn patient began to cry and angrily protest

his dressing change as soon as Jean began to assemble the needed equipment. She told him what she had to do and said that if he cooperated, things would go well. The patient did not cooperate and things did not go well. It seemed impossible to debride burn wounds on a moving target. Midway through the dressing change, Jean, herself near tears, threw the forceps she was using to debride loose eschar on the floor and left the room. On the way out she ran into the patient's physician, who asked her what was wrong. She said she just needed to take a break for a few minutes and would be right back.

Jean went quickly to her purse and took out a bottle of Valium, which she carried with her for use at times like this. It had been prescribed by her family doctor whom she had seen recently about trouble sleeping. She took five milligrams and went back to her patient. The physician had finished the debridement that Jean had started, so all she had left to do was to re-dress the patient's burns. Fortunately, that went well.

As Jean had anticipated, working with the comatose man who had been in a car accident two weeks ago was extremely difficult. She struggled to move him from one side of the bed to the other as she changed the linen. Initially, she planned to skip that part of morning care, but then he had a very loose bowel movement. Jean considered asking one of her colleagues for help; however, she wanted to prove herself to them, so she didn't. She struggled for an hour, during which time she had to suction the patient twice, take his vital signs, and restart an IV that had infiltrated. Just as she finished and was about to leave the room to check on her other patient, she realized that this patient had just had another bowel movement which, again, soiled much of the bed. Jean sat down in the chair next to the patient's bed and began to cry. At that moment, the head nurse walked into the room. She had just spoken with the burn patient's physician about Jean's behavior and had come to see if she could be of any help. The smell in the room apprised her of the source of Jean's distress. Putting her hand on Jean's shoulder she said, "You seem to be having a rough day, and it looks like you could use some help. Let's change Mr. Reilley's linen together." When they finished she asked Jean to come to her office.

The head nurse, Alice Reiner, had been working in the ICU for five years, first as a staff nurse, and for the past two years as the head nurse. She knew that float nurses and new staff members were sometimes given the most difficult patients when the day's assignments were made by the charge nurse. She also knew that the staff had been stretched beyond their limits for over a week due to an unusually high census and a high incidence of illness among the nursing staff. After offering Jean a cup of coffee, she said, "Sometimes we're not very sensitive around here to

new people. It seems that you got an assignment that would be difficult for the most experienced ICU nurse to handle alone. I think we need to talk about this at our next staff group therapy session." Jean asked what that was. Alice explained that, because working in an ICU is so stressful, the staff met with the psychiatric clinical nurse specialist once a month to talk about feelings, both about their patients and each other. Jean began to cry and Alice asked her what was wrong.

"I'm not good at talking about feelings. My mother, brother, sister, and I went through family therapy about a year ago after my father died of complications of a coronary bypass procedure." His death had been unexpected, and especially hard on Jean, his youngest daughter and the one closest to him. "The sessions were terrible," Jean continued. "They made me feel worse."

Alice asked Jean if she still thought about her father. Jean said that she did, especially at this time of year, the Christmas season. Her father had died on Christmas Eve. Alice then asked Jean about her mood and her life outside the ICU. Jean told her that for about a month now she had felt "edgy" and not up to socializing. She attributed this to her recent trouble sleeping. She thought her moodiness and crying spells also were due to lack of sleep. She told Alice that her family doctor prescribed Valium, but it hadn't helped. She said that the Valium did help, however, when she took it for feeling edgy.

Alice told Jean that she was concerned about her. She said that she might be depressed and urged her to see a mental health professional. She told Jean that the hospital had an employee-assistance program which could be very useful to her in getting the help that she needed. She also encouraged Jean to attend the next staff therapy session. "A lot of us have been where you are, Jean. Maybe we can help, too. At least we can offer some support when you're here, and try to avoid making life even harder for you right now."

Jean took Alice's advice and visited the employee-assistance office at the end of the shift. She was referred to a nurse psychologist in the community who treated medical professionals for job burnout. Jean also attended the unit's group therapy session later that week. With the head nurse's support, she was able to talk about her feelings as a new member of the staff, as well as her continuing grief over her father's death. Ultimately, the staff came up with and agreed to try a buddy system for new nurses in the ICU. It would involve pairing a new nurse with a seasoned one for at least two weeks after orientation. They vowed to adhere to this system, even on the busiest of days. They also suggested that Jean be the first new nurse to receive this one-on-one orientation, beginning the next day.

Box 25–6 ● Rx for RN's

Two-month-old Alexandra* has been in PICU, the pediatric intensive care unit at the Johns Hopkins Children's Center, for 47 days following cardiac surgery. She is still so desperately ill that her vital signs must be taken every 15 minutes. Alexandra's nurse records them on a graph at the top of her data sheet. Below that, she chronicles the various procedures she performs on Alexandra. Next, she lists the fluids given and taken. The notations started at midnight; now it is 9 a.m., and already the oversized sheet is so full of black ink that it looks like a symphonic score.

Alexandra's bed occupies front and center of two adjoining rooms reserved for the most critically ill. Her tiny body—wired all over, legs splayed and arms outstretched—is but a dot on a landscape littered with space-age equipment, an all-white field through which nurses move swiftly, ministering to their patients. The two doctors who stroll in and stop at Alexandra's bed to confer, with their colorful button-down shirts and rep ties, look almost out of place.

Throughout PICU, bells and beepers are ringing and buzzing, signaling changes in cardiac monitors and ventilators beside the unit's 15 beds. But Ruth Lebet, charge nurse for the day, is still able to single out the piercing alarm of the "red phone."

Lebet rushes to the desk to take the call. A 3-year-old boy, who has fallen off a table and lost consciousness, is on his way to the emergency room. All morning Lebet has been thinking about who will need one nurse all to himself and who can share a nurse, about who is getting better and who is getting worse, and about who will be leaving and making room for someone new. Should he be admitted, this boy is probably, in the parlance of PICU, a "soft hit," meaning he won't require one-on-one nurs-

ing. Lebet knows she can swing it; she has enough nurses, at least for the moment.

But Lebet can remember a time last year when the unit had half its budgeted number of nurses. For several months it was on "fly-by" status 30 percent of the time. That meant many children arriving in helicopters and ambulances were diverted from this, Maryland's designated center for critical pediatric trauma and transplant patients, to other hospitals.

These days, PICU is in a fairly decent, if precarious, holding pattern, with the equivalent of 32 to 38 full-time nurses. It is budgeted for 40. Because of the stress associated with caring for patients like Alexandra, this unit is a tough place to staff. "I'd say the average life span of a PICU nurse is two to three years," says Lebet, adding that many RNs work here for only a year, just to get the prestigious "Hopkins PICU" on their resumes.

The cost of long-term solutions to the nursing crisis goes beyond money. To make the nursing profession attractive to bright, committed people, says [Carolyne Davis, Chair of the Federal Commission on Nursing appointed by Secretary of Health and Human Services, Otis Bowen,] the health care system must squarely confront the chronic ills that have beset nursing: a confused system of education, inequitable compensation, poor professional image, inefficient use of nursing talent, and the uneasy relationship between medicine and nursing. Difficult reforms in each of these areas will be essential to give nursing the professionalism that today's nurses—and today's health care system—demand.

"The crisis in nursing is not just for nursing to resolve but for the entire health care system," [according to Carol Gray, Hopkin's dean of nursing.] "Medicine should support us in pursuing federal dollars, in sup-

continued

*The names of patients have been changed to protect their privacy.

porting federal and state initiatives promoting the financing of education. I'm not asking for anything special, just something that's equitable in terms of supporting nurses as doctors have been supported."

Four-year-old Sarah probably has a mild concussion. She sits erect on her bed, encircled by blankets, wide-eyed and perplexed. As she is pushed out of the emergency room en route to the CT scanner, the ER doctor shakes his head and says, "We can't admit her; we don't have a bed."

"I can find a bed for that kid," says nurse Deborah Krohn from the sidelines. Krohn is a supervisory nurse responsible for juggling beds. When a kid is "crumping," she gets him into PICU; when one is getting better, she keeps her eye on that soon-to-be-empty bed.

Krohn, 34, has been here for 12 years; she knows every corner of the Children's Center, and has resources all over Hopkins Hospital. Yet despite her seniority and experience, a recent annual raise did not even equal a cost-of-living allowance. "I'm at the top of my salary bracket," says Krohn. "The hospital is following a recipe, and I lose out on it."

Krohn is the victim of a wage compression. The range from minimum to maximum wage for the Hopkins staff nurse is $22,672 to $31,000, based on a 40-hour week, right in sync with national figures.

Head nurses are often reluctant to surrender their authority, to "empower" their staff. But [Shirley Sohmer, director of nursing for psychiatry and neurosciences,] points out, "It's silly to think I can have control over 200 nurses. When you go into a critical care unit in the middle of the night and see a nurse caring for someone who's desperately ill, it's ridiculous not to trust these people to govern themselves."

When word spread about head nurse "Ski" Lower's plans for the new eight-bed neurosciences critical care unit on Meyer 7, people were

horrified. "Ski," they would say, "you can't do that. No one does." But Lower turned a deaf ear, plunged in, and built one of the most innovative nursing units at Hopkins Hospital.

On Lower's unit, the primary nurse for each patient is part of a group of six nurses, all of whom help carry out her plans for that patient's care 24 hours a day, seven days a week. The senior clinical nurse in each group is responsible for that group's care. It's a system that promotes consistency of care.

Every six weeks, Lower even pays each group of nurses for four hours to go have dinner together. There's an educational agenda and lots of shop talk, but much of the focus is social. "It's a good catharsis," says Lower. "You can't ask a group of people to work well together if they never get to know each other."

What's more, Lower won't allow her nurses to do tasks that could just as well be done by support staff. If a nurse needs help turning over a heavy patient, she asks an aide, not another nurse. Says Lower, "We never give away the essence of nursing. Never!"

Not surprisingly, the professional practice model is thoroughly ingrained here, but the spirit of autonomy transcends even that. "The unit belongs to the nurses and medical directors. We own the unit. We don't change our standards. This guy [a doctor] likes two dressings; this guy likes none. Forget it. We set the standard, and we make it clear to the physicians what the standard is." When doctors make rounds, the nurse presents the patient to them. "There's no nursing shortage here," claims Lower, adding that since the unit opened in July 1982, only one nurse has left because she was dissatisfied.

Most of all, though, making better use of nurses depends on individual nursing leaders like Lower who are not afraid to take risks. "In the average unit there's a lack of freedom and a lack of support to be creative,"

says Lower. "With the physicians, the patient, the families, and the telephone that's always ringing, the reality of nursing is that it sucks people dry. I believe that the head nurse has to design a unit with an environment that will support the nurse and a philosophy that nurtures her and fills her cup."

The mutual interest of doctors and nurses, of course, is in the patient. "I know this sounds hokey," says [Howard Markel, a senior assistant resident in pediatrics,] "but relationships on the ward are better when physicians support the nurse in what she does. Otherwise things break down." A 1986 study of ICUs in 13 hospitals found that an atmosphere of trust and good communication between unit physicians and nursing staff improved patients' prognoses.

The problems in nursing are deeply ingrained, and any solutions are likely to be painful. But, says Carol Gray, "there's no way out of the dilemma we're in without making major changes. This is absolutely critical. For too long we've been trying to make everyone happy and everyone a part of the decision process. Now decisions will have to be made by committed nursing leaders, and I know that group is out there. We need total change, a global affront."

Source: Swingle, Anne Bennet (1988). Johns Hopkins's Magazine, October, excerpts from pp. 16–22.

Case Study: Nonpsychiatric Setting Jane: A Hostile ICU Patient

Jane, a 5½-year-old child, was admitted to the ICU with forty percent third-degree burns to her neck, chest, upper arms, left leg, and right foot, resulting from playing with matches. An only child, Jane lived with her mother, who was a single parent. According to her mother, Jane was precocious, independent, and somewhat rebellious before her burn. Her major problems were the lack of a father and the disruption associated with relocating five times during the previous year.

Jane underwent excision and grafting of the affected areas four times in three months. Her physical recovery was uncomplicated except for graft loss during week three of hospitalization and gastrointestinal problems (poor appetite, vomiting, stomach pain, belching, and weight loss) throughout her hospital stay.

Jane was anxious and whiny throughout her hospitalization. By the end of week one in the ICU she was angry and depressed. By week two she was agitated and hostile much of the time, regardless of who was present. Jane vigorously protested all nursing procedures and even short separations from her mother. By week three in the ICU, Jane's protests escalated regularly into uncontrollable thrashing and screaming. The staff attempted unsuccessfully to decrease Jane's screaming, especially during dressing change, with time-outs, incentives, and withdrawal of privileges. This high level of protest continued until Jane was discharged from the ICU. Jane's gastrointestinal problems, agitated squirming and scratching, and the difficulty of doing adequate debridement on a moving target, all resulted in greatly delayed healing.

Pediatric, burn, and psychiatric clinicians would probably agree that Jane's hostility and out-of-control behavior was the result of chronic and severe pain and associated anxiety. In her environment (which she perceived as invasive and attacking), Jane only had control of eating and interpersonal interactions. She attempted to protect herself from her "attackers" and to attack them by refusing to eat, vomiting, and making social interaction as aversive as possible. To some degree, Jane was successful. At times, the nurse working with her would become so exasperated that she would cut short the dressing change or take a long break during it in order to get some distance from Jane and deal with her own anger.

It is not difficult to understand Jane's panic and anger. She was a small, helpless individual in an attacking world that was supposed to be helping her. In some ways her response was adaptive; she never gave up and retreated but continued to try to protect herself. Unfortunately, this behavior was also self-destructive since it interfered with and sabotaged her treatment. As a result, Jane's physical and psychological prognosis was poor. Because she continued to resist treatments now being done by her mother at home after discharge, she was vulnerable to skin breakdown and the development of muscle contractures. Both these conditions were likely to exacerbate her hostility as well as her anxiety and depression. If the level of functioning she achieved in the hospital was lost as a result, rehospitalization would be necessary. Jane might also need surgery for muscle contracture release, severe hypertrophic scarring (if she refused to wear the pressure garments designed to prevent it), and regrafting areas of skin breakdown, all of which would involve additional psychological trauma.

A pediatric ICU patient's maladaptive hostile response to his or her injury and its treatment could be prevented or, at some point, successfully treated if a nursing care plan such as the one for Jane is implemented at the start of his or her ICU stay.

Nursing Care Plan for Jane

Nursing Diagnosis	Desired Outcomes	Interventions	Rationale
1. Anxiety	Jane's anxiety, pain, depression, and associated hostility will decrease.	Focus Jane on dressing change rather than try to distract her from it.	Predictability of aversive events, facilitated by focusing the patient on them, telling the patient what is going to happen before it happens, and giving the patient accurate sensory information about aversive events prior to experiencing them will decrease anxiety.
2. Ineffective individual coping	Jane will experience fewer feelings of anxiety during and before dressing change.	Tell Jane what is happening and about to happen at every step of dressing change, and give her as much accurate sensory information as possible.	(Same as above)
3. Powerlessness	Jane will begin to experience more feelings of control over her situation and will avoid developing learned helplessness.	Involve Jane actively in nursing care, especially dressing change, setting limits as necessary. For example, let her remove adherent dressings by herself if she does so within thirty minutes; tell her that if she is not finished in thirty minutes, the nurse will need to assist her.	Maximizing patient control of aversive events such as dressing change will decrease pain and associated anxiety, and prevent or treat related learned helplessness depression. The nurse needs to determine the parameters of patient control with the patient *ahead of time* (e.g., time allowed for removal of dressings) so that limit-setting is not experienced by the patient as loss of control.
		Gradually increase Jane's role and responsibility for her own care as she is able to handle it.	Gradually increasing expectations for self-care will steadily increase Jane's experience of control in her new world without overwhelming her.
		Praise Jane for attempts to help and all adaptive responses to treatment of her burn.	Children, like adults, like to experience success. When they feel successful, as they do with praise from adults, they will be motivated to repeat or continue associated behaviors and will feel good about themselves.

Nursing Diagnosis	Desired Outcomes	Interventions	Rationale
		Schedule daily play session in which Jane's feelings, anxiety, sadness, and anger can be labeled (interpreted) by nurse, and accepted by her as they are played out. Make sure Jane has daily opportunities for active play (for example, with balls, rubber dart gun, or squirt gun) so she has the opportunity to channel adaptively anger about what has happened and is happening to her. Provide play opportunities in which Jane can reenact what has happened to her, possibly reversing roles (she is the nurse and the doll is the patient) in attempt to understand and master her trauma and associated feelings.	Play therapy offers the child the opportunity to master anxiety and work through feelings of grief, guilt, and anger in a setting in which *he* has control and determines the outcome. The child's play offers the nurse the opportunity to understand the child's feelings and give him words for them.
		Ask Jane's mother about what would be an especially rewarding reinforcer staff can deliver whenever she cooperates with care. For example, the nurse might give child special sticker for her collection, or "star" for achievement chart she made and hung in room, whenever she eats or helps with dressing change. Also consider delivering mild aversives (time-outs, withdrawal of T.V. or video-game time) for oppositional, maladaptive, or self-destructive behavior.	Positive reinforcement must be determined on an individual basis. Usually, consistently delivered positive reinforcement is enough to motivate and maintain desired behavior. Mild aversives for undesirable behavior (such as medication refusal), if it is not extinguished with lack of positive reinforcement alone, may need to be added to the behavior program in order to ensure success.

SUMMARY

Patients in intensive care units have a high incidence of psychiatric illness. Although the etiology of this illness is usually multi-factorial, most mental health professionals agree that a patient's emotional response to his or her physical condition and the intensive care setting plays the greatest role in the development of psychopathology. In addition, medical and nursing staffs in intensive care units have a higher incidence of psychiatric illness than their peers in other health care settings. While there are many reasons for this, it is likely that these problems are the result of the highly unpredictable and often uncontrollable atmosphere in the ICU.

Many patients in ICUs are in crisis. The characteristics of an individual in crisis are: 1) decreased ability to maintain perspective, 2) decreased ability to mobilize resources, and 3) decreased ability to solve problems. The nurse who cares for these patients takes a more active, directive stance than she might in other circumstances. She must identify the most pressing problem in the situation and reduce it to manageability by suggesting adaptive responses to the patient and his or her family. She must also be able to identify maladaptive responses when they occur.

Anxiety is the most common emotion among ICU patients and staff. Anxiety in the intensive care unit typically rises as environmental predictability falls. However, by involving the patient actively in his or her own care, the nurse can help reduce this anxiety. Other effective nursing interventions are: 1) encouraging patients to verbalize anxiety, 2) explaining procedures, 3) gradually exposing the patients to feared objects and situations, 4) educating them about the normalcy of anxiety in the ICU, and 5) teaching them to use the physical symptoms of anxiety as stimuli to invoke relaxation exercises.

Patients in the ICU can begin to show signs of clinical depression, which is different from the normal grief associated with loss. This depression is usually best understood in the context of the learned-helplessness model of depression. Thus prevention and treatment of depression in the ICU patient often involves increasing the predictability and controllability of his experiences in the hospital. Since narcotics can increase depression, they should be used with caution and their effects monitored closely.

Occasionally, ICU patients become hostile to their families, other patients, and staff. This hostility probably has its roots in unexpressed anger associated with loss and pain. If the nurse validates the patient's anger, and the anger is channeled adaptively, it is less likely to result in self-destructive behavior. The nurse facilitates adaptive management of anger by setting and enforcing limits—on the patient's behavior, but not on his feelings.

Delirium is a common problem among patients in the ICU. Delirium is the result of impaired functioning of brain tissue. The reversibility of delirium depends on early recognition and treatment. Although some drugs can reduce delirium, the wrong drug can make it worse. Environmental intervention is always necessary for the delirious patient.

Sometimes medical and nursing staff in the ICU experience anxiety, depression, and hostility among themselves. They, like their patients, must deal with constant unpredictability and uncontrollability in the ICU. While group therapy or venting sessions can help staff members, the most important preventive against emotional or psychological chaos in the ICU is effective leadership by the head nurse.

KEY TERMS

intensive care unit

learned helplessness

learned-helplessness model

active and adaptive responses

maladaptive responses

experimental neurosis

stress analgesia

delirium

acute organic brain syndrome

environmental intervention

STUDY QUESTIONS

1. Name the three characteristics of the individual in crisis.

2. What kind of stance does the nurse take with the patient in crisis? Why? What are effective nursing interventions for individuals in crisis?

3. Name five ways in which the nurse can help prevent and treat anxiety in the ICU patient.

4. What is the most important intervention for patients in the ICU who are depressed?

5. How can the nurse help deal with anxiety, depression, and hostility in both herself and her colleagues in the ICU?

REFERENCES

Burgess, A. W., & Baldwin, B. A. (1981). *Crisis intervention theory-practice.* Englewood Cliffs: Prentice-Hall, Inc.

Cassem, N. H., & Hackett, T. P. (1978). The setting of intensive care. In N. H. Cassem & T. P. Hackett (Eds.), *Massachusetts General handbook of general hospital psychiatry.* St. Louis: C. V. Mosby.

Engle, G. (1962). Anxiety and depression-withdrawal: The primary affects of unpleasure. *Int. J. Psychoanal, 58,* 89.

Engle, G., & Reichsman, F. (1956). Spontaneous and experimentally induced depression in an infant with a gastric fistula, a contribution to the problem of depression. *J. Am. Psychoanal Assoc, 4,* 428.

Engle, G. I., & Schmale, A. H. (1972). Conservation-withdrawal. In *Physiology, emotions, and psychosomatic illness*. Amsterdam: Elsevier, Biomedical Press.

Fost, N. C., & Cranford, R. E. (1985). Hospital ethics committees: Administrative aspects. *Journal of American Medical Association, 253*, 2687–2692.

Goldfried, M., & Davison, G. (1976). *Clinical behavior therapy*. New York: Holt, Rinehart and Winston, pp. 112–135.

Grau, J. W., Hyson, R. L., Maier, S. F., Madden, J., & Barchas, J. D. (1981). Long-term stress-induced analgesia and activation of the opiate system. *Science, 213*, 1409.

Kaufman, I. C. (1973). Mother-infant separation in monkeys: An experimental model. In J. P. Scotland & E. C. Senay (Eds.), *Separation & depression*. Washington, D.C.: American Assoc. for the Advancement of Science.

Kavanagh, C. (1981). The concepts of predictability and controllability as applied to the treatment of children with severe burn injury. (Doctoral dissertation, University of Wisconsin.) Ann Arbor: Dissertation Abstracts International.

Kavanagh, C. (1983a). Psychological intervention with the severely burned child: Report of an experimental comparison of two approaches and their effects on psychological sequelae. *American Academy Child Psychiatry, 22*, 145.

Kavanagh, C. (1983b). A new approach to dressing change in the severely burned child and its effect on burn-related psychopathology. *Heart and Lung: The Journal of Critical Care, 12*, 612–619.

Kavanagh, C., & Freeman, R. (1984, May/June). Burn care and the pediatric patient. *PRN Forum, 3*, No. 2.

Kavanagh, C., et al. (1990). Learned helplessness and the pediatric burn patient: Dressing change behavior and serum cortisol and beta endorphin. *Advances in Pediatrics, 37*, July.

Leventhal, D. (1979). Emotion, pain, and physical illness. In C. E. Izard (Ed.), *Emotions and psychopathology*. New York: Plenum Press.

Lewis, J. W., Cannon, J. T., & Liebeskind, J. C. (1980). Opioid and non-opioid mechanisms of stress analgesia. *Science, 208*, 623.

Maier, S. F., Drugan, R, Grau, J. W., Hyson, R. A., Maclenna, A. J., & Moye. (1981) Learned helplessness pain inhibition and the endogenous opiates. In M. D. Zeilier & P. Harzem (Eds.), *Advances in analysis of behavior*. New York: John Wiley & Sons.

Maier, S. F., & Jackson, R. L. (1979). Learned helplessness; all of us were right (and wrong): Inescapable shock has multiple effects. In N. G. Bower (Ed.), *The psychology of learning and motivation*, Vol. 13. New York: Academic Press.

Miczek, K. A., Thompson, M. L., & Shuster, L. (1982). Opioid-like analgesia in defeated mice. *Science, 215*, 1520.

Miller, J. C., Dehen, H., & Cambier, J. (1981). Stress-induced analgesia in humans: Endogenous opioids and nalloxone-reversible depression of pain reflexes. *Science, 212*, 689.

Mineka, S., & Kihlstrom, J. (1978). Unpredictable and uncontrollable events: A new perspective on experimental neurosis. *J. Abnorm. Psychol., 87*, 256.

Murray, G. B. (1978). Confusion, delirium, and dementia. In N. H. Cassem & T. P. Hackett (Eds.), *Massachusetts General handbook of general hospital psychiatry*. St. Louis: C. V. Mosby.

Overmier, J. B., Patterson, J., & Wielkiewisz, R. M. (1980). Environmental contingencies as sources of stress in animals. In N. S. Levine & H. Ursine (Eds.), *Coping and health*. New York: Plenum Press.

Peters, T. J., & Waterman, R. H. (1982). *In search of excellence*. New York: Warner Books.

Physicians desk reference (1987). Oradelle, N. J.: Barnhart, E. R. pub., Medical Economics Co. Inc., p. 1089.

Seligman, M. (1968). Chronic fear produced by unpredictable shock. *Journal of Comparative and Psychological Psychology, 66*, 402–411.

Seligman, M. (1975). *Helplessness: On depression, development, and death*. San Francisco: W. H. Freeman and Co.

Seligman, M. E., Maier, S. F., & Soloman, R. L. (1971). Unpredictable and uncontrollable aversive advents. In F. R. Brush (Ed.), *Aversive conditioning and learning*. New York: Academic Press.

26

PSYCHIATRIC MENTAL HEALTH NURSING WITH THE CHRONICALLY ILL OR DYING PATIENT

NANCY BOHNET

LEARNING OBJECTIVES

After studying this chapter, the student will be able to:

- Describe a historical overview of death.
- List the chronological responses to death.
- Define and describe the stages and phases of dying.
- Identify and describe the dying patient's rights and needs.
- Describe the needs of the dying person's family.
- Describe the role of the nurse caring for the dying patient and his family.

Historical Perspectives

Primitive society
Early civilizations
Biblical times
Middle ages
Nineteenth century
Twentieth century

Death and the Life Cycle

Stages and Phases in Dying

Denial
Anger
Bargaining
Depression
Acceptance

Tasks of Dying

Patient Rights

Pain control

Chronic Illness

Patient Needs

Physical
Social
Financial
Spiritual
Emotional

Family Needs

Education
Support

The Role of the Nurse

Self-awareness
Assessing the patient
Nursing interventions with the dying patient

Case Study: Nonpsychiatric Setting

Summary

HISTORICAL PERSPECTIVES

A nurse may gain increased understanding and empathy with patients who are chronically ill and/or dying by exploring the concept of death and its meaning over time. Throughout history, the idea of death has posed the eternal mystery which is the core of our religious and philosophical system of thought (Feifel, 1965). According to Kubler-Ross (1969), a study of previous cultures reveals that death has always been distasteful to man (and probably always will be). She explains that in our unconscious, death is never possible in regard to ourselves. Since it is inconceivable to imagine an ending of our own life here on earth, death must be due to malicious intervention from the outside. In our unconscious, we can only be killed; therefore, death is associated with a bad act, a frightening happening, something that calls for retribution and punishment (Kubler-Ross, 1969).

Chronic illness has been regarded, in some ways, much like death. It may signal a loss of full, independent functioning or a change in lifestyle that can be, for some, as devastating as the prospect of death itself.

PRIMITIVE SOCIETY

Early man believed that, although death was something that happened, no one ever died completely. Death was merely a transition which enabled people to change from one form to another: the human personality remained embodied in a different form (a ghost). The primitive societies remaining on earth today, such as those in Australia, Africa, and South America, have much the same concept of death as did people thousands of years B.C. (Martocchio, 1982).

EARLY CIVILIZATIONS

The Egyptians had no doubts about the existence of an afterlife. Pyramids of the pharaohs were originally filled with food, chairs, even boats to assist with their activities. Less-important people were also buried with some necessities for life after death. Tombs' contents have revealed that citizens were commonly buried with 365 statues, called *ushabtis,* whose purpose was to provide menial labor, perhaps in the fields (one "servant" for each day of the year).

BIBLICAL TIMES

The concept of an afterlife is not encountered in many of the books of the *Old Testament.* Death is

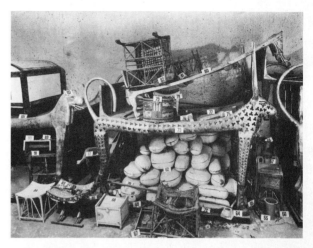

Early civilizations like the Egyptians believed in an afterlife *and* in being ready for it. In the tombs of the pharaohs there are even huge ornate boats to carry the Prince through the "Underworld."

often viewed as a curse and men yearn, in fact, for life after death. The most important idea in the *New Testament* is that of eternal life: Christ's resurrection from the dead testified that all men could expect life after death. For 2,000 years believers have held fast to this concept and gained comfort during life's trials that a better existence awaits them after they die. The early Christians, while espousing the tenet of an afterlife, were preoccupied with the Second Coming. Over time, that belief diminished but people continued secure in the belief that life would continue after earthly existence ceased.

MIDDLE AGES

During the middle ages a number of rituals emerged around the course of dying. People prepared themselves for death by assuming a supine position, their arms folded across their chests. Many religious practices such as confession, blessing, and prayers were carried out. The dying person said goodbye to his friends and loved ones, pardoned those who had wronged him, and asked pardon of those he had injured (Aries, 1981).

NINETEENTH CENTURY

Elaborate customs emerged during the Victorian era concerning death. In the United States the world was considered a wilderness to be suffered as preparation for an eternal home. Mourning periods were lengthy and associated with mourning cards, crepe, and black clothing. Bodies were bathed and cared for by families and friends and then carefully placed in fine cof-

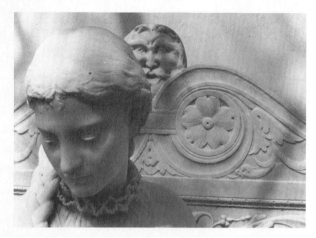

In the nineteenth century, cemeteries were much more ornate than they are today. Statuary depicting the deceased in the prime of life were constant reminders to the living of those who had gone before them, and now rested in the ground beneath them.

fins. After the Civil War, coffins were replaced by caskets (which were not tapered from the shoulders), creating the connotation of a jewel box holding something valuable (Jackson, 1980). Cemeteries were beautifully landscaped and manicured and held a great deal of romantic statuary reminding the living of those who rested in the ground. Constant reminders of dead loved ones were created. Jewelry was fashioned from a deceased person's hair, either braided or coiled. Items from the deceased, such as watch chains, brooches, and bracelets, adorned the living and kept at least a trace of the loved one in everyday view.

Death scenes were popular—lithographs, drawings, and paintings were framed and hung in the parlor depicting the death of a famous person. Early photographers used the new medium to capture the memory of deceased people in their caskets for their families to treasure. The living and dead were intertwined and coexisted comfortably.

TWENTIETH CENTURY

Some writers hold that drastic changes have occurred in the United States in this century in the living-dead relationship. The connection between the world of the dead and that of the living seems to have been severed in many instances (Jackson, 1980). Many Americans no longer live with a belief that death (at least premature death) is a natural part of life. Today, death is often viewed as a social problem. The dying person has become the dying patient. Doctors struggle to avert death in most cases; when it occurs, something has gone wrong (with the patient) to cause this failure. The doctor claims the control of death as his mission in life; perhaps the doctor is the spokesman for society. When death arrives it is usually regarded as an accident, or injustice, a sign of helplessness, or clumsiness that must be coped with (Aries, 1981).

Improved technology, especially life-support systems, has resulted in ever more complex surgical procedures. Antibiotics and vaccines continue to thwart life-threatening conditions. People today die primarily of heart disease, cancer, and accidents, not of the plague, diptheria, or smallpox. Society has become responsible for preventing premature death; health care in the U.S. has become a right, not a privilege (Martocchio, 1982). However, in the 20th century death is almost always seen as premature, in spite of the fact that life expectancy now exceeds 70 years but was only 47 years in the late 1800s.

Jackson (1980) discusses the dichotomizing of the living and dead that has occurred in the past 80–90 years and gives the following rationale for it:

1. *Urbanization.* The mobility of U.S. society means that family and friends are often separated by great distances. After separation, even death diminishes in importance. In large impersonal cities where people don't get to know one another, death means less than it does in small, rural close-knit communities. People die in hospitals and are then transported to funeral parlors—this results in more people having less exposure to death.

2. *Decreased visibility of death.* This has occurred since fewer children die now than in previous centuries. At present, the elderly are the ones who do the dying. They are also considered the least important members of our society. Many have already been segregated in nursing or retirement homes or lately in the new phenomenon—"elder-care life centers."

3. *Depersonalization of cemeteries.* A new kind of burial place has developed in this century. The memorial park has been developed which restricts the use of statuary or monuments to mark graves. Only a flat bronze plaque, one indistinguishable from another, indicates someone's final resting place. Gone, too, is the traditional mound of a burial plot. Diminishing the signs of death also diminishes the presence or intrusion of the dead upon the living.

4. *Abandonment of death as a topic by society.* A culture which no longer supports an afterlife finds natural death and decomposition too horrible to contemplate or discuss.

It is hard to face death calmly. Dying is viewed as gruesome, lonely, and mechanical. People are removed from their own environment and placed in institutions; they are then treated as if they had no rights to choices regarding their care (Kubler-Ross, 1969). In fact, 80 percent of deaths occur in institutions. Altogether, the dying are treated badly. They are avoided and isolated, which makes dying a long and lonely process (Simpson & Doyle, 1981). Hospital personnel have defined an "acceptable style of facing death" as the death of the man who pretends that he is not going to die (Aries, 1981). Most assuredly, this myth makes it easier for all concerned since, for most people (including health care professionals), death is an uncomfortable topic.

According to Kubler-Ross, death is the key to the door of life and the denial of death is partly responsible for people living empty, purposeless lives. Living in preparedness for tomorrow or remembrance of yesterday means that today is lost. If we understand that today could be our last, it could open the door to growth (Kubler-Ross, 1975).

TABLE 26–1 Chronological responses to death

Age	Concerns
Birth–two years	Aware of discomfort Loss and separation anxiety
Two years–four years	Aware that things have an end Separation means loss of love
School age	Death seen as punishment Death permanent—magic may reverse
Adolescent	Biological finality of death Psychic immortality
Young Adult	Strives to develop meaning of life Death interrupts life's goals
Adult	Reluctance to die Philosophy of life integrated
Old Age	Affirmation of life Accepts impending death

DEATH AND THE LIFE CYCLE

Children's ideas about death are related to age and cognitive development (see Table 26-1) as well as the influence of family and society (Fetsch & Miles, 1986). Infants have no perception of death. A toddler begins to recognize separation, especially from parents. Death can easily be viewed as separation by a young child and can be devastating.

An older child begins to dream about the future and death is seen as an interference (Pattison, 1978). During adolescence, a child has a firm, often grandiose, grasp of himself as a distinct person, separate from everyone else. This perception of self makes death a real adversary, difficult to accept and easy to deny.

Young adults see death as a disappointment and as unfair. The cessation of life is fraught with frustration. During life's middle years, people are reluctant to die. They have many reasons for not wanting to leave their lives. Old age brings a questioning about the worth of one's existence. Old people reminisce about their lives and strive to find meaning in their pasts (Kalish & Reynolds, 1981). The last phase of life requires one to accept the worth of one's life along with a sense of social, economic, and physical loss (Sayre, 1979), and fear of death is diminished (Feifel & Branscomb, 1973). (See Box 26–1.)

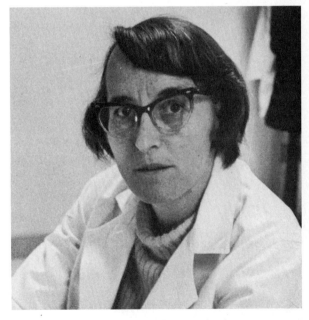

Elizabeth Kubler-Ross. Still famous for her stage/phase theory of the emotional response to the dying process, her work is less referred to in this day of theories of uneven development and emotional responding. Critics of Kubler-Ross have said that we have in the past tended to put such complex processes as emotional development and grief into stages for *our* purposes, for example, the need to organize data, *not* because that is how the data presents itself.

Box 26–1 ● The Legacy of Widowhood

One October evening 21 months ago, my husband and I went out to dinner and to see "La Traviata" at the Metropolitan. We ate at a favorite restaurant and he said that I looked beautiful in my new wool suit. Since my outfit was a decade old, I smiled and thanked him for his compliment: we'd been married for 21 years. During the night, I became a widow.

My husband was only 49 and we never had a chance to say goodbye to each other. Everyone told me that he didn't suffer; there wasn't any time. The police, the emergency crew and the doctors agreed: he'd been struck by "a catastrophic physical event." Like grand opera misplaced from the stage to our bed, death swooped down and stole him; it was as if he'd been assigned a tragic fatal aria of the heart.

The shock, overwhelming, dammed back my tears but could not stop the refrain I was hearing: I'm going to become an old woman. All I could think of was what my husband, now caught in eternity, would think of me. He'd been handsome and passionate, a Roman whose face was classical enough to have been stamped on an ancient coin. His life as a child had been disrupted by a war and I often saw him as fissured; within him were shifting layers of earthiness and artistry, science and history, prejudice and generosity. He was an exceptional man with a sense of adventure for distant places who'd been singled out for the farthest destination one final time.

But as I discovered, I had been singled out, too. Much older widows eagerly embraced me, clairvoyants whispering into my ear. I didn't need their prognostications; I knew them instinctively. Through the great silence of grief, I barely heard them anyway. My husband had disappeared, taking with him his past and my future. I was struck with the conviction that by dying too young, he had aged me overnight. Unwittingly, he had left me a terrible legacy: to be among the first in my college class to choose between coffins and deal with a funeral, to cope with a death notice, will and insurance, to have to tell children who needed their father the two hardest words in the English language: "Daddy died," to settle these matters not for an elderly parent but for the man with whom I'd still been happy to share my bed.

That's one enormous difference between death and divorce, although comparisons were often made to me. Yet I had no conjugal regrets or animosity, just incredulity; I had no flesh and blood to hate, nor even secretly to desire. I wouldn't have that one chance in a million to work things out. I was bringing news from a different front, a more remote posting where most of my contemporaries had never been. I was like my col-

STAGES AND PHASES IN DYING

Pattison (1978) and Kubler-Ross (1969) have both explored death from the perception of the dying. According to Pattison, the first phase or **acute phase** is hallmarked by immobilization and bewilderment. People are suspended in time, feeling both anxious and inadequate. A later phase is called the **chronic phase** and is abundant with fears of the unknown, loneliness, and loss of family and friends. Personal fears are also experienced such as loss of control, suffering and pain, and loss of identity. The last phase, **terminal phase,** is characterized by the patient's withdrawal into himself. Anxiety is diminished, emotional disorganization is evidenced, and the person slowly turns away from the world, experiencing **psychic death.** At any phase, the dying person may be the victim of **sociological death,** which is the separation of himself from others.

Kubler-Ross has identified coping mechanisms exhibited by terminally ill persons as one way to look

lege classmate all those years ago with her unwanted baby: she'd gotten pregnant, gotten married, gotten trapped in a life which the rest of us, safely ensconced in Nietzsche and mixers, knew little about. Nor did we wish to. On a visit to her, we cuddled that baby while averting our eyes from the diapers and bottles and the circles beneath *her* eyes. It was as if we were paying some macabre condolence call; we came to mourn the passing of her youth.

Now I, too, was old. I felt there was something shameful about my condition, inappropriate, abnormal, widowed at the wrong age. There was also shame in my bereavement; perhaps the extreme emotion of grief made me feel as if I'd lost myself along with 21 years of my past. In order to find myself, I had to search for a time when such pain could have been imagined but in fact was impossible, a time when nothing could have hurt so much because not that much had been invested yet. And as I reached back toward what seemed idyllic days, my college classmates, as different in their reactions now as they'd been when I first knew them, reached out to me.

When my husband's obituary appeared in the paper, a friend with whom I'd almost lost touch came to his funeral, treasuring her unbroken life, I think, as much as mourning mine. A real-estate agent, she not only became my friend again but helped me to sell the house my husband had loved. When he heard the news, a continent away, a lawyer's disbelief echoed through the phone: too shocked and scared to guard his tongue, he raged about diet and exercise, as if men who were tough and smart enough didn't die in their prime.

The teacher whose husband had abandoned her years ago sighed, resigned, immediately grasping the breadth of my loneliness. From the Rockies came a letter high on transcendentalism, which I think might have comforted that friend more than me. From the classmate nearby whose own mother had been widowed young came intolerance; too impatient to cope with my grief, he seemed still damaged from an accident of the heart that had happened to his father almost 30 years ago.

But others were more generous, like the friend growing deaf who managed to hear my psychic deafness, while another friend, a Congressman, knew that aid can be apolitical, that one American widow could need help as much as his constituents and far-off archipelagoes. But there was also the friend who'd seen me as the golden girl due for a fall, stern in his belief that everyone pays, that I, too, deserved punishment. When he suggested, several months ago, that I should "grow up," I was furious. For I had not only grown up, grown old, as I had expected, but I had died in my own way and been reborn a different human being.

This new person crawled out weighted with sadness, then, weak in the knees, began walking toward the future. By now I feel like a midlife adolescent, in some ways no different from what I was at 18. Confused, sometimes angry, frightened yet amazed by my shaky independence, I have those same inchoate longings, those wild curiosities and romantic yearnings, that need to find meaning and connection in the world. I remember those feelings in the girl I once was and try to adapt them to a full-grown woman. As a bride, I was led by my parents to the altar; at his unveiling, I was led to my husband's grave. The years in between seem like moments, not decades: two hearts beat together; one tripped; it was over.

He had very dark hair that curled on his neck; I keep remembering the fine Roman shape of my husband's head. But what I know now is that even if we love them inordinately, people are not ours to possess; they are only loaned to us. In fact, we barely own ourselves, and we need to keep re-inventing our lives in order to move along.

Source: New York Times Magazine, July 31, 1988, pp 20–21.

---

at death and dying; she has theorized a series of stages through which the dying move in and out.

DENIAL

Denial, the refusal to admit the truth or accept reality, may be the major defense which can help a person get through the crisis of dealing with death (Paulay, 1977). For some, denial is an important factor in maintaining relationships and helps to cope with un-resolved issues and conflicts (Beilin, 1981). Though seldom used throughout a terminal illness, denial comes and goes as the threat of reality ebbs and flows. Denial helps significant others as well, since they can avoid coming to terms with an uncomfortable issue with the dying person.

The nurse should remember that denial is a very important and vital coping mechanism for everyone. The extent of its use will vary from person to person. There is never any reason to interfere with denial unless it can be replaced with something better such as acceptance. Since it is unlikely that a better replacement can be provided, especially early in the dying process, the general rule is to leave denial intact unless it is causing harm, and be ready to support the person who begins to discontinue its use.

Mrs. G.: A Dying Patient Using Denial

Mrs. G., though physically deteriorating day by day, always talked with the hospice nurse about the trip she planned to take to California as soon as she got over her illness. The nurse had done a thorough assessment of Mrs. G. and her family and recognized that Mrs. G. had a great need to cope by using denial. Her marriage had been precarious for many years. Her husband refused to talk about her illness or the possibility she would not get better. On several occasions Mrs. G. had tentatively broached the subject and Mr. G. had walked away from her. He had threatened to leave her permanently on several occasions in previous years. The couple had two children who were remote—separated both by distance and strained relationships with their parents. It became very obvious to those caring for Mrs. G. that denial was the means by which her husband was dealing with his wife's illness and impending death. An admission of the reality of the situation could cause discomfort for Mr. G. and, as a result, the physical or emotional abandonment of his wife.

ANGER

It is not surprising that people become angry when they are faced with dying. When one's life is interrupted by a terminal illness, **anger** is a natural reaction. It can be difficult for others to deal with though, especially when it is displaced. The nurse must understand why and how people feel angry and not take their moods and outbursts personally. If a patient lashes out in anger out of proportion to a statement or situation, the nurse may respond to the tirade by saying, "Has this been a particularly difficult day?" or "Would you like to talk about the pain you're feeling?" Anger is also a natural emotion for the patient's loved ones to feel, including anger at the one who is dying. Who does not feel anger when death is about to end the life of someone dear?

BARGAINING

Having vented anger and denied that death was probable, people frequently try **bargaining**, such as making a deal with God, doctors, or fate for an extension of life. Can it be that better behavior, good works, or diligent prayer might postpone death?

DEPRESSION

Depression is caused by the sense of great loss one feels when encountering death. When the losses are itemized the list is lengthy, including loss of body parts, finances, job, as well as everything and everyone loved. Depression is certainly a normal reaction and one that can be expected, as well as treated.

ACCEPTANCE

When a person is no longer using denial or stuck in anger and has sufficiently mourned his impending losses, he may begin to experience **acceptance,** the ability to contemplate life's end with quiet expectation. This stage is not a happy one; in fact, it may be devoid of feelings and pain. However, a person is able to come to terms with death by accepting it. This acceptance can lead to a newly experienced sense of the value of life and the desire to make it more meaningful (Paulay, 1977).

Kubler-Ross's view of the process of dying has existed for nearly twenty years, during which time it has been invaluable to the many health care professionals who work with dying patients, nurses in particular. Today, however, there are several other theories to aid nurses and other professionals in their work with dying patients and their families. These include crisis theory and principles of crisis intervention (see Chapter 18 on psychological crises), personality theory (see Chapter 12 on personality disorders), and family systems theory (see Chapter 21 on families).

TASKS OF DYING

The dying have a limited time period, ending in death, in which they must make arrangements and accommodations. Affairs need to be put in order, including the appropriate transfer of property through a will (Noyes & Clancy, 1977). Other tasks can be divided into emotional and physical categories. Accommodating oneself to one's own loss requires introspection and meditation, and both require effort. The most important task a dying person has is to cope effectively with impending death. This involves planning for what time is left and making important decisions such as where to die and whether to speed up the process (see Chapter 28 on ethical considerations in psychiatric mental health practice).

Mrs. L.: A Dying Patient

Mrs. L. was a 66-year-old married woman dying of multiple myeloma. Though her disease was advanced, her condition remained stable and she was hospitalized for studies and tests to determine the current extent of disease. Early one morning an oncologist and nurse visited Mrs. L. during rounds. She asked the doctor to promise her one thing before he left the room. Obligingly, the physician agreed and asked for her request. Mrs. L. said, "Doctor, please promise me that you won't send me home. I can't possibly die at home, I must die here." The young doctor was taken off guard and said "My goodness, we're certainly not ready to talk about that yet, you're doing well." After leaving the room, the doctor asked the nurse to return later to look into what was going on with the patient. The nurse went back, sat in a chair close to Mrs. L.'s bed and said, "Let's talk about what you said to Dr. P. about dying here in the hospital. Do you feel like that will happen soon?" Mrs. L. informed the nurse that she felt she was indeed going to die very soon (in spite of the favorable test results) and that it would be impossible for her husband to care for her at home. She said that Mr. L. experienced urinary problems following a prostatectomy two years earlier. He had continuous urgency, frequency, and dribbling which had resulted in his confinement to home. This complication had resulted in Mr. L.'s becoming tense, anxious, and extremely labile. His wife's perception was that he would be physically and emotionally unable to provide terminal care for her in their home. Fearing for her husband and perhaps also for herself, Mrs. L. wanted to remain in the hospital for a few days to die. The physician ordered more lab work and scans and Mrs. L. slipped quietly into a coma, dying four days later as she desired and predicted.

PATIENT RIGHTS

Every dying person has rights which the nurse must both understand and protect. First and foremost is the right to be treated respectfully and dealt with honestly. Questions such as "how long do I have?" also mean "what quality of life do I have?" (Sternburg, 1982). Death is frequently not the most important issue troubling the fatally ill. When confronted with the assault of liver disease which causes deteriorating health, the patient realizes how far he or she has come from former good health. He or she encounters one unpleasant symptom after another, which diminishes the quality of day-to-day experiences. His or her capacity to function as a worker, parent, or spouse is compromised. The most important question is not just how *long* shall the patient live, but what level of *well-being* is compatible with life for this patient? Many feel that these criteria must be established by the patient (Koenig, 1980).

Noyes and Clancy (1977) also state that a dying person has the right to be taken care of. We know that fear of abandonment ranks high among fears of the dying. However, merely staying with the patient is inadequate. Patients have the right to expert symptom control, especially pain management, as information to treat pain adequately is readily available in this day and age. Though 50 percent of terminally ill cancer patients experience no pain, we know that fear of pain is of utmost concern to these patients. (See Box 26–2.)

PAIN CONTROL

A great deal has been learned about **pain control** and the assessment and management of pain in dying patients. It is necessary to assess the patient carefully for the parameters of pain location, quality, and quantity, in addition to the chronological aspects of pain such as duration, onset, and frequency. The possibility of alleviating any precipitating factors is also ascertained. The nurse needs to remember that the goals of pain management are: 1) to erase the memory of pain; 2) to keep the patient comfortable yet not sedated; 3) to prevent pain from recurring; 4) to alleviate side effects of analgesics; 5) to keep the patient as comfortable as he desires using the means he wishes (Amenta & Bohnet, 1986).

To achieve these goals means using the appropriate medication for the type and degree of pain. Bone pain, for example, would be managed with a prostaglandin inhibitor such as ASA or a nonsteroidal anti-inflammatory drug (NSAID) such as ibuprofen. Pain associated with muscle spasms would best be combatted with a muscle relaxant such as Valium. The patient who has a combination of pains, which is frequently the case, often needs a combination of drugs, each specific to the type of pain. Adequate dosages are titrated according to the patient's response and needs and are based on knowledge of onset, duration, and oral-parenteral ratios. There is no magic formula that will help all patients. Each individual's pain must be individually assessed and managed.

The nurse must understand the patient's wishes regarding pain control. Using a scale of 0–10 the

**Box 26–2 ●
Determining How Much
Care Society Owes the
Dying**

. . . When and to what extent doctors should use the many death-thwarting machines and techniques available today. In a pluralistic society that values life and individual choice, what are the limits? How much should society spend to extend by a few days or months a life that would otherwise end sooner? Which patients should get such care at public expense? Andrew H. Malcolm, a reporter for *The New York Times*, discussed the subject separately with three experts. Following are excerpts from the interviews.

Age Should Not Be Sole Standard

People age differently. Instead of using age as an absolute criteria we should use the potential of the individual to benefit physically, mentally and socially from our medical intervention.

Take an AIDS patient with severe dementia and kidney problems. Do we put him on a kidney machine to keep him going another two or three months when the underlying terminal disease is progressing and the outcome is inevitable? I think not. But do we fight an early AIDS patient's pneumonia to get him another six or 12 months? I wouldn't hesitate to do that.

I have eight patients in their 70's and 80's with chronic arthritis.

There's no cure. They are mentally sharp, writing books, whatever, but they suffer miserably. They may see themselves at times as burdens on their kids. I can't cure their disease. But I think our system ought to take care of these folks—physical therapy, nerve stimulators, ultrasound. The total cost per year: about $1,000.

How about an elderly woman with a terrible heart attack and severe breathing difficulties? I do everything—respirator, coronary care aortic balloon pump, the works. If she survives till morning, we'll do a cardiac catheterization. I don't know what she would want; patients don't like to discuss problems in advance.

By morning she has consumed $5,000 in medical services. And someone says, "Is this an appropriate use of resources?" She's 85, had a good life and I'm filling up a bed with a high-tech patient. Is that humane or wasteful? Frankly, if she dies next month, we'll look back and say she's one of those consuming so much of society's resources in the last few months of life. Was that a vain attempt?

At what point does my critically ill but maybe salvageable patient become a terminally ill and unsalvageable one? I don't know. You don't know. Nobody knows.

Dr. Mark Siegler, professor of medicine and director of the Center for Clinical Medical Ethics at the University of Chicago.

---

nurse asks the patient to describe his pain today and where he wishes to be. Contrary to popular belief, not everyone wants to be totally pain free. Some people want to have a minimal amount of pain—rated at 1–2 rather than at 0. This is because they feel that sensing some pain means they're still alive. People may fear pain medications used regularly will cause addiction. The nurse can explain that this is a myth. People whose pain diminishes typically request less or no pain medication once pain relief is established. The amount of medication should be established by the patient so that he achieves desired pain relief and maximum alertness and control.

Though this information is not new, many professionals are not familiar with it, causing patients to be underdosed or improperly medicated. It is essential that nurses understand current principles of pain management and provide this information to other health-care professionals, patients, and their families. Outdated perceptions about analgesia may prevent patients from obtaining the relief from pain that is currently possible, for example, through a self-administered morphine drip.

Health care professionals may be unaware of the high doses of narcotics that may be necessitated to alleviate pain. No one knows how high a dose of

No Blank Checks on Life Expectancy

Our health care system must face up to setting limits and the elderly pose a particular problem. They will double to 60 million in 25 years; those over 85 will triple. Forty percent of doctor's visits now involve those over 65. Thirty percent of Medicare is spent on 5 percent of its enrollees.

We are very soon going to have to set limits on patient choices, doctors' choices and providers' choices because the possibility of medical progress is unlimited for curing disease, stalling death, relieving disabilities. The possibility of paying for that progress is, however, very limited. One study projects Medicare deficits over $100 billion a year by 2020.

Other countries have been far more successful in controlling health costs because they are willing to accept stronger government involvement, like Canada. And other countries are less enamored of endless medical progress. They're more prepared to accept illness and death.

I don't want to go backward, just maybe not go forward quite so fast. We already do a pretty good job with life expectancy and we can't keep writing blank checks forever. Some say, "I want to live to 100. If it takes an organ transplant, why not?" I say that's understandable. We should relieve suffering, provide a reasonably adequate life span. But it's not reasonable to expect your neighbor to underwrite every possible piece of medical technology that might extend your life by a few days or months. You ought to be free to pay for that yourself.

We now say it is reasonable for a parent to expect us to develop and use our costly technology to save their premature infant down to one pound. Maybe it's not reasonable to push that limit down to a half-pound. At some point, we must say enough is enough.

Daniel Callahan, director of the Hastings Center, a group in Hastings-on-Hudson, N.Y., that studies ethical problems; author of "Setting Limits: Medical Care in an Aging Society."

In America, Death Is a Dirty Word

There's a distinct change going on in the public perception. Many people have a far greater fear of what doctors are going to do to them than what doctors can do for them.

I treat many dying patients. Before discussing any treatment, the first thing they always want is agreement not to do too much. They'll say point blank "I never want to be on a respirator," or "Promise me you won't make me go to a hospital if I don't want to." That's especially true for my serious cancer, stroke and AIDS patients.

They also want assurance that the doctor will call it quits when the patient wants to call it quits. They're more fully aware of their rights today. After all, a patient's illness is the patient's property, not the doctor's. Now patients demand the right to make the decisions. That's radically different from just 10 years ago.

The reason is simply that a greater fraction of the population has had a direct experience with some marvelous medical intervention and tragedy. "My mom was 85, a vegetable and they kept her on a machine." Everybody has a story like that. People are finally becoming aware that we don't live forever.

In this country, death is such a dirty word. We all act like we're going to live forever. We don't discuss death or our desires in the event of serious illness. Yet there's one constant of life for all of us: statistically, the death rate is one per person. What strikes me about our system is that more people are afraid of how they are going to die than the fact that they are going to die. How did the medical profession get to where people are so afraid of us?

Dr. Jack B. Weissman, infectious disease specialist, Columbia-Presbyterian Medical Center, New York City.

Source: *The New York Times*, June 9, 1988. Reprinted with permission.

---

morphine may be given safely. Patients have been administered morphine 1000 mg. and higher by mouth every few hours. When such a dose has been titrated carefully to counteract pain, there has been no evidence of respiratory depression. Very high doses of morphine have also been administered intravenously, in excess of 500 mg. per hour, again without respiratory depression. Extremely high doses are not routine, however, as most patients have their pain adequately controlled with 10–30 mg. p.o. every four hours.

Most pain can be controlled using oral medications. If the oral route is not appropriate or tolerated, rectal, vaginal, sublingual, and buccal routes can be tried to provide the patient with comfortable administration. Injections should always be considered as the last resort; what to use if all else fails to provide analgesia. By whatever means, pain must be controlled. If not, death will be welcome (Koenig, 1980). (Also see Chapter 13 on psychophysiological disorders for more on the importance of pain relief.)

Predictable pain relief leads to hope. If pain is controllable, so may be the illness. Everyone needs hope. The dying are no exception. A person has hope as long as he lives: hope of celebrating the next birthday; hope of mending relationships; hope of seeing a child born or married (Taylor & Gideon, 1982). Someone's hope may be to see the spring flowers bloom once more or to eat a favorite specially prepared food. Acknowledging that a person is dying does not take away hope. As a result of renewed hope, the question becomes "How do I want to live the rest of my life?" One likely answer is: "without pain."

CHRONIC ILLNESS

Chronic illness is described as impairments or deviations from normal which have one or more of the following characteristics:

- Permanency.
- Residual disability.
- Nonreversible pathologic alterations (often causal).
- Requires a long period of supervision, observation or care, often by specialists (Martocchio, 1982).

In many respects a chronic disabling illness can be likened to the process of dying. There are similar patterns of ups and downs, and highs and lows, leading to an overall decline. Physical disability eventually affects the patient's ability to cope. Physical disability can also cause social displacement. Chronically ill persons find themselves suspended between the present and the future. It becomes difficult for them to make long-range plans, and a change in lifestyle slowly occurs. A chronically ill person may feel great sorrow at his loss of what was once mastery over living (Martocchio, 1982). Corollaries between the perceptions and needs of chronically ill persons and their dying counterparts are many.

PATIENT NEEDS

PHYSICAL

Research reveals that dying people experience an average of five and one-half symptoms in the last thirty-five days of life (Mor, 1986). Along with pain, people are troubled by shortness of breath, dysphagia, and anorexia. Careful palliation of these symptoms is mandated. As physical condition declines, there is an increase in untoward symptoms and in cognitive impairment. Dying can be very uncomfortable without appropriate interventions.

Physical comfort measures, in addition to symptom control for pain, nausea, vomiting, and anorexia, should be provided for the dying. People are interested in their appearance and good grooming helps morale immensely. A shower or tub bath along with hair shampooing and shaving does wonders for a person's comfort and self-esteem. Certainly it is impossible to feel comfortable or valued if one is unkempt and odorous.

SOCIAL

The dying, like most people, have the need to maintain their life roles as long as possible (Taylor, 1983). Whether at work or at home, it is fulfilling and rewarding to function competently in a familiar role. Thus a mother might wish to care for her child, prepare meals, and do light housekeeping even though others might view the tasks as burdensome and tiring.

Judy: A Dying Mother

Judy, dying at 34 from ovarian cancer, had one four-year-old preschool child. Her husband mixed the prescribed intravenous solutions and placed Judy on the hyper-alimentation pump as soon as he came home from work. The fluids infused all night and Judy's husband capped the central lines before leaving for work in the morning. This permitted Judy to have the necessary freedom to manage her house and mother her child for the next 8–9 hours. Her fondest hope was to live for six months so that she could best prepare her only daughter for the start of kindergarten. She held the child, sang to her, and allowed her to help with simple cooking and cleaning. Judy lived until Christmas, three months after school started, and was comforted by the knowledge she had remained capable in her chosen role as a loving wife and mother until she died.

FINANCIAL

Dying has the potential to create many financial difficulties. If a person is no longer able to work, income may be drastically diminished. Many people have either no or inadequate insurance coverage to deal with the high costs of being ill. Basic expenses include medications and supplies, doctors' and visiting nurses' bills, and equipment rental. It is the fortunate minority who have no difficulty handling these expenses.

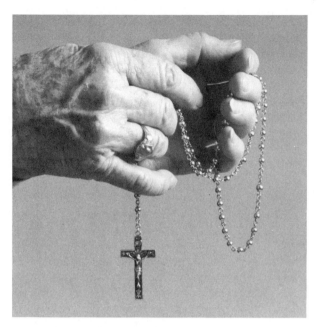

Spiritual strength and comfort can be garnered by the patient from prayer and meditation.

SPIRITUAL

The spiritual area of patient need is frequently unmet especially if nurses view the patient's **spirituality,** his philosophy of life and death and their meaning to him, and his relationship to the universe and God, as "private" or if the visiting clergyman is presumed to be responsible for this aspect of patient care. Spirituality and religion are not the same. A Roman Catholic attends Mass and receives the sacraments as religious practices, but the spiritual aspect of his life involves much more. Dying people may have spiritual concerns that require assistance from the nurse. While the nurse may help explore and support the patient's spiritual quest, attempts to convert the patient to a particular religion are never appropriate. Spiritual strength and comfort can be garnered by the patient from prayer, meditation, and religious practices or readings. Each individual has a unique spiritual self and has the right to be assisted in obtaining spiritual solace.

EMOTIONAL

A lifetime of behavior is embodied in the dying person. People typically approach death as they do life, without suddenly changed behavior. Those who have avoided confrontation throughout life will probably continue to avoid it. Stoics are likely to remain stoic. People who would rather not know what to expect in the future will probably opt for that choice as they die (Martocchio, 1982). On the other hand, many people are definitely more comfortable knowing in advance what may lie in store. (Also, see Chapter 25 on psychiatric mental health nursing with the patient in intensive care regarding the role of predictability in mental health.) In *A Way to Die* the Zorzas (1980) report a conversation a hospice volunteer had with the Zorzas's dying daughter, Jane, a young woman in her twenties.

> "There's only one thing that worries me. I wish I knew what it was going to be like—dying, I mean. I'm a bit scared of that, but I suppose nobody knows. . . ."
>
> Julie (the volunteer) replied, "I think I can tell you. You'll go to sleep and slip away without even waking up. I've watched a lot of people while they died and that's what will probably happen to you."
>
> Jane was content. Now, free of the constraints of the future, free of possible disciplines that she would resent and probable defeats that might crush her, she had only to deal with the present, and it was manageable, limited, under control. She seemed to have no fear left in her.

Importantly, the nurse must remember that the dying person has choices, including how much and what kind of information he or she wishes to receive at any time.

Pattison (1978) states that each person's unique coping abilities and philosophy of death assist him in achieving what for him is an appropriate death. Patients have the need to face death without emotional disintegration and must reconcile the reality of their lives with what they hoped to achieve. In addition, the dying have the need to preserve relationships and to be accepted despite impending death.

The nurse assisting the dying person knows that her efforts at helping him are *normal,* not special, and that death is a normal part of life, not pathology. Helping the dying often means *being,* not *doing* (Pattison, 1978). Similarly, when the nurse doesn't know what to say, she can say how she feels; for example, "I can see that this is a very difficult time for you and I'd like to help if I can, but I'm not sure what would be helpful. Would it help if I just stayed with you for a while?"

FAMILY NEEDS
EDUCATION

Research with the families of patients dying at home has found that nursing behaviors directed toward the patient are more helpful than behaviors directed toward the families (Skorupka & Bohnet, 1982). This study also indicated that family members designated as caregivers give high priority to making sure the patient's physical and emotional needs are met. Thus the family members need education, for example, in technical skills to care competently for the dying patient. It is up to the nurse to provide specific information and skills training for family members, enabling them to participate in a significant way with their loved one and helping them to maintain their relationship with the patient until death. (See Box 26–3.)

When a patient is dying in an institution, the family may not be able to be as actively involved in physical care. However, education and information provided by the nurse in a caring way decreases their anxiety. Telling a husband why his wife has a Foley catheter, suction apparatus, or IV answers questions he may be reluctant to ask, while decreasing his feelings of isolation and loss of control.

SUPPORT

When a patient dies at home the family assumes a very large task. Martocchio (1986) states:

> The psychic costs of home care to the family, despite noble intentions and heroic efforts, may be substantial. Even with the best of programs, anxiety and depression may pervade the home: there may be preoccupation with chores or dread of awakening or returning home to find the dying person dead or not dead. The fatiguing role turns joys to conflicts and produces changes in family relationships. The family may feel more like victims than caregivers.

When dying is prolonged, in any setting, the dying person may become less and less involved in decisions regarding family or personal interests. The family perceives this behavior as protective; the patient feels as if he is already dead. A family may actually finish mourning before the patient dies and may be unable to be of help to him, having prepared too well. Family members may feel resentful of the time and money spent in hospitalization and visiting. They may even take on the patient's role in the family, not allowing him to reenter, should he stabilize or improve. Knowing that families have the potential to treat a patient as though he has died before phys-

ical death occurs, can help the nurse recognize this when it happens. This behavior should be pointed out to the family and the consequences explored. The family should also be helped to understand the underlying reason for their behavior. Respite from their burden may be a possible solution and may be provided through volunteer caregivers or paid help which allows the family to have some freedom. (Also see Chapter 21 on psychiatric mental health nursing with families.)

THE ROLE OF THE NURSE
SELF-AWARENESS

Nurses who care for people who are dying must first become, themselves, comfortable with death. In essence, this means coming to terms with one's own mortality. By exploring her own values, and feelings about the meaning of life as well as death, the nurse can develop a personal philosophy. Questions such as "Why am I here?" and "What is life all about?" must be explored and answered personally to the best of her ability and satisfaction. She may master feelings about her own death and the deaths of patients through religion, active participation in the process of dying, and the identification and expression of associated anxiety, anger, and grief (McKitrick, 1981–1982).

Increased comfort with death can be arrived at by identifying why, first of all, death causes discomfort. Today, there are many seminars on death and dying to assist the nurse striving to understand and deal with feelings about death. There are also many professionals (social workers, psychiatrists, and psychologists, as well as other nurses who work with the dying) whom nurses can learn from and go to for support as they strive to increase the awareness and skills needed to work with this patient population (Joseph, 1983).

ASSESSING THE PATIENT

Dying patients should be assessed to determine their problems and needs—physical, spiritual, and emotional. Realistic and measurable goals for care should be established with the patient's participation, and nursing interventions should be aimed at achieving these goals.

The nurse approaches the dying patient with concern about his present physical, emotional, and spiritual status, helping him to realize that his present state is more important than dying (Koenig, 1980).

Box 26–3 ● The Hospice Movement

The Contemporary Hospice Concept in the United States

The modern hospice is not a place, a building, or an institution; it is a concept. It is a collection of ideas and attitudes informing an array of services based on a holistic philosophy of living and dying. . . . It is a programmatic approach to the search for a meaningful treatment of terminally ill patients and their families that unites contemporary science, belief, and caring. Since its goal is to prolong meaningful living, not physiological dying, no active, curative therapies are undertaken. In short, the goal of all hospice care is palliation, or making the patient comfortable. A presumed component of that comfort is that the patient will be as much like himself or herself as possible, with personality not warped or obtunded by social isolation, drugs, treatments, equipment, or the environment.

The medical cornerstone of the modern hospice is relief of physical pain and other disturbing symptoms through the sophisticated use of state-of-the-art pharmacologic and other pain- and symptom-control techniques. The object is to balance analgesia with alertness—to relieve pain without causing drowsiness. That accomplished, patients can get on with controlling their remaining life, time, and choices as much as possible.

Modern hospice care also provides active support for the families of the patient. In order for patients to be as much themselves as possible throughout the living while dying period, they must have the opportunity of remaining a part of their families if that is desired and possible. Patients and families are helped, when necessary, to communicate through the barriers that impending death might impose. Support of family members during their anticipatory grief and regular, organized bereavement care after the death of the patient is also provided.

Spiritual care for both patients and families is another necessary part of any bona fide hospice program. All persons approaching their deaths in a conscious and forthright way deserve the opportunity to examine the dimensions of meaning, relatedness, forgiveness, and transcendence that this powerful life event inevitably brings to the fore.

Hospice services are available in the home as well as in inpatient settings when such are needed for either symptom stabilization or pain control for the patient or respite for the family. Inpatient settings that accommodate the hospice philosophy are notable for their homelike atmosphere and relaxation of traditionally rigid institutional rules about visiting for friends, family, children, even pets.

In order to provide and coordinate these varied services around the clock, an interdisciplinary team of professionals is required. Volunteers are almost without exception a part of the team. The resources of built-in staff support and the time to use them are necessary to help all these people work at melding themselves into an efficiently caring community.

Source: Amenta, M. O. (1986) *Nursing care of the terminally ill,* Boston: Little, Brown, & Co. pp 49–64.

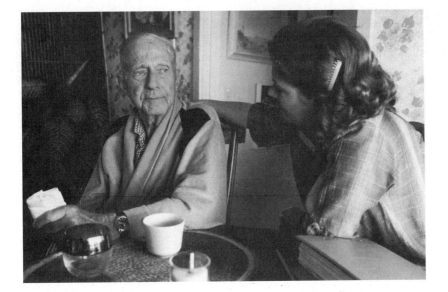

It is important to determine what the patient knows and wants to know about his condition in order to provide relevant information to him, abiding by his choice to know much or little. Before talking with the patient about his death, the nurse should first ask about his life; questions about what is important to this person regarding his life, primary relationships, and his work can help the nurse get to know the *patient* who is dying. Additionally, the nurse should determine any fears the patient might have about death (Koenig, 1980). It is only possible to allay specific fears when the nurse knows what they are.

John: A Patient Who Fears Death

John expressed his fear of death. The nurse asked him to tell her what most frightened him about it. He told her that his father had died 20 years earlier of the same cancer in a great deal of pain. He did not fear the possibility of pain as much as he did losing control and crying out, thus not behaving "like a man" which was what his father did. The nurse explained that pain management today would be very different than when his father died. He would be in control of the dose and frequency of pain medication, titrating it to his specific needs while remaining alert and comfortable. This information had an immediate impact and allayed John's first and foremost fear.

The importance of expert physical care and symptom management has already been emphasized. Emotional care is also important and should be provided in an open and supportive manner. Dying patients are usually receptive to signs of overt affection and appreciate being touched (Baldonado & Stahl, 1982). Sometimes a pat or hug says or accomplishes a lot more than words ever could.

Peter: A Dying Patient with AIDS

Peter laid on his bed appearing cachectic and very ill; he was dying of AIDS. The nurse recognized that conversation would cause him undue exertion so she merely greeted him, sat down next to his bed, and reached for his hand to hold in her own. Peter smiled, tears running down his cheeks. He whispered to the nurse that everyone seemed afraid of him and he was grateful for her presence and for the touch of another human being. It was clear that her actions meant a lot to him.

Dying with dignity results from the participation and autonomy of the patient throughout the dying process, and his ability to make choices about his own death. It is also important that the patient feel that he is not alone and that his family loves him and will miss him (Simonton, 1984). If a patient wants to share his fears and feelings, it is comforting for him to learn that the nurse will listen to what he has to say and try to understand what he is going through. It is often not necessary for the nurse to say very much except perhaps "It's really hard, isn't it?" but the message conveyed is one of "I care about you."

When a patient is so agitated about impending death that he threatens harm to himself or to others, a psychiatric consultation is warranted. Though this is a rare occurrence, the nurse should know how to get assistance from a mental health professional as soon as possible.

NURSING INTERVENTIONS WITH THE DYING PATIENT

Several principles will assist the nurse in comforting and supporting dying patients. Garfield (1976) stresses that the care of the dying is a formidable task requiring shared responsibility among health-care professionals. Knowledge should be provided so that a person's expectations and limitations imposed by disease are realistic and based on factual information.

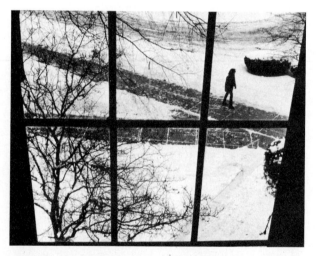

In her work with the dying, the nurse is likely to become more aware of her own spiritual self. Perhaps it had become lost to her until now. She needs to spend time with it, feel what it is and how it affects her as an individual, as a partner, as a nurse, and as a nurse who works with the dying patient and his or her family.

The patient's self-esteem must be preserved. (It can be enhanced when the patient feels understood.) Because it is difficult to work with dying people, monitoring one's emotions and feelings is critical. It is counterproductive for the nurse to allow her own emotional font of well-being to become depleted. Periodically, it is necessary for the nurse to rejuvenate and replenish herself by distancing, reflection, and introspection.

One of the most important nursing interventions is **advocacy,** support or defense of the patient and his rights. Nurses find themselves requesting, often demanding, better measures for symptom management, requesting respite from troublesome treatments, and consulting with other members of the health-care team on behalf of the dying patient. The nurse who intercedes skillfully with a variety of professionals, family, or others, fulfills the role of patient advocate and is likely to make a vital difference in the patient's comfort and, ultimately, quality of life.

People who are dying should be treated with the respect due them at any time of their lives. However, as previously discussed, the dying may be ignored, isolated, or treated as if they are already dead. The nurse needs to be sensitive to this possibility and intervene as appropriate in order to ensure quality of life to a dying patient.

Importantly, patients should be given an opportunity to talk about themselves. A therapeutic relationship develops when the nurse accepts an individual as he is, along with his anxieties, anger, and depression, without judgment, remembering this patient's feelings are as unique as he is. (See Chapter 7 on the nurse as therapist.)

It is sometimes helpful for the nurse to engage the dying patient in **life-review therapy,** a technique which involves a mental process characterized by a progressive return to past experiences, especially unresolved conflicts (Lewis & Butler, 1974). That is, the nurse guides the patient's reflections to explore, reorganize, resolve, and reintegrate troublesome and preoccupying thoughts and feelings. The purpose of this process is to make sense of past experiences, and to come to terms with and accept them. The nurse facilitates the process and helps a person take a positive view of the life he's lived and himself (Wysocki, 1983). Ideally, short 20–30 minute sessions can take place once or twice a week for 8–10 weeks. The luxury of over two months to engage in life review may not be a possibility, however, and the nurse may need to prioritize the patient's conflicts and focus on the most troublesome in the time available. It would also be appropriate to enlist the help of a mental-health professional in this situation.

Jean: A Dying Patient

Jean was in the last phase of her life, dying of lung cancer. Though she was kept physically comfortable,

We all need to be touched, even held at times. Here the nurse is so tuned in to the patient's feeling state that, for a few moments, nothing else exists. Her eyes tell the story. She sees inside the patient, not invasively, but as one human being to another. And she wants to be *with* her, and "hold her"—with those eyes.

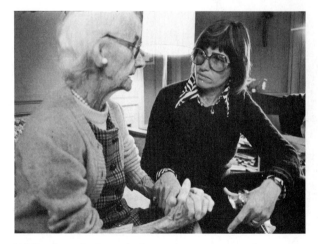

While there isn't such dramatic eye-contact here—or the affective attunement (Stern, 1985)—the nurse is truly there for the patient. She's sitting and listening, and covering the patient's wringing hands with her own large and steady one. The result: the patient talks, and talks, and talks. She's had a lot to say for *years*. It now feels safe to say it. And someone is listening.

she was emotionally distressed since she was unable to come to terms with a decision made years ago. At age 20, Jean had given birth to a baby boy. Marrying the child's father was impossible and Jean, prodded by her mother, gave the child up for adoption without ever seeing or holding him. She was now struggling with this decision and wondered if it had been made in haste due to her mother's pressure. Jean's nurse made arrangements for subsequent visits to gather the facts of Jean's life up to her present illness. Jean gradually unfolded her life history following the child's birth. She had gone on to finish college, had worked as an architect for 20 years, and had never had a serious relationship with another man. As she opened the doors to her life, Jean gradually realized that since the child's birth occurred in 1955, it would have been difficult for both her and the child if the child had been raised out of wedlock. As she remembered society in the 1950s, Jean knew that an unwed mother and her child would not have been accepted. The "anything goes" attitude of this decade definitely did not prevail in those days. The child would have been taunted and perhaps shunned for something over which he had no control. Jean had been looking at the unwed mothers and their children of today and felt she had made a poor choice. Only by consciously reviewing her life and times was she able to resolve the dilemma. Jean accepted the correctness of her decision and believed that her mother had positively influenced her. For this she was both pleased and grateful and had reason to believe her son had also benefited from the choice.

Another intervention used to facilitate emotional well-being in the dying patient is **logotherapy,** which involves enhancing the individual's feeling that life has meaning and purpose. In this way the nurse assists the patient in dealing with his impending death by understanding that he may live as meaningful a life as is possible with his remaining abilities in the time he has left (Hutzell, 1986).

The nurse, then, provides emotional support by helping the patient deal with loss by planning and allocating the time remaining to him (Kalish, 1980).

Common psychosocial problems experienced by the dying are concern about the inability to have a future and the mandate to end long-range planning. Despite these losses, however, patients may be emotionally comforted when their affairs are in order, when they are surrounded with caring friends and family, and when their symptoms (physical and psychological) have abated. They also benefit from being allowed to remain in control of their life and death as much as is possible, and to be involved in decisions related to death and the process of dying. When a nurse enables a patient to do this, while helping him to affirm his life, both the art and science of nursing is practiced.

> Death must simply become the discreet but dignified exit of a peaceful person from a helpful society that is not torn, not even overly upset by the idea of a biological transition without significance, without pain or suffering, and ultimately, without fear (Aries, 1981).

Case Study: Nonpsychiatric Setting

Alice was a 35-year-old, white, married mother of a boy, age six, and a girl, age eight. She lived with her children and husband in an urban two-story, comfortable, well-kept home.

After being in the hospital for five days, Alice left in the middle of the night against medical advice (without her physician's agreement). She feared that she would die soon and could no longer tolerate being separated from her children.

Two years ago Alice had discovered a lump in her right breast. She sought medical advice immediately and after a staging workup she was diagnosed as having breast cancer with bone and liver metastases. Following a radical mastectomy, chemotherapy was started. The disease continued to progress and Alice's chemotherapy was changed to a new protocol which controlled the cancer for a brief period of two months. The last three months before her hospitalization saw rapid growth of metastatic lesions and a steady downward decline in Alice's physical and emotional status. The chemotherapy resulted in troublesome side effects, such as bone marrow depression, nausea, weight loss, alopecia, and various infectious processes ranging from herpes zoster to thrush of the mouth, throat, and vagina. When Alice was hospitalized for five days of tests and chemotherapy administration, investigative studies revealed advancing disease in spite of the course of chemotherapy and Alice decided to stop treatment. Her husband supported her decision but her children were not informed of either the seriousness of their mother's condition or of her decision to discontinue chemotherapy. Prior to leaving the hospital, Alice had become agitated and anxious at about 2:00 A.M. She called her husband to come and take her home. He called her physician who tried to talk Alice out of her decision, but she remained adamant. Since the doctor was unable to dissuade Alice, her husband came for her.

Alice's mother died at 48 from breast cancer as had her maternal grandmother at 56 years of age. Alice's husband, Tom, is a high school principal in a large urban school. Their children are both in school. Bobby is in first grade and his sister, Mary, is a third grader.

Personal History

Alice was an only child; her mother gave birth to her at age 35 and died of breast cancer when Alice was a teenager. Alice's father died of a stroke five years ago. Alice was in good health throughout her childhood, which she described as uneventful and pleasant. Adolescence was a difficult period for Alice since her mother died and she was raised by her grieving father, who never remarried. She did well in school and had many friends but did not date until graduation from high school. Alice and Tom met at the state college they both attended, dated, became engaged their senior year, and married shortly after they graduated with degrees in education. Alice taught grade school for five years and then retired to have a family. Tom taught high school and was promoted to principal in another school three years ago. They both wanted a family and were elated about parenthood.

Current Social Situation

Tom and Alice lived in a comfortable home in a well-kept neighborhood at the time of her diagnosis and were in good shape financially. Their children attended school three miles from home and were on spring break when Alice left the hospital and returned home.

Physical Examination

1. *General description.* With her doctor's and husband's encouragement, Alice agreed to involvement with a visiting nurse. On her first home visit the day after Alice left the hospital, the nurse found Alice huddled in bed wearing a nightgown and socks. She appeared anxious and frightened. Although she had lost her hair, she wore neither wig nor head covering. Her children hovered outside her room while, trembling, their mother spoke in a whisper.

2. *Gastrointestinal.* Alice's physical problems at that time included anorexia, a constant problem during chemotherapy over the past three months. Her mouth was reddened and sore from a yeast infection. She had bowel problems, and her enlarged liver caused discomfort when palpated.

3. *Genitourinary.* Alice had been troubled with a urinary-tract infection. She was experiencing urgency, frequency, and dysuria. She walked 30 feet each way from her bed to the bathroom at least once an hour.

4. *Cardiovascular.* Alice's pulse was regular and rapid at 120/minute. Her blood pressure was 135/90. Her heart rate was regular with no abnormal sounds.

5. *Respiratory.* Alice's respirations were shallow and rapid at 26/minute. She complained of chest pain on inspiration. Lung sounds were difficult to obtain, but there were no rales or rhonchi.

6. *Reproductive.* The surgical site of Alice's mastectomy was well healed. The yeast infection was still present in her vagina and vulva.

7. *Pain.* Alice complained of bone pain in her right shoulder and humerus as well as her lower vertebrae. The stomatitis and vaginitis also caused discomfort. Her urinary-tract infection resulted in dysuria. She had codeine for pain but only took one 30 mg pill once or twice a day, and was reluctant to do this since it caused her to be nauseated.

8. *Emotional status.* Alice was agitated as a result of her pain and accompanying anxiety. She said she was miserable physically as a result of the yeast infections, UTI, and bone pain. She also admitted exhaustion from the frequent trips to the bathroom, lack of sleep, and emotional upheaval. She was most worried, however, that she would soon die and that her children would feel abandoned by her. Although she and Tom had told the children about her illness, they had not discussed her death with them. Alice had wanted to protect them from this painful fact since they were so young.

9. *Insight and judgment.* Alice had an excellent understanding of her physical status and prognosis. She wanted assistance from the nurse, however, in providing information to her children and planning for her care and death at home.

Nursing Diagnoses

Anticipatory grieving
Powerlessness
Anxiety
Discomfort
Altered nutrition: less than body requirements
Altered family processes

Nursing Care Plan for Alice

Nursing Diagnosis	Desired Outcomes	Interventions	Rationale
1. Anticipatory grieving of both Alice and family related to imminent death and loss of future together.	Enhanced coping. Alice and family will verbalize love, sadness over impending loss, goodbyes, and last wishes.	Encourage Alice to vent her sadness and offer emotional support.	Listening to Alice's feelings ascertains areas of greatest concern.
		Assist Alice and Tom in communicating about Alice's death to their children.	Parents need guidance in talking about death to young children.

Nursing Diagnosis	Desired Outcomes	Interventions	Rationale
		Encourage Alice and Tom to engage the children in a family conference within 48 hours.	Alice is actively dying; conference must be held within two days if Alice is to participate.
		Meet with the children to offer support and answer questions about death and loss.	Children feel isolated and fearful. Need reassurance and answers from nurse.
		Help Alice make funeral and burial plans. Include children in planning.	Eliciting Alice's preferences helps her feel in control.
2. Powerlessness related to dependence on others for care, weakened state, and loss of control.	Alice will make decisions regarding her care to regain a sense of control of her life.	Encourage Alice to conserve physical energy so that remaining time is quality time. Discuss possibility of Foley catheterization so that Alice might conserve energy now used for bathroom trips.	Indwelling catheter would eliminate bathroom visits to void.
		Offer choices regarding hospital bed, bedside commode, or walker.	Choices involve active patient participation, show respect, and help patient regain a sense of control.
		Instruct Alice in medication administration; leave meds and logs at bedside so that Alice may self-administer as long as possible.	Alice needs to feel in control because of its pain-killing and antidepressant properties.
		Offer Alice personal care assistance by home health aide.	Clean body and hair will enhance Alice's feeling of well-being, self-esteem, and attractiveness to her family.
		(Also see nursing interventions for nursing diagnosis #4 related to pain control.)	
3. Anxiety related to impending death.	Alice will understand that death does not have to be painful and will experience decreased anxiety about it.	Provide factual description of the physical parameters of this patient's dying process.	Providing realistic description of death to Alice will diminish anxiety-promoting fantasies.
		Assure Alice that everything possible will be done to make her comfortable, and she will not be alone.	Prevents fears of abandonment and discomfort.

Nursing Diagnosis	Desired Outcomes	Interventions	Rationale
		Reassure Alice that her children will be helped to understand that their mother is not abandoning them, and supported emotionally.	Assurance of children's well-being will comfort Alice.
		Suggest pastoral counseling for the family.	This type of counseling may enhance spiritual solace and comfort.
4. Discomfort related to terminal disease process: 1) Pain related to bone metastasis. 2) Stomatitis, vaginitis, cystitis secondary to depressed immune system. 3) Dyspnea related to lung metastasis.	Minimized physical discomfort	Assess parameters of bone pain. Obtain order for oral Morphine and ASA. Evaluate pain relief and adjust Morphine dosage and route of delivery in collaboration with the patient and her physician. Start Pericolace and MOM with MS.	MS should be given on a regular schedule to prevent the development of severe pain. ASA is a prostaglandin inhibitor and is specific for bone pain. Narcotics cause constipation so bowel regimen must be instituted with regular narcotic schedule.
		Obtain order for Nizoral, Mylanta-Benadryl-Xylocaine (M-B-X). Obtain order for Bactrim. Instruct Alice in oral care comfort measures.	Nizoral is specific for infections in mouth and vagina, Bactrim combats bladder infection. M-B-X will promote healing and comfort in sore mouth. Good oral care will promote comfort and appetite.
		Elevate head of bed. Obtain order for oxygen. Assist Alice in relaxation therapy techniques. (See Chapter 25 for specifics.)	Elevation of head relieves pressure on diaphragm and eases breathing as does oxygen and relaxation.
		Obtain order for MS suppositories if Alice is unable to swallow or comatose and in pain.	MS suppositories are absorbed at the same rate as the oral dose.
5. Altered nutrition: less than body requirements.	Optimal intake for comfort. Prevention of dehydration.	Assist Alice in making choices to increase fluid intake to 1000 cc/day.	Increased fluid will promote bladder comfort and prevent dehydration.
		Keep preferred chilled fluids with increased calories at bedside along with ice chips.	Alice is not able to consume much food so calories may be provided with milkshakes, Ensure, fruit nectar drinks.
		Encourage family to offer fluids frequently.	Family participation in provision of comfort.

Nursing Diagnosis	Desired Outcomes	Interventions	Rationale
		Apply K-Y jelly (or Vaseline) to lips.	It is important to promote mouth comfort and fluid intake. K-Y will prevent dry lips from becoming cracked, sore, and a potential entry site for life-theatening bacterial organisms.
6. Altered family processes.	Alice and Tom will be able to talk with each other and the children about Alice's anticipated death and what the future will be like without her.	Talk with Alice and Tom together about their perceptions of how the children are coping with the anticipated death of their mother, and what the children will need in the immediate future, after Alice dies.	Alice and Tom need to be reassured that their children receive accurate information about their mother's condition to eliminate anxiety and fear which could lead to lifelong grieving.
		Assist Alice and Tom with mobilizing resources to meet future family needs (at the time of Alice's death and in the first few months afterwards).	Alice will be comforted in the knowledge that her family will be adequately cared for.
		Offer Alice and Tom assistance in talking with their children, or talk with Alice and Tom about the children's probable concept of death and developmental needs at this time as they go through their mother's death and the initial adjustment period afterwards. (Also see Table 26–1 and Chapter 22 on child psychiatry.)	The children need simple factual information about what is happening. Parents need to talk to children together as a family to decrease the anxiety in the system. Parents should not be surprised if the younger, normally egocentric, child responds with: "Who will be my mommy then?"

SUMMARY

People have responded to and coped with death in various ways at different times in history. The living and dead experienced a peaceful coexistence in the Victorian Age, but drastic changes have occurred in this century. The ultimate consequence of the modern view of death is that it is no longer viewed as natural or normal. Because of this, the dying are often isolated, ignored, and abandoned.

People have differing concepts of death, which are related to their differences—stage in the life cycle, culture, and so on. Their ability to cope effectively is enhanced by moving through various stages such as denial, anger, bargaining, depression, and acceptance in their own style and in their own time.

The dying patient has to move through a somewhat predictable psychological process. This process can be facilitated when the nurse is aware of patient/family needs, and their coping mechanisms, support systems, and resources.

Patients who are dying have rights which nurses must both understand and ensure. These include the rights to respectful treatment, honesty, expert symptom management, freedom from fear of abandonment, and hope.

Patient needs include maintenance of life roles as long as possible and promotion of physical and emotional comfort. Spiritual and financial concerns must also be assessed and addressed. Families must be helped to participate in the physical and emotional care of their dying loved one.

Nurses who care for dying patients are encouraged to familiarize themselves with that phase of life through self-exploration, education, and experience. Nursing interventions focus on promoting comfort and quality in all aspects of the patient's life.

Assessing patient/family needs, identifying problems and initiating appropriate interventions, and ongoing evaluation of physical and psychological care affirm that death is a part of life. The art and science of nursing can facilitate a comfortable, peaceful transition from life to death for both patient and family.

KEY TERMS

acute phase	acceptance
chronic phase	pain control
terminal phase	chronic illness
psychic death	spirituality
sociological death	premortem dying
denial	advocacy
anger	life-review therapy
bargaining	logotherapy
depression	control

STUDY QUESTIONS

1. Name three reasons why death is not regarded as a normal part of life in this century.

2. What are the stages of dying identified by Kubler-Ross?

3. Describe the differences in concept of death between a five-year-old child and an adult of 35.

4. List the general needs of a dying patient and his family.

5. What are three nursing interventions which may assist a patient who is fearful of dying?

6. Describe how caring for dying persons can be rewarding.

REFERENCES

Amenta, M., & Bohnet, N. (1986). *Nursing care of the terminally ill.* Boston: Little, Brown.

Aries, P. (1981). *The hour of our death.* New York: Alfred A. Knopf.

Baldonado, A., & Stahl, D. (1982). *Cancer nursing: A holistic multidisciplinary approach,* 2nd Ed. Garden City, New York: Medical Examination Publishing Co.

Beilin, R. (1981). Social functions denial of death. *Omega, 12,* 25.

Beisser, A. (1979). Denial and affirmation in illness and health. *Am. J. Psychiatry, 136,* 1026.

Brunner, L., & Suddarth, D. (1986). *The Lippincott manual of nursing practice,* 4th Ed. Philadelphia: J. B. Lippincott, pp. 919–20.

Feifel, H., Ed. (1965). *The meaning of death.* New York: McGraw-Hill.

Feifel, H., & Branscomb, A. (1973). Who's afraid of death? *Journal of Abnormal Psychology, 81,* 282.

Fetsch, S., & Miles, M. (1986). Children and death. In M. Amenta & N. Bohnet, *Nursing care of the terminally ill.* Boston: Little, Brown and Co.

Garfield, C. (1976). Foundations of psycho-social oncology: The terminal phase. *Front. Rad. Onc, 11,* 180.

Hutzell, R. (1986). Meaning and purpose in life: Assessment techniques of logotherapy. *The Hospice Journal, 2,* 37.

Jackson, C. (1980). Death shall have no dominion: The passing of the world of the dead in America. In R. Kalish (Ed.), *Death and dying: Views from many cultures.* Farmingdale, N.Y: Baywood Pub. Co.

Joseph S. (1983). Interview: Elisabeth Kubler-Ross, M.D. *The Coordinator, 2,* 28.

Kalish, R. (1980). The onset of the dying process. In R. Kalish (Ed.), *Death, dying transcending.* Farmingdale, N.Y.: Baywood Pub. Co.

Kalish, R., & Reynolds, D. (1981). *Death and ethnicity: A psychocultural study.* Farmingdale, N.Y.: Baywood Publishing Co.

Koenig, R. (1980). Dying vs. well being. In R. Kalish (Ed.), *Caring relationships: The dying and the bereaved.* Farmingdale, N.Y.: Baywood Pub. Co.

Kubler-Ross, E. (1969). *On death and dying.* New York: Macmillan Co.

Kubler-Ross, E. (1975). *Death: The final stage of growth.* Englewood Cliffs, N.J.: Prentice-Hall, Inc.

Lewis, M., & Butler, R. (1974, November). Life-review therapy: Putting memories to work in individual and group psychotherapy. *Geriatrics,* 165–173.

McKitrick, D. (1981–1982). Counseling dying clients. *Omega, 12,* No. 2.

Martocchio, B. (1982). *Living while dying.* Bowie, MD: R. J. Brady Co.

Martocchio, B. (1986). Agenda for quality of life. *The Hospice Journal, 2,* 11.

Mor, V. (1986). Assessing patient outcomes in hospice: what to measure? *The Hospice Journal, 2,* 17.

Noyes, R., & Clancy, J. (1977). The dying role: Its relevance to improved patient care. *Psychiatry, 40,* 41.

Pattison, E. M. (1978). The living-dying process. In C. Garfield, *Psychosocial care of the dying patient.* New York: McGraw-Hill Book Co.

Paulay, D. (1977). Slow death: one survivor's experience. *Omega, 8,* 173.

Quinn, S. (1984). Elderly in hospice. *American Journal of Hospice Care, 1,* 27.

Sayre, J. (1979). Life theories in optimal wellness. In H. Wilson & C. Kneisl, *Psychiatric nursing.* Menlo Park, Calif: Addison-Wesley Publishing Co., pp. 170–216.

Simonton, S. (1984). *The healing family.* New York: Bantam Books.

Simpson, J., & Doyle, D. (1981, October 7). Protracted dying a challenge to the caring team. *Nursing Times,* 1752.

Skorupka, P., & Bohnet, N. (1982). Primary caregivers' perceptions of nursing behaviors that best meet their needs in a home care hospice setting. *Cancer Nursing, 5,* 371.

Sternburg, J., & Scheibel, W. (1982). Terminal care. *J. of Family Practice, 14,* 995.

Taylor, P. (1983). Understanding sexuality in the dying patient. *Nurs. 83, 13,* 54.

Taylor, P., & Gideon, M. (1982). Holding out hope to your dying patient. *Nurs. 82, 12,* 42.

Wilson, H., & Kneisl, C. (1979). *Psychiatric nursing.* Menlo Park, CA: Addison-Wesley Pub. Co., pp. 249–50.

Wysocki, M. (1983, February). Life review for the elderly patient. *Nursing 83,* 47.

Zorza, V., & Zorza, R. (1980). *A way to die.* New York: Alfred A. Knopf.

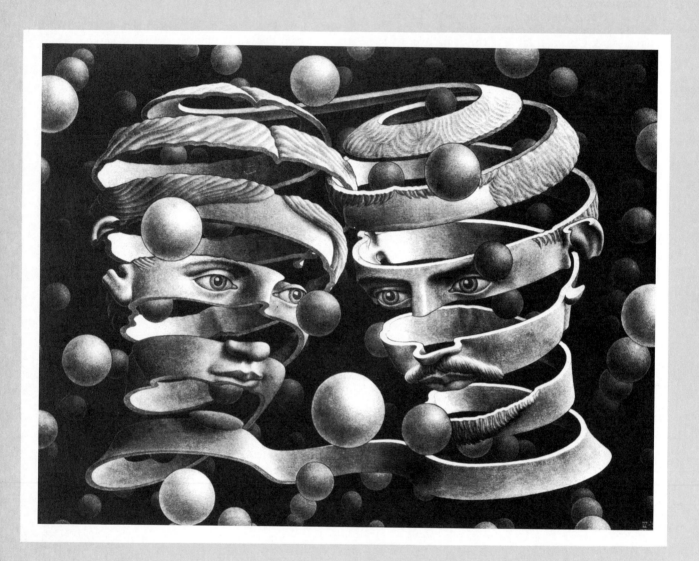

Part Five

PSYCHIATRIC MENTAL HEALTH NURSING PRACTICE ISSUES

27

LEGAL CONSIDERATIONS IN MENTAL HEALTH NURSING PRACTICE

LOUISE B. ZEULI

INTRODUCTION

In the last twenty years, while the practice of nursing has become more technically complicated, the profession of nursing has come to exert an ever-increasing impact on the health care system. With their significantly increasing responsibilities and growing technical expertise, nurses are also experiencing expanded legal accountability. Patients are more acutely aware that nursing decisions are not only important, but essential to their state of health. In addition, patient expectations regarding the outcomes of their health care have increased. Consequently, nurses are being sued more often and being held personally accountable for their independent decisions. Further, the number of theories used to find liability against the nurse is increasing (Herran & Guerrini, 1979).

One of the most significant characteristics of nursing that has enabled it to survive these legal challenges is that it adapts to the changing needs of its patients. The law is similar to nursing in this respect: law responds and adapts to the expectations and attitudes of its society. Society's attitudes toward various values change from time to time in response to external events. The practice of nursing changes to meet the new needs of society. The field of psychiatric nursing is especially affected by the law, because providing health care to the mentally ill has always been an emotional and explosive issue. Even the care of those who have a physical illness with psychological implications can provoke intense conflicts.

Knowledge of nursing principles alone is no longer sufficient to practice psychiatric nursing or, indeed, any type of nursing. Nursing is a profession, and the "hallmark of the professional is knowing the limits of one's professional knowledge" (*Sermchief* v. *Gonzales*, 1983). Knowledge is power or the ability to control one's own practice and those affected by it. As a therapist, the nurse must be acutely aware of not only her patients' rights but her own potential liabilities in the complicated areas of health care and the legal dilemmas and judgment calls that will appear on a daily basis in her practice. Thus, the nurse must be familiar with the law as it pertains to the standards of health care and the political/legal process in the criminal/civil system. An understanding of fundamental legal principles is essential to: 1) ensure that nursing decisions are consistent with appropriate legal principles; 2) provide optimum, safe nursing care; 3) facilitate the protection of patients' rights and promote their interests; and 4) protect the nurse from liability (Rhodes & Miller, 1984).

This chapter begins by identifying the rights which have been granted by state and federal law and the courts to the mentally ill. It then introduces the nurse to the legal system by focusing on basic legal principles, the elements of a malpractice lawsuit, and several areas of the nurse's vulnerability to liability, such as breach of confidentiality, patient suicide, charting responsibilities, involuntary commitment of a patient, and the patient's right to refuse treatment or medication. This information will provide the nurse therapist with a foundation for intelligent, informed decision making for optimum, safe patient care.

PATIENTS' RIGHTS

While the focus of this chapter is on legal principles and responsibilities of the nurse, it is important to recognize that these legal issues revolve around the patient and his rights under the law. Significant variation exists among the states as to the rights mandated by law on behalf of the mentally ill, but there are some commonly accepted rights for persons with mental illness. These rights are summarized in Table 27–1. Among the more important of these are the right to privacy (confidentiality), the right to refuse treatment, and the right of the patient who is in a hospital or institution to maintain communication with persons outside the hospital setting.

Many of these rights have been established in the last twenty years through federal and state legislation as well as through recent court decisions. Some of the more important decisions affecting rights of patients with mental disorders are summarized in Box 27–1.

As discussed in Chapter 5, "The Nurse as Therapist," and in other chapters of this text, nurses are often in a unique position to help patients understand their rights, and, for patients with severe mental illness, to facilitate the safeguarding of these rights. As this chapter will demonstrate, it is essential for the nurse to be aware of the legal ramifications regarding the patient's rights and certain aspects of care. Commitment of a patient to an institution, voluntarily or involuntarily, restraining a patient for his or others' safety, and medicating the patient against his will, are examples of care situations requiring the nurse to be especially observant and to document with care. This will not only help to preserve the patient's rights but will also protect the nurse from potential liability. In addition, the "right" way to handle a situation is not always apparent; often, what can at first seem a strictly legal issue can turn into an ethical dilemma. Deciding when a patient is no longer able to make a decision regarding treatment that is based on reasonable choice (proving incompetence) or when to breach confidentiality and alert a third party of a patient's voiced threat of physical harm are among the many dilemmas facing nurses and other health care providers who work with mentally ill patients. These and other issues are discussed in this chapter and in Chapter 28, "Ethical Considerations in Mental Health Practice."

TABLE 27–1 The mentally ill patient's bill of rights

---

1. The right to be treated with decency and respect.

2. Every right established by the Declaration of Independence and guaranteed by the Constitution of the United States of America as an American citizen.

3. The right to the integrity of your own mind and the integrity of your own body.

4. The right to have treatment and medication administered to you only with your consent and to be given all relevant information regarding said treatment and/or medication.

5. The right to access to your own legal and medical counsel.

6. The right to competent medical care.

7. The right to uncensored communication by telephone, letter, and in person.

8. The right to decent living conditions.

9. The right to retain your own personal property.

10. The right to bring grievance against those who have mistreated you and to be afforded counsel and a court hearing.

11. The right to refuse any drugs and treatments, even if involuntarily committed.

12. The right not to have your character questioned or defamed.

13. The right to request an alternative to legal commitment or incarceration in a psychiatric hospital.

Source: Adapted from Kemp, B., Pillitteri, A., & Brown, P., (1989) *Fundamentals of nursing: A framework for practice* (2nd ed.) Glenview, IL: Scott, Foresman. Modified from *Mental Patient's Bill of Rights*, Mental Patient's Liberation Project.

THE LEGAL SYSTEM: THE NATURE OF LAW AND ITS ORIGINATION

Like the medical field, the legal field has its own language for interprofessional communications. A nonlawyer must become familiar with the basic legal terminology to understand the process of law as well as the foundations upon which the law relies in regulating social conduct. The following discussion of law is comparable to the nurse's first exposure to medicine as a science, for example, physiology and anatomy. As in nursing, legal concepts build upon each other. The nurse must understand the conceptual bases for the legal process so that she can understand how law affects her duties in delivering mental health care.

"Law" has many definitions but the one that will serve this discussion is a rule or method with which phenomena or actions coexist or follow each other. Failure to follow the law may result in sanctions or legal consequences (Black, 1984, p. 1028). Law is derived from two sources: 1) legislative acts, called *statutes;* and 2) decisions by courts or governmental agencies, called *common law* or *administrative rules,* respectively (Prosser & Keeton, 1984). Statutory and common law have equal powers of meaning and enforcement; i.e., they are equally valid and enforceable (Prosser & Keeton, 1984). They both regulate human conduct and are subject to change in a continuing process of growth and modification (Katz, 1979). Laws function to regulate behavior in fulfilling society's needs as those needs are perceived by society itself (Murchisn & Nichols, 1970, p. 9).

Individuals in society have many interests for which they claim protection under the law and which the law acknowledges as worthy of protection. In any society, those interests inevitably conflict and the law is called upon to arbitrate the disputes (Prosser & Keeton, 1984). A legal entity, such as a person, the federal or state government, or a corporation, may seek any one of three general types of legal redress: 1) criminal; 2) administrative; and/or 3) civil.

Criminal law deals with disputes between the federal and/or state government on behalf of the United States residents against persons or entities such as corporations who are accused of committing

Box 27-1 ● Patient Advocacy: Important Court Decisions in Establishing Patient Rights

Several important court decisions in recent years have helped establish certain basic rights for individuals suffering from mental disorders.

Right to treatment In 1972, a U.S. District Court in Alabama made a landmark decision in the case of *Wyatt* v. *Stickney.* The ruling held that a mentally ill or mentally retarded individual had a right to receive treatment. Since the decision, the State of Alabama has increased its budget for treatment of mental health and mental retardation by 300 percent.

Freedom from custodial confinement In 1975, the U.S. Supreme Court upheld the principle that patients have a right to freedom from custodial confinement if they are not dangerous to themselves or others and if they can safely survive outside of custody. In the *O'Connor* v. *Donaldson* decision, the defendants were required to pay Donaldson $10,000 for having kept him in custody without providing treatment.

Right to compensation for work In 1973, a U.S. District Court ruled in the case of *Souder* v. *Brennan* (Secretary of Labor) that a patient in a nonfederal mental institution who performed work must be paid according to the Fair Labor Standards Act. Although a 1978 Supreme Court ruling nullified the part of the lower court's decision dealing with state hospitals, the ruling still applied to mentally ill and mentally retarded patients in private facilities.

Right to legal counsel at commitment hearings The State Supreme Court in Wisconsin decided in 1976 in the case of *Memmel* v. *Mundy* that an individual had the right to legal counsel during the commitment process.

Right to live in a community In 1974, the U.S. District Court decided, in the case of *Stoner* v. *Miller,* that released state mental hospital patients had a right to live in "adult homes" in the community.

Right to refuse treatment Several court decisions have provided rulings and some states have enacted legislation permitting patients to refuse certain treatments, such as psychiatric medications (*Rennie* v. *Klein*), electroconvulsive therapy, and psychosurgery.

References

Memmel v. *Mundy* 75 Wis. 2d 276 (Wis. 1977)

O'Connor v. *Donaldson* 422 U.S. 563 (1977)

Rennie v. *Klein* 476 F. Supp. 1294 (D.N.J. 1979)

Souder v. *Brennan* 367 F. Supp. 808 (D.D.C. 1973)

Stoner v. *Miller* 377 F. Supp. 177 (E.D.N.Y. 1974)

Wyatt v. *Stickney* 344 F. Supp. 373 (1973)

Based on Bernard (1979), National Association for Mental Health (1979), and Mental Health Law Project (1976).

Source: Adapted from Carson, R., Butcher, J., and Coleman, J. (1988). *Abnormal psychology and modern life* (8th ed.). Glenview, IL: Scott, Foresman.

---

crimes. The government's purpose in bringing a criminal action is to compel compliance with its laws. Criminal penalties typically involve punishment, i.e., loss of freedom (prison) and/or a monetary fine (Murchisn & Nichols, 1970, p. 10).

Administrative law involves disputes between a federal and/or state governmental administrative agency and a person, corporation, and/or other business entity on a specific social concern, such as professional licensing, industry, environment, or tax-

ation. Examples of an administrative agency are the Department of Professional Regulation (which oversees the practice of nursing, medicine, pharmacy, and nursing homes), the Interstate Commerce Commission, the Environmental Protection Agency, and the Internal Revenue Service. An administrative agency may obtain remedies against a person, such as suspension or revocation of a license, and/or payment of a monetary fine (Davis, 1972). Nurses are automatically involved in administrative law because they are licensed and regulated by the state. Most states require nurses to participate in continuing education to maintain current licenses. Many states permit nurses to specialize in their practice, such as psychiatric nursing or counseling. All of these situations concern administrative law.

Civil law involves private disputes between private persons, business entities, or sometimes a government entity. They usually seek monetary compensation for the alleged wrong committed against them. They may not seek loss of freedom or a professional license as a penalty; that remedy is available in only criminal law or administrative law, respectively. A suit alleging nursing malpractice is a civil lawsuit.*

Criminal, administrative, and civil law are not mutually exclusive remedies, although they each have their own set of rules and procedures. These categories do not divide human conduct but the law as it regulates society. One act may subject the person to all three actions. For example, if a nurse intentionally administers a medication to which she knows or should have known the patient is allergic, the state may prosecute the nurse for battery in *criminal* court, the Board of Nursing may charge the nurse with violating the Nurse Practice Act in an *administrative action,* and the patient may sue the nurse for money damages in a *civil lawsuit.* The nurse may be found liable in all three actions (Murchisn & Nichols, 1970).

CIVIL LAW AND NURSING: THE ELEMENTS OF A LAWSUIT

Although a nurse may be sued in any one of three types of actions (criminal, administrative, and/or civil), this chapter focuses on civil law, primarily *tort law,* as it affects psychiatric nursing practice. If a nurse is involved in any type of litigation in health care, she is most likely involved in a civil suit. No one satisfactory definition of tort law exists. The generally accepted definition of tort law is that a "tort" is a civil wrong, a breach of duty, other than a contractual or quasi-contractual duty, for which the courts will provide a remedy in the form of damages (usually money). Derived from Latin "tortus" or "twisted," a tort may include assault, battery, inva-

sion of privacy, malpractice, or injury to a person's reputation (Prosser & Keeton, 1984).

The most frequent basis for mental health nursing liability is the *negligent tort,* that is, the nurse has acted negligently (carelessly) in her duties. However, the *plaintiff* (patient or the patient's representative who is suing the nurse) must prove each of four elements to establish the nurse's liability and obtain a monetary damage award: 1) duty; 2) breach of duty; 3) damages (injury); and 4) proximate (direct or legal) causation.

DUTY (RESPONSIBILITY)

The plaintiff must first prove that the nurse owed some specific duty to the patient. Duty has two aspects: 1) that the nurse owed a duty to the person harmed; and 2) that the nurse's conduct should have conformed with the standard of care of a reasonably prudent nurse under the same or similar circumstances. The standard of care is a *minimum* standard below which the prudent psychiatric nurse must not fall in providing patient care. This minimum standard in no way precludes the nurse from maintaining optimum standards. For example, if a nurse provided care to the plaintiff, the nurse owed a duty to the plaintiff to provide safe nursing care. However, in general, if the nurse was not on duty on the particular day of the incident, then she owed no duty to the plaintiff to act one way or the other.

The plaintiff must also prove the standard of care applicable to the nurse's duty, and may do so by using expert testimony and published standards. Such standards may include the Nurse Practice Act, a textbook and/or journals, institutional rules, licensing standards, hospital policies, and/or common sense. Because the standard of care and its breach may be established by a hospital's or other institution's policies and procedures, nurses must be very familiar with the institution's administrative rules (Kelly & Garrick, 1984). Expert testimony is given by an individual recognized by the judge as an expert witness, one who possesses special knowledge, skill, and experience beyond matters generally known by ordinary persons.

These witnesses assist the jury in understanding what the nurse should or should not have done under the circumstances, that is, the applicable standard of care or duty the nurse owed the patient. In earlier years, physicians were frequently used as expert witnesses to establish the applicable nursing standards of care; however, nurse expert witnesses are most commonly and sometimes exclusively used (Rhodes &

---

*Many states use the term "medical malpractice" instead of "nursing malpractice" for not only lawsuits against nurses but also most health care professionals.

Miller, 1984, pp. 119–120). The nurse expert witness must possess the same or similar qualifications as the nurse defendant with regard to type of nursing licensure, experience, certifications and/or skills.

Published standards usually do not create a presumption of the standard of care or duty. They are generally used as guidelines to assist the jury in deciding whether or not the nurse should be liable to the plaintiff. No specific standard of care exists for nurses providing mental health care other than those standards applicable to nurses in general. However, the American Nurses' Association has issued a statement that is suggestive but not binding on the nurse's standard of care (Am. Nurses Assoc., 1973). In general, the nurse's standard of care includes, but is not limited to 1) using assessment and observation skills; 2) being familiar with the drugs, psychotropic or otherwise, being prescribed to patients; 3) documenting completely, accurately and in a timely manner; 4) properly administering medicines; and 5) notifying the physician under appropriate circumstances (Andrede & Andrede, 1979).

A nurse can be held responsible either directly or indirectly for damages to a patient. *Direct liability* occurs when the nurse is liable for *her own* acts. *Indirect or vicarious liability* occurs when the nurse is liable for the acts of *someone else* (Black, 1984). For example, if a charge nurse administers the wrong medication to the patient, she is *directly liable* to that patient, because *she* gave the medication. However, if a student nurse administered the wrong medication *and* the charge nurse was supervising the student that day, the charge nurse is *vicariously liable* for the student nurse's acts. Further, it is possible for the charge nurse to be directly liable *and* vicariously liable to the patient, depending on the fact situation. The charge nurse can be directly liable for her own negligence in supervising the student nurse and vicariously liable for the student nurse's negligence.

BREACH OF DUTY

Once the plaintiff proves the duty that the nurse therapist owes to him, he must then prove a breach of that duty. A *breach of duty* is a deviation from the duty or standard of care owed. Expert and lay persons' testimony may be used to establish that the nurse fell below the minimum standard expected. For example, a nurse who fails to notify the physician that the nurse has observed the patient *unexpectedly* preparing to commit suicide may have breached the standard of care or duty to report that behavior. Expert testimony may be used to establish that the nurse should have notified the physician. Lay testimony, such as from hospital support personnel or the patient's family, may be used to support that the nurse did not notify the physician.

On the other hand, a breach of duty or negligence is not established simply by proof that a certain therapy technique used was not the best. Technique need not be the best; it need only be reasonable (Slovenko, 1981).

DAMAGES (INJURIES)

The third element that the plaintiff must prove to show the nurse's negligence is the injury or *damages* the plaintiff has sustained. Injury or damage may be physical, emotional and/or financial. The jury may award any amount of money that it feels is reasonable under the circumstances. The jury has no guidelines or rules by which it determines an amount to award the plaintiff. However, in general, most courts will not allow suits that claim damages for emotional injury unaccompanied by physical injury (Rhodes & Miller, 1984, p. 122).

PROXIMATE (DIRECT) CAUSATION

The fourth element that the plaintiff must prove is *causation,* i.e., that the breach of duty legally or directly caused the damages. For example, suppose Patient Brown sues Nurse Smith. Patient Brown alleges that the nurse had a duty to 1) observe him and 2) report to the physician any tardive dyskinetic side effects from his medication. Patient Brown alleges that Nurse Smith breached her duty in failing to watch for those effects and report them to the physician, resulting in Patient Brown's permanent neurological deficit (damages). To prove his case and obtain a monetary award, Patient Brown must prove by the greater weight of the evidence (more than fifty percent) that Nurse Smith's breach of her duty was the proximate cause of his neurological deficit; i.e., that had the nurse not failed in her duty, the patient would not have suffered these specific neurological deficits. If it is not proved by the greater weight of the evidence, the nurse defendant is not liable or guilty of negligence. The plaintiff is not entitled to any damages, and, hence, goes without a remedy.

This element of the plaintiff's case can be the most difficult one to prove. However, jury sympathy may sometimes be an overwhelming unmeasurable, uncontrollable, and unpredictable factor that assists the plaintiff, who may not have scientifically proven his case as outlined above but who, nevertheless, obtains a monetary award.

Proving proximate causation in mental health cases may pose an interesting dilemma for the plaintiff. The treatment of mental illness or psychological care in general is not an exact science. For example, despite many years of research, a patient's propensity for dangerousness still cannot be predicted with any accuracy. Also, because of the many types of therapies, a plaintiff would find it nearly an impossible task to prove that the therapist negatively and unprofessionally influenced the patient. Juries may view a plaintiff who has a history of mental illness as incapable of thinking rationally. The plaintiff may need to prove a pattern or scheme of behavior of impropriety by the nurse therapist to establish malpractice (Slovenko, 1981, p. 29).

On the other hand, certain types of actions for which nurse therapists are increasingly found liable do exist but are thus far confined to a limited number of situations. Those situations and the consequences are discussed in the next section.

LIABILITY

Lawsuits against psychotherapists, including psychiatric nurses and nurse therapists, have been relatively limited in the past to certain classic situations for potential liability, such as engaging in sex with the patient. However, the areas of malpractice in psychiatry and mental health are increasing, limited only by the creativity of the attorney representing the patient. This latter observation holds true because, unlike the principles of science, law is a dynamic, political, ethical, and social process. Lawsuits reflect such attitudes about a person's rights to certain remedies because of a wrong committed against the person. If society's attitudes change toward a particular moral or legal view, the standard for health care will change, too. For example, twenty years ago, society did not believe that mentally ill patients had a *constitutional right* to refuse medication. Consequently, a nurse who forced or coerced a patient into taking his antipsychotic medication would not be liable for malpractice or anything else. Such behavior was perceived as not only desirable but absolutely necessary for that patient's well-being. Society believed that force was often necessary to treat a mentally ill patient. Today, due to the court's recognition of the importance of autonomy to patient interests, that same act can subject the psychiatric nurse to a lawsuit for assault and battery, malpractice, and violation of the patient's civil rights. Mentally ill patients have their own constitutional rights, and psychiatric nurses must respect those rights when providing treatment.

Which situations pose the greatest risk to the psychiatric nurse for liability? Is it when the patient commits suicide while in the hospital or after discharge? Is it the situation in which a patient, convicted of a crime, tells the nurse that when he gets out on parole, he plans to kill the witness who assisted in his conviction? Is the nurse subject to liability for dating a current or former patient? Being in any of the above-described circumstances may result in a monetary judgment against the nurse for negligence or malpractice. All of these scenarios, as well as others, are legally dangerous for psychiatric nurses.

SUICIDE

The threat of litigation over suicide continuously poses deep concern to all psychiatric health care providers. Yet one of the most difficult challenges to nurses is assessing a patient's suicidal risk. Nurses also encounter difficulty in differentiating which patients are sincere in their suicide threats from those who are simply trying to manipulate the health care system to their own advantage. Once a patient is admitted to the hospital, judged to be at risk for suicide and on suicide precautions, the full burden rests squarely with the psychiatric nurse for watching that patient, continuously assessing him for suicide potential, and guarding him against suicide opportunities. The liability issues for the nurse are: 1) the foreseeability of the suicidal tendency, and 2) the adequacy of the suicide precautions in view of the patient's suicidal tendency (Slovenko, 1981). Once the patient commits suicide in the hospital, the presumption of the nurse's negligence is difficult to overcome.

What types of nursing behavior could have permitted the suicide and, thus, constituted malpractice? First, nurses frequently fail to follow the physician's orders for suicide precautions (Andrede & Andrede, 1979, p. 173). Second, the nurse may fail to assess adequately the patient's signs of pending suicide, often because she is not closely monitoring the patient. Third, the nurse may have been negligent by not notifying the physician for more stringent suicide precautions. Fourth, the nurse may fail to take the initiative to monitor the patient more closely, regardless of the physician's orders.

What can a nurse do to keep herself keenly aware of the potential problems associated with treating the suicidal patient? As with all treatment, she must be well-acquainted with the underlying disease process. Knowing the signs and symptoms of the underlying problems, its stages, and the predictable, potential consequences cannot be replaced. She must also know and follow the hospital's policies and procedures for these patients. Failure to adhere to administrative rules is more likely to result in not only her own liability but also that of the hospital and physician (Perr, 1978). The nurse should also seek out the supervisor or administrator for assistance and guidance. Communication and cooperation as a team increase her chances of providing a safe environment for the patient.

How does the nurse know when the patient's condition is worsening? Suppose the patient is a criminal, who is charged with first-degree murder and faces the death penalty if convicted. The nurse knows the circumstances but feels that the patient is innocent. The nurse opposes the death penalty. The patient is now verbalizing his thoughts of suicide, possibly to avoid the death penalty. The patient is on a suicide watch requiring visual observation every fifteen minutes. What are the nurse's legal obligations? Should she chart and report the patient's suicidal behavior? The nurse may hesitate to do so, as in her own mind prolonging the patient's life in the hospital may mean that the patient will be put to death for the crime he may have committed.

The nurse should consider a number of factors in the decision-making process with this patient. The nurse must analyze her own motivations and needs. What are this patient's objective behaviors? She should report and chart those behaviors. The nurse may be confused by the temptation to meet her own needs of opposing the death penalty, rather than the patient's needs of safe health care, and thus she may be motivated not to chart and report the patient's suicidal behavior. Is the nurse denying the patient's behavior because she wants to believe in the patient's innocence? Neither of these motivations is appropriate. The nurse has a legal obligation to report to the physician all significant changes in the patient's behavior. The nurse has a legal duty to take the appropriate precautions, especially if the institution has *standing orders*. She does not have the authority to screen the behavior upon which she acts. The nurse must remain objective.

The bottom line is that *the nurse must not be influenced by her own motivations in using her nursing skills and judgment on a patient*. The nurse must distinguish her own personal desires from her legal duties; if she feels that her judgment is cloudy, she should seek guidance from her supervisor. Regardless of the patient's fate in the criminal procedure, the nurse's duty to properly treat that patient is upper-

most. Use of any other approach may result in the nurse's liability.

INVOLUNTARY TREATMENT

Not all suicidal patients are already hospitalized when they are treated by a nurse. The nurse may be working in an outpatient setting and meet a depressed patient who has suicidal thoughts. The patient refuses admission to the hospital. Does the nurse have any legal recourse to obtain treatment for this patient whom she feels needs it?

The law permits a patient to be involuntarily committed to a hospital setting for treatment when the patient poses an imminent danger to himself or others.* This situation is only one instance which can override the patient's constitutional right to refuse treatment. (*O'Connor* v. *Donaldson*, 1975). All states have statutes governing this situation. The statute's guidelines must be followed, because a patient, even though mentally ill, still has the same constitutional rights as the physically ill patient. While it is true that the patient can be involuntarily committed, the time period is limited, after which the patient has the right to refuse further treatment. If the patient does refuse further treatment, court proceedings may be necessary to resolve the situation. It is important to note that even though the law permits involuntary commitment under certain circumstances, it does *not impose* a legal duty on the nurse to take a patient into a custodial setting against the patient's will to protect him from self-destructive tendencies (Paddock v. Chacko, 1988).

LEAST RESTRICTIVE MEANS OF TREATMENT

Some states, such as Florida, permit psychiatric nurses to participate in involuntary commitment process by evaluating the patient's status and documenting the evaluation (Fla. Stat., § 394.463 (2)(a)(3)). The decision to involuntarily commit a patient for treatment must be balanced against the patient's right to have the least restrictive means of treatment used on him (Brooks, 1974, p. 732). "*Least restrictive means of treatment*" is treatment that minimally interferes with the individual's freedom but is still effective (or likely to be effective). This procedure meets the patient's need for treatment, yet also meets the

---

*Fla. Stat. 394.451 et seq. (1987). Florida's "Baker Act" is typical of acts in other states which permits involuntary psychiatric treatment for a limited time without court intervention.

public's need for safety (Brooks, 1974; Guntheil & Appelbaum, 1985). The alternative choices of treatment are as numerous as the community resources permit; for example, outpatient therapy, social programs, alcoholic detoxification, and civil commitment.

The psychiatric nurse's role is extremely important not only in protecting the patient's constitutional rights but also herself, the hospital, and/or physician from liability. While the physician and hospital may have complied fully with their legal obligations, the nurse's negligence in her responsibilities can result in potential liability for not only that one nurse but also the charge nurse, head nurse, director of nursing, hospital administrator, hospital, and various physicians. Direct and vicarious liability may be involved. Why are other personnel implicated? Because the law imposes a duty that people will provide adequate direct and indirect care to a patient. The duty goes all the way to the top administrator.

The nurse's obligations have far-reaching implications, not only for the patient but for all health care providers who interact in the patient's care. The law views the practice of nursing, like all licensed professions, not only as a constitutional right for the practitioner but also a privilege. The public is not in a position to adequately judge the skills of the health care provider. The law through its federal and state legislators and bodies assumes that role and holds the practitioners to their legal duties.

The nurse's role is not an easy one. Most often, the nurse must decide to initiate treatment with little or no time to consult with the supervisor or physician. No single answer will be correct for all situations. However, if the nurse properly supervises the patient, documents her observations, follows the physician's and institution's orders and regulations, and takes the appropriate steps when a problem arises, she has done as much as can be reasonably expected to protect the patient from harm and herself and the administrators from liability. The nurse should remember that she is not legally responsible for *everything* that happens to a patient—only those things that she could have reasonably prevented under the circumstances. For example, legal and psychiatric professionals have grappled with the problem of accurately predicting which people will be dangerous, and thus, should have their freedom restricted. The general consensus seems to be that mental health providers will never be 100 percent accurate in predicting dangerous behavior (Mullen & Norman, 1979).

THE DOCTRINE OF INFORMED CONSENT: THE RIGHT TO CHOOSE AND REFUSE MEDICAL TREATMENT

The *doctrine of informed consent* holds that any patient, whether mentally and/or physically ill, has the constitutional right to make informed decisions about his own medical treatment. Every human being of adult years and of sound mind has a right to determine what shall be done with his own body (*Schloendorff* v. *The Society of New York Hospital,* 1914). This doctrine is a product of two theories in law: 1) negligence and 2) battery (Waltz & Sheuneman, 1969; Katz, 1979).

The doctrine focuses on the physician's duty to disclose material risks to the patient. Emphasis is placed upon the physician's conduct in disclosing rather than the patient's understanding of the content of the disclosed material (Meisel, Roth & Lidz, 1977).

The doctrine consists of three elements: 1) information (knowledge); 2) consent; and 3) competency (Waltz & Sheuneman, 1969, p. 629). Two basic contentions exist: 1) the patient's right to decide his own medical treatment, (Meisel & Kabnick, 1980) i.e., self-determination (Katz, 1979, p. 139) and 2) the physician's traditional, authoritative position to decide the course of medical treatment (Meisel & Kabnick, 1980, p.409). A basic assumption underlies the informed consent doctrine. If a patient must consent to proposed treatment before it can be legally rendered, then the patient may, alternatively, rightly refuse that consent when he so desires. This right to

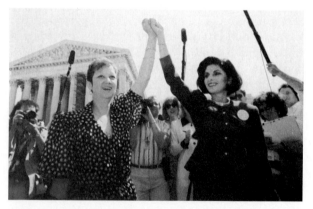

Cases involving the patient's right to refuse treatment and the right to privacy continue to be challenged in our courts, an example of which is *Roe* v. *Wade.*

refuse medical treatment is the counterpart to the informed consent doctrine. The refusal right has been judicially upheld on the basis of the patient's right to privacy (*Roe* v. *Wade*, 1973; *Griswold* v. *Connecticut*, 1965), right to mentation (*Rennie* v. *Klein*, 1979; *Stanley* v. *Georgia*, 1969), freedom from cruel and unusual punishment (*Scott* v. *Plante*, 1976), freedom of religion (*Winters* v. *Miller*, 1971), and procedural due process (*Davis* v. *Hubbard*, 1980).

The right to refuse treatment is controversial in the mental health setting, especially for those who have been involuntarily hospitalized. Some people make the incorrect assumption that a mentally ill person is incapable of making decisions for himself, particularly if involuntarily committed. However, the courts have held that certain constitutional rights of mentally ill persons must be respected, including the right to refuse treatment. Even when the court finds the patient to be mentally ill, this finding "does not raise even a presumption that the patient is incompetent or unable adequately to manage his own affairs; absent a specific finding of incompetence the mental patient retains the right . . . to manage his own affairs." The presumption of competency includes the competency to decide on psychiatrically related treatment (*Winters* v. *Miller*, 1971, pp. 68–71). Furthermore, choosing an unorthodox treatment does not raise the question of incompetency (*Sarasota County Dept. of Soc. Serv.* v. *Hofbauer*, 1979). Former United States Supreme Court Chief Justice Burger phrased it this way:

> Nothing [suggests that] an individual [possesses] these rights only as to *sensible* beliefs, *valid* thoughts, *reasonable* emotions or *well-founded* sensations. [It was intended] to include a great many foolish, unreasonable and even absurd ideas which do not conform, such as refusing medical treatment even at great risks (Katz, 1979, p. 172, n. 110). [*Emphasis added*]

The right to refuse treatment is subject to the state's compelling interest in emergency situations and exercise of its parens patriae power. "Parens patriae," literally "parent of the country," refers traditionally to the role of the state as sovereign and guardian of persons under legal disability. It is a concept of standing utilized to protect those quasi-sovereign interests such as health, comfort, and welfare of the people, general economy of the state, and so on. The parens patriae power in the United States belongs to the individual state (Black, 1984 p. 1003).

To exercise this power, i.e., to overrule the patient's right to refuse treatment, the state must show a strong countervailing interest. Examples include when the individual constitutes a danger to himself and/or others, the physician's exercise of the therapeutic privileges, the patient's waiver of the right, and when the person is declared legally incompetent (Meisel, 1979). However, the presumption of patient competency is still strong. Even institutionalized patients have the right to refuse treatment unless they are declared legally incompetent (*Davis* v. *Hubbard*, 1980).

Through its legal system, society has accepted this type of interference with personal autonomy. The state has an overriding interest in not only preserving health and life but also facilitating health care providers' freedom to practice responsibly and progressively without fear of frequent litigation (*Dunham* v. *Wright*, 1970).

When clinically approaching a patient who refuses medical treatment of any type, the nurse should presume that the patient has the legal competency, and, therefore, the right to refuse treatment. This assumption does not mean that the nurse should make no attempt to deal with the refusal; rather, she should explore the reasons for the refusal. First, do any of the four exceptions to right of refusal exist? Second, what does the refusal truthfully represent? Is it a symptom of the patient's underlying illness, whether medical and/or psychiatric? If so, does the patient need more information or clarification of the reasons for the medical treatment? Are any of the patient's laboratory test results abnormal? Does this refusal represent a worsening of the patient's condition?

Third, the therapeutic alliance approach in which the nurse recruits and allies herself with the healthiest level of the patient's function may be useful. The nurse then appeals to this level in discussing the refusal with the patient. Fourth, the nurse should explore the possibility of causative influences on the refusal. In addition to the therapeutic investigation or intervention, specific influences provoking refusal should be isolated and directly ameliorated. A positive, caring relationship with the patient may help the patient reverse his refusal (Doudera & Swazey, 1982).

Depending on the circumstances, if the patient continues to refuse treatment, consider whether the patient requires involuntary treatment. If so, she should initiate those procedures according to the proper legal outlines for the respective state.

Regardless of the alternatives chosen by the patient or the action taken by the nurse, the patient's constitutional rights to refuse medical treatment must be protected. The nurse should follow all the respective steps taken whether the patient will be involuntarily committed, involuntarily tested, or left as he already is. No simple solution exists to guarantee that the patient receives his maximum rights and maximum benefits. The nurse's role is to facilitate these rights and benefits while she follows all the applicable policies, procedures, and laws.

THE DUTY TO WARN THIRD PARTIES AND THE DUTY OF SPECIAL RELATIONSHIPS/BREACH OF CONFIDENTIALITY

In the controversial case of *Tarasoff* v. *Regents of University of California,* 1976, the California Supreme Court created a new legal duty for therapists. The mental health care provider may be found negligent when she fails to prevent her patient from harming an *identified* third party. In this particular case, a voluntary outpatient, Prosengit Poddar, confided his intention to kill an unnamed girl, readily identified as Tatiana [Tarasoff], to his therapist, Dr. Lawrence Moore, a psychologist employed by the Cowell Memorial Hospital at University of California at Berkeley. After consulting with Dr. Gold and Dr. Yardell, assistant directors at the psychiatry department, Dr. Moore decided that Poddar should be committed for observation in a mental hospital.

Dr. Moore requested by letter that the campus police detain Poddar, which they did briefly. The police released Poddar when he appeared rational and promised to stay away from Tatiana. Dr. Powelson, director at the psychiatry department, then asked the police to return Dr. Moore's letter, directed that all copies of the letter and therapy notes taken by Dr. Moore be destroyed, and ordered no action to place Poddar in a 72-hour treatment and evaluation facility (*Tarasoff* v. *Regents of University of Cal.,* 1976, at 341). Poddar killed Tatiana Tarasoff approximately two months later (*Tarasoff* v. *Regents of Cal.,* 1976, at 339).

In finding that Tatiana's parents *could sue* the psychiatrists and the University of California at Berkeley for their failure to warn Tatiana or others likely to apprise her of the danger, the court outlined its analysis. First, the court had to find that the psychiatrists owed a legal duty to Tatiana. The psychiatrists argued that because Tatiana was not their patient, they owed her no legal duty to warn her of Poddar's in-

tentions and, thus, could have no liability. In rejecting this argument, the court stated:

> We shall explain that defendant therapists cannot escape liability merely because Tatiana was not their patient. When a therapist determines, or pursuant to the standards of his profession should determine, that his patient presents a serious danger of violence to another, he incurs an obligation to use reasonable care to protect the intended victim against such danger (*Tarasoff* v. *Regents of Cal.,* 1976, at 340)

The court balanced several considerations in finding the legal duty:

1. The foreseeability of harm to the [person];

2. The degree of certainty that the [person] suffered injury;

3. The closeness of the connection between the defendant's conduct and the injury suffered;

4. The moral blame attached to the defendant's conduct;

5. The policy of preventing future harm;

6. The extent of the burden to the [therapist] and consequences to the community of imposing a duty to exercise care with resulting liability for breach; and

7. The availability, cost and prevalence of insurance for the risk involved (*Tarasoff* v. *Regents of Cal.,* 1976, at 342).

The most important factor is the first one—foreseeability of harm. This concept means that the victim must be foreseeable, i.e., identifiable.

The legal duty to prevent foreseeable harm, however, arises only in the presence of a special relationship between the therapist and the dangerous person *or* the potential victim. The relationship between the therapist and patient satisfied this requirement in *Tarasoff,* although other relationships, such as between the police and patient, may not. Because Tatiana's parents showed no special relationship between the police and Tatiana, the court ruled that Tatiana's parents could not sue the police.

The court stated in *Tarasoff* that the risk of having therapists warn too frequently was outweighed by the benefit of preventing harm. This duty is no different from a hospital's duty to control violent patient behavior or a doctor's duty to warn a patient of potential problems related to a condition or medication, such as driving a car after taking certain medication. Further, the therapists' inability to predict accurately a patient's dangerousness did not thwart the court. The court reasoned that the therapists' judgment in diagnosing emotional disorders and predicting dangerousness is comparable to other judgments she must make.

The therapist need not be perfect; but she must use the reasonable degree of skill, knowledge, and care ordinarily exercised by other members of her profession under similar circumstances (*Tarasoff* v. *Regents of Cal.*, 1976, at 344, 345).

The court also addressed in *Tarasoff* the therapist's legal duty of confidentiality of all communications relating to treatment. If a patient feels that the information will not be held in utmost confidence, the creation of the very relationship upon which diagnosis and treatment depends will be destroyed. While the court recognized the importance of protecting the patient's privacy rights, it ruled that the public's safety against violent assault must nonetheless be paramount: "The protective privilege ends where the public peril begins." (*Tarasoff* v. *Regents of Cal.*, 1976, at 346, 347).

Lastly, the court gave some guidance on the therapist's procedure for fulfilling the duty to warn. The disclosure should be discreet in order to preserve the patient's privacy vis-à-vis the threatened danger. However, the therapist may be required to warn the intended victim or others likely to apprise the victim of danger or notify the police. In short, the therapist should take the necessary steps under the circumstances (*Tarasoff* v. *Regents of Cal.*, 1976, at 340, 347).

The *Tarasoff* decision spurred other cases which allowed lawsuits against therapists based on the therapist's failure to warn of a patient's threats or violent propensities. Most courts have limited the cause of action to situations in which the patient poses a threat toward a limited, readily identifiable group. For example, the court in *Beck* v. *Kansas University of Psychiatry Foundation,* 1984, permitted a lawsuit for civil rights violation and personal injuries under state law against therapists for failure to warn of a prisoner's violent propensities against hospital emergency room personnel. The prisoner murdered two persons in the emergency room after having been unconditionally discharged by the parole board. Several therapists had treated the prisoner but had failed to give any warnings about his violent behavior. In contrast to *Tarasoff* and *Beck,* courts have not allowed lawsuits when the victim had independent knowledge of the patient's violent propensities (*Matter of Estate of Vottler,* 1982) or when the patient had not made specific threats against readily identifiable victims (*Doyle* v. *United States,* 1982).

An extreme example of this potential liability is illustrated by the case of *Hedlund* v. *Superior Court,* 1983. The patient had warned his psychologists that he intended to harm his former girlfriend. The patient and his former girlfriend had been seeing the psychologists for counseling. During the patient's attack on his former girlfriend, which resulted in her death by shooting, the victim threw herself over her eight-year-old son to protect him. Although the child was not physically injured, he suffered serious emotional and psychological injuries. The issue of the case was whether the child could be compensated for his injuries, even though the perpetrator had made no threats against him.

The court held that the child was a foreseeable and identifiable victim of any attack against his mother. Because of the parent-child relationship and the child's age, a failure to protect the mother could foreseeably lead to her child's harm. The court believed that extending the therapist's duty to persons close to the threatened party was not unreasonable. The court stated that *the therapist should consider the existence of such persons both in evaluating the seriousness of the danger posed by the patient and in determining the appropriate steps to be taken to protect the potential victim* (*Hedlund* v. *Superior Court,* 1983).

Where does the nurse fit into this potential liability picture? Actually, the nurse is an integral link in all the scenarios. The nurse is often the first staff person to see a patient in the emergency room, office, or clinic. The staff nurse spends more time with patients during their hospitalization than any other health care provider. The nurse is often the only regular health care provider for prisoners, whether they are incarcerated in a county jail or state prison. When the nurse takes on an expanded role, she traditionally spends more time with a patient than a physician or physician's assistant.

Because the nurse spends so much time with the patient, she must avail herself of the opportunity to observe him for violent propensities. Since the majority of nurses are female, the nurse may herself experience threats. The nurse must be aware of her unique position, which allows her to know the patient. She must document her observations and use her nursing skills to assess the patient, guard against danger, and prevent herself from being manipulated by the patient. Her failure to do so could put herself in danger personally as well as subject third parties to danger. Finally, because of her responsibilities, the nurse subjects herself, the physician, and other health care providers to liability for negligence. Her notes and memory of the patient may be the only evidence that she and her colleagues have to support their position that they had no duty to warn and/or were not negligent in their treatment of the patient.

TRANSFERENCE THEORY AND SEXUAL MISCONDUCT

Transference is a phenomenon in which the patient projects feelings and attitudes originally connected with significant others early in his life (such as his parents) onto the nurse therapist. This projection results in the patient becoming emotionally dependent on the therapist (*L.L.* v. *Medical Protective Co.,* 1984). The theory is most widely applied to psychiatrists and mental health care providers, although it has been applied in other health care settings (*Hirst* v. *St. Paul Fire & Marine Ins. Co.,* 1984). This relationship makes the patient particularly vulnerable to the therapist's suggestions, for he believes that the therapist always acts in his best interests to make him well. What the therapist perceives as extraneous may be part of the whole relationship with the patient (*Vigilant Ins. Co.* v. *Employer Ins. of Wausau,* 1986).

The nurse therapist should be acutely aware of this power over the patient. Thus, she should totally avoid any compromising positions or situations with the patient, never taking advantage of this relationship. No compromise exists. Some therapists *do* abuse this relationship by seeking out, fostering, and/or engaging in social and/or sexual relationships with their patients. Sometimes a patient initiates the relationship, and the therapist may be responding to his/her patient's sexual advances. Regardless of whether the therapist or patient initiates the social and/or sexual contact, the therapist's engagement in such activity is wrong and clearly unethical and unacceptable. Further, the therapist's conduct is actionable for assault and battery, intentional infliction of emotional distress, and other torts for compensatory and punitive damages. Even though the patient is fully competent, he is viewed as incapable of consenting to the social and/or sexual contact. The therapist is the more knowledgeable person and should not have permitted the interaction (*L.L.* v. *Medical Protective Co.,* 1984). As one court explained:

> A sexual relationship between therapist and patient cannot be viewed separately from the therapeutic relationship that has developed between them. The transference phenomenon makes it impossible that the patient will have the same emotional response to sexual contact with the therapist that he or she would have to sexual contact with other persons.
>
> (*L.L.* v. *Medical Protective Co.,* 1984).

A good example of this abuse is illustrated by the case of *Vigilant Insurance Co.* v. *Employers Insurance Co.,* 1986. The psychiatrist had engaged in sexual activities with several patients during and immediately after therapy sessions. The psychiatrist and one female patient had "primal therapy" sessions during which she and the psychiatrist were nude and the patient lay on the floor, spread-eagle. The alleged purposes of these sessions were to "derepress" the patient's repressed feelings, including those toward her father. The patient and psychiatrist later had intercourse during the "primal therapy" session and frequently after therapy sessions in the bedroom of the psychiatrist's office-apartment. The psychiatrist ordered a different female patient to take off her clothes and lie on the bed while he showered. When she told him that the incident upset her, he said that she would understand when she became well (*Vigilant Ins. Co.* v. *Employers Ins. Co.,* 1986 at 262).

Nurses are in the same legal position as the psychiatrist in *Vigilant.* They may also be the targets of these lawsuits if they engage in sexual conduct with their patients. This conclusion would apply to a nurse who agrees to meet a current or former patient for a date, lives with such a patient, and/or engages in sex. The nurse could also be involved indirectly simply by being aware that another therapist or nurse is partaking in such behavior. In these cases, should the nurse report her observations to the appropriate hospital and state personnel? Does her silence not only condone the therapist's behavior but also make her an accomplice? The answer to these questions is yes; the nurse has a legal duty to report this behavior to the appropriate professional regulatory board (Fla. Stat. §464 et seq., 1989). If criminal charges are filed against the abusing therapist, the nurse could be an accomplice by silence. The nurse's civil liability may not be too far behind (*Malone* v. *Longa,* 1979).

Whether the nurse is involved directly or indirectly in such a situation, she has lost sight of her purpose in being there—objective, patient treatment. Personal involvement by definition means lack of objectivity. The nurse can no longer be an effective therapist and poses more danger to the patient than she provides assistance. She has substituted her own needs for that of the patient's. Regardless of how strongly the patient verbalizes his desire to be close to the nurse, she must maintain the professional aspect of the relationship only.

An example of a nurse being indirectly involved when a therapist is engaging in inappropriate sexual behavior with a patient is when the nurse has observed that the male psychiatrist quickly discharges male patients but obviously prolongs hospitalization for young women. The psychiatrist insists also that no one accompany him into the patients' room for therapy. The female patients have over time complained about unnecessary treatment or hospitalization (Silverberg, 1974). If the nurse becomes aware of the psychiatrist's behavior and/or the women's complaints and does not investigate the situation, she may become the psychiatrist's accomplice by her silence. If the nurse became involved in observing and reporting the psychiatrist's behavior, however, this situation may be prevented (*Roy* v. *Hartogs*, New York Supreme Court, 1976).*

RECORD KEEPING IN NURSING PRACTICE

"Do not take notes" is the title of a section on advice to therapists in a book entitled *The Ethics of Psychoanalysis* by a leading psychiatrist and author, Dr. Thomas Szasz (Szasz, 1965). The book's premise is that historically the practice of psychotherapy has espoused minimal records or notes of the patient's communications or evaluations (Slovenko, 1979, pp. 399, 401). This view has gradually changed over time for a variety of reasons, including: 1) legal; 2) insurance; 3) accountability to the patient; 4) quality assurance; 5) financial reimbursement; and 6) cost containment (Slovenko, 1979, p. 406).

Legal accountability is most likely one of the greatest influences on record-keeping in the entire health care industry. However, potential liability should actually be the impetus for assuring not only quality health care but its documentation as well. Accurate, efficient charting of a patient's history, symptoms, behaviors, and response to treatment should result in better continuity of and optimum safe health care. Those results are the ultimate goals, along with the patient's well-being. However, it could be argued that the record-keeping requirements have become overwhelming, particularly those necessary to satisfy governmental and nongovernmental agency reviews for such things as the Department of Health, Joint Commission on Accreditation of Hospitals, and state licensing boards (Slovenko, 1979, p. 412).

Each medical or business record is a potential legal document. The chart is a story of a patient's med-

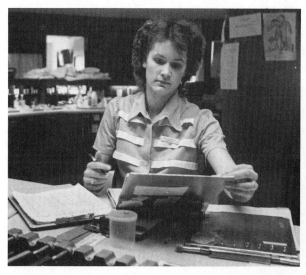

One of the most important aspects of health care delivery in a mental health setting is to accurately record prescribed treatments, why the treatments were ordered, and the resulting effects of those treatments. The nurse should prepare a psychosocial assessment for each patient, from which a treatment plan can be formulated and updated as necessary.

ical life. When the outcome of that life is challenged, the natural inclination is to believe that the chart, which was supposedly written and compiled simultaneously with the respective events, is the most accurate recitation of the events in question. Unfortunately, more often than not, the chart is not much more than an outline of that phase of the patient's life. A basic test used in the legal process in evaluating a chart is: *If it is not in the chart, then it did not happen.* An inadequate record is often considered indicative of poor care, which is used as a fact to establish liability (Slovenko, 1979, pp. 417, 418).

The nurse's notes are often the single most important part of the medical record, because the nurse has the greatest amount of contact with the patient. The notes answer questions such as: How did the patient react to the pain medication? Did the surgical wound show signs of infection, and if so, which signs? Has the patient's mood improved after initiation of antidepression therapy? Were suicide precautions followed? Did the patient consent to voluntary treatment? If the nurse does not chart the answers to these questions, she most likely will not remember the facts several years later when the patient's treatment is at issue in a lawsuit.

If the nurse has no testimony to refute the patient's allegations, then the jury may deduce right-

*After reading of the lawsuit for sexual misconduct, former female patients of the psychiatrist in the *Roy* case came forward to report that the psychiatrist had engaged in sexual intercourse with them, too. Without their testimony, the complainant probably would have lost her suit, as the psychiatrist asserted that she was delusional and he had been impotent for the last ten years.

fully that the plaintiff has met his burden of proof by the greater weight of the evidence. The sole evidence available for the nurse's defense is her own testimony, based on her recollection of the patient. If the nurse does not remember the events, her defense comes down to the type of impression she makes as a witness. That can be a big risk, placing her chances of winning on her perceived credibility by six strangers.

The following rules will help the nurse avoid this dilemma:

1. DO NOT begin charting until you check the name on the patient's chart. DO NOT pull a chart by room number only.

2. DO NOT use notebook paper or pencil. Always use the appropriate nurses' note forms of the institution, and always use ink. Write neatly and legibly in the ink color prescribed.

3. DO read the other nurses' notes on the patient before caring for him and charting your care. You have a better appreciation of changes to observe for the duration of your shift.

4. DO read the physician's orders to double-check medication, intravenous fluids, laboratory tests, X rays, and other treatment modalities. The previous nurse may have missed and/or misinterpreted an order. Compare what has been ordered with what has been given.

5. DO make entries as close to the occurrence or event as possible. Chart at least as frequently as your institution mandates. DO make entries in order of consecutive shifts and days. Write the complete date and time of each entry. Label a late entry as such and the reason for its being late. Date, time, and sign the late entry.

6. DO use concise, descriptive phrases. Begin each phrase with a capital letter and each new topic on a separate line.

7. DO sign each entry and postscript.

8. DO describe each entry and postscript.

9. DO use accepted hospital abbreviations whenever possible.

10. DO document nursing actions taken following indication of a need for action. Chart the patient's responses to the nursing intervention. No purpose will be served if no documentation exists on whether the intervention was successful, or if not successful, why it was not.

11. DO be definite and thorough. The use of "appears" is outmoded. Nurses are authorized to make their own diagnoses. At least chart the patient's major problems and whatever is related to them.

12. DO chart when the physician is in or called. Chart the physician's response or lack of response.

13. DO chart when the family visits and any of their questions or comments.

14. DO chart all signs and symptoms of any substance abuse or use, whether it be alcohol, cocaine, or anything else.

15. DO chart all patient responses to treatment, medication, recommended therapy. DO chart any family resistance to any aspect of the patient's treatment. DO chart also all steps taken by all health care providers in response to the patient's refusal.

16. DO NOT chart "Patient appears to be sleeping or resting" without determining with certainty that the patient is either not in distress or dead. Once you have made that determination, the appropriate charting is "Patient is sleeping; heart rate *60* beats/minute, regular; respiration *16*/minute without difficulty; color pink; skin warm and dry." Chart whatever complies with your institution's policy.

17. DO NOT BACKDATE OR TAMPER WITH NOTES PREVIOUSLY WRITTEN. If and when you learn that you are a defendant or potential defendant in a lawsuit, DO NOT go near or examine the original medical records without your attorney being present. The plaintiff may accuse you of altering the record to cover up your malpractice. If you have not gone near the original medical record, you can dispel this line of attack easily and quickly.

18. DO NOT skip lines between entries. DO NOT leave a space before your signature.

19. DO NOT remove a controlled substance without simultaneously signing out for it AND having another authorized nurse witness AND simultaneously cosign, or whatever your institution requires. DO NOT waste a portion of a controlled substance without simultaneously signing for it, having it witnessed by another authorized nurse, AND having that nurse simultaneously sign as witness.

20. DO NOT chart mere conclusions without describing the events supporting your conclusions.

21. DO NOT use medical terms unless you are sure of their meaning.

22. DO NOT chart procedures in advance.

23. DO NOT wait until the end of your duty that day to chart. DO NOT rely on your memory.

24. DO NOT chart for anyone else, especially for nursing actions performed by another nurse or anyone else.

25. DO NOT throw away nurse's notes which have errors on them. Mark through the error with one

horizontal line and label it, "ERROR." Include the sheet as part of the chart. DO NOT ERASE.

26. DO NOT repeat in your narrative events noted or written on forms in other parts of the chart UNLESS you feel that it is very important. Err on the side of redundancy rather than lose a vital piece of information.

The nurse's adherence to these rules will facilitate the preservation of a complete, accurate, and succinct medical record. If the nurse fails to do so, the nurse expert witness, who has been retained to testify against the nurse defendant, will have as her job to dissect and digest your editorials. While the nurse's shortcomings in charting do not in and of themselves amount to malpractice, the jury nonetheless may have difficulty looking past the chart to the merits of the lawsuit. Further, if the jury discovers that you have altered any medical record in any way, the verdict against the nurse is all but signed and sealed.

Therefore, in contrast to Dr. Szasz's recommendation, DO CHART! The nurse's duty is not to screen the charting entries based on the potential consequences (Slovenko, 1979 pp. 422, 423). You cannot change the facts and fill in after the occurrence. Give yourself and other health care providers the best possible chance to defend yourself in a lawsuit.

MALPRACTICE INSURANCE

Should the nurse purchase *malpractice insurance*? If so, what policy limits should the nurse have? What types of policies are available?

THE DECISION TO PURCHASE

First, whether or not the nurse carries malpractice insurance is her own personal decision. However, the nurse should be aware of both sides of the insurance question. Some believe that if the nurse does not have insurance, she will not be named personally in a lawsuit, but she will be more likely to be named if she does carry it. If the nurse works in an institutional setting, such as a hospital or nursing home, that institution is usually also named in the suit. The plaintiff rightfully presumes that the institution has some sort of malpractice coverage. The plaintiff generally does not legally need to personally name the nurse to reach into the "deep pockets" of the institution's malpractice insurance fund. The general rule is that *unless* the nurse is *directly* and *importantly* in-

volved in a significant event in the lawsuit, she will not be named personally.

If the nurse is named, the institution typically retains its own attorney to represent its and the nurse's interest, as the nurse is most likely an "additional insured" under the institution's policy. In this case, one attorney represents both interests. This arrangement can pose an ethical conflict or dilemma for the attorney *if* some facts are revealed which could put the hospital in an adversarial position to the nurse. If a conflict does arise, the hospital's insurer might hire independent counsel for the nurse, which spares the nurse her own expense. However, the hospital's insurer would be legally within its rights to refuse to defend the nurse under certain circumstances.

The nurse has two choices in a situation like this: 1) to obtain counsel and face possible financial ruin, because these suits usually last a year or more and often cost thousands of dollars in legal fees; or 2) to represent herself. In general, self-representation is not a good idea because the nurse is not trained in the legal field. Attorneys have a saying: "The lawyer who represents herself has a fool for a client." The nurse would be no different.

Another consideration regarding the purchase of insurance concerns having an attorney who represents the nurse and no one else. When an attorney represents the hospital, several nurses, and other employees, many issues arise which can distract the attorney from particular concerns for different clients. Even if no conflict exists among the clients, the attorney may have some logistical problems with multiple representation. However, when the nurse's insurer retains an attorney for the nurse, that attorney has one concern only: the representation of that nurse.

Being named in a lawsuit and not having insurance will mean that the nurse must still pay for representation until her dismissal from the case. Even if the nurse does not have insurance, the plaintiff's attorney may either not believe the nurse or may feel that the nurse's remaining in the suit will tactically give the plaintiff a better chance of receiving compensation from the other defendants. If the nurse is ultimately dismissed from the case, that event could be two or three years and $30,000 or more in legal expenses away.

The purchase of malpractice insurance seems to be the better decision for the nurse's financial well-being. In addition, the nurse has an ethical and legal duty to compensate a patient who has been injured by her malpractice. After all, the nurse's increased responsibility means legal accountability. Why should the patient suffer injury and simultaneously remain uncompensated?

TYPES OF POLICIES AND THEIR LIMITS

If the nurse does purchase insurance, what type of insurance should she buy and what are the limitations on each type? Two main types of malpractice insurance exist: 1) claims-based, and 2) occurrence-based. A claims-based policy provides coverage for only those *claims made* during the policy period. An occurrence-based policy provides coverage for alleged negligence that occurs during the policy period, regardless of when the claim is made.

For example, assume that a policy period extends from January 1, 1990 until January 1, 1991. A former patient makes a claim on February 3, 1991 for an alleged malpractice which occurred March, 1990. Under an occurrence-based policy, because the occurrence (malpractice) took place in March, 1990, which was during the policy period, the nurse would have coverage, assuming that all other conditions of the policy had been fulfilled. Also, no coverage defenses can exist against the insured and no claim for punitive damages can be made. Under a claims-based policy, because the claim was made after the policy had expired, the nurse would not have coverage unless she had purchased other insurance for that period.

The benefit of an occurrence-based policy is that it provides coverage regardless of the amount of time that has passed between the incident and the date the claim is made. The nurse does not have to worry about payment of legal fees or a judgment that is within policy limits. The disadvantage is that the premiums may fluctuate depending on the market and state of health of the industry that is writing malpractice insurance. In a policy that limits liability to "$200,000/$600,000," the "$200,000" indicates that the insurance company will provide payment for any individual claim up to $200,000. The "$600,000" represents that the insurer will pay up to $600,000 total (on all claims) during any given year. Therefore, if a plaintiff successfully sued a nurse for a $500,000 judgment, the insurance company would pay the nurse's attorney's fees and pay $200,000, leaving $300,000 to be paid by the nurse out of her own pocket (Williams, 1981, pp. 87, 88).

Who is covered under the malpractice policy? Most, but not all, policies cover staff nurses and supervisors, administrators, and even nurse midwives or nurse practitioners. Nurses in expanded roles are, however, finding it more difficult to obtain coverage and are at greater risk for being sued.

Certain activities generally are excluded from coverage, regardless of the state in which the nurse practices. Criminal, malicious, or fraudulent acts, or those outside the scope of the nurse's practice are likely to be excluded from coverage.

The nurse should do competitive price and content shopping before purchasing the insurance policy. If she has any questions once she purchases the policy, she should keep the policy and all communications between her and the insurer in a safe place (Arbeiter, 1986, pp. 23, 25, 26).

An insurance policy is a contract between the nurse and the insurer; thus, both parties have obligations under the contract. The nurse's duties generally include, but are not limited to, the duty to cooperate with the company and the duty to rapidly report any claim, potential or otherwise, to the company. The nurse's failure to fulfill her contractual duties could result in a denial of coverage, which in effect means that the nurse would be without any liability policy for protection. Therefore, the purchase of the policy is the first step in protecting the nurse, who must also subsequently cooperate with the investigation and defense of the claim.

JUDGES AND JURIES

The nurse should understand the roles and potential attitudes of judges and jurors when they are faced with a case that involves the medical profession. First, most judges are lay consumers vis-à-vis medicine and nursing; that is, they have no greater understanding of the everyday practice of nursing than any other lay person. Even though the judge is more educated in law than the average juror, he or she does not necessarily know all the principles of nursing or medicine. A nurse who assumes that the judge has greater understanding of nursing or medicine makes a critical mistake. The judge is not necessarily aware of the nurse's functions and may not know that a nurse is obligated legally to question a physician's order, may make her own diagnoses, and may act independently of the physician. A judge does try to be fair to all participants in the legal system, as he or she has sworn to uphold the law; however, the judge may need to be educated about nursing practice like any other lay individual.

Second, educating the public, which necessarily includes jurors, about the role of the nurse has far-reaching potential consequences. Because they focus solely on the jury trial process, the jurors are, on the average, uninformed about nursing in general. Yet the jurors will decide the nurse's fate regarding the liability issue. The jurors only know the information contained in the chart and the nurse's live testimony. This small amount of information alone will assist the jury in its decision-making process. The jurors may never know that the nurse works extremely hard, with long hours and very little time for breaks, or that the nurse makes critical life and death decisions on a daily basis. If the jurors cannot identify with the nurse's position, they may have trouble empathizing with the nurse and understanding the decision she faced at a crucial point in the patient's care.

Nurses must become actively involved as leaders in controlling the fate of their own profession, both in and out of the courtroom. Nurses must learn the sources of the power within their own state and federal governments to influence and control the practice of nursing. Nurses must obtain the assistance of other individuals, nurses and non-nurses, through networking to cooperate in their endeavors. Networking can be accomplished in many ways, but belonging to one's own professional organization is an excellent beginning.

SUMMARY

As professionals with growing responsibilities in the health care arena, nurses are now often being held legally accountable for the care they provide. Because of the potential for misunderstanding and the emotional nature of patient issues involved, nurses working with mentally ill patients must be especially knowledgeable about patients' rights, the nurse's own potential for liability, and the workings of the legal system.

Law is defined as "a rule or method with which phenomena or actions coexist or follow each other." Law is derived from statutes and common law. Three types of legal redress—criminal law, administrative law, and civil law—exist, though the nurse is most likely to be involved in a civil lawsuit based on a negligent tort. Five areas of liability addressed in this chapter include suicide, involuntary treatment, the doctrine of informed consent and the right to refuse medical treatment, the duty to warn third parties, and sexual misconduct.

Record-keeping is one of the most important parts of nursing practice. An accurate record not only helps ensure good patient care, but it may be the single most important document in a legal case involving the nurse. An inadequate record is often considered by judges and juries to be indicative of poor patient care.

The nurse makes her own choice about purchasing malpractice insurance, but going without it may cost her a great deal of money if she is involved in a lawsuit. Finally, if the nurse is knowledgeable about the law and its many facets, such as law-making for professional conduct and regulations, she is less likely to be manipulated by the system.

KEY TERMS

law

statutes

common law

administrative rules

criminal law

administrative law

civil law

tort law

negligent tort

plaintiff

direct liability

indirect (or vicarious) liability

breach of duty

damages

causation

least restrictive means of treatment

doctrine of informed consent

transference

malpractice insurance

claims-based insurance

occurrence-based insurance

STUDY QUESTIONS

1. Identify five patients' rights that have been upheld or established by the courts in the last twenty years.

2. Name and describe briefly the three general types of legal redress.

3. Name and describe briefly the four elements of a lawsuit.

4. Name and describe briefly the five areas of liability.

5. Why is record keeping in nursing practice so important? What are some of the things the nurse can do to improve her record keeping?

6. Name and describe briefly the two different types of malpractice insurance policies. Which would you choose, and why?

REFERENCES

Am. Nurses Assoc. (1973). *Standards of practice,* Kansas City: ANA.

Am. Nurses Assoc. (1976). *Quality assurance workbook,* Kansas City: ANA.

Andrede, P. D. & Andrede, J. C. (1979, Summer). Professional liability of the psychiatric nurse. *The Journal of Psychiatry and Law, 141,* 148. (Summer, 1979).

Arbeiter, J. (1986, May). A buyer's guide to malpractice insurance. *RN, 22.*

Beck v. *Kansas University Psychiatry Foundation* 580 F. Supp. 527 (D. Kan 1984).

Black, H. (1984). *Black's law dictionary,* 4th ed. 1028.

Brooks, A. D. (1974). *Law, psychiatry and the health care system.* Boston: Little, Brown, p. 732.

Davis, K. C. (1972). *Administrative law text,* 3d ed. St. Paul, MN: West Publishing Company, pp. 1, 2.

Davis v. *Hubbard,* 506 F. Supp. 915 (N. D. Ohio 1980).

Doudera, A. E. & Swazey, J. P. (Eds.) (1982). *Refusing treatment in mental health institutions—values in conflict.* Michigan: AUPHA Press.

Doyle v. *United States* 530 F. Supp. 1278 (C. D. Cal. 1982)

Dunham v. *Wright* 423 F. 2d. 940, 942 (3d Cir. 1970).

Ewing, C. P. (1983, Winter). Dr. Death & the case for an ethical ban on psychiatric & psychological predictions of dangerousness in capital sentencing proceedings. *Am. J. Law & Medicine,* 8 (4), 407.

Fla. Stat. §394.451, 394.463 (2)(a), (3) (1989).

Fla. Stat. §464 et seq. (1989).

Greenlaw, J. (1985, June). Definition & regulation of nursing practice: a historical perspective. *Law, Medicine & Health Care, 13* (3), 117.

Griswold v. *Connecticut* 381 U.S. 479, 85 S. Ct. 1678, 14 L. Ed. 2d 510 (1965).

Guntheil, T. G., & Appelbaum, P. S. (1985, April). The substituted judgment approach: Its difficulties and paradoxes in mental health settings, *Law, Medicine & Health Care* 13 (2) 61.

Hedlund v. *Superior Court.* 669 P. 2d 41 (Cal. 1983).

Herran, D. J. & Guerrini, N. E. (1979, Spring). Developing legal trends in psychiatric malpractice. *The Journal of Psychiatry & Law,* 65, 66.

Hirst v. *St. Paul Fire & Marine Ins. Co.* (1984). 683 P. 2d. 440 (Idaho 1984).

Jablonski v. *U.S.,* 712 F. 2d 391 (3d Cir. 1983).

Katz, J. (1979). Informed Consent—A fairy tale? Law's vision. *39 U.P.H.L.Rev. 89,* 137–143.

Kelly, M. E. & Garrick, T. R. (1984, December). Nursing negligence in collaborative practice: legal liability in California. *Law, Medicine & Health Care* 12 (6), 260, 264.

L. L. v. *Medical Protection Co.* 362 N.W. 2d 174, 177 (Wis. 1984).

Malone v. *Longa,* 463 F.Supp. 139 (E.D.N.Y. 1979)

Matter of Estate of Votteler 327 N.W. 2d 759 (Iowa 1982).

Meisel, A. (1979). The exceptions to the informed consent doctrine: Striking a balance between competing values in medical decision-making *2 Wisc. K. Rev.,* 413, 426, 433.

Meisel, A., & Kabnick, L. (1980). Informed consent to medical treatment: An analysis of recent legislation, *U.P.H.L. Rev., 41,* 407, 490.

Meisel, A., Roth, L. H., & Lidz, C. (1977). Toward a model of the legal doctrine of informed consent. *Am. J. Psych., 134,* 285.

Meyers, C. J. (1984, Spring). The legal perils of psychotherapeutic practice (Part II): Coping with "Hedlund" and "Jablonski." *The Journal of Psychiatry & Law,* 187.

Mullen, J. M. & Norman, B. (Summer 1979). Innovations in Forensics: developing criteria for determination of dangerous behavior. *The Journal of Psychiatry & the Law,* 187.

Murchisn, I., & Nichols, T. (1970). *Legal foundations of nursing practice.* London: Collier-MacMillan Ltd.

O'Connor v. *Donaldson* 422 U.S. 563, 95 S. Ct. 2486, 45 L. Ed. 2d 396 (1975).

Paddock v. *Chacko,* 522 So. 2d 410, 412 (Fla 5th DCA 1988).

Perr, I. N. (1978, January). Legal aspects of suicide. *The Journalist Legal Medicine, 49,* 54.

Prosser, W., & Keeton, W. (1984). *The law of torts,* 5th ed. St. Paul, MN: West Publishing Company, p. 17.

Rennie v. *Klein* 462 F. Supp. 1131 (D.N.J. 1978).

Rennie v. *Klein* 476 F. Supp. 1294 (D.N.J. 1979).

Rhoden, N. K. (1985, April). The presumption for treatment: Has it been justified? *Law, Medicine & Health Care, 13* (2), 65.

Rhodes, A. M., & Miller, R. D. (1984). *Nursing and the law,* 4th ed. Rockville, MD: Aspen Systems Corp.

Roe v. *Wade* 410 U.S. 113, 93 S. Ct. 705, 35 L. Ed.2d 147 (1973)

Roy v. *Hartogs* 381 N.Y.S.2d 587 (Sup. Ct. N.Y. 1976).

Sarasota County Dept. of Soc. Serv. v. *Hofbauer* (1970). 393 N.E.2d 1009 (N.Y. 1979).

Schloendorff v. *The Society of New York Hospital* (1914). 211 N.Y. 125, 105 N.E. 92.

Schopp, R. F., & Quattrocchi, M. R. (1984, Spring). Tarasoff, the doctrine of special relationships, and the psychotherapist's duty to warn. *The Journal of Psychiatry & Law, 12,* 13.

Scott v. *Plante* 532 F.2d 939 (3d Cir. 1976).

Sermchief v. *Gonzales,* 660 S.W. 2d 683 (Mo. banc. 1983).

Silverberg, H. M., (1974, Fall). Protecting the human rights of mental patients, *Barrister* 46.

Slovenko, R. (1981, Summer). Malpractice and psychiatry in related fields. *The Journal of Psychiatry & The Law,* 5, 16.

Slovenko, R. (1979, Winter). On the need for record-keeping in the practice of psychiatry. *The Journal of Psychiatry & the Law,* 399.

Stanley v. *Georgia,* 394 U.S. 557, 895 ct. 1243, 22 L.Ed. 2d 542 (1969).

Szasz, T. S. (1965). *The ethics of psychoanalysis.* London: Basic Books.

Tarasoff v. *Regents of Univ. of Cal.,* 551 P.2d at 340 (1976).

Vigilant Ins. Co. v. *Employers Ins. Wausau,* 626 F. Supp. 262 (S.D.N.Y.1986).

Waltz, & Scheuneman (1969). Informed consent therapy. *Nw.U.L.Rev., 64,* 628.

Williams, B.N. (1981, January). Malpractice: How good is your insurance protection? *Nursing '76,* 81, 87.

Winters v. *Miller,* 306 F. Supp. 1158 (E.D.N.Y. 1969), rev'd and rem'd 446 F.2d 65 (2nd Cir.), *cert. den.,* 404 U.S. 985 (1971).

Zeuli, L. B. (1982). The doctrine of informed consent; the right to choose & refuse medical treatment (unpublished).

28

ETHICAL CONSIDERATIONS IN MENTAL HEALTH NURSING PRACTICE

NORMAN FOST

LEARNING OBJECTIVES
After studying this chapter, the student will be able to:

- Discuss why it is difficult to define *disease* as it pertains to mental health and understand the ethical issues that arise around this difficulty.
- Understand the concept of competence and the ethical issues that surround it.
- Understand the concept of paternalism and the conditions under which it is and is not justified.
- Describe the ethical justifications for confidentiality and the situations in which it may be necessary to break confidentiality.
- Discuss the central issues to the nurse acting as "double agent."
- List the variables relevant to efforts aimed at controlling a patient's behavior.
- Describe the ethical issues surrounding suicide intervention or nonintervention.

INTRODUCTION

Every interaction between a health professional and a patient raises ethical questions: Is the patient truly consenting to treatment? Are the benefits of treatment worth the cost? Does the therapist have conflicts of interest? The purpose of this chapter is to sensitize the reader to the range of ethical problems which commonly arise in psychiatric settings, to clarify the meaning of important ethical terms and concepts, and to review the major arguments for familiar positions. This chapter does not recommend solutions to specific clinical problems as any "solution" must be based on the unique circumstances of each situation, institutional guidelines, if any, and the mental health care provider's own value system.

For an introduction to ethical theory as it applies to medical problems in general, the reader is referred to introductory chapters in anthologies on medical ethics (Hunt, 1977; Beauchamp & Walters, 1982; Gorovitz et al., 1983) or general works on principles of biomedical ethics (Beauchamp, 1979). There is also a rapidly growing literature on procedural approaches to resolving clinical ethical dilemmas through such mechanisms as hospital ethics committees (Fost & Cranford, 1985).

This chapter contains a brief review of three conceptual problems: the definition of disease, competence, and paternalism. Then some common clinical-ethical problems—informed consent, confidentiality, conflict of interest, behavior control, and suicide—will be analyzed.

DEFINITION OF DISEASE

Agreement on the definition of *disease* as a general concept, as well as on the criteria for specific diseases, including mental illness, is important for several reasons. First, being sick or diseased provides a person with excuses for some behaviors which would not otherwise be acceptable, such as missing work or even killing someone. Second, a certification that someone is ill facilitates access to certain kinds of assistance, such as financial support for treatment. Third, a diagnosis of some diseases may have adverse consequences for the patient, by leading to involuntary commitment, exclusion from certain types of employment, or other restrictions on his liberty. These issues are particularly important in the field of mental health, where a diagnosis is almost always accompanied by stigmatization.

Despite the importance of the definition of disease, consensus has been elusive (Caplan, Englehardt, & McCartney, 1981). The dictionary defines disease as "any departure from health" (Guralnik, 1979). Health, we are advised, means "physical and mental well-being" or "normality of physical and mental function." These broad criteria would suggest that someone who is tired or angry has a disease. Further, the suggestion that health is equated with normality implies that the abnormally tall or happy person is sick or diseased.

The problem is compounded in psychiatry, where knowledge of specific etiologies is usually lacking, making it more difficult to define diseases using objective criteria (Szasz, 1960). Unlike other diseases, which can usually be equated with disturbance in the structure or measurable function of identifiable organs, mental illnesses are typically not associated with observable abnormalities in any organ.

These ambiguities in defining mental illness have ethical implications for citizens whose behavior or beliefs are unpopular. Governments and organizations, with the support of the medical profession, have long used the concept of mental illness to achieve political ends. Behaviors which are merely deviant or unwelcome, if labeled as diseases, can be more easily controlled. "Drapetomania" for example—an affliction of slaves which caused them to have an irresistible urge to run away (Engelhardt, 1974)—was a disease invented by the medical profession in the eighteenth century to aid slaveowners seeking justification for returning runaway slaves. More recently, the Soviet Union has used psychiatric diagnosis as a justification for imprisonment of political dissidents, in the name of involuntary commitment for treatment.

A modern example of the arbitrariness of defining psychiatric diseases is the disappearance of the entry "homosexuality" between the second and third editions of the Diagnostic and Statistical Manual of the American Psychiatric Association (DSM-II, 1968; DSM-III, 1980) As a result of a close vote, millions of Americans went from a state of being "sick" to one of being "well" overnight.

A more common example of the use of psychiatric diagnosis as an instrument of control arises when critically ill patients refuse life-sustaining medical treatment. Such refusals are often offensive to the medical staff, who seek help from psychiatrists in declaring the patient incompetent, as a justification for ignoring the patient's expressed wishes. A similar practice occurs, in a less formal way, when an individual volunteers to donate his kidney for allegedly altruistic reasons, or even for money. Such individuals are typically labeled as "crazy," without formal evaluation, rather than evaluated on the basis of the complex ethical issues which such offers raise.

Another feature of psychiatric diagnoses is their persistence. Because they are without known causes, and rely on states of mind, which are more difficult to document than diseases due to microbes or cancerous cells, their resolution may be as difficult to document as their presence. The adverse effects of such diagnoses may, therefore, linger long after the manifestations of illness have disappeared (Rosenhan, 1973).

COMPETENCE

A central principle in American medical ethics and health law is the principle of **autonomy,** the right of a competent person to determine what shall be done to his own body. Yet, no one would advocate leaving a clearly incompetent person, such as an infant, to make his own decisions on matters that affect his health in an important way. Therefore, the problem lies in defining competence in a way that does not allow undue interference with individual liberties, yet allows protection of patients in danger of injuring themselves in a way they would later regret.

Mental competence is not global, in the sense of being present or absent. A patient can be competent to do some things, such as driving a car or deciding when to eat, but not others, such as deciding whether to have surgery.

As a practical matter, the definition of competence is primarily a legal issue, since it is the law which sets the limits to permissible interference with a person's autonomy. Unfortunately, there is no consensus, in theory or in practice, on the proper definition. Different notions are used in the mental health field. Roth and his colleagues have analyzed five competing concepts of competence: evidencing a choice, making a reasonable choice, making a choice based on rational reasons, having the ability to understand, and proving understanding (Roth, 1977).

EVIDENCING A CHOICE

This definition of competence requires only that the patient show an ability to choose, regardless of whether the choice is rational, informed, or reasonable. Patients who would be considered incompetent according to this definition include the comatose or catatonic person who shows no preferences at all. It is the most respectful of autonomy and has the advantage of being easy to apply in practice, since it depends primarily on the patient's observable behavior, rather than his thought processes or understanding.

John: A Patient Evidencing a Choice

John, an 82-year-old man in chronic congestive heart failure, malnourished and depressed, did not talk or answer questions. He ate some food put on his tray and took pills, but physically rebuffed attempts by his nurse to draw blood, give injections, or insert a nasogastric tube.

Under the definition of evidencing a choice, John, in the case study, would be considered competent and, therefore, allowed to refuse nasogastric feedings and injections, even if the refusal seemed to be leading to his death.

MAKING A REASONABLE CHOICE

This definition requires that the patient's choice be compatible with prevailing societal notions of what a reasonable person would or should do. It is relatively intolerant of individuals who are outside the mainstream, even though they may have a clear understanding of the nature and consequences of their decisions. This standard maximizes widely shared social goals, such as the preservation of life, at the expense of personal freedom.

Brian: A Patient Making an Unreasonable Choice

Brian, a 45-year-old married man with no children was a lifelong Jehovah's Witness. Because of his religion, he refused a medically necessary blood transfusion, realizing that he would die. His wife supported his decision.

Under the definition of making a reasonable choice, if the doctors and court believe Brian is acting unreasonably, he could be declared incompetent and forced to receive blood.

MAKING A CHOICE BASED ON RATIONAL REASONS

To meet this definition of competence, a patient must convince others that the thought processes that led to his decision were based on valid facts and logical conclusions. It is difficult to implement accurately, since decisions are influenced by so many factors and it is so difficult to know whether the crucial factors were rational ones or not. The definition also gives broad latitude to those who seek to limit patient freedom, since few important decisions in life are based on sound facts or logical thinking.

Mark: A Patient Making a Choice Based on Irrational Reasons

Mark, a 45-year-old homeless alcoholic, was admitted to a hospital emergency room because of pneumonia. Although essential to his treatment, Mark refused antibiotics because he believed they were part of a communist plot.

Mark could be declared incompetent under the definition of making a choice based on rational reasons since his refusal to accept treatment is not based on logical facts.

HAVING THE ABILITY TO UNDERSTAND

According to this definition of competence the patient must have the intellectual ability to understand the proposed treatment, likely benefits and risks, and alternative treatments, as well as the risks of refusing treatment. The actual decision could be based on irrational considerations or religious grounds as long as all aspects of the treatment are understood.

Mary: A Patient Able to Understand

Mary, a 22-year-old woman, was 5 feet 8 inches tall and weighed 62 pounds. She said her hips were too big and she wanted to lose two more pounds. She was in mild congestive heart failure, and her serum potassium was 1.9 mEq/L due to frequent use of ipecac. She was quite lucid and said she understood she was in danger, but it was more important that she lose weight.

Mary would be considered competent under this test, since she has the ability to understand what is at stake and what is necessary, even though she seems to be actually deciding on unreasonable or irrational grounds.

PROVING UNDERSTANDING

This is the most stringent definition of competence, requiring that the patient prove he understands the actual issues involved in the particular decision at hand. The problems with this definition include the difficulty of defining the degree of understanding, and the potentially large numbers of patients who might fail such a test because they cannot demonstrate or prove their understanding.

David: A Patient Without Understanding

David, a 22-year-old mildly retarded man, had appendicitis. The doctor explained to him that there was a small chance of dying from the anesthesia. David repeatedly asked "Whatsat?" He also stated repeatedly that his sister had appendicitis, but outgrew it. He had no objection to surgery, but apparently had no understanding of what was going on. His mother, with whom he lives, advised the doctor to proceed although she did not have legal guardianship of David.

Under the definition of providing understanding, David would presumably be considered incompetent and, therefore, unable to consent to treatment. Since his mother does not have legal guardianship, the doctor would have to seek permission from the court in order to proceed.

In our society, there is a bias toward life and toward treatment in general, so that patients' competence is not questioned as long as they agree or acquiesce to treatment. This means that patients are generally not allowed to refuse treatment unless the treatment's risk/benefit ratio is very unfavorable—that is, the risk is very high, and/or the benefit is very low. This practice is not based on respect for autonomy, but on paternalism, the belief that health care professionals and courts should interfere with a person's liberty when it is for his own good, as defined by those in power.

In summary, there are widely varying notions on competence. Which one is actually used depends largely on the preexisting value system of the person(s) in power. Those who favor autonomy will tend to use an "easy" standard of competence, achievable by a large majority of patients. Those who are inclined toward paternalism, believing that decisions should be based primarily on what is good for patients rather than what they want, will tend toward a "strict" standard, difficult for many patients to meet.

PATERNALISM

Paternalism can be defined as interfering with someone's liberty for the good of that person. Examples of paternalism include lying to a patient to protect him from upsetting news; involuntarily committing a patient to protect him from self-inflicted harm; or sharing confidential information with a family member or employer, without the patient's permission, so that others can be more supportive.

While it may seem self-evident to some healthcare professionals that it is ethically permissible, if not obligatory, to do whatever is for the good of the patient, the problem can be better understood if we imagine what life would be like if everyone with the power to control another took that view. For example, the government could prohibit high cholesterol foods and require daily exercise and reading of good books. Doctors could withhold information at will and do procedures on reluctant patients without informing them or obtaining their consent. Instead, most people are sympathetic with philosopher John Stuart Mill's assertion that

> . . . The sole ends for which mankind are warranted, individually or collectively, in interfering with the liberty or action of any of their number, is self-protection. That the only purpose for which power can be rightfully exercised over any member of a civilized community, against his will, is to prevent harm to others. His own good, either physical or moral, is not a sufficient warrant. (Mill, 1947, p. 9).

This general objection to paternalism is not absolute. There are some situations—such as attempted suicide—when most would agree that interfering with a person's liberty is morally justified. The challenge is to define the conditions which justify such interference.

The simple answer is that it is permissible to interfere with a person's liberty when failure to do so would result in harm. But that allows too much, for many people act in ways that involve risk of harm, such as smoking or failing to exercise. The probability and seriousness of the harm are relevant, but even a decision which will lead to certain death, such as refusal of life-sustaining treatment in an intensive care unit, should not always be opposed (such as when death is imminent anyway or the patient is clearly competent).

Some might argue that it is permissible to interfere with a person's decisions when he seems incapable of acting in his own interests, but that would describe many adults who make decisions that appear to block attainment of their most cherished goals. Examples include the smoker who insists he wants to stop but seems unable to, or the overweight person who insists he wants to lose weight but doesn't. While it might be permissible to put such persons on a behavior-modification program with their informed consent, it would not be permissible to confiscate cigarettes or desserts without their permission.

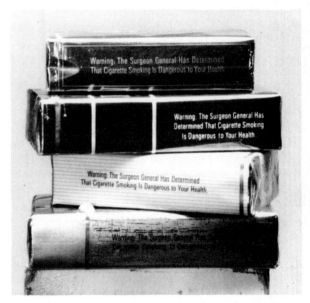

The ethical issue here is one of paternalism versus personal freedom, including the freedom to abuse one's body. Few are willing to give up the freedom to kill themselves in a socially accepted manner in exchange for health and what is said to be a better and longer life. "Control," even if it has gone haywire, will never be given up without a fight. It's too important to maintaining a sense of humanness, not to mention hope.

Some might claim that it is permissible to interfere with a patient's liberty when he seems incompetent. This requires a working definition of incompetence and a reliable means of determining whether the patient meets the definition. The ambiguities of doing this, including the fact that competence is not a global attribute, were discussed earlier. A patient may not be competent to make some decisions such as buying a house, but may be competent to decide whether or not he wants to participate in a nontherapeutic research project.

How, then, can a general rule be developed that would provide guidance in deciding when paternalism is justified? One way is to identify the relevant variables in a situation where paternalism is widely considered to be warranted, such as interference with a suicide attempt. Such an analysis leads to the following general rule:

Paternalism is justified only if all four of the following conditions exist:

1. There is a high risk of serious physical harm.

2. There is a high probability of benefit from interfering.

3. The patient is likely to say "thank you" later.

4. You would want someone to interfere with your liberty if you were in the patient's situation.

Jill: A Patient Refusing Treatment

Jill, a 32-year-old Jehovah's Witness, was refusing a transfusion which was necessary to save her life. The internist in charge of the case asked for a psychiatric consultation because he believed the patient was "crazy" and the decision was not in her long-range interest.

While there is clear risk of harm in the case study, and clear benefit from interfering, Jill is not likely to say "thank you" and paternalism would not be justified according to the general rule discussed above. She is not mentally ill by any DSM-III criteria and is competent in the sense of understanding the consequences of her decision. (There might be other moral reasons for interfering, such as to protect the interests of her dependent children, or to protect the public interest in respect for life.)

With these philosophical themes as introduction, we turn to more pragmatic considerations involving common clinical-ethical dilemmas.

INFORMED CONSENT, REFUSING TREATMENT, AND INVOLUNTARY TREATMENT

Every human being of adult years and sound mind has a right to determine what shall be done with his own body. . . . This is true except in cases of emergency. (*Schloendorff,* 1914).

INFORMED CONSENT

The oldest principle in Anglo-Saxon law is battery, which is a prohibition against unconsented touchings. The modern medical-legal notion of informed consent derives from this principle and serves two functions: to protect patients from harm, and to preserve autonomy. (See Chapter 27 on legal considerations.) Even though the requirement to obtain consent for treatment may result in harm to a patient—as in a Jehovah's Witness's refusal to consent—autonomy is valued above paternalistic protection in American society.

Although there are two familiar exceptions, consent is essential to treatment in mental health settings. The two exceptions are when the patient is dangerous to others, and when he is dangerous to himself. Interfering with the liberty of those who are dangerous to others requires no elaboration as to its ethical justification. The primary purpose of government is to protect citizens from harm. The right to autonomy does not include the right to cause harm to others. The central ethical obligation in such circumstances is to restrict such intrusions to situations of high probability of harm to others. Some observers point to the notorious inaccuracy of predictions of dangerousness (Stone, 1976), generally in the direction of overprediction, and conclude that psychiatrists and other mental-health professionals should not be required to act as state agents in such situations (Szasz, 1963; Chodoff, 1976).

REFUSING TREATMENT

The more controversial examples of treatment without consent involve interventions for the intended benefit of the patient, rather than protection of others. This includes patients who are treated in a way that may be inconsistent with their apparent wishes, for reasons other than saving life itself.

A patient can be covertly compelled to accept treatment by feeling that he has no choice, or by his ignorance of alternatives. Consent must be free and informed to be meaningful. The patient with depression, for example, who ardently seeks help but is not informed that, in addition to drug treatment, talking therapies, behavior therapies, and exercise programs might be helpful, has not truly consented to drug treatment. Similarly, the hospitalized patient who fears that he may be involuntarily committed if he doesn't comply with a suggested program has not freely consented to treatment.

Kathy: An Uninformed Patient

Kathy, a 19-year-old college student, had been diagnosed with anorexia nervosa but was not presently in danger of dying. She was admitted under pressure from her parents. The nurses warned her, under instruction from an authoritarian doctor, that she would be restrained and tube-fed if she did not comply with a recommended diet.

If Kathy is unaware that she cannot legally be forced to submit to treatment, and that she is free to refuse treatment and leave the hospital, then she is being treated without consent. Respect for her as a person and the need for Kathy's informed consent would require an explicit disclosure at the time of admission of the nature of the treatment program, including restrictions of privileges, use of tube feedings, and so on.

Involuntary Treatment

Dan, a 44-year-old man with chronic schizophrenia was recurrently hospitalized in a state institution when he failed to take his antipsychotic medication. When on the medicine, he did well on the outside, where he clearly preferred to live. His doctor wrote an order for an injection of a long-acting drug, even though the patient had clearly refused such treatment.

While there is no clear moral basis for treating Dan without his consent, the moral claim would be that the patient is so confused by his mental disease that he is unable to consent to what his "real" self would want. Involuntary treatment, it could be argued, is the only way to give him what he values most, freedom. The situation is similar to the 5-year-old who refuses an appendectomy for appendicitis;

there is little doubt that the child would consent if he understood all the issues clearly.

Szasz (1974) has argued that involuntary treatment for mental illness is "a form of imprisonment" that should be prohibited. If the basis of involuntary treatment is societal protection, then the criminal statutes that apply to all citizens equally should be used. Regarding commitment for the benefit of the patient, Szasz objects on several grounds. First, he rejects the notion that mental illnesses are diseases, particularly when there is no clear organic disorder that can be treated primarily. He argues that mental illness is a metaphor used "by the state and by psychiatrists as a device for exerting social control over annoying or unconventional people" (Szasz, 1970). In support, he cites the ease and confidence with which psychiatrists declare public figures to be seriously mentally ill: Barry Goldwater was declared a "paranoid schizophrenic"; Woodrow Wilson "close to psychosis"; and Jesus "a born degenerate . . . (with a) fixed delusional system."

Second, he believes that the individual's right to control his own body supersedes any paternalistic interest of the state in doing good for others. Third, he cites extensive historical evidence of the abuse of commitment procedures, ranging from statutes which permitted women to be "detained at the hospital at the request of the husband," to contemporary uses for crass political purposes, such as expediting criminal cases through the use of declarations of psychiatric incompetence (Szasz, 1963).

Proponents of involuntary commitment generally rely on the "best interest" standard as the major justification for involuntary commitment. Chodoff (1976) would restrict such treatment to situations in which three criteria are met: 1) the patient's actions are imminently dangerous, in the physical *or* social sense, to his best interests; 2) the disruptive behavior is due to mental illness; and 3) the condition is treatable and facilities exist to provide treatment. He sees the emphasis on autonomy as resulting in harm to patients, who cannot be protected from their own disability, and who are forced out of institutions into communities with inadequate resources for treatment. He views illness, in some cases, as being more restrictive of liberty than state action.

VOLUNTARY FUTURE COMMITMENT: ULYSSES CONTRACTS

Because of the increasing reluctance to commit patients involuntarily unless they are physically danger-

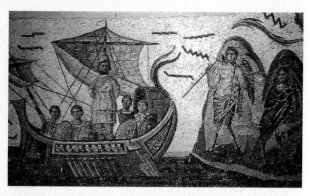

The moral dilemma here: once Ulysses begins asking his men for release, who do they take as the *real* Ulysses? Yesterday's cautious leader or today's tempted Ulysses begging for release?

ous to themselves or others, some patients who can benefit from involuntary treatment have been unable to obtain such treatment. The typical case is the patient with manic-depressive illness who recurrently causes great psychosocial harm to himself and/or his family, but does not qualify for involuntary commitment because he is not physically dangerous. To allow his physician to exercise such authority when the patient becomes manic, some patients have signed **Ulysses contracts**, voluntary future commitment contracts which authorize the physician to deprive the patient of his liberty under specified circumstances (Howell, 1982). (The name is derived from the mythical Greek figure who, in his fear of being tempted by the deadly Sirens, ordered his shipmates to tie him to a mast and ignore all protests to let him go.)

The moral dilemma for Ulysses' shipmates, and for current professionals responsible for such patients, is determining who is the "real" patient: the one who signed a contract months or years ago, or the person presently insisting that he has changed his mind and declines treatment. The legal dilemma is that such patients cannot be detained over their current objection, regardless of prior contracts, unless the civil commitment laws expressly allow for such circumstances. Since the commitment laws have become increasingly restrictive, they do not presently allow such contracts to be recognized.

Those who oppose such contracts emphasize the risk of manipulation by therapists who might pressure patients into signing away their liberties for the convenience and legal protection of the doctor (Dresser, 1982).

CONFIDENTIALITY

The concept of **confidentiality** can be understood from the Latin root of the word—*fidele*—meaning trust. A patient discloses personal information with implicit trust that the doctor, nurse, or other health professional will not reveal it to others. It is as if a promise were made not to reveal anything.

The ethical justifications for the medical custom of confidentiality are twofold. First, there is the utilitarian claim that many fewer people would seek mental health services, or health care of any kind, without such a principle. This would presumably not be in the general societal interest, since for economic considerations alone, society has an interest in the mental well-being of its members. Other benefits of seeking mental health services include avoiding physical impairment and possibly antisocial and self-destructive acts.

In addition, there is a more formal argument in support of maintaining confidentiality: the claim that it is wrong to break a promise, regardless of the consequences. Indeed, the definition of a promise implies that it is a solemn pledge to behave in a certain way, and that the pledge will not be broken simply because it might increase the good of others. If the clinician secretly means "I will not tell anyone what you say, unless there is a net benefit in doing so," that is not what is understood by the psychiatric patient, and could therefore be construed not only as a broken promise, but also as a lie. (See also Box 28–1.)

Like all ethical principles, confidentiality cannot be absolute, overruling all other considerations. Situations arise in which it clearly seems wrong *not* to disclose confidential information. For example, state statutes require reporting suspected child abuse and venereal diseases. The most celebrated case of disclosure of confidential information in the mental health field, California's *Tarasoff* case (Stone, 1976), involved a university student who told his therapist he intended to kill a woman who had rebuffed his amorous feelings. The therapist informed the police, who detained and then released the would-be assailant when he appeared rational and promised to stay away from the woman. Two months later he killed the woman, who had not been informed of his dangerousness or the police action. Her parents brought a negligence action against the therapist and his supervisors.

Those who oppose this duty to break confidentiality when a patient may be dangerous point out that psychiatrists are notoriously inaccurate in predicting violence, particularly when the subject has never actually performed a dangerous act. To avoid liability, the therapist might tend to overpredict, resulting in many unnecessary warnings. This could lead to widespread distrust of mental health professionals, a reluctance to seek help and/or disclose dangerous intentions, and result in a decrease in public safety (Stone, 1976).

No matter how public policy resolves this trade-off between public safety and the interest of the mentally ill in receiving confidential treatment, the therapist may have a moral obligation to inform the patient of his policies and responsibilities. If a report of dangerous intentions will result in disclosure to the police or third parties in danger, the patient is entitled to be informed before he decides whether and how much to trust the therapist.

Sue: A Nurse Observing Possible Child Abuse

Sue, a visiting nurse in a child abuse prevention program, made twice-weekly visits to a high-risk family. She won the mother's trust by being an empathic, nonjudgmental listener. One day the mother told her that she often got very frustrated and shook the crying baby, and sometimes felt like throwing him against the wall.

A typical abuse reporting law would require Sue to report an *injury* which she believed was nonaccidental, but not necessarily the possibility of a future injury. In states which have upheld the *Tarasoff* principle, she might have a duty to protect the child, independent of the child-abuse statute. Morally, her duty to protect the child conflicts with her promise (implied or explicit) to keep her conversations with the mother confidential.

In a situation such as this where the risk of harm to another is high at the beginning of the relationship, the nurse should consider setting a limit to the confidentiality at the outset, preferably with a written contract stating her obligation to take protective measures if she thinks the child is in danger.

THE PROFESSIONAL AS DOUBLE AGENT

Nurses, like all health professionals, frequently have obligations or loyalties to more than one client, and the interests of these clients may conflict. Sometimes these conflicts are obvious, as when the nurse is em-

ployed by an agency, such as a state, which requires reporting of disorders such as AIDS or child abuse, or a company, which may require reporting of impaired workers to management. Sometimes conflicts arise after a contact with a patient is initiated or even terminated, as when a prospective employer of the patient or a litigant in a trial requests psychiatric information.

Perhaps the most common type of double agentry occurs when health professionals care for more than one person in a family. While this "holistic" approach to health care has become widely accepted and may often have benefits for all parties concerned, the nurse must be alert to situations in which it may not be beneficial and may constitute an abrogation of duty to some member of the family.

Judith, a nurse working with a family practitioner, learned that one of her patients—a married man—was having an affair. His wife had made a separate appointment, complaining of headaches and a depressed mood, and stated she was worried that her husband was losing interest in her and might be having an affair. In a separate medical exam the husband was found to have AIDS. He insisted that the information not be disclosed to his wife.

Linda, a nurse in a pediatric office, noticed extensive bruises while weighing a child. Sara, the mother, volunteered that her husband had left her, and she had no outlet from the continuous pressure of caring for the hyperactive 3-year-old child.

Ann, a school nurse, was a paid consultant to an elementary school which wanted her to control the behavior of a brilliant, obnoxious, 7-year-old. Ann thought the child's interests would be best served with an individualized program, but the school did not have the resources to provide it.

Although the clinician's loyalty should be to the primary patient, as these three cases illustrate, it is often unclear who the primary patient is. The philandering husband and his wife are both primary patients. The mother, Sara, seems to expect empathy and support, as if she is the patient instead of her child; and Ann is employed and paid by the school, not by the patient.

In addition to serving more than one family member, and/or third parties such as schools and

Box 28–1 ●
Confidentiality in
Mental Health
Treatment

Patients routinely confide potentially embarrassing or distressing information to therapists. When are therapists obliged to keep it secret, and when must they tell others? Thomas G. Gutheil, MD, co-director of the Program in Psychiatry and Law at the Massachusetts Mental Health Center and Associate Professor of Psychiatry at the Harvard Medical School sheds some light on this question.

Confidentiality is the clinician's obligation not to divulge information to third parties without the patient's permission. (It is distinct from privilege, the right of the patient to prohibit testimony in court about information shared with professionals.) Confidentiality has clinical, ethical, and legal dimensions. Clinically, no patient can be expected to convey the information needed to conduct psychiatric evaluation and treatment without assurances that it will be kept confidential. From an ethical point of view, the right to privacy

demands respect for patients' confidences. Legally, breach of confidentiality is a deviation from the standard of care imposed on all clinicians; it is the third most common basis for lawsuits recorded by the American Psychiatric Association's Malpractice Insurance Trust.

Circle of Confidentiality

The 'circle of confidentiality' within which information about a patient may properly be shared without permission includes supervisors who are in the chain of clinical responsibility, as well as nurses, aides, social workers, and other members of the treatment team from whom secrets should rarely be kept. Certain consultants (for example, a gynecological consultant for a hospitalized psychiatric patient) are also inside the circle, assuming that the patient has given permission for the consultation.

To transmit information outside the circle a release from the patient—

government agencies, the nurse may feel an obligation to another party—herself. How she behaves, and whom she treats as her primary or most important client, may affect her own well-being, including future referrals, continued employment, or criminal prosecution for nonreporting.

There are two central ethical issues in double-agent situations. The first involves confidentiality (see above), and the second involves deception. The nurse who invites a mother to discuss her personal history, which may trigger a report of suspected child abuse, is concealing her mixed motives in exploring such issues.

While one motive may include genuine concern for the well-being of the mother, the hidden one is not just concern for the child, but a conscious intent to call in the authorities if the history obtained crosses a certain threshold. Since the possible consequences for the abusive parent include criminal prosecution, the moral principles which require police officers to give "Miranda" warnings to suspects who may incriminate themselves would also seem to re-

quire mental health professionals to give such warnings to abuse suspects.*

But it is precisely because such warnings would suppress the information which the nurse seeks that she conceals her intent. The nurse, unlike the police officer, has no legal duty to give such warnings, and may feel deception is justified on the moral grounds that the parent's disclosures may be the only persuasive evidence that will provoke an investigation.

Nurses confronted with double-agent dilemmas have the following options:

1. They can avoid them, either by getting out of clinical nursing, or avoiding jobs in which such situations are likely to arise.

2. They can issue the moral equivalent of Miranda warnings to clients. In some settings, this could result

*Under the "Miranda Rule," the U.S. Supreme Court requires police officers to warn suspects of their constitutional rights, including the right to remain silent, since voluntary statements could be used against them in a criminal proceeding.

preferably written but in certain circumstances oral—is normally required. (If the patient is incompetent, a guardian or other substitute must consent to the release). The patient's family and attorney are outside the circle. So are previous therapists and the outside therapist of a hospitalized patient. Of course, it is almost always better to share all information with this therapist; the clinician should make a patient's refusal to do so a major issue in treatment. Minors have no separate right to confidentiality, but the clinician may want to make it part of the agreement before undertaking therapy, especially with adolescents.

The police are also outside the circle; a psychiatric hospital or other mental health institution may not give them information without the patient's permission. An appropriate response to police requests is of the following type: "We cannot tell you whether Mr. X is a patient here, but we can make inquiries, and if there is someone here by that name, we will encourage him to get in touch with you to discuss the matter."

All clinicians should be aware of some exceptions to the rule of confidentiality. Reporting to state agencies is often mandatory for communicable diseases and child abuse. Confidentiality can be breached in certain emergencies, including (in many but not all states) involuntary commitment to a mental hospital. In some jurisdictions confidentiality must be breached to protect a third party endangered by the patient. Information can be transmitted to satisfy insurance requirements when the patient has implicitly agreed to this as part of the insurance contract. A judicial order may also require a breach of confidentiality.

Patients Can Inform

Clinicians too often fail to make good use of the fact that patients can legally tell anyone anything about themselves. Whenever the requirements of confidentiality are unclear, I recommend that the patient do the informing. For example, the patient may be the best person to pass on information to outside clinicians or warn third parties of danger.

In any case, patients should be allowed to read or hear every communication about themselves that leaves the circle of confidentiality. This strengthens the therapeutic alliance by showing the clinician's respect for the patient, and also provides a useful opportunity for discussion and dialogue.

Reprinted with permission from *The Harvard Medical School Mental Health Letter.* (1988). Vol. 4 (9) February p. 8.

in harm, as with abused children, who will either remain undetected due to parental silence, or who will be inadequately supervised by social services, due to the state's inability to prove abuse because of the lack of information from a suspected parent. Further, emotionally troubled adults may be less likely to seek help for impulse control if they are warned that the therapist has duties to other parties which may require disclosure of confidential information.

3. They can, in settings where there is little risk of physical harm, conclude that the duty to the patient warrants either a pledge not to reveal potentially stigmatizing information to third parties, or at least to disclose conflicts of interest prior to establishing a therapeutic relationship (Halleck, 1971).

4. They can act on their perceived primary duties, and then explain, apologize, or justify their double agentry to the aggrieved party afterwards.

5. They can maintain the deception according to their personal ethical analysis, justifying it to themselves. The general principles that might warrant maintaining such a deception include: a high risk of serious physical harm occuring to an innocent person; a reasonable likelihood of benefit, that is, preventing such harm, if the nurse acts as a double agent; and lack of alternatives.

BEHAVIOR CONTROL

All humans, from infancy to senility, attempt to affect or control the behavior of others. No serious ethical issues arise when competent adults control each other's behavior through a written contract, or when a parent rewards a child for work well done. At the other extreme, though, state-ordered psychosurgery for the purpose of controlling political dissidents, or the use of electroconvulsive therapy on involuntarily committed patients raises a variety of ethical concerns. Because the concept of "behavior control" encompasses such an enormous range of human interactions, from a crying baby to assassination, and such a wide range of techniques, from praise to violence, it is difficult to develop general guidelines for ethically acceptable behavior (Macklin, 1981). Still, the following variables are relevant to the ethical acceptability of efforts and techniques to control a patient's behavior in a health-care setting.

COMPETENCE AND CONSENT

Consent may not be a sufficient justification for controlling the behavior of a competent patient, but it is a necessary one. Just as patients have a nearly absolute right to determine what shall be done to their bodies in a physical sense, the patient's interest in autonomy entitles him to determine how his behavior will be manipulated by a health-care professional.

Rose: An Anorexic Denied Visitors Because of Weight Loss

Rose, a 20-year-old woman, was admitted to an eating disorders unit in a general hospital for treatment of severe anorexia nervosa. After a few days of additional weight loss, she was confined to her room and told she could have visitors only if she achieved a specified weight gain.

Assuming Rose's admission in the case study is voluntary, the proposed treatment plan should be discussed with Rose in detail prior to treatment, and, ideally, presented in writing. If there is no plan to have her detained involuntarily, she should be told that, as with any treatment, she is free to withdraw at any time. The treating team could permissibly state, however, that they do not believe the admission will be of likely benefit unless Rose consents to relinquishing considerable control to the treatment team as long as she is in the hospital, i.e., that daily decisions regarding her treatment will not be negotiable.

If a patient is incompetent, whether adult or child, temporarily or permanently, the usual rules for proxy decision making would apply (see Competence on page 1001 and Chapter 27 on legal considerations). When a patient is in an institutional setting involuntarily, treatment programs warrant especially careful consideration. Such patients have double vulnerability, due to their presumed incompetence, and the added risk of being under the control of a powerful institution whose interests may conflict with the patient's, and whose personnel may have no prior relationship of trust and caring.

RISK AND REVERSIBILITY OF THE TECHNIQUE

Clearly, behavior-modification techniques that have no apparent risk—such as education—are less troubling than those which present serious risks. The degree of risk is usually related to the degree to which physical intrusion is involved, so that verbal interactions are generally less problematic than the use of drugs. Direct physical manipulation of the brain, as with electroconvulsive therapy or psychosurgery, is most troublesome of all (Valenstein, 1978; 1980).

Sometimes the categories of risk merge, as in the case of threats to use physical force if the patient does not comply with a mild therapy. Patients may often believe that such force will be imposed, even though the doctor has not made an explicit threat (Breggin, 1964). Similarly, while education appears to have no apparent risk, it can have powerful and irreversible effects if the patient is particularly vulnerable or dependent on the educator, as occurs in "brainwashing" of prisoners or cult members in isolated surroundings.

The risk involved in physical manipulation of the brain is of particular ethical concern because the treatment may interfere with or permanently change the person himself, or that part of the person which is capable of future autonomy. If the purpose of

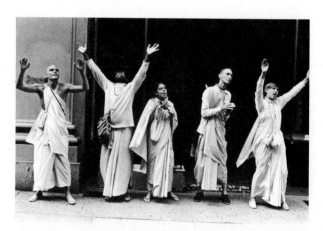

Behavior modification is easy to do, and can be done by most psychiatric practitioners, from social workers to medical directors of psychiatric units. Just because it *can* be done, however, doesn't mean it *should* be done. Is it therapeutic for the patient? Sometimes behavior is modified because of the needs of parents, teachers, or peers. This leads to the patient's feeling loss of control and an increased sense of the need to please others.

treatment is to benefit the patient as a whole person, and not just as a collection of behavior and affect, then treatment which destroys part of that person may undermine its ultimate purpose. Treatment which causes somatic injury, such as hitting, is also of ethical concern, since avoiding harm to others is a fundamental moral obligation, but such injuries do not have the added insult of causing damage to the structures which define the personality.

PRESENCE OF ORGANIC DISEASE

Even risky and irreversible direct intrusions on the brain may be justified when there is a clear organic explanation, such as a brain tumor, for the patient's disability. While brain manipulation or psychosurgery is undoubtedly helpful for some patients with psychiatric disorders whose etiology is unknown, its use in such circumstances is accompanied by concerns that the patient may not have any disease at all, and that the motive for treatment is conflicted with a quest for social control of deviant behavior. The treatment of a patient with a brain tumor and aggressive behavior may also be the result of conflicting motives, but the number of citizens at risk for such interventions is relatively small, making it difficult to support the argument that social control is the sole reason for the therapy.

EXPERIMENTAL TREATMENT

Experimental treatment raises a host of ethical problems in any setting, not just those involving psychiatric patients. The central issue is the conflict of interest the clinician/investigator may have, between the present patient on the one hand, and future possible patients or societal interests on the other. In addition, the benefits and risks of experimental treatment are, by definition, unclear, and the patient is therefore less able to make a rational choice.

This distinction should not obscure the unproven nature of much standard therapy. In many instances a patient's interests may be better served by participating in an experimental study, given the tighter regulation of research, the greater regulatory requirements for extensive disclosure, and the probability that the patient will be monitored more carefully then in standard therapy. Conversely, regulations allow a clinician to use almost any untested and dangerous treatment under the category of "innovative therapy," without the procedural safeguards of institutional review and written consent requirements. The moral obligation to disclose the uncertain nature of benefits and risks would be the same in all treatments, whether experimental or standard.

DENIAL OF BASIC RIGHTS

Even free and uncoerced consent may not be a sufficient reason for embarking on a behavior-modification program, particularly in an institutional setting. For example, manic-depressive patients, while asymptomatic and competent, are not legally allowed to sign away their future liberty by agreeing to future involuntary commitment during a manic phase (Ulysses contract), for the purpose of protecting themselves from psychosocial harm. (Howell, Wikler, & Diamond, 1982). The reason for this is that liberty is considered so valuable, and the risk of coercion by physicians and others so high, that a judgment has been collectively made that, in the long run, the interests of such patients, and society in general, will be better served by not allowing patients to sign away their liberty (Dresser, 1982).

Patients agreeing to behavior-modification programs which entail denial of certain privileges, such as watching television or having visitors, should probably not be allowed to enter into contracts which involve deprivation of food, clothing, or basic privacy needs since such denials of basic human needs may be suspect of being entered under coercive circumstances.

USE OF POSITIVE REWARDS RATHER THAN AVERSIVE STIMULI

A behavior-modification program which offers the patient a chance to be better off, by "winning" benefits beyond basic needs, is preferable to one which threatens him with the risk of being worse off, through the use of painful or other aversive events. This derives partly from the ethical obligation to do no harm, and partly from the duty to avoid coercion, which can be defined as a threat of physical force, or of making a person worse off than he otherwise would be. For example, it would be preferable for a nurse to admit a patient to a room without television, and offer a set in exchange for behavior conforming to expectations than to threaten to take away an existing television set if the patient did not conform. While this distinction might be so subtle as to be meaningless, it becomes clearer if one considers the alternatives of electroshock and candy as incentives for inducing behavior change in a recalcitrant child. The former might be more effective, and even justified for serious refractory disorders, such as those characterized by self-abuse, but would, in general, be less desirable than a program that used positive rewards.

For example, in an experiment, a clinician/investigator used electroshock to induce autistic children to exhibit social behaviors such as hugging (Lovaas, Schaeffer, & Simmons, 1965). This program evoked controversy because: 1) it used very painful stimuli; 2) the subjects were not able to consent; 3) there were unverifiable assumptions about the meaning of the behavior change (it was interpreted as "affectionate" by the observers); 4) there was controversy and ignorance about the cause of the patients' underlying abnormal behavior; and 5) there was ambiguity about whether the behavior change was primarily benefitting the staff or the patients. The investigator defended the technique as being a last resort, since all other conventional and less intrusive therapies failed, and the only other alternative was institutionalization.

SUICIDE

The fundamental ethical question about suicide is whether an individual is morally justified in willfully taking his own life. For the purposes of this book, however, the central questions involve the nurse's duty when confronted with such patients, either to intervene to prevent a possible death, or to assist the patient. For a discussion on the former question, the ethical issues in committing suicide, the reader is referred elsewhere (Brandt, 1975; Battin & Maris, 1983). Before addressing the nurse's responsibility to intervene, some comments about the definition of suicide are necessary.

DEFINITION

There is little doubt that the term suicide—literally "self-killing"—is appropriate when a person actively takes his own life, as by poison, hanging, or gunfire. There is controversy, however, about the use of the term for the more common situation in hospitals, involving the patient who intends to end his life by passive means, such as refusal of life-sustaining medical care.

The overwhelming majority of Americans die in hospitals, and most of these deaths are planned, in the sense that conscious decisions are made by patients and staff to withhold or withdraw life-sustaining treatments, such as resuscitation, mechanical ventilation, or transfusion. Ideally, when competent

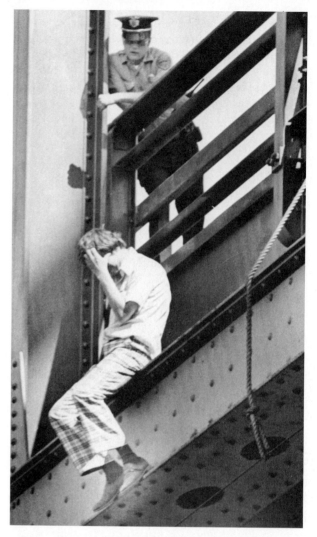

Is it possible to save every potentially suicidal individual? No. Some make mistakes and die rather than hold back and stay safe. They would hate themselves for that. Others choose death and are smart enough to make it happen—even in a locked high-security wing of a hospital or mental institution.

patients are involved, these decisions are made by the patient, in consultation and agreement with the doctor, family, and other health-care providers. Traditionally, these planned deaths have not been considered suicides.

The case of Elizabeth Bouvia (Annas, 1984) challenged this tradition. Ms. Bouvia was a competent adult, suffering from quadriparesis due to progressive neurologic disease. She had lost her husband, a pregnancy, and her job and perceived her future as bleak. She was being kept alive involuntarily by nasogastric feedings and petitioned a court to have the feedings stopped. She claimed the long-established right of a person to control her own body, and argued that refusal of medically administered nutrition was not qualitatively different from administration of other necessities of life, such as blood through intravenous tubing, or air through the tubing of a mechanical ventilator. The courts initially labeled her wish as suicidal, and prohibited the healthcare workers from assisting her. This decision was later overturned on the grounds that there were not morally relevant distinctions between the many medical treatments that keep patients alive and she was allowed to refuse nasogastric feeding.

Others have tried to make distinctions in what is considered suicide on the basis of whether a patient is "terminally ill," so that patients who are not terminal could be considered suicidal if they refuse standard life-sustaining treatment. This runs counter to the legal tradition of allowing patients who are clearly not terminally ill to refuse standard treatments, such as a Jehovah's Witness patient refusing a transfusion. The ambiguity of the phrase "terminally ill" has defied attempts to clarify it in statutory terms, recognizing that definite suicide victims differ from others not in the wish to die, but in the wish to die sooner rather than later.

Even patients who request assistance to end their lives through active means, such as the taking of sedatives or analgesics, which may hasten death, are not always clearly suicidal in the sense that they intend to end their life or hasten their death by such actions. More commonly, the medication is intended to relieve discomfort or pain, with the realization that death may be a consequence. This is not qualitatively different from the patient who accepts toxic chemotherapy or high-risk surgery, with the realization and acceptance that death may result.

Mental health professionals are sometimes recruited to declare a patient suicidal in an effort to compel treatment. For reasons discussed above, the term suicidal should probably be limited to patients whose primary motive is to end their lives through active means. An alternative would be to label the common practice of refusing life-sustaining treatment, typically at the end of life, as justifiable suicide even though that would be so contrary to the customary use of the word as to distort its conventional meaning. (See Box 28–2.)

SHOULD A NURSE INTERVENE?

A nurse who believes that suicide is always immoral would not necessarily feel compelled to intervene, since it is consistent to believe that while a person is behaving immorally, he should be free to make his own decisions. A common position in the abortion debate, for example, is that it is wrong but should be left as a matter of individual choice. Given the high value placed on autonomy in this country, particularly in decisions about health care, it would be reasonable to start with the position that an individual should be left alone. The question then becomes: what reasons would ethically justify intervening in a suicide attempt? Two general reasons are commonly given: preventing harm to the potential victim and preventing harm to others.

PREVENTING HARM TO THE POTENTIAL VICTIM. In general, it would not be justified to interfere with a person's liberty simply for the purpose of preventing harm from coming to him. The arguments against such a broad concept of paternalism were reviewed earlier, acknowledging that preventing serious physical harm might be justified if certain conditions were met: namely, there was a high likelihood of benefit from interfering; the patient was likely to appreciate the intervention; and the intervener would want to be similarly treated if he were in the patient's position. It is precisely because these conditions are generally met in the case of the attempted suicide that there is broad consensus in favor of intervention.

Another way of formulating this argument is to claim that intervention does not interfere with the patient's autonomy at all, because he doesn't really want to die anyway. Numerous studies support the view that attempted suicide is most commonly "not an attempt to die, but a communication in an effort to improve one's life" (Rubinstein, Moses, & Lidz, 1958), i.e., a call for help. Only about 1 percent of those who attempt suicide die within the first year after an attempt, and 5–15 percent in 15 years. Even though this rate is higher than the mortality rate in the general population, in the absence of other information, such as explicit discussions showing a persistent wish to die, it would be probable that a person attempting suicide did not really want to die.

Some would also claim that it is permissible to intervene when the person attempting suicide is suffering from mental illness, arguing that such a person has not truly chosen to die but has been driven to the act by forces outside of his true self. There are three problems with this position:

1. Mental illness is difficult to define, and/or it may be difficult to determine whether the patient is/was suffering from mental illness at the time of the suicide attempt (Szasz, 1974).

Box 28–2 ● Disclosing HIV Positive Test Results to a Suicidal Male

Report of a Case

The patient is a 45-year-old black male. He admits to using IV drugs up until two years ago but denies recent IV drug use or that he shared needles during the time of his drug use.

This individual had worked as a messenger, but found that he was growing too tired to do the work. He complains of recent weight loss of about ten pounds, but relates this to the increased physical exercise related to his job. He says that he drinks alcohol quite often because "it helps [him] to forget [his] troubles." He denies any support system, saying that he has had trouble with maintaining intimate relationships and that he is estranged from his family. He denies any interest in sexual activity. He lives in a men's shelter and finds this arrangement adequate.

He presents himself to the nurse clinician for HIV testing. The man expresses a desire for testing because of his knowledge about drug use and HIV transmission, his weight loss, and increasing fatigue. He says that if he tests positive, his living arrangements will have to change because he would not feel comfortable at the shelter. A condition for living at the shelter is employment; he feels that if he is HIV positive, he would not be able to work. This misconception is clarified but he still persists in his need to move.

On physical examination, the nurse clinician identifies that the patient has enlarged cervical lymph nodes, thrush, and a skin rash. He is occasionally short of breath, but denies having a cough; he is in no acute distress. The nurse tries to prepare him for the possibility that he is HIV positive, but he says that he is not ready to hear this information. HIV testing is requested and he is instructed to return in three weeks for the results. He also is referred to the social worker because he does not have health insurance and because of his housing situation. He keeps the appointment with the social worker.

He returns in three weeks but the results are not available because of a problem with the Department of Health and the clinic procedures. The nurse clinician explains this problem to him and provides an atmosphere in which he can share his feelings. He says that the prior three weeks have been "hell." He admits to increased alcohol intake, dreaming about being dead, and increased anxiety. He says that if he had received the news that he was HIV positive, he planned to take the train, "find an abandoned building, and inject an overdose of drugs." He adds that he planned to make this trip without any identification, so he would be just another "John Doe." The nurse clinician speaks with him for about one hour, and he seems clear about

---

2. There may be no causal connection between the mental illness and the suicidal act; the patient may have attempted suicide for reasons unrelated to his mental illness.

3. Some mental illnesses may constitute an excellent reason for suicide; namely, severe, unremediable suffering with no prospect of relief.

PREVENTING HARM TO OTHERS. Suicide is often intended to cause distress to others. In addition to emotional injury to survivors, which may be profound and long-lasting, there may be economic hardship and the loss of parenting for dependent children. While it would clearly be desirable to prevent such injuries, the question is whether the nurse's duty to these individuals supercedes her duty to the patient.

In general, the duty to the primary patient takes precedence. A health professional may not breach this duty simply because others would benefit. To do so would violate the implied promise of confidentiality. While it might be desirable to help others, it is not clear that the nurse has any duty to do so. Duty arises out of mutual agreements, or special relationships. If the nurse has no special relationship with

this plan to kill himself if he were HIV positive. He has an appointment with the social worker that afternoon, and the nurse encourages him to keep the appointment. The nurse makes another appointment to discuss results in one week.

The patient returns after lunch to see the social worker, but there is confusion with the appointment and he is sent away.

After he leaves, the nurse clinician consults with the psychiatrist about the case and the best way to approach the patient when he returns for results. The psychiatrist requests more information about the patient regarding history of suicidal attempts or intent and history of depression or other psychiatric illnesses. The history of unstable interpersonal relationships, effective instability, a pattern of manipulative behavior, impulsiveness, inability to sustain consistent work behaviors, and multiple substance abuse suggest the diagnosis of a personality disorder. This opens the possibility of the suicidal threat being part of the pattern of manipulative behavior. The fact that the patient engages in some degree of bargaining and is planning for the future indicates that he has already started the process of adjusting to the possibility that he may be HIV positive. The patient is asking himself if his efforts to improve himself and reintegrate into society are worth the

effort if he has an HIV positive result.

The patient breaks his follow-up appointment. He calls two weeks later to say that he is now ready for "good news." The nurse clinician explains that she is not giving him any news over the phone and makes a subsequent appointment for him the following Tuesday. He says that he is feeling fine and is going for a job interview the following day. The nurse wishes him luck with the interview. The nurse and the social worker, in consultation with the psychiatrist, plan to meet with the patient during his next appointment which he subsequently breaks.

Comment

The ethical dilemma facing the health care providers here is, should the client be told that his HIV test results are positive? By telling him, is the provider giving him the key element to implement his suicide plan? On the other hand, if the results are withheld because of the client's suicide plan, what reason could be given for not revealing expected information? Does an adult have the right to know his test results?

The change between the patient's initial satisfaction with his living arrangement in the shelter and disinterest in sexual activity to his assertion that he was feeling fine and

planning to go to a job interview the next day indicates that the possibility that he might attempt suicide is not as high as it would have seemed at the first interview. He has an alcohol abuse history, no social support, and a suicide plan that he identified after being tested for HIV. He has tested positive HIV. However, in light of the behavior change, his bargaining, and his planning for the future with respect for employment, he should be given his results along with counseling to support him through this difficult period. Depending upon the evaluation at the time he presents for results, the scope of supportive services that he will need can be identified.

It is most helpful to use a multidisciplinary approach when working with a patient such as this man. Through collaboration, the health care providers can discuss the issues presented by the individual and arrive at a plan that is tailored to the patient's needs. The patient still does not know that he is HIV positive. When he chooses to learn his results, he will be given the information that he indicates he has the ability to integrate.

Source: Nokes, K. M., & Cerra, L. (1989). AIDS Patient Care, August, 1989, pp. 6–7.

these strangers, and has not contracted to care for them, there is no apparent source for a duty to protect their welfare. When the suicide is for a serious cause, such as unrelenting and irremediable suffering, it is even less clear why the suffering of the family should take precedence over that of the suicidal patient.

There is at least one circumstance in which the patient's well-being may be secondary to others; namely, when loyalty to the patient will cause death or serious disability to others. It is unlikely that a completed suicide would threaten the lives of others.

The nurse herself is one other person whose life may be seriously affected by a completed suicide and whose welfare should therefore be considered. There may, for example, be legal liability for allowing a patient under supervision to complete a suicide. While a nurse may choose to "go the extra mile" and risk damage to her career by breaking the law, it would not be reasonable to consider her duty to the patient to include law breaking. The nurse's duty to herself, therefore, would constitute one instance of justifiable interference with the patient's right to commit suicide.

SUMMARY

Every interaction between a nurse and her patients raises ethical questions. Questions even surround the definition of disease itself, especially with regard to mental illness, which often has fewer objective criteria than other illnesses.

In contemporary medical ethics, a patient has the right to liberty and autonomy; in other words, a competent person has a right to determine what will be done to his own body. However, *competence* must be defined; and different people define it differently. There are five basic definitions of *competence:* 1) evidencing a choice; 2) making a reasonable choice; 3) making a choice based on rational reasons; 4) having the ability to understand; and 5) proving understanding.

Paternalism also arises as an ethical issue in psychiatric care. Paternalism is interfering with a person's liberty for his own good. Paternalism may be justified only under the following conditions: 1) if there is a high risk of serious physical harm; 2) if there is high probability of benefit from interfering; 3) if the patient is likely to say "thank you" later; and 4) if the nurse would want someone to interfere with her liberty if she were in the patient's situation.

The modern medical concept of informed consent is based on the old Anglo-Saxon principle of battery. Consent serves two purposes: 1) to protect patients from harm and 2) to preserve autonomy. However, the right to autonomy does not include the right to cause harm to others.

Confidentiality is an important part of mental health care. The ethical justifications for confidentiality are twofold: first, fewer people would seek treatment without it; and second, society has an interest in the well-being of its members. On occasion, a nurse may have to break confidentiality, particularly if it is to warn an identified party of a patient's violent intentions (as illustrated by the *Tarasoff* case).

The nurse may have to act as a "double agent" in some cases. For example, she may be caring for more than one person in a family, or may have to answer to a school or government agency regarding the behavior of her patient. The two central ethical issues that arise when the nurse acts in this capacity are confidentiality and deception. As a "double agent," the nurse has several options: 1) she can avoid these situations; 2) she can issue the moral equivalent of Miranda warnings to the patients involved; 3) she can act on her perceived primary duties and justify them to the aggrieved parties later; 4) she can maintain the deception, justifying it only to herself.

In the health-care setting and, often, the school, the nurse will confront issues of behavior control. The relevant variables in this issue are as follows: 1) competence and consent; 2) risk and reversibility of the technique; 3) presence of organic disease; 4) treatment is established and proven; 5) denial of basic rights; and 6) use of positive rewards rather than aversive stimuli.

Finally, one of the most critical situations in which a nurse must face ethical issues involves dealing with the suicidal patient. She may have to decide whether or not to intervene (using the criteria for justified paternalism) and if so, how.

KEY TERMS

autonomy

paternalism

competence

Ulysses contract

confidentiality

double agent

STUDY QUESTIONS

1. Why is it difficult to define the term *disease?* Give two examples of how the concept of disease has been used for political or social control of people.

2. What are the five "definitions" of *competence* as it pertains to mental health care?

3. Under what four conditions is paternalism justified?

4. What is the ethical basis of confidentiality?

5. What are the two central ethical issues that the nurse must face when she is in a "double agent" situation?

REFERENCES

Annas, G. J. (1984). When suicide becomes brutality: The case of Elizabeth Bouvia. *Hastings Center Report, 14,* 20–21, 46.

Battin, M. P., & Maris, R. W. (1983, Winter). Suicide and ethics: *Suicide and Life-Threatening Behavior, 13,* 4.

Beauchamp, T. L. & Childress, J. F. (1979) *Principles of biomedical ethics.* Oxford Press, NY.

Beauchamp, T. L., & Walters, L. (1982). *Contemporary issues in bioethics,* 2nd ed. New York: Wadsworth Pub. Co.

Brandt, R. B. (1975). The morality and rationality of suicide. In S. Perlin (Ed.), *A handbook for the study of suicide.* New York: Oxford.

Breggin, P. (1964). Coercion of voluntary patients in an open hospital. *Arch Gen Psych, 10,* 173–181.

Caplan, A. L. Engelhardt, H. T., & McCartney, J. J. (1981). *Concepts of health and disease: Interdisciplinary perspectives.* Reading MA: Addison-Wesley Pub. Co.

Chodoff, P. (1976, May). The case for involuntary hospitalization of the mentally ill. *Am J Psych, 133,* 496–501.

Cooper, A. E. (1982, July 23). Duty to warn third parties. *JAMA, 248,* 431–432.

Daley, D. W. (1975, July). *Tarasoff* and the duty to warn. *San Diego Law Rev, 12,* 932–951.

Diagnostic and Statistical Manual of Mental Disorder. 2nd ed. (1968). New York: American Psychiatric Association.

Diagnostic and Statistical Manual of Mental Disorder, 3rd ed. (1980). New York: American Psychiatric Association.

Dresser, R. (1982). Ulysses and the psychiatrist: A legal and political analysis of voluntary committment contract. *Harvard Civil Rights and Civil Liberty Law Review, 16,* 777–854.

Engelhardt, H. T. (1974, Summer). The disease of masturbation: values and the concept of disease. *Bull Hist Med, 48,* 234–248.

Fost, N., & Cranford, R. (1985, May 10). Hospital ethics committees: administrative aspects. *J Am Med Assn,* 2687–2692.

Gorovitz, S., Macklin, R., Jameton, A. et al (Eds.) (1983). *Moral problems in medicine.* Englewood Cliffs, N.J.: Prentice-Hall.

Greenburg, D. F. (1974). Involuntary psychiatric commitments to prevent suicide. *NY Univ Law Rev, 49,* 227–245.

Guralnik, D. B. (1979). *Webster's new world dictionary of the American language,* 2nd College Edition. Cleveland, Ohio: World Pub. Co.

Halleck, S. L. (1971). Privacy and social control. In S. L. Halleck, *The politics of therapy.* New York: Jason Aronson, Inc.

Howell T., Wikler, D., & Diamond, R. J. (1982). Is there a case for voluntary commitment? In T. L. Beauchamp, & L. Walters, *Contemporary issues in bioethics.* 2nd ed. New York: Wadsworth Pub. Co.

Hunt, R., & Arras, J. (1977). *Ethical issues in modern medicine.* Palo Alto, CA: Mayfield Pub. Co.

Lovaas, O. I., Schaeffer, B., & Simmons, J. Q. (1965). Building social behavior in autistic children by use of electric shock. *J Exp Res in Personality, 1,* 99–109.

Macklin, R. (1981). *Man, mind and morality: The ethics of behavior control,* Englewood Cliffs, NJ: Prentice-Hall.

Mill, J. S. (1947). *On liberty,* edited by C. V. Shields. New York: Liberal Arts Press.

Rosenhan, D. L. (1973). On being sane in insane places. *Science, 179,* 250–258.

Roth, L. H., Meisel, A., & Lidz, C. W. (1977). Tests of competency to consent to treatment. *Am J Psych, 134,* 279–284.

Rubinstein, J., Moses, N., & Lidz, C. W. (1958). On attempted suicide. *AMA Arch Neur & Psych, 79,* 103.

Schloendorff v. *NY Hospital* (1914). 211 NY 127, 105 NE 92.

Spitzer, R. L. (1975). On pseudoscience in science, logic in remission, and psychiatric diagnosis: A critique of Rosenhan's "On being sane in insane places." *J Abnl Psychol, 84,* 442–452.

Stone, A. A. (1976, December). The Tarasoff decisions: suing psychotherapists to safeguard society. *Harvard Law Rev, 90,* 358–378.

Szasz, T. (1960). The myth of mental illness. *American Psychologist, 15,* 113–118.

Szasz, T. (1963). *Law, liberty and psychiatry: An inquiry into the social uses of mental health practices.* New York: Macmillan.

Szasz, T. (1965). *Psychiatric justice.* New York: Macmillan.

Szasz, T. (1970). *Ideology and insanity.* New York: Doubleday.

Szasz, T. (1974). *The myth of mental illness.* New York: Harper and Row.

Valenstein, E. S. (1978, July). Science fiction fantasy and the brain. *Psychology Today, 12,* 29–31, 37–39.

Valenstein, E. S. (1980). *The psychosurgery debate: Scientific, legal and ethical perspectives.* San Francisco: Freeman.

GLOSSARY OF TERMS

A

Abuse Physical or verbal assault which may include physical and emotional neglect, and forced sexual contact, or sexual contact between adult and child.

Acceptance In the context of death and dying, acceptance is the last of five stages defined by Kübler-Ross. The dying person may come to terms with death, though not with particular happiness, and resolve to make his or her remaining time more meaningful.

Accommodation The cognitive process through which new information causes a reorganization of previously existing cognitive structures. In reference to culture, the recognition of cultural group differences, with no attempt to remove or diminish the differences.

Acculturation The exchange of cultural values and patterns that occurs as a result of first-hand contact between individuals of different cultures (usually a minority group takes on the values of the dominant group).

Acting out Maladaptive behaviors a patient uses to deal with feelings in order to keep them out of conscious awareness.

Active and adaptive responses Responses to crisis that are in the affected person's best interests. By communicating effectively with family members, thoroughly assessing their needs, enlisting other professional services such as a social worker or other nurses and physicians, and offering ongoing support to both the patient and his or her family, the nurse can help guide a patient and family who are in crisis to make such positive responses.

Activity theory A theory founded by Robert Havighurst that posits that older people are similar in their response to the aging process, and that the relationship between the individual and society in old age is little different from that during the younger, more productive years of life.

Acute confusional states A form of organic brain dysfunction characterized by abrupt onset of disturbances in sleep-wake cycles, psychomotor behaviors, emotional responses, and attention span.

Acute phase In the context of death and dying, as defined by Pattison and Kübler-Ross, the first phase in which the dying person experiences immobilization and bewilderment as he or she prepares for death.

Acute organic brain syndrome Impaired functioning of brain tissue due to metabolic, traumatic, neoplastic, vascular, hematologic, hypoxic, endocrine, or toxic events such as drug reactions or withdrawal from alcohol.

Administrative law A form of law that deals with disputes between a federal and/or state governmental administrative agency and a person, corporation and/or other business entity on a specific social concern, such as professional licensing, industry, environment, or taxation.

Administrative rules Decisions made by courts or governmental agencies, that are designed to regulate human conduct and are subject to change in a continuing process of societal growth and modification.

Advocacy Support or defense of the patient and his or her rights. This may involve demanding better measures of symptom management, requesting respite from troublesome treatments, and consulting with other members of the health-care team.

Affective display The communication of feelings or emotions through body language.

Age-stratification theory A theory that conceptualizes society as comprising strata based on age and explains why societies respond as they do to older people. Whereas the elderly are accorded high status in countries such as Japan and India, some Western societies such as the United States tend to shun and devalue the elderly.

Ageism A concept similar to racism, in which society tends to stereotype all older people in negative terms that have little or no basis in reality, such as assuming that all the elderly are bad-tempered and set in their ways.

Aggression Forceful physical or verbal behavior intended (consciously or unconsciously) to injure or destroy.

Agnosia The inability to recognize stimuli through any of the senses typically involved in doing so.

Agoraphobia Literally, "fear of the market place." In psychiatric terms, a frequently incapacitating fear of open spaces, and inability to function independently outside the home.

Alcoholic dementia A poorly understood defined dementia associated with alcohol abuse, probably related to irreversible toxic damage to the cortex, primarily the temporal lobes.

Alcoholics Anonymous (AA) A worldwide organization run by volunteer recovering alcoholics, whose philosophy of alcoholism is summarized by the Twelve Steps and Traditions. The program subscribes to the belief that alcoholism is a disease and insists on the need for abstinence. The process of the program takes place in regular meetings and contacts with other AA members.

Alcoholism A condition of being addicted to alcoholic beverages. The alcoholic cannot control his or her intake of alcohol and feels unable to function without it.

Alexithymia The inability to express or recognize one's emotions.

Altruistic suicide A form of suicide motivated by the rigid obedience to customs or rules of a society, as when a person feels it is nobler to die than to bring shame onto his or her family.

Alzheimer's disease The most prevalent type of senile

dementia. It may be classified as senile dementia, Alzheimer's type (SDAT), or primary degenerative dementia (PDD). A chronic organic mental disorder, Alzheimer's entails loss of previously acquired intellectual abilities, which interferes with an individual's social or occupational function. Symptoms include memory disturbance and impairment of abstract thinking, judgment, and impulse control, which leads to personality change.

Anger In the context of death and dying, anger is the second of five stages defined by Kübler-Ross. The dying person and family members may lash out in anger out of proportion to a statement or situation as they deal with the crisis of approaching death.

Anhedonia The inability to experience pleasure, as seen in a child with persistent depression.

Anomia Loss of the ability to name objects. Individuals may compensate by describing the objects.

Anomic suicide A form of suicide motivated by an abrupt severance or change in the relationship between an individual and his or her society. The death of a friend or spouse or loss of a job could lead to suicidal despondency.

Anorexia nervosa A severe disturbance in one's body image, characterized by deliberate starvation with the intention of becoming as thin as possible.

Anticholingergic side effects Systemic side effects produced either by antipsychotic or anticholinergic medications. These may include peripheral (or autonomic) nervous system reactions such as dry mouth, blurred vision, decreased gastric motility, and drying of bronchial secretions; or CNS reactions such as memory problems, confusion and loss of concentration.

Antipsychotic medications Also called neuroleptics, these drugs control and prevent psychotic symptoms, possibly by regulating excessive dopamine levels in the brain.

Antisocial personality disorder The acting out of personal conflicts as a means of avoiding anxiety and unpleasant feelings. The individual does not assume responsibility for his or her actions and does not trust others.

Anxiety A feeling of apprehension, tension, or uneasiness, often accompanied by autonomic responses such as increased respiration and heart rates in anticipation of danger, the source of which is largely unknown or unrecognized.

Anxiety management training A short-term means of reducing tension by combining relaxation techniques with biofeedback.

Anxiety neurosis Also known as anxiety state, anxiety neurosis consists of two forms: panic disorder and generalized anxiety.

Anxiety state Also called anxiety neurosis, anxiety state consists of two forms: panic disorder and generalized anxiety.

Aphasia Loss of a previously possessed facility of language comprehension or speech that cannot be explained by neurological defects.

Apraxia Loss of a previously possessed ability to carry out purposeful movements in the absence of paralysis.

Assertiveness training A form of therapy that teaches assertive behavior. Through role playing, positive reinforcement, and modeling in a controlled group setting, the individual learns to stand up for his or her rights without violating other people's rights.

Assimilation The end-result of acculturation, in which groups and individuals become absorbed into a dominant group's cultural tradition.

Associative learning Learned behavior paired with a reinforcer (reward) that increases the frequency of the event.

Attachment bond A close emotional relationship formed early in life between a child and primary caregiver, which most theorists consider necessary for normal emotional and psychological development.

Attribution theory Concerned with an individual's attempts to "make sense" of events by assigning responsibility to internal-external, stable-unstable, or global-specific factors.

Autism A developmental disability appearing during the first three years of life. Symptoms include disturbances in physical, social, and language skills; abnormal responses to sensations; and abnormal ways of relating to people, objects, and events.

Auto-immune hypothesis A speculative biochemical theory that suggests that there may be an abundance of antibodies accumulated in the limbic system of the schizophrenic individual.

Automatic reactions An individual's response to and interactions with others, based on previous experience.

Automization of behaviors The principle that the unconscious contains learned and instinctive behaviors that allow a person to function expeditiously, such as driving, playing the piano, dancing, or interpreting the radar screen in an air traffic control tower without making a determined effort to do so.

Autonomy The right of a competent person to determine what shall be done to his or her own body.

Avoidant personality disorder A pervasive pattern of social discomfort, fear of negative evaluation, and timidity in which the individual is easily hurt by criticism, avoids significant interpersonal contact, and exaggerates potential physical dangers and risks.

Awareness The spontaneous sensing of what is going on inside oneself; "getting in touch" with feelings by allowing experience to come into consciousness.

B

Bargaining In the context of death and dying, bargaining is the third of five stages defined by Kübler-Ross. The dying person may feel that he or she can make a deal with God, doctors, or fate for an extension of life, hoping that good behavior, good works, or diligent prayer might postpone death.

Basic therapy Therapy in which therapist works with selected patients in structured, goal-directed sessions as part of an overall treatment program, most frequently within a psychiatric mental health setting over a period of time.

Battered child syndrome Medical diagnosis characterized by multiple traumatic lesions of the bones and soft tissues of young children, often accompanied by subdural hematomas, and willfully inflicted upon the child by an adult. May include mental injury.

Behavioral theory Theory focusing on the relationship between environment and behavior, and the importance of the effect of *conscious* motivation on action (action vs. response). Behavioral theory posits that all behavior, normal and pathological, is learned and reinforced by positive or the removal of negative consequences. A more complex definition has come to include an organism's "readiness" to learn at critical periods of development.

Benign senescent forgetfulness A mild, nonprogressive cognitive dysfunction. Refers to an apparent extended course of the forgetfulness phase of Alzheimer's disease.

Binge eating Rapid consumption of a large amount of food in a discrete period of time.

Biogenic-amine theory A theory that the etiology of major depression is underactivity of nerve cells whose neurotransmitters are the biogenic amines (such as serotonin and norepinephrine).

Biological model Theory used to explain psychopathology (such as depression) that emphasizes physical, biochemical, and neurological causes (in this case, catecholamine deficiency) and methods for treatment.

Biopsychosocial model An integrated approach to understanding human behavior that suggests that all mental and physical illnesses have biological, psychological, and social components.

Blackout A form of amnesia in which a person is unable to recall a period of time during a drinking episode, although he or she experienced no impairment of consciousness or alteration in function at the time.

Blaming An ineffective communication pattern that involves an incongruent double message, with the verbal and nonverbal messages saying different things. The "blamer" disagrees with everything and everyone, seeking to dominate others despite his or her inner feelings of loneliness and failure.

Blood alcohol assay A breath test that measures by mg/percent ratios the level of alcohol in a person's bloodstream. For legal purposes, in many states a level of 0.1 percent is considered evidence of intoxication, while levels of 0.35 percent and greater are considered life-threatening.

Body language Also called *kinesics,* this is communication through facial expressions, gestures and posture, and general body movements.

Borderline personality organization A subgroup of personality disorders in which the individual exhibits a lack of a cohesive and well-integrated sense of self, often becoming overwhelmed by powerful feelings of anger and anxiety.

Brazelton Neonatal Assessment Scale An assessment process developed by T. Berry Brazelton that assesses the newborn's integrative behavioral processes in response to a variety of stimuli.

Breach of duty A deviation from the duty or standard of care owed by the health professional to the patient.

Brief psychodynamic therapy Time-limited therapy that enables patients to "work through" problems by becoming aware of how unconscious assumptions based on earlier events continue to dictate present, unwanted behavior.

Briquet's syndrome Also known as *somatization disorder.* A pattern of multiple somatic complaints involving a variety of physiological systems. Characterized by a complicated history of repeated medical complaints, a wide variety of symptoms such as headaches and fainting spells, and symptoms severe enough to have led to medication or visits to a physician.

Bulimia nervosa A severe disturbance in one's body image, characterized by episodic binging on enormous quantities of food, followed by purging with vomiting, laxatives, and occasionally diuretics.

C

Case management A system of health assessment, planning, service procurement/delivery/coordination, and monitoring, through which multiple service needs of patients are met.

Catastrophic reaction Irritability associated with refusal to answer questions about situations or events that are not recalled, coupled with attempts to physically leave the difficult situation.

Causation The direct result of breach of duty. Causation must be proved by sufficient evidence in order for the health professional to be found guilty of negligence.

Chaotic family A disruptive interactional pattern in which there are extreme violations of the boundaries between parents and children, such as sexual abuse.

Childhood depression Similar to adult depression with "correction" for developmental level. The child may display a markedly diminished interest in almost all activities, fatigue or insomnia, lack of appetite and weight loss or gain, feelings of worthlessness, and recurrent thoughts of death or suicide.

Chronic illness Impairments or deviations from normal that are characterized by permanency, residual disability, nonreversible pathological alterations, and the need for a long period of supervision by specialists.

Chronic mental illness Illness that is characterized by vulnerability to stress, deficits in coping skills and meeting ADL needs, dependency, difficulties in interpersonal relationships, and difficulties in finding or maintaining a job. May involve progressive deterioration, especially without professional intervention.

Chronic phase As defined by Pattison and Kübler-Ross, the second phase of dying in which the dying person experiences fears of the unknown, loneliness, and loss of family and friends.

Civil law A form of law that deals with private disputes between private persons, business entities, or sometimes a government entity. A suit alleging nursing malpractice is a civil lawsuit.

Classical conditioning Learning that occurs through pairing a conditioned stimulus, such as a loud noise, with an unconditioned stimulus, such as a small toy. The result is likely to be fear of the toy when presented alone.

Classical psychoanalysis Open-ended therapy that aims at helping patients discover their unconscious motivations for maladaptive behavior through reenactment of old conflicts with important individuals in their life.

Clear sensorium Mental clarity, unimpaired consciousness.

Clouded sensorium Impairment of mental clarity associated with delirium. The individual appears confused or bewildered, may have difficulty with concentration or attention, and is not oriented to time, place, and situation. Misperceptions of stimuli may be manifested as hallucinations.

Coding Expressing the meaning of a message in words or nonverbal language.

Cognitive functions The intellectual functions of memory and language, carried out by the cerebral cortex.

Cognitive restructuring A treatment based on cognitive therapy, in which the therapist encourages the depressed person to identify his or her errors in thinking, to associate these errors with depressed feelings, and to replace these errors with self-enhancing thoughts.

Cognitive theory Psychosocial theory of human behavior that examines the internal changes and mental operations people use to process information.

Cohesive personality A realistic sense of self, which integrates both desirable and undesirable aspects.

Common law Decisions made by courts or governmental agencies, that are designed to regulate human conduct, and are subject to change in a continuing process of societal growth and modification.

Competence The ability of the patient to understand intellectually a proposed treatment, likely benefits and risks, and alternative treatments, as well as the risks of refusing treatment.

Computed tomography (CT) A diagnostic procedure that involves scanning the brain in close detail.

Computing An ineffective communication pattern that involves an incongruent double message, with the verbal and nonverbal messages saying different things. The "computer" appears calm, cool and logical at all times, concealing feelings of vulnerability and need.

Conduct disorder A disturbance of conduct lasting at least six months, during which behaviors such as running away, deliberately destroying others' property, and using physical force on others may be present.

Confabulation Spontaneous and unconscious fabrication of stories in response to questions about experiences that cannot be recalled, in order to hide memory loss.

Confidentiality A concept based on the Latin root of the word *fidele,* meaning "trust." A patient discloses personal information with the implicit trust that the doctor or nurse will not reveal it to others.

Confrontation A special therapeutic technique that changes a patient's cognitive distortions into representations of reality while allowing the patient to maintain his personal integrity. By remarking that some people have to lose everything before they realize they are alcoholics, a therapist can help an alcoholic relinquish denial that he has a problem, and become aware of his need for treatment.

Confused thinking and social withdrawal A subgroup of personality disorders in which an individual is isolated emotionally from other people and may display strange behavior that reinforces the isolation.

Confusional phase The second phase of Alzheimer's disease, in which the patient becomes increasingly dysfunctional. Memory loss, problems with orientation in familiar environments, and difficulty with speech become evident.

Congruent Refers to the ideal matching of feelings and awareness with behavior that is consistent, based on an individual's experiences. When infants are hungry, they will usually express *congruent* behavior by crying to be fed.

Conjoint therapy Individual therapy in a couple or family format. Individual issues, as well as those affecting the relationship, are identified and worked through.

Containment A concept of therapy used with rape victims that consists of providing a safe and noncritical environment for the expression of feelings. Containing behaviors include empathy, willingness to address painful information, and educating family members about the nature of the rape crisis to enable them to be truly supportive of the victim.

Contingency management A means of reinforcing desired behavior by rewording it.

Continuity theory A theory that emphasizes the uniqueness of the individual's response to the aging process, which is based on the complex interplay between biological, psychological, and social characteristics and experiences that result in certain habits, preferences, and activities that remain relatively stable over time.

Continuous amnesia The failure to recall events during a specific time period through the present.

Conversion disorder The conversion of emotional distress or unconscious conflict into a physical symptom, such as paralysis of the hands in place of experiencing underlying helplessness.

Coprolalia Uncontrolled swearing and uttering of obscenities, a symptom of Tourette syndrome.

Counselor An aspect of the nurse's role that involves providing verbal guidance and support in crises as well as long-term care.

Countertransference Conscious or unconscious feelings that a therapist develops towards a patient, such as special concern, sexual attraction, anger, or resentment. Such feelings, if not recognized, can lead to a distorted view of the patient.

Cranial nerves The twelve nerves that emerge from the central nervous system within the brain: olfactory, optic, oculomotor, trochlear, trigeminal, abducent, facial, acoustic, glossopharyngeal, vagus, accessory, and hypoglossal.

Craving The feeling an addict has when he or she is in proximity to a drug or alcoholic drink, particularly in the context of previous use. Craving revolves around environmental cues associated with the pleasurable emotions and relief from tension previously evoked by the drug.

Criminal law A form of law that deals with disputes between the federal and/or state government, on behalf of United States residents, against persons or entities (such as corporations) accused of committing crimes. Criminal penalties typically involve punishment, i.e., loss of freedom and/or monetary fine.

Crisis intervention A brief, active, and collaborative therapy that utilizes the individual's own coping abilities and resources within the family, health care setting, and community.

Cultural subordinates A subgroup of people who experience powerlessness and have internalized the attributes of inferiority assigned to them by the dominant culture in which they live.

Culturally sensitive An understanding and awareness of the historic, economic, social, political, and cultural factors associated with individual and institutional racism.

Cyclothymic disorder A mild form of bipolar disorder, characterized by shorter and more manageable duration of symptoms of mood disturbance.

D

Damages Physical, emotional and/or financial injury that must be proved in order for the plaintiff to be awarded monetary compensation.

Data deficits Gaps in information that result from people's tendencies to generalize from specific past experience to all experience.

Defense mechanisms Unconscious intrapsychic processes used to maintain the individual's feelings of adequacy and avoid conscious or unconscious conflict and anxiety.

Those include denial, rationalization, and sublimation, among others.

Dehumanization of victims The viewing of victims as nonhuman objects, in order to be able to commit a violent act against them.

Deinstitutionalization A mental health movement begun in the early 1960s and based on the principle that patients can receive more humane and therapeutic care in the community than in mental hospitals.

Delirium Impaired functioning of brain tissue due to metabolic, traumatic, neoplastic, vascular, hematologic, hypoxic, endocrine, or toxic events such as drug reactions or withdrawal from alcohol.

Delusions Unfounded beliefs that are held to be true, even in the face of contradictory evidence.

Dementia phase The third, late phase of Alzheimer's disease, in which the patient's dysfunction is obvious even to the casual observer. He or she requires assistance with activities of daily living, and close supervision to prevent wandering or safety hazards such as leaving the stove on.

Dementia Chronic organic mental disorder (irreversible).

Dementia paralytica A rapidly progressive but now rarely seen dementia in the late stage of advanced syphilis, characterized by personality changes (possibly due to frontal lobe involvement), poor hygiene, and grandiose delusions.

Denial An unconscious defense mechanism used to block emotional conflict or allay anxiety so it does not reach conscious awareness. In the context of death and dying, denial is the first of five stages defined by Kübler-Ross. Denial may be a major defense that can help the dying person get through the crisis of dealing with death, but may block open communication with his or her family.

Denver Developmental Screening Test The most commonly used screening instrument in the United States. This test quickly identifies developmental delays in children who can then be referred for more thorough assessment.

Dependence Behaviors, cognitions, and other symptoms that indicate a lack of control of substance use and continued use of the substance despite negative consequences. The dependent (or "addicted") person experiences physiological symptoms of tolerance and withdrawal.

Dependent personality disorder An individual's inability to function without heavy reliance on a forceful or dominant significant other, even when that person is abusive.

Depersonalization A multisensory experience in which the individual's sense of self is altered, and he perceives parts of his body as increased or decreased in size or altered in form. Depersonalization can also involve the experience of being outside of one's own body, serving as a defense mechanism to protect the individual from an emotion, idea, or feeling.

Depot medications Long-acting medications that help control severe psychotic symptoms and are especially useful when maintenance therapy is indicated.

Depression Emotional state characterized by feelings of worthlessness, dejection, loss of hope, and sadness. In the context of death and dying, depression is the fourth of five stages defined by Kübler-Ross. The dying person and family members may experience a sense of great loss and discouragement.

Depressogenic model A theoretical model that describes the etiology and maintenance of depression.

Derealization A perception that the external environment has changed or become unreal. The individual describes perceptions that indicate objects in the environment have changes in size and shape, and may think that others have become unreal.

Desensitization In reference to sex therapy, a step-by-step behavioral program that encourages the nonorgasmic individual to explore and become familiar with areas of the body that are pleasurable, in order to learn what will help him or her achieve orgasm.

Detoxification The process of chemical withdrawal from an abused substance. A substitute substance is given to the patient in order to prevent the more severe forms of withdrawal, and the patient's condition is monitored regularly.

Developmental models A category of nursing theories (such as Hildegard Peplau's model [1952]) that focus on the process of psychological growth and maturation.

Diathesis-stress concept A biomedical model of psychosomatic illness that incorporates a diathesis (a weakness or physical predisposition) with stress as a trigger of illness.

Direct-liability Refers to a health professional's responsibility for her own acts.

Discrimination Overt and unfavorable action that results in unfavorable and disenfranchising treatment against a group or individual because of race, ethnicity, or religion, depriving people of economic, political, and/or social opportunities.

Disengagement theory A theory that states that aging entails an inevitable withdrawal of the individual from society, and of society from the individual, in later years of life.

Dissociation A defense mechanism that operates unconsciously to separate and detach emotional significance from an idea or experience. In dissociative disorders, the individual may experience an altered state of consciousness, reduced or increased sensory input, relaxation of critical mental faculties, and changes in body chemistry such as hypoglycemia, dehydration, seizures, and severe headaches.

Dissociative disorders A group of five psychiatric disorders in which there is a disturbance in identity, memory, and consciousness.

Distracting An ineffective communication pattern that involves an incongruent double message, with the verbal and nonverbal messages saying different things. The "distractor" attempts to cover feelings of uncertainty with hyperactivity, going in all directions at once and assuming that no one really cares.

Disturbances in communication The inability to communicate about communication, as when individuals deny their communication and develop problems in order to avoid communication.

Disulfiram A drug, used in the treatment of alcoholism, that blocks the breakdown of acetaldehyde in the liver and allows it to accumulate, thus causing a person to have a very unpleasant reaction when attempting to consume alcohol.

Doctrine of informed consent The patient's constitutional right to make informed decisions about his or her medical treatment, based on two theories in law: 1) *neg-*

ligence and 2) *battery*. A physician is legally required to disclose material risks of any treatment to the patient, after which the patient will decide whether to accept or refuse that treatment.

Dogmatic receiver The individual who imposes personal needs, values, and feelings on the communication and/or interprets it in a narrow, stereotypical way.

Dominant goal An unrealistic goal obsessively pursued by an individual who seeks gratification.

Dominant other An influential person to whom the depressed individual turns for his or her sense of self-worth and well-being.

Dopamine hypothesis A theory that behaviors manifested in schizophrenics are specifically related to an excess of dopamine activity in the limbic system.

Double agent A situation in which the nurse has obligations or loyalties to more than one client, and the interests of these clients may conflict. A typical example of double agentry occurs when health professionals care for more than one person in a family. The nurse must be alert to situations in which this type of "holistic" care may result in an abrogation of duty to some member of the family.

Double-bind theory A theory developed by Bateson et al., describing a situation in which a person receives a nonverbal message that conflicts with a verbal communication. The person receiving these conflicting messages is left unable to respond without experiencing some level of punishment, putting him or her in a "no-win" position.

Drive theory of aggression A motivating force toward death that causes the person to release violent urges in ways that are both self-destructive and destructive of others. Intervention requires a rechanneling of the violent urges toward less destructive means.

Dyspareunia Painful coitus that may be due to infection, tumors, certain types of contraceptive devices, or sexual inhibitions.

Dysphoria Unhappiness as a result of a low rate of positive reinforcement with little or no rewards or satisfactions.

Dysthymic disorder Also called "depressive neurosis." Depressive reaction, e.g., due to a chronic unconscious conflict or to an identifiable event such as loss of a loved person or cherished possession.

E

Ego One of the three major divisions in the psychoanalytic model of the psychic apparatus, the others being the *id* and the *superego*. The ego represents the sum of certain mental mechanisms, such as perception and memory, and specific *defense mechanisms*. It mediates between the demands of primitive instinctual drives (the id), of internalized parental and social prohibitions (the superego), and of reality.

Ego functions Elements in the ego's part of the psychic apparatus, such as the individual's sense of reality and control of drives, that are responsible for his or her overall adaptation to the environment. Bellak and others believe that these functions exist in all people, and that knowledge about them will help the nurse determine the theory behind various disorders. The twelve ego functions are as follows.

1. *Reality testing*—a sense of self and the world as real.
2. *Judgment*—understanding of the consequences of one's behavior.
3. *Sense of the world and of self*—sense of the world and of one's self as separate.
4. *Regulation*—having control of drives, affects, and emotions, and the ability to delay gratification.
5. *Object relations*—relationships with others; the ability to love and to form attachments.
6. *Thought processes*—ability to conceptualize and use appropriate abstract thinking.
7. *Adaptive regression in service of the ego (ARISE)*—ability to be creative and demonstrate flexibility.
8. *Defensive functioning*—use of defense mechanisms; the extent to which these defensive mechanisms are used flexibly or rigidly and their success or failure. Determines whether they are preserving mental health or illness.
9. *Stimulus barrier*—ability to differentiate between external and internal stimuli.
10. *Autonomous functioning*—ability to function independently.
11. *Mastery competence*—how effectively the person interacts with his or her environment without relying on maladaptive patterns established early in life.
12. *Synthetic integrative functioning*—integration of a variety of ego functions that allows for thinking, learning, and judgment among others.

Ego psychology A theory built on Freud's work, that views a person's ego as being driven by his id (instinct) and by his superego (who the person would like to be.) In ego psychology, depression is considered the result of an intolerable "credibility gap" between a person's superego and ego.

Ego states Roles or moods wherein a person may have different feelings, experiences, and behaviors at different times, depending on the situation. In an individual with a dissociative disorder, his or her behavior in a given situation becomes a separate ego state, i.e., with a complete identity of its own.

Egoistic suicide A form of suicide motivated by an individual's unbearable loneliness and perceived or real isolation from society. Most suicides in the United States belong to this category.

Electroconvulsive therapy (ECT) A form of therapy used to ameliorate a patient's symptoms of severe depression and/or delusional thinking when pharmacological measures have proved ineffective. ECT involves the application of electrical current to the mildly anesthetized patient's brain, resulting in controlled seizures followed by a post-anesthetic period of calm wakefulness.

Electrolyte abnormalities Changes in electrolyte balance that cause a variety of delirious conditions.

Emergency An unforeseen event that requires immediate action. The stress that builds up in an individual as a result of numerous predicaments and emergencies can cause a crisis situation, depending on his or her ability to cope.

Emotional incontinence Extreme instability of mood. Includes excessive emotional reactions to humor, sadness, frustration, etc., accompanied by rapid mood changes.

Empathic listening Listening that conveys genuine concern for the feelings of another through the use of body language.

Empathy The ability to put oneself emotionally in someone else's place and feel what another person feels.

Encephalopathy Acute organic brain disorder.

Enhanced striving A behavior in which a victim strives obsessively towards a goal to compensate for feelings of powerlessness, such as the anorexic patient's fierce perfectionism and overriding need to control her eating.

Enmeshment An interactional pattern characteristic of some families with anorexic children, in which there is a lack of clear boundaries between the subsystems. Although a facade of harmony is maintained, problems are deflected onto the child and the family becomes locked into a rigid, unchanging pattern of behavior.

Environmental intervention A means of reversing the delirium experienced by patients in intensive care units by changing aspects of the patient's daily treatment routine. The visually stimulating bright lights and lack of day-and-night orientation, the management of other patients in crisis (code resuscitation), complicated machinery, and constant coming and going of staff and family members can cause a patient to become uncontrollably agitated. Environmental intervention can include moving the patient to a dark room, using soft lights, and limiting the number of staff members involved.

Esteem support Feedback from others that a person is valued and accepted.

Excitement phase The first phase of the sexual response cycle identified by Masters and Johnson. Males experience penile erection and an increase in pulse, respirations, and blood pressure. Females experience breast enlargement and nipple erection as well as increased pulse, respirations, and blood pressure.

Exhibitionism The act of obtaining sexual gratification from publicly exposing the genitals to others.

Experimental neurosis A specific type of learned helplessness, in which the patient develops cognitive, affective, and somatic disturbances due to exposure to unpredictable and uncontrollable aversive events, such as painful burn treatments. Symptoms include agitation followed by lethargy and depression, feeding disturbances, decreased ability to learn new associations between responses and outcomes, and chronic anxiety.

Expressed emotions (EE) Emotions expressed by the schizophrenic individual's family members that can have a profound effect on the ill person's ability to succeed outside the hospital milieu.

Extensional level of abstraction The concrete or non-verbal experience of the object a symbol stands for.

Extinction-trial behavior A frustratingly repetitive behavior in a depressed individual that eventually alienates those around him or her.

Extrapyrimidal side effects Parkinsonian central nervous system reactions caused by the administration of high-potency antipsychotic medications.

Extraversion Direction of interest toward external events and objects rather than the self and ideas (opposite of *introverson*).

Extropunitive Victim behavior that is directed outward toward others, such as competitiveness and the excessive need to control others.

F

Factitious disorder with physical symptoms (see Munchausen syndrome)

Family phobia systems Hidden fears that may exist in each family. These may be covered over by symptoms displayed by one family member as a response to life crises.

Family system The complex patterns of interaction between family members, and their influence on how an individual perceives himself or herself.

Family systems theory A theory that views a person within the context of his or her family as a whole. The family is viewed as having a structural hierarchy consisting of parents as executive subsystem and children as sibling subsystem, with a clearly defined boundary between the two. Conflicts between the parents are ideally resolved within their subsystem. If the boundaries between the two subsystems become blurred, neuroses may occur in either group.

Family therapy A form of interpersonal therapy focusing on relationships within the family.

Feedback The selective *positive* or *negative* response to one or more aspects of a message.

Female sexual arousal disorder Persistent, partial, or complete failure to attain or maintain the lubrication-swelling response of sexual excitement until completion of the sexual activity.

Fetishism An individual's recurrent and intense sexual arousal to an inanimate object, such as clothing, or to body parts, such as feet, that are neither primary nor secondary sexual organs.

Folk medicine The traditional healing arts of a particular cultural group that are used to treat its members as a defense against the hostility of the world at large. This may include witchcraft, belief in supernatural healing, rituals, and traditional medicines.

Forgetfulness phase The first phase of Alzheimer's disease, in which the patient remains functional while forgetting names and specific details about daily experiences. During this phase, he or she will often be aware of his or her memory difficulty.

Fragmentation A pathological defense mechanism in which the individual is unable to perceive himself and others as whole people, only as discrete characteristics such as physical traits, roles, and judgments.

Frontal symptoms Symptoms related to dysfunction of the frontal lobes of the brain. Affected frontal lobe functions may include judgment, reasoning, social sense, personal hygiene, motivation, emotional regulation, and bowel or bladder control. These symptoms may be difficult to differentiate from functional psychiatric illnesses such as depression or personality disorders.

Frotteurism Sexual behavior in which gratification is achieved by rubbing or pressing against women, usually in public places.

Frustration-aggression theory A theory proposed by behaviorists Dollard, Miller, and others that conceptualizes a reservoir of aggressive energy seeking a violent outlet if goal-directed behavior is blocked or interrupted.

Fully functioning person One who is open to experience and has the psychological freedom to be himself or herself in this world, and is therefore perceived as open, honest, genuine, and worthy of trust.

G

Gender identity disorder The psychological disequilibrium associated with an incongruence between biological sex assignment and subjectively experienced gender.

General adaptation syndrome A theory that postulates that there is a general stress reaction that is similar for all individuals, and that the same series of physiological events is produced whenever an individual is stressed.

Generalized amnesia The failure to recall events associated with the individual's entire life. The occurrence of this is relatively rare.

Generalized anxiety disorder Disorder in which a person experiences diffuse feelings of apprehension and physiological symptoms, including motor tension, autonomic hyperactivity, apprehension, and vigilance.

Geriatric mental health A specialized field of research inquiry and clinical practice that examines the biological, socioeconomic, and psychological needs of the elderly, based on an expanded knowledge of older people and the aging process.

Graded exposure A means of treating a phobic individual by gradually exposing him or her to that which produces anxiety and fear.

Guided fantasy A technique that asks the patient to provide a narrative about an imagined exposure to the object of his or her phobia, and with the guidance of the therapist, gradually imagines overcoming fear of the object.

H

Habituation A decrease in strength of response when a stimulus is presented repeatedly (see *nonassociative learning*).

Hallucinations A sensory perception in the absence of an actual external stimulus. May occur in any of the senses.

Healthy role model An example of good mental health set by the nurse in order to help patients learn healthy ways of responding to conflicts. By demonstrating a positive, realistic attitude, maintaining a professional physical appearance, and responding to stress and fatigue in a mature manner, the nurse becomes a model of mental health for others.

Hepatic encephalopathy A cause of delirium progressing to coma, most commonly seen in alcoholics with severe liver disease.

High-potency medications One of two classifications of neuroleptics. The high-potency medications are used to prevent the unpredictable exacerbation of psychotic symptoms, but produce significant CNS side effects such as tremors, shuffling gait, motor retardation, and drooling.

Histrionic personality disorder A pervasive pattern of excessive emotionality and attention-seeking that begins in early adulthood and includes extreme self-centeredness, the constant need for approval, inappropriate seductiveness, and excessive emotion over minor events.

Holistic approach A therapeutic approach in which the nurse cares for a patient's physical and emotional needs, taking into account the "whole person" interacting with his or her environment.

Homelessness A state of poverty into which many deinstitutionalized mentally ill persons can fall, in which they lack an address, stable environment, money, and self-esteem.

Homeostasis The tendency of organisms to maintain equilibrium and resist change. In reference to family functioning, refers to the maintenance of living patterns in a family system form one generation to the next.

Humanistic approach Psychological model stressing the inherent goodness in each individual as well as the potential for maximum growth and fulfillment.

Hypermasculinity An extreme of male behavior, in which strong cultural messages dictate that men be emotionally restricted, possessive, and achievement-oriented, to the exclusion of their own needs.

Hyperthyroidism Thyroid hormone excess, an often overlooked cause of a relatively chronic dementia. Signs of hyperthyroidism include anxiety, heat intolerance, tachycardia, and tremor.

Hypoactive desire disorder Persistent or recurrently deficient or absent sexual fantasies and desire for sexual activity.

Hypochondriasis Complaints of symptoms that cannot be confirmed by medical examination or laboratory procedures.

Hypomania Also called "cyclothymic" disorder. A mild form of bipolar disorder, with less intense mania alternating with depressive episodes.

Hypothyroidism Thyroid hormone deficiency, a commonly overlooked cause of chronic dementia. Signs of hypothyroidism include depression, weight gain, cold intolerance, and skin and hair changes.

I

I-P reflex Automatic and predictable interpersonal reflexes to specific stimuli, similar to a physiological knee-jerk reaction. The I-P reflex is based on established patterns of behavior and previous experiences, as when one person smiles and says "good morning," and the other person usually returns the greeting automatically.

Iatrogenic A pathological condition unwittingly precipitated, aggravated, or induced by the health care providers. Iatrogenic organic brain syndrome in elderly patients with underlying dementias or mild cognitive dysfunctions may be produced by anticholinergic medications, sedatives, and steroids.

Identification That process in which a person modifies his behavior in an effort to design himself after another person, whom he admires, holds in high esteem, and wishes to use as a model for himself.

Incest Sexual relations between family members, usually considered taboo in most societies.

Incongruent Behavior that appears confusing, deceptive, and controlling, due to an individual's unawareness or deliberate suppression of certain feelings.

Incorporation A process in which an idea is not separated or differentiated from an act or deed. The individual indiscriminately takes a part or all of another person or thing and uses its components to gratify and/or upset his own impulses, sensations, feeling, and thoughts.

Indirect (or vicarious) liability Legal responsibility for the acts of someone else, such as a nurse for a student nurse or nursing assistant.

Inertia An object's lack of motion or inability to change direction when moving. A patient experiencing inertia may resist getting up for activities or may have difficulty stopping a task once begun (see *Perseveration*).

Informational support The informational help an individual receives in defining, understanding, and coping with life's difficulties.

Informing In reference to communication theory, the technique of listening and being aware of hidden feelings in a patient's statements or questions. If a patient reveals anxiety when asking a question such as "Could I wake up during my surgery?", the nurse can help the patient deal with that anxiety by responding, "I wonder if you are frightened about anesthesia during your surgery."

Inhibited female orgasm Persistent or recurrent delay in, or absence of, orgasm in a female following a normal sexual excitement phase during sexual activity.

Inhibited male orgasm Persistent or recurrent delay in, or absence of, orgasm in a male following a normal sexual excitement phase during sexual activity.

Inhibition Unconscious restraint of impulse or desire.

Integrative functions Identity, memory, and consciousness.

Intensive care unit A highly specialized hospital unit for patients who are in physical crisis and have poor vital signs caused by trauma, overdose, serious illness, or postoperative complications. Outside of the psychiatric ward, the intensive care unit contains patients with the most psychological problems in the hospital, owing to the high anxiety level and prevalent air of urgency, danger, and impending crisis.

Intentional level of abstraction The verbal level of labeling an object, which can become increasingly generalized and abstract. A woman named Marilyn may be labeled as a cancer patient or, in more abstract terms, as a 56-year-old woman with bowel cancer, a patient, or simply Case Number 221—a label far removed from the real person whom the nurse will encounter.

Interaction models A category of nursing theories (such as King's Conceptual Theory for Nursing) that emphasizes social arts and relationships, focusing on the individual's perceptions of other people, the environment, situations, and events.

Intermittent explosive disorder A disruptive and violent behavior characterized by several discrete episodes of loss of control of aggressive impulses resulting in serious assaultive acts or destruction of property.

Internalization The processes an individual utilizes when transforming real or imaginary interactions that occur in the external environment into inner guidelines, regulations, and self-governance mechanisms.

Internalizing The taking on of an externally imposed value and treating it as one's own.

Interpersonal approach A psychiatric theory that focuses on the relationships, first with parents and later with others, that the child forms during the socialization process.

Interpersonal communication Communication that takes place between two people or in a small group.

Interpersonal or person-centered therapy Therapy that focuses on the patient's interpersonal relationships by examining the feelings experienced in his or her relationship with the therapist.

Intervention When used in association with the treatment of alcoholics, the first phase of some treatment programs that involves assembling the alcoholic's family, friends, coworkers, and significant others, and asking each person to tell the patient what his or her experiences with the patient's drinking have meant to him or her. The patient is protected from being totally overwhelmed by the confrontation and instead is guided toward constructive action, such as seeking counseling or joining Alcoholics Anonymous.

Intrapersonal communication The processing of information internally or "talking to oneself."

Introjection A type of internalization in which objects loved or hated are taken in, becoming part of the self.

Intropunitive Victim behavior that is directed inward toward the self, such as internalizing and personalizing conflicts, resulting in depression.

Introspection Self-observation; examining (and often reporting on) one's feelings.

Introversion Preoccupation with one's inner world of experience and concepts, accompanied by a lack of interest in external events (opposite of *extraversion*.)

In vivo desensitization A treatment method focusing on real-life situations that adheres to the principle that exposure to a feared situation will ultimately result in decreased anxiety. In treating premature ejaculation, for example, the man is encouraged to simply lie with his partner until he feels free of anxiety, and then gradually increase the degree of sexual interaction until a satisfactory amount of stimulation can be sustained prior to ejaculation.

K

Korsakoff's psychosis Psychosis usually associated with chronic alcoholism, characterized by subacute delirium and a marked degree of short-term memory impairment.

L

Labeling or interpreting maladaptive responses The identification of responses by family members that are not in the patient's best long-term interest, such as parents who withdraw emotionally from their terminally ill child. The nurse should gently communicate to the parents the need for changing their behavior, and intervene as needed.

Lacunar infarcts Multiple, small thrombotic strokes, mostly in small vessels. Although usually too small to produce clinical symptomatology when they occur, lacunar infarcts will result in clinical deficits if they accrue over the years, and will be visible on a cranial CT scan.

Language function The ability to comprehend language and express oneself verbally.

Law A rule or method with which phenomena or actions coexist or follow each other.

Learned helplessness Theory developed by Seligman to describe depression that occurs when a person realizes he cannot control the aversive outcome of a situation.

Learned helplessness model of depression Theory that has been used as a rationale for promoting predictability and control of aversive events for patients undergoing painful medical treatments.

Learning theory The theory that forms the foundation of all behavioral treatment and research. Learning theory posits that all behavior is learned directly or indirectly and has biological and survival value. The tension induced by a stressful situation produces a "fight-or-flight" response which includes tachycardia, increased blood pressure, and raised muscle tone. This raises the level of preparedness, alertness, and ability to cope with a fear-producing situation.

Least restrictive means of treatment The treatment to which an involuntarily committed patient is entitled that minimally interferes with the individual's freedom but is still effective.

Lethality The potential risk of successful self-annihilation in a suicidal situation, based on whether the patient's suicide plan is specific, well-thought-out, and easily implemented, or a vague threat based on extreme despondency.

Leveling Congruent communication that "represents a truth of the person at a moment in time," involving a whole response with body, senses, and feelings working together.

Life-review therapy A technique that involves a mental process characterized by a progressive return to past experiences, especially unresolved conflicts. The therapist facilitates the process and helps a person take a positive view of his or her life and self.

Lithium The drug of choice for treating bipolar disorders, lithium is thought to help stabilize the patient's moods by altering the level of enzymes and catecholamines in the central nervous system.

Localized amnesia The failure to recall all events surrounding a specified time period. This is the most common type of amnesia.

Locus of control An individual's perceived control over his or her ability to change or influence a particular health outcome.

Logotherapy A nursing intervention used to facilitate emotional well-being in the dying patient, which involves enhancing the individual's feeling that his life has meaning and purpose.

Low-potency medications One of two classifications of neuroleptics. The low-potency medications are used regularly in low doses to modify psychotic symptoms and facilitate the therapeutic effects of higher doses in the presence of severe psychotic symptoms. Side effects can include dry mouth, urinary retention, and sedation.

M

Major depression A mood disorder characterized by sustained, intense, depressive symptoms.

Male erectile disorder One of two sexual arousal disorders in which the male experiences inability to achieve or maintain an erection well enough, or long enough, for vaginal penetration and until the sexual activity is complete.

Malingering Reporting of false or grossly exaggerated physical symptoms in an attempt to gain some recognizable goal such as avoiding work.

Malpractice insurance Insurance carried by medical care providers that provides financial coverage for them in the event that successful litigation is brought against them. Two main types of malpractice are (1) *claims-based insurance,* which provides coverage for only those claims made during the policy period, and (2) *occurrence-based insurance,* covering alleged negligence that occurs during the policy period, regardless of when the claim is made.

Manager An aspect of the nurse's role that requires maintaining the therapeutic milieu or environment by providing a safe, comfortable, pleasant physical facility and a supportive living environment. The nurse manages the patient's schedule, protects him or her from volatile situations, and oversees the course of treatment.

Mania Mood disorder characterized by a sense of elation or euphoria. Like depression, mania varies in duration, intensity, and frequency.

Masturbation Manual self-stimulation for the purpose of achieving sexual gratification.

Maturational crisis Any event that is related to the normal growth and development process, such as becoming a parent, conflicts during adolescence, and retirement.

Meaning In communication theory, the content of a message, which can be communicated on two levels. On the first level the meaning is *cognitive;* it is the literal content of the words of the message. On the second level the communicators define their relationship by indicating their perceptions of themselves and their listeners. The *affective* or emotional aspect of communication may reinforce or change the literal meaning of a message.

Medicaid A federal-state welfare program designed to provide medical care to the poor of all ages.

Medicare A health insurance program that pays a substantial portion of the costs of hospital and physician services for individuals aged 65 and over, for certain disabled persons under age 65, and for persons with end-stage renal disease.

Medigap Supplemental medical insurance for the aged for services not covered by Medicare.

Medroxyprogesterone acetate (MPA; Depo-provera) A female hormone that causes reversible chemical castration.

Melting pot A metaphor for the blending of different minority groups into the larger dominant group, in which the submerging of cultural differences is encouraged.

Mental maps A person's perception of reality, his map of his world.

Mental-status exam The assessment of an individual's general appearance and behavior, affective range, thought processes, and thought content.

Mentally frail elderly Some elderly over the age of 75, who because of the accumulation of various continuing problems often require one or several supportive services in order to cope with activities of daily living.

Metabolic encephalopathies Mental status changes, most commonly due to organic mental disorders, caused by a number of systemic illnesses, including electrolyte abnormalities, hepatic encephalopathy, thyroid disorders, vitamin deficiencies, iatrogenic causes, or sedative-hypnotic withdrawal syndrome.

Metacommunication The nonverbal aspect of a message, or "communication about the communication," that may have a different impact than the literal words. Metacommunication is conveyed by the communicator's tone of voice and body language.

Metamodel A linguistic tool used to tie language to experience by addressing the ways people limit and distort experience. The nurse can ask such questions as who, what, and how, to draw out specific information and help the patient begin to understand his or her mental map.

Methadone A drug, used in the treatment of narcotics addiction, that prevents withdrawal symptoms and abolishes the craving for narcotics. A drawback to methadone use is the addict's need for daily oral doses, often for life.

Minnesota Multiphasic Personality Inventory (MMPI) A complex questionnaire-based test that assesses the individual's personality structure and diagnostic classification. It contains clinical scales and indices that measure nine dimensions of the patient's personality and behavior.

Minority group A cultural group that exists within the larger dominant cultural group and often is subjected to differential treatment. The largest minority groups in the United States are African-Americans, Hispanics, and Asians.

Mirroring   A means of establishing rapport with another person and encouraging his or her trust. By "mirroring" an individual's general posture, eye movements, breathing pattern, and voice tone, the nurse can help that person relax and feel safe.

Model distortions   Limitations of the patient's mental map, as expressed by words such as "always," "never," "all," and "every."

Monitors   Behaviors that may be used consciously or unconsciously to regulate one's own behaviors or the behaviors of others.

Monoamine oxidase inhibitors (MAOIs)   Drugs that inhibit the breakdown of amino acids in many parts of the body, and are used to treat a depressed patient when tricyclic or other medication has proven to be ineffective.

Mood-congruent delusions   Delusions consistent with a manic individual's inflated sense of worth and power, which may take the form of believing he or she has supernatural ability to solve the world's problems.

Mood disorders   Termed "affective disorders" in DSM-II (1980), those disorders that involve a disturbance in mood or affect.

Multi-infarct dementia (MID)   In contrast to primary degenerative dementia, multi-infarct dementia is a disease of the blood vessels rather than the neurons, pathophysiologically characterized by numerous small thrombotic strokes (see *Lacunar infarcts*). MID risk factors are similar to those for hypertension, stroke, diabetes mellitus, and cigarette smoking.

Multiple personality   The presence of two or more distinct personalities or personality states within one person. The dominant personality may or may not know about the others, which may range in number from two to more than one hundred. He or she experiences an altered state of consciousness when subpersonalities emerge.

Munchausen syndrome   Also known as *factitious disorder with physical symptoms*. The patient presents with physical symptoms to such a degree that he or she is able to obtain and sustain multiple hospitalizations and even surgery. The physical signs of illness are voluntarily produced through physiological tampering, such as the ingestion of contaminated substances, in order to gain medical attention.

N

Narcissism   A severe personality disorder that involves a grandiose persona and inability to empathize with the effects of one's behavior on others.

Negative cognitive-set theory   A theory that emphasizes the influence of cognitions on emotions. According to this theory, the depressed person's negative perceptions of self, the world, and the future are responsible for his or her emotional, motivational, and behavioral changes.

Negligent tort   See *tort law*. The negligent tort is a charge of negligence made by a patient or patient advocate against the medical care provider. Proof of negligence must be based on the health provider's duty, breach or dereliction of duty, damages (injury), and proximate (direct or legal) causation.

Neurofibrillary tangles   A particular type of neuronal degeneration that is a characteristic, histopathological feature of Alzheimer's disease and other cerebral disorders.

Neuroleptics   Also called antipsychotic medications, these drugs control and prevent psychotic symptoms.

Neurosis   An emotional disturbance with varying levels of maladaptive responses to anxiety, but with no loss of contact with reality.

Nonassociative learning   A stimulus-induced response that can become weaker *(habituation)* or stronger *(sensitization)* with repetition of exposure.

Normal pressure hydrocephalus   A type of dementia caused by decreased reabsorption of cerebrospinal fluid, often due to trauma, hemorrhage, or meningitis, which leads to enlargement of the lateral ventricles of the brain. The classic symptoms of normal pressure hydrocephalus are dementia, incontinence, and gait problems.

Norms   Standards of behavior, achievement, or other, based on measurements of a large group; used for comparison to an individual.

Nurse therapist   A more specific definition of the nurse's role as caregiver, in which the nurse demonstrates a good understanding of psychopathology and has the ability to use selected tools for assessing mental illness. The nurse therapist uses at least one basic therapy modality as well, such as interpersonal theory or learning theory.

Nursing diagnoses   Hypotheses of actual or potential health problems that are formulated by the nurse through ongoing assessment.

Nursing process   The systematic process by which the nurse assesses, analyzes, plans, implements, and evaluates the effectiveness of interventions for a particular patient. The overall purpose of the nursing process is to promote, maintain, restore, or enhance the health of the individual (or family or community).

Nurturing behavior   When used in health care, a non-threatening approach to patients, which includes providing support and comforting them, as well as caring for their physical needs.

O

Object-relations   Melanie Klein's theory that emphasizes the child's need to integrate good and bad experiences into one love object, the mother, in order to have a balanced perception of other objects (people) later in life.

Obsessive-compulsive behaviors   Compulsive repetition of behaviors, such as repeatedly checking that doors are locked at night or washing one's hands, used by organically impaired individuals as a maladaptive attempt to cope with anxiety.

Obsessive-compulsive disorder   An anxiety disorder characterized by *obsession,* which can be defined as recurrent, persistent thoughts that feel alien to the individual but are not attributable to an external source, and *compulsion,* which compels the individual to undertake an act despite feelings that it is senseless.

Open receiver   In communication theory, the individual who emphathizes with the message sender by attempting to take his or her position and to understand that person's perspective.

Operant conditioning   Type of learning in which a spontaneous behavior is reinforced and thereby becomes more likely to occur.

Opiate receptors   Highly specific sites on the surfaces of cells in the central nervous system, especially in the limbic area and nerve pathways, to which narcotic substances bind, changing the permeability of the cell membrane to ions. The membrane then changes its electrical characteristics or activates the cyclic AMP system, thus influencing chemical reactions within the cell.

Organic mental disorders Disorders in which mental changes are caused by a specific structural or chemical central nervous system lesion.

Organizational communication Public communication or communication with large groups.

Orgasmic phase The third phase of the sexual response cycle identified by Masters and Johnson. Orgasm lasts a few seconds, during which the individual experiences sexual release through vasoconstriction and myotonia. Males ejaculate seminal fluid by a series of contractions in the penis, prostate, and seminal vesicles. Females experience contractions in the clitoral body, vagina, and uterus.

Orientation Awareness of appropriate time, place, and situation.

Orientation phase The beginning stage of the therapeutic nurse-patient relationship, in which goals are established based on assessment, structuring the relationship, and establishing rapport.

Overprotective family An interactional pattern characteristic of some families with children with eating disorders.

P

Pain control Process by which pain is assessed and treated. Planning for pain control, in which the patient actively participates, must take into account not only the patient's pain, but the associated emotional, social, spiritual, and financial components. Emotional support is crucial. Treatment includes medication as well as noninvasive methods such as relaxation therapy, massage, and distraction.

Panic disorder Characterized by unpredictable, acute attacks of anxiety that are not specific to a particular situation. The individual suffering from panic disorder often experiences intense apprehension and various physical manifestations such as dyspnea, palpitations, and dizziness.

Paralanguage The level of communication that consists of all aspects of spoken communication except the words themselves. This includes vocal pitch and tone, rate of speech, nasality, mannerisms such as giggles or stuttering, and varying degrees of forcefulness.

Paranoid personality disorder A pervasive and unwarranted tendency to interpret the actions of people as deliberately threatening or harmful.

Paraphilias One of two groups of sexual disorders in which sexual arousal occurs in response to objects or situations that are not part of normative arousal-activity patterns and that in varying degrees may interfere with the capacity for reciprocal, affectionate sexual activity.

Paraphrasal A technique of active listening that involves the repetition back to the patient in succinct phrases what the nurse understands him or her to say, such as "You are very angry," and "You feel right now that you are angry enough to kill your lover."

Paraphrasia Use of inappropriate words, or of senseless and inappropriate combinations of words. In progressive dementia, e.g., Alzheimer's, paraphrasia may progress to loss of spontaneous speech and increasing muteness.

Passive-aggressive personality disorder A pervasive pattern of passive resistance to demands for adequate social and occupational performance, or a pattern in which a person who has agreed to complete a task expresses anger indirectly by dawdling or deliberately sabotaging the task.

Paternalism A practice of interfering with someone's liberty for the good of that person. In the context of mental health, examples of paternalism include lying to a patient to protect him or her from upsetting news, involuntarily committing a patient to protect him or her from self-inflicted harm, or sharing confidential information with a family member without the patient's permission.

Patient advocate The aspect of the nurse's role that involves acting as the patient's ally in the struggle for mental health by speaking up for the patient's rights and needs.

Patriarchal hierarchy A cultural framework in which there is a concentration of power at the top of a vertical social structure (hierarchy), with concentration of power in the hands of males (patriarchy).

Pedophilia A form of sexual pathology in which the individual is erotically aroused by and seeks sexual gratification from children. This may be hetero- or homosexual in nature; one of the most damaging variants is father-daughter incest.

Perceptions An individual's representation of his or her feelings about outside events.

Perfect family Used in the description of families with anorexic or bulimic children; refers to an interactional pattern in which expectations of female family members are strong yet inconsistent. The women are expected to demonstrate career success but behave in a traditional feminine manner by refraining from anger, assertiveness, or independence.

Perseveration The inability to inhibit repetitive behaviors, such as brushing teeth, walking, or uttering certain phrases.

Personality disorder A deeply ingrained, inflexible, maladaptive pattern of relating to, perceiving, and thinking about the environment and the self that is of sufficient severity to cause significant impairment in adaptive functioning or personal distress.

Personalizing The taking on of events in a given situation as if they were directed at oneself personally.

Perversion Deviation from the normal.

Phobia A persistent, obsessive, and irrational fear of an object or situation that results in its avoidance.

Physical abuse Violence directed at another individual, usually in anger or frustration but also, possibly, for sexual pleasure or ego gratification.

Placating An ineffective communication pattern that involves an incongruent double message, with the verbal and nonverbal messages saying different things. The "placater" lacks a sense of self-worth and is ingratiating, submissive, and eager to please others.

Plaintiff The party who is bringing suit against another party. In the context of nursing, it is the patient or patient's representative who sues the nurse for negligence.

Plateau phase The second phase of the sexual response cycle identified by Masters and Johnson. Males and females experience an increase in sexual tension and, if sexual stimulation continues, a level of excitement close to orgasm.

Pleasuring Learning to give sensual pleasure to a partner through observation, verbal communication, and experimentation with various forms of touching.

Polysubstance abuse The abuse of several substances,

causing overlapping intoxication syndromes that are difficult to evaluate on the basis of physical signs and symptoms alone.

Post-traumatic stress disorder A severe anxiety reaction to an extremely traumatic event, such as physical assault, combat duty, or man-made disasters.

Pragmatics of communication A theory that states that behavior is equal to communication as a means of influencing and evaluating others.

Punctuation sequence The order of exchange in communication, or the cause-and-effect relationship between information being communicated.

Predicament A situation that is unpleasant, dangerous, or embarrassing. When coupled with emergencies in an individual's life, predicaments can cause mounting stress in an individual and lead to a crisis situation.

Prejudice A state of mind, including a prejudged set of feelings and attitudes based on emotions rather than rationality, about an entire group of people.

Premature ejaculation Persistent or recurring ejaculation with minimal sexual stimulation or before, upon, or shortly after penetration and before the person wishes it.

Premortem dying Treating the dying person as if he or she had already died.

Presenting problem The chief complaint, whether physical or psychological, that has motivated the patient to seek medical help. Always necessitates interviewing the patient in order to obtain important factual and intuitive information.

Pressured speech Frantic, jumbled speech in the manic individual as he or she struggles to keep pace with racing thoughts.

Primary degenerative dementia (PDD) Chronic mental disorder, commonly called senile dementia, in which there is a deterioration of previously acquired intellectual abilities, leading to memory disturbance and impairment of abstract thinking, judgment, and impulse control. See *Alzheimer's disease*.

Primary gain A process by which the patient gains relief from an emotional conflict through the use of a defense mechanism and its reinforcement from the outside world.

Primary prevention Measures used to find and remove conditions that might contribute to mental illnesses, as well as fostering those positive conditions that contribute to mental health.

Primary symptoms The actual cognitive symptoms of the organic mental disorder, i.e., intellectual deficits and their direct results. The severity of these symptoms mirrors the severity of the organic mental disorder itself. Symptoms respond largely to definitive treatment of the organic mental disorder as well as environmental manipulation.

Primary therapy Therapy in which the nurse with specialized training (or primary therapist) has major responsibility for the patient's individual and environmental therapy, in the context of in-patient or out-patient treatment.

Projective personality test A test that uses visual stimuli to elicit a response from a patient. The experienced clinician then "interprets" the patient's response, searching for a pattern of underlying tendencies and/or hidden psychopathology in the patient. Among them are the following:

1. *Rorschach Personality Test*. The Rorschach Test consists of cards containing abstract "ink blot" pictures that are interpreted by the patient according to his or her perception.

2. *Thematic Apperception Test (TAT)*. This test consists of twenty pictures showing individuals in ambiguous but striking circumstances. Based on the psychological significance of the patient's response, central issues and conflicts may be revealed.

3. *Sentence Completion Test (SCT)*. This test consists of 75 to 100 sentence stems such as "I like ——," and "My greatest fear ——." Clinicians view the patient's responses for major patterns and affective tone, which may give insight into a patient's unique situation.

4. *Draw-a-Person Test*. The patient is asked simply to draw a person. Information about the patient's body image and feelings about himself are often revealed.

5. *Bender-Gestalt Test*. A test that can be helpful in the detection of organic brain disease. The patient is asked to copy patterns from memory, one at a time, or to recall as many patterns as possible after a short time interval. Inferences about the patient's personality and visual and motor function can be made from these rendered patterns.

Proxemics The study of the perception and use of space that individuals find most comfortable for communication. Spatial distances between individuals vary from less than twelve inches to several feet, depending on the cultural background of the participants.

Pseudobulbar palsy A neurological condition resembling parkinsonism, resulting from frontal lobe impairment or damage.

Pseudodementia Syndrome masquerading as dementia (not an organic syndrome), characterized by abrupt onset, rapid progression, and history of depression with symptoms such as hopelessness, sleep or appetite disturbances, and guilt.

Psychiatric history One of two major components of the traditional psychiatric nursing interview. Includes the patient's name, age, marital status, occupation, and past history of hospitalizations and episodes that required treatment. A family history, psychosocial history, and personal history can also help the nurse identify patterns of behavior that will be targeted for treatment. The nurse helps the patient explore his or her presenting problem and reasons for seeking treatment. Additional information may be gathered from the patient's family, friends, and other mental health personnel, with the patient's permission.

Psychiatric/mental health assessment Information compiled by the nurse concerning the patient's general behavior, cognitive functioning, mood or affect, and thought content. Parameters of the psychiatric assessment include an appraisal of the nurse's own emotional reactions to the patient (*Countertransference*).

Psychic death A psychological and spiritual separation from the world that may be experienced by a dying person before actual physical death takes place.

Psychoanalytic model The Freudian-based theory of the unconscious and its structure (id, ego, and superego) used to explain psychopathology.

Psychoanalytic or psychodynamic theory Proposes that bringing the *unconscious* motivations of human behavior into conscious awareness will decrease symptoms.

Psychogenic amnesia The sudden inability to recall important personal information when there is no organic disorder present.

Psychological crisis Circumstances that create psychological disequilibrium in a person; these circumstances constitute an important problem for the individual that he can, for the time being, neither escape nor solve with his customary problem-solving resources.

Psychomotor retardation The slowing down of body movement in a depressed individual, ranging from difficulty in changing his or her position to catatonia—the complete inability to move.

Psychopathology Psychologically motivated behavior that is inappropriate for the individual's environment, and therefore characterized as "abnormal." Also used to describe the study of mental or emotional disorders.

Psychosexual development Specific stages of development that progress from infantile to mature sexuality.

Psychosis A severe mental disorder in which a person's ability to think, respond, remember, communicate, interpret reality, or behave appropriately is sufficiently impaired as to interfere grossly with the capacity to meet the ordinary demands of life.

Psychosocial network An approach that focuses on the sum total of all persons with whom an individual has a relationship, including family, friends, neighbors, coworkers, employers, and significant others.

Psychosocial theory As developed by Erik Erikson and expanded by others, a framework focusing on the interaction between the self and the social environment. Erikson described the process of development in stages as determined by the individual's orientation toward self and others; the conflicts encountered in each stage are resolved through the successful achievement of developmental tasks, such as trust versus mistrust in the infant or autonomy versus dependence in the toddler.

Psychosomatic or psychophysiological disorders Psychiatric disorders in which patients have valid physical complaints despite absence of demonstrable tissue damage or impairment.

Psychotherapy Therapy that involves exploring thoughts and feelings within a therapeutic relationship directed at increasing the patient's self-understanding and alleviating psychological distress or injury.

Psychotic depression A severe depression that involves delusions and/or hallucinations, indicating that the individual has lost touch with reality.

Pyschogenic fugue A massive amnesia in which the individual attempts to take flight from whatever is overwhelming, threatening, or unacceptable. The individual is unable to recall personal information about his or her old identity and assumes a new one.

Q

Quasi-communication Behaviors that stimulate other individuals, such as heightened intensity of eye contact, tone of voice, and "preening." Although not seductive or overtly sexual, quasi-communication attempts to regulate communication by keeping individuals attentive, alert, and ready to relate.

R

Rape-trauma syndrome Two phases of significant physical and emotional symptoms that may be experienced by a rape victim for some time following the assault. In the first phase, the victim may display a controlled calm masking fear and anger, and suffer from bodily soreness, sleep and appetite disturbances, and intense fear, guilt, and shame. In the second phase, the victim may resume a minimal level of daily functioning, suffer from nightmares about the attack, and experience phobias such as fear of crowds or fear of sex.

Reactive attachment disorder of infancy Also known as *nonorganic failure to thrive.* The infant exhibits markedly disturbed social relatedness in most contexts, as evidence by persistent failure to initiate and respond to social interactions and lack of playfulness and vocalizations.

Reality-based therapy An approach to therapy in which the nurse provides objective reality for the patient by distinguishing subjective stimuli (those coming from within by the patient) from objective stimuli, which can be validated with the five senses and experienced by others within the environment.

Reality orientation A strategy devised to deal with impaired cognition, which relieves disorientation by increasing a person's awareness of himself and his relationship to his immediate environment.

Reality principle In psychoanalytic theory, refers to the gradual development of the ability to modify instinctual desires (represented by the *Pleasure principle*) according to demands of the external world (society).

Reality testing An essential ego function allowing an individual to evaluate the external environment objectively and to differentiate it from the internal world.

Reality therapy When used with depressed patients, a therapy based on the premise that the person is in control of the depression and can relinquish passive behavior and learned helplessness in favor of control, independence, and power in life situations. The patient is encouraged to clarify his or her wants and goals, and, with the therapist, formulates a flexible plan of eliminating nonhelpful behavior.

Redundancy Also called *repetition,* provides a bridge between the known and the unknown and helps the individual define and structure new ideas or concepts.

Regression Defense mechanism involving a retreat to a less mature level of thought or action in an attempt to avoid anxiety and cope with stress.

Regulation The process of limiting and controlling behaviors that are considered unacceptable to society. A person may self-regulate behaviors or attempt to regulate the behaviors of others.

Relationships In communication theory, refers to the interaction between people that can be communicated through nonverbal behavior. How they face each other, whether the arms are relaxed or folded or the head is raised or lowered, indicates how open each person is to the other's ideas or whether he or she feels dominant or submissive to the other person.

Relaxation therapy A method of reducing tension and maladaptive responses to stress by teaching the individual to relax major muscle groups.

REM latency test The measurement of time that elapses between initially falling asleep and the onset of REM (rapid eye movement) sleep as a means of evaluating sleep disturbances in patients with borderline personality disorder.

Reminiscing therapy Encouraging the aging or demented individual to discuss past experiences as a positive life review, promoting his or her self-esteem.

Remotivation therapy   Therapy based on the assumption that many symptoms of confusion are iatrogenic consequences of institutional living. This therapy is designed to treat symptoms of mild confusion, apathy, withdrawal, and inactivity.

Repression   Defense mechanism by which unpleasant, anxiety-producing thoughts and desires or intolerable memories are kept out of conscious awareness.

Resistance   A behavior exhibited by a patient who struggles against change, both consciously and unconsciously, and who simultaneously seeks and rejects help. The patient may use any number of defense mechanisms and deny that he or she has a problem.

Resolution phase   The fourth phase of the sexual response cycle identified by Masters and Johnson. Both males and females experience loss of bodily tension and return to the unstimulated state.

Respite programs   Admission of a chronically ill patient to tertiary care facilities for a few days or weeks, several times per year, in order to allow family members a rest from constant home care.

Response prevention   An approach to treating individuals with obsessive-compulsive disorder that combines graded real-life exposure with modeling and positive reinforcement for refraining from the obsessive behavior and teaches people around the patient to help block the obsessive behavior with appropriate responses and treatment exercises.

Retrograde amnesia   Impairment in memory of events occurring before a significant event, such as trauma or onset of the causative disease.

Revictimization   The exacerbation of a rape victim's original trauma, caused by societal attitudes and misunderstandings in which the victim is blamed for provoking the attack.

Rigidity   Simplification of the environment by decreasing the number of possible changes, as a primary adaptive coping mechanism. A patient with ever-decreasing cognitive abilities will insist that things always be done in the way to which he or she is accustomed.

S

Safety signals   A concept that identifies specific environmental cues that indicate the absence of danger and enable an individual to feel less anxious, such as the presence of a trusted person or sight of familiar landmarks.

Schizoid personality disorder   A pervasive pattern of indifference to social relationships and a restricted range of emotional experience and expression, in which the individual rarely displays strong emotions and chooses solitude over companionship.

Schizophrenia   A large group of psychotic disorders, manifested by characteristic disturbances of language and communication, thought, perception, affect, and behavior that last longer than six months.

Schizophreniform disorder   A disorder in which the clinical features are the same as schizophrenia but the duration is more than one week but less than six months. Schizophreniform disorder has a better prognosis than schizophrenia.

Schizotypal personality disorder   A relatively new definition in DSM-III-R that describes the healthier end of the schizophrenic spectrum. The schizotypal individual is severely disturbed and displays bizarre behavior that lacks the features of frank schizophrenic psychosis, such as hallucinations or delusions.

Second-generation antidepressants   Medications containing four-ring structures that are options to the use of tricyclic antidepressants. These newer drugs have been observed to have an earlier onset of action than the tricyclic antidepressants, but their effectiveness is not significantly superior to the older drugs.

Secondary gain   An indirect reward or benefit, such as attention or sympathy, derived from an illness.

Secondary prevention   Measures focusing on detecting and treating existing mental health problems at the earliest possible stage.

Secondary symptoms   Adaptive or maladaptive responses that patients make to their psychiatic illness. These symptoms, such as denial, are highly variable with individuals, may not correlate with the severity of the disorder, and may be more responsive to environmental manipulation than primary symptoms.

Sedative-hypnotic withdrawal syndrome   A cause of severe delirium, commonly due to alcohol withdrawal, but also seen in barbiturate and benzodiazepine withdrawal. Agitated delirium is often accompanied by visual hallucinations, tachycardia, hypertension, tremor, and seizures.

Selective amnesia   The failure to recall some specific events, while remembering others, during a circumscribed time period.

Self   That which makes an individual unique in character, inherent potential, and worth. The concept of self embraces an individual's dimensions and purposes, ambitions, and ideals.

Self-concept   An individual's organized pattern of self in awareness, and what he or she means when using the words "I" or "me."

Self-disclosure   An honest and congruent means of communication, involving the revealing of relevant aspects of one's experience, including personal thoughts, feelings, and values.

Self-esteem   A general attitude toward the self regarding one's worth that influences mood and behavior.

Self-image system   That part of the personality born out of the influences of significant others on a person's sense of self.

Self-monitoring   A therapeutic technique used in the treatment of eating disorders in which the patient keeps track of his or her binging and purging, and identifies triggers that precipitate them, in order to find alternative behaviors for reducing inner tension.

Self-psychology   A theory grounded in traditional psychoanalytic theory, which asserts that the primary goal of psychotherapy is to have the patient feel understood.

Self-regulation   A person's ability to identify needs, manage impulses, tolerate frustration, organize a need-gratifying response, and delay gratification.

Semantic ill-formedness   An indication of the limitation of an individual's mental map. Ill-formed sentences may reflect a person's perceived lack of choice in thoughts or emotions and distorted views of other people's actions.

Senile   Pertaining to old age. Refers to an illness occurring in persons older than 60 years, e.g., senile cataracts.

Senile plaques   A characteristic histopathological feature of Alzheimer's disease. Plaques are areas of partial necrosis in the cerebral cortex.

Senility Old age. A common misnomer for organic mental disorders.

Sensate focus Attention to touch as a vital part of personal relating through which feelings can be conveyed. Used in sexual therapy to enhance sexual feelings and overcome sexual dysfunction.

Sensitization An increased stress response that occurs when a stimulus becomes stronger (see *Nonassociative learning*).

Sensory deprivation Confusion, disorientation, and possibly hallucinations as a result of a lack of normal stimulation and an excess of abnormal stimulation, such as happens in the intensive care setting owing to lack of orientating clues such as windows; artificial lighting; round-the-clock tube feeding; and constant change of personnel.

Separation anxiety disorder The specific trauma of separation from an attachment figure (usually the mother) leading to significant distress and dysfunction due to the associated activity. The child may resist going to school, and develop physical symptoms such as headaches and vomiting in order to stay home.

Separation-individuation A developmental process in which the child gradually evolves from complete dependence on the mother for satisfaction of needs to having a rudimentary capacity to self-regulate in the absence of the mother or other caretaker.

Sexual aversion disorder Persistent or recurrent extreme aversion to, and avoidance of, all or almost all genital sexual contact with a sexual partner.

Sexual dysfunction Inhibition in the sexual appetite or inhibition of the psychophysiological changes necessary to complete the sexual response sequence.

Sexual masochism The achievement of sexual satisfaction from receiving physical or psychological pain. The individual derives pleasure from being humiliated, beaten, bound, or tortured.

Sexual sadism The achievement of sexual satisfaction from inflicting psychological or physical suffering on others.

Simple phobia The persistent, irrational fear and avoidance of a particular object or situation. All phobics who do not meet the diagnostic criteria for agoraphobia or social phobia fall into this category.

Situational crisis Events that are precipitated by unanticipated stress, such as the death of a loved one, acute physical or mental illness, and any type of serious physical or psychological trauma.

Social-learning theory Based on the premise that learning takes place through the interdependence of person, environment, *and* behavior.

Social network theory A theory that focuses on human beings as social animals and views them within the context of their relationships with society.

Social phobia Characterized by fear and avoidance of situations in which the individual may feel he is to be scrutinized by others or expected to perform a particular social role or activity, such as public speaking or being in crowds.

Social relationships Emotional bonds of varying intensity and duration that children form with parents and others. According to Bowlby, if these relationships are frequently disrupted early in life, the children's later psychological development may be profoundly affected.

Social-skills training A phase of behavioral therapy that is designed to increase the depressed individual's social interactions by strengthening his or her social skills. The nurse positively reinforces the patient's successful social interaction activity and focuses discussion on how that success can be carried over to other social interactions.

Socializing agent The social aspect of the nurse's role, in which he or she encourages the patient to develop skills in conversation and participation in group activities, as well as good table manners and personal grooming.

Sociocultural context Cultural beliefs, values, and behaviors that constitute an individual's environment.

Sociological death A sense of isolation and separation from other people that may be experienced by the dying person, not necessarily by his or her choice.

Somatic Pertaining to the body.

Somatization Preoccupation with bodily needs and functions. Multiple and recurrent physical complaints such as loss of appetite, difficulty with bowel movements, dizziness, headaches, and heart palpitations can mask an underlying depression.

Somatoform disorders A group of disorders in which there are physical complaints and apparent physical distress but little or no evidence of tissue damage or impairment.

Specific-organ vulnerability A hypothesis that when an individual is under stress, the weakest link in the biological chain, or the most vulnerable organ, is affected. For example, a person with a predisposition to excess secretion of acid in the stomach lining may develop ulcers when under stress.

Spirituality An individual's philosophy of life and death and their meaning, and his or her relationship to the universe and God.

Splitting A pathological defense mechanism in which the individual tries to contain the anxiety generated by emotional decompensation (see *Fragmentation*). Perceptions of self and others are split into categories of "all good" and "all bad."

Statutes Legislative acts that are designed to regulate human conduct and are subject to change in a continuing process of societal growth and modification.

Stimulate-organism-response-consequence (SORC) A summary of variables identified by Goldfried and Sprofrin that are explored in a behavior assessment. They are as follows:

1. *Stimulus*. Environmental variables that precede the target behavior.
2. *Organisms*. The person with all his or her unique variables, such as physiological states, personality, and past experiences.
3. *Response*. The target or problematic behavior.
4. *Consequences*. Events that follow the target behavior.

Stimulus control A therapeutic technique often used with eating disorders in which a patient distracts herself from behaviors that trigger the need to binge, finding an alternative means of coping. This may include a pleasant reward such as exercising or listening to music.

Strange-Situation Assessment A method of judging attachment in the older toddler, developed by Ainsworth et al., which involves observation of the toddler's affect and behavior when separated from and reunited with his mother. The quality of the child's response to this stress provides insight into the type and intensity of the parent-child attachment that has developed in the shared family environment.

Stress   Tension, strain, or pressure that may result from numerous predicaments and emergencies in an individual's life. Stressful situations may carry the potential of becoming crises, depending on the individual's ability to cope with them.

Stress analgesia   A clinical phenomenon associated with learned helplessness, in which passivity and withdrawal characterize an individual's response to uncontrollable aversive events. Although it appears to be a physiological adaptation to the stressful event, the extreme passivity and conservation of energy involved in stress analgesia poses difficulties for the individual in future problem solving and leads to nutritional and social deprivation.

Stress inoculation   A treatment that involves instructing the individual on the physiology of anxiety, teaching coping skills, and rehearsing the use of these coping skills.

Substance abuse   A maladaptive pattern of substance (drug or alcohol) use that presents health hazards to the abuser but that does not meet the criteria for dependence.

Suicide ideation   Suicidal thoughts or attempts on the part of the patient as a form of escape from depression.

Sundowning   A phenomenon in which an organically impaired individual functions well in the daytime but is unable to cope with the environment at night. He or she may become confused, disoriented, or psychotic owing to loss of visual orientation in the dark.

Survival mechanisms   Behaviors used by cultural subordinates in which survival (physical or emotional) is or is perceived to be threatened.

Susto   A spanish term for anxiety reaction that is believed to be brought about by the evil eye, witchcraft, bad air, or black magic, and may result in "soul loss." Symptoms may include headaches, vomiting, tremors, sweating, and motor retardation.

Syndrome   A cluster of symptoms that a person experiences during a mood change that continues for a designated period of time. The cluster of symptoms involves cognitive, motivational, physical, and behavioral changes.

Systematic desensitization   Wolpe's technique of treating simple phobia, based on teaching the individual to relax and then asking him or her to imagine the components of the phobia on a graded hierarchy, working up from the least fearful to the most fearful.

Systems model   A framework (such as Rogers' system of unitary man) for looking at human behavior that emphasizes the person in his or her environment. When used to guide nursing assessment, actual and potential problems are identified that may interfere with the organization and interaction of the parts and the elements of the system.

T

Teacher   An aspect of the nurse's role that involves keeping the patient informed of his rights, providing accurate information about the patient's particular condition and course of treatment, and helping the patient enhance his social interaction and rehabilitation skills.

Terminal phase   As defined by Pattison and Kübler-Ross, the phase in which the dying person experiences withdrawal from the world, diminished anxiety, and emotional disorganization as he or she prepares for death.

Termination phase   The culmination of the therapeutic nurse-patient relationship, in which issues that have surfaced are reviewed and the patient is encouraged to re-enter the world to cope with situations that previously caused anxiety.

Tertiary prevention   Measures aimed at reducing the severity of a mental health problem and helping a person live at his or her highest functional capacity.

Therapeutic community   A protected and controlled environment that resembles community living rather than a psychiatric ward. Patients are encouraged to develop socialization skills, and become more self-reliant. They receive job training and individual counseling and may share housekeeping and administrative duties with the staff.

Therapeutic match   A relationship between a therapist and patient in which they share compatible views, values, and culture, enhancing their understanding of each other.

Therapeutic nurse-patient relationship   The interaction between the nurse and patient, which requires that the nurse present himself or herself in a professional manner, focus on the patient, encourage the patient to express his or her feelings, and provide a supportive environment for the patient. This applies to *all* nursing settings, not just those involved in the care of psychiatric patients.

Tolerance   The need for increasing amounts of a drug to produce the desired effect.

Topographical model of the mind   Freud's division of the mind into three components: id, ego, and superego.

Tort law   Derived from the Latin *tortus* meaning "twisted," tort law deals with a civil wrong or a breach of duty for which the courts will provide a remedy in the form of damages (usually money). This may include assault, battery, invasion of privacy, malpractice, or injury to a person's reputation.

Tourette syndrome   A disorder due to a neurochemical vulnerability that may cause a person to experience recurrent tics, attention span deficits, and uncontrolled speech.

Transference   The unconscious assignment to others of certain feelings and behavioral predispositions as a result of early experiences with significant people in one's life (i.e., family).

Transsexualism   A sexual practice in which individuals undergo surgical procedures in order to achieve gender reassignment. Transsexuals often feel a persistent sense of discomfort and inappropriateness with their anatomical sex, and a wish to be rid of their particular genitals so that they might acquire those of the opposite sex.

Transvestism   Recurrent, intense sexual urges and sexually arousing fantasies involving cross-dressing.

Tricyclic antidepressants   Medications that, in chemical form, include three-ring structures, and that are often used to alleviate physical symptoms associated with depression.

Trisomy 21 (Down's syndrome)   A form of mental retardation caused by an extra chromosome; formerly known as mongolism owing to the characteristic widely spaced eyes, moon face, and tongue-thrust.

U

Ulysses contract   A voluntary future commitment contract signed by a patient who may recurrently cause psychosocial harm to himself and/or his family, but who does not qualify for involuntary commitment because he is not physically dangerous. The contract authorizes the physician to deprive the patient of his liberty under specified circumstances.

Unconscious mind Factors that, according to Freud, motivate an individual's thoughts, feelings, and behavior without that person's awareness.

Unipolar depression A mood disorder characterized by sustained, intense depressive symptoms.

V

Vaginismus A persistent, involuntary muscle constriction of the outer third of the vagina, which prohibits penetration. It may be caused by extreme performance anxiety or previous sexual trauma.

Values An individual's beliefs about self-worth, behavior, other people, events, and other things that are important to him.

Values clarification An approach to discovering and developing values. This process has three components: thinking about one's values, recognizing true feelings or awareness of the self, and acting upon one's values.

Values indicators Behaviors including beliefs, goals, attitudes, interests, feelings, and aspirations that are inconsistent with an individual's true values. For example, one may claim to value honesty and return a lost wallet, but do nothing when undercharged at a grocery store. Honesty may be a values indicator for a person, but he or she may not always act accordingly.

Victim behaviors Survival behaviors used by victims of crime, economic and social oppression, discrimination, and violence. The victim uses adaptive techniques such as giving in to the demands of an abusive husband in order to protect her children. Victim behaviors reflect and reinforce feelings of powerlessness and helplessness.

Violence Destructive aggression that inflicts physical damage on persons or property.

Visuospatial orientaton Refers to visual perception of spatial relationships. A person without this will have difficulty in finding his or her way in unfamiliar surroundings.

Vitamin B$_{12}$ deficiency A cause of organic brain syndrome, seen in patients with gastrointestinal conditions such as pernicious anemia, malabsorption syndromes, and malnourishment.

Voyeurism The seeking of sexual gratification from looking at sexual objects or sexually arousing situations, such as people undressing or having intercourse.

W

Wernicke-Korsakoff syndrome Organic mental disorder caused by chronic alcohol abuse, seen in advanced alcoholism. Components of the syndrome include *Wernicke's encephalopathy* and *Korsakoff's psychosis*.

Wernicke's encephalopathy A component of Wernicke-Korsakoff syndrome, characterized by ataxia, gaze palsies, and diplopia.

Withdrawal (psychological) A pathological retreat from people or the world of reality.

Withdrawal (substance) A syndrome precipitated by abrupt discontinuance of a substance that the individual has regularly used. In addition to a hangover or craving for a drug, there are signs and symptoms specific to the lack of the addictive substance.

Working phase The second stage of the therapeutic nurse-patient relationship, the goals of which are developing insight into the patient's feelings and helping the patient change his or her behavior.

World view An open-mindedness with regard to a variety of cultural/ethnic perspectives, based upon an individual's acculturation and accommodation.

INDEX

Page numbers followed by g *indicate glossary entries.*

A

Abnormal behavior, popular views of, 29
Abreaction, 231
Abstraction
  extensional level of, 79
  intentional level of, 79
Abstract thinking, 112–13
Abuse, 1018g. *See also* Child abuse;
  Elder abuse; Sexual abuse
Acceptance, as stage of dying, 960, 1018g
Accommodation, 138, 812, 1018g
Acculturation, 138, 1018g
Acquired immune deficiency
  syndrome (AIDS), 567
  and confidentiality, 359–60
  crisis related to, 678–79
    and children, 679–80
    nursing management of, 680–83
  disclosure of positive test to
    suicidal patient, 1014–15
  and education, 569
  and mental health, 770–71
  patient care in, 358–59
  patient dying with, 968
  sources of information about, 571
Acting out, 1018g
  as defense mechanism, 31, 437
  and substance abuse, 546
Active and adaptive response, to
  intensive care unit patient in
  crisis, 923, 1018g
Activity theory, of aging, 866–67, 1018g
Acute confusional states, 872, 1018g
Acute dystonia, 339
Acute organic brain syndrome,
  1018g. *See also* Organic brain
  disorders
Acute phase, of dying, 958, 1018g
Adapin, 289
Adaptive regression in service of the
  ego (ARISE), 116–17, 1023g
Adaptive value, of emotion, 23
Addictions nursing, 553
Adjustment disorder, 51
Administrative law, 983–84, 1018g

Administrative rules, 982, 1018g
Adolescents
  assessing, 827
  pregnancy of, 828
  substance abuse of, 538
Adolescent suicide. *See also* Suicide
  assessment of, 697–98
  description of, 696, 697
  epidemiology of, 696–97
  theories of, 698–99
Adult Children of Alcoholics, 456
Adult hospitalized population,
  access of, to psychiatric
  mental health care, 3–4
Advocacy, and nursing intervention
  with dying patient, 969, 1018g
Affect, in mental-status examination,
  110
Affective display, 80, 1018g
Affect problem, 313
African Americans. *See* Black
  Americans
Ageism, 867–68, 1018g
Age-stratification theory of aging,
  867, 1018g
Aggression, 1018g
  drive theory of, 901–2
  frustration-aggression theory of,
  901–2
Aging, 863–64. *See also* Elderly;
  Geriatric mental health
  differentiating normal from
    abnormal processes of, 874–75
  and sexual expression, 582–83
  theories of, 866–68
Agnosia, 119, 1018g
Agoraphobia, 225, 1018g
  case history of, 226
  safety signals, 225–26
  treatment for, 226–27
AIDS. *See* Acquired immune
  deficiency syndrome
Akathisia, 414
Al-Anon, 543, 545
Alateen, 545
Alcohol, 531, 532
  and sexual dysfunction, 583–84
  withdrawal syndromes in, 534–35

Alcohol abuse, 523
  relationship between, and mood
  disorders, 542
Alcohol consumption
  in depression, 263
  in mania, 268
  by men, 768
  by women, 537
Alcoholic dementia, 1018g
  assessment of patients with, 398–99
  case history of, 392
  treatment of, 399
Alcoholics Anonymous (AA),
  543–45, 1018g
Alcoholism, 523, 527, 1018g
  and Adult Children of Alcoholics,
  456
  case history of, 546
  disease concept of, 527
  among elderly, 539
Alexithymia, 471–72, 1018g
Alienation
  from others, 762–63
  from self, 763
  from work, 761–62
Allergies, 222
Aloofness, in schizophrenia, 322
Altered states of consciousness
  (ASC), variables associated
  with, 622
Altruism, 437
Altruistic suicide, 687, 1018–19g
Alzheimer's disease, 50, 313, 872,
  1019g
  assessment of patients with, 393,
  395, 875–78
  case history of, 383, 385, 389,
  391, 394
  epidemiology of, 392–93
  families' responses to, 396
  symptoms of, 875–76
  theories of etiology of, 395
  treatment of, 395–96, 881
Ambivalence, 313
American Nurses Association
  definition of nursing, 176
    Standards of Psychiatric and

1037

ISBN 0-397-54852-4

90000

9 780397 548521